MEDICAL MANAGEMENT OF THE SURGICAL PATIENT

edited by

MICHAEL F. LUBIN, MD
Associate Professor of Medicine
Emory University School of Medicine
Atlanta, Georgia

H. KENNETH WALKER, MD
Professor of Medicine
Emory University School of Medicine
Atlanta, Georgia

ROBERT B. SMITH III, MD
Professor of Surgery
Head, General Vascular Surgery
Emory University School of Medicine
Atlanta, Georgia

with 94 contributors

MEDICAL MANAGEMENT OF THE SURGICAL PATIENT

third edition

J. B. LIPPINCOTT COMPANY
PHILADELPHIA

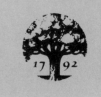

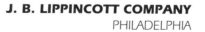

Acquisitions Editor: **RICHARD WINTERS**
Assistant Editor: **MELISSA JAMES**
Associate Managing Editor: **GRACE R. CAPUTO**
Production Manager: **CAREN ERLICHMAN**
Production Coordinator: **DAVID YURKOVICH**
Senior Design Coordinator: **KATHY KELLEY-LUEDTKE**
Interior Designer: **MARIA S. KARKUCINSKI**
Cover Designer: **SUZANNE BENNETT**
Indexer: **SANDRA SCHROEDER**
Compositor: **PINE TREE COMPOSITION, INC.**
Printer/Binder: **COURIER/WESTFORD**

6 5 4 3 2 1

Library of Congress Cataloging-in Publication Data

Medical management of the surgical patient/edited by Michael F.
    Lubin, H. Kenneth Walker, Robert B. Smith; with 94 contributors.—
    3rd ed.
        p. cm.
    Includes bibliographical references and index.
    ISBN 0–397–51318–6 (alk. paper)
    1. Surgery—Complications. 2. Diseases—Complications.
3. Therapeutics, Surgical. I. Lubin, Michael F., 1947–
II. Walker, H. Kenneth (Henry Kenneth), 1936–   III. Smith,
Robert B., 1933–
    [DNLM: 1. Intraoperative Care. 2. Intraoperative Complications.
3. Postoperative Care. 4. Postoperative Complications. 5. Surgery,
Operative. WO 178 M488 1995]
RD98.M43 1995
617′.01—dc20
DNLM/DLC
for Library of Congress   94–34549
                                                            CIP

3rd Edition

∞ This paper meets the requirements of ANSI/NISO Z39.48–1992 (permanance of paper).

We gratefully dedicate this book to our secretaries—Joanne Boykin, Harriet Eason, Michele Banfield, and Brian Hage—who worked tirelessly through the stresses and strains of the production process. Without their help, this project would have been impossible to complete.

CONTRIBUTORS

THOMAS M. AABERG, MD, FACS
Professor and Chairman
Department of Ophthalmology
Emory University School of Medicine
Emory University Hospital
Atlanta, Georgia

MARY J. ALBERT, MD
Assistant Professor of Orthopaedic Surgery
Emory University School of Medicine
Atlanta, Georgia

JOSEPH D. ANSLEY, MD
Associate Professor of Surgery
Emory University School of Medicine
Staff Surgeon and Chair
Hyperalimentation Committee
Grady Memorial Hospital
Atlanta, Georgia

ALEXANDER P. AUCHUS, MD
Assistant Professor of Neurology and Geriatrics
Emory University School of Medicine
Atlanta, Georgia

ROY A.E. BAKAY, MD
Professor of Neurological Surgery
Emory University School of Medicine
Emory University Hospital
Atlanta, Georgia

DANIEL L. BARROW, MD
Associate Professor and Vice Chairman
Department of Neurosurgery
Emory University School of Medicine
Emory University Hospital
Atlanta, Georgia

THOMAS P. BRANCH, MD
Assistant Professor of Orthopaedic Surgery
Chief, Sports Medicine Section
Emory University Hospital
Crawford W. Long Memorial Hospital
Grady Memorial Hospital
VA Medical Center
Atlanta, Georgia

C. MICHAEL CAWLEY, MD
Resident Physician
Department of Neurosurgery
Emory University School of Medicine
Atlanta, Georgia

HARRY S. CLARKE, JR., MD, PhD
Assistant Professor of Surgery (Urology)
Emory University School of Medicine
The Emory Clinic
Atlanta, Georgia

AUSTIN R.T. COLOHAN, MD
Professor of Neurosurgery
Emory University School of Medicine
The Emory Clinic
Atlanta, Georgia

MARK W. CONNOLLY, MD
Peachtree Cardiovascular Group
Atlanta, Georgia

J. ROBIN DeANDRADE, MD, FRCS(ENG IC), FACS
Professor of Orthopaedic Surgery
Emory University School of Medicine
The Emory Clinic
Atlanta, Georgia

STEVEN M. DEVINE, MD
Assistant Professor of Medicine
Department of Medicine
Section of Hematology/Oncology
Emory University School of Medicine
Atlanta, Georgia

THOMAS F. DODSON, MD
Associate Professor of Surgery
Emory University School of Medicine
The Emory Clinic
Atlanta, Georgia

CHARLES A. DUNCAN, MD
Associate Professor of Medicine
University of Texas Health Science Center at San Antonio
Medical Director, Medical Intensive Care Unit
University Hospital
San Antonio, Texas

JAMES R. ECKMAN, MD
Professor of Medicine
Division of Hematology–Urology
Assistant Professor
Division of Human Genetics
Emory University School of Medicine
Director, Georgia Comprehensive Sickle Cell Center
Grady Memorial Hospital
Atlanta, Georgia

BRUCE L. EVATT, MD
Chief, Hematologic Diseases Branch
Centers for Disease Control and Prevention
Atlanta, Georgia

DAVID V. FELICIANO, MD
Professor of Surgery
Emory University School of Medicine
Chief of Surgery
Grady Memorial Hospital
Atlanta, Georgia

CHARLES M. FERGUSON, MD
Assistant Professor of Surgery
Harvard Medical School
Associate Visiting Surgeon
Massachusetts General Hospital
Boston, Massachusetts

LAMAR L. FLEMING, MD
Professor and Chairman
Department of Orthopaedic Surgery
Emory University School of Medicine
Emory University Hospital
Atlanta, Georgia

MICHAEL R. FRANKEL, MD
Assistant Professor of Neurology
Emory University School of Medicine
Chief of Neurology
Grady Memorial Hospital
Atlanta, Georgia

NIALL T.M. GALLOWAY, FRCS, MB, CʜB
Assistant Professor of Surgery (Urology)
Emory University School of Medicine
The Emory Clinic
Atlanta, Georgia

JAVIER GARCIA-BENGOCHEA, MD
Lyerly Neurosurgical Group
Jacksonville, Florida

NORMAN GITLIN, MD
Professor of Medicine
Emory University School of Medicine
Chief of Hepatology
Emory University Medical Center
Atlanta, Georgia

STEVE GOLDSCHMID, MD
Associate Professor of Medicine
Emory University School of Medicine
Chief, Gastroenterology and Endoscopy
VA Medical Center
Atlanta, Georgia

JOHN PARKER GOTT, MD
Assistant Professor of Surgery
Emory University School of Medicine
Emory University Hospital
Crawford W. Long Memorial Hospital
Atlanta, Georgia

SAM D. GRAHAM, JR., MD
Professor of Surgery (Urology)
Emory University School of Medicine
Chief, Section of Urology
The Emory Clinic
Atlanta, Georgia

ROBERT C. GREEN, MD
Assistant Professor of Neurology
Director, Neurobehavioral Program
Emory University School of Medicine
Chief of Neurology
Wesley Woods Center
Atlanta, Georgia

WILLIAM G. GRIST, MD
Assistant Professor of Otolaryngology
Emory University School of Medicine
Chief of Surgery
VA Medical Center
Atlanta, Georgia

GERALD S. GUSSACK, MD
Associate Professor of Otolaryngology
Emory University School of Medicine
Directory of Residency Education
Emory University Hospital
Henrietta Egleston Children's Hospital
Atlanta, Georgia

W. DALLAS HALL, MD
Professor of Medicine
Emory University School of Medicine
Atlanta, Georgia

JOHN G. HELLER, MD
Assistant Professor of Orthopaedic Surgery
Emory University School of Medicine
Atlanta, Georgia

JOHN D. HENRY, JR., MD
Assistant Professor of Orthopaedic Surgery
Emory University School of Medicine
Crawford W. Long Memorial Hospital
Chief, Orthopaedic Surgery
VA Medical Center
Atlanta, Georgia

SEAN P. HERON, MD
Resident in Surgery (Urology)
Emory University School of Medicine
The Emory Clinic
Atlanta, Georgia

MARC C. HOCHBERG, MD, MPH
Professor of Medicine
University of Maryland School of Medicine
Baltimore, Maryland

TRAVIS C. HOLCOMBE, MD
Attending Surgeon
Phoenix Integrated Surgical Residency
Good Samaritan Hospital
Phoenix, Arizona

ERIC G. HONIG, MD
Associate Professor of Medicine
Emory University School of Medicine
Chief, Pulmonary Services
Grady Memorial Hospital
Atlanta, Georgia

IRA A. HOROWITZ, MD
Associate Professor of Gynecology and Obstetrics
Director, Gynecologic Oncology
Emory University School of Medicine
Atlanta, Georgia

WILLIAM C. HORTON, MD
Assistant Professor of Orthopaedic Surgery
Emory University School of Medicine
Emory Spine Center
Atlanta, Georgia

JORGE L. JUNCOS, MD
Assistant Professor of Neurology
Emory University School of Medicine
Co-Director, Movement Disorder Program
Emory University Hospital
The Emory Clinic
Atlanta, Georgia

M.J. JURKIEWICZ, MD, FACS, FRACS(HON)
Professor of Surgery
Emory University School of Medicine
Attending Surgeon
Division of Plastic Surgery
Emory Affiliated Hospitals
Atlanta, Georgia

ALEXANDER G. JUSTICZ, MD
Fellow in Cardiothoracic Surgery
Emory University School of Medicine
The Emory Clinic
Atlanta, Georgia

VAHAN S. KASSABIAN, MD
Assistant Professor of Surgery (Urology)
Emory University School of Medicine
The Emory Clinic
Atlanta, Georgia

DEEPAK KIKERI, MD
Assistant Professor of Medicine
Department of Medicine
Renal Section
Emory University School of Medicine
Atlanta, Georgia

SUZY L. KIM, MD
Assistant Professor of Medicine
Division of Digestive Diseases
Emory University School of Medicine
Atlanta, Georgia

JOHN G. KRAL, MD, PHD
Professor of Surgery
State University of New York Health Sciences Center
  at Brooklyn College of Medicine
Director of Vascular/General Surgery
Kings County Hospital Center
Brooklyn, New York

DAVID A. KRENDEL, MD
Associate Professor of Neurology
Emory University School of Medicine
Emory University Hospital
Atlanta, Georgia

ALI F. KRISHT, MD
Chief Resident
Department of Neurosurgery
Emory University Hospital
Atlanta, Georgia

H. MICHAEL LAMBERT, MD
Associate Professor of Ophthalmology
Baylor College of Medicine
Houston, Texas

RUTH M. LAWRENCE, MD
Professor of Clinical Medicine
Division of General Medicine
Department of Internal Medicine
University of California, Davis, School of Medicine
University of California, Davis, Medical Center
Sacramento, California

VALERIE A. LAWRENCE, MD
Associate Professor
University of Texas Health Science Center
Audie L. Murphy Memorial Veterans Hospital
University Hospital
San Antonio, Texas

PEDRO F. LOPEZ, MD
Assistant Professor of Ophthalmology
University of Southern California School of Medicine
Attending Physician
Doheny Eye Institute
Los Angeles, California

MICHAEL F. LUBIN, MD
Associate Professor of Medicine
Emory University School of Medicine
Atlanta, Georgia

ALAN B. LUMSDEN, MD
Assistant Professor
Emory University School of Medicine
Emory University Hospital
Atlanta, Georgia

BRUCE C. MACKAY, MD
Atlanta Neurological Institute, P.C.
Atlanta, Georgia

KAMAL A. MANSOUR, MD
Professor of Surgery
Emory University School of Medicine
The Emory Clinic
Atlanta, Georgia

JOHN E. McGOWAN, JR., MD
Professor of Pathology and Laboratory Medicine
Emory University School of Medicine
Director, Clinical Microbiology
Grady Memorial Hospital
Atlanta, Georgia

GENO J. MERLI, MD
Clinical Professor of Medicine
Jefferson Medical College of Thomas Jefferson University
Vice Chair, Department of Medicine
Director, Division of Internal Medicine
Thomas Jefferson University Hospital
Philadelphia, Pennsylvania

JOHN O. MEYERHOFF, MD
Assistant Professor of Medicine
Johns Hopkins University School of Medicine
Clinical Assistant Professor of Medicine
University of Maryland School of Medicine
Clinical Scholar in Rheumatology
Sinai Hospital of Baltimore
Baltimore, Maryland

JOSEPH I. MILLER, JR., MD
Professor of Surgery
Division of Cardio-Thoracic Surgery
Emory University School of Medicine
Emory University Hospital
Crawford W. Long Memorial Hospital
Piedmont Hospital
Atlanta, Georgia

SAM NASSER, MD, PHD
Associate Professor of Orthopedics
Wayne State University School of Medicine
Chief of Orthopedic Surgery
VA Medical Center
Detroit, Michigan

MARK S. O'BRIEN, MD, FACS, FAAP
Chief, Neurosurgery Section
Egleston Children's Hospital at Emory
Atlanta, Georgia

DAVID A. OLSON, MD
Assistant Professor of Surgery
Emory University School of Medicine
Atlanta, Georgia

JEFFREY J. OLSON, MD
Assistant Professor of Neurosurgery
Emory University School of Medicine
Emory University Hospital
Atlanta, Georgia

NELSON M. OYESIKU, MD
Assistant Professor of Neurosurgery
Emory University School of Medicine
Emory University Hospital
Atlanta, Georgia

TED PARRAN, JR., MD, FACP
Assistant Clinical Professor of Medicine and Family Medicine
Case Western Reserve University School of Medicine
St Vincent's Charity Hospital
Rosary Hall
Cleveland, Ohio

VIJAY M. PATEL, MD
Pulmonary Fellow
Department of Medicine
Division of Pulmonary Diseases and Critical Care
Emory University School of Medicine
Grady Memorial Hospital
Atlanta, Georgia

JEFFREY R. PINE, MD
Associate Professor of Medicine
Division of Pulmonary and Critical Care Medicine
Emory University School of Medicine
Emory University Hospital
Atlanta, Georgia

OWEN S. REICHMAN, MD
Assistant Professor of Surgery
Division of Otolaryngology
Emory University School of Medicine
Atlanta, Georgia

ANDREW REISNER, MD
Neurological Institute of Kentucky
Louisville, Kentucky

JAMES M. RIOPELLE, MD
Professor of Anesthesiology
Louisiana State University Medical Center
Assistant Director, Department of Anesthesiology
Charity Hospital at New Orleans
Medical Center of Louisiana
New Orleans, Louisiana

JAMES R. ROBERSON, MD
Associate Professor of Orthopedics
Emory University School of Medicine
Emory University Hospital
Atlanta, Georgia

ATEF A. SALAM, MD
Professor of Surgery
Emory University School of Medicine
Emory University Affiliated Hospitals
Atlanta, Georgia

TAREK A. SALAM, MD, FRCS
Assistant Professor of Surgery
Ain Shams University School of Medicine
Ain Shams Specialty Hospital
Cairo, Egypt

THOMAS E. SEAY
Atlanta Cancer Care Center
Atlanta, Georgia

JOHN GRAY SEILER III, MD
Assistant Professor of Orthopaedic Surgery
Director, Orthopaedic Surgery Training Program
Emory University School of Medicine
Atlanta, Georgia

ROGER SHERMAN, MD
Whitaker Professor of Surgery
Department of Surgery
Emory University School of Medicine
Atlanta, Georgia

JACK L. SIEGEL, MD
Jordan-Young Institute
Norfolk, Virginia

GERALD W. STATON, JR., MD
Professor of Medicine
Emory University School of Medicine
Crawford W. Long Memorial Hospital
Atlanta, Georgia

SIDNEY F. STEIN, MD
Associate Professor of Medicine
Department of Internal Medicine
Division of Hematology and Oncology
Emory University School of Medicine
Atlanta, Georgia

JAMES P. STEINBERG, MD
Assistant Professor of Medicine
Division of Infectious Diseases
Emory University School of Medicine
Associate Chief of Medicine
Crawford W. Long Memorial Hospital
Atlanta, Georgia

ALAN STOUDEMIRE, MD
Professor, Department of Psychiatry and Behavioral Sciences
Emory University School of Medicine
Director, Medical-Psychiatry Unit
Emory University Hospital
Atlanta, Georgia

ROBERT H. STRAUSS, MD
Assistant Professor of Medicine
Division of Digestive Diseases
Emory University School of Medicine
Director, Gastrointestinal Oncology
Emory University Hospital
Atlanta, Georgia

SUMNER E. THOMPSON III, MD, MPH
Professor of Medicine
Emory University School of Medicine
Director, HIV/AIDS Program
Chief, Infectious Disease
Grady Memorial Hospital
Atlanta, Georgia

GEORGE T. TINDALL, MD
Professor and Chairman
Department of Neurosurgery
Emory University School of Medicine
Chief, Neurosurgery
Emory University Hospital
Atlanta, Georgia

SUZIE C. TINDALL, MD
Professor of Neurosurgery
Emory University School of Medicine
The Emory Clinic
Atlanta, Georgia

JOHN S. TURNER, JR., BS, MD
Chief, Division of Otolaryngology
Professor of Surgery
Emory University School of Medicine
Chief, Otolaryngology
Emory University Hospital
Atlanta, Georgia

ROBERT M. WALTER, JR., MD
Professor of Internal Medicine
Division of Endocrinology and Metabolism
University of California, Davis, School of Medicine
University of California, Davis, Medical Center
Sacramento, California

J. PATRICK WARING, MD
Assistant Professor of Medicine
Emory University Hospital
Atlanta, Georgia

HOWARD M. WEITZ, MD
Clinical Associate Professor of Medicine
Jefferson Medical College of Thomas Jefferson University
Director, Clinical Cardiology
Division of Cardiology
Department of Medicine
Thomas Jefferson University Hospital
Philadelphia, Pennsylvania

CLIFFORD R. WHEELESS, JR., MD, FACS
Associate Professor of Gynecology and Obstetrics
Johns Hopkins University School of Medicine
Director, Gynecology Oncology
Director, Residency Education
Baltimore, Maryland

THOMAS E. WHITESIDES, JR., MD
Professor of Orthopedics
Emory University School of Medicine
Emory University Hospital
Atlanta, Georgia

CAROLYN F. WHITSETT, MD
Associate Professor of Pathology and Laboratory Medicine
Emory University School of Medicine
Director, Blood Bank and Transfusion Service
Crawford W. Long Hospital
Atlanta, Georgia

JOHN R. WINGARD, MD
Professor of Medicine
Emory University School of Medicine
Director, BMT/Leukemia Program
Emory University Hospital
Atlanta, Georgia

MICHAEL A. WITT, MD
Assistant Professor of Surgery (Urology)
Emory University School of Medicine
Emory University Hospital
Atlanta, Georgia

PREFACE

The production of the third edition of *Medical Management of the Surgical Patient* has been particularly satisfying. It marks the coming of age of a book whose first edition was born of necessity as a local answer to common but unaddressed problems. The second edition was an update of the information in the first edition with some new topics added; it remained essentially an Emory University effort.

This third edition is different. In the original publication, we asked our colleagues at Emory to provide us with their best ideas on how to treat patients with medical illnesses since so little objective information was available; our surgical colleagues provided information on surgical procedures that were prevalent at the time. Since 1982, however, a great deal of work has been done in many areas of perioperative consultation. In addition, there are now nationally recognized experts in a number of areas.

To update the text and take advantage of this expertise, we sought out authorities in the field wherever possible. This has clearly allowed the information in the current edition to come from a national, rather than regional, perspective. In areas in which recognized experts were not available, we have again relied on our colleagues at Emory, who we believe to be as capable as anyone of delivering clinical care, gathering pertinent information, and communicating that information to others.

Virtually the entire text of the medical sections has been rewritten. We have maintained our vision that *Medical Management of the Surgical Patient* should be an extensive, usable, well-documented reference book. Many authors are new and have written their chapters based on current information; previous authors have substantially revised or rewritten their chapters. In addition, a number of new chapters we believed important have been included. The areas they cover include HIV infection and AIDS, and patients who abuse drugs and alcohol. In addition, the section on perioperative deep venous thrombosis and pulmonary embolus has been greatly expanded.

The cardiology sections have been entirely revised to reflect the many studies performed to determine the best ways to evaluate patients with heart disease who need surgery. New therapies for perioperative problems, such as adenosine use in supraventricular tachycardia, have been added. There have been many studies about the evaluation and care of patients with pulmonary disease, and the corresponding chapters reflect the knowledge gained from them. Substantial changes in the care of patients needing nutritional support have occurred, and this chapter has been updated.

In Part 2, we have continued our plan to provide up-to-date information about surgical procedures, the usual postoperative course, and common postoperative complications. Various surgical techniques have been developed, changed, and abandoned. Chapters on all areas of surgical care have been rewritten to reflect these advances.

We are gratified by the success of the first two editions of *Medical Management of the Surgical Patient*. This edition makes a quantum leap over those first two editions because of both the great explosion of objective information available and our ability to recruit superb and nationally known experts to convey that information. The academic and financial rewards for this kind of work are small at best, and we are grateful to our contributors for their willingness to participate. They are making a major contribution to patients and their care.

We are particularly indebted to J. B. Lippincott for publishing this third edition. The company's support, hard work, and forbearance have been greatly appreciated. In addition, we thank Cathy Alden for editorial support.

Finally, we would like to thank our readers; we have worked hard to provide you with a thorough, well-supported, clinically useful book that will help you provide superb care. It is our hope that your uncountable hours caring for patients have been made easier by our efforts.

Michael F. Lubin, MD
H. Kenneth Walker, MD
Robert B. Smith III, MD

INTRODUCTION

The interchange between physicians discussing a patient's case has been mentioned in written history since ancient Greece. From the time of Hippocrates, physicians have been encouraged to seek consultation on difficult cases when they were in doubt. They were urged not to be jealous of one another but to realize their own limitations and to use the knowledge of their colleagues to help. "Nor, among physicians, do those who treat by diet envy those who employ surgery, but they even call each other into consultation and commend one another."[1] It is clear, however, that there were disagreements in those days: "Physicians who meet in consultation must never quarrel or jeer at one another."[2] There were also "wretched quarrelsome consultations at the bedside of the patient, with no consultant agreeing with another, fearing he might acknowledge a superior."[3]

Over the next 25 centuries, consultation has had its ups and downs. Much of what was written had to do with the etiquette and ethics of the interaction. In medieval Europe, little changed from ancient times. Physicians were encouraged to ask colleagues for help if needed and to refrain from criticizing each other in front of nonphysicians.

In the 14th century, patients were warned against consulting large numbers of doctors because there would be "endless disagreements and different suggestions" and "the patient [would] suffer from lack of care."[4] The doctor could call in another physician for consultations, but the treatment should be administered by the one knowing most about the case. Physicians, curiously enough, were warned about consulting with other physicians. "It is better if he have good excuses that he may refuse their demands. He may feign an injury, or illness, or some other likely excuse. But if he accepts their demands let him make a covenant for his work and make it beforehand.... Clearly advise the other leech that he will give no definite answer in any case

until he has seen the sickness and the symptoms of the patient."[4] At least the last is sound advice.

The 17th and 18th centuries brought out the best and the worst in physicians. In Italy, Julius Caesar Claudinius wrote, "There is no part of a Physician's Office more illustrious than Consultation, because by it alone unlearned physicians are known from the Learned.... And there is nothing that brings greater advantage to the Sick."[5] Contrast this with the following: "On December 28, 1750, Drs. John Williams and Parker Bennett, of Jamaica, having become involved in a wrangle about their respective views on bilious fever, came to blows, and, the next day, proceeded to a desperate hand-to-hand combat with swords and pistols, which ended fatally for both. It is said that Johann Peter Frank was so disgusted with the behavior of doctors in consultation that he advised the calling in of the police on all such occasions."[6] Again, in contrast to the brutish behavior in the British colony, John Gregory wrote that "consultation, when required, is to be conducted in a gentlemanly manner. The chief concern is to be the relief of the patient's suffering and not personal advancement. That is, the duty to one's patients takes precedence over personal and professional differences."[7]

During the 18th century, there had been (and would continue to be) a great deal of competition between practitioners. At the turn of the 19th century, there was much activity in writing about the ethics of medicine, many of which were aimed at avoiding the harmful effect of this competition. Two men in particular bear mention—Johann Stieglitz and Thomas Percival.

In 1798, Stieglitz addressed the problem of the profession's internal difficulties and the distrust they engendered in the public. Many practitioners were afraid to admit their need for help and thus avoided consultation with more knowledgeable physicians. He encouraged consultation for the good of the patient while exhorting the consultants to treat the consulting physicians as colleagues and with respect that would only improve the public's view of the profession.

In 1803, Percival published *Medical Ethics*, a few years after he had been requested to write on the subject by his fellow physicians. Much of the book was devoted to the etiquette of professional interaction, and consultation was addressed in much the same manner as in centuries past: consultation should be obtained to help the patient; no jealousy, competition, or patient stealing should be tolerated; conflict in front of patients was to be avoided at all costs. It is a tribute to the relative timelessness of Percival's work that much of it was used almost verbatim in the AMA Codes of Ethics in 1847, 1911, and 1912.

In the late 1800s, another problem surfaced in England. A great gap had appeared between the eminent consultants and general practitioners. Although the former, because of superior knowledge and prestige, were able to command high fees from wealthy clients, they apparently continued to see less well-to-do patients for the same fees that were being charged by the general practitioners. This attracted business to the consultants but left the ordinary physicians with much less work and poor incomes. The result, as could have been anticipated, was ill feeling between the groups. The conflict was of such consequence that the *British Medical Journal* in 1872 was moved to comment entirely against the "great consultants," who they believed should charge higher fees. This would decrease the burden of the overworked consultants and distribute the workload and the income in a more reasonable manner.

There was great fear among the general practitioners of sending their patients to consultants, because often these patients remained in the care of the more prestigious men whose care was considered better and whose fees were identical. Thus, the patients had no incentive to return to their practitioners. Therefore, in 1886, the Association of General Practitioners was established to try to regulate the relations between these opponents.

In the United States, meanwhile, another problem was developing. In the mid-1800s, many states repealed their laws regulating medicine, resulting in a large influx of quacks and cults. Because of this, a code of ethics restricting competition among doctors was adopted by the medical profession. This code condemned practitioners who did not have orthodox training, who claimed secret medications, and, importantly for consultants, who offered special abilities. (They may have actually had special abilities.) Although the code did much to discourage unqualified practitioners, as medical practice moved into the 20th century, it allowed ill feeling to exist between general practitioners and a growing group of medical "specialists."

A number of other negative results surfaced. Because the code forbade consultations with unlicensed physicians, if a patient insisted on a consultation with an outsider, the legitimate physician was forced to withdraw from the case, leaving the patient in the hands of these unqualified people. The rules also provided an opportunity for exclusion of even qualified physicians, and in the late 1800s, women, blacks, and those who were trying to specialize were at times subjected to these consultation bans.

In the 20th century, laws have again been passed reducing the numbers of unqualified practitioners. The International Code of Ethics encourages consultation in difficult cases. The attainment of equal status by osteopathic physicians is an interesting sidelight to these ancient struggles to protect patients and the profession.

Today, the problem is entirely different. In previous centuries, consultation was requested from a physician who, although similarly trained, was thought to be more knowledgeable overall. Even 60 years ago, in "uncomplicated" cases, consultation was generally considered unnecessary. The doctor who took care of the patient was the doctor who did the surgery, attended to preoperative and postoperative care, and continued to do the "primary care" long after.

For the past few decades, however, as medical knowledge has mushroomed and physicians have specialized and subspecialized, these tasks have been divided and subdivided. This division of labor has helped the great advances in medicine in the United States, but it also has created some special problems.

The proliferation in consultative medicine has allowed patients to have a large number of experts taking care of each separate part of an illness. The internist asks the cardiologist to consult on myocardial infarctions; the cardiologist asks the endocrinologist to consult on patients with diabetes; the surgeon asks the internist for help on patients with hypertension and congestive failure. Although this accumulation of expertise is impressive and would seem to lead to the best care possible, it can, and not infrequently does, lead to conflicting orders, incompatible medications, and conflicts between consulting physicians. Unfortunately, these conflicts are at times perceived by the patients and can cause unnecessary insecurity, fear, and anger.

These kinds of problems are common in the perisurgical patient who has complicating medical problems before surgery or who develops complications afterward. The surgeon frequently needs to have medical support to help with the complicated problems of preoperative and postoperative care. Unfortunately, the internist's knowledge of the surgical procedures, the recovery course, and complications is often scanty. This sets up a situation in which each physician has knowledge that the other needs to take optimal care of the patient.

The advantages of the primary care physician, although they should be obvious, have been lost in the tangle of subspecialization. This physician can be either the internist or the surgeon. The important concept is that the responsibility for the integration of therapies falls to that one physician because he or she is most familiar with *all* aspects of the patient's case. All other physicians must function as advisors (consultants) to the primary care provider.

The consultant's role can be a difficult one. It is imperative that the primary physician be aware of and approve of all therapy, and therefore feel free to accept and reject the advice of the consultant. Rejection is, thankfully, an unusual occurrence. Under ideal circumstances, it is best for the consultant to discuss all recommendations with the primary physician before they are written in the chart. In this way, information can be exchanged, theories can be discussed, and a mutually satisfactory plan of treatment can be formulated. This avoids the confusion, anger, and mistakes that can occur when the consultant writes recommendations that the primary doctor believes are improper. It is a rare occurrence indeed when the consultant must institute therapy without discussion; this should be done only in an emergency situation, when delay would cause harm to the patient.

Another area of potential difficulty for the consultant is in discussing plans and diagnoses with patients who are exquisitely sensitive to any discrepancy, real or perceived, between physicians. This can cause misunderstanding and anxiety for the patient, and can require an immense amount of explanation by the primary physician to reestablish the patient's trust, to help him or her understand what is happening, and to allay his or her fears.

In general, it is best for the consultant to communicate treatment plans through the primary physician. When asked, the consultant can give the patient the broad outline of possibilities to be presented to the primary doctor. The consultant should always make it clear that the final decision about what is to be done will be made by the primary physician and the patient.

There seem to be five basic principles behind optimal patient care. The first is the one-patient/one-doctor principle of primary care, or the "final common pathway" to integrate therapies as discussed above. Second, the primary doctor and consultant should trust each other. There needs to be a feeling between them that each one is able to provide something important to the patient's care. Third, communication is indispensible. If the physicians take the time to talk to one another, confusion, irritation, anger, and mistakes can be avoided. The fourth principle is really a corollary of the third, and that is cooperation. It is the natural extension of communication: if two physicians can talk to each other and each one trusts the other's judgment and knowledge, they will be able to cooperate, even in areas of disagreement, in taking the best care of the patient.

The final principle that ties the others together is etiquette. As in all human interactions, the way people deal with each other may be as important as the content of the interaction. A brilliant consultation, handled in a brusque and rude manner may be no more useful than no consultation at all. Controversial or optimal therapies begun before consultation with the primary physician will make further interaction difficult. Finally, and worst of all, improper therapy instituted erroneously or because of inadequate information not only will harm the physicians' relationship but may harm the patient as well.

The art of consultation is one that involves many aspects of interaction. The primary physician and the patient must feel that the consultant is concerned not only with the hard scientific facts of the patient's care from the specialist's viewpoint but with optimal overall management. The request for consultation is not a carte blanche for management; it is a request for advice in treating some part of the patient's illness. Thus, the consultant should feel like an invited guest in someone's house, not the master of ceremonies.

M.F.L.

References

1. Plutarch, Moralia 486C. Quoted by Amundsen DW. Ancient Greece and Rome. In: Reich WT, ed. Encyclopedia of bioethics, vol 3. London, Free Press, 1978:935.
2. Plutarch. Percepts 8. Quoted by Amundsen DW. Ancient Greece and Rome. In: Reich WT, ed. Encyclopedia of bioethics, vol 3. London, Free Press, 1978:935.
3. Pliny the Elder. Natural history 29, 5, 11. Quoted by Amundsen DW. Ancient Greece and Rome. In: Reich WT, ed. Encyclopedia of bioethics, vol 3. London, Free Press, 1978:935.
4. Welborn MC. The long tradition: a study in fourteenth century medical deontology. Quoted by Cate JL, Anderson EN, eds. Medieval and historiographical essays in honor of James Westfall Thompson. Chicago, University of Chicago Press, 1938:352–354.
5. Julius Caesar Claudinius. Quoted by White AF. Clinical medicine. In: Debus AG. Medicine in seventeenth century England. Berkeley, University of California Press, 1974:114.
6. Williams J, Bennett P. Essays on bilious fever, London, 1752. Quoted by Garrison FH. An introduction to the history of medicine. Philadelphia, WB Saunders, 1922:405.
7. McCullough LB. Britain and the U.S. in the eighteenth century. In: Reich WT, ed. Encyclopedia of bioethics, vol 3. London, Free Press, 1978:961.

CONTENTS

PART 2
SURGICAL PROCEDURES AND THEIR COMPLICATIONS

MEDICAL MANAGEMENT OF THE SURGICAL PATIENT

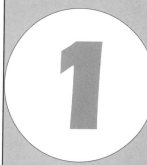

PERIOPERATIVE CARE OF THE SURGICAL PATIENT

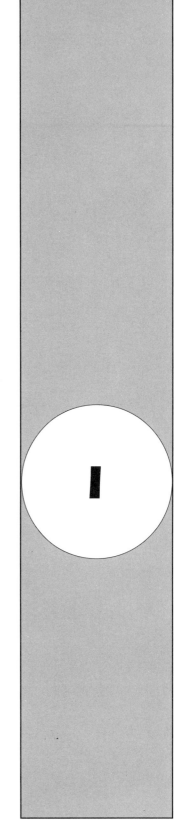

SECTION

I

ANESTHESIA

Medical Management of the Surgical Patient, Third Edition,
edited by Michael F. Lubin, H. Kenneth Walker, and Robert B. Smith III.
J.B. Lippincott Company, Philadelphia, PA © 1995.

CHAPTER

1

ANESTHETIC CARE

James M. Riopelle

Medical consultants provide important information and advice to anesthesiologists attending seriously ill patients. Not all of these consultants have had sufficient training in anesthesia, however, to permit them to anticipate the practical problems that anesthesiologists may encounter when attempting to implement their recommendations.

Medical consultants are often asked to see patients who have developed unusual medical problems either during or immediately after operation. Their evaluation of these problems can be hampered by a lack of familiarity with relatively common anesthesia-mediated physiologic perturbations.

The purpose of this chapter is to help medical consultants advise anesthesiologists both before and after surgery. Standard anesthetic practice is outlined first in the hope that aware internists will find it easier to discover ways of prescribing medical care for coexisting disease within its framework. Some of the more frequently occurring medical problems that can develop as a consequence of anesthetic administration are reviewed next so that internists who visit patients immediately after operation are alert to their presence. Finally, an attempt is made to persuade medical consultants of the at least occasional usefulness of direct, two-way communication between themselves and anesthesiologists.

THE ANESTHESIOLOGIST'S OBJECTIVES

Whether anesthesiologists are administering general anesthesia or regional anesthesia with intravenous sedation, their goals are as follows:

- To alleviate anxiety before operation
- To provide freedom from pain and anxiety and to ensure lack of patient movement during operation
- To reduce pain to the greatest degree compatible with safety after operation
- To maintain physiologic homeostasis and avoid anesthetic complications throughout the hospital stay

THE ANESTHESIOLOGIST'S METHODS

PREANESTHETIC DATA BASE

Before they actually administer anesthesia for elective surgical procedures, anesthesiologists collect basic clinical data. Main sources of information are patients' medical records and problem-oriented histories and physical examinations. Figure 1-1 provides an example of a preanesthetic data base. Abnormalities discovered during data collection

Date _____ Allergies _____ Ward Vital Signs

Time _____ Medications _____ BP _____ T _____

Consents _____ Pre-Op Diagnosis _____ P _____ Wt _____

_____ Proposed Procedure _____ R _____ Ht _____

DATE	TEST	RESULT	DATE	TEST	RESULT
_____	Hct	_____	_____	Urine	
_____	WBC	_____ /mm³	_____	CXR	
_____	Platlets	_____ /mm³	_____	EKG	
_____	PT	Patient _____ sec	_____	Chem	
		Control _____ sec			
_____	PTT	Patient _____ sec	_____	ABGs	
		Control _____ sec			
_____	Crossmatch _____ units		_____		

Na _____ mEq/L   K _____ mEq/L   BUN _____ mg/dL
Cl _____ mEq/L CO_2 _____ mEq/L   Glucose ___ mg/dL
pH _____ pCO_2 _____ torr pO_2 _____ torr
HCO_3 _____ mEq/L   Saturation _____ % FiO_2 _____

CHECKLIST FOR SYSTEM REVIEW   EXPLAIN ALL "YES" ANSWERS BY NUMBER

Yes No

1. ☐ ☐ Alcohol
2. ☐ ☐ Drug Abuse
3. ☐ ☐ Anemia/Sickle Cell
4. ☐ ☐ Coagulopathy (or family history)
5. ☐ ☐ Transfusion/Reaction
6. ☐ ☐ Diabetes
7. ☐ ☐ Thyroid Disease
8. ☐ ☐ Cortisone Within 1 Year
9. ☐ ☐ Seizures
10. ☐ ☐ Blackouts
11. ☐ ☐ Stroke
12. ☐ ☐ Paralysis
13. ☐ ☐ Back or Neck Injury/Disease
14. ☐ ☐ Current URI
15. ☐ ☐ Lung Disease
16. ☐ ☐ Cough
17. ☐ ☐ Asthma/Croup
18. ☐ ☐ Smoking
19. ☐ ☐ Dyspnea
20. ☐ ☐ Heart Disease

Yes No

21. ☐ ☐ Reduced Exercise Tolerance
22. ☐ ☐ Chest Pain/Tightness
23. ☐ ☐ Myocardial Infarction
24. ☐ ☐ High Blood Pressure
25. ☐ ☐ Palpitations
26. ☐ ☐ Murmur
27. ☐ ☐ Liver Disease/Hepatitis/Jaundice
28. ☐ ☐ Kidney Disease
29. ☐ ☐ Eye Disease/Rx/Contact Lenses
30. ☐ ☐ Nose Bleeds
31. ☐ ☐ Dentures/Caps/Loose Teeth
32. ☐ ☐ Previous Surgery/Anesthesia
       (Review old chart for Date/
        Agent/Problems)
33. ☐ ☐ Other Hospitalization(s)
34. ☐ ☐ Family History Anesthesia
       Complication/Death
35. ☐ ☐ Currently Pregnant
36. ☐ ☐ Recent P.O. Food or Drink
       (Emergencies)

PHYSICAL EXAM
1. General Appearance
2. Airway (Jaw, Teeth, Neck)
3. Respiratory
4. Circulatory (Pulses, Allen's Test)
5. Cardiac
6. Neuro   _____ MD
7. Other   _____ SRNA

Date _____ ASA Status _____   Approved by:
Time _____ Choice of Anesthesia: _____ MD
                                                                 _____ CRNA

FIG. 1-1. Preanesthetic assessment form.

prompt further investigation to define the presence and severity of diseases relevant to anesthetic administration. The brevity of the history and physical examination sections indicates that anesthesiologists do not primarily seek to discover new diseases but to ensure awareness of all those that are already known. Throughout the data collection process, anesthesiologists specifically search for information that relates to the use of anesthetic agents and techniques with which they have had the most consistently favorable experience.

After completing the data base, American anesthesiologists usually grade patients' perioperative risk using the American Society of Anesthesiologists Physical Status Classification (Table 1-1).[1] The next step, which is taken either implicitly or explicitly, is to sift through all the patient information that has been reviewed and assemble the "pertinent positives" into an anesthetic problem list.

ANESTHETIC PROBLEM LIST

Similar to internists, anesthesiologists are concerned with such patient information as drug allergies, hydration status, cardiac reserve, and pulmonary function. Certain aspects of patient anatomy, physiology, or pathology are likely to be of disproportionate interest to anesthesiologists, however. Examples include (1) head and neck anatomy associated with potentially difficult tracheal intubation or mask ventilation, (2) pseudocholinesterase deficiency responsible for prolonged paralysis after a previous anesthetic episode, and (3) strabismus (which may predispose patients to the development of malignant hyperthermia).

Table 1-2 is an example of an anesthetic problem list for a complicated obstetric patient.

TABLE 1–1. American Society of Anesthesiologists Physical Status Classification

Class	Description
1	Normal healthy patient
2	Patient with mild systemic disease
3	Patient with a severe systemic disease that limits activity but is not incapacitating
4	Patient with an incapacitating systemic disease that is a constant threat to life
5	Moribund patient not expected to survive 24 hours with or without an operation
E	In the evaluation of emergencies, the number is preceded with an E

(ASA Physical Status Classification List, 1964, is reprinted with permission of the American Society of Anesthesiologists, 520 N. Northwest Highway, Park Ridge, IL 60068-2573)

TABLE 1–2. Example of an Anesthetic Problem List: A 14-Year-Old Patient Scheduled for Urgent Cesarean Section

Patient refuses regional anesthesia
Receding chin (possible difficult intubation)
Severe preeclampsia
 Systemic arterial hypertension (diastolic blood pressure 110 mmHg on admission)
  Treatment: $MgSO_4$ infusion
  Treatment: intravenous bolus of hydralazine
 Dehydration/oliguria → Resolved
 Coagulation function marginal
  Platelet count of 110,000
  Prothrombin time and partial thromboplastin time are normal; fibrinogen of 120
 Generalized edema (possibly difficult intubation)
Anemia
 Prehydration hematocrit of 28%
 Red blood cell indices pending
Type and crossmatch not yet complete
Fetal tachycardia with lack of variability
Premature rupture of membranes
Piped-in oxygen to cesarean section room not working; oxygen source for anesthetic machine is its back-up E-cylinders

ANESTHETIC PLAN

The Timing of the Operative Procedure: Preoperative Optimization

Anesthesiologists are not ordinarily involved in determining the need for surgery. They should ensure, however, that patient medical status has been "optimized" before an elective operative procedure is performed. This is particularly important in patients who have reversible or potentially reversible conditions (eg, bronchospasm, congestive heart failure). Chronic, irreversible diseases also influence surgical outcome and affect anesthetic technique. Once the decision has been made to perform an operation, however, they provide little justification for its postponement.

Elements of the Anesthetic Plan

Many central nervous system depressant drugs given alone or in combination produce unconsciousness and insensibility to pain. Any of several different regional anesthetic techniques may also be suitable for a particular surgical procedure. Whether it is designed for general or regional anesthesia, however, an anesthetic plan is typically organized as follows:

1. Premedication
2. Application of physiologic monitors
3. Preoxygenation (with sedation)

4. Induction
5. Maintenance
6. Emergence
7. Transportation and recovery room care
8. Control of postoperative pain

Contemporary anesthetic plans, especially those designed for general anesthesia, typically involve the administration of drugs from several pharmacologic classes. Table 1-3 lists some of the most important agents in current use.

Premedication. Anesthesiologists' ability to gain the confidence of patients during preoperative visits is more important than is pharmacologic sedation in allaying patient anxiety about an impending anesthetic.[2] Nevertheless, medications of the following types are often administered before operation to create several helpful effects:

> *Anticholinergics:* to reduce oral secretions (and, thereby, the risk of laryngospasm) and to reduce the likelihood of the development of succinylcholine-induced bradycardia
> *Opiates:* to reduce anxiety and physical discomfort
> *Sedatives, often with antiemetic properties:* to reduce anxiety and prevent opiate-induced nausea
> *Nonparticulate antacids or H₂ antagonists:* to reduce gastric acidity and lessen lung damage in the event pulmonary aspiration of gastric contents occurs
> *Certain of patients' usual medications:* to control underlying cardiovascular, pulmonary, endocrine, or other diseases

It has become standard practice to administer, early on the morning of surgery, any medications that patients routinely take to maintain cardiovascular homeostasis, especially antihypertensive and antianginal agents. If a patient who usually takes a cardiac glycoside to control congestive heart failure is scheduled to undergo a major operative procedure, continuous infusion of an inotropic agent such as dopamine or dobutamine is often substituted for perioperative digitalis administration because these β-agonists are more potent and controllable, and because they have less tendency than digitalis to cause ventricular arrhythmias in the event the patient becomes hypokalemic. Patients who are taking digitalis to control the atrial fibrillation rate, however, usually continue to receive a cardiac glycoside throughout their hospital stay.

Medicines to control bronchopulmonary disease, including antibronchospastic agents and glucocorticoids, are administered orally, intravenously, or by inhalation as appropriate.

Attention is also given to the maintenance of perioperative endocrine homeostasis. Because of its long half-life, thyroxine is often omitted on the day of surgery. Patients receiving long-term glucocorticoid therapy, however, continue to take a drug of this class (often in increased dosage). It is commonly recommended that patients receive some fraction of their daily NPH insulin dose on the morning of surgery. Hypoglycemia severe enough to produce convulsions, coma, and brain damage can result from such insulin administration, however, if a dextrose infusion is not started or is interrupted for any reason. Careful monitoring

TABLE 1–3. Drugs Commonly Administered During General Anesthesia

Gases and Volatile Liquids	Mixed opiate agonist-antagonists	Neuromuscular blockers (muscle relaxants)
Oxygen	Nalbuphine (Nubain)	Succinylcholine
Nitrous oxide (N₂O)	Butorphanol (Stadol)	Curare
Halogenated inhalational agents	Buprenorphine (Buprenex)	Metocurine (Metubine)
Halothane (Fluothane)	Dezocine (Dalgan)	Atracurium (Tracrium)
Enflurane (Ethrane)	Opiate antagonist	Mivacurium (Mivacron)
Isoflurane (Forane)	Naloxone (Narcan)	Doxacurium (Neuromax)
Desflurane (Suprane)	Benzodiazepines	Pancuronium (Pavulon)
Injectable Drugs	Diazepam (Valium)	Vecuronium (Norcuron)
Hypnotic (induction) agents	Midazolam (Versed)	Pipecuronium (Arduan)
Thiopental (Pentothal)	Lorazepam (Ativan)	Rocuronium (Zemuron)
Thiamylal (Surital)	Benzodiazepine antagonist	Cholinesterase inhibitors
Methohexital (Brevital)	Flumazenil (Rumazicon)	Edrophonium (Tensilon, Enlon, Reversol)
Etomidate (Amidate)	Dissociatives	Neostigmine (Prostigmine)
Propofol (Diprivan)	Ketamine (Ketalar,	Pyridostigmine (Regonol, Mestinon)
Opiates	Ketacet)	Antimuscarinics
Morphine	Neuroleptic (major tranquilizer)	Atropine
Meperidine (Demerol)	Droperidol (Inapsine)	Scopolamine
Fentanyl (Sublimaze)		Glycopyrrolate (Robinul)
Sufentanil (Sufenta)		
Alfentanil (Alfenta)		

of the intravenous line is exceedingly important in these patients.

The administration of patients' usual psychiatric medications on the morning of surgery (and throughout the hospital stay) has been a matter of individual discretion, with the exception of monoamine oxidase A inhibitors such as tranylcypromine, phenelzine, pargyline, and isocarboxazid. These long-acting drugs can interact with the commonly prescribed analgesic, meperidine (Demerol), to produce convulsions, coma, and cardiovascular instability and, therefore, are usually discontinued at least 2 weeks before operation unless specific anesthetic techniques and postoperative pain control methods are to be used.[3–6]

Monitoring. Anesthesiologists monitor both the functioning of their own equipment and their patients' responses to anesthesia and surgery. The main goals of such monitoring are (1) to improve the precision with which drugs, parenteral fluids, blood products, and ventilation can be titrated to patients' needs; and (2) to facilitate early detection of the occurrence of critical events (eg, esophageal intubation and breathing circuit disconnection) that result in serious injury or death if they are not quickly rectified. Table 1-4 lists some of the anesthetic monitors in common use. Anesthesiologists are not restricted to such measurements, however, and may arrange for the performance of any other indicated diagnostic tests (eg, assay of plasma electrolytes, chest radiography, fiberoptic bronchoscopy) before, during, or after operation.

Preoxygenation and sedation. Patients often are given 100% oxygen for several minutes before general anesthesia

TABLE 1–4. Physiologic Variables Monitored During the Administration of Anesthesia

Routine	Optional
Breath sounds (after tracheal intubation)	Urine output
Breath sounds and heart tones (continuously through precordial or esophageal stethoscope)	Output of any other indwelling tubes (nasogastric, pleural, mediastinal, etc.)
Appearance of the surgical field	Arterial blood gases (pH, P_{CO_2}, P_{O_2}), serial
For the progress of surgery	Inhaled nitrous oxide concentration (spectrophotometry)
For cyanosis	Exhaled nitrogen concentration (spectrophotometry)
For an estimation of blood loss	Transcutaneous P_{O_2}
Peak ventilation pressure (gauge)	Transcutaneous P_{CO_2}
Ventilatory compliance	Cardiac electrical activity
Manually by the anesthesia reservoir bag	Multilead monitoring
By gauge during mechanical ventilation	ST segment trending
F_{IO_2} (polarography)	Arterial pressure (invasive): extent of depression with positive-pressure mechanical ventilation (a gauge of intravascular volume status)
Arterial oxygen saturation (pulse oximetry)	Central venous pressure
Respiratory rate	Pulmonary artery pressure (Swan-Ganz catheter)
Inspiratory and expiratory breath P_{CO_2} (spectrophotometry)	Wedge pressure
Tidal volume and minute volume (spirometry)	Left atrial pressure (invasive)
Inhaled anesthetic gas concentration (spectrophotometry)	Cardiac output
Pulse strength (palpation)	Pulmonary artery catheter
Blood pressure (noninvasive)	Noninvasive
Cardiac electrical activity (single-lead electrocardiogram)	Precordial Doppler cardiogram
Operative blood loss	Peripheral arterial flow (Doppler)
Surgical suction	Three-dimensional cardiac wall and valvular motion (transesophageal echocardiography)
Surgical sponges	Mixed venous oxygen tension
Surgical field	Intermittent by blood gas analysis
Concealed (by inference)	Continuously by oximetry
Fluid intake	Blood glucose, serial
Total intravenous fluids	Hematocrit and hemoglobin, serial
Blood products	Platelet count, serial
Temperature	Coagulation (prothrombin time, partial thromboplastin time, activated coagulation time thromboelastography), serial
Core (esophageal)	Cerebral electrical activity (spontaneous and evoked)
Skin	Intracranial pressure
Neuromuscular transmission (peripheral nerve stimulator)	

is induced. This maneuver promotes the exchange of bronchial and alveolar nitrogen for oxygen and thereby creates an internal oxygen reservoir capable of increasing by several minutes the time from the onset of (anesthetic-induced) apnea to the development of arterial oxyhemoglobin desaturation.[7–9] A tightly fitting face mask is necessary to ensure maximum benefit. Because this can cause mild discomfort or claustrophobia, intravenous sedation is usually administered at the same time. Patients receiving regional anesthesia and intravenous sedation often are given oxygen through a nasal cannula.

Anesthetic induction. Because the inhalation of anesthetic gases typically produces surgical anesthesia only after patients have passed through a "stage of excitement" (which may include delirium, combativeness, breath-holding, laryngospasm, or vomiting), the intravenous induction of general anesthesia in adults is now an almost universal practice. The following is a typical general anesthetic induction sequence for healthy patients who have not eaten for at least 6 hours before an elective surgical procedure:

1. Administration of a small dose of a nondepolarizing neuromuscular blocking agent (eg, curare) to reduce succinylcholine-induced muscle fasciculations and, perhaps, postoperative myalgia
2. Administration of an opiate or sympatholytic agent to blunt the stress response (hypertension, tachycardia) that typically occurs after tracheal intubation
3. Rapid intravenous administration of the hypnotic (induction) agent, often a thiobarbiturate
4. Administration of a fully paralyzing dose of succinylcholine or some other neuromuscular blocking drug
5. Intermittent positive-pressure mask ventilation with oxygen
6. Insertion of the endotracheal tube (including verification of correct placement)
7. Continuation of positive-pressure ventilation (often by institution of mechanical ventilation) and adjustment of the delivery rates of inhaled and intravenous anesthetic agents to achieve a surgical level of anesthesia without undue cardiovascular depression
8. Provision for ocular protection and placement of additional monitors (eg, Foley catheter, arterial and central venous lines)
9. Positioning of patients for the operative procedure

General anesthetic induction is a busy time for anesthesiologists. Their attention must shift rapidly between the level of consciousness, the adequacy of neuromuscular blockade, the airway, oxygenation and ventilation, and the cardiovascular system.

In the case of regional anesthesia, induction consists of the performance of one or more nerve blocks. An epidural or paraneural catheter may be inserted to permit the repeated injection or continuous infusion of local anesthetic solution. When general and regional anesthetic techniques are combined, either type of induction can precede the other.

Anesthetic maintenance. The most popular hypnotic agents produce unconsciousness for only a few minutes. Anesthetic drugs (plus oxygen), therefore, must be given to maintain general anesthesia for the duration of the operative procedure. Currently available inhaled agents include nitrous oxide, halothane, enflurane, isoflurane, and desflurane. Benzodiazepines, opiates, barbiturates, and other injectable anesthetic agents (see Table 1-3), especially when they are used in combination, are sufficient to maintain general anesthesia but are more commonly used to supplement inhaled anesthetic agents.

The administration of central nervous system depressant drugs constitutes only a portion of modern anesthetic care. To ensure a motionless operative field and to weaken skeletal muscles that must be retracted to expose the surgical site, neuromuscular blocking agents are also given frequently. Peripheral neural blockade using local anesthetic drugs can be instituted to unconscious patients to reduce their requirement for systemically acting drugs. Anesthesiologists also administer any other medications, intravenous fluids, or blood products that are required to maintain intraoperative and postoperative cardiovascular, pulmonary, endocrine, hematologic, renal, acid–base, and fluid and electrolyte homeostasis.

Anesthetic emergence. When the operative procedure is nearly completed (and provided there is no plan for postoperative mechanical ventilation), the administration of anesthetic agents is discontinued. Before patients awaken, any weakness related to residual effects of nondepolarizing neuromuscular blocking agents is reversed using the combination of a cholinesterase-inhibiting and an antimuscarinic drug (see Table 1-3). Hypertension and tachycardia severe enough to require pharmacologic control are common during emergence from general anesthesia. Patients may struggle vigorously, particularly if endotracheal tubes are in place. Removal of the tubes to calm patients can provoke laryngospasm. If patients inhale vigorously during the time that the glottis is closed, negative-pressure pulmonary edema can result.

Occasionally, unconsciousness or weakness persists long after anesthetic agent administration has ceased. The time required for patients to awaken from general anesthesia can sometimes be shortened by the intravenous injection of a specific pharmacologic antagonist such as naloxone or flumazenil or of a general analeptic agent (stimulant) such as aminophylline, caffeine, physostigmine, or doxapram. The administration of such agents can unmask severe pain at the operative site or produce hypertension, tachycardia, myocardial ischemia, pulmonary edema, nausea, vomiting, seizures, or postoperative renarcotization. Such side effects have discouraged the routine use of these drugs to speed the return of consciousness.

Transportation and recovery room. Patients whose endotracheal tubes have been removed can be transported to the recovery room once they are judged to be able to maintain and protect an airway and to breathe adequately while en route. Other patients are probably best transported with their endotracheal tubes in place. Positive-pressure ventilation is not discontinued if spontaneous ventilatory adequacy is at all dubious. Vigilance cannot be relaxed during transportation even if patients are fully awake because regurgitation, choking, laryngospasm, flailing, apnea, and cyanosis occasionally occur without warning. Supplementary oxygen should be administered to many patients during conveyance to the recovery room.[10,11]

During the early part of the recovery room stay, the adequacy of the airway, breathing, and circulation is assessed repeatedly. Renarcotization and dangerous respiratory depression can occur during this period, particularly in patients who have received substantial doses of intravenous anesthetic agents and those who were given narcotic antagonists, benzodiazepine antagonists, or analeptic drugs. Parenteral opiates are administered intravenously in small increments because their respiratory and central nervous system depressant effects are enhanced by the residual presence of anesthetic drugs. Respiratory embarrassment resulting from incompletely reversed or eliminated neuromuscular blocking drugs can also first become apparent in the recovery room.

Good recovery room care entails the observation and treatment of patients for any adverse effects of surgery as well as anesthesia. Of paramount importance in this regard is the early detection of concealed hemorrhage. This diagnosis is usually suspected when unexplained hypotension repeatedly responds to the intravenous administration of large volumes of crystalloid or colloid solutions and serial hematocrit measurements demonstrate a precipitous decline.

Once basic life functions have been ensured, attention is shifted to the treatment of patients' coexisting medical illnesses.

Control of postoperative pain. Anesthesiologists, more often now than in the past, participate in efforts to control postoperative pain that occurs after patients have left the recovery room. This is especially true if the postoperative analgesic regimen includes neuraxially (spinally or epidurally) administered opiates or local anesthetics. Regional analgesic techniques can improve postoperative pulmonary function and promote early mobilization but are labor-intensive (and, therefore, expensive) and not without their

own special risks. Surgical complications such as a leaking bowel anastomosis can be more difficult to detect in patients receiving neuraxial analgesia. When this occurs, definitive surgical treatment is correspondingly delayed. Anticoagulant or thrombolytic agents probably should not be administered to patients receiving spinal or epidural analgesia because they increase the likelihood of development of a compressive epidural hematoma and permanent paraplegia.[12,13]

Choosing the Anesthetic Plan

In designing an anesthetic plan, anesthesiologists consider many factors, including the following:

- Prevailing standards of care
- Training and personal experience in anesthetizing similarly ill patients for the planned surgical procedure
- Skill, speed, methods, and preferences of the operating surgeon
- Recommendations from patients' primary physicians and any consultants
- Nature of the facility where the operation is being performed (eg, hospital with intensive care unit versus freestanding surgical center)
- Patient's own wishes

The dominance of personal considerations in this list partly explains the cornucopia of anesthetic techniques now in use. Customizing the anesthetic plan is a matter of pride to anesthetists but often a source of confusion to others.

ROLE OF THE MEDICAL CONSULTANT IN ANESTHETIC CARE

Medical consultants may be asked to provide advice regarding surgical patients' medical care or to manage certain aspects of such care either before or after operation.

PREOPERATIVE CONSULTATION

Administering general anesthetics to surgical patients is in many ways similar to resuscitating victims of combined severe central nervous system depressant drug overdose and penetrating trauma. A spinal or epidural anesthetic creates (at least temporarily) the same physiologic alterations as does acute spinal cord injury. Even when they are caring for healthy patients, therefore, anesthesiologists must devote a significant amount of their time and attention to protecting patients from iatrogenic harm. Experienced medical consultants understand this and seek to help anesthesiologists incorporate the management of patients' medical problems into anesthetic techniques with which anesthesiologists are skilled and comfortable.

Anesthetic Choice

Some medical consultants evaluating surgical patients before operation believe it to be their duty to specify the type of anesthetic that should be administered. Those who choose to recommend a particular anesthetic typically favor regional anesthesia based on their assumption that local anesthetic injection is safer than general anesthetic administration in medically compromised patients. Retrospective and prospective studies of the safety of general versus regional anesthesia conducted during the past half century provide little support for this notion, however.[14-19] It is true that general anesthesia is not without important risks, even in healthy patients. It should not be forgotten, however, that neuraxial (spinal or epidural) anesthesia, because of its associated sympathetic blockade, can cause hypotension as sudden, profound, and refractory to treatment as is ever seen after general anesthetic induction. Well-intentioned advice to anesthesiologists to avoid general anesthesia can also create practical difficulties. It is not at all unusual, for example, that a regional technique must be abandoned and a contingency plan for general anesthesia implemented for reasons such as the following:

- Last-minute patient refusal of regional anesthesia
- Inability of patients to cooperate with the performance of the block
- Discovery of local infection at the site of proposed local anesthetic injection
- Discovery of the presence of a coagulopathy or a decision by the surgeon to institute (or potentially institute) anticoagulation or thrombolysis
- Discovery of preoperative hypotension (which is likely to be worsened by spinal or epidural anesthesia)
- Intraoperative occurrence of hypoventilation or arterial oxygen desaturation sufficient to require tracheal intubation, mechanical ventilation, positive end-expiratory pressure, tracheal suction, or other respiratory care
- Inadequate quality or duration of action of the nerve block
- Uncontrollable anxiety or deliriousness of patients

POSTOPERATIVE CONSULTATION

Medical consultants who are asked to see patients for the first time during the early postoperative period should first determine whether the matter is urgent, particularly if patients are still in the recovery room. A consultation requested during the immediate postoperative period is usually either a request for help in managing the medical care of patients whose emergency surgery precluded earlier consultation, or a request for assistance in diagnosing or treating a new problem (frequently a surgical or anesthetic complication).

When medical consultants are called to the recovery room to help in diagnosis, they should remember that anesthesiologists determine the cause of most intraoperative and postoperative problems without aid. Because such routine postanesthetic problems are precisely those with which medical consultants usually have the least familiarity, they can often save time (and occasionally embarrassment) by first learning which possible diagnoses the anesthesiologists have considered. Important information can also sometimes be obtained from surgeons, nurse anesthetists, recovery room nurses, patients' families, and even patients themselves.

Several relatively common immediate postanesthetic problems are summarized in Table 1-5. The first step in resolving the differential diagnosis of many such problems is to rule out (or in) the presence of arterial hypoxemia, because calamity awaits patients in whom serious hypoxia has been overlooked. The detection of arterial oxygen desaturation has been greatly facilitated by the routine use of pulse oximetry in the recovery room.

The cause of many puzzling postoperative medical problems is eventually traced to exaggerated, prolonged, or unusual reactions to anesthetic drugs. Medical consultants can find the names and dosages of all drugs administered during an anesthetic episode on patients' anesthetic records. With a little practice (and some initial assistance from anesthesiologists), consultants can quickly become adept at interpreting the information in this important document.

Extreme caution must be taken before making a diagnosis of brain death in patients who have recently received a general or regional anesthetic. Central nervous system alterations produced by hypothermia, barbiturates, other general anesthetic agents, and even local anesthetic drugs (if they reach the brain) can produce findings on neurologic examination and electroencephalography that are indistinguishable from those produced by hypoxic encephalopathy or brain death.

An example of the hazards of disregarding this warning is the following true case of a consulting staff neurologist who received a request from a hospital medical director to examine a patient in the recovery room. Immediately after the performance of a stellate ganglion block, the patient had developed total spinal anesthesia, undoubtedly as the result of inadvertent subarachnoid injection of a large volume of local anesthetic solution. When she was examined by the neurologist, the patient required full mechanical ventilation. Continuous intravenous infusion of epinephrine was

TABLE 1–5. Common Intraoperative and Postoperative Problems for Which Medical Consultation May Be Sought With a Partial List of Anesthesia-Related Causes

Problem	Anesthesia-Related Causes
Hypoxia	Inadequate F_{IO_2} Airway collapse or obstruction (often signaled by inspiratory stridor if incomplete) from unconsciousness, residual effects of neuromuscular blocking drugs, airway foreign body, laryngeal edema, tracheal compression from neck or mediastinal hematoma or extravasation of fluids from central line catheter; if an endotracheal tube is present, it may be kinked (sometimes intraorally) or blocked (eg, with blood clot, tenacious bronchial secretions, chewing gum) Hypoventilation (eg, from weakness, pain from thoracic or abdominal incision, ventilator circuit disconnection or leak) Extrinsic or intrinsic disease of lungs or bronchi, such as pneumothorax, pleural effusion, microatelectasis, lobar collapse, aspiration (of blood, gastric contents, or saliva), pulmonary edema, bronchospasm Shock Artefact
Dyspnea	All the causes of hypoxia (many of which can cause dyspnea independent of producing hypoxemia) Hypercapnea Presence of an endotracheal tube, especially one of small diameter Circulatory insufficiency from almost any cause
Pulmonary edema*	Fluid overload (evidence of good systemic perfusion) Congestive heart failure (evidence of poor systemic perfusion) Pulmonary aspiration of gastric contents Negative-pressure pulmonary edema (resulting from laryngospasm after tracheal extubation while patient simultaneously makes vigorous inspiratory efforts) Massive catecholamine overdose (usually topical phenylephrine or epinephrine administered by surgeon)
Hypotension or shock Hypovolemic	Artefact Bleeding Interstitial edema (third-space loss) Inadequate administration of crystalloid colloid, or blood products
Cardiogenic	Hypoxia Myocardial infarction Cardiac tamponade Drug overdose or administration error involving negative inotropic drug (often a general anesthetic or local anesthetic drug)
Obstructive	Cardiac tamponade Pneumothorax Hemothorax Intrapleural infusion of intravenous fluids Venous air embolism Pulmonary thromboembolism Inferior vena caval compression (eg, from supine position during advanced pregnancy)

Distributive	Severe endocrine imbalance
	  Adrenal insufficiency, often from unintentional discontinuation of chronically administered glucocorticoid medication, etomidate administered daily or for long-term sedation by infusion
	  Insulin excess causing profound hypoglycemia
	  Thyrotoxicosis or myxedema
	  Panhypopituitarism
	Vasodilator drug overdose
	Neuraxial local anesthetic block, such as spinal or epidural anesthesia, especially high or "total" spinal anesthesia (spinal anesthesia extending excessively cephalad to produce cervical dermatomal anesthesia with or without diaphragmatic paralysis and with or without unconsciousness)
	Anaphylaxis (or anaphylactoid reaction)—from either drug administration (antibiotics, morphine, curare) or latex exposure

(continued)

TABLE 1–5. (Continued)

Problem	Anesthesia-Related Causes
Hypertension	Hypoxia Hypercapnea Pain Preexisting hypertension Vasopressor drug administration Artefact
Tachycardia	Hypoxia Hypercapnea Hypovolemia (most importantly, from concealed hemorrhage) Pain Anxiety Medications, including vasodilator or chronotropic drugs Shock (or impending shock from nearly any cause—see above) Malignant hyperthermia (temperature rises only after occurrence of tachycardia; confirm diagnosis with blood gas) Artefact See also hypotension or shock (above)
Bradycardia	Profound hypoxia Heart block Myocardial infarction (especially inferior wall) Negative chronotropic drug administration (β-blocker, cholinesterase inhibitor) Bladder distention Severely increased intracranial pressure Artefact
Ventricular arrhythmias	Hypoxia, hypercapnea, hypokalemia, hypomagnesemia, hyperkalemia, such as after massive transfusion in patients with renal insufficiency or transiently (but massively) after the administration of succinylcholine to patients with recent, crush, burn, or upper or lower motor neuron injuries (eg, cerebrovascular accident, paraplegia or quadriplegia, Guillain-Barré or other peripheral neuropathy, tetanus, polio) Myocardial ischemia or infarction Artefact
Chest pain	Hypoxia Surgical procedures involving the thorax Pneumothorax Reflux esophagitis Myocardial ischemia or infarction Pulmonary thromboembolism
Fever	Exogenous heat (hot operating room, heated inspired gases, use of warming lights or warming blanket) Reduced heat loss (eg, from extensive draping of patient, especially with plastic drapes) Malignant hyperthermia (can become manifest up to several hours after operation)—Malignant Hyperthermia U.S.A. hotline: 209-634-4917 Artefact
Oliguria	Hypovolemia Renal insufficiency or failure (may occur acutely from shock or transfusion with incompatible blood) Artefact (eg, anuria from kinked or blocked urinary drainage system or incorrectly inserted Foley catheter)
Dark urine	Myoglobinuria after succinylcholine administration Hemoglobinuria from transfusion of incompatible blood, Foley catheter trauma, dehydration, or hypovolemia
Prolonged time to awakening, coma	Hypoxia Extreme hypercapnea Residual effects of general anesthetic drugs (eg, high doses of short-acting drugs or normal doses of longer-acting drugs such as morphine, droperidol, or ketamine) Hypothermia

(continued)

TABLE 1–5. (Continued)

Problem	Anesthesia-Related Causes
Prolonged time to awakening, coma (cont.)	Hypoxic brain damage Embolic brain damage (arterial thromboembolism, paradoxical embolism of air or thrombus) Intracerebral hemorrhage (eg, from an episode of severe hypertension, especially in an anticoagulated patient) Total spinal anesthesia Tension pneumocephalus (from intraoperative administration of nitrous oxide once air was trapped intracranially) Artefact (eg, profound pharmacologic neuromuscular blockade: differentiate using peripheral nerve stimulator)
Renarcotization	Hypoxia Cessation of effects of antagonist (naloxone or flumazenil) or analeptic drug (caffeine, aminophylline, physostigmine) Reduction in physical or psychologic stimulation of patient with high residual blood opiate level Potentiation of respiratory or central nervous system depressant effects of residual anesthetic drugs (by administration of a second drug, often an antiemetic such as droperidol) Administration of opiate analgesic or other central nervous system depressant drug either intentionally or inadvertently Neuraxial opiate analgesia (may occur 16 hours or more after the administration of spinal or epidural morphine
Delirium	Hypoxia, hypercapnea, hypoglycemia, hyponatremia (especially from massive venous uptake of glycine irrigating solution during transurethral prostate resection) Residual effects of central nervous system depressant drugs Central anticholinergic syndrome (from atropine or scopolamine administration) Dissociative state (from ketamine) Preexisting neurosis or paranoia (unusual in schizophrenia or depression) Psychic trauma (eg, from recall of frightening or painful intraoperative events)

*When comparing *postoperative* pulmonary artery, wedge, and central venous pressures with *intraoperative* pressures, remember that these pressures are often reduced in proportion to general anesthetic "depth," especially when a volatile, halogenated anesthetic agent is being used.

necessary to maintain satisfactory arterial blood pressure. She had areflexia and her pupils were fixed and fully dilated. Without discussing the case with the anesthesiologist, the neurologist concluded that the patient's anesthetic had been complicated by a hypoxic accident. He advised the medical director that the patient was either severely brain damaged or brain dead. Within only a few hours of his pronouncement, however, the effects of the local anesthetic drug abated. The patient's circulatory system stabilized. She awakened, extubated herself, and was found to be completely intact neurologically.

A related problem is that of distinguishing coma from residual motor paralysis (which can last at least a day after the last administered dose of a neuromuscular blocking drug[20]). Weakness (rather than unconsciousness) can be suspected if the circulation is hyperdynamic (suggesting the presence of pain and fear). The presence of neuromuscular blockade can be confirmed by checking (1) the pupillary reactions to light (which are normal in conscious patients with drug-induced paralysis), (2) the muscular response to electrical stimulation of a peripheral motor nerve or the brachial plexus in the axilla, or (3) the electroencephalogram.

Experienced medical consultants who are asked for advice regarding the management of intraoperative or postoperative complications consider, along with all relevant medical issues, the social or medicolegal impact that expressed opinions will have on colleagues' reputations (or on their own reputation if the opinions prove to be erroneous). Before passing judgment in such cases (even if there is no question of negligence), they gather all relevant information with scrupulous thoroughness and tact.

COMMUNICATION BETWEEN INTERNAL MEDICINE CONSULTANTS AND ANESTHESIOLOGISTS

Perhaps because their paths cross infrequently during the course of the average day, internists and anesthesiologists do not communicate as much as they should.[21] Patients' medical records provide a venue for the exchange of ideas between these professionals, but the official nature of this document can inhibit an open and collaborative approach to problem solving. Especially when a problem is novel or complex, direct communication between anesthesiologists and medical consultants (and surgeons) is usually superior and worth some additional trouble to arrange. An example of a common situation in which two-way communication is helpful is that which occurs when a surgeon requests an internal medicine consultation to ensure that the anesthesiologist will judge a patient to be ready to undergo the proposed procedure. Usually, after only a few face-to-face or telephone conversations, physicians who collaborate with each other regularly become familiar with their colleagues' views on most issues of mutual concern.

Occasionally, medical consultants discover that a preoperative consultation that initially appeared to be a straightforward request for an opinion occurs in the context of a dispute between an anesthesiologist and a surgeon. Experienced internists proceed carefully in such cases, first accumulating the relevant clinical data and medical facts and always remaining faithful to their responsibility to help ensure patient safety. Mediation skills can prove useful at such times.

BIBLIOGRAPHY

GENERAL ANESTHESIOLOGY TEXTS

Barash PG, Cullen BF, Stoelting RK, eds. Clinical anesthesia, ed 2. Philadelphia, JB Lippincott, 1992.

Atkinson RS, Rushman GB, Lee J. A synopsis of anaesthesia, ed 10. Bristol, UK, Wright, 1987.

Rogers MC, Covino BG, Tinker JH, Longnecker DE. Principles and practice of anesthesiology. In: Miller RD, ed. Anesthesia, ed 3. St Louis, Mosby–Year Book, 1993.

ANESTHETIZING THE MEDICALLY COMPROMISED PATIENT

Katz J, Benumof JL, Kadis LB, eds. Anesthesia and uncommon diseases: pathophysiologic and clinical correlations, ed 3. Philadelphia, Saunders, 1990.

Stoelting RK, Dierdorf SF, McCammon RL, eds. Anesthesia and co-existing disease, ed 2. New York, Churchill Livingstone, 1988.

Cheng EY, Kay J, eds. Manual of anesthesia and the medically compromised patient. Philadelphia, JB Lippincott, 1990.

COMPLICATIONS OF ANESTHESIA

Brown DL, ed. Risk and outcome in anesthesia, ed 2. Philadelphia, JB Lippincott, 1992.

Gravenstein N, ed. Manual of complications during anesthesia, ed. 2. Philadelphia, JB Lippincott, 1995.

Orkin FK, Cooperman LH. Complications in anesthesiology. Philadelphia, JB Lippincott, 1983.

REFERENCES

1. New classification of physical status (approved by American Society House of Delegates). Anesthesiology 1963;24:111.
2. Egbert LD, Battit GE, Turndorf H, Beecher HK. The value of the preoperative visit by an anesthetist: a study of doctor–patient rapport. JAMA 1963;185:553–555.
3. Orkin FK, Cooperman LH. Complications in anesthesiology. Philadelphia, JB Lippincott, 1983.
4. Vigran IM. Dangerous potentiation of meperidine hydrochloride by pargyline hydrochloride. JAMA 1964;187:953–954.
5. Wells DG, Bjorksten AR. Monoamine oxidase inhibitors revisited. Can J Anaesth 1989;36:64–74.
6. Hirschman CA, Lindeman K. MAO inhibitors: must they be discontinued before anesthesia. JAMA 1988;260:3507–3508.
7. Miles GG, Martin NT, Adriani J. Factors influencing the elimination of nitrogen using semiclosed inhalers. Anesthesiology 1956;17:213–221.
8. Dillon JB, Darsi ML. Oxygen for acute respiratory depression due to administration of thiopental sodium. JAMA 1955;159:1114–1116.
9. Ovassapian A, Meyer RM. Airway management. In: Longnecker DE, Murphy FL, eds. Dripps/Eckenhoff/Vandam introduction to anesthesia, ed 8. Philadelphia, WB Saunders, 1992.
10. Tyler IL, Tantisira B, Winter PM, Motoyama EK. Continuous monitoring of arterial oxygen saturation with pulse oximetry during transfer to the recovery room. Anesth Analg 1985;64:1108–1112.
11. Meiklejohn BH, Smith G, Elling AE, Hindocha N. Arterial oxygen desaturation during postoperative transportation: the influence of the operative site. Anaesthesia 1987;42:1313–1315.
12. James CF. Local and regional anesthesia. In: Gravenstein N, ed. Manual of complications during anesthesia. Philadelphia, JB Lippincott, 1991.
13. Onishchuk JL, Carlsson C. Epidural hematoma associated with epidural anesthesia: complications of anticoagulant therapy. Anesthesiology 1992;77:1221–1223.
14. Arkins R, Smessaert AA, Hicks RG. Mortality and morbidity in surgical patients with coronary artery disease. JAMA 1964;190:485–488.
15. Topkins MJ, Artusio JF Jr. Myocardial infarction and surgery: a five year study. Anesth Analg 1964;43:716–720.
16. Tarhan S, Moffitt EA, Taylor WF, Giuliani ER. Myocardial infarction after general anesthesia. JAMA 1972;220:1451–1454.
17. Steen PA, Tinker JH, Tarhan S. Myocardial reinfarction after anesthesia and surgery. JAMA 1978;239:2566–2570.
18. Brown DL. Anesthetic choice. In: Brown DL, ed. Risk & outcome in anesthesia, ed 2. Philadelphia, JB Lippincott, 1992.
19. Sorenson RM, Pace NL. Anesthetic techniques during surgical

repair of femoral neck fractures: a meta-analysis. Anesthesiology 1992;77:1095–1104.

20. Petersen RS, Bailey PL, Kalameghan R, Ashwood ER. Prolonged neuromuscular block after mivacurium. Anesth Analg 1993;76:194–196.

21. Lee TH, Goldman L. Use and misuse of consultants. In: Rogers MC, Covino BG, Tinker JH, Longnecker DE, eds. Principles and practice of anesthesiology. St Louis, Mosby–Year Book, 1993.

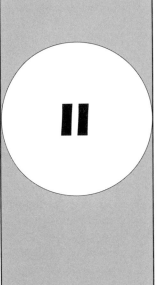

NUTRITION

Medical Management of the Surgical Patient, Third Edition,
edited by Michael F. Lubin, H. Kenneth Walker, and Robert B. Smith III.
J.B. Lippincott Company, Philadelphia, PA © 1995.

NUTRITION

2

Joseph D. Ansley

The nutritional status of surgical patients and the metabolic response to injury are recognized as important factors in wound healing, postoperative complications, infection, and the overall recovery from surgical procedures.[1] Providing appropriate nutritional support to surgical patients can be difficult, however, because surgical diseases and surgical procedures often do not allow the normal oral intake of the nutritionally complete diet that is needed to maintain adequate muscle mass, visceral proteins, and metabolism. Inadequate intake may result from obstructive lesions of the gastrointestinal tract, malabsorption, anorexia related to cancer or other debilitating conditions, postoperative ileus, or the necessity for prolonged bowel rest. The major advance in resolving the problem of inadequate nutritional intake was made by Dudrick and colleagues,[2] who developed a concentrated total parenteral nutrition (TPN) solution that could be administered through the large-caliber, high-flow central veins. This significant development has been followed by two decades of clinical application and additional nutritional research leading to many refinements in the composition of the solutions and to a new understanding of nutritional processes in health and disease.[3–5]

The increased knowledge and interest in nutrition resulting from the development of TPN techniques has stimulated many other nutrition-related activities and specialized research. Some of the most active and productive areas include the biochemical response to traumatic stress,[4] advances in body composition research,[5] the importance of the enteral route of nutrient administration,[6] and the potential for enhancement of the immune system with specialized diets.[7] The processes and knowledge of nutritional support that evolved from parenteral nutrition techniques have resulted in a return to the use of the gastrointestinal tract as the primary method for providing nutrition for surgical or medical patients. The methods of delivery and the dietary compounds in use today have been refined so that enteral nutrition can and should be used in most surgical patients in the perioperative period.[8] Enteral nutrition is less costly, more physiologic, and associated with fewer metabolic or infectious complications than is TPN.[9]

ASSESSMENT OF NUTRITIONAL STATUS

The decision to use specialized nutritional support should be based on nutritional evaluations of patients in conjunction with assessments of the expected course of the surgical diseases or procedures. Patients who are well nourished or only mildly malnourished are unlikely to require specialized nutritional support unless they are unable to resume adequate oral intake within 7 days. Patients who are moderately malnourished can benefit from nutritional support if they will have an inadequate intake for more than 3 to 5 days. Patients who are severely malnourished may benefit from specialized nutritional support for 7 to 10 days before operation. If the urgency of the procedure precludes preoperative therapy, nutritional support should be instituted within 1 to 3 days after operation[10] (Table 2-1).

The nutritional status should be assessed using clinical information from patients' histories and physical examinations supplemented by anthropometric measurements, visceral protein measurements, and immunologic tests when available.[11] In patients with the marasmic form of protein-calorie malnutrition that is associated with starvation, clinical evaluation based on carefully performed histories and physical examinations may be sufficient for nutritional assessment.[12] A history of weight loss greater than 10% over 3 months is significant and has been shown to be of important prognostic value when it is associated with some evidence of physiologic impairment such as weakness, fatigue, or malaise.[13]

Anthropometric tests have been important for nutritional assessment in clinical research studies and for determining the prevalence of malnutrition but may not be helpful in the evaluation of individual patients.[14,15] Preoperative immunologic testing with delayed hypersensitivity skin tests (in combination with other laboratory tests, such as measurement of the albumin level) has been used as a prognostic indicator of postoperative sepsis and death.[16] Because such testing is relatively nonspecific by itself, however, and because there is a 48-hour delay in obtaining results, it is not often used in the evaluation of individual patients. The creatinine-to-height ratio also has been shown to be a sensitive indicator of protein-calorie undernutrition in studies of hospitalized surgical patients[17] and patients with cancer.[18] It requires careful 24-hour urine collection in patients who are stable and is less useful for the evaluation of acutely stressed patients.

Measurement of the visceral proteins (albumin, transferrin, and prealbumin) and determination of the total lymphocyte count are the most useful laboratory tests in diagnosing and classifying the nutritional status in patients with the hypoalbuminemic form of protein-calorie malnutrition. This type of malnutrition is seen most often in hospitalized patients today. It is less clinically recognizable than the marasmic form of malnutrition because weight loss may not be present despite severe depletion of the visceral protein stores.[19] When evaluating visceral protein values, those obtained before surgical intervention, significant stress, or the administration of intravenous fluid or blood have greater prognostic value. Albumin particularly,[20] and transferrin and prealbumin to a lesser degree, are decreased with fluid hydration and the acute stress of trauma.[21] The shorter half-life of prealbumin and retinol-binding protein may make them potentially useful in demonstrating an early response to nutritional therapy, but studies thus far have not shown them to be superior to transferrin and albumin. From a practical standpoint, most hospitalized patients can be properly assessed from a careful history and physical examination combined with measurement of one or more of the visceral proteins (Table 2-2).

Once the need for nutritional support has been determined, calorie and protein requirements must be assessed based on energy expenditure and level of stress. The Harris-Benedict equation for basal energy expenditure (BEE; see Table 2-2) is reliable for initial therapy when the correct stress level modifier is used ($1.2 \times$ BEE for mild stress to $1.75 \times$ BEE for moderate to severe stress).[22] More specific energy requirements can be determined using indirect calorimetry[23] to measure oxygen consumption when the study is performed by trained personnel but this is not routinely available because of its expense and technical limitations.[24] Protein requirements can be estimated from patient weight and level of stress, using 0.8 g/kg for maintenance, 1.5 g/kg for moderate stress, and 2 g/kg for severe stress. Nitrogen balance studies are useful in monitoring patient response to therapy. The 24-hour urine urea nitrogen excretion is used most commonly for this determination, with the addition of a factor of 4 for unmeasured urine nitrogen and extrarenal nitrogen loss. Total urinary nitrogen determination provides a more specific value for nitrogen excretion but is not performed by all clinical laboratories.[25] Newer technologies for determining body composition and nitrogen status are being evaluated using bioelectric impedance[26] and dual-energy x-ray absorptiometry.[27] These tests show promise for use in critically ill patients, in whom nutritional status and nutrient requirements are difficult to assess.[28,29]

INDICATIONS FOR PERIOPERATIVE NUTRITIONAL SUPPORT

The question of when and to whom to provide nutritional support in the perioperative period has still not been definitively answered. A metaanalysis of the safety, effectiveness, and cost of perioperative parenteral nutrition from re-

TABLE 2–1. Indications for Nutritional Intervention in the Perioperative Period*

Inadequate nutrient intake for 7 days in previously well-nourished patient

Inadequate nutrient intake for 5 days in previously well-nourished or mildly malnourished patient with acute stress

Inadequate nutrient intake for 3 days in moderate or severely malnourished patient

Weight loss of over 10% of preillness weight

Preoperative supplementation for 7 to 10 days in severely malnourished patient if surgery can be safely delayed

Therapeutic bowel rest

---

*Significant cardiopulmonary, electrolyte, or acid–base problems should be corrected first in acutely stressed patients to provide the optimal metabolic state for nutrient assimilation.

TABLE 2–2. Nutritional Assessment

	Malnutrition Severity		
	Mild	*Moderate*	*Severe*
Weight loss (%)	<10	10–20	>20
Albumin (g/dL)	<3.5	<3.0	<2.0
Transferrin (mg/dL)	<220	<170	<100
Prealbumin (mg/dL)	<17	<12	<7
Total lymphocyte count (cells/mm³)	<2000	<1500	<1000

Common Equations for Nutritional Assessment

Nitrogen balance $= \dfrac{\text{24-h protein intake}}{6.25} - (\text{24-h urine urea nitrogen} + 4)$

Modification of the Harris-Benedict equation for basal energy expenditure (in kcal)
    Women: 655 + (9.6 × weight [in kg]) + (1.7 × height [in cm]) – (4.7 × age [in years])
    Men: 66   + (13.7 × weight)   + (5 × height)   – (6.8 × age)

Ideal body weight estimation
    Women: 100 lb + 5 lb for each inch over 60
    Men: 106 lb + 6 lb for each inch over 60

ports published through 1986 did not indicate a benefit for unselected patients undergoing major surgery, but did suggest that nutritional support would be helpful in subgroups at high risk, such as severely malnourished patients.[30] A recent Department of Veterans Affairs cooperative study that randomly assigned patients to receive TPN or standard nutrition before operation reached a similar conclusion. The study showed similar rates of major postoperative complications in both groups but more infectious complications in those patients receiving TPN who were well nourished or only mildly malnourished before operation. In contrast, patients receiving TPN who were severely malnourished before operation had fewer noninfectious complications and were the only subgroup to benefit from the nutritional therapy.[31] A later economic analysis from this same trial, however, found that there was no decrease in the cost of care for any subgroup of patients receiving TPN.[32]

Another recent appraisal of this controversy reviewed both perioperative enteral nutrition and perioperative TPN, and concluded that perioperative nutritional support in properly selected groups of patients with overt malnutrition can be medically effective and reduce morbidity and mortality.[33] In an additional recent randomized study of the effect of postoperative parenteral nutritional support, no effect on outcome was demonstrated in 60% of unselected surgical patients. In the remaining patients, there was an increase in morbidity and mortality related to complications of underfeeding and also to complications of overfeeding, which occurred in similar numbers of intravenously fed patients.[34]

These studies should not be used to negate the value of perioperative nutritional support but to indicate that patients should be selected for such therapy based on careful preoperative nutritional assessment and consideration of the expected stress factors related to the disease or procedure and the expected time before adequate oral nutrition can be provided. In addition, patients should receive the method and type of nutritional support that is associated with the fewest complications and lowest cost while providing the most effective and physiologic nutritional repletion.

METHODS OF NUTRITIONAL SUPPORT

ENTERAL NUTRITION

Nutritional support should be given through the gastrointestinal tract whenever possible because of the benefits of maintaining gastrointestinal structure and function and of enhancing the utilization of nutrients, as well as because such nutrition is easier and safer to administer and costs less.[10] This can often be accomplished with oral supplements in conscious patients who are capable of swallowing adequate amounts of one of the many palatable nutritional formulas that are available (Table 2-3). Consultation with a dietitian who is knowledgeable regarding the many specialized formulas is important to obtain patient compliance and ensure that the formula used is nutritionally complete and meets patient needs.

If oral supplementation is not possible or adequate in amount, other methods of enteral tube feeding should be used (Table 2-4). Most medical and surgical patients can be fed through nasogastric or nasoenteric tubes using small catheters and appropriate feeding solutions.[35–37] These en-

TABLE 2–3. Common Enteral Nutrition Formulas

Formula	kcal/mL	Protein (g/L)
Oral Supplements		
Intact protein, lactose-free, moderate to high osmolality		
Ensure	1.0	37
Ensure plus	1.5	55
Sustacal	1.0	61
Enteral Tube Feeding		
Intact protein, lactose-free, low to moderate osmolality		
Osmolite	1.0	34
Isocal	1.0	37
Osmolite HN	1.0	42
Promote	1.0	62
Isosource HN	1.2	57
Traumacal	1.5	83
Intact protein, lactose-free, moderate to high osmolality		
Isocal HCN	2.0	75
Nutren 2.0	2.0	80
Magnacal	2.0	35
Intact protein, lactose-free, low osmolality, added fiber		
Ultracal	1.0	44
Jevity	1.0	42
Protein as peptides and free amino acids, lactose-free, low to moderate osmolality		
Criticare	1.0	38
Reabilan	1.3	58
Peptamen	1.0	40
Vital HN	1.0	42
Protein as free amino acids, lactose-free, low fat, high osmolality		
Vivonex TEN	1.0	38
Low protein, lactose-free, low electrolytes		
Travasorb Renal	1.3	17
High branched-chain amino acids, low aromatic amino acids, lactose-free		
Travasorb Hepatic	1.0	26
Intact protein with supplemental arginine, ω-3 fatty acids, mRNA, lactose-free		
Impact	1.0	56

patients are positioned with their right sides down to allow peristalsis to carry the weighted end of the tube into the duodenum and jejunum. Stimulation of gastric peristalsis with metoclopramide or erythromycin has also improved the rate of successful enteral placement of these tubes in some studies.[39] When these techniques are not successful, manipulation under fluoroscopy by an experienced radiologist or endoscopic manipulation by an endoscopist can facilitate proper tube placement into the duodenum.

If prolonged enteral feeding is anticipated, newer procedures that have been developed using endoscopic or radiologic techniques can be used for the placement of percutaneous gastrostomy or gastrojejunostomy feeding tubes.[40,41] Surgeons should consider intraoperative placement of feeding tubes if patients are not expected to be able to resume adequate oral intake within an appropriate length of time after operation or if they have preexisting moderate or severe malnutrition. If enteral feeding is believed to be a temporary measure, surgeons can have anesthetists place nasoenteric tubes into the stomach. Surgeons then can manually thread the tube into the duodenum or jejunum.

Surgeons should also consider placing a Stamm gastrostomy tube or a feeding jejunostomy tube for prolonged enteral feeding. In constructing a jejunostomy, either the needle catheter technique[42,43] or the Witzel technique using a 14F to 16F catheter may be used. With the latter technique, the catheter is less likely to be occluded by the feeding solution and should last longer.[44]

Enteral feeding formulas have been developed that vary in caloric density, protein complexity and content, fat con-

TABLE 2–4. Methods of Enteral Nutritional Support

Oral supplements
    Nutritionally complete
    Modular

Enteral feeding with small-bore tube
    Nasogastric
    Nasoduodenal
    Nasojejunal

Gastrostomy
    Percutaneous endoscopic gastrostomy
    Percutaneous radiologic gastrostomy
    Surgical gastrostomy

Jejunostomy
    Percutaneous gastrojejunostomy
    Surgical needle catheter jejunostomy
    Surgical 14F to 16F tube jejunostomy

Parenteral feeding
    Peripheral intravenous
    Central intravenous

Combined enteral and parenteral feeding

teral feeding tubes usually can be placed successfully by experienced personnel and have been associated with less discomfort and fewer complications than have the large-bore nasogastric tubes used for decompression of the stomach (Table 2-5). In conscious patients with no history of swallowing difficulties or gastroesophageal reflux and for whom the head of the bed can be elevated 30 degrees, flexible small-bore nasogastric feeding tubes can be used to infuse the nutrient solution into the stomach. In patients who are thought to be at higher risk for gastroesophageal reflux and possible pulmonary aspiration, nasoduodenal or nasojejunal tubes should be placed. Some techniques use stylets in the feeding tube, which may help in directing the end of the tube into the duodenum.[38] In other techniques,

TABLE 2–5. Complications of Enteral Feeding

Mechanical (Tube-Related) Complications

Erosion of nares, otitis media, oropharyngeal erosion: incidence decreased by use of small-bore flexible feeding tubes properly placed and affixed to patient's cheek.

Occlusion of tube: incidence decreased by use of mechanical pumps, frequent irrigation of tube with water, and use of prepared commercial formulas.

Pulmonary aspiration: incidence decreased by elevation of head of bed, use of small-bore feeding tubes, frequent checks for increased gastric residual, and use of jejunostomy feedings in patients at high risk for aspiration.

Incorrect placement of feeding tube: obtain radiograph to verify position of tube in gastrointestinal tract before initiating feeding and verify enteric contents frequently by checking residual volume.

Gastrointestinal Complications

Abdominal pain, cramping, nausea, and diarrhea: incidence decreased by slow, stepwise progression in formula infusion rate or concentration; may require change in formula type; also may be related to concomitant medications, particularly antibiotics.

Metabolic Complications

Less frequent than with parenteral nutrition, but patient needs to be monitored for glucose intolerance and electrolyte abnormalities, with particular attention to the need for free water.

---

tent, osmolarity, and cost. Most patients benefit from one of the standard prepared enteral feeding formulas (see Table 2-3). These ready-to-use solutions are polymeric, containing intact protein, complex carbohydrates, long- and medium-chain triglycerides, vitamins, and trace elements. They are low in residue and lactose-free. These formulas are isotonic or slightly hypertonic, with a choice of normal or high nitrogen content, and can be obtained with a caloric content of 1 to 2 kcal/mL. These polymeric formulas are usually tolerated as well as or better than the more expensive elemental or peptide-based formulas.[45,46]

These solutions are administered into the stomach beginning at a rate of 25 to 30 mL/h and increasing by the same amount every 8 to 12 hours until the final desired volume that meets patient needs is reached. If abdominal cramping, diarrhea, or elevated gastric residuals develop, feeding is stopped and resumed later at a lower rate or at a lower concentration of formula (Table 2-6). The efficiency of enteral feeding has been shown to be improved by the use of a protocol for progression of the rate or concentration of the formula.[47] If the feeding tube is in the jejunum, a similar protocol is followed except that it may be necessary to start with a more dilute, half-strength formula to improve tolerance. After the desired volume is obtained, the concentration may be increased to three-quarter strength formula and then to full-strength formula in a stepwise manner. It usu-

ally takes 3 to 5 days to reach the desired volume of the nutrient formula with either technique.

The most common complication of enteral feeding that interferes with provision of the desired nutrient volume is diarrhea. This can usually be controlled by adjusting the rate or concentration of the solution. Adjustments in the formula type may be necessary because some patients are more tolerant of the peptide-based formulas or the peptide/elemental formulas. Other patients tolerate enteral feeding better when fiber is included in the formula.[48] Both medications containing sorbitol that are given with the tube feeding and antibiotics can cause diarrhea. Antibiotic-associated diarrhea frequently results from bacterial overgrowth with *Clostridium difficile,* which requires specific therapy with vancomycin or metronidazole.[48,49] If adjustments in the formula type, osmolarity, or fiber content do not correct the excessive diarrhea (more than three stools per day) and the results of stool cultures and *C difficile* titers are negative, antidiarrheal medications may be instituted cautiously using kaolin-pectin first and then paregoric or loperamide if necessary.[50]

PERIPHERAL PARENTERAL NUTRITION

If the gastrointestinal tract cannot or should not be used for nutritional support, parenteral nutrition is indicated. Patients who require maintenance nutritional therapy for only a short time and in whom fluid volume tolerance is not a concern can be given peripheral parenteral nutrition.[51] Fifteen hundred to 1800 kcal can be provided, along with 50 to 70 mg of protein, electrolytes, and vitamins in 2.5 to 3 L of

---

TABLE 2–6. Protocol for Enteral Tube Feeding

Nasogastric route: Use small-bore, flexible tube (8 F preferred); obtain radiograph after placement to confirm position.

Elevate head of bed at least 30 degrees.

Use feeding pump for continuous feeding.

Begin with full-strength formula at 25 to 30 mL/h and, if tolerated, increase by 25 to 30 mL/h at 12-hour intervals until desired total volume is reached.*

Check gastric residuals every 4 hours; if greater than 100 mL, hold feeding and repeat at hourly intervals until residuals are less than 100 mL before resuming feeding.

Irrigate with 30 to 50 mL of water after each residual check or after any medications are given. (If patient requires additional free water, use greater volumes of water for irrigation.)

If patient experiences diarrhea or intestinal cramping, slow rate of feeding or decrease concentration of formula.

---

*When using hypertonic formulas or feeding into the jejunum with a nasojejunal or jejunostomy tube, diluting the formula to one-half or three-quarter strength may improve tolerance initially. The concentration can then be increased after the desired volume is reached.

intravenous fluid per day. Most of the calories given are derived from a 10% or 20% lipid emulsion that provides 550 to 1000 kcal/500 mL; additional calories are provided by 5% dextrose solution. The protein and electrolyte solution should have an osmolality of less than 900 and is better tolerated in the peripheral venous system when it is given simultaneously with the lipid emulsion.[52] The addition of 5 mg of hydrocortisone may improve the tolerance of the vein to the hyperosmolar solution but is not used uniformly.[51]

Renewed interest in the use of shorter infusions of peripheral parenteral nutrition has resulted in the development of innovative protocols such as that of Stokes and Hill, in which 3 L of a 680-mmol/L solution is given rapidly over an 8-hour period through an 18-gauge short intravenous catheter in the forearm. The catheter is removed after the infusion and rotated to the opposite forearm the next day. They found this method of peripheral parenteral nutrition infusion to be well tolerated and as nutritionally beneficial as TPN. There was no significant increase in thrombophlebitis of the peripheral veins.[53] Combining the dextrose, protein, electrolyte, and lipid emulsion into an all-in-one container for infusion over 24 hours has been found to be safe and to improve peripheral vein tolerance.[51] Waxman and coworkers[54] used a peripheral nutrition solution containing 3% amino acids, 3% glycerol as a lower osmolar energy source (replacing glucose), and electrolytes given simultaneously with a lipid emulsion in patients who had undergone major trauma or surgery. They found that the glycerol caused no adverse effects and that nitrogen balance was maintained near equilibrium.[54]

These peripheral parenteral nutrition solutions may also be used to supplement enteral nutrition when only a low volume or concentration of enteral feeding is tolerated that does not meet patient requirements. Using this approach, patients gain the benefits of the trophic effect of enteral feeding on the intestine and are ensured of receiving adequate total nutrition.[51,52]

TOTAL PARENTERAL NUTRITION

If enteral feeding cannot be used because of an inadequately functioning gastrointestinal tract or if nutritional requirements exceed the amount that can be given by peripheral vein, TPN is indicated. Hyperosmolar concentrated feeding solutions containing dextrose, amino acids, minerals, vitamins, and trace elements can be infused into a large-caliber, high-flow central vein. Techniques for cannulation of the central veins are well described and have low complication rates in experienced hands[55] (Table 2-7). The procedure should be performed in a sterile manner using caps, masks, gowns, gloves, and appropriate skin preparation and draping. The potential technical complications of pneumothorax, arterial puncture, atrioventricular fistula, poor catheter placement, and air embolism[56–59] should be explained to patients, along with the potential for catheter sepsis,[56,60] and appropriate consent should be obtained. The infraclavicular subclavian vein approach is preferred by most physicians because of the greater ability to maintain an intact sterile dressing in this area compared to the neck, where movement is more frequent. Strict maintenance of this hyperalimentation line using specific guidelines for catheter care,[60,61] dressing changes,[62,63] line changes,[64,65] and nursing care[61] are important to reduce technical complications, particularly catheter sepsis. The use of multiple-lumen intravenous catheters for TPN has been controversial but appears to be safe if a standard protocol is followed, maintaining only one lumen for the hyperalimentation fluid.[64,66] Catheter sepsis is a major problem in patients receiving TPN. When it occurs, the catheter should be removed and central venous access obtained at a different site with a new catheter. Because some patients receiving TPN

TABLE 2–7. Complications of Total Parenteral Nutrition

Mechanical (Catheter-Related) Complications
Pneumothorax
Hydrothorax
Arterial injury
Arteriovenous fistula
Cardiac arrhythmias
Air embolism
Vein thrombosis
Pulmonary embolism

Decrease incidence with proper technique of catheter insertion and management. Initial chest radiograph to confirm proper position and detect pneumothorax or pleural fluid. Daily clinical examination with repeated radiograph as indicated.

Sepsis
Bacterial
Fungal

Decrease incidence with proper sterile technique of catheter insertion and catheter care protocol for dressing changes and intravenous tubing changes. Maintain line for total parenteral nutrition only.

Metabolic Complications
Hyperglycemia or hypoglycemia
Electrolyte abnormality
Acid–base disorder
Azotemia
Hyperphosphatemia or hypophosphatemia
Hypermagnesemia or hypomagnesemia
Elevated liver test from hepatic steatosis
Essential fatty acid, vitamin, or trace element deficiency

Decrease incidence with careful adjustments of total parenteral nutrition formula and careful monitoring of fluid balance and laboratory values. Avoid excess dextrose. Obtain blood levels for essential fatty acids, vitamins, and trace elements when total parenteral nutrition is continued for a prolonged time.

TABLE 2–8. Parenteral Nutritional Requirements

Water	1 mL/kcal
Calories	25–35 kcal/kg/d
Carbohydrate	4 mg/kg/min/d
	50%–60% total calories
Fat	20%–30% total calories
Protein	0.8–2.0 g/kg/d
Essential fatty acids	4% total calories
Minerals	
Na^+	60–120 mEq/d
K^+	60–100 mEq/d
Cl^-	60–120 mEq/d
Mg^{2+}	8–10 mEq/d
Ca^{2+}	200–400 mg/d
Phosphorus	300–400 mg/d
Trace elements	
Zinc	2.5–4.0 mg/d
Copper	0.5–1.5 mg/d
Chromium	10.0–15.0 μg/d
Manganese	0.1–0.8 mg/d
Selenium	20.0–40.0 μg/d
Vitamins	
Fat-soluble	
A	3330.0 IU
D	200.0 IU
E	10.0 IU
K	5.0 mg/wk
Water-soluble	
B_1	3.0 mg
B_2	3.6 mg
Pantothenic acid	15.0 mg
Niacin	40.0 mg
B_6	4.0 mg
Biotin	60.0 μg
Folic acid	400.0 μg
B_{12}	5.0 μg
C	100.0 mg

amounts of dextrose, amino acids, minerals, vitamins, and trace elements that can be included in the formula (Table 2-8). This flexibility is limited primarily by the pharmacologic properties of the individual components: their stability in solution and potential incompatibilities that can lead to precipitation. Calcium, phosphorus, and magnesium in particular precipitate if their concentrations are not compatible. It is essential that pharmacists experienced with nutritional support and the compounding of nutrient solutions determine that a formula meets patient needs and supervise the proper compounding of these solutions under sterile conditions to ensure their safety and effectiveness.

Most patients who receive TPN require a balanced-fuel formula, with 20% to 30% of calories from fat, 15% to 20% from protein, and 50% to 65% from dextrose (Table 2-9). Most often, the lipid emulsion is given as a separate infusion either peripherally or centrally, although some hospi-

TABLE 2–9. Total Parenteral Nutrition Formula for a 24-Hour Period

Volume	2000 mL
Dextrose	500 g
Protein	100 g
Sodium	70 mEq
Potassium	80 mEq
Calcium	9 mEq
Magnesium	10 mEq
Phosphorus	24 mM
Chloride	70 mEq
Acetate	207 mEq
MVI-12	10 mL
MTE-4	3 mL
Phytonadione	1 mg
Kilocalories from	
Dextrose	1700 (3.4 × 500)
Protein	400 (4.0 × 100)
TOTAL	2100
If 10% lipid emulsion added	550 (1.1 × 500)
TOTAL	2650

Acetate content varies with different amino acid solutions used.

Adjustments in the amount of protein, electrolytes, and minerals are necessary for special disease states such as renal insufficiency and hepatic insufficiency.

MVI-12 contains recommended amounts of fat-soluble and water-soluble vitamins except vitamin K (phytonadione), which is added separately.

MTE-4 contains the trace elements zinc 5 mg, copper 1 mg, manganese 0.5 mg, and chromium 10 μg. Selenium 20 μg is recommended for long-term total parenteral nutrition.

Protein sources include 8.5% to 10% amino acid solutions such as Travasol, Aminosyn, and Freamine-III. These are mixed in pharmacies with the components listed above.

may have other potential sources of sepsis, it may be acceptable to change the catheter over a guide wire in patients with difficult venous access. The catheter tip is cultured to determine whether infection is present and the intravenous site is moved to a new area only if the culture results are positive.[64] Special intravenous catheters with silver-impregnated cuffs have been developed to reduce the incidence of catheter sepsis but have shown no improvement over the use of standard catheters following a protocol for placement and care after insertion.[67,68]

PARENTERAL SOLUTIONS

The ability to adjust the concentration of the solution given through a central venous catheter provides greater flexibility in the volume that can be administered and in the tals combine all the ingredients into one container for infusion over 24 hours. This total nutrient admixture system may be time-saving and cost-effective from the pharmacy and nursing standpoint. There does not appear to be an increased risk of infection even though an in-line bacterial filter is not used with this method.[69,70] It is especially important that all the components and concentrations of this total nutrient admixture solution be compatible, however, because any precipitation that occurs will be obscured by the lipid emulsion.

MONITORING

Monitoring of the clinical status and laboratory values is important for patients receiving TPN to allow metabolic abnormalities to be recognized and corrected.[71] Patient weight, intake, output, and vital signs must be observed closely each day. The blood glucose level should be determined using a Chemstrip or urine glucose test every 6 hours (or more often) as indicated. Serum electrolyte, phosphorus, magnesium, calcium, creatinine, and blood urea nitrogen levels should be obtained daily for the first 3 or 4 days until they are stable and then every other day or twice a week thereafter. Liver function and serum triglyceride levels should be measured on a weekly basis. A 24-hour urine collection for urine urea nitrogen or total urine nitrogen should be performed so that a nitrogen balance can be calculated weekly (Table 2-10).

Any abnormal test results should be addressed by changing the quantity or concentration of TPN ingredients and in some instances by totally deleting a component. The most common adjustment made is alteration of the dextrose content to correct hyperglycemia; the amount of dextrose can be decreased or insulin can be added to the solution. Other changes in electrolyte and mineral content (particularly potassium, phosphorus, and magnesium) are often necessary because of the increase in metabolic processes, which may result in rapid utilization of these components.[71] The lipid emulsion should be deleted in patients who develop hypertriglyceridemia until their levels return to normal. If triglyceride levels remain high, the lipid emulsion can be given slowly over a 24-hour period once a week to supply essential fatty acids.[72]

When giving the TPN solution, a steady infusion rate should be maintained; if the volume given falls behind, no attempt should be made to catch up. If the solution runs out or if intravenous access is lost, a solution of 5% or 10% dextrose should be infused to prevent the potential danger of hypoglycemia.

During the early experience with TPN, it was generally believed that patients should be fed as much solution as possible. In recent years, however, the potential dangers of overfeeding have been recognized increasingly. One of

TABLE 2–10. Recommended Monitoring for Parenteral Nutrition

Parameter	Frequency
Weight	Daily
Intake and output	On each shift daily
Vital signs	On each shift daily
Urine glucose	Four times daily
Blood tests	
Glucose Electrolytes Blood urea nitrogen Creatinine	Daily until stable, then every other day
Calcium Phosphorus Magnesium	Daily until stable, then twice a week
Alkaline phosphatase Bilirubin	Twice a week
Hemoglobin Triglycerides Albumin Transferrin	Once a week
24-hour urine for urine urea nitrogen to determine nitrogen balance	Once a week

these problems is hepatic steatosis, which is related in most cases to excessive caloric intake, primarily with dextrose.[73-76] Another potential problem of overfeeding with excess dextrose is the associated increase in CO_2 production, which may interfere with the weaning of patients from artificial ventilation and adds an additional physiologic stress.[77]

Some patients receiving prolonged hyperalimentation develop liver test abnormalities that do not respond to adjustments in the amount of dextrose and total calories administered. These patients may benefit from the use of a cyclic hyperalimentation protocol in which the total nutritional requirement is given over 12 to 16 hours and no intravenous nutrition is provided for the remaining 8 to 12 hours. This method is suggested to improve fat mobilization and visceral protein synthesis in the liver by simulating the physiologic meal profile of nutrients.[78] This cyclic hyperalimentation is used in many patients who are receiving hyperalimentation at home. In addition to the potential metabolic benefits, it also has the psychologic benefit of freeing patients from the infusion apparatus for a certain period.

In patients with specific disease conditions, the amount of nutrients in the parenteral solution must be altered to prevent possible toxicity from excessive protein or minerals. Protein, potassium, phosphorus, magnesium, and trace elements often need to be restricted in patients with acute renal insufficiency, and blood levels should be monitored closely to prevent toxicity.[10] In patients who are undergoing dialysis, greater amounts of protein and minerals can be given but blood levels still must be observed closely. Optimal nonprotein calories can be given with concentrated dextrose and lipid emulsions in limited volumes if fluid restriction is necessary.[10]

Patients with hepatic insufficiency need to be monitored for protein intolerance and electrolyte abnormalities. Most patients with liver disease tolerate standard proteins with an appropriate amount of nonprotein calories. In patients with hepatic encephalopathy who do not respond to medical therapy, it may be necessary to use a liver-specific mixture of amino acids with lower aromatic and higher branched-chain amino acids,[10] although the benefit remains controversial.[79]

Patients with cancer are frequently malnourished and may require nutritional support after surgical procedures or during radiotherapy or chemotherapy, but they may not restore lean body mass efficiently.[10,80] Preoperative nutritional therapy may reduce the risk of postoperative complications in properly selected patients who are malnourished but are not terminal and are expected to respond to therapy.[81]

Recent experimental work has examined specific nutrient substances that may improve the efficiency of nutritional repletion in acutely stressed patients. Glutamine supplementation of parenteral nutrition formulas improved nitrogen balance in patients undergoing bone marrow transplantation in one study[82] and may improve the recovery of the intestine from starvation atrophy,[83] but larger controlled trials are needed to determine its efficacy in malnourished catabolic patients. Supplemental therapy with growth hormone accelerated the protein gain in a small group of stable adult patients receiving nutritional therapy, but larger controlled studies in both acute and chronically malnourished patients are necessary to establish the role of growth hormone supplementation in nutritional repletion.[84]

NUTRITIONAL SUPPORT TEAMS

As the provision of nutritional support has become more complex during the past two decades, many hospitals have established nutritional support teams to improve efficiency and reduce complications. These teams bring together the expertise of several different specialty areas. In addition to physicians, the teams should include clinical pharmacists, nurse clinicians with an interest in direct patient care and infection control, registered dietitians, and others with a

special interest in the assessment of nutritional states and the provision of optimal nutrient repletion. A decrease in metabolic and technical complications has been demonstrated when a nutrition support team either provides consultative services or takes over the complete care and provision of nutritional therapy. All members of the team should participate in the evaluation and treatment of patients and in the development of protocols for provision of care. In addition, members can inform their colleagues on the team of new scientific developments and products in their areas of expertise within the expanding field of nutritional support.

REFERENCES

1. Cuthbertson DP. The metabolic response to injury and its nutritional implications: retrospect and prospect. JPEN 1979; 3:108.
2. Dudrick SJ, Wilmore DW, Vars HM, Rhoads JE. Long-term total parenteral nutrition with growth, development, and positive nitrogen balance. Surgery 1968;64:134.
3. Moore FD. Energy and the maintenance of the body cell mass. JPEN 1980;4:228.
4. Gilder H. Parenteral nourishment of patients undergoing surgical or traumatic stress. JPEN 1986;10:88.
5. Hill GL. Body composition research: implications for the practice of clinical nutrition. JPEN 1992;16:197.
6. Kudsk KA, Croce MA, Fabian TC, et al. Enteral versus parenteral feeding: effects on septic morbidity after blunt and penetrating abdominal trauma. Ann Surg 1992;215:503.
7. Alexander JW. Immunoenhancement via enteral nutrition. Arch Surg 1993;128:1242.
8. McClave SA, Lowen CC, Snider HL. Immunonutrition and enteral hyperalimentation of critically ill patients. Dig Dis Sci 1992;37:1153.
9. Heymsfield SB, Bethal RA, Ansley JD, et al. Enteral hyperalimentation: an alternative to central venous hyperalimentation. Ann Intern Med 1979;90:63.
10. A.S.P.E.N. Board of Directors. Guidelines for the use of parenteral and enteral nutrition in adult and pediatric patients. JPEN 1993;17(Suppl).
11. Blackburn GL, Bistrian BR, Maini BS, et al. Nutritional and metabolic assessment of the hospitalized patient. JPEN 1977;1:11.
12. Baker JP, Detsky AS, Wesson DE, et al. Nutritional assessment: a comparison of clinical judgement and objective measurements. N Engl J Med 1982;306:969.
13. Windsor JA, Hill GL. Weight loss with physiologic impairment: basic indicator of surgical risk. Ann Surg 1988;207:209.
14. Bistrian BR, Blackburn GL, Hallowell E, et al. Protein status of general surgical patients. JAMA 1974;230:858.
15. Bistrian BR, Blackburn GL, Vitale J, et al. Prevalence of malnutrition in general medical patients. JAMA 1976;235:1567.
16. Christou NV, Tellado-Rodriguez J, Chartrand L, et al. Estimating mortality risk in preoperative patients using immunologic, nutritional, and acute-phase response variables. Ann Surg 1989;210:69.

17. Bistrian BR, Blackburn GL, Sherman M, et al. Therapeutic index of nutritional depletion in hospitalized patients. Surg Gynecol Obstet 1975;141:512.

18. Nixon DW, Heymsfield SB, Cohen AE, et al. Protein-caloric undernutrition in hospitalized cancer patients. Am J Med 1980;68:683.

19. McClave SA, Mitoraj TE, Thielmeier KA, et al. Differentiating subtypes (hypoalbuminemic vs marasmic) of protein-calorie malnutrition: incidence and clinical significance in a university hospital setting. JPEN 1992;16:337.

20. Dahn MS, Jacobs LA, Smith S, et al. The significance of hypoalbuminemia following injury and infection. Am Surg 1985;51:340.

21. Sun X, Iles M, Weissman C. Physiologic variables and fluid resuscitation in the postoperative intensive care unit patient. Crit Care Med 1993;21:555.

22. Van Way III CW. Variability of the Harris-Benedict equation in recently published textbooks. JPEN 1992;16:566.

23. Cortes V, Nelson LD. Errors in estimating energy expenditure in critically ill surgical patients. Arch Surg 1989;124:287.

24. Campbell SM, Kudsk KA. "High tech" metabolic measurements: useful in daily clinical practice. JPEN 1988;12:610.

25. Konstantinides FN, Boehm KA, Radmer WJ, et al. Pyrochemiluminescence: real time, cost-effective method for determining total urinary nitrogen in clinical nitrogen balance studies. Clin Chem 1988;34:2518.

26. Robert S, Zarowitz BJ, Hyzy R, et al. Bioelectrical impedance assessment of nutritional status in critically ill patients. Am J Clin Nutr 1993;57:840.

27. Going SB, Masset MP, Hall MC, et al. Detection of small changes in body composition by dual-energy x-ray absorptiometry. Am J Clin Nutr 1993;57:845.

28. McClaren DS, Meguid MM. Nutritional assessment at the crossroads. JPEN 1983;7:575.

29. Tellado JM, Garcia-Sabrido JL, Hanley JA, et al. Predicting mortality based on body composition analysis. Ann Surg 1989;209:81.

30. Detsky AS, Baker JP, O'Rourke K, et al. Perioperative parenteral nutrition: a meta-analysis. Ann Intern Med 1987;107:195.

31. The Veterans Affairs Total Parenteral Nutrition Cooperative Study Group. Perioperative total parenteral nutrition in surgical patients. N Engl J Med 1991;325:525.

32. Eisenberg JM, Glick HA, Buzby GP, et al. Does perioperative total parenteral nutrition reduce medical care costs? JPEN 1993;17:201.

33. Campos AC, Mequid MM. A critical appraisal of the usefulness of perioperative nutritional support. Am J Clin Nutr 1992;55:117.

34. Sandstromm R, Drott C, Hyltander A, et al. The effect of postoperative intravenous feeding (TPN) on outcome following major surgery evaluated in a randomized study. Ann Surg 1993;217:185.

35. Bethal RA, Jansen RD, Heymsfield SB, et al. Nasogastric hyperalimentation through a polyethylene catheter: an alternative to central venous hyperalimentation. Am J Clin Nutr 1979;32:1112.

36. Kaminski MV. Enteral hyperalimentation. Surg Gynecol Obstet 1976;143:12.

37. Page CP, Ryan JA, Haff RC. Continual catheter administration of an elemental diet. Surg Gynecol Obstet 1976;142:184.

38. Caulfield KA, Page CP, Pesana C. Technique for intraduodenal placement of transnasal enteral feeding catheters. Nutr Clin Pract 1991;6:23.

39. Annese V, Janssens J, Vantrappen G. Erythromycin accelerates gastric emptying by inducing enteral contractions and improved gastroduodenal coordination. Gastroenterology 1992;102:823.

40. Kadakia SC, Sullivan HO, Starnes E. Percutaneous endoscopic gastrostomy or jejunostomy and the incidence of aspiration in 79 patients. Am J Surg 1992;164:114.

41. Olson DL, Krubsack AJ, Stewart ET. Percutaneous enteral alimentation: gastrostomy versus gastrojejunostomy. Radiology 1993;187:105.

42. Hoover HC, Ryan JA, Anderson EJ, et al. Nutritional benefits of immediate postoperative jejunal feeding of an elemental diet. Am J Surg 1980;139:153.

43. Moore FA, Moore EE, Jones TN, et al. TEN versus TPN following abdominal trauma: reduced septic morbidity. J Trauma 1989;29:916.

44. Weltz CR, Morris JB, Mullen JL. Surgical jejunostomy in aspiration risk patients. Ann Surg 1992;215:140.

45. Ford EG, Hull SF, Jennings LM, et al. Clinical comparison of tolerance to elemental or polymeric enteral feedings in the postoperative patient. J Am Coll Nutr 1992;11:11.

46. Mowatt-Larssen CA, Brown RO, Wojtysiak SL, et al. Comparison of tolerance and nutritional outcome between a peptide and a standard enteral formula in critically ill, hypoalbuminemic patients. JPEN 1992;16:20.

47. Chapman G, Curtas S, Meguid MM. Standardized enteral orders attain caloric goals sooner: a prospective study. JPEN 1992;16:149.

48. Guenter PA, Settle RG, Perlmutter S, et al. Tube feeding-related diarrhea in acutely ill patients. JPEN 1991;15:277.

49. Fekety R, Shah AB. Diagnosis and treatment of clostridium difficile colitis. JAMA 1993;269:71.

50. Eisenberg PG. Causes of diarrhea in tube-fed patients: a comprehensive approach to diagnosis. Nutr Clin Pract 1993;8:119.

51. Payne-James JJ, Khawaja HT. First choice for total parenteral nutrition: the peripheral route. JPEN 1993;17:468.

52. Issacs JW, Millikan WJ, Stackhouse J, et al. Parenteral nutrition of adults with a 900 milliosmolar solution via peripheral veins. Am J Clin Nutr 1977;30:552.

53. Stokes MA, Hill GL. Peripheral parenteral nutrition: a preliminary report on its efficacy and safety. JPEN 1993;17:145.

54. Waxman K, Day AT, Stellin GP, et al. Safety and efficacy of glycerol and amino acids in combination with lipid emulsion for peripheral parenteral nutrition support. JPEN 1992;16:374.

55. Grant JP. Handbook of total parenteral nutrition, ed 2. Philadelphia, WB Saunders, 1992:107–117.

56. Ryan JA, Abel RM, Abbott WM, et al. Catheter complications in total parenteral nutrition. N Engl J Med 1974;290:757.

57. Kashuk JL, Penn I. Air embolism after central venous catheterization. Surg Gynecol Obstet 1984;159:249.

58. Ruggiero RP, Caruso G. Chylothorax: a complication of subclavian vein catheterization. JPEN 1985;9:750.

59. Mukau L, Talamini MA, Sitzman JV. Risk factors for central venous catheter-related vascular erosions. JPEN 1991;15:513.

60. Sitzman JV, Townsend TR, Siler MC, et al. Septic and technical complications of central venous catheterization: a prospective study of 200 consecutive patients. Ann Surg 1985;202:766.

61. Williams WW. Infection control during parenteral nutrition therapy. JPEN 1985;9:735.
62. Maki DG, Ringer M. Evaluation of dressing regimens for prevention of infection with peripheral intravenous catheters. JAMA 1987;258:2396.
63. Hoffman KK, Weber DJ, Samsa GP, et al. Transparent polyurethane film as an intravenous catheter dressing: a meta-analysis of the infection risks. JAMA 1992;267:2072.
64. Eyer S, Brummitt C, Crossley K, et al. Catheter related sepsis: prospective, randomized study of three methods of long-term catheter maintenance. Crit Care Med 1990;18:1073.
65. Cobb DK, High KP, Sawyer RG, et al. A controlled trial of scheduled replacement of central venous and pulmonary-artery catheters. N Engl J Med 1992;327:1062.
66. Pemberton LB, Lyman B, Lander V, et al. Sepsis from triple-vs single-lumen catheters during total parenteral nutrition in surgical or critically ill patients. Arch Surg 1986;121:591.
67. Groeger JS, Lucas AB, Coit D, et al. A prospective, randomized evaluation of silver impregnated subcutaneous cuffs for preventing tunneled chronic venous access catheter infections in cancer patients. Ann Surg 1993;218:206.
68. Babycos CR, Borrocas A, Webb WR. A prospective randomized trial comparing the silver-impregnated collagen cuff with the bedside tunneled subclavian catheter. JPEN 1993;17:61.
69. Ang SD, Canham JE, Daly JM. Parenteral infusion with an admixture of amino acids, dextrose, and fat emulsion solution: compatibility and clinical safety. JPEN 1987;11:23.
70. Campos AC, Palazzi M, Meguid MM. Clinical use of total nutritional admixtures. Nutrition 1990;6:347.
71. Weinsier RL, Bacon J, Butterworth CE. Central venous alimentation: a prospective study of the frequency of metabolic abnormalities among medical and surgical patients. JPEN 1982;6:421.
72. Abbott WC, Grakauskas AM, Bistrian BP, et al. Metabolic and respiratory effects of continuous and discontinuous lipid infusions: occurrence in excess of resting energy expenditure. Arch Surg 1984;119:1367.
73. Sax HC, Talamini MA, Brackett K, et al. Hepatic steatosis in total parenteral nutrition: failure of fatty infiltration to correlate with abnormal serum hepatic enzyme levels. Surgery 1986;100:697.
74. Leaseburge LA, Winn NJ, Schloerb PR. Liver test alterations with total parenteral nutrition and nutritional status. JPEN 1992;16:348.
75. Buchmiller CE, Kleiman-Wexler RL, Ephgrave KS, et al. Liver dysfunction and energy source: results of a randomized clinical trial. JPEN 1993;17:301.
76. Sax HC, Bower RH. Hepatic complications of total parenteral nutrition. JPEN 1988;12:615.
77. Askanazi J, Rosenbaum SH, Hyman AI, et al. Respiratory changes induced by the large glucose loads of total parenteral nutrition. JAMA 1980;243:1444.
78. Maini B, Blackburn GL, Bistrian BR, et al. Cyclic hyperalimentation: an optimal technique for preservation of visceral protein. J Surg Res 1976;20:515.
79. Kanematsu T, Koyangi N, Matsumata T, et al. Lack of preventive effect of branched chain amino acid solution on postoperative hepatic encephalopathy in patients with cirrhosis: a randomized prospective trial. Surgery 1988;104:482.
80. Nixon DW, Lawson DH, Ansley J, et al. Hyperalimentation of the cancer patient with protein-caloric undernutrition. Cancer Res 1981;41:2038.
81. Daly JM, Redmond HP, Gallagher H. Perioperative nutrition in cancer patients. JPEN 1992;16:100S.
82. Ziegler TR, Young LS, Benfell K, et al. Clinical and metabolic efficacy of glutamine supplemented parenteral nutrition after bone marrow transplantation: a randomized, double-blind, controlled study. Ann Intern Med 1992;116:821.
83. Inoue Y, Grant JP, Snyder PJ. Effect of glutamine-supplemented total parenteral nutrition on recovery of the small intestine after starvation atrophy. JPEN 1993;17:165.
84. Byrne TA, Morrissey TB, Gatzen C, et al. Anabolic therapy with growth hormone accelerates protein gain in surgical patients requiring nutritional rehabilitation. Ann Surg 1993;218:400.

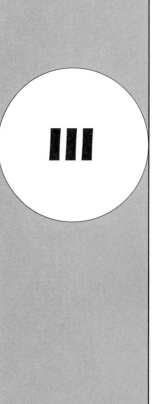

SECTION **III**

PREOPERATIVE TESTING

Medical Management of the Surgical Patient, Third Edition,
edited by Michael F. Lubin, H. Kenneth Walker, and Robert B. Smith III.
J.B. Lippincott Company, Philadelphia, PA © 1995.

CHAPTER

3

PREOPERATIVE TESTING

Michael F. Lubin

The role of preoperative testing has been the subject of much discussion over the last few years. Usually, the following preoperative tests are performed routinely or are considered to be important for many patients:

- Complete blood count
- Platelet count
- Measurement of electrolyte levels
- Determination of creatinine and blood urea nitrogen levels
- Measurement of the prothrombin time and partial thromboplastin time
- Urinalysis
- Electrocardiography
- Chest radiography
- Pulmonary function testing

Subspecialists have frequently encouraged the use of tests in their domain despite data and numerous articles suggesting that they do not aid in the care of many patients. This chapter discusses the reasons for obtaining preoperative tests and their usefulness in various patient groups and provides suggestions for ordering preoperative tests for different types of patients.

Preoperative tests are performed for several reasons. The main indications are to quantify previous disease and to identify new conditions (screening) that may affect the process or outcome of the surgical procedure. Some physicians suggest that routine preoperative tests can serve as an adjunct to health maintenance. In addition, many tests are done in the hope of precluding malpractice suits in case of unsuspected abnormalities.

Routine preoperative screening does not appear to accomplish these goals in many circumstances, however, for many reasons. Studies have shown that as many as 60% of preoperative tests performed on patients undergoing elective surgery could be eliminated without adverse outcome.[1] In addition, many problems with testing often are not considered. Surgery may be delayed by borderline abnormal or false-positive results. Repeating tests and performing other tests that can be invasive and expensive not only may be of no use to patients but may even be harmful. The cost of these unnecessary tests may amount to as much as $24 billion per year.

Finally, rather than preventing malpractice suits, it is more likely that random testing is disadvantageous. It has become clear that the results of tests ordered to prevent malpractice suits are frequently never seen by physicians. If the test results are seen, they are frequently not recorded. If they are seen and recorded, they often are not acted on in any way. Tests that are not seen, recorded, or acted on are a substantial risk. Because textbooks and many articles in consultation medicine support selective ordering of tests, there is greater risk associated with ordering unnecessary tests than with not ordering them.

REVIEW OF THE EFFICACY OF PREOPERATIVE TESTING

CHEMISTRY TESTING

Many studies have been done to examine the usefulness of preoperative testing and all have come to the same basic conclusion: many tests can be eliminated without significantly increasing the risk for healthy patients who are undergoing elective surgery. A few of the major papers on this subject are reviewed here to illustrate the significant points.

Kaplan and coworkers[1] studied a random sample of 2000 patients who underwent tests before elective surgery in an academic medical center. They set criteria for test indications and "action limits" for test results. Action limits were defined as abnormalities that would be expected to trigger a response from the surgical team, not simply results that fell outside the normal range as defined by the laboratory. For example, a hematocrit of 34% in an elderly woman is outside the normal range in the laboratory but generally is not investigated by the surgical team. The lower action limit for hematocrit in this study was set at 30%.

Kaplan's group found that there was no indication for about 60% of the preoperative tests that were performed. Only 3.4% of the results of the entire group of tests fell outside their action limits; 0.36% (10 tests) of these were in the group that would not have been ordered and 0.14% (4 tests) were of potential significance. Despite the potential significance of four of the tests (a platelet count of 101,000/μL, a creatinine level of 1.8 mg/dL, and glucose levels of 203 mg/dL with 1+ ketones and 184 mg/dL with 2+ ketones), however, none were acted on, no changes were made in patient care, and no complications resulted from the abnormalities.

In another study, McKee and Scott[2] evaluated 400 patients admitted for elective surgery. Although 16% of the preoperative tests performed on these patients revealed some abnormality, only 0.013% caused a change in management. Thirteen cases of anemia were addressed; only one complication occurred in this group. None of the biochemical tests required attention. Among 323 electrocardiograms (ECGs) performed, there were 101 abnormalities, only 2 of which warranted any action. One silent myocardial infarction was detected and the patient's procedure was delayed 6 months; digoxin toxicity was noted in another patient and the drug dosage was decreased before surgery. Three hundred twenty-seven chest radiographs were done; 121 were abnormal but only 4 required action. The authors did not indicate the nature of the radiographic abnormalities or the indications for action in this study.

A third retrospective study of preoperative laboratory screening was done by Narr and colleagues at the Mayo Clinic.[3] These investigators evaluated all patients in ASA class 1 (all healthy patients) who were admitted for elective surgery. There were a total of 3782 patients, the oldest of whom was 65 years. The routine tests performed included a complete blood count and measurement of the creatinine, electrolyte, aspartate aminotransferase, and glucose levels. Only 160 patients had abnormal test results. Thirty of these were anticipated by the history and physical examination and 47 were pursued further. The tests were simply repeated in 37 of the patients without further action. Of the 10 patients who were treated, 1 was given potassium and 1 with diabetes was given insulin. There were 5 patients with diabetes who were instructed to lose weight and 3 patients with iron-deficiency anemia. No surgical procedure was delayed and there were no adverse outcomes because of the test results. The Mayo Clinic currently requires no tests before elective surgery on healthy patients younger than 40 years.

COAGULATION TESTS

The efficacy of preoperative coagulation testing has also been evaluated in several studies. Because the results of such tests are rarely abnormal, however, their routine use does not appear to be valuable. The abnormal results that do occur are usually false-positive and revert to normal when the test is repeated. In addition, abnormal results are often ignored by the surgical team.

Rohrer and colleagues[4] evaluated 282 patients who underwent 514 tests. One hundred twenty-three patients were considered to have screening coagulation tests. There were 21 abnormal test results. Three were false-positive results that reverted to normal on repeated testing and 15 were elevated platelet counts and short partial thromboplastin times that were not indicative of coagulopathy. Three test results were suggestive of coagulopathy but were ignored by the surgical team without consequence. Even among patients in whom tests were believed to be indicated, there were few abnormalities. There was an indication for partial thromboplastin time or prothrombin time testing in 159 patients. There were 158 normal prothrombin times; the one abnormality occurred in a patient taking warfarin. There were 10 abnormal partial thromboplastin times, 7 of which were too short and only 3 of which were prolonged. Of the 117 patients in whom a platelet count was indicated, only 20 abnormal test results were obtained. The count was elevated in 17 patients and low in only 3 patients. All the patients with clinically significant coagulopathies had indications for testing.

URINALYSIS

The usefulness of preoperative urinalysis was reviewed by Lawrence and Kroenke in 1988.[5] In a review of 200 cases of elective knee surgery, they found a significant percentage of abnormalities (15%); however, only 29% were addressed in any way. There was no association between the abnormal test results and surgical complications. In reviewing other results from previous papers, the authors found no data that could be interpreted as supporting the use of routine urinalysis.

ELECTROCARDIOGRAPHY

Numerous papers have been published on the usefulness of and indications for preoperative ECGs. There is no consensus regarding who should undergo such testing. Some believe that all patients older than 30 years should have ECGs, whereas others advocate 50 years as the cutoff age. Much of the disagreement is based on the level of risk that the authors are willing to accept without good information.

Numerous abnormalities are found on routine ECGs. They begin to appear in the fourth decade of life and increase substantially at the age of 50 years. Some of the abnormalities are probably of little consequence (eg, premature atrial contractions in a 40-year-old patient) but others carry great significance (eg, silent myocardial infarction in a 60-year-old patient). Unfortunately, the predictive value of the findings in many cases is unknown. As a result, Goldberger and O'Konski have suggested that there is no evidence to support the use of routine ECGs as baseline or screening tests.[6]

Gold and associates[7] evaluated 751 patients undergoing ambulatory surgery. Four hundred fifty-four were younger than 50 years and 134 were older than 60 years. Only 60 patients were in ASA class 3; 633 were in ASA class 1 or 2. Abnormalities were found in 43% of the patients. Twelve complications occurred and the authors believed that a preoperative ECG may have been clinically useful in 6 cases (the criteria for usefulness were exceedingly liberal). They concluded that preoperative electrocardiography is not predictive of postoperative events and suggested that its routine use is probably not indicated in younger, relatively healthy patients who are scheduled for ambulatory surgery.

The prevalence of abnormalities on ECGs in older patients, however, is high. In a study by Seymour and coworkers,[8] only 21% of patients older than 65 years had normal ECG results and 53% had major abnormalities. These authors suggested that preoperative ECGs were useful in elderly patients to identify recent myocardial infarctions and significant arrhythmias before operation and to use for comparison in those patients who required a postoperative tracing. Unfortunately, the ECGs did not predict postoperative cardiovascular events in elderly men and had only limited value in women.

CHEST RADIOGRAPHY

The usefulness of preoperative chest radiographs has also been examined. Tape and Mushlin[9] evaluated 341 patients who were admitted to the hospital for vascular surgery. Seventy-one percent of the patients were men and they had a mean age of 67 years. Forty-two percent were current smokers and 15% never smoked. They found chest radiographs to be useful only in those patients who had indications for the test. Of the 336 patients who had abnormal test results, the results were recorded in only 207 cases. Clinical action was taken in just 9 patients and only 1 patient had useful therapy. In the 8 remaining patients, the abnormal radiograph either resulted in no useful change or had negative effects on the surgery (usually delaying it), and there was one false-negative reading. These authors concluded that routine chest radiography in the absence of clinical indications was of no benefit to patients.

Charpak and colleagues[10] evaluated 3866 patients who underwent 1101 chest radiographs in a protocol designed to limit unneeded tests. Almost 2000 patients were younger than 35 years and about 1000 were older than 55 years. The results of 568 radiographs (52%) were abnormal, 133 (23%) of which were suspected. Only 51 tests had any effect on patient care. Of the other 2765 patients (72%) who did not undergo chest radiographs, the test was believed to have been necessary in only 1 case; by protocol, this patient should have had a film done. No deaths or complications occurred because a chest radiograph was not performed.

PULMONARY FUNCTION TESTING

Good information is available regarding the usefulness of preoperative pulmonary function tests (PFTs). The American College of Physicians[11] developed a position paper in 1990 after reviewing the evidence in the literature. They recommended testing for patients undergoing lung resection to identify those who are at high risk for life-threatening pulmonary complications. They suggested that spirometry and arterial blood gases be used initially, with further testing performed if needed. The position paper suggested that screening PFTs were not necessary for all patients undergoing any other procedure. They recommended that the tests be performed in patients having coronary artery bypass surgery or upper abdominal surgery if there is a history of tobacco use and dyspnea. For all other surgery, PFTs should be performed in those patients in whom there is evidence of underlying lung disease. Another excellent review of the available data by Zibrak and O'Donnell[12] in 1993 came to the same basic conclusions.

REVIEW OF PREVIOUS TESTS

In a unique and thoughtful paper published in 1990, Macpherson and colleagues[13] examined the utility of repeated preoperative testing in patients who had undergone laboratory tests within a year before elective surgery. The tests they evaluated included the complete blood count; sodium, potassium, and creatinine levels; and the prothrombin time and partial thromboplastin time. They found that almost half the tests performed at the time of hospital admission duplicated tests done during the previous year. They also noted that changes in the results of such tests were rare and rarely of clinical importance if the history and physical examination did not suggest a need for repeated testing.

These authors came to the following conclusions:

1. Preoperative screening tests can be done at significant intervals before surgery if there is no indication that the test results may have changed.
2. Test results that are more than 4 months old should be used with caution (their intervals for previous tests ran from 2 to 7 months).

Because the study was conducted on older men, extrapolation of the results to younger populations and to women must be done with caution. In addition, the usefulness of urinalysis, ECGs, chest radiographs, or PFTs was not explored.

STUDIES USING PROTOCOLS TO ORDER TESTS

In light of the information discussed earlier, several studies have been done to determine whether the retrospective findings concerning preoperative testing could be applied prospectively. Blery and colleagues[14] set up a prospective protocol for test ordering in almost 4000 patients admitted to the hospital for surgery. The surgeons and anesthesiologists involved agreed to the protocol. The investigators found that 18% of the tests ordered did not conform to their protocol. Physicians believed that only 0.2% of the tests that were not ordered would have been useful in retrospect. No deaths could be attributed to failure to order a test and the overall mortality rate was no higher than expected. Because morbidity rates also were low, there was no way to determine whether any of the morbidity could be attributed to decreased laboratory testing.

Macario and colleagues[15] conducted a review to determine whether the published information regarding the value of preoperative testing had changed the ordering behavior of physicians. They evaluated more than 2000 patients undergoing surgery in three cities in five different years. They compared the tests ordered in 1979 with those ordered in 1987 and found an overall decrease of almost 7% in the number of tests that were ordered that were not indicated by the history and physical examination. Unfortunately and unexpectedly, however, they also discovered a 12% decrease in the number of tests that were indicated but not ordered. These findings were statistically significant.

These investigators concluded that the change in test ordering behavior was probably not beneficial because patients gain more from the performance of indicated tests than from the avoidance of tests that are not indicated. They suggested that ways should be found to improve preoperative test ordering.

SUGGESTED PROTOCOLS FOR ORDERING PREOPERATIVE TESTS

The information provided in this chapter indicates that few tests should be ordered "routinely." Macpherson[16] has reviewed these data in detail and made recommendations. Everyone who has studied this issue agrees on certain broad points. The following recommendations are based on conclusions that appear to be reasonable extrapolations from the data. Although the recommendations are based on data, substantial areas of uncertainty still remain. The patient populations studied and selection criteria used often differ from those of individual physicians. Generalizing these conclusions to all patients in all settings is not advisable and physicians must exercise their clinical judgment in using the data from these studies.

For patients who are young and healthy, the data clearly indicate that routine tests are of no benefit. Few data exist about older patients who have underlying diseases, and more liberal use of testing is probably indicated in this group. For healthy patients who have no indications for testing in their histories and physical examinations, recom-

TABLE 3–1. Recommendations for Preoperative Testing: Patients Without Indications Undergoing Elective Surgery

Test	Patient Age (years)
Hematocrit	>40
Electrolytes	>60 (major surgery)
Creatinine/blood urea nitrogen	>50
Chest radiograph	>60
Electrocardiogram	>50

TABLE 3–2. Suggested Preoperative Testing: Patients With Indications

Hemoglobin
>40 years
Major surgery
Known anemia
Renal disease
Anticoagulant use
Other underlying diseases known to cause anemia

White Blood Cell Count
Fever
Suspected infection

Platelet count
Suspected bleeding disorder

Prothrombin Time/Partial Thromboplastin Time
Suspected bleeding disorder
Anticoagulant treatment
Liver disease
Malignancy

Electrolytes
>60 years
Major surgery
Major organ system disease
Diuretic use
Diabetes mellitus
Digoxin treatment
Corticosteroid use

Creatinine/Blood Urea Nitrogen
>50 years
Major surgery
Renal disease
Diabetes mellitus
Diuretics
Digoxin treatment

Glucose
Diabetes mellitus
Corticosteroid treatment

Urinalysis
Renal disease
Infection

Chest Radiograph
>60 years
Pulmonary disease
Cardiac disease
Malignancy
High risk for tuberculosis (immigrants)

Electrocardiogram
>50 years
Cardiac disease
Pulmonary disease

mendations are made based on age and are outlined in Table 3-1. No testing is necessary in patients younger than 40 years.

For patients with underlying pathology, certain tests should be ordered to establish a baseline for later comparison, to determine the risks of surgery, and to document unsuspected deterioration from previous function. The necessary tests are determined by the history and physical examination. Table 3-2 outlines some of the major indications for preoperative testing. It is not encyclopedic, however, and there may be other indications for some tests.

REFERENCES

1. Kaplan EB, Sheiner LB, Boeckmann AJ, et al. The usefulness of preoperative laboratory screening. JAMA 1985;253:3576–3581.
2. McKee RF, Scott EM. The value of routine preoperative investigations. Ann R Coll Surg Engl 1987;69:160–162.
3. Narr BJ, Hansen TR, Warner MA. Preoperative laboratory screening in healthy Mayo patients: cost effective elimination of tests and unchanged outcomes. Mayo Clin Proc 1991;66:155–159.
4. Rohrer MJ, Michelotti MC, Nahrwold DL. A prospective evaluation of the efficacy of preoperative coagulation testing. Ann Surg 1988;208:554–557.
5. Lawrence VA, Kroenke K. The unproven utility of preoperative urinalysis. Arch Intern Med 1988;148:1370–1373.
6. Goldberger AL, O'Konski M. Utility of the routine electrocardiogram before surgery and on general hospital admission. Ann Intern Med 1986;105:552–557.
7. Gold BS, Young ML, Kinman JL, et al. The utility of preoperative electrocardiograms in the ambulatory surgical patient. Arch Intern Med 1992;152:301–305.
8. Seymour DG, Pringle R, MacLennan WJ. The role of the routine pre-operative electrocardiogram in the elderly surgical patient. Age Ageing 1983;12:97–104.
9. Tape TG, Mushlin AI. How useful are routine chest x-rays of preoperative patients at risk for postoperative chest disease? J Gen Intern Med 1988;3:15–20.
10. Charpak Y, Blery C, Chastang C, et al. Prospective assessment of a protocol for selective ordering of preoperative chest x-rays. Can J Anaesth 1988;35:259–264.
11. American College of Physicians. Position paper: preoperative pulmonary function testing. Ann Intern Med 1990;112:793–794.
12. Zibrak JD, O'Donnell CR. Indications for preoperative pulmonary function testing. Clin Chest Med 1993;14:227–236.
13. Macpherson DS, Snow R, Lofgren RP. Preoperative screening: value of previous tests. Ann Intern Med 1990;113:969–973.
14. Blery C, Charpak Y, Szatan M, et al. Evaluation of a protocol for selective ordering of preoperative tests. Lancet 1986;1:139–141.
15. Macario A, Roizen MF, Thisted RA, et al. Reassessment of preoperative laboratory testing has changed the test-ordering patterns of physicians. Surg Gynecol Obstet 1992;175:539–547.
16. Macpherson DS. Preoperative laboratory testing: should any tests be routine before surgery? Med Clin North Am 1993;77:289–308.

SECTION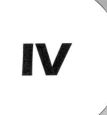

CARDIOLOGY

Medical Management of the Surgical Patient, Third Edition,
edited by Michael F. Lubin, H. Kenneth Walker, and Robert B. Smith III.
J.B. Lippincott Company, Philadelphia, PA © 1995.

CHAPTER

4

CARDIOVASCULAR DISEASE: GENERAL OVERVIEW

Howard M. Weitz

A team approach to patients with cardiovascular disease who undergo noncardiac surgery is the ideal way to expedite perioperative care. It is essential to assess patients' risk of cardiac complications and to identify those risk factors that may be reversed or ameliorated if time allows before surgery. The most likely cardiovascular problems that patients may encounter in the perioperative period should also be anticipated and an approach to these problems planned in advance. The physicians who are responsible for preoperative cardiac risk assessment and perioperative care vary according to locale. In many regions, family physicians, general internists, or cardiologists perform these duties. In other areas, these tasks are performed by surgeons or anesthesiologists. The selection of anesthetic agents as well as their means of administration is typically the domain of anesthesiologists; however, it is essential that surgeons and medical consultants understand the basic cardiovascular and hemodynamic effects of anesthesia.

PHYSIOLOGIC RESPONSE OF THE CARDIOVASCULAR SYSTEM TO SURGERY

Many physiologic changes affect the cardiovascular system in the perioperative period. Most occur as the cardiovascular system attempts to preserve homeostasis in response to the stress of surgery. Although many of these responses are well tolerated and even protective in patients who are free of cardiovascular disease, they may tax patients with compensated or overt cardiac disease. The overall effects on the cardiac system may be viewed as responses that increase myocardial oxygen demand (MVO_2), decrease myocardial oxygen supply, or increase cardiac work.

Increased MVO_2 is common during and after surgery and is of particular concern in patients with coronary artery disease. It often results from an increase in circulating catecholamines that is a consequence of the sympathetic stimulation associated with surgical stress and pain. Hypothermia associated with surgery may also increase MVO_2. It promotes shivering, which increases metabolic activity and decreases the degradation of circulating catecholamines, leading to increased circulating catecholamine levels. Hypoventilation may result in elevations of PCO_2, which is another stimulus of sympathetic activity. Hypertension and tachycardia also occur with increased sympathetic activity and result in increased cardiac work and myocardial oxygen demand.

In addition, several perioperative factors may lead to decreased myocardial oxygen delivery. Hypoventilation and atelectasis may reduce arterial oxygen saturation. Anemia decreases myocardial oxygen delivery. Intravascular volume overload may elevate left ventricular end-diastolic pressure, leading to pulmonary edema with hypoxia. Volume depletion or excessive perioperative vasodilation may lead to hypotension with coronary artery hypoperfusion.

43

Increases in MV_{O_2} or decreases in myocardial oxygen supply may precipitate myocardial ischemia in patients with coronary artery disease, lead to congestive heart failure in patients with impaired left ventricular function or obstruction to left ventricular outflow, or provoke arrhythmias in patients with cardiac electrical instability. Responses that attempt to increase cardiac output may result in congestive heart failure in patients with "fixed" cardiac output (eg, aortic stenosis, severe left ventricular dysfunction).[1]

The goal in the perioperative period is to maintain myocardial oxygen demand, myocardial oxygen delivery, and cardiac work as close to baseline levels as possible.

ANESTHESIA CONSIDERATIONS

General anesthesia offers the best control of the cardiorespiratory system and is typically induced with intravenous agents and maintained with inhaled agents, often in conjunction with intravenous narcotics and skeletal muscle relaxants.

General anesthesia is most often induced by the injection of short-acting barbiturates or benzodiazepines. Barbiturates may impair cardiac performance by a direct negative inotropic effect in addition to peripheral vasodilation. Although there is often compensation in the form of a baroreceptor-mediated sympathetic increase in peripheral vascular resistance, β-blockers may blunt the compensatory sympathetic response and result in hypotension.[2] Cardiac depression may also be exaggerated in elderly or hypovolemic patients. Ketamine is a unique nonbarbiturate induction agent that does not cause significant cardiovascular depression. Although it may depress cardiac contractility directly, it produces sympathetic stimulation that may elevate the blood pressure. This may be beneficial for patients in shock but the sympathomimetic effect may be deleterious for patients with coronary artery disease.[3] Propofol is an intravenous sedative hypnotic agent that is a member of a new class of anesthetic agents known as alkylphenols. It has the shortest action of all the induction agents and can also be used to maintain general anesthesia. For these reasons, it is finding widespread use in outpatient anesthesia. Propofol may lead to transient decreases in blood pressure and cardiac output.[4] Diazepam and midazolam are the benzodiazepines most widely used for anesthesia induction and are associated with minimal cardiac depression.

Inhaled agents are typically used to maintain anesthesia. The most common of these are nitrous oxide, halothane, enflurane, and isoflurane.[5] Although these agents are myocardial depressants, the effect of nitrous oxide, which depresses the myocardium least, is rarely manifest because of compensation by a reflex sympathetic response that results in an increase in peripheral vascular resistance with maintenance of the systemic blood pressure.[6] Halothane has the greatest myocardial depressant effect among these agents and may change cardiovascular hemodynamics by both direct myocardial depression and peripheral vasodilation. The negative inotropic effect of halothane is clinically most significant in the setting of coexisting left ventricular dysfunction; the hypotensive effect is most pronounced in patients who are taking venous or arterial vasodilators (eg, nitrates, hydralazine, angiotensin-converting enzyme inhibitors, calcium channel antagonists) or are intravascularly volume-depleted. Therefore, halothane should be used cautiously in patients in whom hypotension may be particularly hazardous (ie, those who have aortic stenosis or hypertrophic cardiomyopathy with aortic outflow tract obstruction). Halothane also sensitizes the myocardium to catecholamines and may be arrhythmogenic, particularly if hypercarbia is present.[7] This may occur clinically in patients with low cardiac output who require catecholamine inotropic support. Arrhythmias may also occur in patients without organic heart disease and are usually transient. Halothane may also depress sinus node function, leading to bradycardia.

Enflurane and isoflurane are also commonly used halogenated inhaled agents. Enflurane produces more vasodilation than does halothane and may result in a similar degree of direct myocardial depression. Isoflurane produces the least direct myocardial depression of the halogenated agents and is a potent peripheral as well as coronary vasodilator.[8]

The muscle relaxants used in general anesthesia have varied hemodynamic effects. Pancuronium has a vagolytic effect and may increase heart rate and cardiac output. This effect may be antagonized by the use of β-blockers. Metocurine may lower blood pressure but does not result in tachycardia. Succinylcholine may cause bradycardia but otherwise has minimal adverse cardiac effects.[9] Vecuronium and atacuronium are short-acting agents that do not have significant cardiovascular side effects. Quinidine and procainamide may prolong the action of muscle relaxants, resulting in longer perioperative skeletal muscle paralysis.[10]

Opioid analgesics (narcotics) are often used during surgery in conjunction with inhaled anesthetic agents. They may allow the use of lower doses of inhaled agents or may serve in high doses as the primary anesthetic agent in hemodynamically unstable patients. Morphine has been used most widely; its major cardiac side effect is peripheral vasodilation and hypotension resulting from the histamine release that it induces.[11,12] Fentanyl and sufentanil are synthetic opioids that do not lead to histamine release and are not associated with vasodilation or hypotension. They are preferred over morphine for patients who require high-dose narcotic anesthesia and have largely supplanted the role of morphine in anesthesia. Because it is not associated with significant alteration of cardiovascular hemodynamics, the combination of a narcotic (fentanyl) and nitrous oxide is often used in patients with significant left ventricular dysfunction.[11,13] These agents are also used to blunt the stress response during intubation and to minimize the risk of intubation-induced hypertension and arrhythmia.

For patients with cardiac disease who are undergoing noncardiac surgery, no anesthetic agent or technique is without risk. Several studies have found no difference in the rate of cardiovascular complications between regional (spinal, regional, local) and general anesthesia, except that the incidence of perioperative congestive heart failure in patients with histories of heart failure seems to be lower with regional anesthesia.[14–18] Most cardiac complications that are related to noncardiac surgery occur hours to days after patients are given anesthesia. The actual contribution of the anesthetic agent to cardiac morbidity is not well defined. Local anesthesia has been found to be safe in patients with prior myocardial infarction who undergo ophthalmic procedures.[19] For elderly patients undergoing surgical repair of groin hernias, local anesthesia has been found to be associated with a lower risk of cardiac complications than has regional or general anesthesia.[20] Regional anesthesia has also been shown to be associated with a lower risk of perioperative myocardial infarction in patients with prior myocardial infarction who undergo transurethral prostate resection.[21,22]

One anesthetic technique may be preferred over another in a particular case. Regional anesthesia may be favored in patients with myocardial dysfunction because it causes less cardiac and respiratory dysfunction than does general anesthesia. Spinal or epidural anesthesia used for surgery at or above the level of the groin (dermatome T12) inhibits spinal sympathetic outflow. Vasodilation and hypotension may subsequently occur in an unpredictable fashion.[23] The heart rate response to the stress of surgery as well as to hypotension may be attenuated if the cardiac sympathetic nerves are interrupted by the regional anesthetic.[24] Although vasodilation and hypotension are usually well tolerated, they may lead to hemodynamic compromise in patients with "fixed" cardiac output (eg, critical aortic stenosis, severe left ventricular dysfunction) who are unable to increase cardiac output to compensate for hypotension. They are also potentially harmful for patients who require an elevated preload (eg, patients with pulmonary hypertension). For these reasons, general anesthesia is often preferred over spinal anesthesia in this patient population. Finally, the use of general anesthesia may be advisable in anxious and fearful patients to prevent anxiety-induced catecholamine release with subsequent increases in myocardial oxygen demand.

Cardiovascular benefits of epidural anesthesia-analgesia have been suggested. In a small series of patients at high risk for perioperative cardiac complications, Yeager and colleagues[25] found that those who received epidural as well as general anesthesia had a lower incidence of perioperative cardiac complications compared to those who received only general anesthesia followed by postoperative parenteral analgesia with narcotics. This study has been criticized, however, because data collection was not uniform.[26] Preliminary studies also indicate that epidural anesthesia-analgesia may result in fewer cardiac complications in vascular surgery.[27] It has been suggested that this type of anesthesia-analgesia blunts perioperative sympathetic activity and serves an antiischemic function. Epidural anesthesia-analgesia may also modify the postoperative thrombotic response, limiting postoperative increases in coagulation factor VIII and von Willebrand's factor and thereby lowering the incidence of venous and arterial thrombotic events.[28] In contrast, a study of patients who underwent infrainguinal vascular bypass surgery found equivalent rates of cardiovascular complications with epidural and conventional general anesthesia.[18] A pilot study comparing low-dose postoperative analgesia to intensive postoperative analgesia (using continuous sufentanil infusion in patients undergoing coronary bypass surgery) revealed a lower rate of adverse cardiac events associated with the latter approach.[29]

No ideal anesthetic agent is available for patients with cardiac disease who are undergoing noncardiac surgery. General, epidural, spinal, and local anesthesia all have unique risks and benefits. There is great interest in the possibility of using perioperative and postoperative epidural analgesia, often in conjunction with general anesthesia, to decrease the incidence of cardiac complications. Irrespective of the type of anesthesia used and its mode of delivery, it is the ability of anesthesiologists to respond to patients' changing demands during and immediately after surgery that is the principal determinant of cardiac risk.[30]

ASSESSMENT OF CARDIAC RISK

The occurrence of perioperative cardiac complications is influenced by many factors, including the general medical status of patients, the presence and severity of existing cardiovascular diseases, and the type of surgical procedures performed.

A multifactorial approach to risk assessment was initially described by Goldman and colleagues in 1977.[17] A total of 1001 patients older than 40 years who underwent general noncardiac surgery were evaluated. Using univariate analysis, nine risk factors were identified and found to be associated with an increased risk of perioperative cardiac complications:

- Age greater than 70 years
- Myocardial infarction within the preceding 6 months
- The presence of a third heart sound or jugular venous distention

- Important valvular aortic stenosis
- A rhythm other than sinus rhythm or the presence of atrial premature contractions on the preoperative electrocardiogram (ECG)
- More than five ventricular premature contractions per minute before surgery
- Abdominal, thoracic, or aortic surgery
- Emergency surgery
- Poor general medical condition

Multivariate analysis was used to assign "risk points" to each factor (Table 4-1). A point scoring system was devised that allowed the stratification of patients to one of four groups at increasing risk for cardiac complications. The cardiac event end points were myocardial infarction, pulmonary edema, ventricular tachycardia, and cardiac death (Table 4-2).

The multifactorial risk index facilitated cardiac risk assessment using easily obtained, clinically relevant variables. It was suggested that the control or reversal of risk factors could reduce cardiac risk. Several factors were found to be insignificant in the prediction of risk. They were controlled diabetes mellitus, the presence of a fourth heart sound, controlled hypertension with a diastolic blood pressure of 110 mmHg or less, and chronic stable angina. In a subsequent study of 1140 patients, the utility of this index was confirmed. Although the risk for patients in risk classes 1, 2, and 3 was similar to that predicted by Goldman and associates, the risk for those in the high-risk class 4 was about 50% less than described in the initial index.[31] The reason for this improvement is not definitely known, although increased

TABLE 4–2. Correlation of Risk Index With Operative Complication

Class	Points	Life-Threatening Complications* (%)	Mortality (%)
I	0–5	0.7	0.2
II	6–12	5.0	2.0
III	13–25	11.0	2.0
IV	>25	22.0	56.0

*Including myocardial infarction, pulmonary edema, and ventricular tachycardia.
(Goldman L, Caldera D, Nussbaum SR, et al. Multifactorial index of cardiac risk in noncardiac surgical procedures. N Engl J Med 1977;297:845)

perioperative surveillance of high-risk patients as well as the availability of parenteral cardiac medications and invasive hemodynamic monitoring for these patients may have played a role. The use of a multifactorial risk index was also validated by Detsky and colleagues.[32] In addition to those risk factors identified by Goldman, these authors found that Canadian Cardiovascular Society class 3 angina (angina on walking one or two blocks on a level surface or climbing one flight of stairs), class 4 angina (angina with any activity) within 2 weeks before surgery, unstable angina during the 3 months preceding surgery, and pulmonary edema were significant risk factors[32] (Table 4-3).

The reliability of risk stratification indices has been challenged. In a study of men who had known coronary artery disease or were at high risk for coronary artery disease, Mangano and coworkers[33] found that the cardiac risk index did not correlate with the risk of perioperative myocardial ischemia. Postoperative myocardial ischemia was related to the occurrence of adverse cardiac events. Five independent preoperative clinical predictors of postoperative myocardial ischemia were identified:

- Left ventricular hypertrophy on electrocardiography
- A history of hypertension
- Diabetes mellitus treated with medications
- Definite coronary artery disease (previous myocardial infarction, typical angina pectoris, or atypical angina accompanied either by an ischemic electrocardiographic response to exercise or by a myocardial perfusion defect on thallium scintigraphy)
- The use of digoxin

The risk of postoperative myocardial ischemia increased progressively with the number of predictors present. It occurred in 22% of patients with no predictors, in 31% of those with one predictor, in 46% of those with two predictors, in 70% of those with three predictors, and in 77% of those with four predictors[34] (Table 4-4). Until these results are confirmed in large trials, however, multifactorial cardiac risk

TABLE 4–1. Computation of the Cardiac Risk Index

Variable	Points
Age >70 years	5
Myocardial infarction in previous 6 months	10
S_3 gallop or jugular vein distention	11
Important valvular aortic stenosis	3
Rhythm other than sinus or the presence of premature atrial contractions on preoperative electrocardiogram	7
More than 5 ventricular premature contractions per minute at any time before operation	7
Po_2 <60 or Pco_2 >50 mmHg Potassium <3 or HCO_3^- <20 mEq/L Blood urea nitrogen >50 or creatinine >3 mg/dL Abnormal SGOT, chronic liver disease, or patient bedridden from noncardiac cause	3
Intraperitoneal, intrathoracic, or aortic surgery	3
Emergency surgery	4
TOTAL	53

(Goldman L, Caldera D, Nussbaum SR, et al. Multifactorial index of cardiac risk in noncardiac surgical procedures. N Engl J Med 1977;297:845)

TABLE 4–3. Modified Multifactorial Risk Index

Variable	Points
Coronary Artery Disease	
Myocardial infarction within 6 months	10
Myocardial infarction more than 6 months ago	5
Canadian Cardiovascular Society Angina	
Class 3	10
Class 4	20
Unstable angina within 3 months	10
Alveolar Pulmonary Edema	
Within 1 week	10
Ever	5
Valvular Disease	
Critical aortic stenosis	20
Arrhythmias	
Sinus plus atrial premature beats or rhythm other than sinus on preoperative electrocardiogram	5
More than 5 ventricular premature contractions per minute at any time before surgery	5
Medical Status	
Poor general medical status	5
Po_2 <60 or Pco_2 >50	
Potassium <3 or HCO_3 <20 mEq/L	
Blood urea nitrogen >50 or creatinine >3 mg/dL	
Abnormal SGOT	
Chronic liver disease	
Bedridden from noncardiac cause	
Age	
Age > 70 years	5
Operation	
Emergency operation	10

(Detsky AS, Abrams H, McLaughlin J, et al. Predicting cardiac complications in patients undergoing non-cardiac surgery. J Gen Intern Med 1986;1:211)

TABLE 4–4. Risk of Postoperative Myocardial Ischemia in Men With or at High Risk for Definite Coronary Artery Disease

Number of Predictors*	Risk of Ischemia (%)
0	22
1	31
2	46
3	70
4	77

*Predictors: left ventricular hypertrophy on ECG; history of hypertension; diabetes mellitus; definite coronary artery disease (previous myocardial infarction, typical angina pectoris, or atypical angina accompanied by either an ischemic ECG response to exercise or a myocardial perfusion defect on thallium scintigraphy); or use of digoxin.

(Adapted from Hollenberg M, Mangano D, Browner W, et al. Predictors of postoperative myocardial ischemia in patients undergoing noncardiac surgery. JAMA 1992;268:205–209)

3.7 times in those who had known coronary artery disease, and 2.2 times in those who had postoperative myocardial ischemia without unstable angina or myocardial infarction.[36] Therefore, this patient population requires careful cardiac observation in the immediate perioperative period as well as over the long term.

The significance of several of the clinical variables has changed since the initial multifactorial risk index was described in 1977. These variables are discussed in the following sections.

Myocardial infarction within the preceding six months. Patients who have sustained a myocardial infarction within 6 months before undergoing noncardiac surgery are at increased risk for recurrent myocardial infarction during the perioperative period. The incidence of recurrent myocardial infarction has decreased, however. Data from the 1960s and 1970s indicated recurrent myocardial infarction rates of 27% to 37% when surgery was done within 3 months and 11% to 16% when surgery was done within 4 to 6 months of a myocardial infarction. The rate of recurrent infarction was 5% for patients who underwent noncardiac surgery more than 6 months after a myocardial infarction.[37,38] In marked contrast, a study presenting data from the 1980s indicated a recurrent infarction rate of only 5.7% when noncardiac surgery was done within 3 months, 2.3% when it was done within 6 months, and 1.9% when it was done more than 6 months after a myocardial infarction. In this study, most of the patients who sustained myocardial infarctions during the 6 months before they underwent noncardiac surgery were monitored hemodynamically in the perioperative period; observed in intensive care units for 72 to 96 hours after surgery; and treated with intravenous nitrates, β-adrenergic blockers, and vasopressors as clinically indicated.[39] This study has been criticized because it used historical control

indices remain useful tools for the assessment of perioperative cardiac risk.

This study also provided insight into both long-term cardiac outcome and the causes of death in patients with cardiovascular disease after noncardiac surgery. In this group of patients at high risk for cardiac complications, noncardiac causes of death predominated over cardiac etiologies. Patients at highest risk of in-hospital mortality after noncardiac surgery were those with a history of hypertension, severely limited physical activity, and renal dysfunction.[35] Long-term follow-up after noncardiac surgery revealed a significant incidence of adverse cardiac outcomes. The incidence of adverse cardiac events up to 2 years after noncardiac surgery was increased 28 times in patients who had perioperative unstable angina or myocardial infarction, 6.1 times in those who had peripheral vascular disease, 5 times in those who had a history of congestive heart failure, subjects and inadequate subgroup analysis so that specific factors responsible for improved outcome could not be identified.

Pending further controlled studies, we use post–myocardial infarction risk stratification in deciding who may undergo noncardiac surgery. Patients who have uncomplicated courses after myocardial infarction, have preserved left ventricular function, are free of exercise-induced myocardial ischemia documented by exercise electrocardiography, and do not have complex ventricular ectopy have a 1-year cardiac mortality of under 2%. We believe that these patients will have a lower incidence of cardiac morbidity and mortality than initially predicted when they are operated on during the first 6 months after myocardial infarction.

The clinical decision is more complex in patients who do not meet these criteria after myocardial infarction. For patients who require emergency surgery, we often use invasive hemodynamic monitoring in conjunction with parenteral antianginal medications to decrease the ischemic burden. In less emergent settings, nuclear cardiac imaging (ie, dipyridamole thallium imaging) or coronary angiography has been used to better assess the extent of myocardium at risk. If it is clinically indicated, a coronary revascularization procedure, coronary artery bypass grafting, or percutaneous transluminal coronary angioplasty is performed before noncardiac surgery is undertaken (see Chapter 5).

More than five ventricular premature contractions per minute at any time before surgery. The clinical significance of ventricular premature contractions depends on the presence of coexisting cardiac disease. Ventricular premature contractions are a risk factor for sudden death in patients with residual myocardial ischemia or left ventricular dysfunction.[40] Complex ventricular ectopy in the absence of coexisting heart disease is not associated with increased cardiac morbidity or mortality.[41] Perioperative risk stratification indices have not taken this principle into consideration. We believe that healthy patients with premature ventricular contractions and no evidence of structural or ischemic heart disease are probably not at increased risk for cardiac complications in the perioperative period.

Valvular aortic stenosis. The perioperative incidence of significant cardiac morbidity and mortality in a small, selected group of patients with aortic stenosis was significantly less than the 14-fold increase in mortality for patients with aortic stenosis predicted by the initial multifactorial risk index.[42] This was attributed to advances in anesthetic technique and perioperative cardiac monitoring. Because of the small number of patients evaluated in this study, we believe that critical aortic stenosis should continue to be considered a risk factor for perioperative cardiac complications pending further evaluation.

Aortic surgery. In the original multifactorial risk index, aortic surgery was associated with increased cardiac risk, whereas peripheral vascular surgery was not. Only 16.2% of the patients studied in deriving the index underwent vascular surgery. When it was applied only to patients undergoing aortic aneurysm repair, the multifactorial risk index was found to underestimate the incidence of cardiovascular complications in patients thought to be at low risk.[43,44] Pilot studies have also found the incidence of cardiovascular complications to be similar between aortoiliac and infrainguinal vascular repair.[45,46] This higher than predicted incidence of cardiac complications in vascular surgery probably results from the high incidence of significant, often clinically occult coronary artery disease in this patient population.[47] A classic study of patients undergoing elective vascular surgery found that only 8% had normal coronary arteries and that 31% had coronary artery disease that was either inoperable or severe enough to warrant surgical revascularization.[48] Contributing to the risk are the hemodynamic stress and increased demand for myocardial oxygen delivery that accompany vascular surgery.

These inadequacies have led to the development of a risk stratification algorithm that combines clinical factors with radionuclear myocardial imaging (Fig. 4-1). Age greater than 70 years, a history of angina, electrocardiographic evidence of a Q-wave myocardial infarction, a history of ventricular premature contractions that have required medical therapy, and diabetes mellitus that requires medical treatment are risk factors for cardiac complications after vascular surgery.[49] Patients who are physically active and have none of these risk factors are at low risk for cardiac complications and may undergo vascular surgery without specialized cardiac testing. At the opposite extreme are high-risk patients, who have three or more risk factors, exertional angina despite antianginal therapy, unstable angina, or recent myocardial infarction. Elective vascular surgery is usually delayed in this group until the cardiac status is stabilized.

If surgery is deemed mandatory in high-risk patients, coronary angiography is often done to assess the coronary anatomy. A coronary revascularization procedure frequently is performed before major vascular surgery in clinical conditions in which coronary revascularization has been shown to decrease long-term mortality. These include critical left main coronary stenosis, triple-vessel coronary artery disease with left ventricular dysfunction, double-vessel coronary artery disease with severe proximal stenosis of the left anterior descending coronary artery, and severe proximal stenosis of a large left anterior descending coronary artery with demonstrable myocardial ischemia.[50] Although it is clinically useful, this approach has not been tested in prospective, randomized clinical trials.

Patients who have one or two risk factors or who have no risk factors but lead a sedentary life are at intermediate risk for cardiac complications with vascular surgery. For

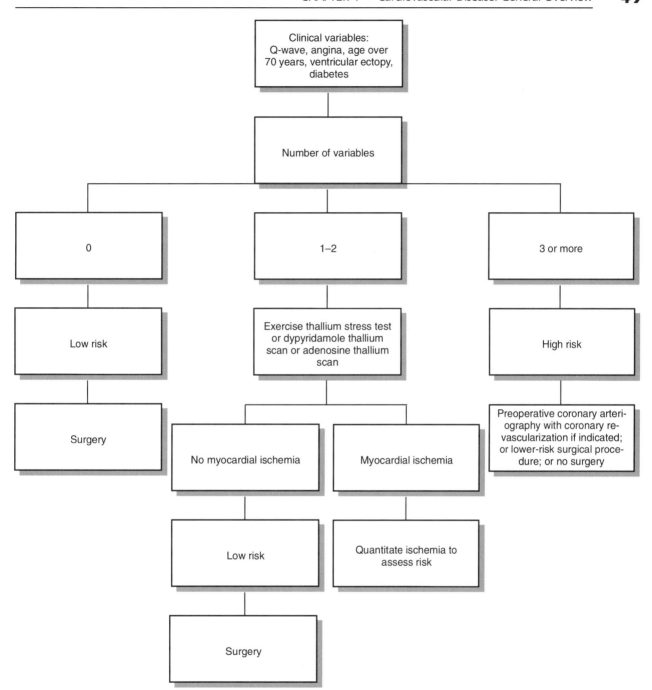

FIG. 4-1. Risk stratification before vascular surgery. (Weitz H. Cardiac risk stratification prior to vascular surgery. Med Clin North Am 1993;77:377–396)

these patients, vasodilator myocardial nuclear imaging with dipyridamole or adenosine is helpful in stratifying risk. Normal results or results indicating a fixed myocardial defect suggest a level of risk similar to that of patients who have no risk factors, with a perioperative cardiac event rate as low as 1%.[51] Normal scan results also predict a low incidence of cardiac complications during the 30 months after vascular surgery.[52] If the study demonstrates myocardial ischemia, the degree of ischemia is measured[53] (Table 4-5). Ischemia in the distribution of more than one coronary artery or involving more than 3 of 15 myocardial segments is suggestive of moderate to high risk, and these patients are evaluated in a fashion similar to patients with three or more risk factors. If patients cannot undergo vasodilator myocardial imaging, other imaging modalities are attempted, such as conventional stress testing, dobutamine echocardiography, arm ergometry thallium scanning, and atrial pacing stress testing. If these studies cannot be performed or their results are indeterminate, 24-hour ambulatory ischemia monitoring may be attempted. Negative study results are associated with a low risk of perioperative cardiac complications. The positive predictive value of these studies is relatively low, however, and further evaluation after positive test results are obtained must be individualized. A recent study identified definite clinical evidence of coronary artery disease and age greater than 65 years as the most important predictors of cardiac complications after abdominal aortic surgery. Contrary to other studies, thallium scanning was not found to be helpful in the prediction of risk.[53a] Further clinical trials are necessary to settle this controversy.

A somewhat different approach is used for patients undergoing carotid endarterectomy. The morbidity and mortality of this procedure are low enough that, for most patients (except those who have angina with daily activity, unstable angina, or recent myocardial infarction), carotid revascularization may proceed without specialized studies to assess the coronary anatomy.[54-57] The risk of combined or sequential procedures exceeds the risk of endarterectomy alone. For patients who have angina at a low work load, unstable angina, or recent myocardial infarction, we usually perform coronary angiography to define the coronary anatomy. If a revascularization procedure is warranted, a combined carotid and coronary artery revascularization procedure is performed.

Pilot studies have indicated that perioperative β-blocking agents as well as epidural analgesia decrease the incidence of perioperative myocardial ischemia during vascular surgery.[27,58]

PREOPERATIVE CARDIAC TESTS

Twelve-lead electrocardiogram. No consensus exists regarding the indications for a preoperative ECG. There is no evidence that a baseline ECG provides significant benefit to warrant its use in all patients. Although the incidence of asymptomatic electrocardiographic abnormalities increases with age, there is no proof that these abnormalities have any impact on the outcome after noncardiac surgery.[59] The most compelling reason for performing a preoperative ECG in asymptomatic patients is to identify silent myocardial infarction. It is also useful in identifying cardiac arrhythmias and ventricular ectopy, which are associated with an increased risk of perioperative cardiac complications if they are combined with structural or ischemic cardiovascular disease. Most of these rhythms, however, are apparent on physical examination. A recent study of the utility of preoperative ECGs in patients undergoing ambulatory surgery found that, although nonspecific electrocardiographic abnormalities were common before surgery, few patients benefited from performance of the test. Some benefit was suggested in patients older than 60 years who were judged to be at least moderate anesthetic risks.[60]

We believe that preoperative ECGs are justified in patients with known cardiac disease or significant cardiac risk factors (eg, hypertension, diabetes mellitus). They may also be of benefit in patients with peripheral atherosclerosis, who frequently have occult coronary artery disease. In addition, a preoperative ECG may be useful to identify the cardiac sequelae that can occur in patients with electrolyte abnormalities as well as those who take noncardiac medications that can affect the cardiovascular system (ie, tricyclic antidepressants, phenothiazines, and anthracycline chemotherapeutic agents). We believe that preoperative ECGs should be performed in patients with histories of cardiac arrhythmias and in patients who are scheduled to undergo

TABLE 4–5. Semiquantitative Analysis of Dipyridamole-Thallium Scans*

Extent of Thallium Redistribution	Predictive Value of Cardiac Event[†] (%)
None	0
≤3 segments	12
≥4 segments	38
1 coronary territory	13
2 or 3 coronary territories	43

*Scoring based on analysis of thallium scan in three standard views with each view divided into 5 segments for a total of 15 segments.
[†]Perioperative cardiac events: unstable angina ≥2 episodes of symptomatic ischemic ECG changes, ischemic pulmonary edema, myocardial infarction, or cardiac death.
(Adapted from Levinson J, Boucher C, Coley C, et al. Usefulness of semiquantitative analysis of dipyridamole-thallium-201 redistribution for improving risk stratification before vascular surgery. Am J Cardiol 1990;66:406–410)

surgical procedures associated with increased risk, such as abdominal, thoracic, or emergency surgery. Although no age-specific guidelines are available, recommendations from the American College of Physicians stated that an ECG may be useful in patients at risk for heart disease (ie, men older than 35 to 40 years and women older than 50 years).[61]

Echocardiography. An echocardiogram with Doppler evaluation may be helpful in selected patients to assess cardiac risk and facilitate perioperative management. This test estimates the severity of aortic stenosis or other valvular lesions, identifies the etiology of heart murmurs, measures left ventricular systolic and diastolic function in patients with congestive heart failure, and identifies structural heart disease in patients with ventricular premature contractions.

Radionuclide ventriculography. Resting radionuclide ventriculography is an alternative means of estimating left ventricular function in patients in whom echocardiographic evaluation is technically inadequate. Several studies have assessed the prognostic value of resting left ventricular function before vascular surgery but no consensus exists.[62]

Exercise stress testing. Exercise-induced myocardial ischemia, especially when it occurs at a low work load, indicates an increased risk of cardiac complications with vascular surgery. Conversely, the absence of inducible myocardial ischemia when the heart rate during exercise reaches or surpasses 85% of the maximal predicted heart rate indicates a low cardiac risk.[63] Only 30% of patients who require vascular surgery are able to exercise sufficiently to perform a valid exercise test.[64] In contrast, routine preoperative exercise stress testing in patients older than 40 years who are undergoing other types of surgery has not been found to be helpful in predicting cardiac risk.[65] In patients 65 years or older, the inability to perform 2 minutes of supine bicycle exercise and raise the heart rate above 99 beats/min (without β-blocking agents) was found in one study to be the strongest predictor of perioperative cardiac complications or death.[66] Most patients who could not exercise were limited by noncardiac causes. It is unclear whether the increased cardiac risk was the result of cardiac factors, poor general medical status, or unidentified causes.

Vasodilator myocardial imaging. Vasodilator myocardial imaging is useful in preoperative risk stratification when a noninvasive physiologic assessment of coronary perfusion is required and patients are unable to perform conventional exercise stress tests.[67] Although it is most commonly used to assess risk before vascular surgery, it also has been found to be helpful in stratifying risk in patients with a high likelihood of coronary artery disease before other major surgery.[51] Dipyridamole and adenosine are the coronary vasodilators most often used. When they are administered intravenously, these agents increase the concentration of cyclic adenosine monophosphate at the coronary artery, resulting in coronary vasodilation. Coronary blood flow in nonobstructed coronary arteries is increased 3 to 5 times and is minimally changed in coronary vessels that are severely stenotic. Radionuclide myocardial scanning is performed in conjunction with administration of the coronary vasodilators. Normal scan results suggest that the myocardial blood supply is preserved. The presence of a myocardial perfusion defect on initial scanning that redistributes on delayed scanning 3 or 4 hours later indicates viable but ischemic myocardium. A fixed radionuclear myocardial defect on initial as well as delayed scanning suggests a myocardial scar. This test is safe and yields results similar to those of exercise stress tests in which patients are able to achieve 85% of their maximal predicted heart rates.[68]

Side effects are common but transient and are of shorter duration when adenosine is used. They include chest pain, headache, and light-headedness. Bronchospasm may be provoked in patients with asthma and myocardial ischemia may occur in those with unstable angina. Therefore, the study is contraindicated in these patients. The effects of adenosine and dipyridamole are antagonized by compounds that contain theophylline (eg, caffeine, theophylline-containing bronchodilators) and these compounds must not be used before the study. Intravenous theophylline is given to reverse sustained side effects of dipyridamole. Adenosine is metabolized during its first pass through the liver and its side effects typically are brief. Negative results on vasodilator myocardial imaging suggest a low likelihood of perioperative cardiac complications in patients undergoing peripheral vascular and major noncardiac surgery, with a negative predictive value of about 98%. Positive results are less helpful because the positive predictive value of cardiac complications is only 16%.[62]

Arm ergometry stress testing and pacing electrocardiography. Arm ergometry stress testing and pacing electrocardiography have limited roles in risk stratification. They are used for patients who require noninvasive evaluation of coronary perfusion but are unable to perform conventional treadmill exercise stress tests or who have contraindications to vasodilator myocardial imaging. Many patients who are unable to perform adequate treadmill exercise are also unable to perform adequate arm exercise. Pacing studies are limited by the risks of transvenous pacemaker insertion, patient intolerance of transesophageal pacemaker placement, and normal development of Mobitz I atrioventricular block before the target heart rate is achieved, even if patients have no evidence of cardiac conduction system disease. Pilot studies suggest that negative results on arm ergometry stress testing or pacing electrocardiography (peak heart rate 85% to 100% of age-predicted maximal heart rate) done in conjunction with thallium myocardial scanning indicate a low likelihood of perioperative cardiac complications in association with vascular surgery. The significance of positive study results is unclear.[69,70]

Ambulatory silent myocardial ischemia monitoring. Silent myocardial ischemia monitoring also shows promise in preoperative risk assessment. It has been used before vascular surgery, and the absence of myocardial ischemia during 24 to 48 hours of continuous ambulatory electrocardiographic monitoring has been shown to have a negative predictive value for perioperative cardiac complications of 99%. The clinical significance of silent preoperative ischemia is less clear. Preoperative silent myocardial ischemia was associated with a 37% incidence of intraoperative and postoperative cardiac events in one study but showed no correlation in another study.[33,71] Because of these discrepancies, we refrain from using preoperative ischemia monitoring to predict risk, with one exception: patients undergoing vascular surgery who require risk stratification but are unable to exercise, undergo vasodilator myocardial imaging, or perform pacing or arm ergometry studies. In these patients, we consider the perioperative risk to be low if the monitor reveals no evidence of myocardial ischemia for 24 to 48 hours.

Other techniques that show promise for preoperative risk stratification, but need further validation, are dobutamine echocardiography, dipyridamole echocardiography, and dobutamine-thallium imaging.[54]

ELDERLY PATIENTS

Many physiologic changes occur in response to aging that have a significant effect on the cardiovascular response to surgery. The resting heart rate and the heart rate response to stress decrease.[72] Because cardiac output is a function of heart rate and stroke volume, it increases in elderly patients in response to stress by increasing the left ventricular end-diastolic volume.[73] In patients with left ventricular dysfunction, decreased ventricular compliance, or intravascular volume overload, this compensatory response may result in congestive heart failure. Baroreceptor responsiveness decreases with increased age and may cause exaggerated hypotension after intravascular volume loss as well as the administration of vasodilators or diuretics. The incidence of sick sinus syndrome and other cardiac conduction disorders is also increased, and occult conduction disorders may be unmasked when β-blockers or calcium channel antagonists are used in the perioperative period. Other cardiovascular changes that may affect cardiac function in the perioperative period are left ventricular hypertrophy with associated decreased left ventricular compliance, elevated left ventricular end-diastolic pressure, and subsequent interstitial edema. In this situation, which often results from long-standing hypertension, left ventricular hypertrophy may cause diastolic left ventricular dysfunction.

Drug metabolism is altered in the elderly. Renal function declines and cardiovascular drugs that are cleared by the kidney (eg, digoxin, procainamide, enalapril) may have increased half-lives. Hepatic blood flow also decreases, leading to delayed metabolism of agents such as lidocaine, propranolol, and verapamil.[74]

MANAGEMENT OF CARDIAC MEDICATIONS IN THE PERIOPERATIVE PERIOD

Perioperative continuation of patients' long-term cardiac medications is often challenging. Many oral medications have no parenteral substitutes. The stress of surgery may render patients' long-term cardiac medical regimens inadequate during the perioperative period. Finally, few controlled studies have evaluated the use of cardiac medications during and after noncardiac surgery. Several guidelines are helpful in attempting to maintain patients' long-term medical therapeutic regimens in the perioperative period.

Nitrates are a mainstay of therapy for patients with ischemic heart disease. Patients who are stable receiving nitrates on a long-term basis typically are given their oral nitrate preparations on the morning of the surgical procedure. Topical nitroglycerin ointment (0.5 to 2 inches) is then applied every 8 hours until oral nitrates are resumed. To replace long-acting transdermal nitrate preparations, nitroglycerin ointment is applied topically every 8 hours to decrease the risk of nitrate tolerance. This dosing schedule allows for a nitrate-free period, decreasing the potential for nitrate tolerance to develop. Nitrates may cause excessive preload reduction and hypotension, which may be exacerbated by intravascular volume depletion and the simultaneous use of other vasodilator medications or anesthetic agents. In some patients, hypotension may occur unpredictably with the initial use of nitrates. For this reason, we recommend that nitrates given initially to decrease the likelihood of perioperative myocardial ischemia be administered well before surgery. For patients who develop myocardial ischemia in the perioperative period that is not alleviated by topical nitrates, intravenous nitroglycerin may be used.

β-Adrenergic blockers are used in the treatment of myocardial ischemia, arrhythmias, and hypertension. Patients who receive β-blockers on a long-term basis should be given oral doses on the morning of their surgical procedure. Long-acting agents such as nadolol or atenolol produce β-blockade for as long as 24 hours. Patients' long-term β-blocker regimens are then restarted 24 hours after surgery if oral intake has resumed. For patients whose gastrointestinal tracts are not functional at that time, the administration of intravenous β-blockers (eg, propranolol, 0.5 to 2 mg every 4 to 6 hours) is begun and continued until the usual long-term oral β-blocker is tolerated. This regimen is often effective for patients who are receiving β-blockers for coronary artery disease or cardiac arrhythmias but may require alteration in patients who take these drugs for hypertension until oral medications are resumed. Labetalol (a test dose of 2.5 to 5 mg intravenously, then an infusion of 20 to 80 mg) may also be given by intravenous infusion at 2 mg/min until the blood pressure is controlled or a total of 300 mg or more has been administered. The short-acting intravenous β-blocker esmolol (at a loading infusion of 500 µg/kg/min for 1 minute followed by a continuous infusion at 50 µg/kg/min) may also control blood pressure in the postoperative period. Patients whose blood pressures are not controlled with these agents may require supplemental antihypertensive agents in addition to intravenous β-blockers until oral medications are resumed.

Intravenous nitroprusside is highly effective in controlling perioperative hypertension but the need for continuous blood pressure monitoring and the risk of cyanate toxicity make its use impractical for more than a few days. Intravenous methyldopa and enalaprilat, given 3 to 4 times daily, are effective in controlling postoperative hypertension, are well tolerated, and may be used without continuous blood pressure monitoring in stable patients. They are useful adjuncts for controlling hypertension in the postoperative period.

Intravascular volume depletion may occur in patients receiving long-term diuretic therapy and places them at risk for hypotension when anesthetic agents that produce vasodilation are administered. Intravascular volume depletion is suggested by the presence of orthostatic changes in the blood pressure and heart rate and should be corrected with fluid administration, if possible, before surgery. Patients who take diuretics may also have hypokalemia or hyperkalemia from potassium-sparing agents. Serum potassium levels should be checked in these patients before surgery. Although the multifactorial cardiac risk index identified preoperative hypokalemia (a potassium level of less than 3 mEq/L) as a cardiac risk, subsequent studies indicate that chronic preoperative hypokalemia in patients who are not taking digoxin is not a risk factor for perioperative arrhythmias. It has been suggested that a chronic serum potassium level of 3 mmol/L or higher is acceptable for anesthesia and surgery, and that chronic asymptomatic hypokalemia as low as 2.5 mmol/L may be adequate in patients who are at low risk for cardiac complications.[75] Hypokalemia has been shown to increase the incidence of cardiac arrhythmias in patients taking digoxin; therefore, perioperative hypokalemia should be corrected in this group.

The abrupt withdrawal of centrally acting antihypertensive agents, which may occur in the perioperative period, may result in a "discontinuation syndrome" characterized by sympathetic overactivity and rebound hypertension.[76] Symptoms may resemble those of pheochromocytoma. Clonidine is the prototype drug of this class. The discontinuation syndrome may occur 8 to 72 hours after clonidine is withdrawn but rarely occurs in patients who receive less than 1.2 mg of clonidine daily. This syndrome may be aggravated by the simultaneous use of propranolol, which blocks peripheral vasodilatory β-receptors, leaving vasoconstrictor α-receptors unopposed.[77] The syndrome may be terminated by resumption of clonidine therapy. If that is not possible because patients cannot resume oral intake, rebound hypertension may be controlled with intravenous nitroprusside or labetalol. Clonidine withdrawal syndrome may be prevented by slow tapering of clonidine therapy before surgery. For patients in whom this is not feasible, transdermal clonidine may be given in the perioperative period. The transdermal clonidine preparation requires about 48 hours to achieve therapeutic drug levels.[78] Therefore, it should be given well in advance of surgery and be administered simultaneously with oral clonidine for about 48 hours. The transdermal preparation maintains therapeutic clonidine levels for as long as 7 days.

Calcium channel antagonists are used to treat angina, hypertension, and arrhythmias. Sustained-release preparations of the calcium channel antagonists that patients have been using may be given on the morning of surgery in an effort to achieve effective drug levels for the next 24 hours. Patients who are capable of oral intake the day after surgery may resume oral calcium channel antagonists. Problems exist, however, in substituting appropriate parenteral formulations for patients who cannot resume oral calcium channel antagonists at this time. The few calcium channel antagonists that are available for parenteral administration often have their primary effect on the cardiac conduction system rather than treating hypertension or angina. Intravenous verapamil has potent negative chronotropic effects and can induce heart block. Intravenous diltiazem is indicated primarily to control the ventricular response in patients with atrial fibrillation and to convert paroxysmal supraventricular tachycardia to sinus rhythm in patients who have atrioventricular nodal reentrant tachycardia. There is no parenteral preparation of nifedipine.

In patients who receive calcium channel antagonists for their antianginal effects, topical or intravenous nitrates may be substituted until oral intake resumes. When calcium channel antagonists are used over the long term to treat coronary artery spasm, sublingual nifedipine may be given acutely to patients who cannot tolerate oral medications to abort an acute attack and every 4 hours to prevent coronary artery spasm. Sublingual nifedipine may cause acute hypotension, however. In patients who take calcium channel antagonists for hypertension, intravenous α-methyldopa or enalaprilat is often effective until oral medications are resumed. Most patients who receive calcium channel antagonists for antiarrhythmic therapy have supraventricular tachycardia. Several parenteral agents may be used to treat supraventricular tachycardia in the perioperative period, including intravenous β-blockers, diltiazem, verapamil, adenosine, and digoxin.

Digitalis glycosides may be given orally on the morning of surgery and then intravenously on a daily basis until patients' long-term oral regimens are resumed. The intravenous administration of these agents increases their bioavailability as much as 20%, and the maintenance parenteral dose may have to be reduced appropriately. To preclude increases in mesenteric or coronary artery vascular tone, intravenous administration should be accomplished slowly over 10 to 15 minutes.

Angiotensin-converting enzyme inhibitors are used to treat hypertension and congestive heart failure. Enalaprilat is the only agent of this class available for parenteral administration and is given intravenously every 6 hours.

PERIOPERATIVE INVASIVE CARDIAC MONITORING

Invasive pulmonary artery pressure monitoring is commonly used in patients who are at increased risk for myocardial infarction during and after operation in an effort to diagnose and treat perioperative myocardial ischemia. Indications for perioperative pulmonary artery pressure monitoring are ill-defined. Myocardial ischemia decreases left ventricular compliance and increases left ventricular end-diastolic pressure, left atrial pressure, pulmonary capillary wedge pressure, and pulmonary artery pressure. If it is extensive, myocardial ischemia may also reduce cardiac output. These hemodynamic consequences may occur before myocardial ischemia is apparent on standard electrocardiographic monitoring or manifest as abnormalities of cardiac hemodynamics.

Although it is attractive in theory, invasive pulmonary artery pressure monitoring has suboptimal sensitivity and specificity for the detection of perioperative myocardial ischemia. Numerous perioperative situations (eg, intravascular volume overload, increased afterload) may result in increased pulmonary artery capillary wedge pressure without associated myocardial ischemia. Similarly, myocardial ischemia may be present without changes in pulmonary capillary pressure. Some clinical studies have found no effect on outcome, whereas others have demonstrated improved outcome in patients who underwent perioperative invasive hemodynamic monitoring. These studies are characterized by small sample size, lack of randomization, and, in some cases, the use of historical case controls.[79] Our approach has been to assess the need for invasive hemodynamic monitoring on an individual basis. Although an effect on outcome has not been proved in large, prospective clinical trials, invasive monitoring may be helpful in managing the cardiac status in patients with left ventricular dysfunction or "fixed" cardiac output (eg, aortic stenosis) who are undergoing major surgery as well as in patients with unstable angina or recent myocardial infarction.

Transesophageal echocardiography (TEE) has been used to assess the presence of intraoperative myocardial ischemia. Ischemic wall motion abnormalities typically precede electrocardiographic evidence of ischemia. TEE is probably the most sensitive real-time indicator of intraoperative myocardial ischemia. Although it is sensitive, the specificity of this technique is poorly delineated. Factors other than myocardial ischemia (eg, increased afterload) may alter left ventricular systolic function and wall motion. Focal ventricular wall motion abnormalities may persist even after local myocardial ischemia has resolved. In a series of high-risk patients undergoing noncardiac surgery, the correlation between intraoperative wall motion abnormalities and postoperative cardiac events was poor.[80] TEE was also found to have little incremental advantage over preoperative clinical data and two-lead intraoperative electrocardiographic monitoring in identifying patients at high risk for perioperative cardiac complications. Other limiting factors of TEE are the high cost of equipment and the need for specialized training for physicians performing and interpreting the studies. TEE is not routinely used for monitoring during noncardiac surgery. Its greatest role is in the intraoperative assessment of cardiac valves before and after valve repair or replacement procedures.

REFERENCES

1. Weitz HH, Goldman L. Noncardiac surgery in the patient with heart disease. Med Clin North Am 1987;71:413–432.
2. Stoelting R. Hemodynamic effects of barbiturates and benzodiazepines. Cleve Clin Q 1981;48:9.
3. Derrer S. Pharmacology of anesthetic agents and muscle relaxants. In: Breslow M, Miller C, Rogers M, eds. Perioperative management. St Louis, CV Mosby, 1990:89.
4. Stephan H, Sonntag H, Schenk H, et al. Effects of propofol on cardiovascular hemodynamics, myocardial blood flow and myocardial metabolism in patients with coronary artery disease. Br J Anaesth 1986;58:969–975.
5. Bull AP. The anesthetic evaluation and management of the surgical patient with heart disease. Surg Clin North Am 1983;63: 1035–1048.
6. Rose SD, Corman L, Mason D. Cardiac risk factors in patients

undergoing noncardiac surgery. Med Clin North Am 1979;63: 1271.

7. Koehntop D, Liao JC, Van Bergen FH. Effects of pharmacologic alteration of adrenergic mechanism by cocaine, tropolone, aminophylline, and ketamine on epinephrine induced arrhythmias during halothane-nitrous oxide anesthesia. Anesthesiology 1977;46:83–93.

8. Reiz S, Balfors E, Sorensen MD, et al. Isoflurane: a powerful coronary vasodilator in patients with coronary artery disease. Anesthesiology 1983;59:91–97.

9. Wells P, Kaplan J. Optimal management of patients with ischemic heart disease for noncardiac surgery by complementary anesthesiologist and cardiologist interaction. Am Heart J 1981; 102:1029.

10. Rogers MC. Anesthetic management of patients with heart disease. Mod Concepts Cardiovasc Dis 1983;52:29.

11. Stanley TH. Hemodynamic effects of narcotics. Cleve Clin Q 1981;48:22.

12. Moss J, Rosow CE. Histamine release by narcotics and muscle relaxants in humans. Anesthesiology 1983;59:330–339.

13. Logue R, Kaplan J. The cardiac patient and noncardiac surgery. Curr Probl Cardiol 1982;7:2.

14. Arkins R, Smessaert AA, Hicks RG. Mortality and morbidity in surgical patients with coronary artery disease. JAMA 1964;190: 485–488.

15. Sapala J, Ponka J, Duvernoy W. Operative and nonoperative risks in the cardiac patient. J Geriatr Soc 1975;23:529.

16. Tinker JH. Perioperative myocardial infarction. Semin Anesth 1982;1:253–263.

17. Goldman L, Caldera D, Nussbaum SR, et al. Multifactorial index of cardiac risk in noncardiac surgical procedures. N Engl J Med 1977;297:845–850.

18. Rivers SP, Scherr LA, Sheehan E, et al. Epidural versus general anesthesia for infrainguinal arterial reconstruction. J Vasc Surg 1991;14:764–768.

19. Backer C, Tinker J, Robertson D, et al. Myocardial reinfarction following local anesthesia for opthalmic surgery. Anesth Analg 1980;59:257–262.

20. Nehme A. Groin hernias in elderly patients. Am J Surg 1983;146:257.

21. Erlik D, Valero A, Birkhan J, et al. Prostatic surgery and the cardiovascular patient. Br J Urol 1968;40:53–61.

22. McGown SW, Smith G. Anesthesia for transurethral prostatectomy: a comparison of spinal intradural analgesia with two methods of general anesthesia. Anaesthesia 1980;35:847–853.

23. Phero JC, Bridenbaugh PO, Edstrom HH, et al. Hypotension in spinal anesthesia. Anesth Analg 1987;66:549–552.

24. Yeager M. Pro: regional anesthesia is preferable to general anesthesia for the patient with heart disease. J Cardiothorac Anesth 1989;3:793–796.

25. Yeager MP, Glass D, Neff R, et al. Epidural anesthesia and analgesia in high risk surgical patients. Anesthesiology 1987;66: 729–736.

26. Beattie C. Regional anesthesia is not preferable to general anesthesia for the patient with heart disease. J Cardiothorac Anesth 1987;3:797–800.

27. Tuman K, McCarthy R, March R, et al. Effects of epidural anesthesia and analgesia on coagulation and outcome after major vascular surgery. Anesth Analg 1991;73:696–704.

28. Steele S, Slaughter T, Greenberg C, et al. Epidural anesthesia and analgesia: implications for perioperative coagulability. Anesth Analg 1991;73:683–685.

29. Mangano D, Siliciano D, Hollenberg M, et al. Postoperative myocardial ischemia: therapeutic trials using intensive analgesia following surgery. Anesthesiology 1992;76:342–353.

30. Goldman L, Braunwald E. General anesthesia and noncardiac surgery in patients with heart disease. In: Braunwald E, ed. Heart disease. Philadelphia, WB Saunders, 1992:1708–1720.

31. Zeldin R. Assessing cardiac risk in patients who undergo noncardiac surgical procedures. Can J Surg 1984;27:402.

32. Detsky A, Abrams H, McLaughlin J, et al. Predicting cardiac complications in patients undergoing non-cardiac surgery. J Gen Intern Med 1986;1:211.

33. Mangano DT, Browner WS, Hollenberg M, et al. Association of perioperative myocardial ischemia with cardiac morbidity and mortality in men undergoing noncardiac surgery. N Engl J Med 1990;323:1781–1788.

34. Hollenberg M, Mangano DT, Browner WS, et al. Predictors of postoperative myocardial ischemia in patients undergoing noncardiac surgery. JAMA 1992;268:205–209.

35. Browner WS, Li J, Mangano DT, et al. In-hospital and long-term mortality in male veterans following noncardiac surgery. JAMA 1992;268:228–232.

36. Mangano DT, Browner W, Hollenberg M, et al. Long-term cardiac prognosis following noncardiac surgery. JAMA 1992;268: 233–239.

37. Tarhan S, Moffitt E, Taylor W, et al. Myocardial infarction after general anesthesia. JAMA 1972;220:1451.

38. Steen P, Tinker J, Tarhan S. Myocardial reinfarction after anesthesia and surgery. JAMA 1978;239:2566.

39. Rao T, Jacobs K, El-Etr A. Reinfarction following anesthesia in patients with myocardial infarction. Anesthesiology 1983;59: 499.

40. Multicenter Postinfarction Research Group. Risk stratification and survival after myocardial infarction. N Engl J Med 1983; 309:331–336.

41. Kennedy H, Whitlock J, Sprague M, et al. Long term follow up of asymptomatic health subjects with frequent and complex ventricular ectopy. N Engl J Med 1985;312:193.

42. O'Keefe J, Shub C, Rettke S. Risk of noncardiac surgical procedures in patients with aortic stenosis. Mayo Clin Proc 1989;64: 400–405.

43. Jeffrey C, Kunsman J, Cullen D, et al. A prospective evaluation of cardiac risk index. Anesthesiology 1983;58:462–464.

44. McEnroe CS, O'Donnell T, Yeager A, et al. Comparison of ejection fraction and Goldman risk factor analysis to dipyridamole-thallium 201 studies in the evaluation of cardiac morbidity after aortic aneurysm surgery. J Vasc Surg 1990;7:497–504.

45. Cambria R, Brewster D, Abbott W. The impact of selective use of dipyridamole thallium scans and surgical function on the current morbidity of aortic surgery. J Vasc Surg 1992;15:43–51.

46. Krupski W, Layug E, Reilly L, et al. Comparison of cardiac morbidity between aortic and infrainguinal operations. J Vasc Surg 1992;15:354–365.

47. Orecchia P, Berger P, White C, et al. Coronary artery disease in aortic surgery. Ann Vasc Surg 1988;2:28–36.

48. Hertzer N, Beven E, Young J, et al. Coronary artery disease in

peripheral vascular patients: a classification of 1000 coronary angiograms and results of surgical management. Ann Surg 1984;199:223–233.

49. Eagle K, Coley C, Newell J, et al. Combining clinical and thallium data optimizes preoperative assessment of cardiac risk before major vascular surgery. Ann Intern Med 1989;110:859–866.

50. Guidelines and indications for coronary bypass graft surgery. A report of the American College of Cardiology/American Heart Association Task Force on Assessment of Diagnostic and Therapeutic Cardiovascular Procedures. J Am Coll Cardiol 1991;17:543–589.

51. Lette J, Waters D, Champagne P, et al. Prognostic implications of a negative dipyridamole-thallium scan: results in 360 patients. Am J Med 1992;92:615–620.

52. Hendel RC, Whitfield S, Villegas BJ, et al. Prediction of late cardiac events by dipyridamole thallium imaging in patients undergoing elective vascular surgery. Am J Cardiol 1992; 70:1243–1249.

53. Levinson J, Boucher C, Coley C, et al. Usefulness of semiquantitative analysis of dipyridamole-thallium 201 redistribution for risk stratification before vascular surgery. Am J Cardiol 1990;66:406–410.

53a. Baron JF, Mundler O, Bertrand M, et al. Dipyridamole thallium scintigraphy and gated radionucleotide angiography to assess cardiac risk before abdominal aortic surgery. N Engl J Med 1994;330:663–669.

54. Weitz HH. Cardiac risk stratification prior to vascular surgery. Med Clin North Am 1993;77:377–396.

55. Mackey W, O'Donnell T, Callow A. Carotid endarterectomy in patients with intracranial vascular disease: short term risk and long term outcome. J Vasc Surg 1989;10:432–438.

56. Rihal C, Gersh B, Whisnant J, et al. Influence of coronary heart disease on morbidity and mortality after carotid endarterectomy: a population based study in Olmsted County, Minnesota (1970–1988). J Am Coll Cardiol 1992;19:1254–1260.

57. Yeager R, Moneta G, McConnell D, et al. Analysis of risk factors for myocardial infarction following carotid endarterectomy. Arch Surg 1989;124:1142–1145.

58. Pasternack P, Grossi E, Baumann F, et al. Beta blockade to decrease silent myocardial ischemia during peripheral vascular surgery. Am J Surg 1989;158:113–116.

59. Goldberger A, O'Konski M. Utility of the routine electrocardiogram before surgery and on general hospital admission: critical review and new guidelines. Ann Intern Med 1986; 105:552–557.

60. Gold BS, Young ML, Kinman JL, et al. The utility of preoperative electrocardiograms in the ambulatory surgical patient. Arch Intern Med 1992;152:301–305.

61. Sox HC Jr. Common diagnostic tests: use and interpretation. Philadelphia, American College of Physicians, 1987:334–335.

62. Gersh B, Charanjit S, Rooke T, et al. Evaluation and management of patients with both peripheral vascular and coronary artery disease. J Am Coll Cardiol 1991;18:203–214.

63. Cutler BS, Wheeler HB, Paraskos JA, et al. Applicability and interpretation of electrocardiographic stress testing in pa-

64. McPhail N, Calvin JE, Shariatmadar A, et al. The use of preoperative exercise testing to predict cardiac complications after arterial reconstruction. J Vasc Surg 1988;7:60–68.

65. Carliner NH, Fisher ML, Plotnick GD, et al. Routine preoperative exercise testing in patients undergoing major noncardiac surgery. Am J Cardiol 1985;56:51–57.

66. Gerson M, Hurst J, Hertzberg V, et al. Cardiac prognosis in noncardiac geriatric surgery. Ann Intern Med 1985;103:832–837.

67. Wong T, Detsky AS. Preoperative cardiac risk assessment for patients having peripheral vascular surgery. Ann Intern Med 1992;116:743–753.

68. Lette J, Waters D, Lassonde J, et al. Multivariate clinical models and quantitative dipyridamole-thallium imaging to predict cardiac morbidity and death after vascular reconstruction. J Vasc Surg 1991;14:160–169.

69. Macpherson DS, Conroy W, Grund F. Arm ergometry thallium-201 cardiac imaging in the vascular surgery patient. Clin Res 1991;39:581A.

70. Stratmann HG, Mark AL, Walter KE, et al. Preoperative evaluation of cardiac risk by means of atrial pacing and thallium 201 scintigraphy. J Vasc Surg 1989;10:385–391.

71. Raby KE, Goldman L, Creager M, et al. Correlation between preoperative ischemia and major cardiac events after peripheral vascular surgery. N Engl J Med 1989;321:1296–1300.

72. Rosberg B, Rosberg B, Wulff K. Hemodynamics following normovolemic hemodilution in elderly patients. Acta Anaesthesiol Scand 1981;25:402–406.

73. Rodeheffer R, Gerstenblith G, Becker L, et al. Exercise cardiac output is maintained with advancing age in healthy human subjects: cardiac dilatation and increased stroke volume compensate for a diminished heart rate. Circulation 1984;69:203–213.

74. Wenger NK. Cardiovascular disease in the elderly. Curr Probl Cardiol 1992;17:618–624.

75. Restrick LJ, Huddy N, Hoffbrand BI. Diuretic-induced hypokalemia and surgery: much ado about nothing? Postgrad Med J 1992;68:318–320.

76. Houston M. Abrupt cessation of treatment in hypertension: consideration of clinical features, mechanisms, prevention and management of the discontinuation syndrome. Am Heart J 1981;102:415–430.

77. Bailey R, Neale T. Rapid clonidine withdrawal with blood pressure overshoot exaggerated by beta blockade. Br Med J 1976;1:942–943.

78. MacGregor T, Matzek K, Keirns J. Pharmacokinetics of transdermally delivered clonidine. Clin Pharmacol Ther 1985;38:278–284.

79. Tuman K. Pulmonary artery catheterization and outcome in patients with cardiovascular disease. Anesthesiol Rev 1989;16:34–41.

80. London M, Tubau I, Wong M, et al. The "natural history" of segmental wall motion abnormalities in patients undergoing noncardiac surgery. Anesthesiology 1990;73:544–555.

Medical Management of the Surgical Patient, Third Edition,
edited by Michael F. Lubin, H. Kenneth Walker, and Robert B. Smith III.
J.B. Lippincott Company, Philadelphia, PA © 1995.

CHAPTER

5

CORONARY ARTERY DISEASE

Howard M. Weitz

It has been estimated that of the 25 million patients who undergo noncardiac surgery each year in the United States, 3 million have either multiple coronary risk factors or known coronary artery disease (CAD). Together with the additional 4 million surgical patients who are older than 65 years, this group accounts for 80% of the 1 million patients each year who sustain perioperative cardiac morbidity and mortality.[1] CAD causes or is indirectly related to most of the cardiac complications that occur after noncardiac surgery.[2]

PATHOPHYSIOLOGY OF PERIOPERATIVE MYOCARDIAL ISCHEMIA AND INFARCTION

The pathophysiology of perioperative myocardial ischemia has been discussed by Massie and Mangano.[2] Although more than one mechanism may be operative in any one patient, the classic scenarios for perioperative myocardial ischemia are as follows:

- Increased myocardial metabolic demand that cannot be met, which is most common in patients with either critical coronary artery stenoses or occluded coronary arteries with myocardium at risk supplied by collateral vessels
- Myocardial ischemia resulting from decreased oxygen delivery associated with hypotension, coronary vaso-

spasm, or diminished oxygen-carrying capacity related to anemia
- Coronary artery occlusion with an abrupt decrease in the myocardial oxygen supply caused by perioperative coronary thrombosis

Patients with histories of myocardial infarctions (MIs) without further myocardium at risk of infarction may experience perioperative congestive heart failure as a result of infarct-related left ventricular dysfunction.

CORONARY ARTERY DISEASE AS A CARDIAC RISK FACTOR

Numerous risk factor indices have been described to assess the risk of cardiac complications in noncardiac surgery. For the most part, evidence of CAD (eg, angina pectoris, prior MI), factors associated with CAD (eg, advanced age, cardiac arrhythmias, severe hypertension), or evidence of the complications of CAD (eg, signs of heart failure) have been associated with an increased risk of perioperative cardiac complications.

The multifactorial cardiac risk index developed by Goldman, which assessed cardiac risk in patients 40 years or older who underwent noncardiac surgery, suggested that evidence of CAD (eg, MI in the previous 6 months), risk factors for CAD (eg, age greater than 70 years), and evidence of complications of CAD (eg, signs of left ventricular dysfunction such as S_3 or jugular vein distention, more than five ventricular premature contractions per minute at any time before surgery) were markers for perioperative cardiac complications. Several risk factors for CAD, including controlled diabetes mellitus, a history of smoking, and hypertension with a diastolic blood pressure less than 110 mmHg, were found not to be risk factors for perioperative cardiac complications. The risk of such complications also was not increased significantly by the occurrence of an MI more than 6 months before the surgical procedure or the presence of chronic stable angina. It must be noted that patients with unstable angina were excluded from the analysis.[3] The multifactorial index was found to be less helpful in predicting cardiac risk in patients who underwent aortic surgery.[4]

Detsky and colleagues modified the multifactorial risk index to include the type of surgical procedure performed and the severity of the CAD (manifested by angina class) in the risk assessment.[4a] They verified that a history of MI within 6 months, the presence of a cardiac arrhythmia, and patient age greater than 70 years were risk factors for perioperative cardiac complications. These authors also found that patients with unstable angina during the 3 months before surgery and those with Canadian Cardiovascular Society class 3 angina (angina that occurs on walking one or two blocks on a level surface or climbing one flight of stairs under normal conditions and at a normal pace) during the 2 weeks before surgery were at a risk level similar to that of patients who had sustained MIs within the previous 6 months. Patients with Canadian Cardiovascular Society class 4 angina (inability to carry on any physical activity without angina) had twice the risk of those with class 3 angina.

The utility of these indices has been questioned in patients who have known CAD or are at high risk for CAD. In an evaluation of 474 men who fall into these categories, Mangano[5] found that the multivariate cardiac risk indices did not correlate with perioperative ischemic events. The only factor that did correlate with postoperative cardiac death, MI, unstable angina, congestive heart failure, or ventricular tachycardia was postoperative myocardial ischemia. Predictors of postoperative myocardial ischemia in this study were a history of definite CAD, left ventricular hypertrophy by electrocardiogram, a history of hypertension, diabetes mellitus, and use of digoxin. In a subsequent paper, the authors stated that these predictors were markers of more serious CAD.[6] Landesberg[7] confirmed the relationship between postoperative myocardial ischemia and cardiac complications in patients undergoing vascular surgery and found postoperative ischemia of long duration (more than 2 hours) to be the factor most significantly associated with adverse cardiac outcome.

Mangano postulated that left ventricular hypertrophy is a marker of increased cardiac risk because it typically occurs in patients with hypertension who may also have ac-

celerated atherosclerosis. Left ventricular hypertrophy may also represent a situation in which increased left ventricular mass raises myocardial oxygen demand without a corresponding increase in coronary artery blood flow. The presence of diabetes mellitus was thought to be a risk factor because of its strong association with atherosclerosis.

Ashton and associates[8] proposed a preoperative risk stratification scheme based predominantly on a patient's probability of having CAD, supported by the belief that coronary atherosclerosis is a necessary condition for perioperative MI. In their study, the risk of perioperative MI was proportional to the likelihood of the presence of CAD. Patients with known significant CAD (ie, those with typical angina, prior MI, previous coronary artery bypass surgery, or documentation of significant CAD by prior cardiac catheterization) were found to have a 4% incidence of perioperative cardiac complications. Patients at intermediate risk (ie, those without evidence of CAD but with coronary atherosclerosis elsewhere, such as peripheral vascular disease or prior stroke) had a 0.8% incidence of perioperative cardiac complications. In addition to the presence of CAD, patient age greater than 75 years, the presence of peripheral vascular disease, and heart failure were noted to be independent risk factors for perioperative MI.[8]

Fleisher[9] proposed that the severity of CAD symptoms is as important in assessing cardiac risk as the surgical procedure is in provoking perioperative myocardial ischemia. He believes that patients with histories of recent non–Q-wave MIs are probably at greater risk of perioperative cardiac complications than are those who have sustained Q-wave MIs because of the greater overall rate of recurrent infarction after non–Q-wave infarction.

INCIDENCE AND PRESENTATION OF PERIOPERATIVE MYOCARDIAL ISCHEMIA

Most postoperative MIs occur during the first 3 days after surgery, with some series reporting a peak from the third to fifth postoperative days.[3,5,10] In a study of men who had CAD or were at risk for it, Mangano and associates found that preoperative myocardial ischemia (detected by electrocardiographic monitoring) was common. It occurred in 27% of patients, equally divided between those with known CAD and those at risk for CAD. Intraoperative myocardial ischemia was similar in incidence and severity to preoperative ischemia, suggesting that surgery is not as stressful as previously believed.

The incidence and severity of perioperative myocardial ischemia were found to be greatest during the first 48 hours after surgery. The cause of this postoperative phenomenon is not known and may be multifactorial. Mangano[11] noted a significant increase in heart rate in the postoperative period that may have increased myocardial oxygen demand. Other investigators, however, have detected no link between elevated postoperative heart rate and myocardial ischemia.[7] Possible potentiators of postoperative myocardial ischemia include increased circulating catecholamine levels, changes in fluid balance, hypoxia, alteration of body temperature, hypertension, hypotension, platelet activation, hypercoagulability, and sleep deprivation.[11]

Perioperative myocardial ischemia and infarction are often silent. In Mangano's study of postoperative myocardial ischemia, 94% of ischemic episodes were not associated with anginal pain. Other investigators have found that MI occurring after noncardiac surgery is not associated with chest pain in 20% to 70% of cases. Possible reasons for the absence of chest pain include a residual effect of anesthetics and analgesics, and altered pain perception resulting from competing somatic stimuli (eg, incisional pain).[11]

Perioperative myocardial ischemia and infarction indicate the potential for adverse cardiac events long after surgery. Mangano[12] found that patients with postoperative myocardial ischemia had a 2.2-fold increase in the rate of adverse cardiac outcome during the first 2 years after surgery. Patients who sustained postoperative MIs had a 20-fold increased risk for subsequent cardiac complications, particularly during the first 6 months after surgery.

DOES PREOPERATIVE CORONARY ARTERY REVASCULARIZATION REDUCE THE RISK OF CARDIAC COMPLICATIONS?

No prospective, randomized studies have been conducted to evaluate the efficacy of preoperative coronary artery revascularization in reducing perioperative risk. A protective effect of previous coronary artery bypass surgery has been suggested. Pooled data from studies that used historical control subjects reveal that, of 2000 patients who underwent noncardiac surgery, the rate of postoperative infarction was significantly lower in those who underwent previous coronary artery bypass surgery (0% to 1.2%) than in those who did not (1.1% to 6%).[1] In addition to the perioperative benefit, Hertzer[13] noted a late benefit that he attributed to perioperative coronary revascularization. In a group of patients who underwent coronary artery bypass surgery before aortic aneurysm repair, survival 5 years after aneurysm surgery was similar to that of patients with trivial coronary disease.

In other studies, the overall benefit of preoperative myocardial revascularization has been less clear. Data from the Coronary Artery Surgery Study reveal higher perioperative mortality in nonrandomized patients who underwent noncardiac surgery without preceding coronary surgery (2.4%) than in those who had preceding coronary surgery (0.9%). The operative mortality for coronary artery bypass surgery

was 1.4%. Therefore, the combination of coronary surgery followed by noncardiac surgery was no less risky than was noncardiac surgery alone in medically treated patients.[14] The risk of coronary artery bypass surgery should be included in the overall risk assessment.

It has been suggested that percutaneous transluminal coronary angioplasty reduces perioperative cardiac morbidity when it is performed before noncardiac surgery. The few studies that have assessed this technique, however, were nonrandomized and based on historical control subjects.[15,16]

The durability of the myocardial revascularization procedure must be considered in the preoperative evaluation. The occlusion rate of saphenous vein bypass grafts is 12% to 20% at 1 year, 20% to 30% at 5 years, and 40% to 50% at 10 years after coronary artery bypass surgery. The coronary restenosis rate after coronary angioplasty is 25% to 35% during the first 6 months after the procedure. Histories of angina should be obtained from patients who have undergone myocardial revascularization. If the patients are sedentary, angina may be absent even if restenosis has occurred. Noninvasive evaluation of myocardial perfusion should be considered in patients at risk who are undergoing major noncardiac surgery.

PATIENTS WHO HAVE HAD PREVIOUS MYOCARDIAL INFARCTIONS

The last 20 years have witnessed a decline in the incidence of perioperative MI. In a series of patients who underwent surgery at the Mayo Clinic during 1967 and 1968, the rate of recurrent infarction was 37% in those who underwent operation within 3 months of a previous MI. This rate decreased to 16% when surgery was performed 4 to 6 months after MI and leveled out at 5% when the MI occurred more than 6 months before surgery.[17] Similar results were obtained in a series of patients who underwent general surgery in 1974 and 1975. The rate of recurrent infarction was 27% when surgery was done within 3 months of MI, 11% when it was done 4 to 6 months after MI, and 5% when it was done more than 6 months after MI.[10]

These results formed the foundation for the practice of delaying noncardiac surgery for 6 months after MI. Rao[18] documented a dramatic decrease in the risk of infarction. In patients who underwent perioperative invasive hemodynamic monitoring with aggressive treatment of adverse changes in hemodynamic parameters, the rate of recurrent MI when noncardiac surgery was done within 3 months of MI was only 5.7%. For those in whom surgery was performed 4 to 6 months after MI, the rate of recurrent infarction was 2.3%. This study has been reevaluated and the decreased rate of recurrent infarction has been confirmed.[19]

The reason that the rate of recurrent MI has decreased is

not precisely known. It is probably related to increased physician awareness of the complications to which these patients are predisposed leading to more intense perioperative care. In addition, advances have occurred in cardiac monitoring and cardiac medical therapy.

The risk of cardiac complications after MI can be best evaluated by assessing left ventricular function and determining the extent of myocardium that is at risk for perioperative ischemia. Patients who have uncomplicated courses after MI and who have no evidence of left ventricular dysfunction or of myocardial ischemia on exercise testing have a cardiac mortality rate of under 2%. In contrast, the 1-year mortality is increased in patients who have left ventricular dysfunction or inducible ischemia after MI. Although this has not been studied in clinical trials, we believe that patients who have sustained an MI and do not have left ventricular dysfunction or exercise-induced ischemia have less cardiac morbidity and lower mortality when they undergo operation during the first 6 months after their MI.

PATIENTS WITH CHRONIC STABLE ANGINA

Patients who are physically active and have chronic stable angina as their only risk factor are at low cardiac risk during noncardiac surgery.[20] Patients who are maintained on antianginal regimens should receive appropriate antianginal therapy in the perioperative period. β-Blockers are continued up to the time of surgery. For prolonged effect, a long-acting preparation (ie, nadolol or atenolol) may be given on the morning of surgery. If patients are unable to resume oral intake 24 hours after surgery, β-blockers may be given intravenously (eg, propranolol, 0.5 to 2 mg every 1 to 6 hours). Either a continuous propranolol infusion or an infusion of the short-acting β-blocker, esmolol, also may be used. Oral β-blocker therapy is resumed as soon as possible after surgery.

Patients who are receiving long-term treatment with calcium channel antagonists are usually given a long-acting oral preparation on the morning of surgery. If they are unable to resume oral intake 24 hours after surgery, we generally add intravenous or topical nitrates to the regimen. The only calcium channel antagonists available for intravenous use are verapamil and diltiazem. Because their effect is primarily antiarrhythmic when they are given intravenously, we do not use these agents as primary antiischemic therapy for patients who are unable to take oral medications. Patients who receive calcium channel antagonists for the treatment of coronary artery spasm are given topical or intravenous nitrates if they cannot take oral calcium channel antagonists. Sublingual nifedipine is given if coronary artery spasm occurs despite nitrate therapy. The use of intra-

venous verapamil for refractory perioperative coronary artery vasospasm has been reported.[21]

PATIENTS WITH UNSTABLE ANGINA

Unstable angina is a significant risk factor for perioperative cardiac complications. If possible, noncardiac surgery should be delayed while a medical antianginal regimen is titrated and coronary arteriography with coronary revascularization is performed, if indicated. If evaluation and stabilization cannot be accomplished and the noncardiac surgery is essential, our approach has been to use parenteral antianginal medications (eg, β-blockers) to decrease myocardial oxygen demand in the perioperative period. If significant intravascular volume shifts are anticipated, invasive hemodynamic monitoring is used.

Perioperative MI is often linked to postoperative myocardial ischemia, and most ischemic episodes are clinically silent. Continuous electrocardiographic monitoring to detect myocardial ischemia may be used in high-risk patients to maximize antiischemic medical therapy. The effect that treating postoperative myocardial ischemia has on the occurrence of perioperative MI has not been evaluated.

Patients who remain unstable despite maximum medical therapy and who are not candidates for coronary artery revascularization before noncardiac surgery should be considered for intraaortic balloon counterpulsation to decrease myocardial ischemia. The intraaortic balloon pump improves the ratio between myocardial oxygen supply and demand. It increases aortic diastolic pressure, which augments coronary artery blood flow and reduces aortic pressure in systole to decrease afterload. Georgeson,[22] using decision analysis techniques, has shown that patients who are most likely to benefit from the intraaortic balloon pump are those who are at exceptionally high risk of life-threatening cardiac complications or cardiac death related to a noncardiac surgical procedure. This may include patients with severe CAD in whom myocardial revascularization is not possible because of the extent of their CAD, coexisting disease processes, or the emergent nature of their noncardiac surgery. One of the greatest limiting factors in the use of the intraaortic balloon pump is the risk of peripheral vascular complications (eg, femoral artery occlusion).

PATIENTS WHO EXPERIENCE PERIOPERATIVE MYOCARDIAL INFARCTION

Acute MI in the perioperative period presents unlike MI in other settings. Most patients do not experience angina. Common symptoms and signs include dyspnea, confusion, new onset of congestive heart failure, arrhythmia, and hypotension. In patients with diabetes, perioperative MI may be manifest by hyperglycemia.

Thrombolytic therapy is indicated for most patients with acute MIs but should not be used in the majority of patients who have undergone recent surgery. Although it is not known exactly how soon after surgery it is safe to use thrombolytic agents, any operation within the previous 2 weeks that could be a source of uncontrollable bleeding with thrombolytic therapy is an absolute contraindication to its use. Recent surgery more than 2 weeks before thrombolytic therapy has also been suggested as a relative contraindication to its use, and the choice must be made on an individual basis.[23] We perform urgent cardiac catheterization and percutaneous coronary angioplasty when thrombolytic agents cannot be used in perioperative patients with evolving acute MIs.

In the absence of contraindications, aspirin is administered during the acute phase of MI. Its use has been shown to decrease early mortality from MI by as much as 21%.[24]

β-Blockers given to patients with acute MIs decrease excessive reflex activation of the sympathetic nervous system, which may increase myocardial ischemia, platelet aggregation, and arrhythmia. These agents have been shown to reduce postinfarction morbidity and mortality.[25] Therefore, in the absence of contraindications, we administer β-blockers to all patients except those at the lowest risk. Contraindications to the use of β-blockers in the perioperative period include significant bradycardia or hypotension, moderate to severe left ventricular dysfunction, heart block, and severe chronic obstructive lung disease.

The role of calcium channel antagonists in the primary treatment of acute postoperative MI is limited. They are used primarily to treat postinfarction angina or coronary artery spasm. There is no well-established evidence that they decrease postinfarction mortality.

Recent evidence indicates that patients who are given angiotensin-converting enzyme inhibitors early after MI have improved 6-month survival. If these agents are tolerated, they should be administered to patients who sustain perioperative MIs.[26,27]

Nitroglycerin is effective in decreasing the pain of acute ongoing myocardial ischemia. It is also beneficial when MI is complicated by congestive heart failure or pulmonary edema. Whether the use of nitrates decreases mortality after MI is controversial. The typical starting dose for nitroglycerin is 5 to 10 μg/min for most patients with perioperative MIs. The dose is increased by 5 to 10 μg/min every 5 to 10 minutes. During titration, continuous monitoring of vital signs is essential. Although titration end points for nitroglycerin vary between individual patients, recent guidelines suggest the following: (1) control of symptoms or a decrease in mean arterial blood pressure of 10% in patients with normal blood pressure or 30% in patients with hypertension (never a systolic blood pressure of less than 90 mmHg); (2) a maximum increase in heart rate of more than 10 beats/min but usually not greater than 110 beats/min; and (3) a decrease in pulmonary artery end-diastolic pressure of 10% to 30%. For most patients, the final nitrate dose is less than 200 μg/min.[23]

REFERENCES

1. Mangano DT. Perioperative cardiac morbidity. Anesthesiology 1990;72:153–184.
2. Massie B, Mangano D. Assessment of perioperative risk: have we put the cart before the horse? J Am Coll Cardiol 1993;21:1353–1356.
3. Goldman L, Caldera D, Nussbaum SR, et al. Multifactorial index of cardiac risk in noncardiac surgical procedures. N Engl J Med 1977;297:845–850.
4. Jeffrey C, Kunsman J, Cullen D, Brewster D. A prospective evaluation of cardiac risk index. Anesthesiology 1983;58:462–464.
4a. Detsky A, Abrams H, McLaughlin J, et al. Predicting cardiac complications in patients undergoing non-cardiac surgery. J Gen Intern Med 1986;1:211.
5. Mangano DT, Browner WS, Hollenberg M, et al. Association of perioperative myocardial ischemia with cardiac morbidity and mortality in men undergoing noncardiac surgery. N Engl J Med 1990;323:1781–1788.
6. Hollenberg M, Mangano D, Browner W, et al. Predictors of postoperative myocardial ischemia in patients undergoing noncardiac surgery. JAMA 1992;268:205–209.
7. Landesberg G, Luria M, Cotev S, et al. Importance of long-duration postoperative ST-segment depression in cardiac morbidity after vascular surgery. Lancet 1993;341:715–719.
8. Ashton C, Petersen N, Wray N, et al. The incidence of perioperative myocardial infarction in men undergoing noncardiac surgery. Ann Intern Med 1993;118:504–510.
9. Fleisher L, Barash P. Preoperative cardiac evaluation for noncardiac surgery: a functional approach. Anesth Analg 1992;74:586–598.
10. Steen P, Tinker J, Tarhan S. Myocardial reinfarction after anesthesia and surgery. JAMA 1978;239:2566.
11. Mangano D, Hollenberg M, Fegert G, et al. Perioperative myocardial ischemia in patients undergoing noncardiac surgery: I: incidence and severity during the 4 day perioperative period. J Am Coll Cardiol 1991;17:843–850.
12. Mangano DT, Browner W, Hollenberg M, et al. Long-term cardiac prognosis following noncardiac surgery. JAMA 1992;268:233–239.
13. Hertzer N, Young J, Beven E, et al. Late results of coronary bypass in patients with infrarenal aortic aneurysms: the Cleveland Clinic study. Ann Surg 1987;205:360–367.
14. Foster E, Davis K, Carpenter J. Risk of noncardiac operation in patients with defined coronary artery disease: the Coronary Artery Surgery Study (CASS) Registry experience. Ann Thorac Surg 1986;41:42.
15. Huber K, Evans M, Bresnahan J, et al. Outcome of noncardiac

operations in patients with severe coronary artery disease successfully treated preoperatively with coronary angioplasty. Mayo Clin Proc 1992;67:15–21.

16. Allen J, Helling T, Hartzler G. Operative procedures not involving the heart after percutaneous transluminal coronary angioplasty. Surg Gynecol Obstet 1991;173:285–288.

17. Tarhan S, Moffit E, Taylor W, Giuliani E. Myocardial infarction after general anesthesia. JAMA 1972;220:1451.

18. Rao T, Jacobs K, El-Etr A. Reinfarction following anesthesia in patients with myocardial infarction. Anesthesiology 1983;59: 499.

19. Shah K, Kleinman B, Sami H, et al. Reevaluation of perioperative myocardial infarction in patients with prior myocardial infarction undergoing noncardiac surgery. Anesth Analg 1990; 71:231–235.

20. Goldman L. Cardiac risks and complications of non-cardiac surgery. Ann Intern Med 1983;98:504.

21. Nussmeier N, Slogoff S. Verapamil treatment of intraoperative coronary artery spasm. Anesthesiology 1985;62:539.

22. Georgeson S, Combs A, Eckman M. Prophylactic use of the intra-aortic balloon pump in high risk cardiac patients undergoing noncardiac surgery. Am J Med 1992;92:665–678.

23. Gunnar R, Bourdillon P, Dixon D, et al. Guidelines for the early management of patients with acute myocardial infarction. J Am Coll Cardiol 1990;16:249–292.

24. ISIS-2 Collaborative Group. Randomized trial of intravenous streptokinase, oral aspirin, both or neither among 17187 cases of suspected acute myocardial infarction. Lancet 1988;2:349–360.

25. Yusuf S, Collins R, Lewis J, et al. Beta blockers during and after myocardial infarction: an overview of the randomized trials. Prog Cardiovasc Dis 1985;27:335–371.

26. ISIS-4 Collaborative Group. Randomised study of oral captopril in over 50,000 patients with suspected acute myocardial infarction. Circulation 1993;88:I-894.

27. Swedberg K, Held P, Kjekshus J. Effects of early administration of enalapril on mortality of patients with acute myocardial infarction. N Engl J Med 1992;327:678–684.

Medical Management of the Surgical Patient, Third Edition,
edited by Michael F. Lubin, H. Kenneth Walker, and Robert B. Smith III.
J.B. Lippincott Company, Philadelphia, PA © 1995.

CHAPTER

6

VALVULAR HEART DISEASE AND HYPERTROPHIC CARDIOMYOPATHY

Howard M. Weitz

MITRAL STENOSIS

Mitral stenosis in adults is almost always a result of rheumatic fever. Rheumatic valvulitis causes scarring of the mitral valve leaflets, with fusion of the commissures as well as the subvalvular apparatus. Rare causes of nonrheumatic mitral stenosis include carcinoid syndrome, systemic lupus erythematosus, rheumatoid arthritis, and idiopathic calcification of the mitral valve annulus with extension to the mitral leaflets (which is almost always restricted to the elderly).

In normal adults, the mitral valve area is 4 to 6 cm^2. Mitral stenosis is critical when the valve area is reduced to 1 cm^2. As mitral valve leaflet fusion progresses, left atrial pressure increases to maintain left ventricular filling and a diastolic transvalvular pressure gradient exists between the left atrium and ventricle. Increased left atrial pressure leads to increased pulmonary vascular pressure. Conditions that decrease diastolic filling time (eg, tachycardia) as well as those that increase cardiac blood flow across the mitral valve (eg, physical exercise, fever) further increase left atrial and pulmonary vascular pressure.[1] The pressure gradient across the mitral valve is proportional to the square of the transvalvular flow rate. Therefore, modest increases in transvalvular flow result in significant increases in the pressure gradient.[2] The onset of atrial fibrillation with the loss of the atrial contribution to ventricular filling as well as decreased diastolic filling time associated with a rapid heart rate may also lead to increased left atrial pressure. Pulmonary hypertension occurs as mitral stenosis progresses. Although pulmonary venous and arterial hypertension is usually reversible after mechanical correction of mitral stenosis, advanced disease is often associated with mitral regurgitation, hypertrophy of the pulmonary vasculature, and an irreversible component of pulmonary hypertension. Right ventricular pressure overload may occur as a consequence of pulmonary hypertension.

The clinical findings of mitral stenosis result from inability of the left atrium to empty normally and from pulmonary venous and arterial hypertension. Progressive dyspnea that is worse during exertion, paroxysmal nocturnal dyspnea, and orthopnea are common. Hoarseness may occur and is caused by compression of the left recurrent laryngeal nerve by the enlarged left atrium and pulmonary artery. Fatigue resulting from decreased cardiac output characterizes late disease. Atrial fibrillation commonly accompanies mitral stenosis and is the result of persistently elevated left atrial pressure and left atrial dilation as well as involvement of the left atrium by rheumatic carditis. Patients with atrial fibrillation are at high risk for intracardiac thrombus formation with subsequent systemic embolization. The risk of embolization increases with increased size of the left atrium and atrial appendage as well as with decreased cardiac output.

Physical findings of mitral stenosis include an accentuated first heart sound that decreases in intensity as stenosis worsens and a high-pitched opening snap heard after the second heart sound that is caused by opening of the stenotic but pliable mitral valve. As mitral stenosis progresses, left atrial pressure rises and the interval between the second heart sound and the opening snap shortens. When valve mobility is lost, the opening snap disappears. A low-pitched diastolic rumble is heard at the apex and its duration correlates with the severity of stenosis. Patients in whom sinus rhythm is preserved may have presystolic accentuation of this murmur.

Echocardiography is particularly useful in patient evaluation. It confirms the diagnosis, allows for an estimation of valve orifice area, and, with the use of Doppler techniques, facilitates an approximation of the transvalvular pressure gradient. Doppler echocardiography may also document the presence of mitral regurgitation, which coexists in as many as 40% of patients with mitral stenosis, as well as other valve abnormalities.

Therapy is based on the severity of symptoms. Patients with minimal symptoms often respond to diuretics; those with atrial fibrillation respond to control of the ventricular response with digoxin, β-blockers, or calcium channel antagonists. Because survival is decreased when symptoms are more than mild, the presence of moderate symptoms in the setting of severe mitral stenosis (mitral valve area less than 1 cm^2/m^2 body surface area) is an indication for valvuloplasty or valve replacement. In patients whose valves have minimal calcification, good leaflet mobility, little involvement of the subvalvular apparatus, and minimal or no regurgitation, balloon mitral valvotomy has become the treatment of choice for severe symptomatic mitral stenosis. Procedural mortality is under 1%. Although long-term follow-up results are not available, this procedure is expected to be similar to open mitral commissurotomy and to provide relief from severe mitral stenosis for as long as 10 years. Balloon mitral valvotomy is contraindicated in patients with left atrial thrombi. If these patients otherwise meet the criteria described earlier, open mitral commissurotomy is the mechanical procedure of choice.[3] If they do not meet these criteria, mitral valve replacement should be performed.

Intravascular volume status and heart rate are key factors that require attention in patients undergoing noncardiac surgery. Volume overload must be prevented because further increases in left atrial pressure may result in pulmonary edema. Conversely, excessive volume depletion or preload reduction may decrease left atrial volume too much, with subsequent decreases in the left ventricular filling pressure and cardiac output. Perioperative tachycardia may impair left ventricular filling and can be treated with β-blockers, intravenous diltiazem, or digoxin in patients who have atrial fibrillation with rapid ventricular response. Because of the significant hemodynamic alterations that occur with relatively small volume shifts in patients with severe mitral stenosis, invasive hemodynamic monitoring of the pulmonary capillary wedge pressure should be considered if perioperative volume changes are anticipated. Infective endocarditis antibiotic prophylaxis for indicated procedures is necessary.

MITRAL REGURGITATION

Mitral regurgitation may be caused by one or more abnormalities of the structures that comprise the mitral valve apparatus: the anterior and posterior valve leaflets, chordae tendineae, papillary muscles, and mitral valve annulus. It may also result from poor alignment of a structurally normal valve apparatus or from mitral annular dilation, both of which are caused by left ventricular dysfunction or dilation. Common causes of mitral apparatus dysfunction are rheumatic valve disease or infective endocarditis that may involve the valve leaflets, myxomatous degeneration leading to chordal rupture, and coronary artery disease with myocardial ischemia resulting in papillary muscle dysfunction. Numerous cardiac illnesses may cause dysfunction or dilation of the left ventricle, including dilated cardiomyopathy and coronary artery disease. The mitral valve apparatus may also be distorted as a result of systolic anterior motion of the valve caused by hypertrophic cardiomyopathy.[4] Rare causes of mitral regurgitation include mitral annular calcification (usually limited to the elderly) and involvement of the mitral valve by systemic lupus erythematosus. Degeneration of the mitral valve may also be seen in patients receiving long-term hemodialysis as well as those with the antiphospholipid syndrome.

The pathophysiology of mitral regurgitation depends highly on whether the regurgitation occurs on an acute or a chronic basis. Acute mitral regurgitation is characterized by sudden increases in left atrial volume and pressure as blood is ejected back into the left atrium during systole. This often results in pulmonary edema. Overall total left ventricular stroke volume is increased by many factors, including decreased afterload, increased left ventricular end-diastolic volume, and increased left ventricular contractility resulting from increased sympathetic activity.[3] The total left ventricular ejection fraction (forward and regurgitant) is increased in patients with preserved left ventricular function and should be greater than 55%. A "normal" ejection fraction of 50% to 55% in these patients gives the appearance that ventricular function is preserved but is really evidence for significant left ventricular dysfunction. In chronic mitral regurgitation, the ventricle slowly dilates and accommodates significant increases in blood volume without significant increases in left ventricular end-diastolic pressure. Thus, pulmonary congestion is initially prevented. Although patients may be stable for long periods, chronic left ventricular volume overload eventually leads to left ventricular dysfunction with decreased ejection fraction, decreased cardiac output, elevated left ventricular filling pressure, and pulmonary congestion.

In otherwise healthy persons, the sudden onset of fulminant heart failure with the presence of an apical holosystolic murmur strongly suggests acute mitral regurgitation resulting from chordal rupture. Congestive heart failure in patients with inferior myocardial infarctions indicates the possibility of papillary muscle dysfunction. Sudden respiratory distress after a febrile illness suggests acute mitral regurgitation caused by ruptured chordae or valve leaflet perforation due to infective endocarditis. In the presence of acute mitral regurgitation, patients usually have sinus tachycardia and nondisplaced hyperdynamic left ventricular apical impulses. An apical systolic murmur begins with S_1 but often ends before S_2 as left atrial and left ventricular pressures equalize and valvular regurgitation ceases. In chronic mitral regurgitation, the left ventricular apical impulse is displaced because of left ventricular dilation. A holosystolic blowing murmur is heard at the apex and radiates to the axilla. A third heart sound is common and does not necessarily indicate the presence of left ventricular dysfunction. It may occur solely as a result of early diastolic filling.[5] A left parasternal lift and accentuated pulmonic component of the second heart sound suggest coexistent pulmonary hypertension.

Echocardiography is a particularly useful diagnostic test. It usually provides a measure of the degree of regurgitation as well as an estimate of left ventricular chamber size and function. It often identifies the component of the mitral valve apparatus that is responsible for valvular regurgitation.

Surgical repair or replacement of the mitral valve is indicated in patients with severe acute mitral regurgitation. Vasodilators such as intravenous nitroprusside may help stabilize patients who are awaiting surgery by decreasing both afterload and the volume of regurgitant blood.

For patients with chronic mitral regurgitation, it is often difficult to determine when valve repair or replacement should be performed. The risks and benefits of surgery must be weighed. Because of its associated hazards, surgery should not be performed too early. The life-style changes that may be necessary after the placement of a valve prosthesis are significant as well. Surgery that is delayed so long that significant left ventricular dysfunction occurs, however, carries unacceptable risks. Complicating patient assessment and follow-up is the fact that the afterload reduction and increased preload that accompany mitral regurgitation may mask left ventricular dysfunction, which becomes apparent only after surgical correction.[6]

When surgery is undertaken, an attempt should be made to repair rather than replace the valve. The papillary muscle—chordae unit has been found to play a role in preserving left ventricular contractility. Patients who undergo mitral valve repair typically have lower perioperative mortality and better postoperative left ventricular function than do those who undergo valve replacement. Another benefit of mitral repair is that long-term anticoagulant therapy is often unnecessary. Patients with mitral valve calcification and scarring as well as those with severe myxomatous degeneration of the valve and chordae are usually not candidates for valve repair.[7]

It is generally agreed that surgery is indicated for patients who experience symptoms with less than ordinary activity and for those who experience symptoms with heavy exertion despite aggressive medical therapy. Controversy exists regarding the timing of surgery in asymptomatic patients, however. It is essential that their left ventricular function be tracked. Patients with preserved left ventricular function (ie, a left ventricular ejection fraction greater than 70%) can be observed. Those with left ventricular ejection fractions between 55% and 70% should undergo measurement of the left ventricular ejection fraction as well as indices of left ventricular systolic function (eg, end-systolic volume index) about every 6 months. Surgery should be performed before significant ventricular dysfunction occurs (ie, the left ventricular ejection fraction is less than 50% or the end-systolic volume index is greater than 50 mL/m²) or pulmonary hypertension develops.[8] The risk of surgery is often prohibitive in patients with severe mitral regurgitation and severe left ventricular dysfunction. In these cases, medical therapy with diuretics, digoxin, and afterload-reducing agents often results in symptomatic improvement.

The status of left ventricular function is a major determinant of perioperative complications in patients with mitral regurgitation who undergo noncardiac surgery. We believe that patients with chronic severe mitral regurgitation should undergo noninvasive assessment of left ventricular function before noncardiac surgery. If the ejection fraction is not greater than normal, as would be expected with preserved left ventricular function, we consider the use of invasive hemodynamic monitoring in the perioperative period if significant intravascular volume shifts are anticipated. Patients with mitral regurgitation tolerate afterload reduction well in the perioperative period. Agents that increase afterload (ie, vasopressors) increase the amount of regurgitant blood and their use should be avoided if possible. Infective endocarditis prophylaxis for indicated procedures is necessary.

MITRAL VALVE PROLAPSE

Mitral valve prolapse (MVP) is a condition in which one or both mitral valve leaflets extend above the mitral annular plane during systole and prolapse into the left atrium. The degree of valve abnormality varies greatly, ranging from relatively normal valves with only intermittent prolapse to markedly abnormal valve structures with valve leaflet thickening, redundancy, and regurgitation. MVP occurs in about 3% of the population and has a female predominance.[9]

Most persons with MVP are asymptomatic. Some have symptoms that are unrelated to the valve abnormality. These symptoms may be associated with autonomic dysfunction and include chest pain, palpitations, and dizziness.[10]

The diagnosis is usually made on hearing the classic mid-systolic click and, in patients with mitral regurgitation, a mid to late systolic murmur. Conditions that decrease the size of the ventricle (ie, the Valsalva maneuver or dehydration) cause the valve to prolapse earlier, in which case the click is heard closer to S_1 and the intensity and duration of the murmur may be greater. The diagnosis can be confirmed by echocardiography.

The risk of infective endocarditis is the greatest concern for patients with MVP who are undergoing noncardiac surgery. The risk of developing endocarditis has been estimated to be 1 in 1400 in patients who have MVP and mitral regurgitation, 35 times greater than in those who have MVP alone.[11] The American Heart Association recommends that patients with MVP and mitral regurgitation receive infective endocarditis antibiotic prophylaxis for specific procedures (see later).

It has been suggested that patients with MVP have a slightly higher incidence of cardiac arrhythmias. The etiology is unclear and the risk of serious arrhythmias is low. These arrhythmias respond to treatment with β-adrenergic blockers. Patients who have dizziness with MVP often have decreased blood volume.[12] The onset of this symptom in the perioperative period should prompt an assessment of volume status and the administration of fluids if indicated.

AORTIC REGURGITATION

Aortic regurgitation may be caused by processes that affect the aortic valve leaflets (eg, rheumatic fever, infective endocarditis, congenital bicuspid aortic valve) or the aortic root (eg, systemic hypertension, cystic medial necrosis, Marfan syndrome, aortic dissection). Eighty percent of cases that come to medical attention are chronic and the remainder are acute.

Chronic aortic regurgitation is accompanied by left ventricular dilation and a gradual, progressive increase in left ventricular end-diastolic volume with only an initial slight increase in left ventricular end-diastolic pressure. The dilated left ventricle facilitates the rapid return of blood back to the ventricle during diastole, resulting in decreased pe-

ripheral arterial diastolic pressure. Left ventricular stroke volume, comprised of both forward and regurgitant blood flow, is increased. The heart rate usually remains normal. This compensation often permits patients to remain asymptomatic even with severe aortic regurgitation. The combination of increased stroke volume and decreased diastolic blood pressure explains several of the classic physical findings of chronic aortic regurgitation: wide pulse pressure, water-hammer pulse (brisk pulse upstroke with rapid collapse), de Musset's sign (head-bobbing during systole related to increased stroke volume), and Quincke's pulse (visible nail bed capillary pulsations).

Acute aortic regurgitation, in contrast, is characterized by the abrupt regurgitation of blood into a normal left ventricle leading to a sudden increase in left ventricular volume and marked elevation of left ventricular end-diastolic pressure. Compensatory mechanisms do not occur as in chronic aortic regurgitation. The heart rate increases, cardiac output decreases, and peripheral vasoconstriction occurs. The wide pulse pressure of chronic aortic regurgitation is not present and systolic blood pressure may decrease. Acute heart failure and pulmonary edema are common. Because of the absence of chronic compensation, the classic physical findings of chronic aortic regurgitation are not present.

Acute aortic regurgitation may rapidly progress to intractable heart failure. Therefore, it is an indication for urgent aortic valve replacement. In contrast, chronic aortic regurgitation may be associated with minimal or no symptoms for years. Determining whether to operate on these patients is often difficult. Aortic valve replacement is indicated for patients with symptomatic aortic regurgitation and for asymptomatic patients with severe aortic regurgitation accompanied by left ventricular dysfunction.

Controversy exists regarding the timing of valve replacement in asymptomatic patients with severe regurgitation and normal left ventricular function. There is no evidence that early aortic valve replacement in these patients prolongs survival. It is well documented that aortic valve replacement in patients with severe left ventricular dysfunction is associated with increased mortality.

The goal, therefore, is to observe asymptomatic patients with normal ventricular function closely with serial measurements of ventricular function and to perform aortic valve replacement when either symptoms or early left ventricular dysfunction occurs. There is evidence that perioperative morbidity and mortality are related to preoperative left ventricular function and size.[13] Many asymptomatic patients should undergo aortic valve replacement when they show evidence of either a decline in the left ventricular ejection fraction (resting left ventricular ejection fraction less than 50%) or left ventricular dilation (left ventricular end-systolic dimension greater than 55 mm as calculated by M-mode echocardiography).[14]

In noncardiac surgery, operative risk correlates more

closely with the status of left ventricular function than with the degree of aortic valve regurgitation. Vasopressors that raise peripheral vascular resistance may increase the degree of regurgitation and must be used cautiously. Bradycardia is associated with increased diastolic filling time, which raises the magnitude of regurgitant volume by lengthening the period during which regurgitation may occur. In contrast to patients with aortic stenosis, patients with aortic regurgitation typically tolerate vasodilation well, often with an increase in cardiac output. Caution must be exercised to prevent excessive decreases in already lowered diastolic pressure in an effort to preclude reductions in coronary artery perfusion pressure. Infective endocarditis antibiotic prophylaxis for indicated surgical procedures is necessary.

AORTIC STENOSIS

In adults, clinically significant aortic stenosis is usually the result of degenerative calcification of otherwise normal tricuspid aortic valves. When aortic stenosis manifests in adults younger than 50 years, it is usually a result of calcification and fusion of a congenital bicuspid aortic valve. Even when it is severe, aortic stenosis remains clinically silent for many years. The onset of symptoms indicates that patients are at risk for sudden cardiac death. In patients with untreated symptomatic aortic stenosis, the occurrence of angina or syncope indicates a potential survival of only 2 to 3 years. The onset of congestive heart failure is more ominous and suggests the likelihood of death within 1 to 2 years.[15] Sudden death is rare in patients with asymptomatic, hemodynamically significant aortic stenosis (ie, aortic gradient greater than 50 mmHg and aortic valve area less than 0.75 cm^2).[16]

The classic physical findings of significant aortic stenosis are a low-amplitude and slow-rising carotid pulse pressure (pulsus parvus and tardus), a sustained apical impulse, a crescendo–decrescendo harsh systolic murmur heard at the second right intercostal space radiating to the carotids and precordium, an S$_4$, and diminished intensity of the aortic component of the second heart sound. As the degree of aortic obstruction increases, the systolic murmur peaks later in systole and the intensity of the aortic component of the second heart sound decreases and may even disappear.

The absence of these classic findings does not rule out the presence of critical aortic stenosis. The intensity of the heart murmur may decrease as the left ventricle fails. The carotid pulse findings may be altered in elderly patients with noncompliant peripheral vasculatures. Doppler echocardiography may be required before surgery to estimate the severity of aortic stenosis as well as the status of left ventricular function.

Adults with critical aortic stenosis (ie, an aortic valve area less than 0.75 cm^2) should undergo aortic valve replacement once they experience symptoms (eg, angina, presyncope, syncope, congestive heart failure) or manifest evidence of left ventricular dysfunction without symptoms. Fifty percent of adults with critical aortic stenosis and angina have significant coronary artery disease that may require revascularization at the time of aortic valve replacement. Five-year survival after aortic valve replacement is excellent and patients with left ventricular dysfunction often experience marked improvement in ventricular function.

Because the operative risk exceeds the risk of sudden death in patients who have asymptomatic critical aortic stenosis with normal left ventricular function, aortic valve replacement is typically not performed. Balloon aortic valvuloplasty has been described as a nonsurgical means of decreasing the degree of aortic obstruction in aortic stenosis. The immediate and long-term results of this procedure have been disappointing. Although the aortic valve area initially may be increased up to 60%, many patients with severe aortic stenosis still have significant aortic stenosis after the procedure. Mortality or major morbidity occurs in as many as 13% of patients who undergo balloon aortic valvuloplasty, and aortic valve restenosis occurs in 50% of patients within 6 months.

This technique has a limited role in patients with aortic stenosis who require noncardiac surgery. We reserve it for patients with critical aortic stenosis and either congestive heart failure or shock who require urgent noncardiac surgery. It may also be considered before noncardiac surgery in patients with hemodynamic compromise as a result of aortic stenosis who are not candidates for aortic valve replacement.[17,18]

Aortic stenosis was the only valvular heart abnormality found by Goldman[19] to be associated with an increased risk of perioperative cardiac complications or death. Patients with critical aortic stenosis had a 13% cardiac perioperative mortality, compared to an overall cardiac mortality of 1.9%. Other studies that have examined the multifactorial risk index have confirmed aortic stenosis to be a risk factor for perioperative cardiac complications.[20,21] O'Keefe[22] reported a small series of patients with moderate or critical aortic stenosis who underwent elective noncardiac surgery. Although no deaths occurred, 10% of the patients had significant perioperative hypotension that was transient in all but one case. Local anesthesia was used in about half the cases and was not associated with any cardiac complications. The overall lower than expected complication rate was attributed to effective preoperative identification of aortic stenosis as well as careful perioperative anesthesia monitoring and management.

One of the hemodynamic consequences of severe aortic stenosis is a "fixed" cardiac output resulting from left ventricular outflow tract obstruction. Patients are unable to increase cardiac output in response to the stress of surgery and there is decreased left ventricular compliance related to left ventricular hypertrophy. Patients become markedly dependent on adequate preload. Hypovolemia and the vasodilation that may accompany spinal anesthesia or vasodilators are tolerated poorly and may result in profound hypotension. The onset of atrial fibrillation with loss of the atrial contribution to ventricular filling may also lead to severe hemodynamic compromise.

We believe that the perioperative approach to patients with aortic stenosis must be individualized and based on the severity of the aortic stenosis, patients' symptoms, left ventricular function, and the anticipated hemodynamic demands of the surgical procedure. All patients with aortic stenosis should receive bacterial endocarditis antibiotic prophylaxis if indicated.[23] Patients with asymptomatic critical aortic stenosis who have preserved left ventricular function are monitored closely during the perioperative period. Invasive hemodynamic monitoring is used if the surgical procedure is associated with significant fluid shifts or changes in preload or afterload. Patients with symptomatic critical aortic stenosis or aortic stenosis associated with severe left ventricular dysfunction should undergo aortic valve replacement before noncardiac surgery if possible. If the noncardiac surgery cannot be delayed or if the patients are not candidates for aortic valve replacement, the risks and benefits of aortic valvuloplasty are considered. If patients are not candidates for aortic balloon valvuloplasty and surgery is absolutely necessary, it is performed under the guidance of invasive hemodynamic monitoring. The use of vasodilators and anesthetic techniques that may cause vasodilation is avoided if possible.

HYPERTROPHIC CARDIOMYOPATHY

Hypertrophic cardiomyopathy is a myocardial abnormality in which the left ventricle is hypertrophied in the absence of a secondary cardiac or systemic process that is capable of causing hypertrophy.[24] It is characterized by left ventricular diastolic dysfunction. In some patients, the hypertrophy involves the interventricular septum out of proportion to the rest of the ventricle. This variant is termed *asymmetric septal hypertrophy* and may result in left ventricular outflow tract obstruction. About 25% of patients with hypertrophic cardiomyopathy have evidence of left ventricular outflow tract obstruction. Patients with this feature are said to have hypertrophic obstructive cardiomyopathy and share some of the features of aortic stenosis.[25] Hypertrophic cardiomyopathy is genetically transmitted in about half of all patients and occurs spontaneously in the remainder. A unique variant is found in the elderly and is characterized by severe concentric left ventricular hypertrophy, a small left ventricular cavity, and left ventricular outflow tract obstruction.[26]

One of the physiologic features of hypertrophic cardiomyopathy is left ventricular diastolic dysfunction; this occurs in most patients and results from myocardial hypertrophy with subsequent impaired ventricular relaxation. Diastolic filling pressures are increased. Dynamic left ventricular systolic outflow tract obstruction results if septal hypertrophy and systolic anterior motion of the mitral valve toward the interventricular septum occur. The outflow tract gradient is labile and may be provoked by factors that increase contractility (ie, catecholamines) as well as by reductions in preload and afterload. Myocardial ischemia may be present in the absence of epicardial coronary artery disease. This is a result of several factors, including thickening of the intramyocardial coronary arteries and increased myocardial oxygen demand imposed by the hypertrophied left ventricle.[24]

The clinical course of hypertrophic cardiomyopathy is variable and ranges from absence of symptoms in most patients to sudden death. Of those who are symptomatic, most have dyspnea or angina. Dizziness, presyncope, and syncope are common in patients who have hypertrophic obstructive cardiomyopathy. Risk factors for sudden death include young age (childhood or adolescence), a family history of sudden death (particularly in young siblings), syncope, and ventricular arrhythmias.[27]

Physical findings reflect the presence of diastolic dysfunction and, in patients with hypertrophic obstructive cardiomyopathy, a dynamic provocable left ventricular outflow tract obstruction. A left ventricular lift and S_4 are common. The jugular venous pulse may exhibit a prominent "a" wave. In hypertrophic obstructive cardiomyopathy, the arterial pulses are brisk and may have a double peak or bisferiens configuration. The classic murmur of hypertrophic obstructive cardiomyopathy is harsh and crescendo–decrescendo, and is heard between the apex and left sternal border. It radiates to the precordium in a fashion similar to the murmur of aortic stenosis but does not radiate to the carotid arteries. The dynamic nature of the outflow tract obstruction may be demonstrated by the effect of certain maneuvers. Murmur intensity increases with maneuvers that decrease preload, with the Valsalva maneuver, with standing, and with the administration of amyl nitrite. Increasing afterload by squatting or administering phenylephrine decreases the intensity of the murmur. The murmur of mitral regurgitation also is frequently present.

Echocardiography is helpful in confirming the diagnosis and, with Doppler studies, can determine whether outflow tract obstruction is present. Typical findings are left ventricular hypertrophy, hyperdynamic left ventricular function, and septal hypertrophy out of proportion to ventricular hypertrophy. There is also systolic anterior motion of the mitral valve in patients with asymmetric septal hypertrophy.

Treatment of asymptomatic patients is controversial. β-Blockers and calcium channel antagonists have been suggested to delay disease progression and decrease the risk of sudden death but have not been studied in large-scale trials. Amiodarone has been shown in small trials to increase the survival of asymptomatic patients with nonsustained ventricular tachycardia. For those with hypertrophic cardiomyopathy and preserved left ventricular function, β-blockers and verapamil are effective in decreasing symptoms, principally by enhancing diastolic filling. Preload and afterload reduction are indicated for patients with severe left ventricular systolic dysfunction. Septal myotomy-myectomy or mitral valve replacement is effective in selected patients whose symptoms are refractory to medical therapy.[28] Atrioventricular sequential pacing reduces the outflow tract gradient by inducing paradoxical motion of the interventricular septum and has been suggested as an alternate approach for symptomatic patients who are refractory to medical therapy.[29]

In the perioperative period, care must be taken to prevent worsening of the dynamic left ventricular outflow tract gradient in patients with hypertrophic obstructive cardiomyopathy. Drugs that increase myocardial contractility (eg, catecholamines, digoxin) may increase the gradient and should not be used. Other factors that may lead to hemodynamic instability include excessive preload reduction by volume depletion or vasodilation, loss of sinus rhythm with loss of the atrial contribution to ventricular filling that is important for patients with diastolic left ventricular dysfunction, and tachycardia with reduced diastolic filling time. Because of the risk of hypotension, spinal anesthesia should not be used.[30] For patients whose surgeries are associated with intravascular volume shifts, invasive hemodynamic monitoring is recommended. Hypotension that occurs during or after surgery should be treated with fluid administration. If that is insufficient, peripheral vasoconstrictors such as phenylephrine hydrochloride should be used to raise the blood pressure.[31] Halothane and enflurane are commonly recommended for maintenance anesthesia because of their negative inotropic and chronotropic properties.[32]

INFECTIVE ENDOCARDITIS PROPHYLAXIS

Infective endocarditis prophylaxis is indicated for patients with specific cardiac structural abnormalities who are at risk for bacteremia resulting from the disruption of mucosal surfaces colonized with bacteria. It is estimated that, even if endocarditis prophylaxis were completely effective, under 10% of cases of bacterial endocarditis could be prevented. Reasons include the fact that the organisms targeted by currently recommended antibiotic regimens, *Streptococcus*

viridans and enterococcus, account for only 50% of all cases of endocarditis, and only 25% of patients with *S viridans* endocarditis and 40% of those with enterococcus endocarditis develop their infection after procedures for which prophylaxis could have been given. Only half of all patients with endocarditis have a cardiac condition that would have made them candidates for antibiotic prophylaxis.[33]

Antibiotic prophylaxis is recommended for patients with high-risk cardiac lesions (eg, prosthetic cardiac valves), most congenital cardiac lesions (eg, bicuspid aortic valve, patent ductus arteriosus, cyanotic congenital heart lesions), a previous history of bacterial endocarditis (even in the absence of structural heart disease), rheumatic and other acquired valvular lesions, MVP with mitral regurgitation, and hypertrophic cardiomyopathy. Endocarditis prophylaxis is not recommended for patients with isolated atrial septal defects of the secundum type, MVP without mitral regurgitation, an innocent or physiologic heart murmur, previous rheumatic fever without valve dysfunction, or a cardiac pacemaker. It also should not be used in patients who have undergone surgical repair of a ventricular septal defect without residua more than 6 months earlier, or previous coronary artery bypass surgery.[34]

Antibiotic prophylaxis is indicated for procedures during which transient bacteremia is expected. These include specific dental, oropharyngeal, respiratory tract, genitourinary, gastrointestinal, gynecologic/obstetric, and general surgical procedures. Prophylactic antibiotic regimens are directed specifically toward the most likely infecting organism, which is *S viridans* in dental and upper respiratory tract procedures and enterococcus in genitourinary and gastrointestinal procedures.

TREATMENT OF PATIENTS WITH PROSTHETIC HEART VALVES

Major considerations for patients with mechanical heart valves who are receiving anticoagulants include the risk and prevention of valve thrombosis as well as the possibility of thromboembolic phenomena that may occur when anticoagulants are withheld in the perioperative period. Few trials describe the rates of prosthetic valve thrombosis in patients who are not receiving anticoagulants. Overall, the risk of thromboembolism is higher in patients with valve prostheses in the mitral versus the aortic positions. Although data are scant, the incidence of valve thrombosis is probably greatest in patients who are not receiving anticoagulants and who have pivoting disc valves (Björk-Shiley, Lillehei-Kaster), and are lowest in patients who have ball valves (Starr-Edwards) or leaflet valves (St. Jude).[35]

For most patients, it is safe to discontinue warfarin therapy 2 or 3 days before surgery and reinitiate it as soon as possible after the procedure (usually within 2 or 3 days).[36] If patients are unable to resume taking oral medications within this time frame, full-dose heparin anticoagulation is provided and continued until warfarin can be given again. For patients who are at high risk for thromboembolism without anticoagulant therapy (eg, those with tilting disc valves in the mitral position), we recommend the administration of full-dose heparin when warfarin therapy is discontinued before operation. Heparin administration is discontinued 6 to 8 hours before surgery and started again as soon as hemostasis is stable in the postoperative period. Heparin is given until a therapeutic level of anticoagulation has been achieved with warfarin. Levels of warfarin that prolong the International Normalized Ratio to 2.5 to 3.5 are generally recommended.[37] Dental extractions can safely be performed with patients at a therapeutic level of anticoagulation.[38] Infective endocarditis prophylaxis is required for specific surgical procedures.

REFERENCES

1. Reichek N, Shelburne JC, Perloff JK. Clinical aspects of rheumatic valvular disease. Prog Cardiovasc Dis 1973;15:491–537.
2. Gorlin R, Gorlin SG. Hydraulic formula for calculation of the area of stenotic mitral valve, other cardiac valves and central circulatory states. Am Heart J 1951;41:1–29.
3. Carabello BA. Mitral valve disease. Curr Probl Cardiol 1993;18:423–478.
4. Wigle ED, Sasson Z, Henderson MA, et al. Hypertrophic cardiomyopathy: the importance of the site and the extent of hypertrophy: a review. Prog Cardiovasc Dis 1985;28:1–83.
5. Folland ED, Kriegel BJ, Henderson WG, et al. Implications of third heart sounds in patients with valvular heart disease: the Veterans Affairs Cooperative Study on Valvular Heart Disease. N Engl J Med 1992;327:458–462.
6. Assey ME, Spann JF Jr. Indications for heart valve replacement. Clin Cardiol 1990;13:81–88.
7. Kirklin JW. Mitral valve repair for mitral incompetence. Mod Concepts Cardiovasc Dis 1987;56:7–11.
8. Crawford MH, Souchek J, Oprian CA, et al. Determinants of survival and left ventricular performance after mitral valve replacement: Department of Veterans Affairs Cooperative Study on Valvular Heart Disease. Circulation 1990;81:1173–1181.
9. Devereux RB, Brown WT, Kramer-Fox R, et al. Inheritance of mitral valve prolapse: effect of age and sex on gene expression. Ann Intern Med 1982;97:826–832.
10. Gaffney FA, Karlsson ES, Campbell W, et al. Autonomic dysfunction in women with mitral valve prolapse syndrome. Circulation 1979;59:894–901.
11. MacMahon SW, Hickey AJ, Wilcken DE, et al. Risk of infective endocarditis in mitral valve prolapse with and without precordial systolic murmurs. Am J Cardiol 1987;59:105–108.
12. Devereux RB, Kramer-Fox R, Kligfield P. Mitral valve prolapse: causes, clinical manifestations, and management. Ann Intern Med 1989;111:305–317.
13. Bonow RO, Lakatos E, Maron BJ, et al. Serial long-term assessment of the natural history of asymptomatic patients with chronic aortic regurgitation and normal left ventricular systolic function. Circulation 1991;84:1625–1635.
14. Errichetti A, Greenberg JM, Gaasch WM. Is valve replacement indicated in asymptomatic patients with aortic stenosis or aortic regurgitation? Cardiovasc Clin 1990;21:199–210.
15. Ross J Jr, Braunwald E. Aortic stenosis. Circulation 1968;38 (Suppl 5):V61.
16. Pellikka PA, Nishimura RA, Bailey KR, et al. The natural history of adults with asymptomatic, hemodynamically significant aortic stenosis. J Am Coll Cardiol 1990;15:1012–1017.
17. Hayes SN, Holmes DR, Nishimura RA, et al. Palliative percutaneous aortic balloon valvuloplasty before noncardiac operations and invasive diagnostic procedures. Mayo Clin Proc 1989;64:753–757.
18. Cribier A, Letac B. Percutaneous balloon aortic valvuloplasty in adults with calcific aortic stenosis. Curr Opin Cardiol 1991;6:212.
19. Goldman L, Caldera DL, Nussbaum SR, et al. Multifactorial index of cardiac risk in noncardiac surgical procedures. N Engl J Med 1977;297:845–850.
20. Detsky AS, Abrams HB, McLaughlin JR, et al. Predicting cardiac complications in patients undergoing non-cardiac surgery. J Gen Intern Med 1986;1:211–219.
21. Zeldin RA. Assessing cardiac risk in patients who undergo noncardiac surgical procedures. Can J Surg 1984;27:402–404.
22. O'Keefe JH Jr, Shub C, Rettke SR. Risk of noncardiac surgical procedures in patients with aortic stenosis. Mayo Clin Proc 1989;64:400–405.
23. Dajani AS, Bisno AL, Chung KJ, et al. Prevention of bacterial endocarditis: recommendations by the American Heart Association. JAMA 1990;264:2919–2922.
24. Maron BJ. Hypertrophic cardiomyopathy: interrelations of clinical manifestations, pathophysiology, and therapy (1). N Engl J Med 1987;316:780–789.
25. Wynne J, Braunwald E. The cardiomyopathies and myocarditides: toxic, chemical, and physical damage to the heart. In: Braunwald E, ed. Heart disease: a textbook of cardiovascular medicine. Philadelphia, WB Saunders, 1992;1398–1438.
26. Lewis JF, Maron BJ. Elderly patients with hypertrophic cardiomyopathy: a subset with distinctive left ventricular morphology and progressive clinical course late in life. J Am Coll Cardiol 1989;13:36–45.
27. Leier CV. The cardiomyopathies: mortality, sudden death and ventricular arrhythmias. Cardiovasc Clin 1991;22:275–306.
28. Maron BJ. Hypertrophic cardiomyopathy. Curr Probl Cardiol 1993;18:639–704.
29. Fananapazir L, Cannon RO, Tripodi D, et al. Impact of dual-chamber permanent pacing in patients with obstructive hypertrophic cardiomyopathy with symptoms refractory to vera-

pamil and beta-adrenergic blocker therapy. Circulation 1992;85:2149–2161.

30. Thompson RC, Liberthson RR, Lowenstein E. Perioperative anesthetic risk of noncardiac surgery in hypertrophic obstructive cardiomyopathy. JAMA 1985;254:2419–2421.

31. Weitz HH, Goldman L. Noncardiac surgery in the patient with heart disease. Med Clin North Am 1987;71:413–432.

32. Freilich JD, Jacobs BR. Anesthetic management of cerebral aneurysm resection in a patient with idiopathic hypertrophic subaortic stenosis. Anesth Analg 1990;71:558–560.

33. Molavi A. Endocarditis: recognition, management, and prophylaxis. Cardiovasc Clin 1992;23:139–174.

34. Dajani AS, Bisno AL, Chung KJ, et al. Prevention of bacterial endocarditis: recommendations by the American Heart Association. JAMA 1978;239:738–739.

35. Harker LA. Antithrombotic therapy following mitral valve replacement. In: Duran C, ed. Recent progress in mitral valve disease. London, Butterworth, 1984:340–345.

36. Tinker JH, Tarhan S. Discontinuing anticoagulant therapy in surgical patients with cardiac valve prostheses: observations in 180 operations. JAMA 1978;239:738–739.

37. Stein PD, Alpert JS, Copeland J, et al. Antithrombotic therapy in patients with mechanical and biological prosthetic heart valves. Chest 1992;102:445S–455S.

38. McIntyre H. Management, during dental surgery, of patients on anticoagulants. Lancet 1966;2:99–100.

CHAPTER

7

Medical Management of the Surgical Patient, Third Edition,
edited by Michael F. Lubin, H. Kenneth Walker, and Robert B. Smith III.
J.B. Lippincott Company, Philadelphia, PA © 1995.

CONGESTIVE HEART FAILURE

Howard M. Weitz

Congestive heart failure (CHF) is a syndrome in which cardiac output is insufficient for the body's needs. The many possible causes include valvular and pericardial disease, myocardial dysfunction related to ischemia, infarction, hypertension, and cardiomyopathy. CHF may also be precipitated by noncardiac causes that increase the demand for cardiac output. Common examples that occur in the perioperative period include anemia, fever, and hypoxia. This chapter focuses on myocardial dysfunction, which is the most prevalent cause of CHF in the perioperative period.

CHF is the only major cardiovascular disorder that is increasing in incidence, prevalence, and overall mortality.[1] The incidence and prevalence rise with increasing age; the prevalence of CHF is 2% to 3% in persons older than 65 years and 5% to 10% in those older than 75 years. As the population of the United States ages, the incidence of chronic CHF in patients who undergo noncardiac surgery is likely to increase. The most common cause of CHF is coronary artery disease; hypertension is another major cause.[2] The mortality of patients with CHF is strikingly high, especially in the first few months after diagnosis. Three-month, 1-year, and 8-year survival rates among patients with newly identified CHF are 78%, 65%, and 30%, respectively.[3]

PATHOPHYSIOLOGY

Once valvular lesions, pericardial disease, and noncardiac conditions that increase the demand for cardiac output are ruled out, a primary myocardial abnormality is usually the cause of CHF. About 70% of cases are related to left ventricular systolic dysfunction and the remaining 30% are related to left ventricular diastolic dysfunction.

Impaired left ventricular contractility is the cause of left ventricular systolic dysfunction. Preload and cardiac volume subsequently increase as compensatory responses to increase cardiac output but, as left ventricular function deteriorates, cardiac output cannot increase. Increasing cardiac volume and ventricular pressure result in elevation of the left atrial pressure with subsequent pulmonary venous congestion. Decreased left ventricular contractility leads to decreased cardiac output.

In patients with primary left ventricular diastolic dysfunction, the main abnormality is reduced ventricular compliance. These patients usually have normal or enhanced left ventricular contractile function.[4] The ventricular myocardium is less compliant than normal; increases in preload result in marked elevation of left ventricular end-diastolic pressure with a subsequent rise in pulmonary venous pressure and pulmonary venous hypertension. Left ventricular diastolic dysfunction is characterized by marked sensitivity to changes in intravascular volume. Patients are at risk for marked elevation of ventricular filling pressure in the setting of intravascular volume overload and for hypotension as a consequence of decreased ventricular pressure when intravascular volume is depleted. If patients subsequently develop ventricular systolic dysfunction, these responses can become even more dramatic. The most common cause of ventricular diastolic dysfunction is left ventricular hypertrophy resulting from hypertension. Other, less common, causes include myocardial infiltrative processes such as amyloidosis and restrictive cardiomyopathy.

CONGESTIVE HEART FAILURE AS A CARDIAC RISK FACTOR

Congestive heart failure has been shown to be a predictor of perioperative cardiac complications in some studies. In the classic description of a multifactorial index of cardiac risk in noncardiac surgery, Goldman[5] and colleagues found that two clinical signs that may accompany CHF (jugular venous distention and the presence of a third heart sound) correlate with an increased risk of perioperative cardiac complications.

In a modification of the original multifactorial risk index, Detsky[6] found that alveolar pulmonary edema within 1 week before a noncardiac surgical procedure was a risk factor for perioperative cardiac complications. Compared to other risk factors, it was equivalent to the risk of myocardial infarction within 6 months of noncardiac surgery. A history of pulmonary edema at any time before surgery was noted to impose a somewhat lower risk, similar to that of factors such as age greater than 70 years, myocardial infarction more than 6 months before surgery, poor general medical status, rhythm other than sinus rhythm on the preoperative electrocardiogram, and more than five ventricular premature contractions per minute on electrocardiography before surgery.

In a study of 1487 men older than 40 years who underwent major noncardiac surgery, Ashton[7] found that signs of heart failure (ie, jugular venous distention, presence of a third heart sound, leg edema) noted during the preoperative examination were independently associated with postoperative myocardial infarction. In contrast, in a study of 474 men undergoing noncardiac surgery who either had documented coronary artery disease or were at high risk for it, Mangano and associates[8] found that a history of CHF was not an independent risk factor for perioperative myocardial ischemia. They also noted that postoperative CHF that occurred in the absence of unstable angina or myocar-

dial infarction had no effect on long-term outcome. These authors attributed the long-term absence of adverse cardiac events to the fact that postoperative CHF may result from numerous factors, including coexisting diseases and noncardiac conditions (ie, fluid overload, electrolyte administration, altered pulmonary gas exchange).[9]

RISK FOR THE DEVELOPMENT OF PERIOPERATIVE CONGESTIVE HEART FAILURE

Goldman found the preoperative presence of symptoms and signs of CHF to be the best predictor of the development of perioperative CHF. A history of CHF, which was absent in most of the patients who did develop heart failure, was a less powerful predictor. In a study of patients at higher risk (ie, those with hypertension or diabetes), Charlson[10] found that the risk for postoperative CHF was limited to patients with preoperative symptomatic cardiac disease (eg, previous myocardial infarction, valvular disease, or CHF). Patients with diabetes were at greatest risk, particularly if they had overt cardiac disease. Intraoperative fluctuations of the mean arterial blood pressure (increases or decreases of more than 40 mmHg) were related to increased rates of postoperative heart failure. Finally, in the study by Mangano and associates described earlier, postoperative myocardial ischemia, a history of cardiac arrhythmia, and diabetes were found to predict the development of postoperative CHF.

WHEN DOES PERIOPERATIVE CONGESTIVE HEART FAILURE OCCUR?

In a review of cases of perioperative CHF that occurred during the 1950s and 1960s, Cooperman[11] noted that most cases developed within 1 hour of the cessation of anesthesia, the majority during the first 30 minutes. In a high-risk population of patients with diabetes or hypertension, most of those who developed perioperative CHF did so on the day of surgery or on the second postoperative day.[10] We believe that the risk for postoperative CHF is greatest during two periods. The risk is significantly increased immediately after surgery, probably as a result of hypertension or hypotension, myocardial ischemia, intraoperative fluid administration, sympathetic stimulation, cessation of positive-pressure ventilation, and hypoxia. The second peak occurs 24 to 48 hours after surgery and may be related to the reabsorption of interstitial fluid, myocardial ischemia, and, in some patients, the effects of withdrawal from long-term oral CHF medications.

GENERAL APPROACH TO DIAGNOSIS

In the perioperative period, appropriate CHF therapy is facilitated by determining whether CHF is caused by systolic ventricular dysfunction, diastolic ventricular dysfunction, or a combination of both. Although a cardiac imaging study (eg, echocardiogram, radionuclide ventriculogram, or standard left ventricular angiogram) is necessary to definitively diagnose the presence of left ventricular systolic dysfunction, many clues to the diagnosis of CHF can be found in patients' histories, physical examinations, chest radiographs, and electrocardiograms. CHF in patients with histories of myocardial infarction, cardiomegaly, or S_3 strongly suggests the presence of left ventricular systolic dysfunction. In contrast, CHF in patients with hypertension, S_4, normal heart size on chest radiographs, electrocardiographic evidence of left ventricular hypertrophy, and no histories of myocardial infarction is suggestive of left ventricular diastolic dysfunction. Considerable overlap occurs, however, and patients with CHF may have both systolic and diastolic components to their myocardial dysfunction. Interstitial pulmonary edema may be found in both varieties and does not aid in discrimination. Although the absence of left ventricular systolic dysfunction in patients with CHF suggests that diastolic dysfunction is the cause, a diagnosis of left ventricular diastolic dysfunction ideally requires invasive documentation of increased pulmonary capillary wedge pressure or elevated left ventricular end-diastolic pressure.[4]

GENERAL APPROACH TO THERAPY

The goals of CHF therapy are to alleviate symptoms, preserve left ventricular function, and prolong life. In patients with left ventricular systolic dysfunction, diuretics and vasodilators are used to decrease ventricular preload and reduce pulmonary venous pressure. Venous and arterial vasodilators and angiotensin-converting enzyme (ACE) inhibitors improve cardiac output by reducing cardiac filling pressures and decreasing afterload. Inotropic agents increase cardiac output by directly increasing myocardial contractility.

Digoxin is the only commonly available oral inotropic agent. Its inotropic effect is weak, and a study designed to assess its effect on mortality is in progress. Attempts to develop other oral inotropic agents have been disappointing. The direct-acting venous and arterial vasodilators used in the treatment of CHF are isosorbide dinitrate and hydralazine. Although these agents have been shown to decrease mortality in patients with chronic CHF, the doses used in clinical trials documenting their efficacy were high and led to side effects requiring their discontinuation in numerous patients.[12]

This combination is also inferior to ACE inhibitors in reducing mortality.[13] ACE inhibitors lead to vasodilation by decreasing angiotensin II and aldosterone levels. They have been shown to decrease mortality and to reduce the rate of CHF development in patients with symptomatic left ventricular systolic dysfunction, asymptomatic left ventricular systolic dysfunction, and left ventricular dysfunction after acute myocardial infarction (if they are initiated within 2 weeks of the infarction).[13–15] Low-dose β-blockers have been demonstrated in preliminary studies to promote short-term improvement in patients with CHF caused by left ventricular systolic dysfunction, but definite recommendations regarding their use await further study.

Diastolic left ventricular dysfunction is characterized by abnormal left ventricular compliance, with elevated left ventricular end-diastolic pressure often leading to pulmonary venous hypertension. Therapy is directed toward improving left ventricular compliance and left ventricular relaxation. Agents used include β-blockers and the negative inotropic calcium channel antagonist verapamil. Because hypertension is a major cause of diastolic dysfunction, significant emphasis is placed on its control.

Diuretics, vasodilators, and ACE inhibitors are used to control hypertension and treat acute volume overload but otherwise play a minimal role unless systolic dysfunction is also present. These agents may further complicate the clinical picture by reducing preload excessively, resulting in hypotension. Digoxin may impair ventricular compliance further and is contraindicated except to control the ventricular response in patients with current atrial fibrillation or to aid in maintaining sinus rhythm in patients with previous atrial fibrillation.

APPROACH TO SURGICAL PATIENTS

PATIENTS WITH COMPENSATED CHRONIC CONGESTIVE HEART FAILURE

In patients with compensated chronic congestive heart failure, effort is directed at identifying destabilizing factors (eg, anemia or fever) that may occur in the perioperative period, preventing them if possible, and rendering immediate treatment if they occur. The need for invasive hemodynamic monitoring also must be assessed. Finally, patients' CHF medical regimens must be converted to appropriate parenteral regimens for use until oral intake can be resumed.

Perioperative cardiac mortality depends most on patients' clinical status at the time of surgery. The risk of CHF is greatest if signs of CHF are present at the time of surgery or during the week before the surgical procedure. Patients with chronic CHF are evaluated to determine whether the condition is compensated. If patients are thought to be decompensated, surgery is delayed if possible and attempts are made to achieve medical stabilization. Because the risk imposed by CHF is greatest in patients who have pulmonary edema within 7 days of surgery, we often delay elective surgery for at least 1 week after CHF stabilization.

Although no large-scale, randomized, controlled clinical trials have been performed to assess the impact of perioperative invasive hemodynamic monitoring in patients with histories of CHF who undergo noncardiac surgery, we believe that invasive monitoring provides important hemodynamic data (eg, cardiac output, pulmonary capillary wedge pressure, systemic vascular resistance) that is often helpful in the perioperative period. Therefore, we consider invasive hemodynamic monitoring with a pulmonary artery catheter in the following clinical situations:

* A history of CHF
* Significant left ventricular dysfunction
* Critical aortic stenosis
* Unstable angina
* A recent myocardial infarction in a patient undergoing a surgical procedure associated with significant intravascular volume shifts
* Substantial changes in preload or afterload
* Risk of perioperative myocardial ischemia

For patients with decompensated CHF who require emergent or semiemergent surgery, invasive hemodynamic monitoring may aid in further preoperative cardiac stabilization. Because the risk of postoperative CHF extends beyond the immediate surgical period, invasive hemodynamic monitoring is usually continued for 48 to 72 hours after surgery.

Adjustment of the Long-Term Medical Regimen in the Perioperative Period

Several medications used to treat chronic CHF may cause electrolyte or metabolic abnormalities in the perioperative period. Diuretics may induce intravascular volume depletion, which can predispose patients to hypotension if they are given vasodilator anesthetic agents or spinal anesthesia. Therefore, we monitor for orthostatic changes in blood pressure and pulse during the preoperative physical examination in all patients who receive diuretics. If orthostatic changes are documented, it is important that intravascular volume be replenished before surgery. A similar approach is followed for patients who are being treated with vasodilators.

Preoperative serum potassium levels are obtained in all patients who are receiving diuretics and are corrected before surgery if necessary. Hypokalemia may cause ventricular ectopy; acute potassium loss is probably more arrhythmogenic than is chronic potassium loss. Hypokalemia that does not resolve with potassium supplementation suggests the presence of hypomagnesemia, which also must be corrected before surgery is undertaken. The hyperkalemia that sometimes accompanies the use of potassium-sparing diuretics may cause heart block and other abnormalities of cardiac conduction.

The use of digoxin has been linked to perioperative bradyarrhythmias.[16] We do not begin digoxin therapy before surgery unless patients demonstrate clear indications for its use. For patients who are given digoxin, serial blood levels are measured if renal function declines and the dose is adjusted accordingly. The drug is continued in patients who have been receiving long-term oral digoxin therapy, and is given intravenously when oral intake is suspended. Cardiovascular drugs that may increase digoxin levels in the perioperative period include quinidine, verapamil, and amiodarone.

For patients who are maintained on ACE inhibitors, we often continue to administer the medications until the time of surgery and then give the oral agents again as soon as possible in the postoperative period. Patients' left ventricular function, degree of compensation, dependence on ACE inhibitors, and risk for perioperative CHF determine the need for parenteral ACE inhibitors after surgery until oral intake can be resumed. Patients with moderate to severe ventricular dysfunction who are at high risk for perioperative CHF are given intravenous ACE inhibitors (enalaprilat 0.625 to 1.25 mg every 6 hours) until oral agents can be taken again.

Many patients, particularly those who cannot tolerate ACE inhibitors, take nitrates and hydralazine as vasodilator therapy for CHF. During the time that patients are unable to take oral medications, topical or intravenous nitrates are given. Because of its short duration of action and risk for hypotension, we do not use parenteral hydralazine as a substitute for oral hydralazine. If CHF decompensates while patients being maintained on nitrates and hydralazine are unable to take oral medications, we may discontinue the nitrates and use intravenous nitroprusside for its preload- and afterload-reducing properties. In some cases, if the contraindication to ACE inhibitors is not well defined, we attempt to administer intravenous enalaprilat. In patients who are unable to receive ACE inhibitors, perioperative CHF therapy is centered on diuretics, preload reduction with nitrates, preload and afterload reduction with nitroprusside, digoxin if indicated, and intravenous inotropic agents such as dopamine, dobutamine, and amrinone.

PATIENTS WITH ACUTE CONGESTIVE HEART FAILURE IN THE PERIOPERATIVE PERIOD

Numerous factors may lead to the new onset of CHF or the decompensation of otherwise stable CHF in the perioperative period. Myocardial ischemia or infarction; perioperative volume overload; hypertension with a subsequent increase in afterload; occult valvular heart disease (eg, aortic stenosis, mitral regurgitation); renal failure; anemia; sepsis; pulmonary embolus; pneumonia; and the new onset of atrial fibrillation or flutter with decreased cardiac output may provoke perioperative CHF. In addition, an inadequate medical regimen may precipitate acute CHF in patients with otherwise stable chronic CHF. Medical regimens may be inadequate because of inappropriate medication dosages or inability to substitute orally administered drugs taken on a long-term basis with intravenous equivalents.

Treatment is directed at the primary cause of the acute episode of CHF. If volume overload is present, diuretics are administered. If patients are found to have left ventricular systolic dysfunction, inotropic agents are given to increase myocardial contractility and cardiac output. Intravenous inotropic agents such as dobutamine and dopamine are effective in the short term but must be used cautiously in patients with acute myocardial ischemia or infarction because they may increase myocardial oxygen demand and exacerbate myocardial ischemia. Digoxin is also helpful in the treatment of CHF in patients with left ventricular systolic dysfunction. It is particularly beneficial for patients whose CHF is provoked by atrial fibrillation. It slows the atrial fibrillation ventricular response, thereby prolonging ventricular filling time and decreasing myocardial oxygen demand.

Vasodilator medical therapy may also be used in the perioperative period. Intravenous nitroprusside is the agent of choice for immediate blood pressure control and reduction of afterload in patients with CHF who exhibit hypertension or increased systemic vascular resistance. It is also of benefit when acute perioperative CHF is associated with aortic or mitral regurgitation. It decreases afterload and serves to decrease the regurgitant fraction in patients with these valvular lesions. Its use is limited by the need for continuous blood pressure monitoring and the risk of cyanate toxicity when it is administered for more than a short period.

For patients who require long-term parenteral vasodilator therapy, enalaprilat, an ACE inhibitor that is administered intravenously, is effective in reducing preload and afterload. When patients resume oral intake, oral ACE inhibitors may be substituted. Nitrates are beneficial in the treatment of perioperative CHF when myocardial ischemia is contributing to the condition or when reduction in preload is desired. β-Blockers and calcium channel antagonists should not be given to patients with perioperative CHF caused by left ventricular systolic dysfunction but may prove helpful in patients with left ventricular diastolic dysfunction by promoting left ventricular relaxation and increased compliance.

When patients who have perioperative CHF in the absence of acute myocardial ischemia do not respond to the alleviation of precipitating factors and provision of medical therapy directed at normalizing intravascular volume and cardiac output, the presence of acute pulmonary embolism, sepsis, or other noncardiac causes must be considered.

Ventricular arrhythmias are common in patients who have CHF. Complex ventricular ectopy is a predictor of mortality. The treatment of ventricular arrhythmias in patients with left ventricular dysfunction is controversial. It is generally agreed, however, that the first step is to provide maximal medical therapy for CHF. Empiric antiarrhythmic therapy is not often used because it may have a negative inotropic effect, the available agents have not been demonstrated to decrease mortality in patients with left ventricular systolic dysfunction, and type IA antiarrhythmics may have a proarrhythmic effect and worsen the arrhythmia. There is also evidence that type IC antiarrhythmics may increase mortality in patients with ischemic heart disease and ventricular ectopy. Further discussion of the approach to patients with ventricular ectopy may be found in Chapter 8.

REFERENCES

1. Yamani M, Massie BM. Congestive heart failure: insights from epidemiology, implications for treatment. (Editorial) Mayo Clin Proc 1993;68:1214–1218.
2. Teerlink JR, Goldhaber SZ, Pfeffer MA. An overview of contemporary etiologies of congestive heart failure. (Editorial) Am Heart J 1991;121:1852–1853.
3. Rodeheffer RJ, Jacobsen SJ, Gersch BJ, et al. The incidence and prevalence of congestive heart failure in Rochester, Minnesota. Mayo Clin Proc 1993;68:1143–1150.
4. Goldsmith SR, Dick C. Differentiating systolic from diastolic heart failure: pathophysiologic and therapeutic considerations. Am J Med 1993;95:645–655.
5. Goldman L, Caldera DL, Nussbaum SR, et al. Multifactorial index of cardiac risk in noncardiac surgical procedures. N Engl J Med 1977;297:845–850.
6. Detsky AS, Abrams HB, McLaughlin JR, et al. Predicting cardiac complications in patients undergoing non-cardiac surgery. J Gen Intern Med 1986;1:211–219.
7. Ashton CM, Petersen NJ, Wray NP, et al. The incidence of peri-

operative myocardial infarction in men undergoing noncardiac surgery. Ann Intern Med 1993;118:504–510.

8. Mangano DT, Browner WS, Hollenberg M, et al. Association of perioperative myocardial ischemia with cardiac morbidity and mortality in men undergoing noncardiac surgery: the Study of Perioperative Ischemia Research Group. N Engl J Med 1990; 323:1781–1786.

9. Mangano DT, Browner WS, Hollenberg M, et al. Long-term cardiac prognosis following noncardiac surgery: the Study of Perioperative Ischemia Research Group. JAMA 1992;268:233–239.

10. Charlson ME, MacKenzie CR, Gold JP, et al. Risk for postoperative congestive heart failure. Surg Gynecol Obstet 1991;172: 95–104.

11. Cooperman LH, Price HL. Pulmonary edema in the operative and postoperative period: a review of 40 cases. Ann Surg 1970; 172:833–891.

12. Cohn JN, Archibald DG, Ziesche S, et al. Effect of vasodilator therapy on mortality in chronic congestive heart failure: results of a Veterans Administration Cooperative Study. N Engl J Med 1986;314:1547–1552.

13. Cohn JN, Johnson G, Ziesche S, et al. A comparison of enalapril with hydralazine-isosorbide dinitrate in the treatment of chronic congestive heart failure. N Engl J Med 1991;325:303–310.

14. The SOLVD Investigators. Effect of enalapril on mortality and the development of heart failure in asymptomatic patients with reduced left ventricular ejection fractions. N Engl J Med 1992;327:685–691.

15. Pfeffer MA, Braunwald E, Moye LA, et al. Effect of captopril on mortality and morbidity in patients with left ventricular dysfunction after myocardial infarction: results of the survival and ventricular enlargement trial: the SAVE investigators. N Engl J Med 1992;327:669–677.

16. Goldman L. Supraventricular tachyarrhythmias in hospitalized adults after surgery: clinical correlates in patients over 40 years of age after major noncardiac surgery. Chest 1978;73:450–454.

CHAPTER

8

ARRHYTHMIAS AND CONDUCTION ABNORMALITIES

Medical Management of the Surgical Patient, Third Edition,
edited by Michael F. Lubin, H. Kenneth Walker, and Robert B. Smith III.
J.B. Lippincott Company, Philadelphia, PA © 1995.

Howard M. Weitz

Cardiac arrhythmias are common in the perioperative period but are usually clinically insignificant. In one study using continuous electrocardiographic monitoring, 84% of patients were documented to have at least transient arrhythmias during their hospitalization for surgery. Only 5% of these arrhythmias were clinically important.[1] In another study, Kuner and associates[2] noted a 62% incidence of one or more transient arrhythmias in the perioperative period. The dysrhythmias were primarily supraventricular and consisted predominantly of wandering atrial pacemaker, isorhythmic atrioventricular (AV) dissociation, nodal rhythm, and sinus bradycardia. Ventricular premature contractions were common but paroxysmal ventricular tachycardia was not. Only one study has determined the incidence and clinical significance of perioperative ventricular arrhythmias in men undergoing noncardiac surgery who either have coronary disease or are at high risk for it. O'Kelly[3] found that frequent or major ventricular arrhythmias (more than 30 ventricular premature contractions per hour or ventricular tachycardia) occurred in 44% of the patients who were monitored (21% before operation, 16% during operation, and 36% after operation). Preoperative ventricular arrhythmias were associated with the occurrence of intraoperative and postoperative arrhythmias. These arrhythmias were largely benign, and sustained ventricular tachycardia or ventricular fibrillation did not occur.

The prognostic significance of preoperative cardiac arrhythmias is not well defined. Although multifactorial risk indices have identified preoperative ventricular premature contractions and rhythms other than sinus rhythm on the preoperative electrocardiogram as risk factors for perioperative complications, the risk potential of preoperative ventricular premature contractions has been questioned.[4–6] When these dysrhythmias are markers of underlying cardiac disease, they may indicate a subset of patients who are at increased cardiac risk. Ventricular premature contractions are a risk factor for sudden death in patients who have sustained myocardial infarction and in those who have severe left ventricular dysfunction.[7] Asymptomatic complex ventricular ectopy in healthy patients without evidence of structural or ischemic cardiovascular disease is not associated with an increase in cardiac morbidity or mortality.[8]

We look for evidence of structural or ischemic heart disease, metabolic derangements, and electrolyte abnormalities when preoperative ventricular premature contractions or complex ventricular arrhythmias are identified before surgery. In the absence of these conditions, we do not consider the arrhythmias to be significant risk factors. In patients who have rhythms other than sinus rhythm on their electrocardiograms, we assess the hemodynamic stability and chronicity of the rhythm disorder as well as the presence of any reversible causative factors. In stable patients whose rhythm disorders are asymptomatic and chronic, we typically proceed to surgery if no other significant cardiac risk factors are present.

RISK FACTORS FOR AND CAUSES OF PERIOPERATIVE ARRHYTHMIAS AND CONDUCTION ABNORMALITIES

Risk factors for the development of supraventricular arrhythmias have been described by Goldman[9] and include the following: patient age over 70 years; the presence of preoperative pulmonary rales; and the performance of abdominal, thoracic, or major vascular surgery. The presence of chronic obstructive pulmonary disease and preoperative atrial premature contractions were not found to be risk factors for the development of perioperative supraventricular arrhythmias.

In O'Kelly's study of perioperative ventricular arrhythmias, the presence of preoperative ventricular ectopy was the most significant predictor of intraoperative and postoperative ventricular arrhythmias. Other risk factors were history of congestive heart failure and history of cigarette smoking. Additional causes of perioperative arrhythmias include hypoxia, hypercarbia, and acute hypokalemia.

Sinus tachycardia is common in the perioperative period and often results from catecholamine release precipitated by stress, pain, or anxiety. Hypovolemia or anemia may cause sinus tachycardia as a compensatory response to increase cardiac output. Less common but ominous causes of sinus tachycardia are perioperative congestive heart failure and myocardial infarction. The anesthetic agent ketamine may cause sinus tachycardia as a result of central sympathetic stimulation. Hypercarbia and hypoxemia resulting from inadequate ventilation may cause sinus tachycardia as well as ventricular tachycardia.

Bradycardia is seen frequently during hospitalization for surgery and has numerous causes. Narcotics, with the exception of meperidine, may cause bradycardia by producing central vagal stimulation.[10] Anticholinesterases which are administered to antagonize the effect of nondepolarizing neuromuscular blocking agents by increasing the amount of acetylcholine at the neuromuscular junction, increase acetylcholine at the heart and may result in bradycardia.[11] An imbalance between sympathetic and parasympathetic tone may be produced in patients undergoing spinal or epidural anesthesia if cardiac-stimulating sympathetic fibers are anesthetized. This can occur if the spinal cord is anesthetized at the level of the sympathetic ganglia (T-1 to T-4) or if spinal anesthesia is placed two to six segments distant from this region because the anesthetic agent may migrate or ascending preganglionic sympathetic fibers in the paravertebral chain may be blocked. Unopposed parasympathetic (vagal) activity may occur and lead to peripheral vasodilation and hypotension in addition to bradycardia.[12]

Reflex bradycardia, occasionally associated with heart block and sinus arrest, may occur during many surgical procedures (Table 8-1). It usually is caused by a reflex arc whose efferent limb is the vagus nerve. In addition to bradycardia, this vagally mediated reflex may result in peripheral vasodilation and hypotension. Anesthetic agents such as vecuronium, atracurium, halothane, fentanyl, and succinylcholine may predispose to this reflex.[13] It can be prevented by premedication with an anticholinergic agent such as atropine. If reflex bradycardia does occur, it often can be terminated by discontinuing the procedure or administering anticholinergic agents.

Arrhythmias may be precipitated by medications used specifically during ophthalmic surgery as a result of systemic absorption of eye drops. Ophthalmic atropine has been reported to cause supraventricular tachycardia and

TABLE 8–1. Reflex Bradycardia During Surgery

Surgical Procedure	Afferent Reflex Pathway	Reference
Abdominal manipulation	Celiac plexus	69
Mesenteric traction	?	70
Liver biopsy	Hepatic, celiac plexus	71
Laparoscopy	Parasympathetic stimulation from peritoneal stimulation	72
Ocular stimulation (oculocardiac reflex)	Parasympathetic fibers in the ciliary nerves and the ophthalmic nerve run to the trigeminal nerve, which is adjacent to the nucleus ambiguus, which is the origin of the vagus	13
Maxilla stimulation, zygoma stimulation	Trigeminal nerve	73
Neurosurgery (tentorium manipulation)	Ophthalmic nerve innervates tentorium; reflex similar to oculocardiac reflex	74
Laryngoscopy	Laryngeal stimulation	75
Blepharoplasty	Same as oculocardiac reflex	76

atrial fibrillation, and timolol and pilocarpine eye drops have been reported to cause bradycardia.[14,15]

PATIENTS WITH PREOPERATIVE CARDIAC ARRHYTHMIAS

For patients receiving long-term antiarrhythmic therapy, the nature of the arrhythmia must be determined before surgery, including provocative factors and means of termination. The management of antiarrhythmic therapy is discussed in Chapter 4.

Although the preoperative occurrence of more than five ventricular premature contractions per minute has been identified as a cardiac risk factor for noncardiac surgery, it is probably the presence of coexisting cardiovascular disease that serves as the predominant determinant of risk.[4] We believe that patients who are found to have ventricular ectopy (including more than five ventricular premature contractions per minute, ventricular bigeminy, ventricular trigeminy, and nonsustained ventricular tachycardia) should be evaluated for the presence of underlying heart disease. The evaluation should include an echocardiogram to identify chamber size and function as well as the status of the cardiac valves. Because complex ventricular ectopy may be life-threatening in patients with ischemic heart disease (although it is relatively benign in patients with normal hearts[8]), we also perform a noninvasive assessment of myocardial perfusion (eg, exercise electrocardiogram, vasodilator myocardial imaging) in this patient group.

Patients who are receiving long-term antiarrhythmic therapy to suppress paroxysmal supraventricular tachycardia should be maintained on antiarrhythmic therapy in the perioperative period. Antiarrhythmic agents are given on the morning of surgery, in the form of long-acting preparations if possible. If patients are unable to resume oral intake after surgery, parenteral antiarrhythmic agents are substituted temporarily. Further details are provided in Chapter 4.

If atrial fibrillation is detected during the initial preoperative assessment, further evaluation is recommended to determine the etiology, duration, likelihood of conversion to sinus rhythm, and presence of underlying structural cardiac disease. If the atrial fibrillation is of less than 12 months' duration and does not result from significant conduction system disease, and if the left atrium is not enlarged, cardioversion is often performed.[16] Restoration of sinus rhythm may increase cardiac output up to 30% and significantly decrease the risk of perioperative congestive heart failure during and after surgical procedures. In patients who have been in atrial fibrillation for more than 2 days, anticoagulation with warfarin (International Normalized Ratio [INR] of 2 to 3) should be achieved 3 to 4 weeks

before cardioversion is attempted to decrease the risk of systemic embolization of atrial thrombi.[17] While patients await cardioversion, their ventricular rates should be controlled with digoxin, β-blockers, or calcium channel antagonists. In-hospital cardioversion is then attempted with direct electrical current (85% success rate), intravenous procainamide (about 50% success rate), or oral quinidine (50% to 60% success rate).[18] Anticoagulant therapy with warfarin is continued for 4 weeks after successful cardioversion to decrease the risk of atrial thrombus formation as atrial contractile function resumes and to protect patients from emboli if atrial fibrillation recurs. When anticoagulation is complete after cardioversion, patients may undergo elective surgery. Long-term anticoagulant therapy is considered if atrial fibrillation is related to mitral valve disease or cardiomyopathy, or if patients have histories of systemic thromboembolism.[17]

If chronic atrial fibrillation either is unlikely to convert to sinus rhythm (ie, has lasted more than 1 year or is associated with an enlarged left atrium) or failed to convert after an attempt at conversion, the ventricular response should be controlled before surgery and monitored closely during the perioperative period. Patients with chronic atrial fibrillation (except those younger than 60 years who have no evidence of associated cardiovascular disease ["lone" atrial fibrillation]) should receive anticoagulant therapy with warfarin if no contraindications exist. The INR should be maintained between 2 and 3.[19–22] Anticoagulant therapy usually must be discontinued during the immediate perioperative period but the length of time for which it is safe to withhold this treatment is not known. Thrombi probably take several days to form in the atria, although this process may be accelerated in the setting of mitral valve disease. We recommend that heparin be administered as soon as possible after surgery and that warfarin (Coumadin) be given when patients are able to resume oral intake.

Patients often are found to have asymptomatic ventricular ectopy on preoperative evaluation. The role of ventricular premature contractions as a cardiac risk factor and their relationship to underlying cardiovascular disease have been discussed in Chapter 4. When significant ventricular ectopy is identified in the preoperative period, we first search for a metabolic cause such as hypoxia or hypokalemia. If none is identified, we perform an echocardiogram to assess left ventricular function and, if possible, an exercise stress test or vasodilator myocardial imaging to investigate the possibility that myocardial ischemia is playing a role. In patients with normal left ventricular function and no evidence of inducible myocardial ischemia, asymptomatic ventricular ectopy is usually benign. Patients with severe left ventricular dysfunction or inducible myocardial ischemia as a cause of ventricular ectopy, however, are at significantly increased risk for sudden cardiac death. Cardiac status in these patients is evaluated further with tests such as coronary angiography or invasive electrophysiologic testing, if possible, before noncardiac surgery is performed. The most difficult patients to categorize are those with moderate ventricular dysfunction and significant ventricular ectopy. This group is heterogeneous and the significance of ventricular ectopy as a risk factor during noncardiac surgery has not been studied. We recommend that each case be evaluated on an individual basis and that patients' cardiac rhythms be monitored closely during and after surgery so that appropriate antiarrhythmic therapy can be initiated if malignant or hemodynamically significant ventricular ectopy occurs.

Because prophylactic perioperative antiarrhythmic therapy does not reverse patients' underlying cardiovascular disorders, it is usually reserved for patients with histories of serious ventricular arrhythmias (ie, symptomatic or sustained ventricular tachycardia or "sudden cardiac death"). Many patients will already have undergone evaluation of these arrhythmias, including invasive electrophysiologic testing in some cases. The medical-surgical team must be aware of the results of these investigations before the surgical procedure is undertaken. When prophylactic antiarrhythmic therapy is warranted in the perioperative period, it must be remembered that antiarrhythmic agents increase the frequency and complexity of ventricular arrhythmias in as many as 11% of patients.[23]

Patients who take oral antiarrhythmic agents for the treatment of chronic ventricular ectopy should continue to receive antiarrhythmic therapy in the perioperative period. If type IA antiarrhythmic agents (eg, quinidine, procainamide, disopyramide) are used, the oral medications should be continued. If patients are unable to tolerate type IA oral antiarrhythmic agents, intravenous procainamide may be administered until oral intake is possible again. If patients have prior histories of procainamide intolerance, allergy, or renal insufficiency that may contribute to impaired procainamide clearance, intravenous lidocaine may be administered instead. The half-life of lidocaine may be prolonged and its metabolism impaired as a result of anesthetic-induced reduction of cardiac output or hepatic dysfunction.[24]

Special consideration must be given to patients who take the antiarrhythmic agent amiodarone. This drug is used to treat serious ventricular arrhythmias that are unresponsive to more conventional antiarrhythmic therapy and, in lower doses, to treat supraventricular tachycardia and atrial fibrillation. One side effect of this drug is chronic pulmonary interstitial disease, and acute life-threatening pulmonary complications such as the adult respiratory distress syndrome have been observed in patients undergoing both cardiac and noncardiac surgery. Respiratory failure occurred 16 to 72 hours after surgery and was unrelated to the dose of amiodarone. Amiodarone levels persist in the body for weeks after its use has been discontinued and amiodarone-related postoperative adult respiratory distress syndrome

has been observed in patients who stopped taking the drug 6 days before surgery. The cause of this complication is speculative and may be linked to oxidative lung injury induced by high concentrations of inspired oxygen in the perioperative period. No effective therapy is available for amiodarone pulmonary toxicity and mortality is high. We do not perform elective surgery with general anesthesia in these patients if possible and use the lowest possible concentration of inspired oxygen during and after surgery. Although discontinuation of amiodarone therapy weeks to months before surgery theoretically would be beneficial, this is rarely an option in these patients.[25,26]

IDENTIFICATION AND TREATMENT OF SPECIFIC DISORDERS OF CARDIAC RATE AND RHYTHM

The guiding principle in the treatment of all perioperative cardiac arrhythmias is that the cause of the arrhythmia should be treated and reversed if possible. In the setting of an unstable or life-threatening arrhythmia, medical antiarrhythmic therapy is often instituted while the cause of the arrhythmia is being identified and treated.

Common causes of perioperative arrhythmias are catecholamine release; alterations in autonomic tone; electrolyte abnormalities (eg, acute hypokalemia, hyperkalemia); acid–base disturbances (eg, acidosis, alkalosis); anemia; and acute volume depletion. Less commonly, myocardial ischemia is the cause of serious cardiac arrhythmias or conduction abnormalities. Indications for the treatment of perioperative arrhythmias include hemodynamic instability, myocardial ischemia, and myocardial infarction, or the suspicion that these deleterious consequences may occur if the arrhythmia persists.

SINUS TACHYCARDIA

Sinus tachycardia is the most common perioperative rhythm abnormality and is almost always benign. It is characterized by a heart rate between 100 and 160 beats/min. The electrocardiogram demonstrates a regular rhythm with a normal P wave before each QRS complex. The QRS complex is normal unless patients have myocardial ischemia, aberrant ventricular conduction, or conduction abnormalities. The most common causes of sinus tachycardia are pain, hypovolemia, anemia, hypoxia, fever, and hypercarbia. Treatment is directed at the inciting factor. Patients with coronary artery disease may develop myocardial ischemia as a result of increased heart rate and increased myocardial oxygen demand. β-Adrenergic blockers may be beneficial in this instance to decrease the heart rate and alleviate myocardial ischemia while the underlying cause of the sinus tachycardia is being treated.

ATRIAL PREMATURE CONTRACTIONS

Atrial premature contractions are of minor clinical significance but may be harbingers of supraventricular tachycardia or atrial fibrillation. They arise in the atria at a site other than the sinus node and, therefore, are represented on the electrocardiogram by a P wave that has a different configuration and occurs earlier in the cardiac cycle than does a normal P wave. Atrial premature contractions typically produce a normal QRS complex. If the premature contraction arrives at the ventricular conduction tissue when it is still refractory and has not fully repolarized, however, it may cause no QRS complex or one that is abnormal as a result of aberrant ventricular conduction. The aberrant QRS complex usually is of right bundle-branch block morphology because the refractory period of the right bundle is longer than that of the left bundle.

ATRIAL FLUTTER AND ATRIAL FIBRILLATION

Perioperative atrial flutter and atrial fibrillation are infrequent but are the most common perioperative supraventricular arrhythmias that require therapy. Controversy exists regarding the efficacy of digoxin in the prevention of perioperative supraventricular tachycardia in high-risk patients.[27–29] We refrain from using digoxin for arrhythmia prophylaxis. There is a lack of evidence from rigorously designed studies that prophylactic digitalization is of benefit in preventing perioperative supraventricular arrhythmias; there is also a risk that metabolic stress, catecholamine release, hypoxia, and electrolyte abnormalities may predispose to digitalis toxic arrhythmias.

The treatment of perioperative atrial flutter or fibrillation is dictated by patients' hemodynamic stability and the presence of myocardial ischemia or congestive heart failure. In patients who are unstable as a result of the arrhythmia, the immediate goal is to restore sinus rhythm, usually by direct current (DC) cardioversion. If the arrhythmia is well tolerated, the initial plan is to control the ventricular response. If patients remain in atrial flutter or fibrillation and are hemodynamically stable, conversion to sinus rhythm may be attempted under elective conditions.

Atrial flutter is caused by atrial reentry; the atrial rate is usually 250 to 350 beats/min. Conduction block occurs at the AV node, resulting in a ventricular rate of 150 beats/min. Flutter waves with a saw-tooth configuration are seen on the electrocardiogram and represent atrial electrical activity. In hemodynamically stable patients, control of the atrial flutter ventricular response may be achieved with β-blockers; calcium channel antagonists (eg, verapamil, diltiazem); or digoxin. Atrial flutter is often resistant to attempts at conversion to sinus rhythm using antiarrhythmic medications. Synchronized DC cardioversion with low energy (ie, 25 to 50 J) is usually effective in restoring sinus rhythm and is the treatment of choice in hemodynamically unstable patients. Atrial overdrive pacing is an alternative effective method of rhythm conversion.[30,31]

Atrial fibrillation is characterized by chaotic atrial activity with the atria beating at 300 to 600 beats/min. No P waves are seen on the electrocardiogram and the ventricular rhythm is irregularly irregular. If the AV node and cardiac conduction system are normal and patients are not receiving medications that impair cardiac conduction, the ventricular rate is typically 150 to 200 beats/min. During the postoperative period, acute hypovolemia may precipitate atrial fibrillation.[32] Other reversible causes in the immediate postoperative period are hypoxia, acute pulmonary embolism, anemia, and fever.

When acute perioperative atrial fibrillation precipitates myocardial ischemia, congestive heart failure, or hypotension, emergency DC cardioversion is indicated to restore sinus rhythm. Patients should be given sedatives before cardioversion if the procedure is not emergent. Typical drugs used in this setting are diazepam, midazolam, barbiturates, etomidate, ketamine, and methohexital. Synchronized DC cardioversion, with or without analgesic agents (eg, fentanyl, morphine, meperidine) is performed initially using 100 J. If this is unsuccessful, cardioversion is repeated at 200, 300, and 360 J.[33]

If patients are hemodynamically stable and do not have myocardial ischemia or congestive heart failure, medical attempts at conversion to sinus rhythm may be made. Volume replacement in dehydrated patients, reversal of hypoxia, and correction of electrolyte abnormalities or anemia may restore sinus rhythm. An attempt should be made to slow the ventricular response; numerous drugs may be administered intravenously in the perioperative period, including β-blockers (eg, esmolol, propranolol, metoprolol) and calcium channel antagonists (eg, verapamil, diltiazem).[34–36] Although digoxin is effective in controlling the ventricular rate in chronic atrial fibrillation, its effectiveness in acute atrial fibrillation is controversial.[16] Conversion to sinus rhythm may occur after the ventricular rate is controlled. If atrial fibrillation persists, intravenous procainamide or oral quinidine is successful in restoring sinus rhythm in as many as 60% of cases.[18,37]

Caution must be exercised in the use of antiarrhythmic agents. Type IA antiarrhythmics may provoke ventricular arrhythmias in patients with atrial fibrillation. A recent metaanalysis of patients with coronary artery disease and atrial fibrillation found that, although quinidine was more effective than placebo in maintaining sinus rhythm, its use resulted in a three-fold increase in mortality compared to placebo.[38] For this reason, we administer antiarrhythmic agents in the setting of continuous electrocardiographic monitoring and discontinue their use after conversion is achieved. If sinus rhythm is not restored after 24 to 48 hours of a therapeutic trial, drug administration is discontinued. Some patients may require antiarrhythmic agents for long-term therapy to prevent recurrent hemodynamically significant atrial fibrillation. In these cases, the risk that they impose must be carefully weighed against their benefits.

If atrial fibrillation persists for more than 2 days, an atrial thrombus may form. Although treatment is individualized, these patients should be considered for anticoagulant therapy while they await pharmacologic or electrical cardioversion.[17]

PAROXYSMAL SUPRAVENTRICULAR TACHYCARDIA

Paroxysmal supraventricular tachycardia (PSVT) is characterized by the sudden onset of a rapid rhythm with a rate of 150 to 250 beats/min, usually after an atrial premature contraction. It is often the result of a reentrant circuit in the AV node using slow and fast pathways within the node. Typically, the antegrade limb of the reentrant circuit is a slow-conducting pathway and the retrograde limb is a fast-conducting pathway. During tachycardia, the atria are depolarized simultaneously in a retrograde fashion at the time of ventricular depolarization. Because of this concurrent depolarization, a QRS complex is evident but retrograde P waves are not seen on the electrocardiogram. The QRS complex is usually normal, although aberrant ventricular conduction with a "wide" QRS complex may be found.[39] If patients are hemodynamically unstable or have angina or congestive heart failure as a result of the tachycardia, immediate synchronized DC cardioversion should be performed. PSVT is usually sensitive to DC cardioversion and responds to 50 J. Shocks at higher energy levels should be administered in a sequential fashion (eg, 100, 200, 300, and 360 J) if lower energy levels produce no response. If the QRS complex is wide and the rhythm has not definitely been proved to be supraventricular, it should be treated as ventricular tachycardia.[33]

If patients are hemodynamically stable during PSVT with a narrow QRS complex, vagal maneuvers or medical therapy may terminate the arrhythmia. Vagal maneuvers slow conduction through the AV node by increasing parasympathetic tone. This often terminates the arrhythmia by disrupting the reentrant circuit that is necessary to sustain the tachycardia. The most effective vagal maneuver is the Valsalva maneuver (54% termination rate). This may be impossible to perform in the perioperative period, however, because of the inability of patients to cooperate.[40] Carotid sinus massage has a success rate of 17% on the right and 5%

on the left, and is the most useful vagal maneuver in the perioperative period. It must be performed using electrocardiographic monitoring, and intravenous atropine and antiarrhythmic drugs should be available in the event that advanced heart block or arrhythmias occur. Carotid sinus massage should not be used in elderly patients or in those with carotid bruits or known cerebrovascular disease because of the risk of stroke.

If vagal maneuvers are unsuccessful or contraindicated and patients remain hemodynamically stable, intravenous adenosine should be administered. This agent is the initial drug of choice for the conversion of hemodynamically stable PSVT and is successful in more than 90% of cases. Adenosine should be given as a 6-mg rapid infusion over 1 to 3 seconds. If conversion is not achieved after 1 or 2 minutes, an additional 12-mg rapid infusion should be given. If this also is unsuccessful, 2.5 to 5 mg of verapamil should be administered intravenously over 2 minutes (2 to 4 mg over 3 or 4 minutes in the elderly), with a second dose of 5 to 10 mg administered in 15 to 30 minutes if the PSVT persists. If PSVT still is not converted to sinus rhythm, other drugs such as digoxin, diltiazem, β-blockers, and type IA antiarrhythmics may be considered. Atrial overdrive pacing and DC synchronized cardioversion may become necessary. If patients become hemodynamically unstable during attempts at conversion to sinus rhythm using medical therapy, DC cardioversion should be performed promptly.

MULTIFOCAL ATRIAL TACHYCARDIA

Multifocal atrial tachycardia (MAT) is an automatic arrhythmia characterized by an atrial rate greater than 100 beats/min with organized, discrete, nonsinus P waves with at least three different forms in the same electrocardiographic lead.[41] It is usually associated with severe pulmonary disease and often accompanies critical illness. When the initial onset of MAT occurs in the perioperative period, respiratory failure, pneumonia, and congestive heart failure are common causes. Therapy centers on treating the pulmonary, cardiac, or other acute illness that led to the onset of the arrhythmia.[42] When MAT persists despite these maneuvers, additional medical therapy may be indicated if the arrhythmia is hemodynamically significant (ie, contributing to hypotension, congestive heart failure, or myocardial ischemia). Intravenous magnesium may be helpful in patients with hypomagnesemia or hypokalemia. β-Blockers may be effective in decreasing the ventricular rate but must be used with extreme caution, if at all, in patients with reversible airways disease or congestive heart failure. For patients with bronchospastic lung disease, verapamil or diltiazem may be used instead of β-blockers to decrease the ventricular response. Digitalis preparations are rarely effective in the treatment of MAT. Aminophylline, even at therapeutic levels, may aggravate the tachycardia by increasing the atrial rate and the number of ectopic atrial beats.[43] MAT is usually resistant to DC cardioversion as well as to therapy with quinidine, lidocaine, and procainamide.[41]

VENTRICULAR PREMATURE CONTRACTIONS AND NONSUSTAINED VENTRICULAR TACHYCARDIA

No specific medical therapy is indicated for patients who develop asymptomatic, hemodynamically insignificant ventricular premature contractions or nonsustained ventricular tachycardia in the perioperative period. The cause of these dysrhythmias should be determined and the provoking factors corrected if possible. Common causes of acute ventricular arrhythmias in the perioperative period include acute myocardial ischemia, hypoxia, hypokalemia, and hypomagnesemia. Right heart catheters may cause ventricular irritability and ectopy as a result of trauma to the right ventricular outflow tract in patients who require these devices to aid in hemodynamic monitoring during the perioperative period. This should resolve on repositioning or removal of the monitoring catheter.

No well-studied data are available regarding the treatment of symptomatic or hemodynamically significant nonsustained ventricular tachycardia that develops acutely in the perioperative period. It is our approach to conduct an immediate search for a reversible etiology. We often cautiously initiate medical antiarrhythmic therapy with agents such as intravenous lidocaine or procainamide in these patients. These medications are used for only a short period and under carefully monitored conditions because of their risk for provoking arrhythmias and lack of evidence for long-term benefit.[38] Special precautions must be taken when antiarrhythmic agents are used in the perioperative period. Lidocaine clearance is impaired in the setting of hepatic dysfunction and in the presence of anesthetic-induced decreased cardiac output. Central nervous system toxicity from lidocaine is characterized by confusion, delirium, or stupor and may be obscured by the effects of anesthetic or analgesic agents in the perioperative period. Procainamide clearance may be delayed in elderly patients and in those with decreased renal blood flow.

SUSTAINED VENTRICULAR TACHYCARDIA AND VENTRICULAR FIBRILLATION

Patients who develop sustained ventricular tachycardia or ventricular fibrillation in the perioperative period should be treated according to the Advanced Cardiac Life Support protocol. The treatment of patients with hemodynamically stable sustained ventricular tachycardia is outlined in Fig-

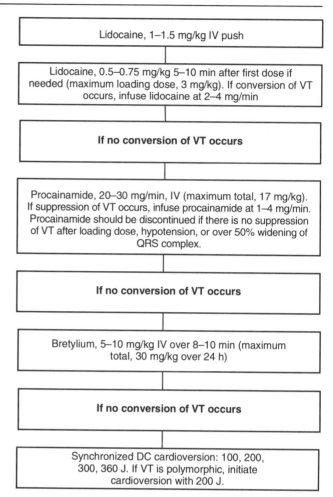

FIG. 8-1. *Treatment of perioperative, hemodynamically stable ventricular tachycardia (VT). (Adapted from Emergency Cardiac Care Committee and Subcommittees, American Heart Association. Guidelines for cardiopulmonary resuscitation and emergency cardiac care. III Adult advanced cardiac life support. JAMA. 1992;268:2199–2241)*

ure 8-1. Patients who have ventricular fibrillation or hemodynamically unstable ventricular tachycardia should undergo DC cardioversion starting at 200 J. If the arrhythmia persists, successive increases in electrical energy should be administered (ie, 300 J and then 360 J). Readers are referred to the Advanced Cardiac Life Support guidelines for further information.[33]

WIDE-COMPLEX TACHYCARDIA

Supraventricular tachycardia may occasionally be accompanied by aberrant ventricular conduction, resulting in a wide QRS complex. It is often difficult to differentiate wide-complex supraventricular tachycardia with aberrancy from ventricular tachycardia. Although criteria have been developed to aid in distinguishing these arrhythmias, the American Heart Association recommends that ill patients with wide-complex tachycardia be treated as if the tachycardia were ventricular tachycardia.[33,44] Therefore, lidocaine is the initial drug of choice for patients who are hemodynamically stable. If tachycardia persists after lidocaine loading and patients remain hemodynamically stable, intravenous adenosine should be administered. This is usually effective in converting PSVT to sinus rhythm and produces little harm in patients with ventricular tachycardia. It should be given intravenously as a 6-mg infusion over 1 to 3 seconds and, if tachycardia persists, as a 12-mg infusion over 1 to 3 seconds. If hemodynamically stable wide-complex tachycardia is still present, patients should be treated with intravenous procainamide (20 to 30 mg/min; maximum dose, 17 mg/kg). If that regimen is unsuccessful, intravenous bretylium (5 to 10 mg/kg over 8 minutes) may be given. If these agents do not restore sinus rhythm or if patients develop hemodynamic instability, synchronized cardioversion should be used. It is essential that verapamil not be given to patients with wide-complex tachycardia of unknown origin because it may accelerate the heart rate and cause hypotension in patients with Wolff-Parkinson-White syndrome or ventricular tachycardia.

PERIOPERATIVE CONDUCTION ABNORMALITIES

In the perioperative period, sinus bradycardia and a Mobitz I type of second-degree AV block are common. Mobitz I AV block is a progressive prolongation of the PR interval until a P wave is not conducted to the ventricles. The P wave that follows is conducted to the ventricles with a PR interval that is shorter than the PR interval that was associated with the last conducted P wave. These conduction abnormalities usually result from enhanced vagal tone and, if they are hemodynamically significant, typically respond to 0.5 to 1 mg of intravenous atropine.

A Mobitz II type of second-degree AV block (a fixed PR interval with P wave conduction to ventricles blocked on a constant [eg, 2:1, 3:1, 4:1] or variable basis) is usually caused by diffuse disease of the conduction system distal to the AV node. Many patients with this conduction disturbance are at high risk for progression to complete heart block, and a means of providing temporary-demand cardiac pacing should be available in the event this occurs. New-onset Mobitz II AV block in the perioperative period should initiate a search for myocardial ischemia or myocardial infarction.

Third-degree AV block occurs when no atrial impulses reach the ventricles. An associated ventricular rate of 40 to 60 beats/min with normal-appearing QRS complexes suggests that the escape rhythm is originating at the level of the AV node. This type of heart block may result from enhanced vagal tone; medications that depress AV nodal conduction (eg, β-blockers, digitalis preparations); and, less commonly, AV nodal ischemia. It is often reversible and may respond to the administration of intravenous atropine or the discontinuation of offending pharmacologic agents. If complete heart block is associated with a ventricular escape rate of 20 to 40 beats/min and the QRS complex is wide, the escape rhythm is originating from the ventricles. This strongly suggests the presence of extensive conduction system disease and warrants the placement of a cardiac pacemaker.[45]

Chronic bifascicular block (ie, right bundle-branch block with either left anterior hemiblock or left posterior hemiblock, or left bundle-branch block) rarely progresses to advanced hemodynamically significant heart block in the perioperative period. In eight studies evaluating a total of 339 patients with chronic bifascicular block, only 1 patient developed perioperative complete heart block. This was transient and occurred during endotracheal intubation. Given these findings, the insertion of a temporary transvenous pacemaker is not indicated for this patient population.[46-50]

Possible exceptions are patients with preexisting left bundle-branch block who are undergoing perioperative pulmonary artery catheterization. Transient right bundle-branch block, which is well tolerated in normal patients, may occur in as many as 5% of patients who undergo pulmonary artery catheterization.[51] Transient complete heart block has been reported in patients with preexisting left bundle-branch block who have developed acute right bundle-branch block related to this procedure.[52,53] Given the potential for this significant complication, a method for pacing the left ventricle should be available in the event complete heart block develops in this clinical setting. A temporary pacemaker should be inserted before surgery if patients meet the criteria for permanent implantation and a pacing device has not been implanted (Table 8-2).

MANAGEMENT OF PERMANENT CARDIAC PACEMAKERS

Permanent pacemakers should be tested before and after surgery. The most significant pacemaker problem in the perioperative period is pacemaker inhibition resulting from electrocautery-induced electromagnetic interference. Most VVI pacemakers are inhibited by electromagnetic interference. This may be prevented by programming the pacemaker to a fixed-rate mode or by placing a magnet over the pacemaker generator, which causes the pacemaker to fire at

TABLE 8-2. Indications for Implantation of Cardiac Pacemakers

Complete heart block (permanent or intermittent) associated with:
  Symptomatic bradycardia
  Congestive heart failure
  Arrhythmia requiring drugs that suppress escape rhythm
  Documented asystole ≥3 seconds or escape rate less than
    40 beats/min
Second-degree atrioventricular block with symptomatic
  bradycardia
Bifascicular block with intermittent complete heart block with
  symptomatic bradycardia
Symptomatic bifascicular block with intermittent type II second-
  degree atrioventricular block
Sinus node dysfunction with documented symptomatic
  bradycardia
Persistent, advanced second-degree atrioventricular block or
  complete heart block after acute myocardial infarction

(Adapted from Frye R, Collins JJ, DeSanctis RW, et al. Guidelines for permanent pacemaker implantation. Circulation 1984;70:331A)

a fixed rate. Other measures include placing the electrocautery ground plate as far away from the pacemaker as possible, not using cautery in the vicinity of the pacemaker generator and lead, and limiting the frequency and duration of
electrocautery to no more than 1-second bursts at least 10
seconds apart.[54] In addition to inhibiting pacemaker function, electromagnetic interference may reprogram the pacemaker or permanently damage the pulse generator. Because there is no industry-wide standardized response to
electromagnetic interference, it is important that data regarding the individual pacemaker response to electromagnetic interference be obtained from the pacemaker manufacturer.[55] Magnetic resonance imaging may also cause
pacemaker malfunction and is contraindicated in patients
with permanent pacemakers.[56]

A relatively recent advance in pacemaker technology is
the "rate-adaptive" pacemaker system. It has been devised
to facilitate a change in heart rate in response to a change in
the desired cardiac output. Various biologic parameters
have been used to trigger heart rate responses, including
patients' levels of physical activity, body temperature, and
minute ventilation. Although no studies are available regarding the management of these pacemaker systems in the
perioperative period, intraoperative hyperventilation has
been reported to cause pacemaker-induced tachycardia in
patients with pacemakers that are responsive to changes in
minute ventilation. It has been suggested that these pacemakers be reprogrammed to exclude the rate-responsive
function before patients undergo surgery involving intraoperative hyperventilation (eg, neurosurgery).[57]

PATIENTS WITH AUTOMATIC IMPLANTABLE CARDIOVERTER-DEFIBRILLATORS

For patients who have survived sudden cardiac death attributed to ventricular tachycardia, the automatic implantable cardioverter-defibrillator (AICD) is an effective
means of preventing death. Experience with the AICD in
patients undergoing noncardiac surgery is limited. A
physician familiar with the devices should assess AICD
function before and after noncardiac surgery. AICD function also may be adversely affected by perioperative
electromagnetic interference (ie, electrocautery). Finally,
patients with AICDs usually have significant left ventricular dysfunction, often with ischemic heart disease, and
require close observation during the perioperative
period.[58]

SPECIAL CARDIAC RHYTHM AND CONDUCTION PROBLEMS IN THE PERIOPERATIVE PERIOD

LONG-QT SYNDROME

The long-QT syndrome is characterized by a prolonged QT
interval when corrected for heart rate, malignant ventricular arrhythmias (classically the torsades de pointes form of
ventricular tachycardia), and the risk of sudden death. It
may occur as an idiopathic form (congenital with deafness
[autosomal recessive Jervell and Lange-Nielsen syndrome],
congenital without deafness [autosomal dominant Ro-
mano-Ward syndrome], sporadic without deafness) or be
acquired as a result of a drug or metabolic abnormality
(Table 8-3).

The approach to patients in the perioperative period depends on whether the long-QT syndrome is idiopathic
(congenital) or acquired. Idiopathic long-QT syndrome is
adrenergic-dependent, and ventricular arrhythmias are typically provoked by sympathetic stimulation (ie, pain, fear,
physical exertion).[59] Patients with idiopathic long-QT syndrome who have one or more risk factors for syncope or
sudden cardiac death should receive long-term maximal β-
blockade.[60] Risk factors for syncope or sudden cardiac
death include congenital deafness, female sex, history of
syncope or sudden cardiac death, and prior torsades de
pointes or ventricular fibrillation. Left cervicothoracic sympathectomy, permanent cardiac pacing, or the placement of
an implantable cardiac defibrillator have been suggested
for patients who have recurrent syncope despite maximal
β-blockade.[61]

For patients with idiopathic long-QT syndrome, we pro-

TABLE 8–3. Causes of Acquired Long-QT Syndrome

Antiarrhythmic Drugs
Type IA antiarrhythmic drugs (quinidine, procainamide, disopyramide)
Amiodarone
Sotalol

Noncardiac Drugs
Phenothiazines
Tricyclic and tetracyclic antidepressants
Antihistamines (H$_1$ type such as astemizole, terfenadine)
Antibiotics (erythromycin)

Metabolic and Electrolyte Disorders
Hypokalemia
Hypomagnesemia
Nutritional disorders (starvation, liquid protein diets)

Central Nervous System Disorders
Subarachnoid hemorrhage
Intracerebral hemorrhage
Head trauma
Encephalitis

(Adapted from Ben-David J, Zipes D. Torsades de pointes and proarrhythmia. Lancet 1993;341:1578)

vide perioperative β-blockade to blunt the adrenergic response to surgery. β-Blockers also shift the rate-adjusted QT interval to the normal range, which may contribute to their efficacy. We do not use anesthetic agents that may prolong the QT interval, such as succinylcholine, propofol, enflurane, or halothane.[62] Although isoflurane has been demonstrated to prolong the QT interval in normal patients, it shortens the QT interval in patients with the long-QT syndrome and has been proposed as an acceptable anesthetic agent for this patient group.[63] Thiopental also has been reported to prolong the QT interval in normal patients but to have no adverse effect in patients with long-QT syndrome.[64] Finally, we minimize sympathetic stimulation and provide adequate sedation to blunt the adrenergic response to surgery.

In patients who have acquired long-QT syndrome, we discontinue administration of the offending drug or correct the metabolic or electrolyte abnormality before undertaking surgery.

Despite these measures, malignant ventricular arrhythmias may still occur in the perioperative period. The treatment of ventricular ectopy is the same for idiopathic and acquired long-QT syndrome. Intravenous magnesium sulfate, 1 to 2 g over 1 or 2 minutes, followed by the same dose infused over 1 hour is often effective in restoring regular rhythm. Immediate ventricular pacing should be used if magnesium sulfate is ineffective. Intravenous isoproterenol may be used cautiously to increase the heart rate and sup-

press the ventricular arrhythmia until temporary ventricular pacing is achieved. If these measures cannot be attempted or are unsuccessful, external defibrillation should be performed.[65]

PATIENTS WITH CARDIAC TRANSPLANTS WHO REQUIRE NONCARDIAC SURGERY

Cardiac physiology is altered after cardiac transplantation. Because the transplanted heart is denervated, cardiac reflexes mediated by the autonomic nervous system are blunted or absent. As a result, heart rate abnormalities may be seen in the perioperative period. The resting heart rate is higher than normal but the heart rate response to stress is less than that of an innervated heart. When the heart rate does increase as a result of stress, it does so gradually in response to increased circulating catecholamines. Reflex tachycardia does not occur in response to vasodilation or volume loss. The effect of certain cardiac drugs on cardiac conduction is altered. Agents that affect the heart indirectly through their action on the autonomic nervous system are generally ineffective. Therefore, the chronotropic effect of atropine is absent, as is the AV nodal inhibitory effect of digoxin. The antiarrhythmic efficacy of β-blockers and verapamil is unchanged. The transplanted heart becomes overly sensitive to adenosine, and reduced doses (ie, one-third to one-half lower than those given to patients with intact cardiac innervation) should be used when this drug is administered to control arrhythmias.[66,67]

BRADYARRHYTHMIAS AFTER ACUTE SPINAL CORD INJURY

Acute injury to the cervical spinal cord is frequently accompanied by clinically significant bradyarrhythmias and, in some cases, hypotension. Acute autonomic dysfunction is thought to be the cause. Sympathetic nerves exit the spinal cord in preganglionic fibers at the first through fourth thoracic levels. With a complete cervical spinal cord lesion, sympathetic control from higher centers is interrupted. Parasympathetic control, which is mediated by the vagus nerve, is unaffected by spinal cord interruption. The clinical picture, therefore, is one of unopposed parasympathetic activity in the setting of markedly reduced sympathetic activity. Sympathetic stimulation with low-dose isoproterenol has been used in several patients for the treatment of clinically significant bradyarrhythmias. In one series, these cardiovascular abnormalities were found to resolve within 14 days of acute cervical spinal cord injury. The reason for resolution is not known but may be related to adaptive sympathetic disinhibition (ie, loss of reflex sympathetic inhibitory control from higher centers or increase in the number and function of adrenergic receptors).[68]

REFERENCES

1. Marchlinski F. Arrhythmias and conduction disturbances in surgical patients. In: Goldman D, ed. Medical care of the surgical patient. Philadelphia, JB Lippincott, 1982:59–77.
2. Kuner J, Enescu V, Utsu F, et al. Cardiac arrhythmias during anesthesia. Dis Chest 1967;52:580–587.
3. O'Kelly B, Browner WS, Massie B, et al. Ventricular arrhythmias in patients undergoing noncardiac surgery: The Study of Perioperative Ischemia Research Group. JAMA 1991;268:217–221.
4. Goldman L, Caldera DL, Nussbaum SR, et al. Multifactorial index of cardiac risk in noncardiac surgical procedures. N Engl J Med 1977;297:845–850.
5. Zeldin R. Assessing cardiac risk in patients who undergo noncardiac surgical procedures. Can J Surg 1984;27:402–404.
6. Detsky AS, Abrams HB, McLaughlin JR, et al. Predicting cardiac complications in patients undergoing non-cardiac surgery. J Gen Intern Med 1986;1:211–219.
7. Multicenter Postinfarction Research Group. Risk stratification and survival after myocardial infarction. N Engl J Med 1983;309:331–336.
8. Kennedy HL, Whitlock JA, Sprague MK, et al. Long-term follow-up of asymptomatic healthy subjects with frequent and complex ventricular ectopy. N Engl J Med 1985;24:193–197.
9. Goldman L. Supraventricular tachyarrhythmias in hospitalized adults after surgery: clinical correlates in patients over 40 years of age after major noncardiac surgery. Chest 1987;73:450–454.
10. Sebel PS, Bovill JG. Opioid analgesics in cardiac anesthesia. In: Kaplan JA, ed. Cardiac anesthesia. Orlando, Grune & Stratton, 1987:67–123.
11. Marymount JH, O'Connor BS. Postoperative cardiovascular complications. In: Veder JS, Spiess BD, eds. Post anesthesia care. Philadelphia, WB Saunders, 1992:42.
12. Underwood SM, Glynn CJ. Sick sinus syndrome manifest after spinal anaesthesia. Anaesthesia 1988;43:307–309.
13. Doyle DJ, Mark PW. Reflex bradycardia during surgery. Can J Anaesth 1990;37:219–222.
14. Merli GJ, Weitz H, Martin JH, et al. Cardiac dysrhythmias associated with ophthalmic atropine. Arch Intern Med 1986;146:45–47.
15. Mishra P, Calvey TN, Williams NE, et al. Intraoperative bradycardia and hypotension associated with timolol and pilocarpine eye drops. Br J Anaesth 1983;55:897–899.
16. Pritchett EL. Management of atrial fibrillation. N Engl J Med 1992;326:1264–1271.
17. Laupacis A, Albers G, Dunn M, et al. Antithrombotic therapy in atrial fibrillation. Chest 1992;102:426S–433S.
18. Fenster PE, Comess KA, Marsh R, et al. Conversion of atrial fibrillation to sinus rhythm by acute intravenous procainamide infusion. Am Heart J 1983;106:501–504.
19. Petersen P, Boysen G, Godtfredsen J, et al. Placebo-controlled, randomised trial of warfarin and aspirin for prevention of thromboembolic complications in chronic atrial fibrillation: the Copenhagen AFASAK study. Lancet 1989;1:175–179.
20. The Boston Area Anticoagulation Trial for Atrial Fibrillation Investigators. The effect of low-dose warfarin on the risk of stroke in patients with nonrheumatic atrial fibrillation. N Engl J Med 1990;323:1505–1511.
21. Stroke Prevention in Atrial Fibrillation Study: final results. Circulation 1991;84:527–539.
22. Connolly SJ, Laupacis A, Gent M, et al. Canadian Atrial Fibrillation Anticoagulation (CAFA) Study. J Am Coll Cardiol 1991;18:349–355.
23. Velebit V, Podrid P, Lown B, et al. Aggravation and provocation of ventricular arrhythmias by antiarrhythmic drugs. Circulation 1982;65:886–894.
24. Fenster PE, Perrier D. Applications of pharmacokinetic principles to cardiovascular drugs. Mod Concepts Cardiovasc Dis 1982;51:91–96.
25. Greenspon AJ, Kidwell GA, Hurley W, et al. Amiodarone-related postoperative adult respiratory distress syndrome. Circulation 1991;84(Suppl 3):407–415.
26. Tuczu M, Maloney JD, Sangani F, et al. Effects of amiodarone therapy on acute post-operative period of cardiac surgical patients. J Am Coll Cardiol 1986;7(Suppl A):91A.
27. Vanik PE, Davis HS. Cardiac arrhythmias during halothane anesthesia. Anesth Analg 1968;47:299–307.
28. Juler GL, Stemmer EA, Connolly JE, et al. Complications of prophylactic digitalization in thoracic surgical patients. J Thorac Cardiovasc Surg 1969;58:352–360.
29. Bergh NP, Dottori O, Malmberg R. Prophylactic digitalis in thoracic surgery. Scand J Resp Dis 1967;48:197–200.
30. Camm J, Ward D, Spurrell R. Response of atrial flutter to overdrive atrial pacing and intravenous disopyramide phosphate, singly and in combination. Br Heart J 1980;44:240–247.
31. Morganroth J, Horowitz LN, Anderson J, et al. Comparative efficacy and tolerance of esmolol to propranolol for control of supraventricular tachyarrhythmia. Am J Cardiol 1985;56:33F–39F.
32. Salem DN, Chuttani K, Isner JM. Assessment and management of cardiac disease in the surgical patient. Curr Probl Cardiol 1989;14:167–224.
33. Emergency Cardiac Care Committee and Subcommittees, American Heart Association. Guidelines for cardiopulmonary resuscitation and emergency cardiac care. Part III. Adult advanced cardiac life support. JAMA 1992;268:2199–2241.
34. Waxman HL, Myerburg RJ, Appel R, et al. Verapamil for control of ventricular rate in paroxysmal supraventricular tachycardia and atrial fibrillation or flutter: a double-blind randomized cross-over study. Ann Intern Med 1981;94:1–6.
35. Ellenbogen KA, Dias VC, Plumb VJ, et al. A placebo-controlled trial of continuous intravenous diltiazem infusion for 24-hour heart rate control during atrial fibrillation and atrial flutter: a multicenter study. J Am Coll Cardiol 1991;18:891–897.
36. Salerno DM, Dias VC, Kleiger RE, et al. Efficacy and safety of intravenous diltiazem for treatment of atrial fibrillation and atrial flutter: the Diltiazem–Atrial Fibrillation/Flutter Study Group. Am J Cardiol 1989;63:1046–1051.
37. Borgeat A, Goy JJ, Maendly R, et al. Flecainide versus quini-

dine for conversion of atrial fibrillation to sinus rhythm. Am J Cardiol 1986;58:496–498.

38. Salerno DM. Quinidine: worse than adverse? Circulation 1991;84:2196–2198.

39. Haines DE, DiMarco JP. Current therapy for supraventricular tachycardia. Curr Probl Cardiol 1992;17:411–477.

40. Mehta D, Wafa S, Ward DE, et al. Relative efficacy of various physical manoeuvres in the termination of junctional tachycardia. Lancet 1988;1181–1185.

41. Kastor JA. Multifocal atrial tachycardia. N Engl J Med 1990;322: 1713–1717.

42. Scher DL, Arsura EL. Multifocal atrial tachycardia: mechanisms, clinical correlates, and treatment. Am Heart J 1989;118: 574–550.

43. Habibzadeh MA. Multifocal atrial tachycardia: a 66 month follow-up of 50 patients. Heart Lung 1980;9:328–335.

44. Brugada P, Brugada J, Mont L, et al. A new approach to the differential diagnosis of a regular tachycardia with a wide QRS complex. Circulation 1991;83:1649–1659.

45. Tremblay DR, Fischer RL, Caouette CJ, et al. Arrhythmias in the PACU: a review. Crit Care Nurs Clin North Am 1991;3:95–108.

46. Bellocci F, Santarelli P, Di-Gennaro M, et al. The risk of cardiac complications in surgical patients with bifascicular block: a clinical and electrophysiologic study in 98 patients. Chest 1980;343:8.

47. Berg GR, Kotler MN. The significance of bilateral bundle branch block in the preoperative patient: a retrospective electrocardiographic and clinical study in 30 patients. Chest 1971;59:62–67.

48. Gertler MM, Finkle AL, Hudson PB, et al. Cardiovascular evaluation in surgery: I: Operative risk in cancer patients with bundle branch block. Surg Gynecol Obstet 1954;99:441–450.

49. Kunstadt D, Punja M, Cagin N, et al. Bifascicular block: a clinical and electrophysiologic study. Am Heart J 1973;86:173–181.

50. Venkataraman K, Madias JE, Hood WB Jr. Indications for prophylactic preoperative insertion of pacemakers in patients with right bundle branch block and left anterior hemiblock. Chest 1975;68:501–506.

51. Sprung CL, Pozen RG, Rozanski JJ, et al. Advanced ventricular arrhythmias during bedside pulmonary artery catheterization. Am J Med 1982;72:203–208.

52. Abernathy WS. Complete heart block caused by the Swan-Ganz catheter. Chest 1974;65:349.

53. Thomson IR, Dalton BC, Lappas DG, et al. Right bundle-branch block and complete heart block caused by the Swan-Ganz catheter. Anesthesiology 1979;51:359–362.

54. Simon AB. Perioperative management of the pacemaker patient. Anesthesiology 1977;46:127–131.

55. Shapiro WA, Roizen MF, Singleton MA, et al. Intraoperative pacemaker complications. Anesthesiology 1985;63:319–322.

56. Hayes DL, Holmes DR Jr, Gray JE. Effect of 1.5 tesla nuclear magnetic resonance imaging scanner on implanted permanent pacemakers. J Am Coll Cardiol 1987;10:782–786.

57. Madsen GM, Andersen C. Pacemaker-induced tachycardia during general anaesthesia: a case report. Br J Anaesth 1989;63:360–361.

58. Carr CM, Whiteley SM. The automatic implantable cardioverter-defibrillator: implications for anaesthetists. Anaesthesia 1991;46:737–740.

59. Jackman WM, Friday KJ, Anderson JL, et al. The long QT syndromes: a critical review, new clinical observations and a unifying hypothesis. Prog Cardiovasc Dis 1988;31:115–172.

60. Moss AJ, Schwartz PJ, Crampton RS, et al. The long QT syndrome: a prospective international study. Circulation 1985;71: 17–21.

61. Ben-David J, Zipes DP. Torsades de pointes and proarrhythmia. Lancet 1993;341:1578–1582.

62. Richardson MG, Roark GL, Helfaer MA. Intraoperative epinephrine-induced torsades de pointes in a child with long QT syndrome. Anesthesiology 1992;76:647–649.

63. Medak R, Benumof JL. Perioperative management of the prolonged Q-T interval syndrome. Br J Anaesth 1983;55:361–364.

64. Wilton NC, Hantler CB. Congenital long QT syndrome: changes in QT interval during anesthesia with thiopental vecuronium fentanyl and isoflurane. Anesth Analg 1987;66: 357–360.

65. Emergency Cardiac Care Committee and Subcommittees, American Heart Association. Guidelines for cardiopulmonary resuscitation and emergency cardiac care. Part III. Adult advanced cardiac life support. JAMA 1992;268:2199–2241.

66. Ellenbogen KA, Thames MD, DiMarco JP, et al. Electrophysiological effects of adenosine in the transplanted human heart: evidence of supersensitivity. Circulation 1990;81:821–828.

67. O'Connell JB, Bourge RC, Costanzo-Nordin MR, et al. Cardiac transplantation: recipient selection, donor procurement, and medical follow-up: a statement for health professionals from the Committee on Cardiac Transplantation of the Council on Clinical Cardiology, American Heart Association. Circulation 1992;86:1061–1079.

68. Lehmann KG, Lane JG, Piepmeier JM, et al. Cardiovascular abnormalities accompanying acute spinal cord injury in humans: incidence, time course and severity. J Am Coll Cardiol 1987;10:46–52.

69. Rocco AG, Vandam LD. Changes in circulation consequent in manipulation during abdominal surgery. JAMA 1957;164:14–18.

70. Seltzer JL, Ritter DE, Starsnic MA, et al. The hemodynamic response to traction on the abdominal mesentery. Anesthesiology 1985;63:96–99.

71. Sullivan S, Watson WC. Acute transient hypotension as complication of percutaneous liver biopsy. Lancet 1974;1:389–390.

72. Doyle DJ, Mark PW. Laparoscopy and vagal arrest. Anaesthesia 1989;44:448.

73. Robideaux V. Oculocardiac reflex caused by midface disimpaction. Anesthesiology 1978;49:433.

74. Hopkins CS. Bradycardia during neurosurgery: a new reflex? Anaesthesia 1988;43:157–158.

75. Podolakin W, Wells DG. Precipitous bradycardia induced by laryngoscopy in cardiac surgical patients. Can J Anaesth 1987; 34:618–621.

76. Matarasso A. The oculocardiac reflex in blepharoplasty surgery. Plast Reconstr Surg 1989;83:243–250.

Medical Management of the Surgical Patient, Third Edition,
edited by Michael F. Lubin, H. Kenneth Walker, and Robert B. Smith III.
J.B. Lippincott Company, Philadelphia, PA © 1995.

CHAPTER

9

POSTOPERATIVE CHEST PAIN AND SHORTNESS OF BREATH

Geno J. Merli
Michael F. Lubin

Chest pain and shortness of breath are frequently encountered medical problems in the postoperative period. The time at which they appear after surgery is important in determining their cause. This chapter reviews the possible causes for these presenting symptoms.

MYOCARDIAL INFARCTION

Chest pain in the postoperative period is always worrisome because of the possibility of myocardial infarction (MI). This concern is well founded. Mortality rates are 30% to 50% for a first perioperative MI and even higher for subsequent MIs in the perioperative period. Although no data are available concerning specific treatment in this situation, standard therapy for MI is likely to be helpful.

The incidence of postoperative MI is under 1% in patients who have no history of coronary disease compared to 6% in those with a history of previous MI. The incidence of postoperative MI has been reported to peak between 3 and 5 days after surgical procedures.[1] More recently, this peak has been found to occur as early as 24 to 48 hours after surgery.[2,3]

Two groups of patients appear to be at greatest risk for postoperative MIs and probably sustain the largest number of postoperative MIs as well: those with clinically diagnosed coronary artery disease and those with significant peripheral vascular disease.[4]

Diagnosing postoperative MI can be difficult. Incisional pain, gastrointestinal or respiratory complications, and sedative and pain medications may obscure symptoms. Pain typical of MI is commonly absent when MI occurs after surgery; many patients do not have chest pain. In Becker's study,[3] only 40% of patients had chest pain as a presenting complaint and in Charlson's study,[2] only 30% of patients with electrocardiographic (ECG) changes experienced chest pain.

Because chest pain does not occur in many patients, physicians must be aware of several other symptoms and signs that suggest the possibility of MI, including new or worsening heart failure, hypotension, arrhythmias, and even altered mental status, particularly in the elderly.

Patients' histories take just a few minutes to elicit and may be life-saving if either MI or ischemia is present. Chest pain does not always occur but is still a common symptom. Ischemic pain is generally described as heavy or pressing, or as a constriction in the substernal area. It may be spread over a large area of the chest and is rarely localized. The pain may radiate down the left arm or both arms. It is not influenced by position and may be associated with nausea, vomiting, weakness, diaphoresis, and, at times, the urge to defecate. The physical examination also can be helpful. The presence of overt heart failure with distended neck veins, rales, and an S_3 gallop in patients without other causes of heart failure is strong evidence of a postoperative MI. A new arrhythmia is also suggestive.

The ECG can provide helpful information but may also cause confusion. It cannot be emphasized too strongly that the absence of ECG changes in patients with chest pain does not rule out the diagnosis of cardiac ischemia or infarction. Many patients with acute MIs initially have normal ECGs, and many postoperative patients have ECG changes in the absence of MIs. If the ECG is normal, unchanged, or reveals nonspecific changes, clinicians must evaluate the possibility of MI on the basis of patients' histories, physical examinations, and other findings (ie, hypotension, arrhythmias). In the final analysis, it is important to protect patients and to admit those with suspicious findings to an intensive care area to rule out the possibility of MI.

Measurement of the creatine phosphokinase or CPK-MB levels also may be helpful. Although enzyme changes can be informative, these are basically retrospective tests and patients must be observed before the results become available. In addition, in Charlson's study,[2] many patients with mildly to moderately elevated levels, including CPK-MB levels above 5%, had no symptoms or signs of MI and no ECG changes. It appears that some patients with elevated CPK-MB levels after surgery do not have MIs. A recent paper by Adams and colleagues[5] suggests that cardiac troponin I may be a better biochemical marker of perioperative myocardial infarction with better sensitivity and specificity than creatine kinase MB. This test is just becoming available, and its usefulness and accuracy will need to be evaluated on a large scale.

All levels of information should be correlated in making the diagnosis of postoperative MI. Patients with suggestive symptoms, signs, and ECG changes clearly have MIs, whereas those with elevated creatine phosphokinase levels in the absence of the other criteria probably do not. Charlson and colleagues[2] have suggested several levels of diagnosis.

PULMONARY EMBOLISM

Pulmonary embolism is another serious cause of chest pain and is one of the leading causes of death in postoperative patients who have not received prophylaxis for deep venous thrombosis. Episodes of pulmonary embolism usually occur between 3 and 7 days after surgery. Patients with risk factors such as previous deep venous thrombosis or pulmonary embolism, long procedures, or older age who are undergoing high-risk operations such as orthopedic procedures have the greatest potential for the propagation of proximal clot and a higher incidence of pulmonary embolism.[6]

The most clearcut cause of chest pain in patients with pulmonary embolism is pulmonary infarction, but this occurs in under 10% of cases. The pain is pleuritic (ie, sharp or sticking pain that increases with respiration and is usually unaffected by position). Patients with pulmonary infarction often have hemoptysis. Many patients who have pulmonary embolism but do not have pulmonary infarction also have chest pain, which also may be pleuritic in nature.

Physical examinations in patients with documented pulmonary embolism may be entirely normal, although tachycardia is usually present. An increased pulmonic component of the second heart sound and, rarely, a right-sided S_3 may be heard. If pulmonary infarction has occurred, a pleural rub can often be detected. A few rales frequently are heard in the affected area.

The diagnosis of postoperative pulmonary embolus is addressed in more detail in Chapter 15, but some basic principles are mentioned here. Laboratory examination may be helpful. The ECG often shows only a sinus tachycardia; the QRS axis may be shifted to either the right or the left. Arterial blood gas levels usually, but not always, reveal significant hypoxia and a respiratory alkalosis with a low $P{CO_2}$. The chest radiograph may show basilar atelectasis but this is common in postoperative patients. If pulmonary infarction has occurred, there may be a dense infiltrate. It is important that pulmonary infarction be differentiated from a new bacterial pneumonia. Significant fever, cough, and sputum production point toward a diagnosis of pneumonia, although these may occur with pulmonary embolism as well.

GASTROESOPHAGEAL REFLUX

Gastroesophageal reflux is a common medical problem and a frequent cause of esophagitis in the postoperative period. The condition may be exacerbated by prolonged recumbency, abdominal surgery, medications, and the use of a nasogastric tube. It is a common cause of postoperative chest pain.

Substernal burning with water brash or regurgitation is common after surgery. These symptoms may occur at any time after operation, and gastroesophageal reflux should be suspected in patients with previous symptoms and those with prior histories of the problem. There also are infectious causes of esophagitis, including diabetes, malnutrition, acquired immunodeficiency syndrome, and debility. Drugs such as calcium antagonists, sedatives, and anticholinergic agents decrease lower esophageal sphincter pressure and may exacerbate gastroesophageal reflux in the postoperative period.[7]

PERICARDITIS

Pericarditis is an infrequent cause of chest pain in the postoperative period. It is seen mainly in patients undergoing cardiopulmonary bypass procedures. The characteristic pain of pericarditis is sharp, stabbing, and located in the midchest. It may be exacerbated by changes in position, especially lying down or twisting the trunk, and is usually relieved by sitting up and leaning forward. On physical examination, there is often an audible pericardial rub, although many patients have a brief rub or none at all. The rub may have one, two, or three components.

Pericarditis is usually an expected postoperative complication. It is usually seen immediately after the procedure and results from direct pericardial irritation. The postpericardiotomy syndrome generally occurs 1 to 3 weeks after the procedure and is probably immunologically mediated. Pericarditis may also be seen in the postoperative period in patients with acute or chronic renal failure.

SHORTNESS OF BREATH

Shortness of breath is another common postoperative complaint. It may be associated with many conditions, ranging from benign problems such as anxiety to life-threatening problems such as heart failure. A discussion of pulmonary causes of shortness of breath is presented in Chapter 15.

The symptom of shortness of breath must be differentiated from the physiologic derangement of hypoxia. Although they commonly occur together, either may be present without the other. In patients with emphysema or restrictive lung disease, for example, the resting PaO_2 may be relatively normal. Shortness of breath is common in such patients because the work involved in breathing with stiff lungs is greatly increased. In young patients with pneumonia, however, a significant degree of hypoxia may be present without any shortness of breath because the work of breathing may not be appreciably increased in young, otherwise healthy patients.

CONGESTIVE HEART FAILURE

Congestive heart failure occurs at two distinct times after surgery. Seventy percent of patients develop pulmonary edema within the first hour after reversal of anesthesia. Intraoperative fluid overload is the cause in most cases, although postoperative hypertension, anesthetic-induced myocardial dysfunction, and termination of positive-pressure ventilation are also important factors.[8] Congestive heart failure also occurs 24 to 48 hours after surgery because of the mobilization of interstitial fluid.[8] Although most cases of postoperative congestive heart failure result from volume overload, acute MI can also be the cause.

SUPRAVENTRICULAR TACHYCARDIA

Perioperative arrhythmias are common and occur in as many as 80% of patients during anesthesia and surgery.[9] These arrhythmias are not usually significant and include a wandering atrial pacemaker, atrioventricular dissociation, nodal rhythm, and sinus bradycardia. Under 5% of perioperative arrhythmias are clinically important.

Supraventricular tachycardia must be considered as a postoperative cause for shortness of breath. Narrow-complex supraventricular tachycardia, atrial fibrillation, and atrial flutter are the most important considerations. Appropriate intervention to correct the hemodynamic changes induced by these rhythms is necessary.

REFERENCES

1. Goldman L, Caldera D, Nussbaum S, et al. Multifactorial index of cardiac risk in noncardiac surgical procedures. N Engl J Med 1977;297:845–850.
2. Charlson ME, MacKenzie CR, Ales KL, et al. The post-operative electrocardiogram and creatine kinase: implications for diagnosis of myocardial infarction after non-cardiac surgery. J Clin Epidemiol 1989;42:25–34.
3. Becker RC, Underwood DA. Myocardial infarction in patients undergoing noncardiac surgery. Cleve Clin J Med 1987;54:25–28.
4. Ashton CM, Petersen NJ, Wray NP, et al. The incidence of perioperative myocardial infarction in men undergoing noncardiac surgery. Ann Intern Med 1993;118:504–510.
5. Adams JE, Sicard GA, Allen BT, et al. Diagnosis of perioperative myocardial infarction with measurement of cardiac troponin I. N Engl J Med 1994;330:670–674.
6. Hull R, Raskob G, Hirsch J. Prophylaxis of venous thromboembolism: an overview. Chest 1986;85:379–383.
7. Gordon S, Chatzinoff M, Peiken S. Medical care of the surgical patient with gastrointestinal disease. Med Clin North Am 1987; 71:433–452.
8. Cooperman L, Price H. Pulmonary edema in the operative and postoperative period: a review of 40 cases. Ann Surg 1970;172: 883–891.
9. Goldman L. Supraventricular tachyarrhythmias in hospitalized adults after surgery. Chest 1978;73:450–454.

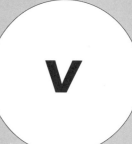

HYPERTENSION

Medical Management of the Surgical Patient, Third Edition,
edited by Michael F. Lubin, H. Kenneth Walker, and Robert B. Smith III.
J.B. Lippincott Company, Philadelphia, PA © 1995.

CHAPTER

PREOPERATIVE AND POSTOPERATIVE HYPERTENSION

10

W. Dallas Hall

PREOPERATIVE HYPERTENSION

Hypertension is one of the most common disorders of adult patients undergoing elective or emergency surgery.[1] Table 10-1 summarizes seven studies that have assessed patient outcome with regard to the presence or absence of preoperative hypertension.[2–9] Operative mortality ranged from 0% to 17%, and patient outcome depended on the population studied, the type of surgical procedure done, and the era in which the surgery and anesthesia were performed. The fact that patients with severe and uncontrolled hypertension could survive major surgery was established in the 1930s and 1940s, when mortality in such patients was noted to be 3.6% after thoracolumbar sympathectomy.[3]

In general, patients with hypertensive heart disease are at considerably greater risk than are patients with uncomplicated hypertension.[5,6] Goldman and colleagues[8,9] correlated multiple risk factors with adverse cardiac outcome in 1000 adult patients undergoing major noncardiac surgery. They defined adverse cardiac outcome as cardiac death, or nonfatal but life-threatening cardiac complications, and found that it was not significantly associated with a history of hypertension or with preoperative hypertension alone. Common target organ manifestations of hypertension (congestive heart failure or renal impairment with a blood urea nitrogen level exceeding 50 or a creatinine level greater than 3 mg/100 mL), however, predicted adverse cardiac outcome. Hence, one reasonably accepted conclusion is that

mortality from anesthesia and surgery among patients with hypertension is considerably higher in those who have target organ complications (hypertensive heart disease, congestive heart failure, or renal impairment) than in those who do not. When the hypertension is not severe and target organ damage is not present, the data are less conclusive. Goldman and Caldera[10] found no significant increase in the incidence of adverse effects from relatively uncomplicated and untreated hypertension when the preoperative diastolic blood pressure was 110 mmHg or less.

The risks of hypertension are particularly manifest in patients with underlying heart disease.[11,12] Four large series indicate a 4% to 8% risk of postoperative myocardial infarction in groups of cardiac patients undergoing nonthoracic surgery[13–16] (Table 10-2). The risk of acute myocardial infarction in the immediate postoperative period is greater for these particular patients with preoperative hypertension and is increased further for patients with recent myocardial infarction (occurring within the past 6 months). Moreover, the 28% to 69% mortality of postoperative myocardial infarction greatly exceeds that of myocardial infarction in nonsurgical patients.

EVALUATION

Proper evaluation of patients with preoperative hypertension should center on a careful search for evidence of target organ damage. Routine preoperative laboratory tests

95

TABLE 10–1. Anesthesia and Surgery in Patients With Hypertension: Mortality in Seven Large Series, 1953–1978

Authors and Year	Type of Surgery	Number of Patients	Patients Seen	Mortality Rate
Smithwick and Thompson, 1953[2]	Splanchnicectomy	1266	Severe high blood pressure	2.5% overall; 11% if grade IV high blood pressure
Dana and Ohler, 1956[3]	Major noncardiac	101	Heart disease	0% in patients with high blood pressure
Nachlas et al, 1961[4]	Elective and emergency nonthoracic	165	Heart disease	10.5%
Skinner and Pearce, 1964[5]	Major noncardiac	766	Heart disease	13% if hypertensive heart disease
Stahlgren, 1961[6]	Elective and emergency abdominal	102	Age ≥70 years	16.6% if hypertensive heart disease
Benson et al, 1968[7]	Closed mitral valvuloplasty	1595	Age <60 years	9.7% in 124 patients with high blood pressure; 4.6% in 1265 patients with normal blood pressure
Goldman et al, 1977, 1978[8,9]	Major noncardiac	1001	Age >40 years	5.9%

should include, at a minimum, a complete blood count, urinalysis, and determinations of the serum potassium and serum creatinine levels. In addition, a chest radiograph and an electrocardiogram (ECG) should always be performed before surgery in adult patients, especially the elderly.[17–19]

Heart

Left ventricular hypertrophy is the hallmark of hypertensive cardiovascular disease and signals an increased risk of congestive heart failure and coronary artery disease. Left ventricular hypertrophy may be manifested by a sustained precordial apical impulse on physical examination, or it may be apparent on the chest radiograph or the ECG. Evidence of congestive heart failure includes distended neck veins, an S_3 gallop, pulsus alternans, and changes on the chest radiograph. Such evidence constitutes one of the strongest predictors of increased operative morbidity and mortality.[9] Hypertension is the leading cause of congestive heart failure; the Framingham study reported a 5-year survival of about 50% for patients with hypertension and congestive heart failure.[20] Thus, heart failure is a prognostic marker that may influence the decision to proceed with cer-

TABLE 10–2. Postoperative Myocardial Infarction After Noncardiac Surgery in Patients With Underlying Cardiac Disease

Authors and Year	Type of Surgery	Number of Patients	Underlying Cardiac Disease	Postoperative Myocardial Infarction	Comments
Tarhan et al, 1972[13]	Nonthoracic	422	Past MI	6.6%	10 of the 28 patients (36%) with acute postoperative MIs had preoperative high blood pressure
Mauney et al, 1970[14]	Major, excluding cardiac valve	360	Abnormal ECG (ischemia, LVH, LBBB)	8.3%	17 of 30 patients (56%) with postoperative MIs had hypertensive heart disease
Steen et al, 1978[15]	Noncardiac	587	Past MI	6.1%	17 of 181 patients (9.4%) with preoperative high blood pressure had postoperative reinfarction
Ashton et al, 1993[16]	Noncardiac	319	Past MI, angina, positive angiogram, or past CABPG	4.1%	7 of 15 men with perioperative MIs had histories of high blood pressure

MI, myocardial infarction; LVH, left ventricular hypertrophy; LBBB, left bundle-branch block; CABPG, coronary artery bypass graft.

tain surgical procedures. The ECG should be evaluated for the presence of premature ventricular contractions and premature atrial contractions, because an increased risk of cardiac death has been noted in surgical patients who have more than five premature ventricular contractions per minute and in those who have premature atrial contractions on the preoperative ECG.[8,9]

Kidneys

Renal failure in patients with hypertension is usually caused by nephrosclerosis, although primary renoparenchymal disease should be suspected if the urinalysis reveals proteinuria, hematuria, or pyuria. Serum creatinine levels greater than 1.5 mg/100 mL in adults generally indicate some degree of renal insufficiency. Levels in the range of 1.2 to 1.4, however, are often abnormal in patients with a small muscle mass, pregnant women, and the elderly. Even mild degrees of renal insufficiency may be associated with an adverse surgical outcome. Any degree of renal failure can limit the body's ability to excrete salt, water, potassium, or drugs that are cleared primarily by the kidney.

Brain

Patients with chronic hypertension have a defect in the autoregulation of cerebral blood flow.[21] Unlike patients with normal blood pressure, in whom normal brain perfusion is maintained with mean arterial pressures as low as 60 mmHg, patients with chronic hypertension often have reduced cerebral blood flow if the mean arterial pressure falls below 110 to 120 mmHg. Therefore, the documentation of chronic hypertension may indicate an exaggerated risk for any intraoperative hypotension. A careful neurologic examination is necessary to detect residual damage from a previous stroke. The carotid arteries should also be auscultated, although there is no evidence that preoperative detection of a carotid bruit is associated with an increased risk of postoperative stroke.[22]

Careful examination of the fundi can reveal hypertensive hemorrhages or exudates that imply severe hypertension with its associated surgical and anesthetic risks, regardless of the blood pressure reading. Hypertensive retinal hemorrhages and exudates also signal an increased likelihood of damage in other organs, such as the heart and kidney.

SCREENING FOR PHEOCHROMOCYTOMA IN SELECTED PATIENTS

Special attention must be given to preoperative screening for pheochromocytoma, because anesthesia and surgery are associated with a mortality rate of 50% or higher in patients undergoing various surgical procedures in the presence of unsuspected pheochromocytoma.[23] Fortunately, this condition is rare and generally causes headaches, palpitations, and excessive sweating. Measurement of the urinary metanephrine level is the most sensitive and useful screening test.[24] A ratio of metanephrine (in micrograms) to creatinine (in milligrams) higher than 1.0 suggests that further diagnostic tests are necessary before nonemergency surgical procedures are undertaken. The possibility of pheochromocytoma always must be considered when patients with hypertension complain of headaches, palpitations, or sweating, or have labile blood pressures or tachyarrhythmias before operation.

TREATMENT OF PATIENTS RECEIVING ANTIHYPERTENSIVE MEDICATIONS

Therapy in patients with adequate blood pressure control usually should be continued until the day of surgery. In those with poor medical control of their hypertension, nonemergency surgery should be postponed pending further reduction in the blood pressure. Control is inadequate in patients with diastolic pressures exceeding 110 mmHg, and many prefer that these pressures be reduced to less than 100 mmHg. The adequacy of blood pressure control generally should be determined by obtaining a series of blood pressure readings over 12 to 24 hours rather than a single reading the night before or the morning of elective surgery. Minor adjustments of the drug dosage improve control in most patients.

Diuretics

Diuretics further reduce the already low plasma volume of most patients with essential hypertension.[25] During chronic therapy, the plasma volume returns toward normal, although it remains somewhat low. Considerable losses of intravascular volume can occur during surgery, exaggerating the risks of hypovolemia in patients with hypertension who are receiving diuretics. Decreases in extracellular fluid volume during surgery correlate with the extent of surgical trauma, independent of blood loss.[26] These observations led to the general principle of preoperative volume expansion to prevent hypotension after induction, anesthesia, and surgery.[27]

The antihypertensive effect of the thiazide diuretics usually lasts for 1 to 4 weeks after therapy is discontinued.[28] In most patients with controlled hypertension and no heart failure, chronic diuretic therapy may be discontinued cautiously a few days before surgery. Additional volume expansion may still be required in the immediate preoperative period.

Hypokalemia is a relatively frequent complication of diuretic therapy. It is undesirable in patients who are scheduled for surgery for three reasons: (1) possible potentiation of the effects of muscle relaxants, (2) an increased risk of arrhythmias, and (3) an increased occurrence of paralytic ileus.

Hypokalemia raises the resting membrane potential of muscle cells and potentiates the action of nondepolarizing muscle relaxants.[29] The hypokalemia-mediated increase in resting membrane potential is also associated with a relative resistance to the usual action of acetylcholine such that hypokalemia may simulate the effects of low-dose muscle relaxants. Some patients experience repeated curarization or respiratory depression when hypokalemia develops in the immediate postoperative period, particularly when relatively large doses of *d*-tubocurarine are required during prolonged or complicated surgery.[30] Potassium has an anticurare effect and can restore the response of curarized muscle to nerve stimulation. Thus, prolonged muscle paralysis or respiratory depression resulting from the use of nondepolarizing agents in patients with hypokalemia may be reversed after the administration of intravenous potassium chloride.[31] The response to muscle relaxants, however, depends on many variables other than the serum potassium concentration.[32] Therefore, it is not possible to predict that patients with hypokalemia will exhibit increased sensitivity to nondepolarizing muscle relaxants. Variable responses have also been observed after the use of depolarizing muscle relaxants (eg, succinylcholine) in patients with hypokalemia.

Patients receiving potassium-sparing diuretics may occasionally have elevated concentrations of serum potassium. Preoperative hyperkalemia is of particular concern, because cardiac asystole is possible if additional potassium is liberated into the serum. The administration of succinylcholine can increase serum potassium levels by 0.2 to 0.5 mEq/L.[33]

Many types of arrhythmias have been associated with hypokalemia and reversed after the administration of potassium, including atrial and ventricular premature contractions, atrial flutter, ventricular bigeminy, ventricular tachycardia, and ventricular fibrillation.[34–37] By far the most common are atrial or ventricular premature contractions. Hypokalemia may rarely be associated with a particular form of ventricular tachycardia known as torsades de pointes. This arrhythmia is characterized by paroxysms of tachycardia in which the QRS axis undulates in different directions, unlike the alternate-beat directional changes of bidirectional ventricular tachycardia.[36] Hypokalemia sensitizes the myocardium to the arrhythmogenic effects of digitalis, and supraventricular, junctional, or ventricular rhythms can occur with alarming frequency in patients with hypokalemia who are receiving digitalis.

Hypokalemia reduces intestinal tone and promotes the development of abdominal distention and paralytic ileus.[38,39] Lans and colleagues[40] reported significant abdominal distention with absent or markedly diminished bowel sounds in 31 of 309 surgical patients who had hypokalemia (serum potassium level less than 3.7 mEq/L) without evidence of bowel obstruction. The clinical signs may be confused with postoperative peritonitis or intestinal obstruction. Decompression by nasogastric suction may be ineffective and worsen the state of potassium depletion. Marked dilation and perforation of a normal cecum has been observed,[41] as has postoperative evisceration.[40] Lowman[39] observed significant radiographic improvement after potassium replacement therapy in 18 patients with hypokalemia who had postoperative ileus.

Reserpine

Early reports indicated impaired circulatory responses during anesthesia and surgery in patients with hypertension who were receiving maintenance therapy with *Rauwolfia* compounds.[42] Subsequent controlled trials involving a larger number of patients revealed no increase in the relative risk of hypotension in patients receiving reserpine compared with those with untreated hypertension or those who stopped taking reserpine before operation.[43] There is no reason to discontinue reserpine therapy in patients with hypertension who have adequate blood pressure control before surgery.

Methyldopa

Methyldopa (Aldomet) appears to lower the alveolar concentration of halothane necessary to maintain a given plane of anesthesia.[44] The effect is dose-related and has also been noted with reserpine and clonidine. Methyldopa generally may be taken until the time of surgery, because a residual pressure-lowering effect usually persists for at least 48 hours after its use is discontinued.[45] Acute increases in blood pressure are usually not observed on the day of surgery in patients with hypertension who received their usual doses of methyldopa the evening before.

α-Blockers

Doxazosin (Cardura), prazosin (Minipress), and terazosin (Hytrin) cause selective inhibition of postsynaptic α-receptors.[46,47] No specific adverse effects of α-blockers have been reported in conjunction with anesthesia or surgery.

Hydralazine

Hydralazine (Apresoline) is a direct vasodilator that generally is used in oral doses ranging between 25 and 100 mg twice a day. Peripheral vasodilation is usually associated with a reflex tachycardia that may provoke ischemic symptoms in patients with underlying coronary artery disease. Concomitant use of sympatholytic agents or β-blockers blunts the reflex tachycardia and associated adverse effects. The hypotensive effect of chronic hydralazine therapy dissipates 12 to 24 hours after use of the drug is discontinued. Hydralazine may be administered parenterally, in which case it is wise to begin with low doses (5 mg) to prevent the marked hypotension and reflex tachycardia that are occasionally observed after larger initial doses.

Minoxidil

Minoxidil (Loniten) is a potent direct vasodilator that generally is used in oral doses of 5 to 20 mg daily. Associated adverse effects of fluid retention and reflex tachycardia usually require the concomitant administration of β-blockers and loop diuretics. During maintenance therapy, the hypotensive effect of minoxidil often lasts for 24 to 72 hours or longer after use of the drug is discontinued.

β-Blockers

Viljoen and associates[48] first described myocardial depression, bradycardia, intraoperative cardiac failure, and poor responsiveness to sympathomimetic amines in five patients with advanced coronary artery disease who received propranolol up to the day of cardiac surgery. Others noted a decrease in cardiac output and heart rate and an increase in central venous pressure when either selective or nonselective β-blockers were given intravenously to healthy young women after anesthetic induction for minor gynecologic surgery.[49] Because of this myocardial depressant effect, they advised against the injudicious use of β-blockers for control of arrhythmias during anesthesia and surgery. These and other observations led to the recommendation in the early 1970s that β-blocker administration generally should be discontinued 24 to 48 hours before surgical procedures.[50]

Subsequent reports, however, documented no increased risk associated with the continuation of propranolol therapy until the time of cardiac surgery.[51] Moreover, abrupt discontinuation was found to be associated with a higher risk of arrhythmias, worsening angina, myocardial infarction, and death in patients with symptomatic coronary artery disease.[52] Hence, data suggest that maintenance therapy generally should be continued before operation, with the last dose given between 10:00 PM the evening before and 8:00 AM the day of anticipated surgery.[53,54]

Many different β-blockers have been shown to be effective in blocking dysrhythmias provoked by catecholamines, endotracheal intubation, or surgical stimulation.[55,56]

Stone and associates[57] reported the results of monitoring for myocardial ischemia during anesthesia and surgery in patients with uncomplicated hypertension who were receiving atenolol (long-term therapy in 14 patients and a single dose of 50 mg 2 hours before induction in 30 patients), long-term diuretic therapy (7 patients), or no antihypertensive therapy (39 patients). Myocardial ischemia was detected during anesthesia and surgery in 11 of 39 untreated patients, 4 of 7 diuretic-treated patients, and none of 44 atenolol-treated patients.

Clonidine

Clonidine (Catapres) dosage schedules less frequent than twice a day are inappropriate because certain patients may demonstrate an exacerbation of high blood pressure within 18 to 36 hours if use of the drug is discontinued abruptly.[58] Clonidine withdrawal syndrome is suggested by the presence of tachycardia, extreme levels of blood pressure, and a short interval during which the blood pressure increases after therapy is discontinued. When the last dose of clonidine is given on the day before operation, markedly elevated blood pressures can be seen on the morning of anticipated surgery, particularly if the operation has been delayed until late morning or early afternoon. Bruce and coworkers[59] recommend the administration of oral clonidine on the morning of surgery. This order must be implemented carefully because it conflicts with a simultaneously written order of "nothing by mouth after midnight." The transdermal clonidine patch requires about 48 hours for the onset or offset of its effect on blood pressure.

Kaukinen and associates[60] observed that hypertensive crisis was relieved by the repeated administration of clonidine in 2 of 10 patients in whom dosages of 0.1 to 0.3 mg three times a day were discontinued before the morning of surgery. No hypertensive crises were observed in 10 patients in whom clonidine therapy was continued using intramuscular injection* on the day of surgery. These results again suggest that oral maintenance therapy with clonidine should be continued without interruption on the morning of operation. Therapeutic approaches to clonidine-withdrawal hypertension include the reinstitution of clonidine therapy and the administration of sodium nitroprusside, phentolamine, or prazosin.

Calcium Channel Blockers

Calcium channel blockers are antihypertensive drugs that cause vasodilation by inhibiting intracellular transport of calcium through specific calcium channels.[61] The calcium channel blockers available in the United States are listed in Table 10-3, along with their usual starting doses. In general,

---

*Parenteral preparations of clonidine are not available in the United States.

TABLE 10–3. Calcium Channel Blockers

Generic Name	Trade Name	Usual Dose Range
Amlodipine*	Norvasc	5–10 mg qd
Diltiazem	Cardizem	30–120 mg tid
	Cardiazem SR	60–80 mg bid
	Cardiazem CD	180–360 mg qd
	Dilacor XR	180–480 mg qd
Felodipine*	Plendil	5–20 mg qd
Isradipine*	DynaCirc	2.5–10 mg qd
Nicardipine*	Cardene	20–40 mg tid
	Cardene SR	30–60 mg bid
Nifedipine*	Adalat	10–40 mg tid
	Procardia	10–40 mg tid
	Procardia XL	30–120 mg qd
Verapamil	Calan	40–240 mg bid
	Isoptin	40–240 mg bid
	Verelan	120–480 mg qd
	Calan SR	120–480 mg qd

*Dihydropyridine type of calcium channel blocker.

the dihydropyridines are more potent peripheral vasodilators than are diltiazem and verapamil but may cause more headaches, tachycardia, flushing, and edema. Sinus bradycardia and heart block are more common with diltiazem and verapamil. Data are available with regard to the use of calcium channel blockers in the perioperative setting.[62,63]

Angiotensin-Converting Enzyme Inhibitors

Angiotensin-converting enzyme (ACE) inhibitors block angiotensin-converting enzyme, thereby causing vasodilation by inhibiting the formation of the pressor substance, angiotensin II. The ACE inhibitors available in the United States are listed in Table 10-4, along with their usual starting doses. In addition to their antihypertensive efficacy, other useful features of ACE inhibitors include their beneficial effects on congestive heart failure, regression of left ventricular hypertrophy, and reduction of the rate at which renal failure progresses in patients with diabetes.[64] The most common adverse effect of ACE inhibitors is a dry cough. Few data are available regarding their use in perioperative settings.

THERAPY FOR PATIENTS WITH UNTREATED HYPERTENSION

Rationale for Treatment

Untreated patients with confirmed hypertension, particularly those with evidence of target organ damage, should receive therapy to control their blood pressures before sur-

gery.[1,65] The rationale for therapy is based primarily on the increased operative risks for patients with poorly controlled hypertension and on the need for protection from the risks of major blood pressure fluctuations during anesthesia and surgery.

Both cardiac output and blood pressure fall during steady-state anesthesia in patients with normal blood pressure, patients with untreated hypertension, and patients with treated hypertension.[66] Patients with untreated hypertension, however, experience greater absolute reductions in peripheral resistance and arterial pressure, often associated with electrocardiographic evidence of myocardial ischemia and dysrhythmias. Similar responses are observed in patients with hypertension who receive treatment but still have uncontrolled blood pressure before surgery. Thus, adverse circulatory changes in response to anesthesia are related to the preoperative blood pressure level rather than to the presence or absence of antihypertensive therapy. Continuous intraoperative monitoring of blood pressure and myocardial ischemia is appropriate for many patients with hypertension.[67]

Ryhänen and coworkers[68] have confirmed the increased cardiovascular lability and accentuated blood pressure fluctuations in patients with untreated hypertension compared with those with treated hypertension. Preoperative therapy reduced maximum fluctuations of blood pressure from 103.3/57.5 mmHg in the untreated group to 64.3/32.8 mmHg in the treated group.

Patients with untreated hypertension often exhibit marked reductions in blood pressure during anesthesia induction and significant blood pressure lability throughout the remainder of the anesthetic and surgical course.[69] The clinical significance of these major fluctuations during anesthesia and surgery should not be underestimated. Studies have shown an associated increase in the risk of general complications,[70] renal complications,[71] perioperative cardiac complications,[72] acute myocardial infarction,[14,15] post-

TABLE 10–4. Angiotensin-Converting Enzyme Inhibitors

Generic Name	Trade Name	Usual Dose Range*
Benazepril	Lotensin	10–40 mg qd
Captopril	Capoten	12.5–50 mg bid
Enalapril	Vasotec	2.5–40 mg qd
Fosinopril	Monopril	10–40 mg qd
Lisinopril	Prinivil/Zestril	5–40 mg qd
Quinapril	Accupril	5–80 mg qd
Ramipril	Altace	1.25–20 mg qd

*Diuretic doses should be reduced before starting ACE inhibitor administration whenever possible to prevent excessive hypotension. These are renally excreted, so the total daily dosage should be reduced with serum creatinine of 2.5 mg/dL or higher.

operative pulmonary edema, and cardiac death.[8,9] Although hypotension is a more common and feared complication than is hypertension, there is a two-fold risk of myocardial infarction in patients with heart disease who experience marked increases in systolic blood pressure lasting 10 minutes or more.[15]

Selection of Appropriate Drug Therapy

Whether to institute therapy for uncontrolled preoperative hypertension is no longer the question; the problem is selecting the most appropriate antihypertensive drugs to regulate blood pressure before surgery. Standard therapeutic regimens often begin with diuretic therapy, yet acute volume depletion is not desirable for usual surgical patients with no evidence of volume overload. Moreover, thiazide diuretics require days to weeks for optimal reduction of blood pressure, and loop diuretics such as furosemide effectively reduce volume but have only a minimal acute effect on blood pressure.[73] Accordingly, diuretics are not a logical first choice for preoperative antihypertensive therapy unless patients exhibit signs of excess volume. Clonidine is also undesirable because of potential problems with exacerbation of blood pressure elevation during the period that oral intake is restricted. The remaining choices for initial therapy are primarily β-blockers, calcium channel blockers, or ACE inhibitors.

Initial therapy with β-blockers may be appropriate if there is no relative or absolute contraindication to their use (ie, bronchospasm, heart failure, insulin-dependent diabetes, bradycardia, heart block, or active peripheral vascular disease). Adverse cardiovascular effects from β-blockers are most common with the initial use of low doses in patients older than 50 years.[74] Initial therapy with a calcium channel blocker or ACE inhibitor is also appropriate, and the recommended dosage schedules are provided in Tables 10-3 and 10-4, respectively. If blood pressure cannot be satisfactorily controlled with one of the many therapeutic options, it is often preferable to reschedule elective surgery pending the implementation of effective antihypertensive therapy.

Hypertensive Crisis

Emergency surgery is sometimes necessary in adult patients with severe and uncontrolled hypertension. In this high-risk circumstance, preoperative blood pressure control may require the administration of potent antihypertensive agents. Table 10-5 summarizes the parenteral antipressor drugs used to treat hypertensive crises. Also included are the recommended initial doses for adults, onset and duration of action, and prominent adverse effects.

Intramuscular hydralazine is often used, beginning with 5 mg and increasing to 10 or 15 mg as necessary. Its onset of action is within 10 to 30 minutes, and its duration of action is 2 to 6 hours. The two largest risks that accompany the use of parenteral hydralazine are a marked reduction in blood pressure (especially in patients with volume depletion) and precipitation of angina and myocardial ischemia in patients with underlying coronary disease. This latter risk is related to reflex tachycardia and increased myocardial oxygen demand, and it is attenuated by the concomitant administration of effective doses of β-blockers when there is no contraindication to their use.

Intravenous methyldopa may be used, beginning with a piggyback infusion of 250 to 500 mg over 15 minutes or more. Its onset of action is usually slow (2 or 3 hours) and its duration is variable (6 to 18 hours). Marked lethargy is a common side effect of repeated intravenous doses.

Labetalol is an α/β-blocker (selective α-blockade and nonselective β-blockade) that is generally safe and effective for use in hypertensive crises.[75] For bolus therapy, a dose of 20 mg can be infused over a 2-minute period, followed at 15-minute intervals by 40- to 80-mg doses as needed. Labetalol infusions have largely replaced the use of hydralazine because they do not cause reflex tachycardia. Labetalol should not be administered to patients in whom the use of β-blockers is contraindicated.

Sodium nitroprusside is a potent, direct-acting vasodilator that must be administered by intravenous infusion in an intensive care setting, where the rate of infusion can be monitored and regulated constantly.[76] Nitroprusside therapy may be initiated by mixing 50 mg of the drug into 250 mL of 5% dextrose in water (D_5W) with an initial infusion rate of 0.3 to 0.5 µg/kg/min and a maximum infusion rate of 8 µg/kg/min. Its onset of action is immediate, and its duration of action is about 2 to 5 minutes. Plasma cyanide levels may increase four-fold or more in patients receiving prolonged doses[77] and can be reduced by the infusion of 25 mg/h of hydroxocobalamin.[78]

Nitroglycerin may also be infused at an initial rate of about 32 µg/min. The infusion of nitroglycerin has advantages over nitroprusside in certain patients and settings, although the pressure-lowering effect of nitroglycerin is much less than that of equivalent doses of nitroprusside.[79]

The only oral drugs with an onset of action rapid enough to reduce blood pressure within 1 to 2 hours or less are the calcium channel antagonists. Nifedipine in particular has been used in this setting because of its predominant effect on the peripheral vasculature. In some series, a single oral dose of 10 to 20 mg reduced blood pressure by an average of 69/27 to 58/27 mmHg in patients with marked elevations.[80,81]

Sublingual administration is neither necessary nor advisable if patients can swallow. The duration of the hypotensive effect varies from as few as 2 to as many as 8 hours; some patients experience reflex tachycardia.

TABLE 10–5. Parenteral Drugs That May Be Useful in Preoperative and Postoperative Hypertension

Drug	Route of Administration	Mixture	Initial Adult Dose	Onset	Duration	Major Side Effects
Nitroprusside*	IV drip	50 mg in 250 mL D5W protected from light and changed q12h	20 µg/min (0.3–0.5 µg/kg/min)	Immediate	2–5 min	Nausea, acidosis, muscle twitching, cyanide toxicity
Nitroglycerin*	IV drip	50-mg/10-mg ampules	31 µg/min (0.5 µg/kg/min)	Immediate	2–5 min	Headache, tachycardia, methemoglobinemia, infusion phlebitis
Hydralazine*	IM	20 mg/mL ampules of 1 mL each	5–15 mg	10–30 min	2–6 h or more	Tachycardia, palpitations, headache, myocardial ischemia
Methyldopa	IV drip IV infusion	25–50 mg in 500 mL saline 50-mg/mL vials of 5 mL each	0.2–0.5 mg/min 250–500 mg in 100 mL D5W given over 30 min	10–15 min 2–3 h	6–18 h	Drowsiness, stupor
Labetalol	IV infusion	5-mg/mL ampules of 20 mg each	0.5 mg/min; increase as necessary to a maximum of 2 mg/min	5–10 min	About 4 h (variable)	Bronchospasm
Enalaprilat	IV minibolus	1.25 mg/mL in a 2-mL vial	1.25 mg in 5 min, followed by 1.25 mg q6h if effective	5–15 min	≥6 h	Excessive hypotension; rarely, angioedema, hyperkalemia, or acute renal failure
Phenotolamine*	IV bolus	5 mg/vial	0.5–1 mg	Immediate	3–10 min	Nausea, tachycardia, coronary insufficiency

*Propranolol in intravenous bolus doses of 0.5–2 mg or esmolol infused at 24 mg/min is generally adequate to reduce the reflex tachycardia associated with peripheral vasodilation.

POSTOPERATIVE HYPERTENSION

PREVALENCE AND MECHANISM

A report from Gal and Cooperman[82] led to increased recognition of the entity that is now referred to as postoperative hypertension. Blood pressure readings obtained in the recovery room that exceeded 190/100 mmHg were noted in 60 (3.3%) of 1844 patients after several different general surgical procedures. Over 80% of the pressor responses occurred in the first 30 minutes after operation, although the onset was sometimes delayed for 60 to 90 minutes. Preoperative hypertension, usually with evidence of target organ damage, was present in 35 of the 60 patients, but the remaining 42% of patients had no history of hypertension before the postoperative elevation. Subsequent reports have emphasized the peculiarly frequent occurrence of postoperative hypertension after many vascular surgical procedures, specifically coronary artery bypass, aortic valve surgery, and carotid endarterectomy.

Coronary Bypass Surgery

Estafanous and coworkers[83] reported a postoperative diastolic blood pressure reading of 100 mmHg or higher (or a 30-mmHg increase above the preoperative systolic or diastolic blood pressure) in 34 (33%) of 102 patients undergoing myocardial revascularization but in only 4 (3.7%) of 107 patients undergoing general surgical procedures. There was no significant difference in the occurrence of postoperative hypertension between patients who previously had normal blood pressures and those who had hypertension. Preoperative antihypertensive therapy did not necessarily protect against postoperative pressor responses.

Whelton and colleagues[84] noted postoperative elevation of the mean arterial blood pressure in 32 (61%) of 52 patients undergoing coronary artery bypass surgery. The elevation in blood pressure was associated with an increase in total peripheral resistance and a fall in cardiac output. The pressor response was observed more frequently in patients who had received propranolol (especially in higher doses) up to 6 to 8 hours before surgery. The authors suggested that unopposed α-adrenergic stimulation (ie, from norepinephrine) in the presence of residual β-adrenergic blockade may be the mechanism responsible for the increased blood pressure. Further support for an α-adrenergic–mediated mechanism for the hypertension is provided by the observation that hypertension after coronary artery bypass surgery responds therapeutically to unilateral stellate ganglion blockade[85] or to α-adrenergic–inhibiting drugs such as phentolamine.[86]

Several investigators have also suggested a pathogenetic role for the renin–angiotensin system based on the elevation of plasma renin activity and angiotensin II levels after cardiopulmonary bypass[87,88] and the reduction in blood pressure and peripheral resistance after the administration of a converting enzyme inhibitor that blocks the formation of angiotensin II.[89] Others have found neither elevated levels nor maximal increases in plasma renin activity during periods of postoperative blood pressure elevation.[84,90] Moreover, the hypertension also responds to direct vasodilators such as nitroprusside, which increase plasma renin activity.[91]

Peterson and Brown[92,93] have identified afferent sympathetic fibers that travel with the left inferior cardiac and pericoronary nerves and cause an increase in blood pressure when stimulated. James and associates[94] have further described a chemoreceptor located near and supplied by the left main coronary artery. Stimulation of the chemoreceptor area evokes a marked increase in blood pressure. These coronary pressor reflexes may be involved in the hypertension that is associated with coronary artery surgery, although postoperative hypertension occurs with similar frequency regardless of the specific artery bypassed.[84]

Aortic Valve Surgery

About one third of patients who undergo aortic valve replacement develop transient and predominantly systolic hypertension in the early postoperative period, presumably as a result of high cardiac output generated by the unleashed hypertrophied left ventricle.[95,96] Moreover, patients with aortic valve homografts, especially men older than 50 years who have predominant aortic regurgitation, have a high incidence of chronic hypertension and an increased risk of homograft failure if hypertension is not treated during the years after valve replacement.[97]

Carotid Artery Surgery

Carotid endarterectomy is associated with a high incidence of postoperative hypertension.[98] Hypertension occurring after endarterectomy is associated with an increase in the risk of neurologic worsening or stroke. Preoperative antihypertensive therapy, however, has not been documented to reduce the incidence of acute postoperative stroke.[99]

Approximately half of all patients with hypertension demonstrate increases in carotid baroreceptor sensitivity and improvements in blood pressure after carotid recanalization. Those with unchanged baroreflex sensitivity have continued blood pressure variability requiring frequent adjustment of their antihypertensive therapy.[100]

ACUTE THERAPY

Increases in blood pressure documented in the recovery room are most often associated with anxiety and pain as anesthesia dissipates and patients begin to regain consciousness. Bolus doses of 2 to 5 mg of morphine, small doses of fentanyl, or 1- to 2-mg doses of chlorpromazine usually reduce the blood pressure. Arterial blood gas measurements should be obtained again if there is any question of hypercarbia or hypoxia. Overdistention of the bladder has been associated with average blood pressure increases of 28/14 mmHg and should be relieved.[101,102] Striking elevations of blood pressure mimicking pheochromocytoma can occur in response to urethral, bladder, or rectal stimulation in patients with spinal cord injury, especially those with high thoracic and cervical cord lesions.[103,104]

Modest elevations in blood pressure usually resolve within the first 1 to 3 hours after operation. More severe elevations require parenteral antihypertensive therapy if they persist despite adequate ventilation, relief of pain, and bladder drainage. Intravenously administered methyldopa, nitroprusside, nitroglycerin, labetalol, esmolol, enalapril, phentolamine, and chlorpromazine have all been used successfully in specific settings.

Once postoperative hypertension has been controlled and patients are discharged from the recovery room, the surgical team and its consultants must monitor and actively regulate the blood pressure over the ensuing hours and days.

LONG-TERM THERAPY

In patients with chronic hypertension, oral medication regimens can be gradually reinstated within 24 to 72 hours after surgery. Lesser amounts of therapeutic agents are often effective in reducing blood pressure, and occasional patients with hypertension maintain normal blood pressure levels throughout the postoperative period. The nonspecific effect of blood pressure reduction after major surgical procedures was first described by Volini and Flaxman.[105] Subsequently, Osmundson[106] documented an average reduction in blood pressure of about 25/18 mmHg during the first 10 postoperative days in patients with untreated hypertension; however, the blood pressure tended to return to hypertensive levels within 2 to 4 weeks after surgery.

Other patients demonstrate persistent postoperative hypertension before oral antipressor therapy can be resumed. Parenteral therapy is indicated, and selection of the most appropriate agent is based on the clinical setting. When there is evidence of excessive volume, small doses (10 to 40 mg) of intravenous furosemide usually potentiate the effect of most other parenteral antihypertensive drugs.

Hypertension is the single most important risk factor for stroke or congestive heart failure and one of the most important risk factors for myocardial infarction and renal failure. Control of hypertension may have a major effect on the long-term risks of patients who have undergone successful coronary bypass surgery.[107] Accordingly, primary care phy-

sicians, anesthesiologists, and surgeons must ensure long-term control of blood pressure lest the hard work and successful results of the operative procedure be negated by interim morbidity or recurrence of the original condition.

REFERENCES

1. Prys-Roberts C. Hypertension and anesthesia: fifty years on. Anesthesiology 1979;50:281–284.
2. Smithwick RH, Thompson JE. Splanchnicectomy for essential hypertension: results in 1266 cases. JAMA 1953;152:1501–1504.
3. Dana JB, Ohler RL. Influence of heart disease on surgical risk. JAMA 1956;162:878–880.
4. Nachlas MM, Abrams SJ, Goldberg MM. The influence of arteriosclerotic heart disease on surgical risk. Am J Surg 1961;101:447–455.
5. Skinner JF, Pearce ML. Surgical risk in the cardiac patient. J Chron Dis 1964;17:57–72.
6. Stahlgren LH. An analysis of factors which influence mortality following extensive abdominal operations upon geriatric patients. Surg Gynecol Obstet 1961;113:283–292.
7. Benson H, Ellis LB, Harken DE. The effect of preoperative systemic blood pressure on closed mitral valvuloplasty. Am Heart J 1968;75:439–448.
8. Goldman L, Caldera DL, Nussbaum SR, et al. Multifactorial index of cardiac risk in noncardiac surgical procedures. N Engl J Med 1977;297:845–850.
9. Goldman L, Caldera DL, Southwick FS, et al. Cardiac risk factors and complications in noncardiac surgery. Medicine (Baltimore) 1978;57:357–370.
10. Goldman L, Caldera DL. Risks of general anesthesia and elective operation in the hypertensive patient. Anesthesiology 1979;50:285–292.
11. Charlson ME, MacKenzie CR, Gold JP, et al. The preoperative and intraoperative hemodynamic predictors of postoperative myocardial infarction or ischemia in patients undergoing noncardiac surgery. Ann Surg 1989;210:637–648.
12. Mangano DT. Perioperative cardiac morbidity. Anesthesiology 1990;72:153–184.
13. Tarhan S, Moffit EA, Taylor WF, et al. Myocardial infarction after general anesthesia. JAMA 1972;220:1451–1454.
14. Mauney FM, Ebert PA, Sabiston DC Jr. Postoperative myocardial infarction: A study of predisposing factors, diagnosis and mortality in high-risk group of surgical patients. Ann Surg 1970;172:497–503.
15. Steen PA, Tinker JH, Tarhan S. Myocardial reinfarction after anesthesia and surgery. JAMA 1978;239:2566–2570.
16. Ashton CM, Petersen NJ, Wray NP, et al. The incidence of perioperative myocardial infarction in men undergoing noncardiac surgery. Ann Intern Med 1993;118:504–510.
17. Geraci JM, Rosen AK, Ash AS, et al. Predicting the occurrence of adverse events after coronary artery bypass surgery. Ann Intern Med 1993;118:18–24.
18. Boghosian SG, Mooradian AD. Usefulness of routine preoper-

ative chest roentgenograms in elderly patients. J Am Geriatr Soc 1987;35:142–146.

19. Weitz HH. Noncardiac surgery in the elderly patient with cardiovascular disease. Clin Geriatr Med 1990;6:511–529.

20. Kannel WB, Castelli WP, McNamara PM, et al. Role of blood pressure in the development of congestive heart failure: the Framingham study. N Engl J Med 1972;287:781–787.

21. Strandgaard S, Olesen J, Skinhøj E, et al. Autoregulation of brain circulation in severe arterial hypertension. Br Med J 1973;1:507–510.

22. Ropper AH, Wechsler LR, Wilson LS. Carotid bruit and the risk of stroke in elective surgery. N Engl J Med 1982;307:1388–1390.

23. Samaan HA. Risk of operation in a patient with unsuspected pheochromocytoma. Br J Surg 1970;57:462–465.

24. Kaplan NM, Kramer NJ, Holland OB, et al. Single-voided urine metanephrine assays in screening for pheochromocytoma. Arch Intern Med 1977;137:190–193.

25. Tarazi RC, Frohlich ED, Dustan HP. Plasma volume in men with essential hypertension. N Engl J Med 1968;278:762–765.

26. Shires T, Williams J, Brown F. Acute change in extracellular fluids associated with major surgical procedures. Ann Surg 1961;154:803–810.

27. Barry KG, Mazze RI, Schwartz FD. Prevention of surgical oliguria and renal-hemodynamic suppression by sustained hydration. N Engl J Med 1964;270:1371–1377.

28. Tarazi RC, Dustan HP, Frohlich ED. Longterm thiazide therapy in essential hypertension: evidence for persistent alteration in plasma volume and renin activity. Circulation 1970;41:709–717.

29. Feldman SA. Effect of changes in electrolytes, hydration and pH upon the reactions to muscle relaxants. Br J Anaesth 1963;35:546–551.

30. Feldman SA. An interesting case of recurarization. Br J Anaesth 1959;31:461–463.

31. Quilliam JP, Taylor DB. Antagonism between curare and the potassium ion. Nature 1947;160:603.

32. Savarese JJ, Philbin DM. Cardiovascular effects of neuromuscular blocking agents. Int Anesthesiol Clin 1979;17:13–54.

33. Koide M, Waud BE. Serum potassium concentrations after succinylcholine in patients with renal failure. Anesthesiology 1972;36:142–145.

34. Siegel D, Hulley SB, Black DM, et al. Diuretics, serum and intracellular electrolyte levels, and ventricular arrhythmias in hypertensive men. JAMA 1992;267:1083–1089.

35. Giangiacomo J, Klint R. Atrioventricular conduction disturbances with hypokalemia in renal tubular acidosis. J Electrocardiol 1974;7:273–274.

36. Krikler DM, Curry PV. Torsade de pointes, an atypical ventricular tachycardia. Br Heart J 1976;38:117–120.

37. Cohen JD, Neaton JD, Prineas RJ, et al. Diuretics, serum potassium and ventricular arrhythmias in the Multiple Risk Factor Intervention Trial. Am J Cardiol 1987;60:548–554.

38. Webster DR, Henrikson W, Currie DJ. The effect of potassium deficiency on intestinal motility and gastric secretion. Ann Surg 1950;132:779–785.

39. Lowman RM. The potassium depletion states and postoperative ileus. Radiology 1971;98:691–694.

40. Lans HS, Stein IF Jr, Meyer KA. Diagnosis, treatment, and prophylaxis of potassium deficiency in surgical patients: analysis of 404 patients. Surg Gynecol Obstet 1952;95:321–330.

41. Muggia AL. Perforation of the cecum associated with hypokalemic ileus. Am J Gastroenterol 1972;57:169–171.

42. Coakley CS, Alpert S, Boling JS. Circulatory responses during anesthesia of patients on *Rauwolfia* therapy. JAMA 1956;161:1143–1144.

43. Katz RL. Hazardous effects of drugs in hypertensive patients scheduled for elective surgery. Cardiovasc Med 1978;3:1185–1205.

44. Miller RD, Way WL, Eger EI II. The effects of alpha-methyldopa, reserpine, guanethidine and iproniazid on minimum alveolar anesthetic requirement (MAC). Anesthesiology 1968;29:1153–1158.

45. Weil MH, Barbour BH, Chesne RB. Alpha-methyldopa for the treatment of hypertension: clinical and pharmacodynamic studies. Circulation 1963;28:165–173.

46. El-Etr AA, Glisson SN. Alpha-adrenergic blocking agents. Int Anesthesiol Clin 1978;16:239–246.

47. Koch-Weser J, Graham RM, Pettinger WA. Drug therapy: prazosin. N Engl J Med 1979;300:232–236.

48. Viljoen JF, Estafanous FG, Kellner GA. Propranolol and cardiac surgery. J Thorac Cardiovasc Surg 1972;64:826–830.

49. Stephen GW, Davie IT, Scott DB. Haemodynamic effects of beta-receptor blocking drugs during nitrous oxide/halothane anaesthesia. Br J Anaesth 1971;43:320–325.

50. Schwartz AJ, Wollman H. Anesthetic considerations for patients on chronic drug therapy: L-dopa, monoamine oxidase inhibitors, tricyclic antidepressants and propranolol: American Society of Anesthesiologists refresher course in anesthesiology. 1976;4:99–111.

51. Kaplan JA, Dunbar RW, Bland JW Jr, et al. Propranolol and cardiac surgery: a problem for the anesthesiologist? Anesth Analg 1975;54:571–578.

52. Miller RR, Olson HG, Amsterdam EA, et al. Propranolol withdrawal rebound phenomenon. Exacerbation of coronary events after abrupt cessation of antianginal therapy. N Engl J Med 1975;293:416–418.

53. Kaplan JA. Cardiac anesthesia. New York, Grune & Stratton, 1979:178.

54. Edwards WJ. Preanesthetic management of the hypertensive patient. N Engl J Med 1979;301:158–159.

55. Prys-Roberts C, Foëx P, Biro GP, et al. Studies of anaesthesia in relation to hypertension. V. adrenergic beta-receptor blockade. Br J Anaesth 1973;45:671–681.

56. Jewell WH. Eraldin in anaesthesia: clinical trials results. Acta Cardiol 1972;16:109–118.

57. Stone JG, Foëx P, Sear JW, et al. Risk of myocardial ischaemia during anaesthesia in treated and untreated hypertensive patients. Br J Anaesth 1988;61:675–679.

58. Brodsky JB, Bravo JJ. Acute postoperative clonidine withdrawal syndrome. Anesthesiology 1976;44:519–520.

59. Bruce DL, Croley TF, Lee JS. Preoperative clonidine withdrawal syndrome. Anesthesiology 1979;51:90–92.

60. Kaukinen S, Kaukinen L, Eerola R. Preoperative and postoperative use of clonidine with neurolept anaesthesia. Acta Anaesthesiol Scand 1979;23:113–120.

61. Kaplan NM. Calcium entry blockers in the treatment of hypertension. JAMA 1989;262:817–823.

62. Adler AG, Leahy JJ, Cressman MD. Management of perioperative hypertension using sublingual nifedipine. Arch Intern Med 1986;146:1927–1930.

63. Iyer VS, Russell WJ. Nifedipine for postoperative blood pressure control following coronary artery vein grafts. Ann R Coll Surg Engl 1986;68:73–75.

64. Hall WD. Hypertension in the elderly with a special focus on treatment with angiotensin-converting enzyme inhibitors and calcium antagonists. Am J Cardiol 1992;69:33–42E.

65. Vertes V, Goldberg G. The preoperative patient with hypertension. Med Clin North Am 1979;63:1299–1308.

66. Prys-Roberts C, Meloche R, Foëx P. Studies of anaesthesia in relation to hypertension. I. Cardiovascular responses of treated and untreated patients. Br J Anaesth 1971;43:122–137.

67. Jain U. Perioperative cardiovascular monitoring: new developments and controversies. Cardiovasc Rev Rep 1993;14:40–43.

68. Ryhänen P, Saarela E, Hollmén A, et al. Blood pressure changes during and after anaesthesia in treated and untreated hypertensive patients. Ann Chir Gynaecol 1978;67:180–184.

69. Bookallil MJ. Anaesthesia in the hypertensive patient. Drugs 1974;8:84–86.

70. Nachlas MM, Abrams SJ, Goldberg MM. The influence of arteriosclerotic heart disease on surgical risk. Am J Surg 1961;101:447–455.

71. Charlson ME, MacKenzie CR, Gold JP, et al. Preoperative characteristics predicting intraoperative hypotension and hypertension among hypertensives and diabetics undergoing noncardiac surgery. Ann Surg 1990;212:66–81.

72. Chamberlain DA, Edmonds-Seal J. Effects of surgery under general anaesthesia on the electrocardiogram in ischemic heart disease and hypertension. BMJ 1964;2:784–787.

73. Tarazi RC, Dustan HP. Hemodynamic effects of diuretics in hypertension. In: Lieban H, Brod J, eds. Contributions to nephrology, vol 8. Mechanisms and recent advances in therapy of hypertension. Basel, S Karger, 1977:162–170.

74. Greenblatt DJ, Koch-Weser J. Adverse reactions to propranolol in hospitalized medical patients: a report from the Boston Collaborative Drug Surveillance Program. Am Heart J 1973;86:478–484.

75. Wilson DJ, Wallin JD, Vlachakis ND, et al. Intravenous labetalol in the treatment of severe hypertension and hypertensive emergencies. Am J Med 1983;75:95–102.

76. Reves JG, Sheppard LC, Wallach R, et al. Therapeutic uses of sodium nitroprusside and an automated method of administration. Int Anesthesiol Clin 1978;16:51–88.

77. Vesey CJ, Cole PV, Linnell JC, et al. Some metabolic effects of sodium nitroprusside in man. BMJ 1974;2:140–143.

78. Cottrell JE, Casthely P, Brodie JD, et al. Prevention of nitroprusside-induced cyanide toxicity with hydroxocobalamin. N Engl J Med 1978;298:809–811.

79. Stetson JB. Intravenous nitroglycerin: a review. Anesthesiol Clin 1978;16:261–298.

80. Bertel O, Conen D, Radü EW, et al. Nifedipine in hypertensive emergencies. Br Med J 1983;286:19–21.

81. Given BD, Lee TH, Stone PH, et al. Nifedipine in severely hypertensive patients with congestive heart failure and preserved ventricular systolic function. Arch Intern Med 1985;145:281–285.

82. Gal TJ, Cooperman LH. Hypertension in the immediate postoperative period. Br J Anaesth 1975;47:70–74.

83. Estafanous FG, Tarazi RC, Viljoen JF, et al. Systemic hypertension following myocardial revascularization. Am Heart J 1973;85:732–738.

84. Whelton PK, Flaherty JT, MacAllister NP, et al. Hypertension following coronary artery bypass surgery: role of preoperative propranolol therapy. Hypertension 1980;2:291–298.

85. Tarazi RC, Estafanous FG, Fouad FM. Unilateral stellate block in the treatment of hypertension after coronary bypass surgery: implications of a new therapeutic approach. Am J Cardiol 1978;42:1013–1018.

86. Roberts AJ, Niarchos AP, Case DB, et al. Coronary artery bypass hypertension: comparison of responses to nitroprusside, phentolamine and converting enzyme inhibitor. Circulation 1977;56(Suppl 3):59.

87. Taylor KM, Morton IJ, Brown JJ, et al. Hypertension and the renin-angiotensin system following open heart surgery. J Thorac Cardiovasc Surg 1977;74:840–845.

88. Roberts AJ, Niarchos AP, Subramanian VA, et al. Systemic hypertension associated with coronary artery bypass surgery: predisposing factors, hemodynamic characteristics, humoral profile, and treatment. J Thorac Cardiovasc Surg 1977;74:846–859.

89. Niarchos AP, Roberts AJ, Case DB, et al. Hemodynamic characteristics of hypertension after coronary bypass surgery and effects of the converting enzyme inhibitor. Am J Cardiol 1979;43:586–593.

90. Robertson D, Michelakis AM. Effect of anesthesia and surgery on plasma renin activity in man. J Clin Endocrinol Metab 1972;34:831–836.

91. Fahmy NR, Mihelakos PT, Battit GE, et al. Propranolol prevents hemodynamic and humoral events after abrupt withdrawal of nitroprusside. Clin Pharmacol Ther 1984;36:470–477.

92. Peterson DF, Brown AM. Pressor reflexes produced by stimulation of afferent fibers in the cardiac sympathetic nerves of the cat. Circ Res 1971;28:605–610.

93. Brown AM. Coronary pressor reflexes. Am J Cardiol 1979;44:849–851.

94. James TN, Hageman GR, Urthaler F. Anatomic and physiologic considerations of a cardiogenic hypertensive chemoreflex. Am J Cardiol 1979;44:852–859.

95. McQueen MJ, Watson ME, Bain WH. Transient systolic hypertension after aortic valve replacement. Br Heart J 1972;34:227–231.

96. Koppes GM, Jones FG. Systolic hypertension after aortic valve replacement. Cardiovasc Med 1978;3:567–569.

97. Layton C, Monro J, Brigden W, et al. Systemic hypertension after homograft aortic valve replacement: a cause of late homograft failure. Lancet 1973;2:1343–1347.

98. Lehv MS, Salzman EW, Silen W. Hypertension complicating carotid endarterectomy. Stroke 1970;1:307–313.

99. Satiani B, Vasko JS, Evans WE. Hypertension following carotid endarterectomy. Surg Neurol 1979;11:357–359.

100. Hirschl M, Kundi M, Hirschl MM, et al. Blood pressure responses after carotid surgery: relationship to postoperative baroreceptor sensitivity. Am J Med 1993;94:463–468.

101. Lapides J, Lovegrove RH. Urinary vesicovascular reflex. J Urol 1965;94:397–401.

102. Albert SN, Pehlivanian Z, McClure R. Urinary bladder distention: a cause of hypertension during anesthesia. Anesth Analg 1971;50:794–797.

103. Mathias CJ, Frankel HL. Autonomic failure in tetraplegia. In: Bannister R, ed. Autonomic failure: a textbook of clinical disorders of the autonomic nervous system. Oxford, Oxford University Press, 1983:453–488.

104. Kurnick NB. Autonomic hyperreflexia and its control in patients with spinal cord lesions. Ann Intern Med 1956;44:678–686.

105. Volini IF, Flaxman N. The effect of nonspecific operations on essential hypertension. JAMA 1939;112:2126–2128.

106. Osmundson PJ. Preoperative and postoperative management of patients with hypertension. Med Clin North Am 1962;46:963–969.

107. Lutz JF, Hall WD. The influence of systemic arterial hypertension on the course of patients with coronary atherosclerosis. In: Hurst JW, ed. Clinical essays on the heart, vol 3. New York, McGraw-Hill, 1984:25–38.

SECTION

PULMONARY CARE

Medical Management of the Surgical Patient, Third Edition,
edited by Michael F. Lubin, H. Kenneth Walker, and Robert B. Smith III.
J.B. Lippincott Company, Philadelphia, PA © 1995.

RESPIRATORY COMPLICATIONS OF SURGERY AND ANESTHESIA: OVERVIEW

Valerie A. Lawrence
Charles A. Duncan

Respiratory complications are among the most common causes of postoperative morbidity and mortality.[1–4] The true incidence of pulmonary complications depends on the criteria used to define complications and on the type of surgery performed, ranging from as low as 5% to as high as 80% for upper abdominal procedures in some series.[2,3] In other series, the reported incidence of complications after upper abdominal and thoracic surgery varies from 20% to 40%,[5] doubling in cigarette smokers[6,7] and approaching 70% in patients with chronic obstructive pulmonary disease (COPD).[8] The criteria used to define complications in different studies have a significant effect on these estimates.[9] Some authors do not report any criteria for complications, others include clinically unimportant microatelectasis or arterial blood gas changes without clinical correlates as complications, and still others focus on severe complications (eg, respiratory failure or ventilator dependence).[9]

Atelectasis (from the Greek *ateles*, meaning imperfect, plus *ekatasis*, meaning expansion) is the most common postoperative respiratory complication, occurring in essentially all patients who undergo general anesthesia. Besides general anesthesia, risk factors for atelectasis include diaphragmatic dysfunction after thoracic and upper abdominal operations and inadequate respiratory and cough efforts due to pain, narcotics, and bed rest. The severity of the condition can range from clinically insignificant involvement of a small group of airways and alveoli to complete collapse of a bronchopulmonary segment or lung (macroatelectasis).

Other common respiratory complications include retained tracheobronchial secretions; bronchospasm; bronchitis and pneumonia; hypoxemia with or without hypercapnia; pulmonary hypertension, cor pulmonale, and right ventricular failure; pulmonary embolism; and respiratory failure requiring mechanical ventilation.

Infection, especially nosocomial pneumonia, often results in mortality or severe morbidity in patients who have undergone surgery. Both atelectasis and impaired mucociliary clearance promote colonization of the airways with bacterial organisms and subsequent development of pneumonia. Infection can be caused by either gram-positive or gram-negative bacteria. If patients are significantly immunocompromised from either underlying diseases or therapeutic agents that impair host defenses, they may develop infection with opportunistic organisms such as those of the genus *Candida.* Sepsis originating from an infected site other than the lung can cause or significantly contribute to respiratory failure by producing the adult respiratory distress syndrome.

Most respiratory complications result from a combination of alterations in normal ventilatory pattern, impaired removal of secretions, and progressive atelectasis. Normal resting ventilation has a tidal volume of about 6 to 8 mL/kg, varying according to body size, with spontaneous sighs to near total lung capacity every 5 to 10 minutes. Sighs are essential for maintaining alveolar inflation. Without periodic sighs, gradual alveolar collapse may begin within 1 hour as a result of decreased surfactant activity, reduced lung volumes, and abnormal gas distribution. Because surfactant maintains the surface tension of alveoli, reduced function promotes airway closure, atelectasis, and abnormal gas distribution. With progressive atelectasis, alveoli are perfused but not ventilated, intrapulmonary shunting develops with a decrease in the PaO_2, lung compliance decreases, and the work of breathing increases. Alveolar collapse and its sequelae may be reversed by periodic deep breaths.

In most patients undergoing upper abdominal and thoracic surgery, changes of microatelectasis develop routinely, may not be clinically apparent, and usually peak 2 or 3 days after operation. If no other complications develop, the pulmonary status should return to normal within several days. In high-risk patients, microatelectasis may progress to pneumonitis or to diffuse, clinically detectable atelectasis that can involve an entire lobe or lung.

Clinical evidence of complications includes dyspnea, fever, purulent secretions, and rapid shallow respirations with an ineffective cough response. Accompanying laboratory signs may include infiltrates or segmental atelectasis on chest radiographs, abnormal arterial blood gas levels, and leukocytosis. Respiratory complications, however, may have a subtle presentation. For instance, elderly patients with COPD who develop postoperative chest infections may not demonstrate fever, leukocytosis, or radiographic infiltrates. If tracheobronchial secretions become viscid and difficult to expectorate, and if the cough mechanism is depressed, purulent sputum with an exacerbation of bronchitis may not be readily apparent.

The development of postoperative respiratory complications is related to several factors: respiratory pathophysiology of surgery and anesthesia, preexisting respiratory disease, type of operation, depressed mucociliary activity, duration of anesthesia, advancing age, obesity, smoking, and general physical and mental condition.

RESPIRATORY PATHOPHYSIOLOGY DURING AND AFTER SURGERY

Characteristic alterations that occur in all patients within hours of major surgery, with both general and spinal anesthesia, include monotonous shallow breathing with loss of spontaneous deep breaths; decreased functional residual capacity (FRC), residual volume, expiratory flow, and compliance; increased work of breathing; and altered ventilation–perfusion ratios resulting in a 10% to 30% decrease in PaO_2.[10] These changes usually are not clinically significant and progress to overt complications only when lung volumes are severely decreased.

Of the different lung volume compartments measured by pulmonary function testing, the most important in relation to postoperative course are vital capacity, tidal volume, and FRC. *Vital capacity* is the volume of air resulting from a maximal exhalation after a maximal inspiratory effort and is highly dependent on voluntary effort. *Tidal volume* is the amount of air exchanged during a breathing cycle. *FRC* is the volume of air remaining in the lungs after a normal tidal exhalation. It represents the point at which forces expanding the chest wall are balanced by the inward elastic recoil of the lung parenchyma.

Regional differences in lung expansion can be explained by the interaction of the pleural pressure gradient and the static pressure-volume curve of the lung. In the upright position, there is a gravity-dependent gradient in pleural pressure down the lung, with more negative pressure toward the apex. Gradients in pleural pressure cause regional differences in distending pressures in the airways and alveoli and help explain regional differences in gas distribution.

As lung volume increases during inspiration, dependent alveoli expand more for a given pressure change than do apical alveoli. Because of these lesser distending pressures, alveoli in dependent regions are considerably smaller than are apical alveoli at lower lung volumes. Surfactants in the alveoli decrease surface tension and make smaller alveoli more distensible than larger alveoli. Thus, during normal breathing, inspired gas is preferentially distributed to alveoli in the dependent regions, provided the airways in these regions are open at the beginning of inspiration.[11] If dependent alveoli and airways are closed at the beginning of inspiration, inspired gas is preferentially distributed to superior regions because alveoli here expand before the critical opening pressure of basilar airways is exceeded.[12] In patients undergoing surgery in the supine position, the pleural pressure gradient is the vertical distance from the ventral to the dependent dorsal side and is sufficient to generate differences in regional distensibility between superiorly located alveoli and dependent dorsal alveoli. During tidal breathing, the inspired gas is again preferentially distributed to alveoli in dependent regions, provided the alveoli and airways in this region are open at the beginning of inspiration. Because pulmonary blood flow is highly dependent on gravity, it is greater in dependent lung regions. Therefore, when airways are closed in these regions at the beginning of inspiration, there is increased ventilation to the superior lung regions, resulting in increased ventilation–perfusion mismatch and the likelihood of arterial hypoxemia.

In healthy persons, regardless of their age, all regions of the lung are open at a full inspiration (total lung capacity). As lung volume decreases during expiration, airway closure occurs first in the dependent lung regions, where the distending pressures are less and the volume change is greater. With advancing age, there is an increased tendency toward airway closure caused by progressive decreases in the elastic recoil pressure of the lung.[13,14] In the upright position, a significant number of airways tend to close above the FRC in patients who are 65 years and older. With a change from the upright to the supine position, the FRC decreases about 20% and the tendency toward airway closure remains about the same and further exceeds the FRC.[15]

With premature airway closure and its influence on the regional pattern of gas distribution, ventilation is reduced, leading to a reduced ventilation–perfusion ratio and decreased PaO_2 in the supine position. If airways remain closed throughout inspiration during and after operation, gas in air spaces distal to the point of closure is gradually absorbed by the blood. The result is atelectasis.[16] Combined with decreased mucociliary clearance and bacterial colonization, atelectasis increases the chance of infection. The reexpansion of collapsed airways requires higher distending pressures. Consequently, if high pressures and volumes are not used, inspired gas tends to be preferentially distributed to the already patent airways and atelectatic areas do not reexpand.

Numerous factors favor premature airway closure and atelectasis. Nonpulmonary factors include supine position, obesity, increased abdominal girth (eg, ileus, pneumoperitoneum, ascites), breathing at low lung volumes, bindings around the chest and abdomen, incisional pain, sedative or narcotic drugs, prolonged effect of paralyzing drugs, muscle weakness, poor nutrition, immobility, and excessively high concentrations of oxygen for prolonged periods. Pulmonary factors favoring premature airway closure and atelectasis include interstitial edema, loss of surfactant with air space instability, airway obstruction due to inflammation with swelling of bronchial and interbronchial tissue, constriction of bronchial smooth muscle, and retained secretions.

Abdominal distention and vigorous expiratory efforts may reduce overall lung volume and thereby enhance the tendency toward premature airway closure. If patients are not turned adequately, the same lung regions remain dependent and at relatively low volumes. Muscle paralysis, general debility, the use of narcotics, and pain interfere with spontaneous sighing and coughing. The use of oxygen in higher concentrations than normal promotes atelectasis because of the rapid absorption of oxygen by surrounding tissues, especially in areas distal to partially obstructed airways. High concentrations of oxygen can also deplete surfactant, which leads to instability and collapse of alveoli.[17,18] Consequently, higher concentrations of oxygen promote airway closure and atelectasis, and reduce matching of ventilation to perfusion. Physicians should use the lowest possible percentage of inspired oxygen for adequate oxygenation.

PREEXISTING RESPIRATORY DISEASE

The incidence of postoperative respiratory complications is increased among patients with COPD. This incidence is difficult to estimate, however, because many relevant studies have been retrospective or poorly designed, and the diagnosis of pulmonary complications has been based on variable criteria.[9] Stein and colleagues[8] demonstrated an increase in the incidence of postoperative respiratory complications from about 3% in patients with normal preoperative pulmonary function to 70% in those with abnormal results on spirometry and clinical histories of lung disease. Other than "100 patients admitted for surgical procedures," however, no selection criteria are provided; the pulmonary status and reason for referral for preoperative pulmonary evaluation are not clear. Thirty-seven patients were excluded because of refusal to participate, "lack of surgical indication," or contraindication to surgery because of cardiac or pulmonary disease (5 patients). Thus, results are presented for only 63 patients. Criteria for postoperative pulmonary complications are not provided and outcome assessment was apparently not blinded to preoperative pulmonary status.[9] A more recent prospective study found a two-fold increase in the incidence of postoperative pulmonary complications in patients with histories of COPD or smoking.[4] A retrospective cohort study attempted to further clarify the surgical risk of COPD by comparing 26 patients with severe COPD (forced expiratory volume less than 50% predicted) who were undergoing thoracic and major abdominal surgery and were matched by age and type of operation to 52 patients with mild to moderate COPD and 52 patients with no COPD.[19] The patients with severe COPD had rates of cardiac, vascular, and minor pulmonary complications similar to those of patients with mild, moderate, or no COPD, but had higher rates of serious pulmonary complications (23% versus 10% versus 4%, $P = .03$) and death (19% versus 4% versus 2%, $P = .02$). All deaths and cases of ventilatory failure occurred in patients with severe COPD who were undergoing coronary artery bypass surgery.

Although COPD is associated with a greater risk for pulmonary complications, its magnitude is unclear, especially given the use of current surgical techniques and supportive technology. Furthermore, the role of preoperative spirometry in accurately predicting pulmonary complications is unproven. A critical review of the evidence regarding the predictive value of preoperative spirometry found it to be flawed and conflicting.[9]

TYPE OF SURGERY

The nearer the incision is made to the diaphragm, the greater will be the reduction in postoperative pulmonary function. Expiration is passive during tidal breathing; with increased airway resistance, however, as in patients with COPD, the upper abdominal muscles of expiration are used. Consequently, the degree of surgical abdominal muscle injury influences the rate of postoperative pulmonary complications. In addition, upper abdominal surgery causes diaphragmatic dysfunction that is not solely attributable to pain.[20–22]

Operations associated with an increased risk of pulmonary complications, in descending order of frequency, are thoracic operations with lung resection; thoracic operations without lung resection (eg, coronary bypass); upper abdominal procedures; lower abdominal procedures; and nonthoracic nonabdominal surgery.[23–25]

DEPRESSION OF MUCOCILIARY ACTIVITY

One of the most important consequences of general anesthesia and surgery is the depression of mucociliary transport. In normal lungs, the amount of mucus secreted by the mucous membranes lining the airways is small and the action of cilia covering these membranes is sufficient to transport mucus up into the pharynx. The mucociliary clearance system extends to the level of the terminal bronchiole. More peripherally, phagocytosis by alveolar macrophages and lymphatic drainage are the clearance mechanisms for small particles.

The use of cuffed endotracheal tubes and dry anesthetic gases depresses mucociliary clearance by altering ciliated epithelium, changing the rheologic properties of mucus, and, at times, promoting excessive mucus secretion. These factors may be potentiated by preoperative fasting and the inhibition of bronchial gland secretion by atropine. Mucociliary transport may be slowed or even halted for as long as 6 days after operation, and this effect correlates with the duration of the operation. Lack of coughing and deep breathing during and after surgery results in the retention of mucus in the airways and is associated with an increased incidence of lobar and segmental atelectasis. All these factors promote colonization and invasion of the lower respiratory tract by bacteria that usually reside in the upper airway. These risks are enhanced by diseases that promote increased tracheobronchial secretions (eg, bronchiectasis, acute and chronic bronchitis, and asthma).

DURATION OF ANESTHESIA

In an older study, anesthesia lasting longer than 3½ hours was associated with higher rates of atelectasis and other complications.[3] A more recent trial of interventions to prevent postoperative complications confirms this associa-

tion,[23] as does a study of operative risk in patients with severe obstructive lung disease.[24] It is not clear whether this effect is the result of prolonged anesthesia itself or of more complicated protracted surgery. The type of anesthetic method used (spinal or general) does not seem to affect the incidence of postoperative complications.

AGE

Advancing age is associated with increases in postoperative atelectasis and hypoxemia in some studies[19,23,26] but not others.[24,27] The explanation may lie partially in the type of patients studied. Two studies in which age was not found to be a risk factor focused on patients with chronic lung disease. Lung disease may be such a strong risk factor that it may mask the effect of age. Thus, age may be a more important risk in groups of patients in whom lung disease is not prominent. In such groups, the elderly may be particularly vulnerable because of progressive age-related loss of the lung's elastic recoil, with a resultant increase in FRC and a greater tendency for airway closure to occur in the tidal breathing range. The result is increased ventilation–perfusion mismatching and hypoxemia, particularly in the supine position.

OBESITY

Obesity consistently has been shown to increase pulmonary operative risk.[28–30] Because it reduces chest wall compliance and increases the work of breathing, morbid obesity may result in respiratory failure in the absence of all other risk factors and may intensify postoperative dysfunction. Mild to moderate obesity, however, may not significantly increase pulmonary risk. In one study, weight/height ratios less than 0.7 were not associated with an increased risk of pulmonary complications.[31] Although obesity itself may not contraindicate surgery, it is associated with conditions such as hypertension and cardiopulmonary dysfunction that may increase operative risk.[30]

SMOKING

Cigarette smoking is associated with an increase in tracheobronchial secretions and bronchitis as well as depressed mucociliary clearance. Several studies have found heavy smoking (more than 20 cigarettes per day) to be associated with a higher incidence of postoperative pulmonary complications.[6,7,32,33] In one study, sputum production of greater than 60 mL in 24 hours identified patients who were at higher risk for pulmonary complications.[34] Smoking cessation immediately before surgery does not appear to significantly reduce risk. A study of patients undergoing coronary artery bypass surgery found that risk was reduced only among patients who ceased smoking 2 months before surgery.[35]

GENERAL MENTAL AND PHYSICAL CONDITION

Patients' general medical conditions, including their nutritional status, are important factors influencing perioperative management and complications but the place of training and nutritional supplements in improving operative outcome in patients with COPD is unclear. In a recent metaanalysis, respiratory muscle training was found to improve strength but not to significantly improve exercise capacity or quality of life.[36] In studies that controlled training intensity, however, significant improvement occurred in both functional status and respiratory muscle strength.[36] Whether such training can reduce postoperative pulmonary complications has not been studied.

A poor nutritional state results in a depressed ventilatory response, prolonged healing, and respiratory muscle weakness.[37,38] In a small, randomized trial of patients with emphysema who weighed less than 90% of their ideal body weights, those who received oral nutritional supplements for 4 months experienced significant weight gain, improved walking distance, and increased strength in handgrip and expiratory muscles.[39] Whether these results are important for patients with lung disease who are undergoing surgery remains to be studied. A multicenter, randomized trial of total parenteral nutrition in surgical patients at veterans' hospitals found that 8 days of preoperative total parenteral nutrition was not beneficial overall; however, the specific question of such therapy in patients with COPD was not addressed.[40]

Patients' emotional stability and anxiety levels help determine their pain perceptions and pain thresholds in the postoperative period.[41,42] Postoperative pain promotes a monotonous breathing pattern and suppresses the cough response. Analgesic requirements can be reduced 50% or more by providing careful instructions and enhancing communication and rapport between patients, physicians, therapists, and especially nurses.[43,44]

Numerous patient, surgical, and anesthetic factors affect pulmonary operative risk. To prevent complications and improve the risk–benefit ratio of surgery, internists who provide perioperative care must be aware of these factors and their importance in preoperative risk assessment and perioperative management.

REFERENCES

1. Bartlett RH, Brennan ML, Gazzaniga AB, Hanson EL. Studies on the pathogenesis and prevention of postoperative pulmonary complications. Surg Gynecol Obstet 1973;1367:925–933.
2. Pontoppidan H. Mechanical aids to lung expansion in non-intubated surgical patients. Am Rev Respir Dis 1980;122:109–119.
3. Latimer RG, Dickman M, Day WC, et al. Ventilatory patterns and pulmonary complications after upper abdominal surgery determined by preoperative and postoperative computerized spirometry and blood gas analysis. Am J Surg 1971;122:622–632.
4. Garibaldi RA, Britt MR, Coleman ML, et al. Risk factors for postoperative pneumonia. Am J Med 1981;70:677–680.
5. Bartlett RH, Gazzaniga AB, Geaghty TR. Respiratory maneuvers to prevent postoperative pulmonary complications. JAMA 1973;224:1017–1021.
6. Collins CD, Drake CS, Knowelden J. Chest complications after upper abdominal surgery: their anticipation and prevention. BMJ 1968;1:401–406.
7. Laszlo G, Archer GG, Darrell JH, et al. The diagnosis and prophylaxis of pulmonary complications of surgical operation. Br J Surg 1973;60:129–134.
8. Stein M, Koota GM, Simon M, Frank HA. Pulmonary evaluation in surgical patients. JAMA 1962;181:765–770.
9. Lawrence VA, Page CP, Harris GD. Preoperative spirometry before abdominal operations: a critical appraisal of its predictive value. Arch Intern Med 1989;149:280–285.
10. Celli BR. Perioperative assessment and management of the patient with pulmonary disease. In: Merli GJ, Weitz HH, eds. Medical management of the surgical patient. Philadelphia, WB Saunders, 1992;1301.
11. Milic-Emili J, Henderson JA, Dolovich MB, et al. Regional distribution of inspired gas in the lung. J Appl Physiol 1966;21: 749–759.
12. Sutherland PW, Katsura T, Milic-Emili J. Previous volume history of the lung and regional distribution of gas. J Appl Physiol 1968;25:566–574.
13. Wahba WM. Influence of aging on lung function: clinical significance of changes from age twenty. Anesth Analg 1983;62: 764–776.
14. Holland J, Milic-Emili J, Macklem PT, et al. Regional distribution of pulmonary ventilation and perfusion in elderly subjects. J Clin Invest 1968;47:81–92.
15. Leblanc P, Ruff F, Milic-Emili J. Effects of age and body position on "airway closure" in man. J Appl Physiol 1970;28:448–451.
16. Ford GT, Guenter CA. Toward prevention of postoperative pulmonary complications. Am Rev Respir Dis 1984;130:4–5.
17. Markello R, Winter P, Olszowka A. Assessment of ventilation perfusion inequalities by arterial-alveolar nitrogen differences in intensive care patients. Anesthesiology 1972;37:4–15.
18. Shapiro BA, Cane RD, Harrison RA, Steiner MC. Changes in intrapulmonary shunting with administration of 100% oxygen. Chest 1980;77:138–141.
19. Kroenke K, Lawrence VA, Theroux JF, et al. Postoperative complications after thoracic and major abdominal surgery in patients with and without obstructive lung disease. Chest 1993;104:1445–1451.

20. Simonneau G, Vivien A, Sartene R, et al. Diaphragm dysfunction induced by upper abdominal surgery. Am Rev Respir Dis 1983;128:899–903.

21. Ford GT, Whitelaw W, Rosenal TW, et al. Diaphragmatic function after upper abdominal surgery in humans. Am Rev Respir Dis 1983;127:431–436.

22. Dureuil B, Vires N, Contineau JP, et al. Diaphragmatic contractility after upper abdominal surgery. J Appl Physiol 1986;61:1775–1780.

23. Celli BR, Rodriguez K, Snider GL. A controlled trial of intermittent positive pressure breathing, incentive spirometry, and deep breathing exercises in preventing pulmonary complications after elective surgery. Am Rev Respir Dis 1984;130:12–15.

24. Kroenke K, Lawrence VA, Theroux JF, Tuley MR. Operative risk in patients with severe obstructive pulmonary disease. Arch Intern Med 1992;152:967–971.

25. Mohr DN, Jett JR. Preoperative evaluation of pulmonary risk factors. J Gen Intern Med 1988;3:277–287.

26. Davis AG, Spence AA. Postoperative hypoxemia and age. Anesthesiology 1972;37:663–664.

27. Tarhan S, Moffitt EA, Sessler AD, et al. Risk of anesthesia and surgery in patients with chronic bronchitis and chronic obstructive pulmonary disease. Surgery 1973;74:720–726.

28. Gould AB Jr. Effect of obesity on respiratory complications following general anesthesia. Anesth Analg 1962;41:448–452.

29. King DS. Postoperative pulmonary complications: statistical study based on two years' personal observation. Surg Gynecol Obstet 1933;56:43–50.

30. Pasulka PS, Bistrian BR, Benotti PN, Blackburn GL. The risks of surgery in obese patients. Ann Intern Med 1986;104:540–546.

31. Bermudez M, Rodriguez K, Celli B. Is weight an independent risk factor in the development of postoperative pulmonary complications after abdominal surgery? Am Rev Respir Dis 1987;135:211.

32. Chalon J, Tayyae MA, Ramanathan S. Cytology of respiratory epithelium as predictor of respiratory complications after operation. Chest 1975;67:32–35.

33. Warner MA, Divertie MB, Tinrer JH. Preoperative cessation of smoking and pulmonary complications in coronary artery bypass patients. Anesthesiology 1984;60:380–383.

34. Gracey DR, Divertie MB, Didier EP. Preoperative pulmonary preparation of patients with chronic obstructive pulmonary disease: a prospective study. Chest 1979;76:123–129.

35. Warner MA, Offord KP, Warner ME, et al. Role of preoperative cessation of smoking and other factors in postoperative pulmonary complications: a blinded prospective study of coronary artery bypass patients. Mayo Clin Proc 1989;64: 609–616.

36. Smith K, Cook D, Guyatt GH, et al. Respiratory muscle training in chronic airflow limitation: a meta-analysis. Am Rev Respir Dis 1992;145:533–539.

37. Doekel RC Jr, Zwillich CW, Scoggin CH, et al. Clinical semistarvation: depression of hypoxic ventilatory response. N Engl J Med 1976;295:358–361.

38. Arora NS, Rochester DF. Respiratory muscle strength and maximal voluntary ventilation in undernourished patients. Am Rev Respir Dis 1982;126:5–8.

39. Rogers RM, Donahoe M, Constantino J. Physiologic effects of oral supplemental feeding in malnourished patients with chronic obstructive pulmonary disease. Am Rev Respir Dis 1992;146:1511–1517.

40. The Veterans Affairs Total Parenteral Nutrition Cooperative Study Group. Perioperative total parenteral nutrition in surgical patients. N Engl J Med 1991;325:525–532.

41. Dalrymple DG, Parbrook GD, Steel DF. Factors predisposing to postoperative pain and pulmonary complications: a study of female patients undergoing elective cholecystectomy. Br J Anaesth 1973;45:589–598.

42. Parbrook GD, Steel DF, Dalrymple DG. Factors predisposing to postoperative pain and pulmonary complications: a study of male patients undergoing elective gastric surgery. Br J Anaesth 1973;45:21–33.

43. Egbert LD, Battit GE, Turndorf H, Beecher HK. The value of the preoperative visit by an anesthetist: a study of doctor–patient rapport. JAMA 1963;185:553–555.

44. Egbert LD, Battit GE, Welch CE, et al. Reduction of postoperative pain by encouragement and instruction of patients: a study of doctor-patient rapport. N Engl J Med 1964;270:825–827.

Medical Management of the Surgical Patient, Third Edition,
edited by Michael F. Lubin, H. Kenneth Walker, and Robert B. Smith III.
J.B. Lippincott Company, Philadelphia, PA © 1995.

PREOPERATIVE RESPIRATORY EVALUATION

Valerie A. Lawrence
Charles A. Duncan

An effective preoperative evaluation should identify factors that increase the risk of postoperative complications. If the history or physical examination suggests significant pulmonary or cardiac disease, further diagnostic tests may be indicated. Once risk factors have been identified, the management plan can focus on minimizing risks and preventing complications. The following factors should be addressed: the risks of the surgical disease, any pulmonary disease, and the planned operation; the reversibility of preoperative pulmonary problems; and management plans for treating existing pulmonary disease, minimizing further loss of respiratory reserve, preventing pulmonary complications, and monitoring patients during the hospital stay.

HISTORY

Because respiratory disease increases the risk of postoperative pulmonary complications, physicians should obtain a careful history to detect its presence and make some quantitative assessment of disability. Specific points that should be assessed include pack-years of cigarette smoking; cough (paroxysmal or productive) and amount of sputum production; symptoms and history of obstructive lung disease (eg, bronchitis, emphysema, asthma); airway disease such as cystic fibrosis and bronchiectasis or recurrent pneumonias,

particularly in the same lung region; environmental or occupational exposure; prior surgery and associated respiratory difficulty; old chest injuries; use of pulmonary or cardiac medications; and wheezing, dyspnea, and exercise tolerance.[1,2] Patients who engage in vigorous exercise usually have good respiratory reserve.

PHYSICAL EXAMINATION

General inspection of patients may yield signs of significant respiratory disease. The respiratory rate should be measured while patients are unaware. Tachypnea (more than 24 breaths/min) suggests an underlying abnormality. Asymmetry of the chest wall may be present in patients with kyphoscoliosis or unilateral loss of underlying lung volume. One specific indicator of significant obstructive disease is the typical hunched posture of severe chronic obstructive disease that is characterized by placement of the hands on the knees and use of accessory muscles for breathing, including intercostal retraction, scalene muscle recruitment, tracheal descent, and upper rib cage inspiratory motion.[3] An inability to speak in complete sentences between breaths demonstrates limited respiratory capacity. A careful chest examination should also be performed. Decreased breath sounds, tracheal deviation, dullness to percussion,

117

localized wheezing, stridor, changes in vocal fremitus, and rales all suggest the presence of abnormalities that may merit further investigation before surgery. Jugular venous distention, hepatojugular reflux, increased intensity of P_2, and a right-sided gallop all suggest right-sided cardiac dysfunction that may be due to pulmonary disease. Other physical findings that may suggest pulmonary disease include clubbing, hypertrophic pulmonary osteoarthropathy, edema, and altered mentation.

Simple bedside maneuvers can suggest the presence of significant obstructive lung disease. With the forced expiratory maneuver, patients forcibly expire while the physician listens with a stethoscope over the trachea. Audible air movement after 4 to 6 seconds indicates significant obstruction.[4] Simply asking patients to walk down the hall with physicians also gives some indication of their exercise tolerance.

An old study reported that the quality of a preanesthesia cough is predictive of postoperative pulmonary complications.[5] Apparently blinded to medical history or findings of physical examination and chest radiography, anesthesiologists asked 1821 "unselected, roughly consecutive" surgical patients to cough immediately before anesthesia was administered. The cough was evaluated "at a normal conversational distance" by multiple examiners and classified as normal (dry and clear) or abnormal. Abnormal coughs were either wet (mild to marked, depending on the persistence of adventitial sounds) or dry but paroxysmal. With this simple test, the quality of the cough had a sensitivity for postoperative pulmonary complications of 81%, a specificity of 86%, and positive and negative predictive values of 78% and 89%, respectively. The likelihood ratio for an abnormal cough was 5.8%. Thus, the quality of early morning coughs in mildly sedated patients should be further tested as a predictor of postoperative pulmonary complications.

CHEST RADIOGRAPHY

Several studies have shown that routine screening preoperative chest radiographs have a low yield, even in high-risk populations, for identifying abnormalities that are new, delay surgery, or change the perioperative management plans.[6,7] Their continued routine preoperative use is a significant waste of health care resources.[7] Preoperative radiographs should be obtained only to answer specific questions and provide usable information that will affect perioperative management. Specifically, it is reasonable to obtain preoperative chest radiographs for evidence of new or changing lung disease on the basis of signs or symptoms, or if patients are at high risk for postoperative pulmonary complications.[6]

ARTERIAL BLOOD GASES AND PH LEVEL

The purpose of testing arterial blood gases before surgery is two-fold: to assess the degree of gas exchange abnormality and to define patients' baseline levels. Arterial blood gases usually should be obtained in patients with clinical evidence of cardiopulmonary dysfunction. Identifying patients with hypoxemia and, particularly, hypercapnia is important, especially if upper abdominal or thoracic surgery is planned. In addition, other factors in the postoperative period can potentiate hypoventilation, including diaphragmatic dysfunction, narcotics, paralysis or partial paralysis of the respiratory muscles, and chest wall and abdominal pain.

Postoperative pulse oximetry or blood gases may be particularly useful in the first several hours after surgery. With frequent monitoring, subtle problems in oxygenation and ventilation can be detected before obvious clinical signs are apparent. The ventilatory status should be characterized before blood gases are interpreted because recent suction, inhalation therapy, or breathing exercises can affect Pa_{O_2}.

When preoperative blood gases are adequate in patients with abnormal lung function, physicians should consider whether ventilation can be reasonably well sustained after operation in the face of increased demands. Before operation, patients may already be near their maximum ventilatory and oxygenation abilities. If the need is suggested by symptoms of dyspnea on exertion, low-normal Pa_{O_2} levels, or abnormal results on lung examination or spirometry, a stress test can be used to assess ventilatory reserve. In the stress test, oxygen saturation is measured continuously with an oximeter, or periodically with assessments of the Pa_{O_2} from an indwelling arterial catheter, while patients are on treadmills performing graded programs of physical exercise.

PULMONARY FUNCTION TESTING

Although the history and physical examination are the cornerstones of the preoperative evaluation, pulmonary function testing is often used to document the presence of respiratory dysfunction and to measure its severity. Spirometry is used most often and has many virtues: it accurately diagnoses the presence and severity of obstructive lung disease and is noninvasive and fairly inexpensive.[8,9] As a result of spirometry's accuracy in diagnosing obstructive disease and the association between chronic obstructive disease and pulmonary complications of surgery, physicians frequently assume that spirometry predicts the likelihood of postoperative pulmonary complications in individual patients with lung disease. The value of spirometry in accurately predicting pulmonary operative risk for individual patients, however, is unproven. A critical appraisal of the evidence regarding the predictive value of spirometry for postoperative pulmonary complications after laparotomy found the evidence to be conflicting and the methodology of most studies to be significantly flawed.[10] Spirometry is probably overused, wasting a significant amount of health care resources.[11] Although spirometry is very sensitive in diagnosing obstructive disease, it is poorly sensitive in assessing individual operative prognosis. No single spirometric variable consistently correlates with risk and there is no degree of disease that absolutely contraindicates nonthoracic surgery.

Many patients with poor spirometric function can be navigated successfully through surgery, as evidenced by a recent study of postoperative pulmonary complications in patients with severe obstructive lung disease.[12] This study is the largest thus far of postoperative pulmonary and cardiac complications in patients with severe lung disease. Using explicit criteria for minor and major pulmonary complications, the authors examined 89 patients with severe chronic obstructive lung disease who were undergoing 107 operations of various types. Pulmonary complications occurred in 60% of coronary artery bypass operations and 56% of major abdominal operations compared to 27% of more peripheral operations using general or spinal anesthesia and 16% of procedures using regional or local anesthesia. Complication rates were also related to the duration of operation: less than 1 hour, 4%; 1 to 2 hours, 23%; 2 to 4 hours, 38%; and more than 4 hours, 73%. The most serious complications were six deaths and two cases of nonfatal ventilatory failure. Notably, five of the deaths occurred in patients undergoing coronary artery bypass grafting compared with the one death that occurred after 97 other operations (50% versus 1%). Thus, severe lung disease is not an absolute contraindication to necessary noncardiac surgery.

A well-done, randomized clinical trial is the best way to determine the value of spirometry in predicting, and thereby preventing, postoperative pulmonary complications. Such a trial may never be done because it would require a large sample and involve a high cost. For now, physicians should be aware that a forced expiratory volume in 1 second (FEV_1) of less than 1 L or an elevated PCO_2 appears to be associated with especially high risk. Even though the risk is increased with severe obstructive disease, recent evidence suggests that the greatest increase in mortality is primarily associated with thoracic operations.[12–14] Maximal voluntary ventilation, in which patients are asked to breathe as deeply and rapidly as possible, has been suggested as the single best predictive spirometric variable because it tests a combination of airflow and lung volume, in addition to patient understanding, motivation, cooperation, and strength.[15,16] Patients should be able to double their resting minute ventilation when performing this test.

Diagnostic spirometry may be indicated only for patients with significant smoking histories or clinical evidence of obstructive disease who have not previously undergone spirometric testing. Because no clinical trial has adequately evaluated the role of perioperative inhaled bronchodilators for patients with chronic obstructive disease who have no evidence of bronchospasm, clinicians should decide whether they are likely to use bronchodilators regardless of evidence of bronchospasm. Spirometry does not yield additional usable information if clinicians use these drugs as empiric prophylaxis in patients who have no evidence of bronchospasm. For patients undergoing thoracotomy, exercise spirometric testing may help in assessing respiratory function and operative risk.

EVALUATION FOR LUNG RESECTION

About 70% of patients undergoing lung resection for bronchogenic carcinoma have significant chronic obstructive lung disease. Two basic questions must be asked: (1) Can the patients tolerate the loss of lung or damage to the chest wall or diaphragm? (2) Will the surgery benefit the patients?

Routine spirometry should be performed and arterial blood gases measured; if the results of these studies are within normal limits, more specific tests are usually not necessary. Generally, patients with FEV_1 levels greater than 2 L can tolerate pneumonectomy. In patients with FEV_1 levels less than 2 L, quantitative lung scanning of perfusion and ventilation is performed to predict more accurately the amount of functional lung that will remain after resection.[17–19] Other, more invasive methods of assessing operability include bronchospirometry (in which patients are intubated with double-lumen tubes and individual lung spirometry is assessed),[20] exercise testing,[21,22] and temporary unilateral pulmonary artery occlusion (which can be accomplished by placing a balloon catheter in the pulmonary artery of the lung to be resected and occluding pulmonary blood flow).[23,24]

EVALUATION OF EMERGENCY SURGICAL PATIENTS

Patients with problems that require emergency surgery are frequently at greater risk for the development of postoperative respiratory complications than are those who undergo elective surgery. Many have sustained major trauma; others have hemorrhage, shock, sepsis, peritonitis, and aspiration of gastric contents. All these situations are associated with pulmonary injury and the adult respiratory distress syndrome.[25] Consequently, surgeons are often operating on high-risk patients and must take specific measures to identify preexisting lung disease and to formulate plans designed to maximize lung function and minimize postoperative complications.

To facilitate operative management, preexisting pulmonary disease should be identified if possible before patients are taken to the operating room. After surgery, weaning from assisted ventilation and extubation must be done carefully because these patients have limited respiratory reserve and may develop respiratory failure. Patients with chronic obstructive lung disease have a propensity to retain carbon dioxide and to develop respiratory acidosis when they are given high levels of supplemental oxygen. Therefore, they should receive controlled oxygen therapy with either nasal cannulas at low flow levels or Venturi masks.

Maintaining adequate delivery of oxygen to all body tissues is essential to adequate patient recovery. Evidence of adequate end-organ oxygen delivery is represented by adequate mentation, renal function, and urine output. Decreased oxygen delivery can result from inadequate saturation of circulating hemoglobin with oxygen (hypoxemia), a decreased level of hemoglobin (anemia), or inadequate cardiac output (which can have several causes). Monitoring of central venous pressure is useful in guiding volume replacement in cases of hemorrhagic shock or acute volume loss[26,27] but often fails to reflect left-sided cardiac function.[28-30] Pulmonary artery catheters classically have been used to guide fluid management, primarily by determination of pulmonary artery occlusion pressures.[31] This concept is being challenged increasingly and no adequate studies exist that demonstrate true improvement in patient outcome.[32-35] The use of pulmonary artery catheters to provide optimal tissue oxygen delivery has proved to be of benefit in perioperative patients when oxygen delivery is likely to be impaired.[33-35] Measurement of mixed venous oxygen saturation by oximetry reflects both oxygen delivery and consumption and can be performed continuously with pulmonary artery catheters that include a fiberoptic probe.[36,37]

CONCLUSION

The incidence of postoperative pulmonary complications is greater in patients with preexisting lung disease and is especially high after abdominal and thoracic surgery. Patients who are more likely to develop these problems can often be identified through careful preoperative evaluation. Emergency surgery carries especially high risk. A planned program of continuing treatment before and after surgery can often prevent or reduce respiratory dysfunction.

REFERENCES

1. Hodgkin JE. Preoperative assessment of respiratory function. Respir Care 1984;29:496–503.
2. Mohr DN, Jett JR. Preoperative evaluation of pulmonary risk factors. J Gen Intern Med 1988;3:277–287.
3. Stubbing DG, Mathur PN, Roberts RS, Campbell EJ. Some physical signs in patients with chronic airflow obstruction. Am Rev Respir Dis 1982;125:549–552.
4. Fishman AP. A first approach to the patient with respiratory signs or symptoms. In: Fishman AP, ed. Pulmonary diseases and disorders. New York, McGraw-Hill, 1980:3–28.
5. Greene BA, Berkowitz S. The preanesthetic induced cough as a method of diagnosis of preoperative bronchitis. Ann Intern Med 1952;37:723–732.
6. Tape TG, Mushlin AI. How useful are routine chest x-rays of preoperative patients at risk for postoperative chest disease? J Gen Intern Med 1988;3:15–20.
7. Roizen MF. Preoperative evaluation. In: Miller RD, ed. Anesthesia, ed 4. New York, Churchill Livingstone, 1994:827–882.
8. Tisi GM. Pulmonary physiology in clinical medicine. Baltimore, Williams & Wilkins, 1980:79–95.
9. Gass GD, Olsen GN. Preoperative pulmonary function testing to predict postoperative morbidity and mortality. Chest 1986;89:127–135.
10. Lawrence VA, Page CP, Harris GD. Preoperative spirometry before abdominal operations: a critical appraisal of its predictive value. Arch Intern Med 1989;149:280–285.
11. Lawrence VA, DeNino LA, Averyt E, et al. Preoperative spirometry before laparotomy: blowing away dollars. Clin Res 1992;40:586A.
12. Kroenke K, Lawrence VA, Theroux JF, Tuley MR. Operative risk in patients with severe obstructive pulmonary disease. Arch Intern Med 1992;152:967–971.
13. Grover FL, Hammermeister KE, Burchfiel C. Initial report of the Veterans Administration Preoperative Risk Assessment Study for Cardiac Surgery. Ann Thorac Surg 1990;50:12–26.
14. Hammermeister KE, Burchfiel C, Johson R, Grover FL. Identification of patients at greatest risk for developing major complications at cardiac surgery. Circulation 1990;82(Suppl 5):380–389.
15. Gaensler EA, Cugell DW, Lindgren I, et al. The role of pulmonary insufficiency in mortality and invalidism following surgery for pulmonary tuberculosis. J Thorac Surg 1955;29:163–187.
16. Boysen PG, Block AJ, Moulder PV. Relationship between preoperative pulmonary function tests and complications after thoracotomy. Surg Gynecol Obstet 1981;152:813–815.
17. Rogers RM, Kuhl DE, Hyde RW, et al. Measurement of the vital capacity and perfusion of each lung by fluoroscopy and macroaggregated albumin lung scanning: an alternate to bronchospirometry for evaluating individual lung function. Ann Intern Med 1967;67:947–956.
18. Olsen GN, Block AJ, Tobias JA. Prediction of post-pneumonectomy pulmonary function using quantitative macroaggregate lung scanning. Chest 1974;66:13–16.
19. Kristersson S, Lindell SE, Svanberg L. Prediction of pulmonary function loss due to pneumonectomy using ^{133}Xe-radiospirometry. Chest 1972;62:694–698.

20. Neuhaus H, Cherniack NS. A bronchospirometric method of estimating the effect of pneumonectomy on the maximum breathing capacity. J Thorac Cardiovasc Surg 1968;55:144–148.

21. Smith TP, Kinasewitz GT, Tucker WY, et al. Exercise capacity as a predictor of post thoracotomy morbidity. Am Res Respir Dis 1984;129:730–734.

22. Reichel J. Assessment of operative risk pneumonectomy. Chest 1972;62:570–576.

23. Sloan H, Morris JD, Figley M, Lee R. Temporary unilateral occlusion of the pulmonary artery in the preoperative evaluation of thoracic patients: preliminary report. J Thorac Surg 1955;30: 591–597.

24. Olsen GN, Block AJ, Swenson EW, et al. Pulmonary function evaluation of the lung resection candidate: a prospective study. Am Rev Respir Dis 1975;111:379–387.

25. Fowler AA, Hamman RF, Good JT, et al. Adult respiratory distress syndrome: risk with common predispositions. Ann Intern Med 1983;98:93–97.

26. Cohn JW, Tristiani FE, Khatri IM. Studies in clinical shock and hypotension: VI: Relationship between left and right ventricular function. J Clin Invest 1969;48:2008.

27. Weil MH, Shubin H, Rosoff L. Fluid repletion in circulatory shock: central venous pressure and other practical guides. JAMA 1965;192:668.

28. Forester JS, Diamond G, McHugh TJ, et al. Filling pressures in the right and left sides of the heart in acute myocardial infarction: a reappraisal of central venous pressure monitoring. N Engl J Med 1971;205:190.

29. James PM, Myers RT. Central venous pressure monitoring: misinterpretations, abuses, indications, and a new technique. Ann Surg 1972;175:693.

30. Bell H, Stubbs D, Pugh D. Reliability of central venous pressure as an indicator of left atrial pressure: a study of patients with mitral valve disease. Chest 1971;59:169.

31. Conners AF Jr, McCaffree DR, Gray BA. Evaluation of right heart catheterization in the critically ill patient without myocardial infarction. N Engl J Med 1983;308:263–267.

32. Robin ED. The cult of the Swan-Ganz catheter: overuse and abuse of pulmonary flow catheters. Ann Intern Med 1985; 103:445.

33. Finch CA, Lenfant C. Oxygen transport in man. N Engl J Med 1972;286:407.

34. Snyder JV. Assessment of systemic oxygen transport. In: Snyder JV, Pinsky MR, eds. Oxygen transport in the critically ill. Chicago, Year Book Medical Publishers, 1987:179–198.

35. Shoemaker WC, Appel PL, Kram HB, et al. Prospective trial of supranormal values of survivors as therapeutic goals in high-risk surgical patients. Chest 1988;94:1176.

36. Divertie MB, McMichan JC. Continuous monitoring of mixed venous oxygen saturation. Chest 1984;85:423.

37. Gettinger A, DeTraglia MC, Glass DD. In vivo comparison of two mixed venous saturation catheters. Anesthesiology 1987; 66:373.

Medical Management of the Surgical Patient, Third Edition,
edited by Michael F. Lubin, H. Kenneth Walker, and Robert B. Smith III.
J.B. Lippincott Company, Philadelphia, PA © 1995.

CHAPTER

13

PERIOPERATIVE RESPIRATORY MANAGEMENT

Valerie A. Lawrence
Charles A. Duncan

After careful preoperative evaluation, the prevention and treatment of postoperative pulmonary complications involves both preoperative and postoperative care. Perioperative respiratory management may include cessation of cigarette smoking; use of bronchodilators; clearance of secretions; provision of respiratory physiotherapy; administration of preoperative antibiotics; education of patients; use of breathing exercises, including incentive spirometry; institution of oxygen therapy; and prophylaxis of thromboembolism. The prophylaxis, diagnosis, and treatment of venous thromboembolism are discussed in Chapters 15 and 22.

CESSATION OF CIGARETTE SMOKING

Smoking more than 20 cigarettes per day is associated with a four-fold increase in the incidence of postoperative atelectasis. This complication is attributed to an increase in tracheobronchial secretions, a reduction in mucociliary clearance, and the consequent obstruction of airways with an internal diameter of less than 2 mm. Dysfunction of small airways in smokers has been documented but does not seem to be singularly related to an increase in the incidence of postoperative problems if the results of spirometry are normal.

Patients undergoing coronary artery bypass have fewer

complications if they stop smoking before surgery, but only when abstinence is sustained for 2 months.[1] Physicians should use this evidence, along with behavioral programs and nicotine withdrawal prophylaxis (ie, sustained-release skin patches, chewing gum), to help patients stop smoking for 2 months before elective surgery and hopefully maintain long-term abstinence.

BRONCHODILATORS

Patients should be free of wheezing whenever possible before anesthesia is induced. Bronchodilators should be given to patients with signs and symptoms of obstructive airway disease and to those who have an increase in tracheobronchial mucus. Data suggest that many patients may respond to bronchodilator medication in the laboratory if they are tested with sufficient frequency. Therefore, bronchodilators should not be withheld because of lack of reversibility on one test occasion.[2] Clinicians often use bronchodilators empirically because they are rarely harmful and may be helpful, and because pulmonary function tests are not always useful in determining a positive response.

Drugs commonly used as bronchodilators include β-adrenergic agonists, ipratropium bromide or atropine, corticosteroids, and aminophylline. It is being recognized increasingly that inflammation is the physiologic basis of asthma.[3] In addition, an association has been noted between chronic continuous β-agonist therapy and an increased death rate, as well as a possibly greater decline in the forced expiratory volume in 1 second.[4,5] As a result, inhaled steroids are considered the primary drug for long-term therapy, whereas aerosolized β-adrenergic agents are the first drug used in the acute treatment of airflow obstruction. β-Agonists relax bronchial smooth muscle by increasing intracellular levels of cyclic adenosine monophosphate and improving mucociliary transport.[6] The oral administration of β-agonists is associated with an increase in the side effects of tremulousness and tachycardia. Subcutaneous administration can cause significant dysrhythmias and should not be used in adults, especially those with cardiovascular disease.[6]

Ipratropium bromide, a derivative of atropine that is not systemically absorbed when given by inhalation, is an effective bronchodilator in patients with chronic obstructive lung disease.[7,8] Both atropine and ipratropium block cholinergic receptors and relax smooth muscle by decreasing intracellular levels of cyclic guanosine monophosphate, which is an intracellular messenger that promotes smooth muscle constriction. These drugs can be administered through metered-dose inhalers, with or without space devices, or through hand-held nebulizers driven by compressed air. The particle size of the inhalant is smaller and reaches distal airways better when metered dose inhalers are used but many patients do not use these canisters appropriately, even after proper instruction.[9] Hand-held nebulizers are often used in acute situations because patients in distress often experience difficulty with metered dose inhalers.[8] The use of spacing devices into which metered doses are injected before inhalation can improve drug delivery.

Theophylline had been considered the primary drug in the treatment of obstructive airway disease but is being challenged increasingly because of serious side effects, including dysrhythmias, seizures, and even death.[10,11] Warning symptoms of nausea or tremulousness may not precede the development of toxicity. Theophylline clearance also is altered by many other drugs and is influenced by the severity of illness. Theophylline should not be used in the perioperative period unless significant benefit is anticipated. Serum levels of theophylline should be maintained in the range of 5 to 15 mg/L to minimize toxic effects. Whether therapy with aminophylline, which improves diaphragmatic contractility, can improve diaphragmatic function after surgery and thereby reduce the incidence of pulmonary complications has not been studied.

Corticosteroids should be given to patients with asthma and to some patients with chronic obstructive lung disease.[12-15] Improvement in lung function should be documented by spirometry in all patients receiving long-term systemic corticosteroid therapy, because most patients have a sense of well-being when they are taking corticosteroids, even in the absence of true clinical improvement. Inhaled corticosteroids are preferred because of their lower incidence of side effects.

Patients who are receiving maintenance corticosteroid therapy and those who have taken corticosteroids for more than 1 week during the year preceding surgery should be given stress doses of corticosteroids, because the stress of surgery may unmask adrenal insufficiency. Patients who are taking at least 1500 μg/d (more than 12 puffs per day) of aerosolized corticosteroids such as beclomethasone should probably be given perioperative corticosteroids.[16] Parenteral corticosteroids (100 mg of hydrocortisone) are given several hours before surgery and again in the immediate postoperative period. For emergency surgery, 100 to 300 mg of hydrocortisone should be given intravenously every 8 hours until patients are stable. For elective surgery, a cosyntropin test can be performed or steroids can be administered empirically. Numerous regimens are outlined in the literature but no rigorous comparisons have been done. For major elective procedures, a standard regimen is 100 mg of hydrocortisone given at midnight before or on the morning of surgery and then every 8 hours through the first postoperative day, followed by 50 mg every 8 hours the second day, 25 mg every 8 hours the third day, and then the elimination of one dose each day as long as patients remain stable. For minor procedures, 50 mg of hydrocortisone may be given before surgery and then every 8 hours for two or three doses, followed by rapid tapering of the dosage. Intramuscular administration should not be used because of unreliable absorption and difficulty in tapering agents that have longer action (eg, dexamethasone).

NONINVASIVE MONITORING OF RESPIRATORY STATUS

Oximetry is being used increasingly as a noninvasive monitoring technique to detect changes in arterial oxygen saturation. A recent review of the literature found that pulse oximetry is an acceptably accurate noninvasive monitor of arterial oxygenation.[17] In contrast, capnography has not proven to be an accurate monitor of arterial CO_2 but can provide relevant information regarding systemic perfusion and dead-space ventilation in critically ill patients.[17]

CLEARANCE OF SECRETIONS AND RESPIRATORY PHYSIOTHERAPY

Tracheobronchial secretions and irritation should be minimized before surgery. The clearance of secretions may be improved by delivering mist aerosols of normal saline solution through an ultrasonic nebulizer 15 to 20 minutes after the administration of an inhaled bronchodilator. Numerous drugs, such as *N*-acetylcysteine, diluted sodium bicarbonate, and alcohol, have been given by inhalation to loosen bronchial secretions. No trials have demonstrated the efficacy of any of these agents and they all irritate the airways. It appears that *N*-acetylcysteine may be beneficial only when it is applied directly to mucus plugs through bronchoscopy.

The most effective techniques for clearing secretions are deep-breathing and coughing maneuvers. When patients cannot initiate coughs, nasotracheal suction may help clear secretions. Fiberoptic bronchoscopy is not indicated in the routine clearance of secretions. In patients who have poor coughs, localized accumulation of secretions in lobes or segments, or the possibility of foreign bodies in the lungs, however, this may be the only method of clearance.

Although no study clearly addresses this issue, it is considered prudent to postpone surgery for 6 weeks after an episode of pneumonia or bronchitis. This recommendation is based on the fact that lung function does not return to baseline levels for at least 6 weeks after a lower respiratory tract infection. The usual recommendation to postpone elective surgery for 10 days to 2 weeks after upper respiratory tract infections also is not based on prospective trials but on reports of persistent airway hyperreactivity after upper respiratory tract infection in children.

PREOPERATIVE ANTIBIOTICS

The value of prophylactic perioperative antibiotics in patients with chronic obstructive lung disease is unproved. Any evidence of clinical deterioration in these patients, however, suggests tracheobronchial infection as the underlying cause. Empiric broad-spectrum antibiotics are indicated and postponement of surgery should be considered.

PATIENT EDUCATION

Respiratory maneuvers should be taught before surgery so that effective therapy can be initiated after surgery. Patient understanding and cooperation are essential if postoperative breathing exercises are to prevent or minimize respiratory complications. Patients should be told why the maneuvers are necessary and be taught appropriate deep-breathing exercises and proper coughing. They should become familiar with the exercises and with respiratory care equipment before surgery while they are alert, free of pain, and unencumbered with restrictive dressings and tubes. Such training can reduce anxiety, improve cooperation after surgery, and provide familiar goals for the postoperative course.

LUNG EXPANSION TECHNIQUES AND PREVENTION OF ATELECTASIS

Breathing exercises, including incentive spirometry, are of special benefit to patients with diffuse obstructive pulmonary disease, providing improved ventilation by increasing diaphragmatic breathing and overcoming some obstruction to airflow on expiration. They increase the ability to empty the lungs, improve the efficiency of breathing, and prevent postoperative pulmonary complications.[19] One of the simplest techniques is to take a deep breath through the nose and exhale through pursed lips slowly and evenly while contracting the abdominal muscles. Physical therapists and respiratory therapists are usually well versed in breathing exercises, and the importance of their role cannot be emphasized too strongly.

Respiratory maneuvers to prevent alveolar collapse should be designed to provide maximal alveolar inflation and maintain a normal functional residual capacity. The optimal respiratory maneuver, therefore, is one in which maximal inspiratory pressure is produced and maintained for as long as possible to achieve the largest possible inhaled volume. A major postoperative concern is the inability to take a maximal inspiratory breath. Procedures and devices that have been recommended to achieve high alveolar filling pressures include forced expiratory maneuvers associated with coughing and deep breathing; expiration against resistance (eg, blow bottles); intermittent positive-pressure breathing machines; voluntary sustained maximal inspiratory maneuvers with incentive spirometers; and continuous positive airway pressure using a face mask.

Many studies have compared the efficacy of these methods in preventing postoperative pulmonary complications. End points have included successful prevention of atelectasis, hypoxemia, and loss of lung volume. Intermittent positive-pressure breathing, initially thought to be promising, has no proven benefit. Blow bottles and blowing into gloves and balloons also provide no benefit. Methods aimed at sustaining inspiration and inflation, including incentive spirometry, deep-breathing exercises, and continuous positive airway pressure using a face mask, are thought to be more effective in preventing respiratory complications.[19–21] No single method has emerged as the procedure of choice. Choosing techniques is probably not as important as is motivating patients, educating patients regarding the desired goals, and having experienced personnel (especially respiratory therapists and nurses) provide encouragement and supervision.[19] No difference was noted in the incidence of pulmonary complications in a trial of incentive spirometry and chest physiotherapy.[22] Incentive spirometry may be preferable because it is less labor-intensive and, therefore, less expensive. The value of the various lung expansion techniques has been discussed in detail elsewhere.[23]

RESPIRATORY MUSCLE STRENGTH

The place of training and nutritional supplements in improving operative outcome in patients with chronic obstructive lung disease is unclear. A recent metaanalysis found that respiratory muscle training improved strength but did not significantly improve exercise capacity or quality of life.[24] In studies that controlled training intensity, however, significant improvement was noted in both functional status and respiratory muscle strength.[24] Whether such training can reduce postoperative pulmonary complications has not been determined.

Respiratory muscle weakness can also result from malnutrition. In a small randomized trial of patients with emphysema who weighed less than 90% of their ideal body weights, intensive oral nutritional supplementation for 4 months produced significant weight gain, improved walking distance, and increased strength in handgrip and expiratory muscles.[25] Whether these results are important for patients with lung disease who are undergoing surgery remains to be studied. A multicenter randomized trial of total parental nutrition in surgical patients at 10 veterans' hospitals was unable to address the specific value of such therapy in patients with chronic lung disease.[26]

MISCELLANEOUS MANEUVERS

Supplemental oxygen is indicated in the treatment of patients with pulmonary disease whenever significant hypoxemia is present. Controlled oxygen administration, with adequate humidification when indicated, rarely produces ventilatory depression or toxicity.

Because remaining supine for prolonged periods reduces both functional residual capacity and expiratory reserve volume, frequent changes in position during the postoperative period are important.[27] When it can be tolerated, a more vertical position allows the diaphragm to descend more freely during inspiration because the abdominal contents do not tend to push against it. Whenever possible, early ambulation is beneficial.

Narcotic analgesics increase the risk of postoperative pulmonary complications because they reduce the ventilatory response to hypoxia and hypercapnia in healthy persons.[28]

Although they are necessary, restrictive bandages, dressings, and chest tubes may interfere with deep breathing. Studies in healthy volunteers whose chests were strapped with adhesive tape showed that total lung capacity decreased and respiratory frequency increased, favoring alveolar collapse. These changes were reversed within minutes after the strapping was removed.[29]

TREATMENT OF COR PULMONALE

Cor pulmonale results from precapillary pulmonary hypertension, which is usually caused by alveolar hypoxia and acidemia. Treatment, therefore, is aimed at reversing the alveolar hypoxia with supplemental oxygen and the acidemia with improved alveolar ventilation. Bronchodilators, bronchial hygiene, and oxygen therapy are used to reduce airway obstruction, hypercapnia, and hypoxemia; to improve cardiac function; and to decrease pulmonary vascular resistance and the work of the right ventricle. Patients with combined left- and right-sided heart failure benefit from angiotensin-converting enzyme inhibitors and digitalis but these drugs are not useful in isolated right heart failure or cor pulmonale from lung disease. Digitalis also is not helpful for multifocal atrial tachycardia.

Perioperative respiratory management is a multifaceted endeavor in all patients but profoundly so in patients with pulmonary disease. Diligent attention to risk evaluation and the use of supportive care techniques allows most patients to survive beneficial noncardiac surgery. Compared to the assessment of cardiac risk before noncardiac surgery, however, the evaluation of pulmonary operative risk has not been well studied using sound methods and designs. Informed clinicians should be aware of this discrepancy and anticipate better information in the future.

REFERENCES

1. Warner MA, Offord KP, Warner ME, et al. Role of cessation of smoking and other factors in postoperative pulmonary complications: a blinded prospective study of coronary artery bypass patients. Mayo Clin Proc 1989;64:609–616.
2. Anthonisen NR, Wright EC. Bronchodilator response in chronic obstructive pulmonary disease. Am Rev Respir Dis 1986;133:814–819.
3. Barnes PJ. A new approach to the treatment of asthma. N Engl J Med 1989;321:1517–1527.
4. Spitzer WO, Suissa S, Ernst P, et al. The use of beta-agonists and the risk of death and near death from asthma. N Engl J Med 1992;326:501–506.
5. Van Schayck CP, Dompeling E, Van Herwaarden CL, et al. Bronchodilator treatment in moderate asthma or chronic bronchitis: continuous or on demand? BMJ 1991;303:1426–1431.
6. McFadden ER. Clinical use of beta-adrenergic agonists. J Allergy Clin Immunol 1985;76:352–356.
7. Baigelman W, Chodish S. Bronchodilator action of the anticholinergic drug, ipratropium bromide, as an aerosol in chronic bronchitis and asthma. Chest 1977;71:324–328.
8. Gross NJ, Skorodin MS. Role of parasympathetic system in airways obstruction due to emphysema. N Engl J Med 1984;311:421–425.
9. Shim C, Williams MH Jr. The adequacy of inhalation of aerosol from canister nebulizers. Am J Med 1980;69:891–894.

10. Bertino JS, Walker JW. Reassessment of theophylline toxicity. Arch Intern Med 1987;147:757–760.

11. Greenberg A, Piraino BH, Kroboth PD, Weiss J. Severe theophylline toxicity. Am J Med 1984;76:854–860.

12. Kaliner M. Mechanisms of glucocorticoid action in bronchial asthma. J Allergy Clin Immunol 1985;76:321–329.

13. Albert RK, Martin TR, Lewis SW. Controlled clinical trial of methylprednisolone in patients with chronic bronchitis and acute respiratory insufficiency. Ann Intern Med 1980;92:753–758.

14. Mandella LA, Manfreda J, Warren CP, Anthonisen NR. Steroid response in stable chronic obstructive pulmonary disease. Ann Intern Med 1982;96:17–21.

15. Kerstjens HAM, Brand PLP, Hughes MD, et al. A comparison of bronchodilator therapy with or without inhaled corticosteroid therapy for obstructive airways disease. N Engl J Med 1992;327:1413–1419.

16. Smith MJ, Hodson ME. Effects of long term inhaled high dose beclomethasone diproprionate on adrenal function. Thorax 1983;38:676–681.

17. Technology Subcommittee of the Working Group on Critical Care, Ontario Ministry of Health. Noninvasive blood gas monitoring: a review for use in the adult critical care unit. Can Med Assoc J 1992;146:703–712.

18. Bendixon HH, Egbert LD, Hedley Whyte J, et al. Respiratory care. St Louis, CV Mosby, 1965.

19. Celli BR, Rodriguez KS, Snider GL. A controlled trial of intermittent positive pressure breathing, incentive spirometry, and deep breathing exercise in preventing pulmonary complications after abdominal surgery. Am Rev Respir Dis 1984;130:12–15.

20. Ricksten SE, Bengtsson A, Soderberg C, et al. Effects of periodic positive airway pressure by mask on postoperative pulmonary function. Chest 1986;89:774–781.

21. Stock MC, Downs JB, Gauer PK, et al. Prevention of postoperative pulmonary complications with CPA incentive spirometry, and conservative therapy. Chest 1985;87:151–157.

22. Hall JC, Tarala R, Harris J, et al. Incentive spirometry versus routine chest physiotherapy for prevention of pulmonary complications after abdominal surgery. Lancet 1991;337:953–956.

23. Celli BR. Perioperative respiratory care of the patient undergoing upper abdominal surgery. Clin Chest Med 1993;14:253–261.

24. Smith K, Cook D, Guyatt GH, et al. Respiratory muscle training in chronic airflow limitation: a meta-analysis. Am Rev Respir Dis 1992;145:533–539.

25. Rogers RM, Donahoe M, Costantino J. Physiologic effects of oral supplemental feeding in malnourished patients with chronic obstructive pulmonary disease. Am Rev Respir Dis 1992;146:1511–1517.

26. The Veterans Affairs Total Parenteral Nutrition Cooperative Study Group. Perioperative total parenteral nutrition in surgical patients. N Engl J Med 1991;325:525–532.

27. Meyers JR, Lembeck L, O'Kane H, et al. Changes in functional residual capacity of the lung after operation. Arch Surg 1975;110:576–583.

28. Weil JV, McCullough RE, Kline JS, et al. Diminished ventilatory response to hypoxia and hypercapnia and morphine in normal man. N Engl J Med 1975;292:1103–1106.

29. Caro CG, Butler J, DuBois AB. Some effects of restriction of chest cage expansion on pulmonary function in man: an experimental study. J Clin Invest 1960;39:57–83.

Medical Management of the Surgical Patient, Third Edition,
edited by Michael F. Lubin, H. Kenneth Walker, and Robert B. Smith III.
J.B. Lippincott Company, Philadelphia, PA © 1995.

CHAPTER

14

ADULT RESPIRATORY DISTRESS SYNDROME AND MULTIPLE ORGAN DYSFUNCTION

Jeffrey R. Pine
Gerald W. Staton, Jr.

HISTORY

In modern medical literature, the adult respiratory distress syndrome (ARDS) was described in 1967 in the classic article by Ashbaugh and associates.[1] As early as 1927, however, Osler's textbook, *The Principles and Practice of Medicine*, described the pulmonary problems associated with sepsis as follows: "uncontrolled septicemia leads to frothy pulmonary edema that resembles serum, not the sanguinous transudative edema fluid seen in dropsy or congestive heart failure."[2] Clearly, the observation had already been made that the edema fluid in the setting of sepsis was highly proteinaceous, implying an understanding that the permeability of the alveolar-capillary membrane was altered.

DEFINITIONS

The adult respiratory distress syndrome is an acute lung injury characterized by certain clinical and physiologic responses resulting from direct lung damage (eg, aspiration, toxic fumes, pneumonia) or systemic inflammatory states (eg, trauma, sepsis, other tissue injuries). During the past three decades, a partial understanding has developed concerning the pathogenesis and interrelationships of the seemingly diverse clinical disorders that produce ARDS.

Although new treatment techniques such as ventilators, defibrillators, and fluid resuscitation have led to longer survival, complicating "syndromes" have developed with names like *sepsis syndrome, hypermetabolic syndrome,* and *multiorgan failure syndrome.* Over time, several facts have become obvious:

1. These "syndromes," as well as ARDS, are derived from a common pathophysiology and are best viewed as a basic injury response with considerable clinical overlap.[3,4]
2. Although acute lung dysfunction is frequently (but not always) the initial and more notorious sequela, it is only part of more diffuse organ damage that may be subtle or overt.[3,4]
3. Prognosis can be reliably predicted by defining the initiating etiologic event and the extent of damage to other organs.[5]

ARDS was first defined as a catastrophic pulmonary or nonpulmonary event followed by severe respiratory distress with interstitial chest radiographic infiltrates progressing to consolidation.[6] Key physiologic parameters were severe hypoxemia (an arterial oxygen tension of less than 50 mmHg with an inspired oxygen fraction greater than 0.6 due to a large intrapulmonary shunt) and a stiff (noncompliant), edematous lung produced by leaky pulmonary capillaries. As researchers and clinicians searched for a better understanding of the way in which a multitude of disorders produced a final common pathway, old nomenclature gave way to an expanded definition of ARDS.[7,8] This new definition includes three components: (1) lung injury and its severity, (2) initiating and associated clinical disorders, and (3) dysfunction in other organs. The new definition includes less severe degrees of lung injury associated with less hypoxemia and ranks the severity of lung injury. ARDS is said to be present when the lung injury score exceeds 0.1 (Table 14-1). This score can change dramatically as ARDS worsens or improves. Nonetheless, it is useful for research purposes and clinical prognosis in certain types of lung injury (ie, aspiration of gastric contents [see later]). The cur-

TABLE 14–1. Components of the Lung Injury Score

Component	Value
Chest Roentgenogram Score	
No alveolar consolidation	0
Alveolar consolidation in 1 quadrant	1
Alveolar consolidation in 2 quadrants	2
Alveolar consolidation in 3 quadrants	3
Alveolar consolidation in all 4 quadrants	4
Hypoxemia Score	
$Pao_2/Fio_2 \geq 300$	0
Pao_2/Fio_2 225–299	1
Pao_2/Fio_2 175–224	2
Pao_2/Fio_2 100–174	3
$Pao_2/Fio_2 < 100$	4
Respiratory System Compliance Score (when ventilated; mL/cm H_2O)	
≥ 80	0
60–79	1
40–59	2
20–39	3
≤ 19	4
Positive End-Expiratory Pressure Score (when ventilated; cm H_2O)	
≤ 5	0
6–8	1
9–11	2
12–14	3
≥ 15	4

The final value is obtained by dividing the aggregate sum by the number of components that were used.

Score	
No injury	0
Mild to moderate injury	0.1–2.5
Severe injury (adult respiratory distress syndrome)	>2.5

(Murray JF, Matthay MA, Luce J, et al. An expanded definition of the adult respiratory distress syndrome. Am Rev Respir Dis 1988;138:720)

TABLE 14–2. Clinical Disorders Associated With Adult Respiratory Distress Syndrome*

Sepsis
Liquid aspiration (gastric contents, hydrocarbons)
Pneumonia (with or without bacteremia)
Trauma (fat emboli, lung contusion, nonthoracic trauma)
Shock (any cause)
Drugs (overdose, chemotherapeutic, idiosyncratic)
Acute pancreatitis
Inhaled toxins (smoke, oxygen, chemicals)
Hematologic disorder (disseminated intravascular coagulation, massive transfusion, thrombotic thrombocytopenic purpura)
Acute liver failure
Cardiopulmonary bypass
Burns
Head injury or increased intracranial pressure†
Pulmonary hemorrhage
Amniotic fluid embolism, eclampsia
Air emboli
Massive pulmonary emboli†
Reexpansion pulmonary edema†
Radiation
Uremia (questionable; more likely fluid overload)
Leukemia (leukostasis)
Transplantation (pulmonary rejection, bone marrow transplantation)
  Drugs: OKT-3, colony-stimulating factors, cyclosporine
Anaphylaxis
Paraquat
Lymphangiogram dye
Upper airway obstruction†
Heat stroke
High-altitude pulmonary edema†
Near-drowning†

*Can also be associated with systemic inflammatory response syndrome.
†These disorders may involve different initial mechanisms, producing fluid formation and ultimately leading to protein-rich edema.

rent definition requires a careful, continuous search for associated clinical disorder(s) and the development of other organ dysfunction. Table 14-2 lists the different disorders that have been associated with ARDS.

A consensus conference recently was convened to standardize the terminology[9] (Table 14-3). The term *systemic inflammatory response syndrome* (SIRS) describes a similar response to various insults (eg, sepsis, trauma) and the term *multiple organ dysfunction syndrome* describes subsequent altered organ function, of which ARDS may be one component. Although several points deserve emphasis, particularly the fact that infection with or without bacteremia can initiate the SIRS, many other causes may produce an identical clinical response. Furthermore, hypotension or shock is not absolutely necessary to produce organ dysfunction.[9,10] The lung is one of many organs that can fail, either alone or

TABLE 14–3. Definitions of Sepsis and Associated Syndromes

Bacteremia: Presence of viable bacteria in the blood

Sepsis: Systemic response to infection, manifested by two or more of the following conditions:
 Temperature over 38°C or under 36°C
 Heart rate over 90 beats/min
 Respiratory rate over 20 breaths/min or $Paco_2$ below 32 mmHg
 White blood cell count over 12,000/μL, below 4000/μL, or over 10% immature
  (band) forms

Sepsis-induced hypotension: Systolic blood pressure below 90 mmHg or a reduction of 44 mmHg or more from baseline in the absence of other causes of hypotension

Septic shock: Sepsis-induced hypotension despite adequate fluid resuscitation along with the presence of perfusion abnormalities that may include, but are not limited to, lactic acidosis, oliguria, or an acute alteration in mental status. Patients who are receiving inotropic or vasopressor agents may not be hypotensive at the time that perfusion abnormalities are measured.

Systemic inflammatory response syndrome (SIRS):* Systemic inflammatory response to a variety of severe clinical insults. The response is manifested by two or more of the following conditions:
 Temperature over 38°C or under 36°C
 Heart rate over 90 beats/min
 Respiratory rate over 20 breaths/min or $Paco_2$ below 32 mmHg
 White blood cell count over 12,000/μL, below 4000/μL, or over 10% immature
  (band) forms

Adult respiratory distress syndrome: Hypoxemia, decreased compliance, and radiographic infiltrates from acute lung injury induced by many causes (see Table 14–2); may be part of SIRS and associated with other organ failure

Multiple organ dysfunction syndrome: Presence of altered organ function in an acutely ill patient such that homeostasis cannot be maintained without intervention

---

*The clinical manifestations of SIRS and sepsis are identical. When it is associated with infection, SIRS is termed *sepsis.* The committee recommended avoiding the terms *septicemia* and *septic syndrome.*
(American College of Chest Physicians/Society of Critical Care Medicine Consensus Conference. Modified from Bone RC, Balk RA, Cerra FB, et al. Definition for sepsis and organ failure and guidelines for the use of innovative therapies in sepsis. Chest 1992;101:1644)

in combination with other organs, and case presentations vary in a dynamic continuous fashion both in time course and in extent of organ failure (Fig. 14-1). As with all definitions, some difficulties arise (ie, ARDS can be superimposed on chronic lung disease or cardiogenic pulmonary edema, both of which can produce infiltrates and hypoxemia). For practical purposes, a tentative diagnosis of ARDS can be made in the setting of acute lung injury with increased hypoxemia and chest radiographic infiltrates associated with an obvious predisposing clinical disorder. Clinical judgment should then guide appropriate testing to rule out other diagnoses, such as fluid overload, cardiac failure, or pulmonary emboli.

INCIDENCE AND EPIDEMIOLOGY

The incidence of ARDS is difficult to establish because many patients have mild acute lung injury and are never classified as having ARDS. In 1977, using the older, more restrictive definition, it was estimated that 150,000 cases (0.6 per 1000) occurred in the United States, with an estimated mortality rate of 50% to 60%.[11] Two more recent studies reported incidence rates about 10 times lower (0.02 to 0.05 per 1000).[12,13] The differences in these estimates may be related to variations in the definitions used and the populations studied.

The incidence of ARDS varies dramatically among the numerous disorders with which it is known to be associated. Reported incidence rates vary between studies but may reflect differences in the patient populations surveyed and the definitions used for underlying diseases.[14,15] ARDS is seen in as many as 40% of all patients with sepsis, which is its most common precipitating condition. ARDS also occurs in 30% to 36% of patients with aspiration of gastric contents. In contrast, it develops in only 5% to 8% of patients with long-bone fractures and fat emboli.

PATHOPHYSIOLOGY

PATHOLOGY

Pathologists describe ARDS as *diffuse alveolar damage,* a descriptive term for the nonspecific but predictable sequence of changes that occurs in affected patients.[16] The causative agent or process usually cannot be determined from the histopathologic pattern. In addition, the process can resolve at any point in the progression described later.

The histologic appearance of diffuse alveolar damage varies depending on the amount of time that has elapsed between the precipitating event and the biopsy or autopsy. Three stages are generally recognized: an acute exudative phase (0 to 7 days); a subacute proliferative or organizing phase (7 to 14 days); and a chronic phase (more than 14 days).

The acute exudative phase is characterized at its earliest point by interstitial and intraalveolar edema, neutrophilic infiltration, hemorrhage, and fibrin deposition. A mixture of fibrin and cellular debris from sloughed cells is laid down on the alveolar surface to form the so-called hyaline membranes that are prominent 3 to 7 days after injury. The

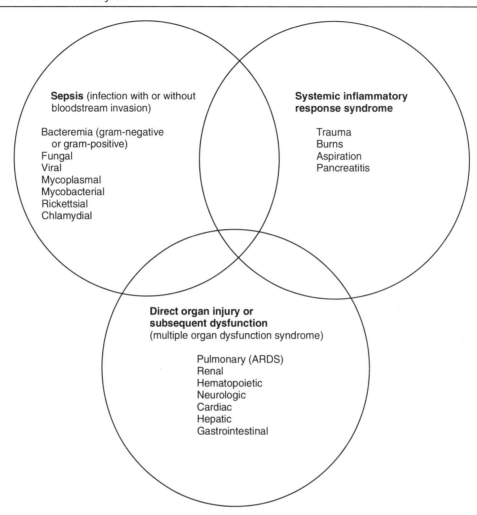

FIG. 14-1. Sepsis or systemic inflammatory response syndrome can produce organ dysfunction through direct damage or systemic mediators and inflammation. Systemic inflammatory response syndrome is termed sepsis when an infection source is known.

alveolar lining cells that have sloughed leave a denuded basement membrane that is important in subsequent repair or fibrosis. An interstitial infiltrate of inflammatory cells becomes more pronounced about 7 days after injury and persists through the proliferative phase.

In response to the denuded basement membrane, type 2 pneumocytes proliferate (days 3 to 7), producing a pattern of alveolar lining cell hyperplasia. In patients who go on to resolution, these proliferating cells ultimately differentiate into type 1 pneumocytes, restoring the epithelial side of the alveolar-capillary wall and returning gas exchange toward normal.

The proliferative or organizing phase of ARDS is charac-

terized by interstitial inflammation and loose fibroblast proliferation, initially in the interstitium, which invades into alveolar spaces through gaps in the basement membrane and produces areas of intraalveolar fibrosis. During this phase, the hyaline membranes disappear by phagocytosis or organization and the exudate is incorporated into intraalveolar plugs of proliferating fibroblasts.

The chronic phase of ARDS is characterized by areas of intense fibrosis, focal emphysema, and pulmonary vascular obliteration. Histologically, this phase of the disease may appear similar to idiopathic pulmonary fibrosis. In contrast to idiopathic pulmonary fibrosis, however, the chronic phase of ARDS improves over time if patients survive.

PATHOGENESIS

The mechanisms leading to ARDS have been studied extensively in the last 25 years but still are not entirely known. The two key sites of injury early in the process are the endothelium of the pulmonary capillary bed and the alveolar epithelium.

The endothelium of the pulmonary capillaries is probably the earliest site of injury in ARDS produced by sepsis and other systemic disorders. Circulating mediators stimulated by endotoxin, such as activated complement fragments,[17] tumor necrosis factor, and other cytokines released from monocytes[18] and coagulation factors, activate neutrophils and platelets, resulting in aggregation and embolization of the pulmonary vasculature.[19] Intravascular aggregates of neutrophils and platelets obstruct local blood flow and reduce the effective volume and surface area of the capillary bed. Platelets release prostaglandins such as thromboxane A_2 and may, along with local obstruction, contribute to the pulmonary hypertension often seen in affected patients.[20] The neutrophils adhere to the endothelium, releasing injurious oxidants, proteolytic enzymes, and arachidonic acid metabolites. This results in endothelial cell dysfunction and destruction, with denuding of the endothelial side of the basement membrane.[21,22] Endotoxin may also injure the endothelial cells directly.[23] Intravascular macrophages sequestered in the pulmonary vascular bed have secretory capabilities similar to those of neutrophils and may play a role in this injury, possibly explaining the development of ARDS in patients with neutropenia.[24,25] Increased permeability of the membrane allows plasma and cells to leak into the interstitial spaces of the lung and ultimately into the alveoli. Similar microvascular damage occurs throughout the body, explaining the multiorgan dysfunction associated with this syndrome.

The second site of injury in early ARDS is the alveolar epithelium. The alveolar epithelium is critically important to normal lung physiology because the tight junctions between cells prevent interstitial fluid from entering the alveolar space. These cells have an active, possibly β-agonist–sensitive sodium transport system that may help to remove fluid from the alveolar space,[25a] and the type 2 cells produce surfactant. Within hours of acute lung injury, type 1 pneumocytes die, denuding the alveolar side of the basement membrane. The exact cause of this phase of lung injury is not known, although neutrophils and activated alveolar macrophages are present in the alveolar spaces early in the course and probably play a role.[26] Elastase and other proteolytic enzymes from neutrophils and macrophages have been found in the bronchoalveolar lavage fluids of patients with ARDS.[27,28] The plasma that leaks from the vasculature contains several antiproteolytic proteins, but these may be inactivated by oxidants generated by the inflammatory cells, allowing the enzymes to be locally active.[29] Oxidants such as hydrogen peroxide, and superoxide or hydroxyl radicals can also act directly to injure cells.[30] In addition, the macrophages produce procoagulant substances, such as tissue factor and factor VII, which activate the coagulation factors that have leaked into the interstitial and alveolar spaces, producing fibrin.[31] Fibrin is an inhibitor of surfactant and, along with other cellular debris, produces the hyaline membranes seen in the early stages of ARDS.[32]

Once the acute lung injury has occurred, the lung attempts to repair itself. The success or failure of this process is crucial to patient survival. Studies suggest that the critical factor is the severity of the injury to the epithelial side of the alveolar capillary membrane. The type 2 epithelial cells begin to proliferate early in the process, attempting to recover the denuded basement membrane. If the basement membrane is not too severely damaged, the type 2 cells are more likely to be successful. Once the basement membrane has been repaired, the epithelial pneumocytes may play a role in removing the fluid and other debris from the alveolar space and in synthesizing new surfactant. In time, the new cells differentiate into type 1 cells and return the membrane to the thin structure that is critical to gas exchange.

If the injury to the epithelial membrane and the basement membrane is severe, progressive interstitial and intraalveolar fibrosis ensues. Controlled by growth factors (many from macrophages), and probably using a matrix of fibrin and fibronectin as a framework, fibroblasts invade the exudate, proliferating and synthesizing collagen (type 1), elastin, and other matrix substances.[33] The normal lung architecture is rapidly replaced by acute, progressive fibrosis that can make gas exchange difficult, if not impossible.

PHYSIOLOGIC AND CLINICAL CONSEQUENCES

Alveolar fluid accumulation tends to be an all-or-none phenomenon; once fluid appears, it rapidly floods the alveolar space.[34] Early on, the alveolar-arterial oxygen gradient widens, progressing to hypoxemia with increasing inspired oxygen requirements. In addition, qualitative and quantitative abnormalities of surfactant occur, causing other alveoli to collapse.[35] Flooded and collapsed alveoli produce a pulmonary shunt with poorly oxygenated venous blood crossing into the arterial circulation, which is found in virtually all patients with ARDS.[36] Some patients also develop significant ventilation–perfusion (V/Q) mismatching augmenting the hypoxemia (low V/Q ratios) and impairing carbon dioxide exchange (high V/Q ratios indicate increased physiologic dead space).[36] Occasionally, mild to moderate bronchospasm may be superimposed. Mild to moderate elevation in pulmonary vascular resistance is common as a result of vascular obstruction and vasoregulatory changes.[37,38]

Early clinical manifestations are respiratory distress with rapid, shallow breathing, followed by progressive, often refractory hypoxemia and cyanosis. Rales are frequently present early in the course of the disease. The chest radiograph initially may be clear or may show an interstitial or hazy ground-glass appearance. With progression, patchy alveolar infiltrates and consolidation become prominent. These changes are typically nonhomogeneous on computed tomographic scanning, with greater involvement of gravity-dependent areas.[39] Small or, occasionally, moderate exudative pleural effusions are common.[39–41]

As part of the SIRS, increased oxygen consumption associated with progressive gas-exchange abnormalities creates an increasing ventilatory requirement. Coupled with reduced pulmonary compliance (stiff, edematous small lungs), this often results in inspiratory muscle fatigue and respiratory failure. Under these circumstances, the respiratory muscles may utilize over 50% of the total oxygen consumption.[42]

Many metabolic changes occur in the SIRS, previously called the hypermetabolic syndrome, including increased oxygen consumption and intense catabolism as a result of the previously mentioned mediators. The heart responds with increased cardiac output facilitated by a decrease in systemic vascular resistance. Concomitant cardiac disease, particularly in the elderly, may prevent this life-sustaining response, resulting in hypotension. Alternatively, profound decreases in systemic vascular resistance despite high cardiac outputs may produce refractory hypotension.[43] This condition, characterized by increased cardiac output, increased oxygen consumption, and vasodilation with hypotension was previously called warm shock. In addition, circulating myocardial depressant factors can reduce cardiac contractility, even in young, previously healthy patients. The decreased contractility may occur within hours to days, producing profound decreases in the right and left ventricular ejection fractions, which may be as low as 12%. Physiologic compensation requires increased ventricular compliance, thereby producing cardiac dilation to maintain the stroke volume and sustain cardiac output (Fig. 14-2). Individual survival is correlated with this response.[43]

The diffuse nature of the tissue injury in the SIRS leads to another phenomenon that has generated significant controversy. One way to view the disorder that results is to consider the diffuse, ongoing microvascular damage and organ malfunction as the result of a relative inability to engage in normal aerobic metabolism. Capillary injury, edema, and cell damage create impediments to tissue oxygen extraction. Hence, tissue ischemia occurs despite normal or even elevated oxygen delivery.[44,45]

The amount of oxygen delivered to the tissues is the product of the oxygen content of the blood (hemoglobin content and oxygen saturation, the latter determined by lung function) and the amount of blood delivered (cardiac output). The oxygen uptake (tissue utilization) is determined by the adequacy of the amount of oxygen delivered and the patency and vasoregulatory capability of the regional and microvascular beds in distributing blood flow according to tissue metabolic needs. Normally, vasoregulatory distributive changes and enhanced oxygen extraction (in which the tissues remove more oxygen per unit of blood) occur as global oxygen delivery is reduced, thereby providing compensation. If oxygen delivery continues to fall to a critical level, then anaerobic metabolism begins, with progressive organ damage and dysfunction. This is illustrated in Figure 14-3. Also shown is the pathophysio-

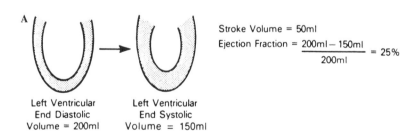

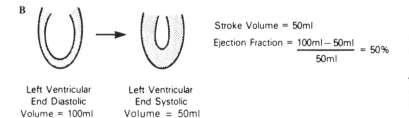

FIG. 14-2. (A) Compensation by ventricular dilatation during acute phase of sepsis (also may occur with SIRS of any cause). (B) After recovery, ejection fraction returns to normal. (Parrillo JE, et al. Septic Shock in Humans. NIH Conference. Ann Intern Med 1990;113:227–242)

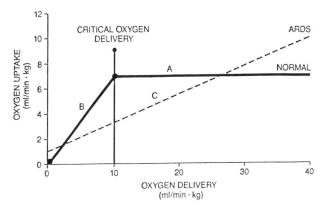

FIG. 14-3. Schematic pathologic relationship between oxygen uptake and delivery that occurs in many (not all) patients with ARDS/SIRS. It is also reported in other disease states. Normally constant oxygen uptake (A) despite variable delivery due to compensatory mechanisms noted in text. (B) critical threshold (cannot compensate further). (C) Like B, dependence of oxygen uptake on delivery but remains dependent over wide levels of delivery in ARDS/SIRS patients. (Dorinsky DM, Gadek JE: Mechanisms of Multiple Nonpulmonary organ failure in ARDS. Chest 1989;96:885–892)

logic response seen in patients with the SIRS/ARDS, in whom this compensatory capability may be lost. In this case, tissue oxygen extraction is dependent on the amount of oxygen delivered, so-called utilization supply/dependency.[46] This implies that enhancing oxygen delivery to supranormal levels can prevent or treat organ dysfunction and reduce mortality.[44,45,47] Debate continues regarding the appropriate techniques for obtaining these measurements, whether oxygen supply/dependency actually is pathologic or physiologic in certain groups of patients, and the best means of providing optimal oxygen delivery for each patient.[48,49]

DETERMINING PROGNOSIS

The causes of death in ARDS are diverse and vary depending on the time course of the illness[50] (Fig. 14-4). Sepsis dominates as a cause of death during the entire course of illness, often associated with vasodilation unresponsive to vasoconstrictors. Other infection, overt or occult, is often present at the time of death.[7,51] Frequent sites of infection are the abdomen, lung, or intravenous lines. Irreversible central nervous system dysfunction and hemorrhagic shock are also common causes of death during the first 3 days of illness, whereas cardiac and respiratory dysfunction are more common later.

Although the degree of lung injury in ARDS is correlated with subsequent outcome, other parameters more accurately predict prognosis. This is not surprising because ARDS is frequently part of the SIRS and results from many different disorders. With state-of-the-art ventilator support techniques, respiratory failure is the cause of death in only 10% (early) to 18% (late) of cases, highlighting the importance of other organ system dysfunc-

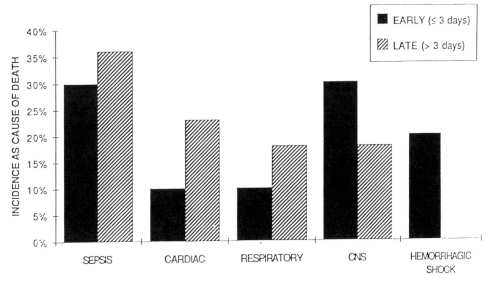

FIG. 14-4. Incidence of several factors as causes of death early (≤3 days) and late (>3 days) after the onset of ARDS. (Adapted from Montgomery B, et al. Causes of mortality in patients with the adult respiratory distress syndrome. Am Rev Respir Dis 1985;132:485–489)

tion, such as hemodynamic failure with refractory shock or progressive renal failure, in producing morbidity and mortality.[7]

Mortality can best be predicted at any given point in time by the number of organs that are failing. Although the term *organ failure* is often used, a better description is *organ dysfunction,* which implies a spectrum of organ damage from mild to severe that has the capacity to improve or deteriorate. Investigators have listed varying criteria to define organ malfunction. Knaus and associates,[5,52] using pooled data from 5677 intensive care unit admissions from several hospitals, demonstrated a consistent mortality rate proportional to the duration of the illness and the number of organs that malfunctioned. An important aspect of this study was that simple, clinically oriented definitions were used to define organ malfunction (Table 14-4). In addition, the type of hospital, its affiliation with a community or a university, and the amount of therapeutic intervention delivered were

---

TABLE 14–4. Definitions of Organ System Failure (OSF)*

If the patient had one or more of the following during a 24-hour period (regardless of other values), OSF existed on that day.

Cardiovascular Failure
(presence of *one or more* of the following):
Heart rate of 54 beats/min or less
Mean arterial blood pressure of 49 mmHg or less
Occurrence of ventricular tachycardia or ventricular fibrillation
Serum pH of 7.24 or less with a $Paco_2$ of 49 mmHg or less

Respiratory Failure
(presence of *one or more* of the following):
Respiratory rate of 5 breaths/min or less, or 49 breaths/min or more
$Paco_2$ of 50 mmHg or more
$(Pao_2 - Pao_2)$ of 350 mmHg or more, where $(Pao_2 - Pao_2) = 713 (Fio_2) - Paco_2 - Pao_2$
Dependent on ventilator on the fourth day of OSF (eg, not applicable for the initial 72 h of OSF)

Renal Failure
(presence of *one or more* of the following)[†]:
Urine ouput of 479 mL/24 h or less, or 159 mL/8 h or less
Serum blood urea nitrogen of 100 mg/100 mL or more
Serum creatinine of 3.5 mg/100 mL or more

Hematologic Failure
(presence of *one or more* of the following):
White blood cells ≤1000/µL
Platelets ≤20,000/µL
Hematocrit ≤20%

Neurologic Failure
Glasgow Coma Score ≤6 (in absence of sedation at any one point in day); sum of best eye opening, best verbal, and best motor responses with responses scored as follows (points):
  Eyes—Open: spontaneously (4), to verbal command (3), to pain (2), no response (1)
  Motor—Obeys verbal command (6), response to painful stimuli: localizes pain (5), flexion-withdrawal (4), decorticate rigidity (3), decerebrate rigidity (2), no response (1), movement without any control (4)
  Verbal—Oriented and converses (5), disoriented and converses (4), inappropriate words (3), incomprehensible sounds (2), no response (1). If intubated, use clinical judgment for verbal responses as follows: patient generally unresponsive (1), patient's ability to converse in question (3), patient appears able to converse (5)

*New terminology would use *organ system dysfunction.*
[†]Excluding patients receiving chronic dialysis before hospital admission.
(Knaus WA, Draper EA, Wagner DP, et al. Prognosis in acute organ-system failure. Ann Surg 1985;202:685)

not found to alter the outcome. As shown in Figure 14-5, the mortality rate rose as the number of failing organs and the length of time since the onset of failure increased. A further increment in mortality was seen in patients older than 65 years.

When a single organ malfunctioned in patients younger than 65 years for more than 5 days, the mortality rate was 27%. In patients older than 65 years, the mortality rate was 48%. Similarly, the malfunction of two organs for 2 days produced 47% and 73% mortality rates, respectively, and the malfunction of three or more organs for 5 days in all age groups was associated with a 97% mortality rate. These data provide a useful reference for further studies of thera-peutic intervention and decision making with patients and their families during catastrophic illnesses.

Although it was not emphasized in this study, other in-vestigators have documented the adverse impact of liver dysfunction on the SIRS.[3,53] When the bilirubin level rises above 8 mg/dL, out of proportion to hepatocellular enzyme or alkaline phosphatase elevation (not attributed to hema-toma, biliary obstruction, or acalculus cholecystitis), the mortality rate approaches 95%. If the liver is the primary organ initiating the SIRS (as may occur with end-stage liver failure of any cause) and ARDS supervenes, the mortality rate is close to 100% unless liver transplantation is per-formed.[54]

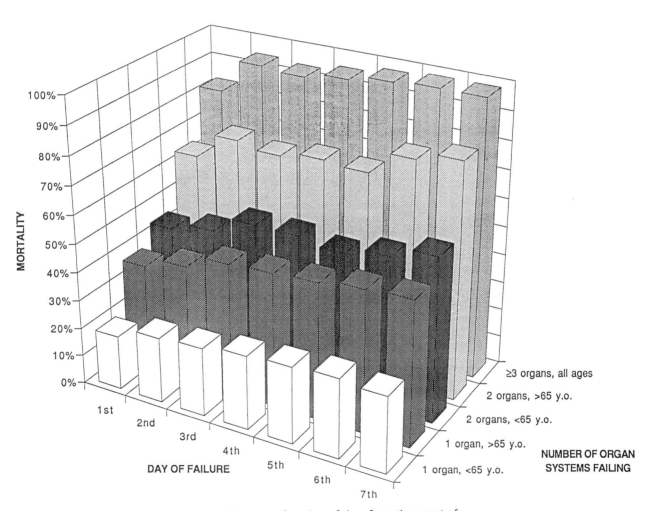

FIG. 14-5. Mortality in multiple organ failure as a function of days from the onset of organ failure, number of organs failing, and age of the patient. The age and number of organs failing relate more to mortality rate than duration of organ failure. (Adapted from Knaus W, Wagner D. Multiple systems organ failure: epidemiology and prognosis. Critical Care Clinics 1989;5:221–232)

Another important predictor of mortality is the acid–base status of patients with ARDS. When the pH level is persistently less than 7.4 and HCO_3^- is less than 20 mEq/dL on the day of onset of ARDS, the mortality rate approaches 85%.[55]

Recently, attention has focused on the gastrointestinal tract as an organ of secondary malfunction and as an effector organ initiating and sustaining the SIRS.[56] After any catastrophic event producing the SIRS, the intestinal flora rapidly change. In addition, there is an increase in mucosal permeability, leading to microbial translocation across the gut wall and augmenting or producing the SIRS.[56,57] The altered flora are also associated with retrograde colonization through the intestines into the stomach, esophagus, nasopharynx, and, finally, the lungs, providing a source for nosocomial infections.

The diffuse nature of the multiple organ dysfunction syndrome is further demonstrated in the nervous system. Not only is the central nervous system affected (see Table 14-4), with altered mentation even progressing to coma, but peripheral nerve damage results in sensorimotor defects that may produce weakness and ventilator weaning difficulty.[58]

In the future, early stratification of patients may improve such that interventional therapy can be applied at an early stage in hopes of improving the chance of recovery. Increasingly sophisticated data banks based on large numbers of patients are being developed. Using the Acute Physiology and Chronic Health Evaluation (APACHE) III score (encompassing Knaus' data), in addition to 17 other physiologic measurements, preexisting illnesses, and patients' ages and diagnoses, computers can now generate reliable daily predictions of mortality.[59] It still is not clear, however, which physiologic variables are independent parameters and should be monitored. Debate also exists regarding the best way to define both the different groups at risk and the nature of organ dysfunction.[60] Whether therapeutic interventions in different APACHE groups will alter outcomes remains uncertain.

DISORDERS THAT FREQUENTLY PRODUCE THE ADULT RESPIRATORY DISTRESS SYNDROME IN SURGICAL PATIENTS

ADULT RESPIRATORY DISTRESS SYNDROME CAUSED BY SEPSIS

The most common cause of ARDS in any series of civilian cases is sepsis. Surgical complications frequently lead to sepsis (eg, abscess or infection of the surgical field, pneumonia, urinary tract infection, intravenous access site infection). In addition, infarcted or traumatized tissues release mediators that can produce the SIRS (see Table 14-2). Sepsis and its consequences have already been discussed (see Definitions and Physiologic and Clinical Consequences).

ADULT RESPIRATORY DISTRESS SYNDROME ASSOCIATED WITH THE ASPIRATION OF GASTRIC CONTENTS

The aspiration of gastric contents is the second most common cause of ARDS in hospitalized patients. Traditionally, three syndromes have been attributed to gastric aspiration: acute lung damage (ARDS), foreign body airway obstruction, and pleuropulmonary infections (eg, pneumonia, abscess, empyema).

Mendelson[61] has been credited with establishing the importance of gastric acidity in producing lung injury. Many animal studies and some anecdotal human data suggest that a pH level of less than 2.5 is necessary to produce lung damage, and that injury increases to a maximum at a pH level of 1.5. Although gastric acidity is clearly a key determinant in lung injury, other studies have shown that high tonicity can also produce extensive damage, explaining why ARDS may result from the aspiration of large volumes of hypertonic enteral nutritional supplements or particulate antacids.[62,63] Small food particles can also produce gas-exchange abnormalities and, subsequently, tiny granulomas.[63–65] In addition, a larger and more diffuse aspirate increases pulmonary impairment. Conditions predisposing to gastric aspiration are altered sensorium (eg, general anesthesia, tracheal intubation, sedation, delirium, seizures, head trauma, cardiopulmonary arrest); and swallowing or gastroesophageal or intestinal disorders (eg, dysmotility, strictures, Zenker's diverticula, fistulas, neuromuscular disease, gastric stasis, intestinal obstruction).[66]

Massive aspiration of gastric contents is a catastrophic event frequently witnessed by anesthesiologists or other medical personnel. Patients who develop ARDS after aspiration have usually inhaled a considerable volume of acidic or particulate fluid (inevitably more than 25 mL and often several hundred milliliters). Aspiration is clinically recognized by the abrupt onset of various combinations of coughing, wheezing, rales, cyanosis, and apnea, associated with interstitial or alveolar infiltrates. Occasionally, patients massively aspirate after emesis, leading to cardiopulmonary arrest.[67] When lung injury follows a single, well-defined lung insult, such as aspiration, the initial severity is well correlated with prognosis. If the arterial–alveolar oxygen tension ratio* is less than 0.5 within a few hours, the mortality rate is 40%; if it is greater than 0.5, the mortality rate is 14%.[67]

Chemical pneumonitis often progresses, with deteriorating pulmonary function and radiographic infiltrates for the

---

*Arterial oxygen tension (PaO_2) is measured by arterial blood gas analysis and the alveolar oxygen tension (PAO_2) is obtained using the alveolar gas equation: $PAO_2 = (PB - 47)FIO_2 - 1.25(PaCO_2)$, where PB = the barometric pressure, FIO_2 = the fractional inspired concentration of oxygen, and $PaCO_2$ = the carbon dioxide tension measured by arterial blood gases.

first 36 to 48 hours. Radiographic resolution occurs over about 4.5 days but may require more than 2 weeks.[67] If acidic fluid is aspirated, polymorphonuclear inflammation appears within 4 hours and progresses over 36 hours to typical ARDS, with hyaline membrane formation by 48 hours and subsequent resolution.[63,65] The aspiration of large volumes of neutral nonparticulate fluid produces acute and possibly severe hypoxemia that rapidly improves within a day without evidence of histologic inflammation.

Preventive measures include elevation of the head of the bed, cautious use of sedation, avoidance of oral and enteral feeding in compromised patients, preoperative use of H_2 receptor antagonists, and careful nasogastric decompression when appropriate. Nasogastric suction and even tracheal intubation, however, do not prevent all cases of aspiration.[63] Once aspiration occurs, supportive therapy is the only treatment. Tracheal suction should be performed immediately after gross aspiration occurs. Bronchoscopy is of no value unless large food particles or foreign bodies are suspected. Alkaline lavage of the airways is not effective because of the rapidity of the acid-tissue neutralization reaction.[65] Steroid therapy may increase the risk of gram-negative pneumonia and has not reduced the mortality of gastric aspiration.[62,66,68]

Antibiotics have no effect on chemical pneumonitis and clinicians are divided as to their efficacy. Aspiration may introduce a bacterial inoculum, producing a clinical picture of stable or improving chemical pneumonitis for the first 48 or more hours followed by increasing infiltrates, fever, an elevated white blood cell count, and respiratory distress. A reasonable approach is to administer antibiotics initially if significant bacterial contamination (ie, poor dental hygiene, obstructed bowel) is suspected. The antibiotics used should be effective against the normal anaerobic oropharyngeal flora, gram-negative aerobes, and against *Staphylococcus aureus* in cases of gastric stasis, bowel obstruction, or intensive care and in sick, hospitalized patients, who are inevitably colonized with these organisms. Antibiotics may be used prophylactically for the first 48 hours or continued for a full course after grossly contaminated aspiration, as dictated by clinical judgment. As in all patients with ARDS, standard oxygen and ventilator therapy may be required (see later).

ADULT RESPIRATORY DISTRESS SYNDROME IN THE SETTING OF TRAUMA

LUNG CONTUSION

Lung contusion occurs after blunt trauma to the chest, with or without rib fractures. Usually within 6 to 24 hours after injury, opacification of the traumatized hemithorax and, sometimes, the contralateral hemithorax (a contrecoup injury) develops, associated with increasing hypoxemia and decreasing compliance.[69] The radiographic abnormalities may lag behind the functional changes by as much as 24 hours, making diagnosis difficult. These changes are produced by interstitial edema with interstitial and intraalveolar extravasation of blood. The extent of lung injury is significantly greater pathologically than is apparent on chest radiography.

FAT EMBOLISM

Fat embolism syndrome also may be a cause of ARDS after injury. The classic syndrome is characterized by multiorgan failure, with central nervous system, renal, and pulmonary dysfunction associated with thrombocytopenia (sometimes with full-blown disseminated intravascular coagulopathy) and petechial skin rash occurring 24 to 48 hours after major long-bone fractures. The incidence of the syndrome increases in parallel with the number and severity of fractures; about 4% of patients with fractured femurs and pelves develop the clinical fat embolism syndrome. Subclinical fat embolism probably occurs in most patients with fractures.[70]

The syndrome is thought to result from the release of marrow elements into venules and lymphatics. This neutral fat undergoes embolization into the lung and other capillary beds, producing mechanical obstruction. Unless the obstruction is massive, little consequence occurs at this stage. In time, however, lipase converts the neutral fat into damaging free fatty acids. The diagnosis is suggested by the occurrence of the clinical syndrome in patients with fractures.

OTHER CONDITIONS ASSOCIATED WITH THE ADULT RESPIRATORY DISTRESS SYNDROME IN SURGICAL PATIENTS

CARDIOPULMONARY BYPASS

For many years, cardiopulmonary bypass was noted to be associated with ARDS. Despite anecdotal reports, however, a review of the current literature reveals that ARDS is unusual after bypass, with an incidence of 1% to 2%.[71] The incidence of less than 2% and mortality rate of 50% have remained unchanged during the past decade. Associated risk factors are age greater than 60 years, prolonged bypass, and the use of ventricular assist devices.[71]

Patients with diabetes who are using insulin preparations containing protamine, patients who are allergic to fish, and patients who have had prior vasectomies are said to have a higher incidence of ARDS after cardiopulmonary bypass.[72,73] Protamine is a protein isolated from salmon fish sperm that is used to reverse anticoagulation after bypass. Presumably, these high-risk patients have antibodies that can cross-react with protamine and produce a reaction similar to anaphylaxis. Although this may occur, a large study demonstrated that it is exceedingly rare.[72,74]

Another cause of lung injury after cardiopulmonary bypass is transfusion reaction. Major blood group mismatches should be extremely rare; however, occasional leukoagglutinin reactions, which are not routinely tested by standard crossmatching techniques, may produce ARDS, particularly among multiparous recipients.[73] Both membrane and bubble pump oxygenators activate complement by the classic and alternate pathways.[73] Activated complement products, however, are frequently found without ARDS in patients who have undergone bypass. Similarly, white blood cell and platelet sequestration has routinely been demonstrated in the lungs of these patients in the absence of ARDS.[75,76]

PANCREATITIS

The development of ARDS after pancreatitis has been regarded as fairly common. When the only risk factor is acute pancreatitis, however, severe ARDS seldom occurs. More often, ARDS develops after septic complications of pancreatitis, such as pancreatic abscesses or infected pseudocysts, and then is a part of sepsis or SIRS.[77] The cause of ARDS associated with acute pancreatitis is uncertain and believed to be related to the release of various pancreatic enzymes that lead to direct lung damage (eg, proteases, free fatty acids, phospholipase A). Hypoxemia is commonly present in pancreatitis and related to many factors (eg, abdominal distention and pain with elevated diaphragms and basilar atelectasis, pleural effusions, vomiting and aspiration, subtle acute lung injury or "full-blown" ARDS).

CURRENT AND FUTURE THERAPY FOR THE ADULT RESPIRATORY DISTRESS SYNDROME

In an excellent review article, Wiener-Kronish[78] and colleagues divided therapy for ARDS into five parts:

- Control of sepsis and its complications
- Improvement of gas exchange and reduction of barotrauma
- Limitation or reduction of pulmonary edema
- Improvement of tissue oxygen delivery
- Reduction of pulmonary and systemic injury.

Both current and potential future therapies are examined here.

CONTROL OF SEPSIS AND ITS COMPLICATIONS

The importance of infection as a cause of ARDS and a source of morbidity and mortality has been emphasized.[79] Unfortunately, our ability to affect this aspect of the syndrome has been limited by difficulties in diagnosing infection early and treating it effectively.

Many cases of ARDS either are or could be prevented by precluding the development of infection or recognizing it early and treating it aggressively. Rapid evaluation of patients with fever, hypotension, altered mental status, or focal signs of infection, along with early, empiric administration of broad-spectrum antibiotics are the key elements of this approach. In addition, maintaining adequate nutrition (especially enteral supplements) may improve the immune system of hospitalized patients, reducing the incidence of infection and improving their ability to combat infection once it is established. Changing or removing foreign bodies such as intravenous and urinary catheters may eliminate these common sources of nosocomial sepsis.

Once ARDS is established, the principles noted above are even more important because these patients have a high incidence of secondary complicating infections that augment and sustain ARDS/SIRS, often resulting in multiorgan failure and death.

Nosocomial pneumonias are common and difficult to detect in the setting of respiratory failure and pulmonary infiltrates. Diagnosing pulmonary infections in the setting of ARDS is notoriously difficult. The growth of bacteria from tracheal aspirates may be the result of colonization or true infection. The presence of new infiltrates, fever, and leukocytosis may suggest the diagnosis but can be related to several complicating problems. Meduri and coworkers[80] have proposed that the culture of sterile lung brushings or bronchoalveolar lavage specimens may play a role in evaluating patients in this situation, but their protocol is expensive and logistically difficult to implement. Further data are required to determine the role of these studies in patients with ARDS before they are used routinely.

The bacterial flora in these infections may arise from the oropharynx or even from the stomach, especially in the setting of therapy with histamine blockers. Whether oral and gastrointestinal tract decontamination with nonabsorbable antibiotics or the use of ulcer and gastrointestinal bleeding prophylaxis that does not decrease the gastric pH will reduce the incidence of these infections has not been conclusively determined.[81] Clinicians must exercise their own clinical judgment in the use of these medications.

One of the difficulties in treating sepsis either before the development of ARDS or multiple organ dysfunction syndrome or after injuries have occurred is that the release of endotoxin seems to continue after and may even be magnified by the administration of antibiotics. Recent studies using monoclonal antibodies directed against endotoxin suggested that these agents may improve the outcome of bacteremia, sepsis, or septic shock and, in certain situations, may be cost-effective.[82,83] Because more recent data have brought into question the conclusions of the original studies, the US Food and Drug Administration has not approved these forms of therapy. Although the rationale behind antiendotoxin therapy is appealing, the use of this extremely expensive medication requires further examination in clinical trials.

IMPROVEMENT OF GAS EXCHANGE AND REDUCTION OF BAROTRAUMA

Studies in animal models and in patients with ARDS have documented significant increases in airway resistance.[84,85] Because some of this increased resistance is probably due to bronchospasm caused by mediators released from inflammatory cells, the administration of inhaled β-agonists and, perhaps, anticholinergic drugs is associated with little risk and may be beneficial.

From the early studies of ARDS, new modes of ventilation have been tried to reduce hypoxemia and even lung edema. Unfortunately, none of these techniques seems to affect the ultimate outcome.

The first method to be studied was positive end-expiratory pressure (PEEP). This was first described in the same paper in which ARDS was reported in 1967.[1] PEEP clearly improved arterial PaO_2, but at the cost of decreased cardiac output in patients with inadequate intravascular volume, resulting in decreased tissue oxygenation. This complication can usually be corrected by the administration of additional fluid or low-dose dopamine (increasing venous return).[86] Some investigators hypothesized that PEEP may be protective against ARDS, but a prospective study in patients at risk showed no benefit.[87] Other investigators used extremely high levels of PEEP in patients with ARDS, producing significant barotrauma.[88] A randomized trial noted no apparent improvement in survival.[89] Currently, moderate levels of PEEP up to a maximum of 20 cm H_2O are advocated, using the minimal amount of PEEP necessary to reduce the fraction of inspired oxygen (FIO_2), preferably to less than 0.5.[90] This goal cannot be accomplished in some patients with severe lung injury, but the role that oxygen toxicity plays in the ultimate outcome has never been completely determined (see later). The only study that has examined the survival of patients with ARDS with and without PEEP noted no difference in survival but did note a longer time from the onset of respiratory failure to death in those who received PEEP.[91]

The second new technique of mechanical support to be studied was high-frequency ventilation. This mode of therapy was thought to cause less pressure-induced injury and

barotrauma. Adequate oxygenation and carbon dioxide removal can be accomplished, but a randomized, prospective trial of a large group of patients with posttraumatic ARDS did not demonstrate a beneficial effect.[92,93] This approach is usually reserved for patients with large bronchopleural fistulas.[94]

In recent years, a return to the pressure-control mode of ventilation for patients with ARDS has been facilitated by the ease with which instantaneous measurements of minute ventilation and tidal volume can be obtained on modern ventilators, and by the use of sedation/paralysis to reduce patient-induced alterations in chest compliance. Often, this mode of ventilation incorporates an inspiratory pause and reversal of the inspiratory-expiratory ratio.[95,96] Although some patients who cannot be adequately oxygenated with conventional volume-controlled ventilation and PEEP can be managed with this new form of ventilatory support, increased barotrauma has been noted.[97] At this point, pressure-control ventilation remains another new mode of mechanical support that has not yet been demonstrated to improve the ultimate outcome in ARDS.

As mentioned, there is an absolute and functional deficiency of surfactant in patients with ARDS.[98] This deficiency differs from that of neonates with neonatal respiratory distress because adults have both decreased production and protein inhibition (especially fibrin) of surfactant. Exogenous surfactant or synthetic surfactant materials resistant to the inhibitory effects of fibrin and other proteins are being investigated.

LIMITATION OR REDUCTION OF PULMONARY EDEMA

Because the primary cause of pulmonary edema in ARDS is increased capillary permeability, elevated pulmonary capillary pressure is associated with further increases in edema and, perhaps, increased mortality.[99] Increases in filling pressures may be caused by the fluids required for hemodynamic resuscitation or by the decreases in cardiac function that are seen in patients with sepsis or SIRS. In addition, many of these patients have decreased colloid oncotic pressure related to reduced serum albumin levels, particularly after several days of illness and after large volume resuscitation, which may increase the edema. The use of hemodynamic monitoring is advocated to control fluid and diuretic administration and keep pulmonary capillary wedge pressures as low as possible while maintaining adequate cardiac output. The administration of colloids or blood products to boost colloid oncotic pressure, although advocated by some, has not altered the outcome of ARDS.

IMPROVEMENT OF TISSUE OXYGEN DELIVERY

During the evolution of ARDS, oxygen delivery to the tissues is often impaired. The combination of hypovolemia, decreased systemic arterial tone, decreased venous return secondary to PEEP, decreased cardiac function, and maldistribution of peripheral blood flow all contribute and may play a role in the subsequent development of multiple organ dysfunction syndrome (see Physiologic and Clinical Consequences).[100] Judicious administration of fluids is often indicated but obviously conflicts with the need to keep filling pressures at a minimum, as noted earlier. Cardiac dysfunction, other causes of hemodynamic compromise, or oliguria may necessitate the administration of fluids or vasoactive agents in selected patients. The appropriate therapy is often best determined by pulmonary arterial catheterization and identification of the hemodynamic defect. The influence of intensive hemodynamic monitoring on the outcome of patients with ARDS remains controversial, however.

Vasodilators such as prostaglandin E_1 have not been shown to improve the outcome and may decrease the PaO_2, probably by reversing hypoxic vasoconstriction in the lung and worsening V/Q mismatching.[101] Another pulmonary vascular dilator, inhaled nitric oxide, may be helpful.[102] The beneficial effect of ensuring maximal tissue oxygen delivery remains controversial (see Physiologic and Clinical Consequences).[103]

ATTENUATION OF PULMONARY AND SYSTEMIC INJURY

The only means of reducing pulmonary injury are to decrease the FIO_2 and minimize barotrauma by careful use of mechanical ventilation. In some severely ill patients, these two goals are contradictory. The data supporting the effects of high FIO_2 in causing lung injury in patients with ARDS are difficult to interpret because the pathology of ARDS and oxygen toxicity are the same. Furthermore, experimental data suggest that sepsis may stimulate the production of oxygen radical–scavenging enzymes that protect against oxygen toxicity. Because of these data, the best approach seems to be to reduce the FIO_2 to less than 1.0 as soon as possible, minimizing the absorption atelectasis that occurs when there is no nitrogen in the alveoli. Further reduction must be balanced against the potential trauma to the lungs caused by high levels of PEEP or by new modes of mechanical ventilation such as inverse-ratio pressure-control ventilation (see earlier).

In 1979, a large trial of extracorporeal membrane oxygenation failed to demonstrate a beneficial effect despite the attractive rationale that "resting" the lung would reduce ventilator-associated injury.[104] New techniques of extracorporeal membrane oxygenation have been developed and are under investigation, with some encouraging early results.[105] A large trial in the United States has not demonstrated a beneficial effect.[106]

In experimental models of ARDS, corticosteroids were found to reduce lung injury. Several prospective trials of steroids at the onset of clinical ARDS failed to document a beneficial effect.[107,108] Three uncontrolled studies in small groups of patients treated later in the course of disease (10 to 14 days during the fibroproliferative phase) have suggested a benefit.[109–111] This mode of therapy cannot be advocated until further prospective, randomized studies have been performed.

LATE PROGNOSIS OF THE ADULT RESPIRATORY DISTRESS SYNDROME

Data regarding the late prognosis in survivors of ARDS are lacking. Inconsistency in defining ARDS and ranking its severity, limited follow-up, and failure to indicate the initial condition producing ARDS have all contributed to the inadequacies of previous studies. Reviews describing the current state of knowledge in this field can be summarized as follows[112,113]:

1. About half of survivors have various degrees of pulmonary impairment.
2. Lung function improves rapidly at first and then slowly for as long as 1 year. Thereafter, any abnormalities are likely to persist.
3. The most common symptom is exertional dyspnea (cough and wheezing also occur occasionally). Cor pulmonale rarely develops. Rales and wheezes may be present but the physical examination generally is normal after 1 year.
4. The chest radiograph usually is normal, although areas of atelectasis, hyperinflation, pneumatoceles, or infiltrates occasionally persist.
5. The most common persistent laboratory abnormality is a decrease in diffusing capacity. Restrictive or obstructive pulmonary function abnormalities as well as hyperreactive airways may be demonstrated on methacholine challenge. Arterial blood gas levels are usually normal. Only occasionally do hypoxemia or hypercapnia persist, and continuous oxygen therapy is rarely required beyond 1 year.

Measurements made after the third day of ARDS that correlate best with subsequent pulmonary impairment are the degree of pulmonary hypertension and the degree of diminution in pulmonary compliance.[112] Surprisingly, ventilator support time, initial inspired oxygen requirement,

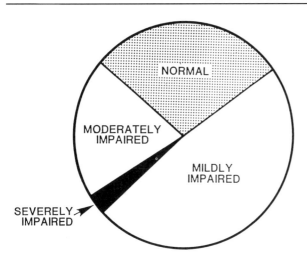

FIG. 14-6. Distribution of pulmonary impairment in survivors evaluated at least 1 year after an episode of ARDS. (Elliott CG. Pulmonary sequelae in survivors of ARDS. Clin Chest Med 1990;11:4)

smoking status, and the initial cause of ARDS do not seem to be related to long-term sequelae.

Figure 14-6 shows the degree of pulmonary impairment in ARDS survivors according to the American Thoracic Society standards for determination of impairment.[113]

Acknowledgment

The authors express their appreciation to Dr. Roland H. Ingram, Jr., and Patsy Hutchinson for their help in preparing this chapter.

REFERENCES

1. Ashbaugh D, Bigelow D, Perry T. Acute respiratory distress in adults. Lancet 1967;2:319–323.
2. Osler W. The principles and practice of medicine, ed 10. New York, D Appleton, 1927.
3. Barton R, Cerra FB. The hypermetabolism: multiple organ failure syndrome. Chest 1989;96:1153–1160.
4. Cerra FB. Multiple organ failure syndrome. Dis Mon 1992;12:847–895.
5. Knaus WA, Draper EA, Wagner DP, et al. Prognosis in acute organ-system failure. Ann Surg 1985;202:685–693.
6. Petty TL. Adult respiratory distress syndrome: definition and historical perspective. Clin Chest Med 1982;13:307.
7. Matthay MA. The adult respiratory distress syndrome. Clin Chest Med 1990;11:575–580.
8. Murray JF, Matthay MA, Luce JM, et al. An expanded definition of the adult respiratory distress syndrome. Am Rev Respir Dis 1988;183:720–723.
9. Bone RC, Balk RA, Cerra FB, et al. Definition for sepsis and organ failure and guidelines for the use of innovative therapies in sepsis. Chest 1992;101:1644–1654.
10. Bone RC, Sibbald WJ, Sprung CL. The AACP-SCCM consensus conference on sepsis and organ failure. Chest 1992;101:1481–1482.
11. Murray J, staff of the Division of Lung Diseases at the Heart, Lung, and Blood Institute. Mechanisms of acute respiratory failure. Am Rev Respir Dis 1977;115:1071–1078.
12. Villar J, Slutsky A. The incidence of the adult respiratory distress syndrome. Am Rev Respir Dis 1989;140:814–816.
13. Webster N, Cohen A, Nunn J. Adult respiratory distress syndrome: how many cases in UK. Anaesthesia 1988;43:923–962.
14. Fowler A, Hamman R, Good J, et al. Adult respiratory distress syndrome: risk with common predispositions. Ann Intern Med 1983;98:593–597.
15. Pepe P, Potkin R, Reus D, et al. Clinical predictors of the adult respiratory distress syndrome. Am J Surg 1982;144:124–130.
16. Katzenstein A, Askin F. Acute lung injury patterns: diffuse alveolar damage, acute interstitial pneumonia, bronchiolitis obliterans—organizing pneumonia. In: Bennington J, ed. Surgical pathology of non-neoplastic lung disease. Philadelphia, WB Saunders, 1990:9–57.
17. Till G, Johnson K, Kunkel R, Ward P. Intra-vascular activation of complement and acute lung injury: dependency on neutrophils and toxic oxygen metabolites. J Clin Invest 1982;69:1126–1135.
18. Beutler B, Cerami A. Cachectin: more than a tumor necrosis factor. N Engl J Med 1987;316:379–385.
19. Malik A. Pulmonary microembolism. Physiol Rev 1983;3:1114–1199.
20. Henderson W. Eicosanoids and lung inflammation. Am Rev Respir Dis 1987;135:1176–1185.
21. Schlag G, Redl H. Morphology of the human lung after traumatic injury. In: Zapol W, ed. Acute respiratory failure. New York, Marcel Dekker, 1985:161–183.
22. Tomashefski JJ, Davies P, Boggis C, et al. The pulmonary vascular lesions of the adult respiratory distress syndrome. Am J Pathol 1983;112:112–126.
23. Meyrick B, Ryan U, Brigham K. Direct effects of E coli endotoxin on structure and permeability of pulmonary endothelial monolayers and the endothelial layer of intimal explants. Am J Pathol 1986;122:140–141.
24. Maunder R, Hackman R, Riff E, et al. Occurrence of the adult respiratory distress syndrome in neutropenic patients. Am Rev Respir Dis 1986;133:313–316.
25. Swank D, Moore S. Roles of the neutrophil and other mediators in adult respiratory distress syndrome. Mayo Clin Proc 1989;64:1118–1132.
25a. Berthiaume Y, Staub N, Matthay M. Beta-adrenergic agonists increase lung liquid clearance in anesthetized sheep. J Clin Invest 1987;79:335–343.
26. Fowler A, Hyers T, Fisher B, et al. The adult respiratory distress syndrome: cell populations and soluble mediators in the air spaces of patients at high risk. Am Rev Respir Dis 1987;136:1225–1231.
27. Lee C, Fein A, Lippmann M, et al. Elastolytic activity in pul-

monary lavage fluid from patients with adult respiratory-distress syndrome. N Engl J Med 1981;304:192–196.

28. Weiland J, Davis W, Holter J, et al. Lung neutrophils in the adult respiratory distress syndrome. Am Rev Respir Dis 1986;133:218–225.

29. Weiss SJ. Tissue destruction by neutrophils. N Engl J Med 1989;320:365–376.

30. Shasby D, Vanbenthuysen K, Tate R, et al. Granulocytes mediate acute edematous lung injury in rabbits and in isolated rabbit lungs perfused with phorbol myristate acetate: role of oxygen radicals. Am Rev Respir Dis 1982;125:443–447.

31. Idell S, Gonzalez K, Bradford H, et al. Procoagulant activity in bronchoalveolar lavage in the adult respiratory distress syndrome: contribution of tissue factor associated with factor VII. Am Rev Respir Dis 1987;136:1466–1474.

32. Seeger W, Stohr G, Wolf HRD, et al. Alteration of surfactant function due to protein leakage: special interaction with fibrin monomer. J Appl Physiol 1985;58:326–388.

33. Raghu G, Striker L, Hudson L, Striker G. Extracellular matrix in normal and fibrotic human lungs. Am Rev Respir Dis 1985; 131:281–289.

34. Staub NC, Naganb H, Pearce ML. Pulmonary edema in dogs, especially the sequence of fluid accumulation in lungs. J Appl Physiol 1967;22:277–290.

35. Lewis JF, Jobe AH. Surfactant and the adult respiratory distress syndrome. Am Rev Respir Dis 1993;147:231–233.

36. Rodriguez-Rosin R. Ventilation–perfusion relationships: pathophysiologic foundation of critical care. Baltimore, Williams & Wilkins, 1993:389–413.

37. Greene R, Zapol WM, Snider MT, et al. Early bedside detection of pulmonary vascular occlusion during acute respiratory failure. Am Rev Respir Dis 1981;124:593–601.

38. Zapol WM, Snider MT. Pulmonary hypertension in severe acute respiratory failure. N Engl J Med 1977;296:476–480.

39. Aberle DR, Brown K. Radiologic consideration in the respiratory distress syndrome. Clin Chest Med 1990;11:737–754.

40. Petty TL. Acute respiratory distress syndrome (ARDS). Dis Mon 1990;1:7–58.

41. Wiener-Kronish JR, Goldstein R, Matthay MA. Pleural effusions are frequently associated with the adult respiratory distress syndrome. Am Rev Respir Dis 1988;137:227A.

42. Field S, Kelly SM, Macklem PT. The oxygen cost of breathing in patients with cardiorespiratory disease. Am Rev Respir Dis 1982;126:9–13.

43. Parrillo JE, Parker MM, Natason C, et al. Septic shock in humans. Ann Intern Med 1990;113:227–242.

44. Shoemaker WC, Appel PL, Kram HB. Role of oxygen debt in the development of organ failure sepsis, and death in high-risk surgical patients. Chest 1992;102:208–215.

45. Tuchschmidt J, Fried J, Astiz M, et al. Elevation of cardiac output and oxygen delivery improves outcome in septic shock. Chest 1992;102:216–220.

46. Dorinsky PM, Gadek JE. Mechanisms of multiple nonpulmonary organ failure in ARDS. Chest 1989;96:885–892.

47. Shoemaker WC, Patil R, Appel PL, et al. Hemodynamic and oxygen transport patterns for outcome prediction, therapeutic goals, and clinical algorithms to improve outcome. Chest 1992; 102:617S–625S.

48. Hankeln KB, Gronemeyer R, Held A, et al. Use of continuous noninvasive measurement of oxygen consumption in patients with adult respiratory distress syndrome following shock of various etiologies. Crit Care Med 1991;19:642–649.

49. Schumacker PT, Samsel RW. Oxygen supply and consumption in the adult respiratory distress syndrome. Clin Chest Med 1990;11:715–722.

50. Montgomery A, Stager M, Carrico C, et al. Causes of mortality in patients with adult respiratory distress syndrome. Am Rev Respir Dis 1985;132:485–489.

51. Niederman MS, Fein AM. Sepsis syndrome, the adult respiratory distress syndrome, and nosocomial pneumonia: a common clinical sequence. Clin Chest Med 1990;11:633–656.

52. Knaus W, Wagner D. Multiple systems organ failure: epidemiology and prognosis. Crit Care Clin 1989;5:221–232.

53. Schwartz DB, Bone RC, Balk RA, et al. Hepatic dysfunction in the adult respiratory distress syndrome. Chest 1989;95:871–875.

54. Matuschak GM, Rinaldo JE, Pinsky MR, et al. Effect of end-stage liver failure on the incidence and resolution of the adult respiratory distress syndrome. J Crit Care 1987;2:162–173.

55. Fowler AA, Hamman RF, Zerbe GO, et al. Adult respiratory distress syndrome: prognosis after onset. Am Rev Respir Dis 1985;132:472–478.

56. Fink MP. Why the GI tract is pivotal in trauma, sepsis, and MOF. J Crit Ill 1991;6:253–273.

57. Fink MP. Gastrointestinal mucosal injury in experimental models of shock, trauma, and sepsis. Crit Care Med 1991;19:627–641.

58. Witt NJ, Zochodne DW, Bolton CF, et al. Peripheral nerve function in sepsis and multiple organ failure. Chest 1991; 99:176–184.

59. Knaus WA, Sun X, Nystrom P, et al. Evaluation of definitions for sepsis. Chest 1992;101:1656–1662.

60. Dorinsky PM, Gadek JE. Multiple organ failure. Clin Chest Med 1990;11:581–591.

61. Mendelson CL. The aspiration of stomach contents into the lungs during obstetric anesthesia. Am J Obstet Gynecol 1946; 52:191–205.

62. Hoyt J. Aspiration pneumonitis: patient risk factors, prevention and management. J Intensive Care Med 1990;5(Suppl): S2–S9.

63. Wynne JW, Modell JH. Respiratory aspiration of stomach contents. Ann Intern Med 1977;87:466–474.

64. Schwartz DJ, Wynne JW, Gibbs CP. The pulmonary consequences of aspiration of gastric contents at pH values greater than 2.5. Am Rev Respir Dis 1980;121:119–126.

65. Wynne JW. Aspiration pneumonitis: correlation of experimental models with clinical disease. Clin Chest Med 1982;3: 25–34.

66. Shapiro MS, Dobbins JW, Matthay RA. Pulmonary manifestations of gastrointestinal disease. Clin Chest Med 1989;10:617–643.

67. Bynum LJ, Pierce AK. Pulmonary aspiration of gastric contents. Am Rev Respir Dis 1976;114:1129–1136.

68. Wolfe JE, Bone RC, Ruth WE. Effects of corticosteroids in the treatment of patients with gastric aspiration. Am J Med 1977; 63:719–722.

69. Wilson R. Trauma. In: Shoemaker W, Ayres S, Grenvik A, et

al, eds. Textbook of critical care. Philadelphia, WB Saunders, 1989:1244.

70. Shier M, Wilson R, Re J, et al. Fat embolism prophylaxis: a study of four treatment modalities. J Trauma 1977;17:621.

71. Messent M, Anaes FC, Sullivan K, et al. Adult respiratory distress syndrome following cardiopulmonary bypass: incidence and prediction. Anaesthesia 1992;47:267–268.

72. Levy JH, Schwieger IM, Zaidan JR, et al. Evaluation of patient at rest for protamine reactions. J Thorac Cardiovasc Surg 1989;98:200–204.

73. Maggart M, Stewart S. The mechanisms and management of noncardiogenic pulmonary edema following cardiopulmonary bypass. Ann Thorac Surg 1987;43:231–236.

74. Levy JH, Zaidan JR, Faraj B. Prospective evaluation of risk of protamine reactions in patients with NPD insulin-dependent diabetes. Anesth Analg 1986;65:739–742.

75. Howard RJ, Crain C, Franzini DA, et al. Effects of cardiopulmonary bypass on pulmonary leukostasis and complement activation. Arch Surg 1988;123:1496–1501.

76. Zimmerman GA, Amory DW. Transpulmonary polymorphonuclear leukocyte number after cardiopulmonary bypass. Am Rev Respir Dis 1982;126:1097–1098.

77. Levine SA, Feinsilver SH, Fein AM. What to do when pancreatitis causes pleuropulmonary complications. J Crit Ill 1990;5:715–734.

78. Wiener-Kronish J, Gropper M, Matthay M. The adult respiratory distress syndrome: definition and prognosis, pathogenesis and treatment. Br J Anaesth 1990;65:107–129.

79. Bell R, Coalson J, Smith J, et al. Multiple organ system failure and infection in adult respiratory distress syndrome. Ann Intern Med 1983;99:293–298.

80. Meduri G, Baselski V. The role of bronchoalveolar lavage in diagnosing nonopportunistic bacterial pneumonia. Chest 1991;100:179–190.

81. Johanson W, Seidenfeld J, De Los Santos R, et al. Prevention of nosocomial pneumonia using topical and parenteral antimicrobial agents. Am Rev Respir Dis 1988;137:265–272.

82. Ziegler E, Fisher CJ, Sprung C, et al. Treatment of gram-negative bacteremia and septic shock with HA-1A human monoclonal antibody against endotoxin: a randomized, double-blind, placebo-controlled trial. N Engl J Med 1991;324:429–436.

83. Schulman K, Glick H, Rubin H, Eisenberg J. Cost-effectiveness of HA-1A monoclonal antibody for gram-negative sepsis. Economic assessment of a new therapeutic agent. JAMA 1991;266:3466–3471.

84. Ploysongsang Y, Rashkin M, Rossi A, et al. Lung mechanics in adult respiratory distress syndrome. (Abstract) Am Rev Respir Dis 1986;133:266.

85. Snapper J, Hutchison A, Ogletre M, et al. Effects of cyclo-oxygenase inhibitors on the alterations in lung mechanics caused by endotoxemia in the unanesthetized sheep. J Clin Invest 1983;72:63–76.

86. Qvist J, Pontoppidan H, Wilson R, et al. Hemodynamic responses to mechanical ventilation with PEEP. Anesthesiology 1975;42:45–55.

87. Pepe P, Hudson L, Carrico C. Early application of positive end-expiratory pressure in patients at risk for the adult respiratory distress syndrome. N Engl J Med 1984;311:281–286.

88. Kirby R, Perloff W, Maki D. High level positive end-expiratory pressure (PEEP) in acute respiratory insufficiency. Chest 1975;67:156–163.

89. Nelson L, Civetta J, Hudson-Civetta J. Titrating positive end-expiratory pressure therapy in patients with early, moderate hypoxemia. Crit Care Med 1981;9:79–82.

90. Carroll G, Tuman K, Braverman B, et al. Minimal positive end-expiratory pressure (PEEP) may be "best PEEP." Chest 1988;93:1020–1025.

91. Springer R, Stevens P. The influence of PEEP on survival in patients in respiratory failure. Am J Med 1979;66:196–202.

92. Macintyre N, Follett J, Deitz J, Lawlor B. Jet ventilation at 100 breaths per minute in adult respiratory failure. Am Rev Respir Dis 1986;134:897–901.

93. Borg U, Stoklosa J, Siegel J, et al. Prospective evaluation of combined high-frequency ventilation in post-traumatic patients with adult respiratory distress syndrome refractory to optimized conventional ventilatory management. Crit Care Med 1989;17:1129–1141.

94. Standiford T, Morganroth M. High-frequency ventilation. Chest 1989;96:1380–1389.

95. Gurevitch M, Van Dyke J, Young E, Jackson K. Improved oxygenation and lower peak airway pressure in severe adult respiratory distress syndrome: treatment with inverse ratio ventilation. Chest 1989;89:211–213.

96. Lain D, DiBenedetto R, Morris S, et al. Pressure control inverse ratio ventilation as a method to reduce peak inspiratory pressure and provide adequate ventilation and oxygenation. Chest 1989;95:1081–1088.

97. Tharratt R, Allen R, Albertson T. Pressure controlled inverse ratio ventilation in severe adult respiratory failure. Chest 1988;94:755–762.

98. Holm B, Matalon S. Role of pulmonary surfactant in the development and treatment of adult respiratory distress syndrome. Anesth Analg 1989;69:805–818.

99. Simmons R, Berdine G, Seidenfeld J, et al. Fluid balance and the adult respiratory distress syndrome. Am Rev Respir Dis 1987;135:924–929.

100. Snell R, Parrillo J. Cardiovascular dysfunction in septic shock. Chest 1991;99:1000–1009.

101. Bone R, Slotman G, Maunder R, et al. Randomized double-blind, multicenter study of prostaglandin E_1 in patients with the adult respiratory distress syndrome. Chest 1989;96:114–119.

102. Rossaint R, Falke K, Lopez F, et al. Inhaled nitric oxide for the adult respiratory distress syndrome. N Engl J Med 1993;328:399–405.

103. Gilbert E, Haupt M, Manadanas R, et al. The effect of fluid loading, blood transfusions and catecholamine infusion on oxygen delivery and consumption in patients with sepsis. Am Rev Respir Dis 1986;134:873–878.

104. Zapol W, Snider M, Hill J, et al. Extracorporeal membrane oxygenation in severe acute respiratory failure: a randomized prospective study. JAMA 1979;242:2193–2196.

105. Gattinoni L, Pesenti A, Mascheroni D, et al. Low-frequency positive pressure ventilation with extracorporeal CO_2 removal in severe acute respiratory failure. JAMA 1986;256:881–886.

106. Morris A, Menlove R, Rollins R, et al. A controlled clinical trial of a new three step therapy that includes extracorporeal CO_2

removal for ARDS. Trans Am Soc Artif Intern Organs 1988;34:48–53.

107. Bone R, Fischer C. A controlled trial of high-dose methylprednisolone in the treatment of severe and septic shock. N Engl J Med 1987;317:653–658.

108. Luce J, Montgomery A, Marks J, et al. Ineffectiveness of high dose methylprednisolone in preventing parenchymal lung injury and improving mortality in patients with septic shock. Am Rev Respir Dis 1988;138:62–68.

109. Ashbaugh D, Maier R. Idiopathic pulmonary fibrosis in adult respiratory distress syndrome: diagnosis and treatment. Arch Surg 1985;120:530–535.

110. Hooper R, Kearl R. Established ARDS treated with a sustained course of adrenocortical steroids. Chest 1990;97:138–143.

111. Meduri G, Belenchia J, Estes R, et al. Fibroproliferative phase of ARDS: clinical findings and effects of corticosteroids. Chest 1991;100:943–952.

112. Elliott CG. Pulmonary sequelae in survivors of the adult respiratory distress syndrome. Clin Chest Med 1990;11:789–800.

113. Ghio AJ, Elliott G, Crapo GO, et al. Impairment after adult respiratory distress syndrome. Am Rev Respir Dis 1989;139:1158–1162.

Medical Management of the Surgical Patient, Third Edition,
edited by Michael F. Lubin, H. Kenneth Walker, and Robert B. Smith III.
J.B. Lippincott Company, Philadelphia, PA © 1995.

CHAPTER

15

POSTOPERATIVE RESPIRATORY COMPLICATIONS

Vijay M. Patel
Eric G. Honig

During the past half century, postoperative pulmonary complications have remained a significant cause of morbidity and mortality in surgical patients. The incidence of these complications ranges from 5% to 80% in various series and is a function of predisposing risk factors as well as the specific operation being performed[1-5] (Table 15-1).

Factors associated with an increased risk for pulmonary complications include the following:

- Type of surgery
- Duration of surgery
- Underlying lung disease
- Smoking history (more than 20 pack-years)
- Obesity
- Nutritional status
- Age greater than 60 years

Preoperative evaluation should be performed to identify these factors and improve patients' risk status. Preoperative respiratory management is discussed elsewhere.

The pathogenesis of pulmonary complications in the postoperative period has been well described.[6] Hypoventilation and reduced lung volumes after anesthesia and surgery combine to produce atelectasis and predispose to respiratory tract infection. Immobility leads to a risk of thromboembolic disease. All these processes contribute to postoperative hypoxemia and can progress to respiratory failure in patients with limited respiratory reserves (Fig. 15-1).

Even with optimal preoperative and perioperative care, some patients develop postoperative hypoxemia, atelectasis, pulmonary edema, pneumonia, pleural effusion, and pulmonary embolism (PE). In this chapter, we discuss the diagnosis and treatment of these complications.

HYPOXEMIA

A low arterial PaO_2 is common after surgery. Hypoxemia is defined as an arterial saturation of less than 90% or a PaO_2 that is 75% or less of the preoperative value. The average PaO_2 drops by 10% to 30% immediately after surgery and returns to baseline 3 or 4 days later. In upper abdominal surgery, arterial oxygen typically decreases by 20% to 30% in the first 48 hours. In nonabdominal, nonthoracic surgery, it decreases by 5% to 10%. Hypoxemia results from changes in lung volumes, ventilation–perfusion (V/Q) mismatching, and shunting. Total lung capacity and each of its subdivisions decrease after thoracic and abdominal surgery but not after extremity surgery. There is a decline of 25% to 50% in vital capacity, residual volume, functional residual capacity, tidal volume, and expiratory flow rates such as forced expiratory volume in 1 second. The decline in lung volumes begins during surgery and progresses for as long as 4 days afterward. It may take 2 weeks or more to re-

TABLE 15–1. Incidence Rate for Postoperative Pulmonary Complications

Complication	Incidence (%)
Atelectasis	
Major atelectasis	
General surgery	42
Thoracic surgery	30
Abdominal surgery	20
Minor atelectasis	20–80
Pneumonia	3–25
Bronchitis	37
Pleural effusion	2–49
Pulmonary embolus	1–5
Hypoxemia	10–30

verse.[7] Restrictive lung volume changes are thought to be a consequence of general anesthesia and muscle relaxants in supine patients. Reflex reduction in central phrenic nerve output secondary to vagal, splanchnic, or sympathetic afferent receptors frequently causes diaphragmatic dysfunction. Stimulation of gastrointestinal viscera during surgical manipulation can result in the cessation of diaphragmatic electrical activity.[1] The decline in lung volumes is not as dramatic after laparoscopic abdominal surgery; laparoscopic cholecystectomy is associated with only a 20% to 25% decrease in forced vital capacity and forced expiratory volume in 1 second.[8]

Patients typically have shallow tidal volumes and increased respiratory rates in the postoperative period. Pain from stretching of the incision or decreased respiratory stimulation from narcotics prevents spontaneous sighing or deep breathing to expand collapsed alveolar units. As the rapid, shallow breathing pattern continues, more alveoli collapse in dependent portions of the lungs. Airway closure may occur at volumes above functional residual capacity. This means that airway closure takes place during tidal breathing and contributes to worsening atelectasis. Dependent airway closure begins as early as 15 minutes after the induction of anesthesia.[9] If it is not corrected by maximal lung inflation, intrapulmonary shunting and V/Q mismatching occurs, resulting in potentially clinically significant hypoxemia.

PULMONARY EDEMA

Pulmonary edema is an increase in the total amount of lung water. It occurs when perialveolar interstitial fluid is formed faster than it can be drained by the pulmonary lymphatics and is a consequence of high intravascular hydrostatic pressures or increased pulmonary capillary permeability. Both forms of pulmonary edema have been shown to disrupt the ultrastructural integrity of the alveolar capillary interface. Pulmonary edema causes an increase in pulmonary vascular resistance, a decrease in functional residual capacity, V/Q mismatching, and an increase in the risk of lung infection. Pulmonary vascular resistance increases because of periarteriolar cuffing by edema fluid. V/Q mismatching is a consequence of peribronchiolar and alveolar compression. Shunting occurs when alveoli collapse or become filled with fluid. A fluid-filled lung is an ideal culture medium for infection.[10]

Pulmonary edema can develop through various mechanisms in surgical patients. Pulmonary hydrostatic pressures are frequently increased because the large volumes of fluid that are given during surgery characteristically reenter the intravascular space on the third or fourth postoperative day. Patients may gain as much as 4 or 5 kg of body weight from intravenous fluid given during and after operation. Patients with underlying heart disease may develop congestive heart failure from volume overload or intraoperative myocardial infarction, producing pulmonary edema. Decreased plasma oncotic pressures may develop when protein from the intravascular compartment is lost into a third-space compartment, as with a postoperative ileus, or as a result of the metabolic response to surgery. If crystalloid solutions, which can equilibrate with the extracellular space, are given rather than colloidal agents such as blood or albumin, extracellular fluid increases and edema results. Pulmonary edema rarely results from an isolated reduction in oncotic pressure, however. Toxic substances such as bacterial endotoxin, lysosomal enzymes, microemboli, fat emboli, or platelet aggregates that are released during surgery or from ischemic tissue are deposited in the pulmonary capillary bed and may produce capillary endothelial damage.

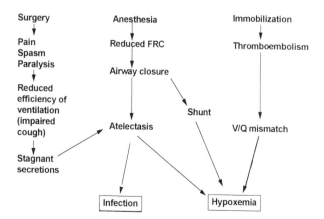

FIG. 15-1. Pathogenesis of major postoperative pulmonary complications. FRC, functional residual capacity.

This damage produces leakage from the capillaries and permeability pulmonary edema.

The diagnosis of pulmonary edema is based on the finding of bilateral rales on physical examination and diffuse fluffy infiltrates on chest radiography. Hydrostatic edema is often associated with perihilar opacity in a butterfly-wing pattern, engorgement of central and hilar blood vessels, Kerley B lines, and an enlarged cardiac silhouette. Jugular venous distention is common. Permeability edema tends to create patchy opacity, with normal cardiac and vascular profiles. A Swan-Ganz catheter may be needed for estimation of left-sided filling pressures to differentiate pulmonary edema caused by volume overload or a cardiac condition from permeability pulmonary edema. Arterial blood gas levels reveal hypoxemia, which may be severe.

Treatment of pulmonary edema involves the correction of contributing underlying problems and scrupulous control of preload. A slightly negative fluid balance has been shown to improve survival in patients with pulmonary edema.[11] Intravascular and extracellular volume can be reduced by the administration of potent diuretics such as furosemide, by hemodialysis, or by hemofiltration in patients with renal failure. The pulmonary capillary wedge pressure should be maintained at the lowest level that does not produce a decrease in the cardiac stroke volume or renal blood flow. Levels of 10 to 14 mmHg usually are sufficient but higher levels may be required in the presence of an abnormally stiff left ventricle. Serum electrolyte levels should be monitored closely to detect hypokalemia or hypernatremia from excessive diuresis. Blood urea nitrogen and urine sodium measurements are helpful indices of the adequacy of renal blood flow. Fluid balance should be monitored closely to prevent significant dehydration. Colloidal agents such as packed red blood cells may be given to patients with anemia. Albumin improves plasma oncotic pressure only briefly and leaks out of damaged capillaries. It is rarely indicated in the treatment of pulmonary edema. Oxygen should be administered to all patients with hypoxia.

ATELECTASIS

Atelectasis is the collapse of a group of alveoli, a small lobule, a segment of a lobe, or, rarely, a whole lung. It is one of the most frequent pulmonary complications in the postoperative period (see Table 15-1). Microatelectasis, which is not visible on radiography but causes hypoxemia, is common. O'Donohue[12] showed that clinically significant atelectasis occurs in 20% of patients undergoing upper abdominal surgery and in 30% of those undergoing thoracic surgery. Atelectasis is clinically important because it leads to increased work of breathing, impaired gas exchange, and a predisposition to infection. Symptoms of acute lobar collapse occur in proportion to the severity of the underlying lung disease. Otherwise healthy patients have few symptoms from lobar collapse, whereas those with chronic lung disease may become significantly hypoxic and tachypneic.

The diagnosis of atelectasis is based on the results of physical examination and chest radiography. Tachypnea; fever; rales; absent, reduced, or bronchial breath sounds in dependent portions of the lungs; decreased resonance to percussion; and reduced movement of the ipsilateral diaphragm may be encountered. The trachea may be shifted to the atelectatic side and mild leukocytosis may be present. The chest radiograph may show increased density in a local segment, displacement of lobar fissures, elevation of the ipsilateral diaphragm, a mediastinal shift toward the side of the collapse, hilar displacement, or compensatory hyperinflation of other lung segments. An air bronchogram indicates that the bronchus feeding the atelectatic segment is patent. It is sometimes difficult to differentiate between atelectasis and pneumonia, especially in the absence of bronchial obstruction. When atelectasis results from an obstructed bronchus, fremitus is decreased and there is dullness to percussion. Auscultation reveals absent or decreased breath sounds.

The treatment of atelectasis is based on two principles: (1) the lungs must be expanded with a transpulmonary pressure sufficient to open collapsed lung units, and (2) stagnant secretions must be cleared. Supplemental oxygen may be necessary to treat hypoxemia. Various therapeutic maneuvers have been used to prevent and treat atelectasis. Treatment techniques include incentive spirometry, deep-breathing exercises, yawning, coughing, chest physiotherapy, and nasal continuous positive airway pressure. In the past, intermittent positive-pressure breathing was also used. Numerous studies have compared different treatment approaches but no consensus exists regarding the best therapy for atelectasis.[12–14]

In the United States, incentive spirometry is used for most surgical patients.[12] In Europe, chest physiotherapy is more common.[15] Typically, incentive spirometry, deep breathing, and coughing are taught before surgery and used afterward. Reducing the frequency and severity of atelectasis in this manner is more effective than is initiating treatment only after complications develop.[7]

When an area of the lung is not ventilated, mucus secreted from the bronchi draining that area becomes thickened and impacted. This makes reexpansion of the alveoli in that segment difficult. Chest physiotherapy and postural drainage help to loosen and clear the mucus. Adequate hydration combined with the use of bronchodilators and mucolytic agents such as acetylcysteine or guaifenesin may help to liquefy and mobilize secretions. Tracheal suction is used to remove mucus that cannot be removed by simple methods. Coughing helps to remove mucus from airways that have been inflated distally. Adequate pain relief is crucial so that patients can cough without discomfort. Excessive sedation with narcotics, however, can depress the respiratory drive and cause shallow respirations, exacerbating atelectasis.

Often, conservative therapy such as incentive spirometry, coughing, chest physiotherapy, bronchodilator therapy, hydration, and occasional use of mucolytic agents and tracheal suction successfully reverses atelectasis in the first 24 to 48 hours.[16] Occasionally, atelectasis must be treated with more aggressive measures. Fiberoptic bronchoscopy is often used to extract mucus plugs, instill mucolytic agents directly into affected areas, and lavage the airways. If an air bronchogram is present in the area of atelectasis, indicating patent central airways and suggesting pneumonia, fiberoptic bronchoscopy is unlikely to be successful.[16] Another method of treating atelectasis is expansion by selective air insufflation of atelectatic areas through a balloon-tipped catheter introduced into the appropriate bronchus under fluoroscopic guidance.[17]

If adequate expansion cannot be accomplished using the described techniques, endotracheal intubation and continuous mechanical ventilation may be indicated.

PNEUMONIA

Pneumonia is a common and life-threatening infection in the postoperative period. The incidence of pneumonia ranges from 3% to 34% after various surgical procedures (Table 15-2). When postoperative infection leads to death, pneumonia is the cause in 38% of cases.[18] Mortality rates are as high as 50% to 70% in patients who develop gram-negative pneumonia, especially with *Pseudomonas*.[19] Risk factors for the development of postoperative pneumonia include the site and duration of surgery, severity of underlying disease, smoking history, underlying nutritional state, and duration of intubation. As noted in Table 15-2, the incidence of pneumonia is highest in thoracic surgery, followed by head and neck procedures and vascular operations. Surgery lasting longer than 3 or 4 hours leads to an increased risk of pneumonia. The highest rates of pneumonia occur in mechanically ventilated patients. The incidence of pneumonia rises as the duration of intubation increases. The incidence of pneumonia is 8% in patients who are intubated 1 or 2 days compared to 45% in those who are intubated longer than 14 days.[20]

Aspiration of bacteria from the oropharynx often leads to the development of pneumonia. Surgical patients and intubated patients have a high rate of oropharyngeal colonization, especially with gram-negative bacilli and staphylococci. The transmission of pathogens on the hands of hospital personnel to patients is a major cause of nosocomial colonization and infection. As many as half of health

TABLE 15–2. Incidence of Postoperative Pneumonia as a Function of Type of Surgery

Type of Surgery	Incidence of Pneumonia (%)
Thoracic	34
Craniotomy	25
Head and neck	25
Coronary artery bypass	21
Cardiac	21
Vascular	20
Cholecystectomy (open)	19
Exploratory laparotomy	18
Colonic	15
Appendectomy	8
Cesarean section	3
Cholecystectomy (laparoscopic)	<1

(Adapted from Horan TC, Culver DH, Gaynes RP, et al. Nosocomial infections in surgical patients in the United States, January 1986–June 1992. Infect Control Hosp Epidemiol 1993;14:73)

care workers have been found to carry gram-negative bacilli or *Staphylococcus aureus* on their hands. Hand-washing has been shown to significantly decrease the incidence of transmission by this route.[20] Often, postoperative patients have nasogastric tubes placed to allow the suction of gastric contents or delivery of nutrition. In addition, they are treated with H_2 blockers and antacids to reduce the incidence of stress ulceration. A rise in the pH level of the stomach has been shown to increase colonization of the stomach by coliform bacteria. These bacteria can then migrate up the nasogastric tube and colonize the pharynx. The use of sucralfate does not alter gastric pH and appears to reduce the incidence of pneumonia.[21] Colonization is also facilitated by direct airway contamination by aerosols, ventilators, and humidifiers; by alteration of normal oral flora with antibiotics; and by reduction in the level of IgA. IgA normally inhibits the adherence of organisms, especially gram-negative bacteria, to the oropharyngeal mucosa. The chance of pneumonia developing is 23% in colonized patients compared to 3% in noncolonized patients.[21] Selective decontamination of the gastrointestinal tract by prophylactic antibiotics has been shown to reduce the rate of pneumonia and other specific infections in the critical care setting but has not been found to significantly improve survival.

Impaired host defenses may contribute to the development of pneumonia after aspiration of bacteria from the oropharynx. Physiologic nasopharyngeal filtration, which traps and filters out microorganisms and particulate debris, is bypassed by endotracheal and nasogastric tubes, allowing infective material to enter the tracheobronchial tree. The cough reflex, the principal means by which the airways are cleared, may be impaired by anesthesia, narcotics, and chest, abdominal, and incisional pain. Mucociliary action clears the smaller airways, which are less effectively cleared by coughing. Anesthetics impair mucociliary action and secretions can plug the small airways if coughing is inadequate. Alveolar macrophages and humoral defense mechanisms are impaired in surgical patients through disturbances such as hypoxia, anemia, malnutrition, and pulmonary edema, allowing the spread of infection.[20]

Bacterial organisms are the most common cause of nosocomial pneumonia. Fungal and viral infections are seen much less often, usually in severely ill and immunocompromised hosts. Table 15-3 lists the incidence of various organisms found in nosocomial pneumonia. Cultures of sputum and tracheal aspirates show polymicrobial growth in over 50% of patients.[19] Gram-negative bacteria are found in 70% of samples and gram-positive organisms are found in 25% to 30%. The most frequently isolated gram-negative bacteria are *Pseudomonas* species. Among gram-positive organisms, *S aureus* is most common. *Candida* is often isolated from cultures but usually reflects colonization rather than true infection. Demonstration of tissue invasion on lung biopsy specimens is necessary before a *Candida* infection is considered clinically significant.[19]

Pneumonia is often extremely difficult to diagnose, especially in ventilator-dependent patients. There may be physical findings of consolidation, rales, rhonchi, fevers, leukocytosis, hypoxemia, and tachypnea; new pulmonary infiltrates on the chest radiograph; and new onset of purulent sputum. These can also be seen in patients with noninfectious pulmonary processes such as atelectasis, pulmonary edema, PE, or infarction. Purulent sputum may arise from oropharyngeal and tracheal colonization. Fevers and

leukocytosis can originate from a nonpulmonary source. Sinusitis is a notoriously common cause of fever in ventilated patients. The following criteria are commonly used for making a diagnosis of ventilator-associated pneumonia:

- Evidence of new or progressive pulmonary infiltrates on the chest radiograph
- New onset of fever (higher than 38°C)
- Purulent tracheobronchial secretions (more than 25 white blood cells, less than 10 squamous epithelial cells per 100× field) with recovery of a pathogenic organism in culture
- Increased peripheral white blood cells (more than 10,000/μL) or neutropenia (less than 4000/μL).[19,22,23]

Despite their widespread use, these criteria are reliable no more than 60% of the time.[24]

Patients in whom pneumonia is suspected should be evaluated with sputum or tracheal samples for Gram stain and cultures, blood cultures, complete blood counts with white blood cell differentials, arterial blood gas determinations, and chest radiographs. Sputum cultures identify the pathogen in half the patients. In the remainder, there is a discrepancy between the results of sputum cultures and samples obtained from the lower respiratory tract by more invasive methods. This discrepancy is believed to be related to the contamination of sputum by oropharyngeal secretions. Delays in plating sputum samples allow bacteria such as *Streptococcus pneumoniae* and *Haemophilus influenzae* to overgrow cultures. Colonization of the oropharynx and the use of antibiotics may alter local bacterial flora and suppress the etiologic pathogen.[20] Blood culture results are positive in only 5% to 15% of patients with pneumonia. Other methods of diagnosing postoperative pneumonia include bronchoscopy with bronchoalveolar lavage and the use of a protected specimen brush to obtain samples from deep areas of the lung. Quantitative bacterial cultures of bronchoscopic specimens are necessary for adequate interpretation. The detection of 10^5 organisms per milliliter of recovered fluid distinguishes a clinically significant infection from colonization, although the presence of intracellular bacteria on spun specimens is highly suggestive, as is the presence of elastin fibers in bronchoscopic specimens. No consensus exists regarding the routine use of bronchoscopy to diagnose pneumonia because its diagnostic specificity and sensitivity are variable and the procedure is not without risk. Open lung biopsy is not used routinely in identifying nosocomial bacterial pneumonia but may be useful for obtaining adequate material for histology and culture in cases involving infection with fungi, cytomegalovirus, and protozoa.[20]

The treatment of pneumonia requires the administration of appropriate antibiotics, the use of pulmonary toilet to clear infected secretions, and the maintenance of host de-

TABLE 15–3. Prevalence of Bacterial Organisms in Nosocomial Pneumonia

Organism	Prevalence (%)
Pseudomonas aeruginosa	10–17
Staphylococcus aureus	10–16
Klebsiella pneumoniae	7–15
Enterobacter sp	10–11
Haemophilus influenzae	8–10
Escherichia coli	5–8
Proteus sp	3–7
Serratia marcescens	4–6
Streptococcus sp	5–6
Fungi	1

(Adapted from Shands JW. Empiric antibiotic therapy of abdominal sepsis and serious perioperative infections. Surg Clin North Am 1993;73:291; and Demling RH, Wolfort S. Early postoperative pneumonia. In: Wilmore DW, Brennan MF, Hasrken AH, et al, eds. Care of the surgical patient, vol 2. Elective care. New York, Scientific American, 1993:1)

TABLE 15–4. Antibiotics Used in the Treatment of Nosocomial Pneumonia

Organism	Antibiotic	Dosage
Staphylococcus	Methicillin	1–2 g q4h
	Oxacillin	1–2 g q4h
	Cefazolin	1 g q6–8h
	Vancomycin	1 g q12h
Haemophilus	Ampicillin	25–50 mg/kg q6h
	Cefuroxime	2–3 g q8h
	Ticarcillin/clavulanate	3.1 g q6h
Klebsiella,	Cefotaxime	1 g q8h–2 g q4h
Enterobacter,	Ceftazidime	1–2 g q8–12h
Escherichea coli	Gentamicin	3–5 mg/kg/d
	Tobramycin	3–5 mg/kg/d
	Ticarcillin/clavulanate	3.1 g q6h
	Imipenem	1 g q6h
	Aztreonam	1–2 g q6–12h
*Pseudomonas**	Gentamicin	3–5 mg/kg/d
	Tobramycin	3–5 mg/kg/d
	Ceftazidime	1–2 g q8–12h
	Imipenem	1 g q6h
	Ofloxacin	0.5 g q12h
	Ticarcillin/clavulanate	3.1 g q6h

*Two drugs advisable.

(Adapted from Demling RH, Wolfort S. Early postoperative pneumonia. In: Wilmore DW, Brennan MF, Hasrken AH, et al, eds. *Care of the surgical patient,* vol 2. Elective care. New York, Scientific American, 1993:1; and Sanford JP. Guide to antimicrobial therapy. Dallas, Antimicrobial Therapy, Inc, 1993:43)

fenses to assist in clearing the infection. Pulmonary toilet measures are the same as those used in the treatment of atelectasis. The antibiotics administered should be effective against the most likely organisms based on the clinical setting, Gram stain findings, and prevalent patterns in the individual hospital. Patients are usually given empiric antibiotic coverage until specific culture results can be obtained. A combination of two or more antibiotics, including an aminoglycoside, is often used for gram-negative pneumonias. Newer antibacterial agents with broad coverage, such as ticarcillin/clavulanate, imipenem/cilastatin, ceftazidime, and aztreonam, may permit the use of a single agent. Because of its high prevalence, *Pseudomonas* must be treated presumptively until culture results are available. Table 15-4 lists the antibiotics typically used in treating nosocomial pneumonia. Appropriate antibiotic therapy may significantly improve survival in these patients, in whom pneumonia is associated with mortality rates as high as 30% to 70%. Mortality is even higher when therapy is inappropriate or superinfections develop.[22] Therefore, it is critical that antibiotic therapy be adjusted once culture and sensitivity results are available.

PULMONARY EMBOLISM

Surgical patients are at increased risk for the development of deep venous thrombosis and PE. About 600,000 patients experience PE each year and about 200,000 die. PE is the third most common cause of death in the United States.[25] Every effort should be made to prevent PE by providing adequate prophylaxis against the development of deep venous thrombosis because this is a preventable complication. Patients often die before a diagnosis is made and therapy can be given. The risk of postoperative thromboembolic events is related to the length of surgery, patient age and previous history of thromboembolic disorders, and the duration of immobility (Table 15-5). Deep venous thrombosis occurs with increased frequency in orthopedic, pelvic, abdominal, and thoracic surgery.[26]

PE and deep venous thrombosis can be difficult to diagnose in extremely ill patients. No component of the history, physical examination, laboratory evaluation, or chest radiograph is specific for this problem. A high index of suspicion must be maintained. Symptoms of PE include dyspnea and pleuritic chest pain. Patients may complain of dull substernal heaviness or tightness along with anxiety and apprehension. Coughing and hemoptysis can occur. Syncope or near-syncope is seen less frequently. Tachypnea is almost universal in PE and tachycardia is frequent (Table 15-6). Patients may have low-grade fevers, rales, prominent pulmonic components of the second heart sounds, and diapho-

TABLE 15–5. Classification of Risk for Postoperative Pulmonary Embolism

High Risk (1%–5%)
Age over 40 y
Surgery lasting more than 30 min
  Major orthopedic surgery
  Pelvic or abdominal cancer surgery
Previous deep venous thrombosis or pulmonary embolism
Plus
Secondary risk factors*

Moderate Risk (0.1%–0.7%)
Age over 40 y
Surgery lasting more than 30 min
Plus
Secondary risk factors*

Low Risk (under 0.01%)
Uncomplicated surgery in patients less than 40 y with no additional risk factors*
Minor surgery lasting less than 30 min in patients over 40 y with no additional risk factors*

*Obesity, immobilization, malignancy, varicose veins, estrogen use, paralysis, and heart failure.

(Modified from Hull RD, Raskob GE, Hirsh J. Prophylaxis of venous thromboembolism: an overview. Chest 1986;89[Suppl]:374S)

TABLE 15–6. Pertinent Findings in Pulmonary Embolus

	Frequency (%)
Symptoms	
Chest pain	85–88
Pleuritic	64–85
Nonpleuritic	6–8
Dyspnea	82–85
Cough	52–53
Hemoptysis	23–40
Syncope	4–20
Signs	
Tachypnea	87–95
Crackles	57–60
Increased S_2P	45–58
Tachycardia	38–48
Fever	42–43

(Adapted from Bell WR, Simon TL, DeMets DL, et al. Clinical features of submassive and massive pulmonary emboli. Am J Med 1977;62:355)

resis. With massive PE, patients have acute cor pulmonale with hypotension and shock. If patients do not have the combination of dyspnea, chest pain, and tachypnea, the likelihood of PE is somewhat reduced. An electrocardiogram should be obtained to rule out myocardial infarction. Electrocardiograms in patients with PE are most often nonspecific but may show sinus tachycardia, T wave inversion, or ST segment inversion in one third to one half of all cases. The classic new $S_1Q_3T_3$ or right bundle-branch block are seen in only 11% of patients with PE. P-pulmonale and right axis deviation are seen in under 5% of cases.[27] Common chest radiographic findings include consolidation of the lung parenchyma, basilar atelectasis, pleural effusions, elevation of the diaphragm, and distention of the proximal pulmonary arteries. Focal oligemia and left or right ventricular enlargement are less common. The chest radiograph can also be completely normal. Arterial blood gas measurements may be misleading. They usually show hypoxemia and hypocarbia with an increased alveolar–arterial oxygen gradient. In 20% of patients with angiographically proven PE, however, the PaO_2 is greater than 80 mmHg. Thus, a normal arterial oxygen tension does not rule out PE. Patients with emboli usually have increased alveolar–arterial oxygen gradients on room air, and normal alveolar–arterial oxygen gradient differences are seen in under 10% of patients with documented PE. A PaO_2 of less than 50 mmHg usually suggests a massive PE.

Transthoracic or transesophageal echocardiography may show a thrombus in the pulmonary trunk, main pulmonary arteries, or right ventricle. There may be right atrial or ventricular dilation and increased pulmonary artery pressure but a normal study does not rule out PE. More re-

cently, levels of d-dimer, a degradation product of cross-linked fibrin, have been used in the detection of PE. Thromboembolism occurs in less than 5% to 10% of cases in the presence of d-dimer levels of 500 ng/mL or lower. Elevated d-dimer levels, however, are less specific and may reflect disseminated intravascular coagulation, liver disease, or other medical conditions.

Once PE is suspected, anticoagulant therapy with heparin should be instituted immediately, unless there are contraindications to its use. A definitive diagnosis should be established. Lung V/Q scanning is the initial noninvasive test used to confirm PE. If the scan is normal with an appropriately low clinical index of suspicion, PE may be safely excluded from active consideration and treatment discontinued. A high-probability scan in the appropriate clinical setting confirms the diagnosis. A low- or intermediate-probability scan is not definitive and further testing is necessary. Figure 15-2 displays the recommended strategy in assessing for PE.[28,29] A pulmonary angiogram is the gold standard for confirming a diagnosis of PE and should be obtained whenever less invasive studies fail to provide a de-

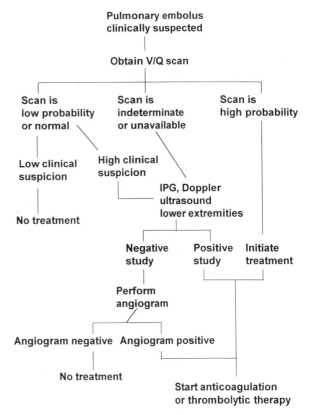

FIG. 15-2. Suggested algorithm for approach to pulmonary thromboembolism in the postoperative setting. IPG, inpedence plethymography.

TABLE 15–7. Differential Diagnosis of Clinical Features of Pulmonary Embolus

Dyspnea
Aspiration
Atelectasis
Pneumonia
Pneumothorax
Pulmonary edema
Bronchitis

Pleuritic Chest Pain
Pneumonia
Pneumothorax
Pericarditis
Chest wall injury
Subdiaphragmatic inflammation

Hemoptysis
Pneumonia
Bronchitis
Pulmonary contusion
Pulmonary neoplasm
Tuberculosis

Right-Sided Heart Failure
Cardiac tamponade
Myocardial infarction
Intracardiac injury

Cardiovascular Collapse
Myocardial infarction
Cardiac tamponade
Sepsis
Pneumothorax
Hypovolemia

finitive diagnosis. Forty to 50% of suspected PE require angiographic confirmation.

Table 15-7 outlines the differential diagnosis of PE. Once a diagnosis of PE is established, heparin administration should be continued at therapeutic doses. Table 15-8 shows suggested dosing regimens for agents used in the treatment of pulmonary thromboembolism.[30] If patients are clinically stable, heparin therapy should be continued for 10 days, adjusted to a partial thromboplastin time of 1.5 to 2.5 times the normal reference value. Anticoagulant therapy with warfarin can be initiated as early as the second day of heparin administration. The prothrombin time should be maintained at an International Normalized Ratio of 3 to 4. Warfarin is administered for 6 to 12 months to prevent recurrence of PE, or longer if risk factors for deep venous thrombosis remain unresolved.[31]

Thrombolytic therapy can be used for rapid lysis of an embolus during the first 24 to 48 hours. Thrombolytic agents should be considered during the first 48 hours after a documented major embolus, especially in the presence of severe hemodynamic or gas-exchange instability. Patients with less than massive PE who have underlying cardiac or pulmonary disease with persistent hemodynamic instability should also be considered for thrombolytic therapy. Agents used include tissue plasminogen activator, streptokinase, and urokinase.

The use of thrombolytic agents may be contraindicated during the postoperative period, although there have been anecdotal reports of successful therapy with heparin or thrombolytic agents immediately after surgery.[32] Table 15-9 lists absolute and relative contraindications to thrombolytic therapy.[33] Bleeding is the major complication of treatment with anticoagulants and thrombolytic agents. Fatal hemorrhage occurs in 1% to 2% of patients and major hemorrhage, requiring transfusion, occurs in 10% to 20%.[33]

If patients develop complications such as bleeding or recurrent emboli while they are receiving adequate anticoagulant or thrombolytic therapy, other options should be considered. These include the placement of a Greenfield filter or a bird's nest filter in the inferior vena cava below the renal veins to block emboli arising from the distal deep venous system. Pulmonary embolectomy is reserved for patients with massive PE who are hemodynamically unstable despite optimal medical therapy or cannot be given anticoagulant therapy.

TABLE 15–8. Recommended Dosage of Anticoagulant and Thrombolytic Therapy in Pulmonary Embolism

	Heparin	Streptokinase	Urokinase	Tissue Plasminogen Activator
Loading dose (intravenous)	10,000 U	250,000 U over 30 min	300,000 U	100 mg over 2 h
Maintenance dose	1000 U/h*	100,000 U/h	300,000 U/h	—
Duration	7–10 days	24 h	12 h	—
Total dose	Variable	2.65×10^6 U	3.9×10^6 U	100 mg

*Keep partial thromboplastin time 1.5–2.5× control. Start warfarin therapy on day 2 after heparin administration is begun. Maintain prothrombin time to an International Normalized Ratio of 3–4.

TABLE 15–9. Contraindications to Thrombolytic Therapy

Absolute Contraindications
Active internal bleeding
Recent (within 2 months) cerebrovascular accident or other active intracranial process

Relative Major Contraindications
Recent (<10 days) major surgery, obstetric delivery, organ biopsy, previous puncture of noncompressible vessel
Recent serious gastrointestinal bleeding
Recent serious trauma

Relative Minor Contraindications
Recent minor trauma, including cardiopulmonary resuscitation
High likelihood of left heart thrombus
Bacterial endocarditis
Coagulation defects, including those associated with hepatic or renal disease
Pregnancy
Age over 75 years
Hemorrhagic diabetic retinopathy
Cerebrovascular accident (nonhemorrhagic)

PLEURAL EFFUSION

Pleural effusions can result from many different problems associated with the postoperative state. Light and George[34] found pleural effusions in 49% of patients after abdominal surgery. Most effusions were small, less than 4 mm thick on decubitus films. Only 10% of patients had effusions thicker than 10 mm. These investigators observed that effusions were mostly ipsilateral to the side of the surgery, occurred primarily in patients undergoing upper abdominal surgery, and were most common among patients who also had atelectasis.

Pleural effusions are usually classified as exudates or transudates and are created when the rate of fluid formation exceeds the rate of drainage. Excessive hydrostatic or decreased oncotic pressures produce increased fluid filtration across the intact capillary walls and result in protein-poor transudates. Breakdown of normal formation-resorption mechanisms caused by damage to the pleural surface or blockage of lymphatics results in protein-rich exudates. The definition of an exudative pleural fluid is based on the following criteria:

- Pleural fluid total protein/serum total protein ratio greater than 0.5
- Pleural fluid lactic dehydrogenase/serum lactic dehydrogenase ratio greater than 0.6
- Pleural fluid lactic dehydrogenase level greater than two thirds of the upper limit of normal for serum lactic dehydrogenase

Any one of these criteria defines an exudate. All three criteria must be absent to define a transudate.[34] The differential diagnosis of postoperative pleural effusions is given in Table 15-10.

Thoracentesis should be performed if patients exhibit evidence of pleural effusions on chest radiographs and the fluids layer to depths greater than 10 mm on decubitus views. Smaller effusions can be monitored with serial chest radiographs and usually resolve spontaneously.

Transudates usually do not require drainage unless they cause respiratory compromise. In the postoperative period, transudates are most often due to congestive heart failure or volume overload. In this situation, correction of the underlying disorder is usually sufficient. Occasionally, patients may have recurrent transudative effusions causing respiratory compromise. In these cases, obliteration of the pleural space (pleurodesis) may be necessary to prevent fluid collection. This is accomplished by draining the fluid completely with a chest tube and instilling an inflammatory agent such as talc, doxycycline, or minocycline, leading to symphysis of the visceral and parietal pleural leaves.

Pneumonia is among the most common causes of postoperative exudates. Most parapneumonic effusions resolve with appropriate antibiotic treatment of the pneumonia but bacteria may invade a sterile effusion and produce a complicated parapneumonic effusion or empyema. Parapneumonic effusions greater than 10 mm in depth should be tapped as early as possible to identify patients who may require drainage of a complicated effusion. Drainage by tube thoracostomy is necessary if the fluid is thick pus or yields bacteria on Gram stain; if the pH level is less than 7.0; or if the pleural fluid glucose level is less than 40 mg/dL. If the fluid has a pH level higher than 7.2, a glucose level greater than 40 mg/dL, and a lactic dehydrogenase level less than

TABLE 15–10. Differential Diagnosis of Postoperative Pleural Effusions

| **Transudates** |
| Congestive heart failure |
| Hypervolemia |
| Hypoproteinemia |
| Ascites |
| Misplaced intravenous catheter |
| Pulmonary embolism (rarely) |
| **Exudates** |
| Pneumonia |
| Pulmonary embolism (usually) |
| Subphrenic abscess |
| Atelectasis |
| Postpericardiotomy syndrome |
| Diaphragmatic contusion |

1000 IU/L, chest tube drainage is not immediately necessary unless organisms are recovered. For intermediate values with a pH level of 7.0 to 7.2, thoracentesis should be repeated in 12 to 24 hours.[35] Chest tube placement is necessary if deteriorating results are noted on repeated thoracentesis. If drainage is delayed, a free effusion may organize into a gelatinous or fibrous peel that will require an open thoracotomy or decortication for resolution.

PE may cause either transudative or exudative effusions. The results of thoracentesis are not specific for PE. Pleural fluid examination usually reveals a clear yellow fluid but the effusion can be bloody. The pleural fluid glucose level is normal and the differential may reveal either polymorphonuclear cells or mononuclear cells.

Subphrenic abscess occurs in 1% of patients undergoing abdominal surgery, leading to an exudative pleural effusion 1 to 3 weeks after operation. Fluid examination usually reveals polymorphonuclear leukocytes. The pleural fluid white blood cell count may reach $50,000/\mu L$, but the effusion rarely becomes infected. The abscess should be identified by thoracoabdominal computed tomography or liver–lung scanning, drainage secured, and appropriate antibiotics administered.[35]

REFERENCES

1. Sykes LA, Boewe EA. Cardiorespiratory effects of anesthesia. Clin Chest Med 1993;14:211–226.
2. Hedenstierna G. Mechanisms of postoperative pulmonary dysfunction. Acta Chir Scand Suppl 1988;550:152–158.
3. Celli BR. Perioperative respiratory care of the patient undergoing upper abdominal surgery. Clin Chest Med 1993;14:253–261.
4. Kroenke K, Lawrence VA, Theroux JF, Tuley MR. Operative risk in patients with severe obstructive pulmonary disease. Arch Intern Med 1992;152:967–972.
5. Wightman JAK. A prospective survey of the incidence of postoperative pulmonary complications. Br J Surg 1968;55: 85–91.
6. Bartlett RH, Brennan ML, Gazzaniga AB, Hanson EL. Studies on the pathogenesis and prevention of postoperative pulmonary complications. Surg Gynecol Obstet 1973;137:925–933.
7. Tisi GM. Preoperative evaluation of pulmonary function: validity, indications, and benefits. Am Rev Respir Dis 1979;119: 293–318.
8. Frazee RC, Roberts JW, Okeson GC, et al. Open versus laparoscopic cholecystectomy. Ann Surg 1991;213:651–653.
9. Roukema JA, Carol EJ, Prins JG. The prevention of pulmonary complications after upper abdominal surgery in patients with noncompromised pulmonary status. Arch Surg 1988;123:30–34.
10. Bartlett RH. Pulmonary insufficiency. In: Wilmore DW, Brennan MF, Hasrken AH, et al, eds. Care of the surgical patient, vol 2. Elective care. New York, Scientific American, 1989.
11. Simmons RS, Berdine GG, Seidenfeld JJ, et al. Fluid balance and the adult respiratory distress syndrome. Am Rev Respir Dis 1987;135:924–929.
12. O'Donohue WJ. National survey of the usage of lung expansion modalities for the prevention and treatment of postoperative atelectasis following abdominal and thoracic surgery. Chest 1985;87:76–80.
13. Celli BR, Rodriguez KS, Snider GL. A controlled trial of intermittent positive pressure breathing, incentive spirometry, and deep breathing exercises in preventing pulmonary complications after abdominal surgery. Am Rev Respir Dis 1984;130: 12–15.
14. Stock MC, Downs JB, Gauer PK, et al. Prevention of postoperative pulmonary complications with CPAP, incentive spirometry and conservative therapy. Chest 1985;87:151–157.
15. Stiller KR, Munday RM. Chest physiotherapy for the surgical patient. Br J Surg 1992;79:745–749.
16. Marini JJ, Pierson DJ, Hudson LD. Acute lobar atelectasis: a prospective comparison of fiberoptic bronchoscopy and respiratory therapy. Am Rev Respir Dis 1979;119:971–978.
17. Susini G, Sisillo E, Bortone F, et al. Postoperative atelectasis reexpansion by selective insufflation through a balloon-tipped catheter. Chest 1992;102:1693–1696.
18. Horan TC, Culver DH, Gaynes RP, et al. Nosocomial infections in surgical patients in the United States, January 1986–June 1992. Infect Control Hosp Epidemiol 1993;14:73–80.
19. Martin LF, Asher EF, Casey JM, Fry DE. Postoperative pneumonia: determinants of mortality. Arch Surg 1984;119: 379–383.
20. Demling RH, Wolfort S. Early postoperative pneumonia. In: Wilmore DW, Brennan MF, Hasrken AH, et al, eds. Care of the surgical patient, vol 2. Elective care. New York, Scientific American, 1989.
21. Craven DE, Steger KA. Nosocomial pneumonia in the intubated patient: new concepts on pathogenesis and prevention. Infect Dis Clin North Am 1989;3:843–866.
22. Shands JW. Empiric antibiotic therapy of abdominal sepsis and serious perioperative infections. Surg Clin North Am 1993;73: 291–306.
23. Meduri GM. Ventilator-associated pneumonia in patients with respiratory failure: a diagnostic approach. Chest 1990;97:1208–1219.
24. Andrews CP, Coalson JJ, Smith JD, Johanson WG Jr. Diagnosis of nosocomial bacterial pneumonia in acute, diffuse lung injury. Chest 1981;80:254–258.
25. Dalen JE, Paraskos JA, Ockene IS, et al. Venous thromboembolism: scope of the problem. Chest 1986;Suppl 89:370S–373S.
26. Hull RD, Raskob GE, Hirsh J. Prophylaxis of venous thromboembolism: an overview. Chest 1986;Suppl 89:374S–383S.
27. Bell WR, Simon TL, DeMets DL. Clinical features of submassive and massive pulmonary emboli. Am J Med 1977;62:355–360.
28. Hull RD, Raskob GE, Hirsh J. The diagnosis of clinically suspected pulmonary embolism: practical approaches. Chest 1986; Suppl 89:417S–425S.
29. The PIOPED Investigators. Value of the ventilation-perfusion scan in acute pulmonary embolism: results of the prospective investigation of pulmonary embolism diagnosis (PIOPED). JAMA 1990;263:2753–2759.
30. Marder VJ, Hirsh J, Bell WR. Rationale and practical basis of

thrombolytic therapy. In: Coleman RW, Hirsh J, Marder VJ, Saljman EW, eds. Hemostasis and thrombosis: basic principles and clinical practice, ed 3. Philadelphia, JB Lippincott, 1994: 1522–1532.

31. Hirsh J, Hull RD. Treatment of venous thromboembolism. Chest 1986;Suppl 89:426S–433S.

32. Kempczinski RF. Surgical prophylaxis of pulmonary embolism. Chest 1986;Suppl 89:384S–388S.

33. Thrombolytic therapy in thrombosis: a National Institutes of Health consensus development conference. Ann Intern Med 1980;93:141–144.

34. Light RW, George RB. Incidence and significance of pleural effusion after abdominal surgery. Chest 1976;69:621–625.

35. Light RW. Postoperative pleural effusion: pathophysiology, clinical importance and principles of management. Respir Care 1984;29:540–546.

36. Sanford JP. Guide to antimicrobial therapy. Dallas, Antimicrobial Therapy, Inc, 1993:43–45.

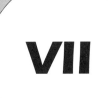

GASTROENTEROLOGY

Medical Management of the Surgical Patient, Third Edition,
edited by Michael F. Lubin, H. Kenneth Walker, and Robert B. Smith III.
J.B. Lippincott Company, Philadelphia, PA © 1995.

CHAPTER

PEPTIC ULCER DISEASE

16

Robert H. Strauss

Peptic ulcer disease is a disorder characterized by periodic exacerbations and remissions. Recent advances have led to an improved understanding of ulcer pathophysiology. For years, the digestive activity of acid as well as pepsin were believed to be the main factors responsible for the formation of ulcers. We are now realizing the importance of protective mechanisms in resisting acid digestion. An imbalance between the digestive and protective factors may result in the formation of ulcers. Although many derangements in the normal physiology of the stomach and duodenum have been identified in patients with ulcers, it remains to be established which of these abnormalities is the most important.

The spectrum of peptic ulcer disease is wide. Some patients with ulcerations have clearcut symptoms, whereas other patients have only symptoms and no identifiable ulcers (nonulcer dyspepsia). Still other patients with ulcers have no symptoms.

EPIDEMIOLOGY

The annual incidence of gastric and duodenal ulcers in the United States is about 500,000 new cases and 4 million recurrences. Peptic ulcer disease is a common cause of morbidity but rarely a cause of death. Postmortem findings indicate that as many as one fourth of men and one sixth of women develop peptic ulcers some time during their lives.

Far fewer patients actually develop symptomatic ulcerations.

The incidence of duodenal ulcer seems to be declining in the United States. Duodenal ulcers are more frequent than gastric ulcers and more common in men than in women. Gastric and duodenal ulcers have overlapping epidemiologic and pathophysiologic features. Patients with duodenal ulcers usually are younger than those with gastric ulcers. The predominance of duodenal ulcers over gastric ulcers in most western countries is changing. Geographic studies indicate that the ratio of duodenal ulcers to gastric ulcers is probably influenced more by environmental than by ethnic factors.

PATHOGENESIS

On average, patients with duodenal ulcers have increased parietal cell mass and acid secretion.[1] Patients with gastric ulcers have normal or decreased acid secretion, which is often associated with decreased mucosal defense. No perfect classification for ulcers exists but the following subgroups have been identified: (1) ulcers caused by massive peptic acid hypersecretion (including those related to Zollinger-Ellison syndrome), (2) ulcers resulting from the ingestion of nonsteroidal antiinflammatory drugs (NSAIDs), (3) ulcers associated with *Helicobacter pylori* infection, and (4) stress ulcers (Table 16-1).

159

TABLE 16–1. Exogenous and Endogenous Factors Associated With the Development of Ulcers

Endogenous
Hydrochloric acid
Pepsin
Bile

Exogenous
Nonsteroidal antiinflammatory
drugs
Helicobacter pylori
?Ethanol
?Nicotine

Physiologic control of acid secretion depends on endocrine (gastrin), neural (cholinergic nerves), and paracrine (histamine) influences. After the ingestion of a meal, the production of acid and pepsin increases as a result of both gastrin release and a vagally mediated cephalic stimulus to the parietal cell. Pepsinogen is secreted by the chief cells in response to gastrin and histamine. In the presence of a low pH, pepsinogen is cleaved to pepsin.

Patients with duodenal ulcers may have an increase in parietal cell mass (1.5 to 2 times above normal). Basal, nocturnal, and maximal acid output can also be elevated in subsets of patients. Because of this, Schwartz' old dictum, "no acid, no ulcer" is still believed to be at least partially true.[2]

Over 95% of patients with duodenal ulcers are infected with *H pylori*, which may cause abnormalities in the acid regulatory process. These patients tend to have elevated serum gastrin responses to meals, among other abnormalities.[3] Patients with gastric ulcers have a lower incidence of *H pylori* infection (60% to 80%). When users of NSAIDs are excluded from this group, however, this figure is higher.

The mucus layer of the gastric and duodenal mucosa is also important. Glycoproteins, which are an important component of the mucosa, form a gel when they are exposed to water. This gel impedes the diffusion of pepsin and creates an unstirred aqueous layer that helps maintain a pH gradient. The secretion of bicarbonate from gastric surface epithelial cells and duodenal mucosa is of vital importance in maintaining a mucosal pH gradient.

Growth factors such as epidermal growth factor and transforming growth factor-α may also play a role in the healing and restitution of the normal mucosa.

Impairment in the production of prostaglandins may be important in mucus depletion. Prostaglandins are endogenous mediators of mucus production. This process may be suppressed in aspirin-induced lesions. Abnormalities in the secretion of bicarbonate in the gastroduodenal mucosa have also been implicated in the formation of duodenal ulcers.

About half of the acid that enters the duodenum is neutralized by bicarbonate secreted by the duodenal mucosa.

The association between NSAIDs and ulcers is dramatic. It has long been known that NSAIDs are a major factor in gastric ulcerations. Data indicate that these agents may also play an important role in duodenal ulcers, especially in regard to bleeding.[4] NSAIDs may cause acute injury by decreasing mucus production and reducing bicarbonate secretion. Prostaglandins also regulate mucosal blood flow, which is important in maintaining the integrity of the mucus barrier.[5] Patients undergoing elective surgery should stop taking NSAIDs in time to allow elimination of the drug; those patients who must take these agents perioperatively should use drugs with short half-lives. More complications related to blood loss occur in patients who take NSAIDs perioperatively than in those who do not.[6]

Cigarette smoking has been linked to both the initiation and the delayed healing of gastric and duodenal ulcers. Smoking increases the incidence of recurrent duodenal ulcers.[7] Some of the adverse effects of cigarette smoking are increased duodenogastric bile reflux,[8] inhibition of pancreatic bicarbonate secretion,[9] decreased duodenal pH,[10] reduced production of salivary epidermal growth factors, and decreased prostaglandin production.[11]

Clinically different from chronic ulcerative lesions are acute upper gastrointestinal erosions and ulcers that may occur in patients that have sustained massive burns, shock, sepsis, and trauma. These lesions are most common in acid-secreting portions of the stomach and often are multiple. Painless gastrointestinal bleeding is a common clinical finding. Erosions and ulcers should be considered when there is a gastrointestinal hemorrhage in the clinical setting of burns, infections, trauma, or shock. Ischemia to the gastric mucosa and injury from acid seem to be of primary importance in the formation of the ulcers. Treatment for the most part is preventive, which includes antacids and H_2 receptive antagonists, but at times, if bleeding is not stopped, surgical approaches are required (Table 16-2).

TABLE 16–2. Indications for Prophylaxis of Stress Ulcers

Medical
Renal failure
Sepsis
Hepatic failure
Respiratory failure

Trauma-Related or Postoperative
Major operative procedures
Major burns
Multiple trauma
Cranial operations
Cardiovascular surgery
Hypovolemic shock

The role of diet in peptic ulcer disease is controversial. Alcohol can cause gastric mucosal damage but abstinence has not been shown to provide a clear benefit. Caffeine may increase gastric acid secretion, yet other substances in the composition of coffee may have greater effects on upper gastrointestinal tract function.

CLINICAL FEATURES

The cardinal manifestation of peptic ulcer is pain. The pain of peptic ulcers involving the stomach and duodenum is frequently described as annoying, gnawing, burning, or aching discomfort, usually present in the epigastrium. Duodenal ulcer pain is generally relieved by the reduction or neutralization of acid that accompanies eating. Pain may be provoked by fasting. This pattern is less typical of gastric ulcers than of duodenal ulcers. The pain of prepyloric or channel ulcers becomes more evident with eating and occasionally is associated with nausea.

Dyspepsia is a term used to describe a symptom complex of epigastric discomfort, bloating, nausea, anorexia, and postprandial distention that is often relieved by either eructation, vomiting, or antacid administration.

Unfortunately, ulcers may also occur without symptoms. Asymptomatic duodenal and gastric ulcers often develop in patients who have been receiving NSAIDs.

In the absence of complications, physical examination is rarely helpful in the diagnosis of peptic ulcer disease.

DIAGNOSTIC TECHNIQUES

The diagnosis of peptic ulcer can be established by demonstrating an ulcer directly through inspection of the mucosa using an endoscope or indirectly through radiographic studies using a contrast agent (usually barium) to coat the gastrointestinal mucosa. Upper gastrointestinal series can detect about 70% to 80% of gastric and duodenal lesions.[12] Some authors state that double-contrast upper gastrointestinal series, which use high-density barium suspension as well as insufflated air, provide a better picture of the mucosal outline and allow the detection of ulcers in a higher percentage of patients.[13] Upper gastrointestinal endoscopy is considered the "gold standard" for the evaluation of suspected gastritis or peptic ulceration as well as the detection of other anatomic abnormalities. Biopsy for histologic examination is also possible, as is therapeutic intervention in selected circumstances. Endoscopy is preferred for the diagnosis of stress erosions; since they are usually too superficial to be seen with barium tests.

In patients in whom perforation is suspected, endoscopic examination with the attendant insufflation of air is contraindicated. Contrast studies using a water-soluble agent should be performed instead. The choice of diagnostic technique also is based on availability as well as cost and physician preference.

GUIDELINES FOR THERAPY

The treatment of peptic ulcer disease has four important goals: (1) to control and alleviate symptoms; (2) to promote healing; (3) to prevent recurrences; and (4) to prevent complications (ie, hemorrhage, obstruction, perforation). The therapies available for the acute treatment of an uncomplicated ulcer alleviate symptoms and promote the healing process in most patients. Approved maintenance therapy also reduces the incidence of recurrences.[14] It remains to be established whether these approaches will also reduce the rate of complications such as hemorrhage, obstruction, and perforation.

Even without specific therapy, most ulcers heal slowly on their own. Although the results of worldwide studies have varied, about 40% of duodenal ulcers can be expected to heal within a period of 4 weeks. Gastric ulcers, especially larger ones, heal more slowly than do duodenal ulcers. Using current regimens (consisting of H_2 blockers, sucralfate, or antacids), most patients with duodenal ulcers experience pain relief within the first 1 or 2 weeks of therapy. About 75% of the ulcers are healed by 4 weeks and 85% to 95% are healed by 8 weeks. If medication use is discontinued after healing and patients are observed closely, most patients have recurrent duodenal ulcer disease after 12 months. Recurrent ulcers may or may not cause symptoms. If patients are given maintenance therapy after their duodenal ulcers have healed, the yearly recurrence rate is reduced by about half.[15] The eradication of *H pylori* infection with antibiotics may reduce the recurrence of duodenal ulcers even more dramatically.[16]

The response of gastric ulcers to treatment is not as well defined as is that of duodenal ulcers. This may result in part from the tendency of physicians to operate on patients with gastric ulcers that are recurrent or slow to heal for fear that the ulcers may be malignant. Gastric ulcers usually heal more slowly than do duodenal ulcers. Treatment should probably be continued until healing is confirmed by either radiography or endoscopy. Gastric ulcers also recur frequently. Relapse rates are probably similar to those of duodenal ulcers. As many as one third of the recurrences may be asymptomatic. No agent has met US Food and Drug Administration approval for maintenance treatment of gastric ulcers. Limited studies of H_2 blockers used in the same dosages as for duodenal ulcers suggest that they are similarly effective in reducing the recurrence of gastric ulcers. The effect of *H pylori* eradication on gastric ulcer relapse also remains to be seen.

SPECIFIC THERAPY FOR PATIENTS WITH PEPTIC ULCER DISEASE WHO ARE UNDERGOING NONRELATED SURGERY

PATIENTS WITH ACUTE ULCERS REQUIRING EMERGENCY SURGERY

Antiulcer regimens should be initiated immediately in patients with documented peptic ulcers who require emergent surgery if adequate therapy has not already been provided. The specific route of administration depends on whether oral medications can safely be used. The choice of one agent over another also depends on previous patient tolerance, availability, cost, and physician preference. As long as oral administration is possible, omeprazole is probably the agent of choice. A single dose inhibits basal and stimulated secretion of gastric acid by more than 90% for 24 hours, even though the elimination half-life of the drug is less than 1 hour. Return of gastric acid secretion to pretreatment levels requires the synthesis of new molecules of H^+-K^+-adenosine triphosphatase. Thus, omeprazole has greater efficacy than do H_2 receptor–blocking drugs, and the administration of a single morning dose completely eliminates intragastric acidity during the late afternoon and evening when relatively poor control is provided by H_2 antagonists. Relatively few side effects have been reported in trials with omeprazole.[17] When oral administration is not possible, it is best to administer intravenous H_2 blockers. If possible, a nasogastric tube should be placed so that the dosage of H_2 blockers can be monitored by serial measurement of the gastric pH level, which should be kept above 3.5.

Complications of peptic ulcer disease during the postoperative period are infrequent but not insignificant. In one study of 143 patients with active ulcer disease, 3 patients required surgical intervention for bleeding or perforation.[18] The incidence of postoperative complications of peptic ulcer disease is not high enough to support the use of prophylactic surgical treatment in patients who are scheduled to undergo extensive operations. Perioperative treatment with antacids or acid inhibition seems prudent, but complications developed in the 3 patients mentioned despite attempts at prophylaxis. Operations in which profound hypotension, sepsis, uremia, and respiratory failure may occur place patients at higher risk for bleeding and perforation. Neurosurgical procedures,[19] aortic artery aneurysm repairs,[20] and cardiac surgery are associated with a higher incidence of ulcer complications.[21] NSAIDs probably should not be administered to patients undergoing such operations. Narcotics should be provided instead for pain control.

PATIENTS WITH ACTIVE ULCERS WHO REQUIRE ELECTIVE SURGERY

Elective surgery should be postponed in patients with active ulcers until these lesions have healed. Healing is encouraged by continuing or initiating one of several accepted therapies. Patients who smoke cigarettes should stop.[22] There is no good evidence that diet has an influence on the rate of ulcer healing. Controversy exists regarding caffeine-containing beverages but these probably should be avoided also. Traditional bland diets are distasteful and no longer prescribed.

PATIENTS WITH CHRONIC ULCER DISEASE OR HISTORIES OF RECURRENT ULCER DISEASE WHO REQUIRE SURGERY

Patients with histories of chronic or recurrent peptic ulcer disease or peptic ulcer symptoms should be treated with H_2 blockers during and after surgery until they return to their baseline status. It is also reasonable to discontinue NSAID use for 7 to 10 days in patients who are scheduled to undergo elective surgery. The drugs used to treat ulcer disease have generally equal efficacy and the choice is based on patients' previous drug experiences and tolerances, potential side effects, the risk of drug interactions, the frequency of administration, and cost. Patients who have been receiving maintenance therapy should be treated again with full-dose therapy before, during, and for some time after their surgical procedures.[23]

PATIENTS WITH HISTORIES OF PEPTIC ULCER DISEASE WHO ARE ASYMPTOMATIC AT THE TIME OF EMERGENT OR ELECTIVE SURGERY

No good study is available that addresses the subset of patients who have histories of peptic ulcer disease but are asymptomatic at the time of emergent or elective surgery. The type of procedure being performed is of paramount importance. Many surgical procedures predispose patients to the formation of "stress ulcerations," whereas others may cause the reactivation or initial expression of chronic peptic ulcer disease.[18] The distinction between "stress ulcerations" and "acute exacerbations of chronic peptic ulcer disease" is not straightforward; these entities differ in their pathogenesis and prognosis. It seems prudent to use the therapeutic regimens outlined earlier in these patients.

DRUGS USED TO TREAT PEPTIC ULCER DISEASE

H₂ BLOCKERS

H₂ blockers are the drugs used most widely to treat peptic ulcer disease.[16] The four agents currently approved (ie, cimetidine, ranitidine, famotidine, and nizatidine) are easy to take, effective, and well tolerated. Intravenous preparations exist and are available for patients who are unable to take oral medications. These agents block the H₂ receptor of the parietal cells and render them less responsive to stimuli. Renal excretion is the major route of elimination of H₂ blockers; therefore, patients with renal insufficiency should receive reduced doses. These agents may be taken once or twice a day. Taken once daily in the evening, these drugs suppress nocturnal acid secretion by over 90% in most patients. Administration twice daily suppresses more daytime secretion and less nocturnal secretion but similar overall secretion during the 24-hour period. Significant data obtained from randomized, controlled trials indicate that numerous regimens of all four H₂ blockers produce healing rates ranging from 70% to 80% after 4 weeks of therapy. By 8 weeks, 80% to 90% of ulcers have healed with therapy.

PROTON PUMP INHIBITORS (OMEPRAZOLE)

Omeprazole acts by suppressing gastric acid secretion, specifically by irreversibly inhibiting the proton pump.[17] It is much more potent than are H₂ blockers. At its usual dose of 20 to 40 mg/d, this drug inhibits 90% of the acid secretion that occurs each day in most patients, causing a state of relative achlorhydria. When gastric acidity is markedly reduced, the G cells secrete increased amounts of gastrin and serum gastrin levels rise. Because of its potency and marked reduction of gastric acidity, omeprazole is more effective than are other agents approved for the treatment of ulcers. It tends to control symptoms and heal ulcers more rapidly than do other drugs. Omeprazole can heal 60% to 90% of duodenal ulcers in 2 weeks and 80% to 100% in 4 weeks.

SUCRALFATE

Sucralfate appears to be as effective as H₂ blockers in healing duodenal ulcers, although its mechanism of action is not well understood.[24] No effect on gastric acidity is noted. This drug is generally considered to be a cytoprotective agent. Little of the drug is absorbed. Sucralfate may reduce the absorption of some other medications, especially phenytoin and warfarin. Occasionally, constipation and nausea may occur.

ANTACIDS

Antacids are effective and relatively safe.[25] Aluminum-based antacids occasionally cause phosphate depletion and may also cause constipation, whereas magnesium-based antacids tend to produce diarrhea. Therefore, a combination of these agents may be necessary to achieve maximum efficacy with the fewest possible adverse effects. Because antacids may bind various drugs within the gut, caution must be exercised in prescribing these agents. Low-sodium antacids should be used for patients on salt-restricted diets.

For antacids to be effective, they should be used in adequate amounts and at proper times to ensure sufficient acid neutralization. Different preparations vary in terms of their potency, the rate at which they neutralize acid, and the length of time they remain in the stomach. Thirty milliliters of a potent antacid taken 1 hour and 3 hours after each meal and 2 hours thereafter until bedtime has been shown to be effective in the treatment of duodenal ulcer disease.[25]

PROSTAGLANDINS

Prostaglandins have many biologic activities.[19] The local production of certain prostaglandins in the gastric mucosa seems to protect its integrity. Synthetic prostaglandins, especially those of the E class, may be useful in the treatment of peptic ulcer disease. Misoprostol (an E₁ analogue) has been shown to reduce the incidence of gastric ulcers in patients taking NSAIDs. Side effects such as diarrhea and abdominal cramping may be disabling, however. It may be advisable to consider the use of misoprostol in patients who require prolonged NSAID therapy. Elderly patients or those with significant histories of peptic ulcer disease should be given this drug.[26]

OTHER MISCELLANEOUS AGENTS

Colloidal bismuth subnitrate is as effective as are H₂ blockers in healing duodenal ulcers. The early recurrence rates of duodenal ulcer disease may be lower when the initial ulcer is healed with colloidal bismuth subnitrate than when it is healed with other agents, presumably because bismuth suppresses *H pylori* infection.

Anticholinergic agents have been used in the past to treat peptic ulcer disease. Because of the limited effectiveness and disturbing side effects of these agents, they are not used often today. Anticholinergic agents reduce as much as 30% to 50% of acid secretion if they are taken appropriately.

Carbenoxolone has been used to treat duodenal ulcers occasionally and gastric ulcers more frequently. Its mechanism of action is unclear but may be cytoprotective, perhaps by decreasing prostaglandin catabolism. This agent may stimulate mucus secretion, decrease mucosal cell loss, and reduce peptic activity. It is not as effective as are other drug regimens and has aldosterone-like activity, which may produce side effects.

REFERENCES

1. Cox AJ. Stomach size and its relation to chronic peptic ulcers. Arch Pathol 1952;54:407.
2. Schwartz K. Uber Penetrienende magen-und jejunal Geschurire. Beitr Klin Chir 1910;76:96.
3. Levi S, Beardshell K, Haddad G, et al. *Campylobacter pylori* and duodenal ulcers: the gastrin link. Lancet 1989;1:1167.
4. Kurata JH, Abbey DE. The effect of chronic aspirin use on duodenal and gastric ulcer hospitalization. J Clin Gastroenterol 1990;12:260.
5. Soll AH, Kurata J, McGuigan JE. Ulcers, nonsteroidal antiinflammatory drugs and related matters. Gastroenterology 1989;96:561.
6. Connelly CS, Parrish RS. Should nonsteroidal antiinflammatory drugs be stopped before elective surgery. Arch Intern Med 1991;151:1963.
7. Korman MG, Hansky J, Eaves ER, et al. Influence of cigarette smoking on healing and relapse in duodenal ulcer disease. Gastroenterology 1983;85:871.
8. Dippy JE, Rhodes J, Cross S. Bile reflux in gastric ulcer: the effect of smoking, metoclopramide, carbenoxolone sodium. Curr Med Res Opin 1973;1:569.
9. Murthy SNS, Dinoso VP, Clearfield HR, et al. Simultaneous measurement of basal pancreatic, gastric acid secretion, plasma gastrin and secretion during smoking. Gastroenterology 1977; 73:758.
10. Murthy SNS, Dinoso VP, Clearfield HR. Acid pH changes in the duodenal bulb during smoking. Gastroenterology 1978;75:1.
11. Quimby GF. Active smoking depresses prostaglandin synthesis in human gastric mucosa. Ann Intern Med 1986;104:616.
12. Montagne JP, Moss AA, Margulis AR. Double-blind study of single and double contrast upper gastrointestinal examinations using endoscopy as a control. AJR 1978;130:1041.
13. Gelfand DW, Orr DJ. Single versus double contrast gastrointestinal studies: critical analysis of reported statistics. AJR Am J Roentgenol 1981;137:523.
14. Isenberg JI, McQuaid KR, Laie LA, et al. Acid peptic disorders. In: Yamada T, ed. Textbook of gastroenterology. Philadelphia, JB Lippincott, 1991:1241–1339.
15. Burgat DW, Chiverton SG, Hank RH. Is there an optimal degree of acid suppression for reducing duodenal ulcers? A model of the relationship between ulcer healing and acid suppression. Gastroenterology 1990;99:345–357.
16. Feldman M, Burton ME. Histamine$_2$-receptor antagonists. N Engl J Med 1990;323:1672–1680.
17. Maton PN. Omeprazole. N Engl J Med 1991;324:965–975.
18. Matthews JB, Tostella BJ, Silen W. Gastroduodenal hemorrhage and perforation in the postoperative period. Surg Gynecol Obstet 1988;1988:389.
19. Chan KM, Mann KS, Lai ECS, et al. Factors influencing the development of gastrointestinal complications after neurosurgery: results of multivariate analysis. Neurosurgery 1989;25: 378.
20. Kanno H, Sakaguchi S, Hachiya T. Bleeding peptic ulcer after abdominal aortic aneurysm surgery. Arch Surg 1991;126:894.
21. Rosen HR, Vlatrakes GJ, Rattner DW. Fulminant peptic ulcer disease in cardiac surgical patients: pathogenesis, prevention, and management. Crit Care Med 1992;20:354.
22. Korman MG, Hans KJ, Eaves ER, Schmidt GT. Influence of cigarette smoking on healing and relapse in duodenal ulcer disease. Gastroenterology 1983;85:871.
23. Strum WB. Prevention of duodenal ulcer recurrence. Ann Intern Med 1986;105:757.
24. McCarthy DM. Sucralfate. N Engl J Med 1991;325:1017–1025.
25. Peterson WH, Sturdevant RAL, Frankl HD, et al. Healing of duodenal ulcers with an antacid regimen. N Engl J Med 1977;297:341.
26. Walt RP. Misoprostol for the treatment of peptic ulcer and antiinflammatory drug–induced gastroduodenal ulceration. N Engl J Med 1992;327:1575–1580.

Medical Management of the Surgical Patient, Third Edition,
edited by Michael F. Lubin, H. Kenneth Walker, and Robert B. Smith III.
J.B. Lippincott Company, Philadelphia, PA © 1995.

CHAPTER

LIVER DISEASE

17

Norman Gitlin

The increasing use of routine screening biochemical tests has resulted in the detection of an apparently increased number of biochemical abnormalities suggestive of hepatic disease in asymptomatic patients. Noninvasive diagnostic radiologic procedures such as ultrasonography, computed tomographic scanning, and nuclear magnetic resonance imaging have also revealed abnormalities ranging from benign hemangiomas to malignancy in asymptomatic patients. More and more patients who require surgery have histories of established hepatic disease or incidentally detected hepatic abnormalities. Many of the abnormalities found in asymptomatic patients do not affect the morbidity or mortality of the proposed surgery. Conditions in this category include Gilbert syndrome, Dubin-Johnson syndrome, small hepatic hemangiomas, and congenital hepatic cysts. Recognition of these entities is imperative to prevent unnecessary investigations and patient anxiety. This chapter focuses on the more serious common hepatic diseases and discusses their presentation, identification, and effect on the course and care of surgical candidates.

LIVER DISEASES EXISTING BEFORE SURGERY

ACUTE DISEASES

Viral Hepatitis

Knowledge and understanding of viral hepatitis has expanded tremendously during the past 15 years. Several viruses commonly infect the liver and cause acute hepatitis.

Infection may be asymptomatic or associated with anicteric or icteric hepatitis that may progress to fulminant hepatic failure, chronic hepatitis, cirrhosis, or hepatocellular cancer. The known hepatitis viruses are hepatitis A virus (HAV), infectious, epidemic hepatitis; hepatitis B virus (HBV), serum hepatitis; hepatitis C virus (HCV), posttransfusion hepatitis; hepatitis D virus (HDV), delta hepatitis; and hepatitis E virus (HEV). The designation non-A non-B (NANB) hepatitis is still retained to account for presumed viral hepatitis that is serologically negative for the other known viruses. This is a diagnosis of exclusion and may include many separate viruses (giant cell hepatitis and a rarer form of fulminant hepatitis). Other causes of acute viral hepatitis include Epstein-Barr virus, cytomegalovirus, herpes simplex virus, hemorrhagic fever virus, Lassa fever virus, and Marburg viral hepatitis.

A classic episode of acute icteric viral hepatitis is separated into four phases: the incubation period, preicteric phase, icteric phase, and convalescence phase. The mean incubation period is 25 days (range, 15 to 45 days) for hepatitis A, 75 days (range, 40 to 180 days) for hepatitis B, and 50 days (range, 15 to 150 days) for hepatitis C. Hepatitis E has yet to be documented in a native American and is found in the Mediterranean area, Asia, Central America, and third world locations. It is transmitted by the fecal-oral route and has an incubation period marginally longer than that of hepatitis A.

The time and mode of exposure to viral hepatitis often is not known and the incubation period cannot be calculated. Patients are asymptomatic during this phase, although results of tests for viral markers may be positive (hepatitis B surface antigen [HBsAg] can be detected as much as 8 weeks before the onset of jaundice). The preicteric phase lasts 3 to 10 days and features nonspecific symptoms such as anorexia, nausea, malaise, lethargy, vomiting, and dull right upper quadrant discomfort (reflecting stretching of the capsule by the inflamed liver).

Other symptoms include myalgia, arthralgia, diarrhea, flulike symptoms, and fever. The last of these is more common in hepatitis A. A nonspecific maculopapular rash may also be present. Rigors are exceptionally rare in viral hepatitis, as are high fever and severe, cramping abdominal pain. Weight loss of 3 to 10 pounds is common. The beginning of the icteric phase is often accompanied by the alleviation of nonspecific symptoms and the onset of jaundice, dark urine, and, often, pruritus. In addition, patients who smoke cigarettes develop a temporary distaste for smoking. Patients usually begin to feel better within 1 to 2 weeks of the onset of jaundice and malaise is frequently the last symptom to disappear. Prolonged jaundice associated with minimal symptoms is suggestive of cholestatic viral hepatitis. Pruritus can be a problem under these circumstances. Rarely, jaundice is the first and only symptom of viral hepatitis; it can mimic a surgical cause of jaundice. About 90% of patients with hepatitis A have an anicteric form of the illness that is not recognized. Antibodies to HAV detected at a later date indicate the previous infection. HBV can have an anicteric presentation in 50% of patients and HCV probably is anicteric in the acute phase in close to 95% of patients. The convalescent phase of viral hepatitis is associated with the resolution of jaundice. Some malaise and a susceptibility to fatigue can persist for weeks and even months after viral hepatitis.

Signs. Signs of acute viral hepatitis include hepatomegaly, hepatic tenderness, and jaundice. The liver is mildly enlarged, smooth, firm, and tender. Splenomegaly is detectable in 15% to 25% of cases. Stigmata of clinical hepatocellular disease (eg, spider nevi, edema, ascites, gynecomastia) are absent.

Laboratory tests. The diagnosis of acute hepatitis is based on the history and biochemical tests. Specific serologic tests make it possible to determine which virus is responsible for the infection (Table 17-1). Characteristic biochemical findings in acute viral hepatitis are marked elevation (10 to 100 times) of the serum aminotransferase, alanine aminotransferase [ALT], and aspartate aminotransferase [AST] levels. The ALT and AST are usually elevated to the same degree but the ALT may be slightly higher. If the elevation is only marginal (less than 10-fold), the presence of other conditions (eg, alcoholic liver disease, drug hepatotoxicity, chronic hepatitis) should be considered. The alkaline phosphatase level and levels of other enzymes suggestive of cholestasis usually are slightly elevated. The prothrombin time is a good index of the severity of acute hepatitis. Slight prolongation (less than 2 seconds) is characteristic of acute hep-

atitis. Marked prolongation that cannot be corrected with vitamin K injections is ominous and suggestive of severe hepatitis with the potential for the development of fulminant liver failure. The serum albumin and globulin levels are essentially unchanged in uncomplicated acute viral hepatitis, as are the complete blood count and the platelet count. A decreasing albumin level is suggestive of subacute hepatic necrosis and is accompanied by ascites and diminution in hepatic size.

Specific serologic tests for HAV include antibody to HAV of the IgM class, which is initially detectable in the serum for 45 to 100 days. Thereafter, IgG antibody is detectable for the remainder of patients' lives. The presence of antibodies to HAV of class IgG alone in the early phases of acute hepatitis indicates previous exposure but no current infection. In acute hepatitis B, HBsAg can be detected in the blood as early as 8 weeks before the onset of jaundice and disappears 12 to 20 weeks after the jaundice becomes clinically apparent. The persistence of HBsAg beyond 20 weeks is indicative of a carrier status or the development of chronic hepatitis. The appearance of antibody to HBsAg after acute hepatitis B is the ideal sequence and indicates a full, uncomplicated recovery.

Hepatitis B core antibodies to IgM are useful in the diagnosis of acute hepatitis B during the "window" phase of the illness, when both HBsAg and antibody to HBsAg are negative. The results of this test are also positive in some patients with chronic HBV infection. In the acute phase of HBV infection, hepatitis B e antigen, HBV DNA, and DNA polymerase may be detected and are indicative of viral replication. Persistence of these markers implies both infectivity and chronicity.

The detection of antibodies to HCV using a second-generation enzyme-linked immunosorbent assay (ELISA) or a radioimmunosorbent assay (RIBA) implies one of the following: (1) acute HCV infection, (2) chronic HCV infection, (3) healthy status after infection, or (4) carrier status. A history, physical examination, and biochemical studies are required to determine patient status. Detection of HCV RNA by polymerase chain reactions is the most reliable diagnostic test of HCV infection available. Quantitation of HCV using branched DNA signal amplification assay provides information of the HCV viral load. If the use of interferon therapy is under consideration, a liver biopsy should be performed to ascertain the severity of the hepatitis. Antibodies to HDV can be used to confirm infection; a rising titer or a high IgM titer indicates current or recent infection.

Transmission and outcome. HAV is transmitted predominantly by the fecal-oral route, although rare episodes of parenteral transmission have been documented.[1] No carrier state occurs and there is no evidence that chronic hepatitis or cirrhosis can complicate HAV. Prolonged cholestasis (lasting months), a relapse of acute hepatitis, and fulminant hepatitis are the major sequelae of HAV.[2] Infectivity of

TABLE 17–1. A Guide to Serologic Testing for Viral Hepatitis

Virus	Test	Interpretation	Comment
A	Anti-HAV		
	Positive IgM	Acute hepatitis A (current)	IgM can be positive for 6 w
	Positive IgG	Post–hepatitis A (full recovery)	to 18 months after acute infections or relapses
B	HBsAg	Carrier or acute B or chronic B	Infectious
	HBsAb	Post–hepatitis B (full recovery)	Not infectious (also seen after vaccination)
	HBcAb	Acute hepatitis, chronic hepatitis or recovery. If HBcAB, IgM positive or with HBsAg positive then it means acute hepatitis B.	
	HBeAg	Indicates infectivity/chronicity	Mostly done for research or treatment studies
	HBV polymerase	Positive means viral replication	Chronicity/infectivity
	HBV DNA	The viral genome that can be detected in the blood or liver	Infectious
C	Anti-HCV	Positive means (1) post-HCV infection; (2) HCV carrier state; (3) acute hepatitis C; or (4) chronic hepatitis C	(1) ELISA test can be false-positive; (2) RIBA or ELISA 2 test is more specific and accurate
	HCV RNA	Positive means active viral replication	Most sensitive test of HCV infection

After HCV infection, it can take 12–52 weeks before acute seroconversion occurs (anti-HCV becomes positive)

D	Anti-HDV		HDV infection *never* occurs unless HBsAg is *also* positive
	IgM	Recent HDV infection	
	IgG	Old HDV infection	
E	Anti-HEV		Rare in the United States
	IgM	Recent HEV infection	
	IgM	Old HEV infection	
Non-A, non-B	Unavailable	Diagnosis by exclusion	Probably includes HFV, HGV, and underdiagnosed or misdiagnosed HCV cases

HAV, hepatitis A virus; HBV, hepatitis B virus; HCV, hepatitis C virus; HDV, hepatitis D virus; HEV, hepatitis E virus; ELISA, enzyme-linked immunosorbent assay; RIBA, radioimmunosorbent assay; HFV, hepatitis F virus; HGV, hepatitis G virus.

HAV associated with fecal viral shedding occurs for a limited period before the onset of jaundice and for about 10 days afterward. Infectivity is rare thereafter, despite an elevated aminotransferase level.

HBV has been identified in tears, saliva, urine, stool, semen, breast milk, serous exudates, and vaginal secretions. Its mode of transmission is predominantly parenteral or venereal. Infection can result from accidental inoculation during surgery by blood or fluids contaminated with HBV.[3,4] Patients who have HBsAg in their blood but no apparent hepatic dysfunction can transmit the illness to the operating staff through a needle stick at the time of surgery.

Other modes of HBV transmission include contaminated needles, syringes, and instruments; intravenous drug abuse; tattooing; ear piercing; acupuncture; shared razors; and blood-sucking vectors such as ticks and bedbugs. HBV is frequently transmitted from infected mothers to their infants during the birth process.[5] This vertical transmission is especially likely if the mother is positive for hepatitis B e antigen as well. Vertical transmission probably accounts for the high prevalence of HBV in third world countries and may also explain the high incidence of hepatocellular cancer in these areas. The outcome of acute hepatitis B is shown in Figure 17-1. Most patients have full recoveries. About 1 in 2000 develops fulminant hepatitis or subacute hepatic failure. Many of these patients die, although liver transplantation is altering this trend. A phase of cholestasis or chronic persistent hepatitis may occur before total recovery in some

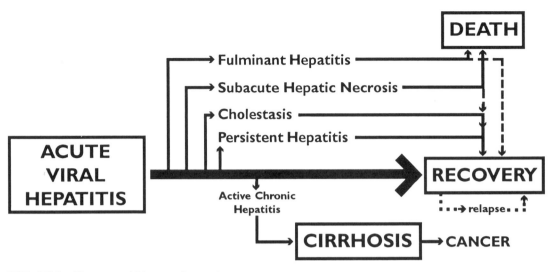

FIG. 17-1. The natural history of acute hepatitis due to HBV.

patients. Others (5% to 8% of men infected with acute HBV) develop chronic active hepatitis that can proceed to cirrhosis, liver failure, or hepatocellular cancer.[6]

The mode of transmission of HCV is unclear.[7–9] A report from the US Centers for Disease Control indicated that 42% of patients acquired their infection through drug abuse using contaminated needles or syringes. Heterosexual exposure accounted for 5% of cases, as did occupational exposure (doctors, nurses, technicians). Blood transfusions accounted for about 4% of infections, dialysis for 1%, and sporadic/cryptogenic or unaccountable transmission for 40%. Unaccountable transmission is a challenge to every epidemiologist. Despite its mild presentation and minimal initial clinical features, HCV infection is complicated by the development of some form of chronic hepatitis in 80% of patients and ultimate progression to cirrhosis, liver failure, or hepatocellular cancer in 20%. There is no correlation between the histologic findings in chronic HCV infection and the duration of the illness, the symptoms, the physical findings, or the results of biochemical tests.

HDV is a small RNA virus that is incapable of infecting cells or replicating on its own.[10] It requires HBV as a "helper" DNA virus and appears to be directly cytopathic.[11] It is universal, being especially prevalent among drug addicts, hemophiliacs, and their sexual partners.[12] It is spread predominantly by the parenteral route. Successful immunization against HBV protects against HDV infection as well because the antibody to HBsAg deprives the HDV of access to the HBsAg. If acute HDV infection occurs in a chronic HBsAg carrier, it is termed *superinfection* and frequently leads to chronic acute hepatitis with the development of cirrhosis and liver failure. Simultaneous acute HDV and acute HBV is termed *coinfection* and is associated with a high incidence of fulminant hepatitis.

Drug Hepatitis

Drug-induced hepatotoxicity accounts for nearly 5% of all patients who are hospitalized for the investigation of jaundice. It also accounts for between 10% and 20% of patients with fulminant hepatic failure. A high index of suspicion is imperative when considering a drug-induced cause for hepatic dysfunction. Drug-induced hepatotoxicity can occur by two mechanisms: from direct hepatotoxins such as salicylates or acetaminophen (a common, dose-related event) or from idiosyncratic hepatotoxins such as halothane (a rare event that is not dose-dependent, probably a hypersensitivity reaction to an intermediate metabolite). The type of injury produced by drugs ranges from acute fulminant hepatitis to insidious asymptomatic cirrhosis.

CHRONIC DISEASES

Alcohol-Related Illness

About 18 million people in the United States have alcohol-related problems. Alcohol abuse is an expensive public health problem. The costs of direct treatment amount to $15 billion per year and total costs, including absenteeism, lost productivity, and industrial accidents, total more than $125 billion per year. About 200,000 deaths per year in this country can be attributed to alcohol abuse. Only 10% of heavy drinkers develop cirrhosis after 10 years, however.[13] The pathogenesis of alcoholic cirrhosis involves factors other than excessive intake. Susceptibility to alcohol-induced liver disease is not clearly understood. Genetic markers may affect susceptibility or impart resistance to the effects of alcohol. Women are more prone to alcohol-induced liver injury than are men and suffer such injury after the ingestion of a lesser amount of alcohol over a shorter period.[14,15] This may be explained in part by decreased alcohol dehydrogenase activity in the gastric mucosa in women resulting in higher blood alcohol levels for the same alcohol intake.[16]

The spectrum of morphologic lesions and clinical presentations attributed to alcoholic liver disease is vast and includes asymptomatic fatty liver; alcoholic hepatitis (with or without cholestasis); alcoholic ketoacidosis; Zieve syndrome (hemolysis, jaundice, hyperlipidemia, and abdominal pain); and cirrhosis (compensated or decompensated). A higher incidence of hepatocellular carcinoma is associated with alcoholic cirrhosis. Combinations of these pathologies often occur simultaneously. Histologic evaluation can be useful in differentiating the conditions. In alcoholic hepatitis, histologic findings include steatosis, necrosis, an inflammatory infiltrate of polymorphonuclear cells, and alcoholic hyaline. The last of these is regarded as nonspecific for alcohol abuse unless it is located predominantly in the centrilobular area. Mallory's hyaline can be found in many liver conditions that are not related to alcohol use.[17] Alcoholic hepatitis can be confused with viral hepatitis. Findings suggestive of alcoholic hepatitis include a modest elevation of the aminotransferase level (less than 10-fold) with an AST/ALT ratio greater than 2, a low albumin level, pyrexia greater than 101°F, and leukocytosis of more than 20,000 cells per microliter. Alcoholic hepatitis associated with cholestasis can mimic a surgical cause of extrahepatic obstructive jaundice. Ultrasonography demonstrating a normal-sized gallbladder, a normal-caliber common bile duct, and no dilation of the intrahepatic ducts is useful in differentiating the two conditions.

The severe form of acute alcoholic hepatitis carries a mortality rate of 40%.[17] Several therapeutic approaches have been evaluated but no consensus exists regarding the optimal technique. Abstinence, nutritional support, corticosteroids, insulin and glucagon, propylthiouracil, and anabolic steroids all have been evaluated. Maddrey and coworkers[18] generated a computer model to assist in predicting the mortality risk in alcoholic hepatitis. The discriminate function is 4.6 (patients' prothrombin times minus control values [in seconds] + bilirubin levels [in mg/dL]). If a total of 32 is exceeded, a high mortality can be anticipated. Corticosteroids have been advocated in the treatment of alcoholic hepatitis. The use of short-term steroid therapy (4 to 6 weeks) is beneficial in patients with severe acute alcoholic hepatitis (ie, patients with encephalopathy).[17–20] In patients with encephalopathy caused by upper gastrointestinal bleeding, however, the use of steroids may be contraindicated.[21] Another study using Maddrey's discriminate function index reported that steroids were beneficial in patients who had severe alcoholic hepatitis or a high index score.[22] None of the studies have shown any beneficial effect of steroids on long-term mortality. The action of steroids in alcoholic hepatitis involves the stimulation of albumin synthesis, the stimulation of appetite, the suppression of collagen and immune mechanisms, the inhibition of cytokines, and the reduction of inflammation. Other therapeutic approaches have included insulin and glucagon, propylthiouracil, colchicine, and nutritional support.[23–27] Colchicine, 1 mg/d for 5 days each week, was prescribed in a study of 100 patients who were followed up for as long as 14 years.[25] Significantly superior 5- and 10-year survival rates were noted compared with the placebo group (75% versus 34% and 56% versus 20%, respectively). In addition, one third of the colchicine-treated patients who underwent biopsies showed histologic improvement. Because of flaws in the matching of treatment and placebo groups, however, the results of this study are not universally accepted.

Alcoholic cirrhosis (old terms include *Laënnec's cirrhosis, portal cirrhosis, nutritional cirrhosis,* and *micronodular cirrhosis*) can progress and decompensate, resulting in jaundice, ascites, encephalopathy, and coagulopathy. Portal hypertension can also develop, with striking splenomegaly, features of hypersplenism, or bleeding portosystemic collaterals (eg, esophageal or gastric varices, hemorrhoids). A useful classification of hepatic reserve using albumin, bilirubin, ascites, encephalopathy, and nutritional status is referred to as the Child's index (Table 17-2). This index can assist in establishing prognoses and selecting patients for shunt decompression surgery or liver transplantation. Alcohol has a direct toxic effect on megakaryocytes, and the platelet count can be as low as 20,000/µL in patients with acute alcoholic intoxication. This rapidly returns to the normal range with abstinence and should not be mistakenly diagnosed as hypersplenism resulting from portal hypertension.

Metabolic Conditions

Several metabolic conditions can be present with hepatic dysfunction. Poorly controlled diabetes mellitus often is associated with an elevated alkaline phosphatase level, reflecting fat and glycogen deposition in the liver; biliary disease with cholelithiasis is also more common. Obese patients, especially those in their mid-fifties, can develop fatty infiltration of the liver, which is referred to as steatonecrosis.[28–31] These patients usually have no symptoms, are overweight, often have diabetes, have hyperlipidemia, and generally admit to only mild social drinking.

TABLE 17–2. Child's Criteria for Hepatic Reserve

	A Minimal Impairment	B Advanced Impairment	C Advanced Impairment
Serum bilirubin (mg/dL)	<2.0	2.0–3.0	>3.0
Serum albumin (g/dL)	>3.5	3.0–3.5	<3.0
Ascites	None	Easily controlled	Poorly controlled
Neurologic status/ encephalopathy	None	Minimal	Advanced, "coma"
Nutrition	Excellent	Good	Poor, "wasting"

Hepatomegaly and mild elevation of the ALT, AST, and alkaline phosphatase levels can occur, and liver histology shows a morphologic picture almost identical to that of alcoholic hepatitis. An incorrect diagnosis may be entertained unless physicians are aware of this entity. A normal prothrombin time, a normal albumin level, a low AST/ALT ratio, and the absence of jaundice can assist in the identification of steatonecrosis. Wilson's syndrome, a metabolic disorder of copper metabolism, can present in teenagers as chronic active hepatitis or even fulminant hepatic failure. Hemochromatosis, an often underdiagnosed condition, can present with hepatic enlargement; deranged biochemistry; and cardiac, endocrine, and musculoskeletal abnormalities.[32] Early recognition and therapy is imperative to prevent serious complications, including hepatocellular cancer.

Chronic Hepatitis (Viral or Immunopathic)

Chronic hepatitis is defined as elevation of the aminotransferase level for more than 6 months and is associated with an inflammatory process (of varying severity) in the liver. Although many conditions can manifest in this way (Table 17-3), this chapter focuses on viral and immunopathic causes of chronic hepatitis. About 5% to 8% of patients develop chronic hepatitis after acute HBV and 80% of patients develop chronic hepatitis after acute HCV. These patients may be asymptomatic or symptomatic, with jaundice, weakness, asthenia, and malaise being the most common symptoms.

The clinical examination is often normal or may reveal jaundice, hepatomegaly, or, occasionally, splenomegaly or cutaneous stigmata of liver disease such as spider angiomas, palmar erythema, and telangiectasia. Results of biochemical testing may suggest chronic liver disease, with elevated aminotransferase, alkaline phosphatase, and bilirubin levels and a low albumin level with a reversed albumin/globulin ratio. Often, the only abnormality is elevation of the aminotransferase level. Immunologic markers of immunopathic chronic active hepatitis such as antinuclear

antibodies and smooth muscle antibodies are highly suggestive of the diagnosis. Histologic findings can vary in severity from mild chronic persistent hepatitis with an inflammatory infiltrate of lymphocytes confined to the portal tracts but maintaining an intact limiting plate, to chronic active hepatitis with an inflammatory infiltrate spreading beyond the portal tract accompanied by piecemeal necrosis, bridging necrosis, and fibrosis.[33] Cirrhosis may complicate this picture.

Cirrhosis

Cirrhosis is the end result of several different conditions. All the conditions that present with chronic hepatitis (see Table 17-3) ultimately may cause cirrhosis. The two cardinal findings in the cirrhotic liver are nodular formation and fibrotic bands. The terms *micronodular, macronodular,* and *biliary cirrhosis* are of little assistance. The major complications of cirrhosis, regardless of its cause, are portal hypertension,

TABLE 17–3. Causes of Chronic Hepatitis

Viral
    Hepatitis B virus
    Hepatitis C virus
Idiopathic
Autoimmune
Medication-related
    Oxyphenisatin
    Isoniazid
    Halothane
Metabolic
    Wilson's syndrome
    Hemochromatosis
    α_1-Antitrypsin deficiency
Miscellaneous
    Primary biliary cirrhosis
    Alcohol

TABLE 17–4. Clinical Stages of Encephalopathy in Liver Disease

Stage	Mortality (%)	Mental Status	Asterixis	
I	25	Slow, irritable, slurred speech, altered affect	Slight	Normal
II	60–80	Lethargic, drowsy, confused	Present	Abnormal
III	75–80	Incoherent, severly confused, sleepy (but able to be roused)	Present	Abnormal
IV	80	Comatose (not able to be roused)	Absent	Abnormal

esophageal varices, splenomegaly, secondary hypersplenism, thrombocytopenia, coagulopathy, ascites, encephalopathy, and jaundice. All these affect the mortality and morbidity of any operation. In addition, surgery can predispose to the development of liver failure, with encephalopathy, jaundice, and ascites being the most common postoperative complications in patients with cirrhosis. These complications are thought to result from a combination of perioperative hypoxia, drug hepatotoxicity, hypokalemia (a recognized potent precipitator of encephalopathy), sepsis and tissue necrosis (releasing an increased nitrogen load), and gastrointestinal bleeding (causing hypotension, hypoxia, and an increased protein load). About 15 g of protein are contained in 100 mL of blood; even without a major hemodynamic change, gut hemorrhage can increase the protein load and precipitate encephalopathy or renal failure. Clinical encephalopathy is divided into four stages (phases; Table 17-4). A preclinical or subclinical form also exists and can be identified through the administration of psychometric tests.[34]

Ascitic fluid in patients with portal hypertension classically has a serum/ascitic albumin gradient of greater than 1.1 g/dL. This distinguishes it from other causes of ascites with lower gradients.[35] Ascitic fluid in patients with cirrhosis is prone to infection because of low opsonic activity and a low complement content. It occasionally is difficult to distinguish spontaneous bacterial peritonitis from secondary surgical peritonitis. The latter requires immediate surgery to correct the precipitating pathology. Several features help differentiate spontaneous bacterial peritonitis from its surgical counterpart; these are outlined in Table 17-5.

Patients with cirrhosis and ascites may develop the hepatorenal syndrome if they undergo an overzealous brisk diuresis or are given nephrotoxic agents (eg, aminoglycosides, cephalosporins). Nonsteroidal antiinflammatory drugs also can precipitate renal failure even when they are prescribed in low doses for analgesia. This action is probably related to their ability to inhibit renal prostaglandins and, consequently, renal perfusion. Patients with cirrhosis are often malnourished and immunocompromised. Susceptibility to infection, with subsequent septicemia and multiorgan failure, is a dreaded complication of surgery in these patients.

TABLE 17–5. Comparison between Ascitic Fluid in Spontaneous Bacterial Peritonitis and Secondary/Surgical Bacterial Peritonitis

Ascitic Fluid	Spontaneous Bacterial Peritonitis	Secondary/Surgical Bacterial Peritonitis
Appearance of fluid	Clear/cloudy	Cloudy/purulent
Single organism	Common	Rare
Multiple organism	Rare	Common
White blood cell count	500–5000/μL	1000–50,000/μL
Protein	<1 g/dL	>2 g/dL
Glucose	Normal	Decreased
pH	7.2–7.4	6.8–7.2
Odor	Nil	Putrid

LIVER DISORDERS CONCURRENT WITH SURGICAL PATHOLOGY

Previously healthy patients without any liver disease can develop jaundice or inflammatory conditions of the intrahepatic biliary system or hepatic parenchyma as a result of neighboring pathology (eg, cholecystitis, cholelithiasis) or as part of systemic sepsis. The primary conditions associated with concurrent liver dysfunction are septicemia, cholecystitis or cholelithiasis, metastatic pyogenic liver abscess, extrahepatic surgical obstructive jaundice, and shock (ischemic hepatitis).

Patients with gram-negative bacterial septicemia, regardless of the source, can develop jaundice with a cholestatic biochemical profile.[36] The pathogenesis of the jaundice is uncertain; it may reflect microductal edema as a consequence of hypersensitivity to a protein in the circulating bacteria. Recognition of this entity and treatment of the sepsis and primary pathology is all that is required for the jaundice to resolve.

Acute cholecystitis with or without cholelithiasis can be complicated by ascending cholangitis and hepatic pyogenic abscesses. Bacteremia in the portal system as a result of appendicitis, diverticulitis, or colitis also can cause pyogenic hepatic abscesses. Once such pathology is suspected, ultrasonography is used to confirm the diagnosis and assist in planning the appropriate treatment. Jaundice resulting from extrahepatic obstructive pathology (eg, cancer, stricture, impacted calculus) is usually self-evident and treated with surgery. Severe hypotension can cause ischemic hepatitis, with a meteoric rise in the aminotransferase level to 20,000 IU within 72 hours of the initial episode.[37] Equally rapid resolution of the elevated enzyme levels occurs within 7 days provided hypotension and hypoxia do not recur. An elevated bilirubin level (less than 5 mg/dL), marginal elevation of the alkaline phosphatase level, and slight prolongation of the prothrombin time can also occur. No specific therapy is necessary except for the restoration of normal blood pressure to permit hepatic perfusion and eliminate hepatic hypoxia.

The possibility of drug-induced (eg, anesthetic, antimicrobial, or analgesic) hepatic dysfunction resulting from the operation or preoperative care must always be considered in patients with jaundice or abnormal biochemical profiles.

PREOPERATIVE CARE

The preoperative approach to patients with existing liver disease varies according to the nature and severity of the pathology. Awareness of conditions such as Gilbert syndrome and Dubin-Johnson syndrome is all that is required

to prevent perioperative concern and investigation for an elevated bilirubin level. Similarly, knowledge of the presence of a small hepatic hemangioma or congenital cyst precludes postoperative concern in the event a liver mass is reported on sonography or computed tomographic scanning.

ACUTE VIRAL HEPATITIS

Patients with acute viral hepatitis seldom require surgery except in emergency situations. If surgery is believed to be absolutely essential under these rare circumstances, it is important to establish the precise cause of the hepatitis (see Table 17-1) to reduce the risk of infection to the surgeon and operative staff. The severity of the hepatitis also affects the morbidity and mortality of the operation. A careful history designed to elicit risk factors such as parenteral drug abuse, homosexual behavior, sexual promiscuity, previous surgery, transfusions, previous hepatitis or jaundice, occupational risk, and needle-stick exposure should be obtained. The current health status can be determined through a physical examination concentrating on the size of the liver and any features of hepatic decompensation. A complete blood count, a full coagulation profile, and basic hepatic and renal biochemical parameters should be established. These include albumin, globulin, ALT, bilirubin, alkaline phosphatase, creatinine, blood urea nitrogen, and electrolyte levels. Any coagulation abnormalities must be corrected before operation. Intramuscular or subcutaneous vitamin K is effective in patients with good hepatic reserve. Even under ideal circumstances, however, it may take days to correct a prolonged prothrombin time. Such delay is not possible under emergency circumstances, in which case the prothrombin time must be corrected using fresh frozen plasma. Significant thrombocytopenia (less than 80,000 cells/μL) may necessitate the use of platelet transfusions to correct the deficiency.

Reports of surgery performed on patients with acute viral hepatitis have indicated higher mortality and morbidity rates (9.5% and 11.9%, respectively).[38] Complications were more likely in patients undergoing more extensive surgery with prolonged anesthesia. Poor postoperative courses were noted in most patients who underwent cholecystectomy or gastrectomy. If emergency surgery is required, it is advisable to perform the minimal surgical procedure in the shortest time possible (ie, a cholecystotomy should be done rather than a cholecystectomy, and a bleeding ulcer or a perforation should be oversewn rather than performing a vagotomy and pyloroplasty or a partial gastrectomy). Definitive surgery can be scheduled later, when patients' conditions have improved. There is no indication to operate on patients with fulminant hepatic failure unless the surgery relates to the primary liver disease and involves the placement of an intracranial bolt, hepatic transplantation, or a tracheostomy.

CHRONIC VIRAL HEPATITIS

Both elective and emergency surgery can be undertaken in patients with chronic liver disease resulting from viral infections. Many patients with chronic hepatitis caused by HCV are unaware of their illness; they are asymptomatic and have minimal elevation of the aminotransferase level and no abnormal physical findings. As many as 40% of patients with chronic hepatitis caused by HCV have no recognizable source of infection, and only 5% of all patients with HCV infection acquired it from a blood transfusion. The lack of previous surgery or blood transfusion does not exclude a diagnosis of HCV infection. Patients who have well-compensated chronic persistent hepatitis or chronic active hepatitis from either HBV or HCV, with or without cirrhosis, generally fare well in surgery. No specific measures (apart from infectious precautions and those mentioned for acute hepatitis) are necessary.

If the liver disease has progressed to cirrhosis with complications (eg, ascites, jaundice, encephalopathy, recent variceal bleeding), surgery carries considerable risk. Morbidity and mortality are high, regardless of the skill, care, and precision of the surgeon. Morbidity and mortality rates of 30% have been reported for elective surgery in patients with cirrhosis.[39] The operations were performed for biliary tract disease, peptic ulcer disease, and colonic disorders (diverticulitis and carcinoma of the colon). A higher mortality was associated with emergency surgery in patients with cirrhosis (57% versus 10%). These rates were remarkably similar in another study (45% versus 11%).[40] The hepatic reserve as determined by Child's criteria (see Table 17-2) assists in determining operative risk. Hemorrhage, sepsis, and multiple organ failure (especially renal failure) accounted for 87% of the deaths in Garrison's study.[39] Bleeding can occur because of preexisting coagulopathy related to prolongation of the prothrombin time and partial thromboplastin time, thrombocytopenia (secondary to the hypersplenism), and a reduced fibrinogen level. Thrombocytopenia and low fibrinogen levels may reflect disseminated intravascular coagulation caused by sepsis. If sepsis is suspected clinically, blood cultures and other appropriate cultures should be performed. It is important that any severe malnutrition be assessed and corrected before surgery if possible.

CHRONIC AUTOIMMUNE HEPATITIS

Patients with chronic autoimmune hepatitis may require higher steroid dosages during the perioperative period.

ALCOHOLIC LIVER DISEASE

Patients with alcoholic liver disease should be treated in much the same manner as patients with viral hepatitis. Nutrition is often a major factor and should receive special emphasis. Nutritional deficiencies in patients with alcoholic hepatitis are corrected with vitamins, minerals (including the correction of hypophosphatemia), and oral or parenteral nutritional formulas. The use of parenteral branched-chain amino acid solutions or oral formulas has been advocated by some to achieve a rapid positive nitrogen balance without precipitating hepatic encephalopathy. Medium-chain triglycerides can be useful in patients with jaundice; 1 tablespoon four times a day can supply 460 kcal. The use of corticosteroid therapy in alcoholic hepatitis was discussed earlier in this chapter.

Delirium tremens can be devastating in operative patients and prophylaxis should be provided with oxazepam or lorazepam. The development of severe hepatocellular disease has been recognized in patients with chronic alcoholism who are treated with doses of acetaminophen that are at or below the therapeutic range.[41-43] The probable cause of hepatic injury from these nontoxic drug levels is induction by chronic alcohol intake of the cytochrome P-450 11E system, which also converts acetaminophen to a toxic metabolite.[42] The clinical picture under these circumstances is fairly characteristic: mild to moderate jaundice, moderately severe coagulopathy, and strikingly elevated aminotransferase levels inconsistent with either acute alcoholic hepatitis or viral hepatitis.[41-43]

INTRAOPERATIVE CARE

Diligent management of the fluid and electrolyte balance is imperative, as is the prevention of hypotension, hepatic hypoxia, and hypoglycemia. The ailing liver is exquisitely sensitive to hypoxia. Hypokalemia can also precipitate hepatic encephalopathy. The need to prevent stress ulceration may dictate the short-term administration of H_2 antagonists to reduce hydrochloric acid in severely ill patients. During the operation, anesthesia can lower splanchnic and portal blood flow. Inhaled, spinal, and epidural anesthetics reduce hepatic blood flow by 30% to 50% during induction. This can have a detrimental effect on hepatic function, especially in those patients with chronic liver disease who are more susceptible to hepatic hypoxia.[44,45] The hepatotoxic potential of anesthetic agents is also a concern. Halothane can produce hepatotoxicity but is rarely used today. Risk factors such as obesity, female sex, and prior exposure are important.[46] Fluothane, enflurane, and other related agents are far less hepatotoxic. There is no increased risk of hepatotoxicity from halothane or its closely associated anesthetic agents in patients with preexisting liver disease.[47]

Internists should inform anesthetists of patients' conditions so that they can select the best anesthetic agents.

Patients with portal hypertension and ascites avidly retain sodium. Excessive transfusion of blood or fluids can raise the venous pressure and lead to an increase in portal pressure, enhancing the risk of a variceal bleed. Careful attention to fluid administration is critical because fluid overload may cause a variceal bleed or aggravate ascites. Ascites can elevate the diaphragm, resulting in reduced vital capacity, atelectasis, pulmonary edema, or renal complications. During surgery, it may be advisable to monitor venous and cardiac pressures with a Swan-Ganz catheter, which can reduce the risk of hypovolemia-induced hepatic ischemia.

The role of prophylactic antibiotics during surgery is controversial. Oral quinolones are effective against enteric gram-negative bacteria and can be used to reduce the risk of spontaneous bacterial peritonitis. Patients at greater risk for sepsis include those with malnutrition and those with hypersplenism caused by portal hypertension. Cultures of blood, sputum, urine, and ascitic fluid should be performed if sepsis is suspected.

Caution must be exercised in prescribing medications. Some benzodiazepines (eg, oxazepam, lorazepam) are metabolized effectively, even in patients with cirrhosis.[48–51] Other medications, however, that are not metabolized by hepatic phase 1 conjugation (eg, diazepam, chlordiazepoxide) may have potentiated action in patients with cirrhosis. In patients who have undergone previous portosystemic shunt procedures, oral meperidine has increased action because of reduced hepatic extraction and metabolism. In general, opiate analgesics, hypnotics, and sedatives are poorly tolerated by patients with severe liver disease and their use should be limited or avoided. Nonsteroidal antiinflammatory drugs reduce renal prostaglandins and can cause the hepatorenal syndrome in patients with cirrhosis. Ulcerogenic agents such as salicylates and nonsteroidal drugs should not be used in patients with cirrhosis and coagulopathy.

POSTOPERATIVE CARE

All patients with acute hepatitis, chronic hepatitis, or cirrhosis who require emergency surgery should be cared for in an intensive care unit. The most common cause of postoperative mortality is sepsis and multiple organ failure. It is critical that adequate hemostasis be ensured, fluid and electrolyte levels be controlled, and the use of medications that can cause hepatic decompensation be avoided. The urine output should be monitored carefully; if it falls below 30 mL/h, the use of intravenous mannitol may be considered. Careful observation for sepsis, encephalopathy, occult gastrointestinal bleeding, ileus, peritonitis, hypokalemia, and wound infection or dehiscence is recommended. Protein reduction or restriction may be necessary if postoperative encephalopathy occurs. Lactulose, 30 mL/h orally until diarrhea occurs followed by doses two or three times daily, can be effective against encephalopathy. Conditions that may precipitate encephalopathy include infection, tissue necrosis, hypoxia, medications, hypokalemia, and constipation.

Atelectasis with secondary pulmonary infection can occur after surgery and may precipitate encephalopathy. If variceal bleeding occurs during the postoperative period, endoscopy and sclerotherapy or banding should be performed. If these measures are ineffective, the administration of a vasopressin (Pitressin) drip, use of a tamponade esophageal balloon tube, or embolization of the left gastric vein through percutaneous transhepatic catheterization of the portal venous system can be attempted.

Elective and emergency surgery in patients with severe acute hepatitis or chronic liver disease complicated by cirrhosis and features of decompensation carries significant morbidity and mortality. They should be restricted to selected patients in whom surgery is the only option. Several hepatic conditions are regarded as contraindications to elective surgery, including acute viral hepatitis; acute alcoholic hepatitis; fulminant hepatitis; severe chronic hepatitis; Child's class C cirrhosis; coagulopathy (uncorrectable); encephalopathy; and severe, resistant ascites.[52]

REFERENCES

1. Sherertz RJ, Russell BA, Reuman PD. Transmission of hepatitis A by transfusion of blood products. Arch Intern Med 1984;144:1579–1580.
2. Gordon SC, Reddy KR, Schiff L, et al. Prolonged intrahepatic cholestasis secondary to acute hepatitis A. Ann Intern Med 1984;101:635–637.
3. Callender ME, White Y, Williams R. Hepatitis B virus infection in medical and health care personnel. Br Med J 1982;284:324–326.
4. Kunches LM, Craven DE, Werner BG, et al. Hepatitis B exposure in emergency medical personnel. Am J Med 1983;75:269–272.
5. Stevens CE. Perinatal hepatitis B virus infection: screening of pregnant women and protection of the infant. Ann Intern Med 1987;107:412–413.
6. Seeff LB, Koff RS. Evolving concepts of the clinical and serologic consequences of hepatitis B virus infection. Semin Liver Dis 1986;6:11–22.
7. Rassam SW, Dusheiko GM. Epidemiology and transmission of hepatitis C infection. Eur J Gastroenterol Hepatol 1991;3:585–591.
8. Dienstag JL. Hepatitis non-A, non-B: C at last. Gastroenterology 1990;99:1177–1180.
9. Thomas HC. Non-A, non-B hepatitis. Q J Med 1987;246:793–798.

10. Bonino F, Smedile A. Delta agent (type D) hepatitis. Semin Liver Dis 1986;6:28–33.

11. Lefkowitch JH, Goldstein H, Yatto R, et al. Cytopathic liver injury in acute delta virus hepatitis. Gastroenterology 1987;92:1262–1266.

12. De Cock KM, Govindarajan S, Chin KP, et al. Delta hepatitis in the Los Angeles area: a report of 126 cases. Ann Intern Med 1986;105:108–114.

13. Lelbach WK. Organize pathology related to volume and pattern of alcohol use. In: Gibbins RJ, Israel Y, Kalant H, eds. Research advances in alcohol and drug problems. New York, John Wiley & Sons, 1974:93–98.

14. Klatsky AL, Armstrong MA, Friedman GD. Alcohol and mortality. Ann Intern Med 1992;117:646–654.

15. Morgan MY, Sherlock S. Sex related difference among 100 patients with alcoholic liver disease. BMJ 1977;1:939–941.

16. Frezza M, Di Padova C, Pozzato G, et al. High blood alcohol levels in women. N Engl J Med 1990;322:95–99.

17. Maddrey WC. Alcoholic hepatitis: clinicopathologic features and therapy. Semin Liver Dis 1988;8:91–102.

18. Maddrey WC, Boitnott JK, Bedine MS, et al. Corticosteroid therapy of alcoholic hepatitis. Gastroenterology 1987;75:193–199.

19. Reynolds TB, Benhamou JP, Blake J, et al. Treatment of acute alcoholic hepatitis. Gastroenterol Int 1989;2:208–216.

20. Black M, Tavill AS. Corticosteroids in severe alcoholic hepatitis. Ann Intern Med 1989;110:677–680.

21. Inperiale TF, McCullough AJ. Do corticosteroids reduce mortality from alcoholic hepatitis? Ann Intern Med 1990;113:299–307.

22. Ramond MJ, Poynard T, Rueff B, et al. A randomized trial of prednisolone in patients with severe alcoholic hepatitis. N Engl J Med 1992;326:507–512.

23. Trinchet JC, Balkau B, Poupn RE, et al. Treatment of severe alcoholic hepatitis by infusion of insulin and glucagon: a multi-centre sequential trial. Hepatology 1992;15:76–81.

24. Orrego H, Kalant H, Israel Y, et al. Effects of short term therapy with propylthiouracil in patients with alcoholic liver disease. Gastroenterology 1979;76:105–115.

25. Kershenobich D, Vargas F, Garcia-Tsao G, et al. Colchicine in the treatment of cirrhosis of the liver. N Engl J Med 1988;318:1709–1713.

26. Soberon S, Pauley MP, Duplantier R, et al. Metabolic effects of enteral formula feeding in alcoholic hepatitis. Hepatology 1987;7:1204–1209.

27. Achord JL. Malnutrition and the role of nutritional support in alcoholic liver disease. Am J Gastroenterol 1987;82:1–7.

28. Adler M, Schaffner F. Fatty liver hepatitis and cirrhosis in obese patients. Am J Med 1979;67:811–816.

29. Ludwig J, Viggiano TR, McGill DB, et al. Nonalcoholic steatohepatitis. Mayo Clin Proc 1980;55:434–438.

30. Powell EE, Cooksley WGE, Hanson R, et al. The natural history of nonalcoholic steatohepatitis: a follow-up study of forty-two patients for up to 21 years. Hepatology 1990;11:74–80.

31. Diehl AM, Goodman Z, Ishak KG. Alcohollike liver disease in nonalcoholics. Gastroenterology 1988;95:1056–1062.

32. Fairbanks VF, Baldus WP. Hemochromatosis: the neglected diagnosis. Mayo Clin Proc 1986;61:296–298.

33. Johnson PJ, McFarlane IG, Eddleston ALWF. The natural course and heterogeneity of autoimmune-type chronic active hepatitis. Semin Liver Dis 1991;11:187–196.

34. Gitlin N. Subclinical portal-systemic encephalopathy. Am J Gastroenterol 1988;83:8–11.

35. Runyon BA, Montano AA, Akriviadis EA, et al. The serum-ascites albumin gradient is superior to the exudate-transudate concept in the differential diagnosis of ascites. Ann Intern Med 1992;117:215–220.

36. Sikuler E, Guetta V, Keynan A, et al. Abnormalities in bilirubin and liver enzyme levels in adult patients with bacteremia. Arch Intern Med 1989;149:2246–2247.

37. Gitlin N, Serio KM. Ischemic hepatitis: widening horizons. Am J Gastroenterol 1992;87:831–835.

38. Harvill DD, Summerskill WH. Surgery in acute hepatitis: causes and effects. JAMA 1963;184:257–261.

39. Garrison RN, Cryer HM, Howard DA, et al. Clarification of risk factors for abdominal operations in patients with hepatic cirrhosis. Ann Surg 1984;199:648–655.

40. Dobereck RC, Sterling WA, Allison DC. Morbidity and mortality after operation in nonbleeding cirrhotic patients. Am J Surg 1983;146:306–309.

41. O'Dell JR, Zetterman RK, Burnett DA. Centrilobular hepatic fibrosis following acetaminophen-induced hepatic necrosis in an alcoholic. JAMA 1986;255:2636–2637.

42. Seeff LB, Cuccherini BA, Zimmerman HJ, et al. Acetaminophen hepatotoxicity in alcoholics. Ann Intern Med 1986;104:399–404.

43. Maddrey WC. Hepatic effects of acetaminophen. J Clin Gastroenterol 1987;9:180–185.

44. Friedman LS, Maddrey WC. Surgery in the patient with liver disease. Med Clin North Am 1987;71:453–476.

45. Ngai SH. Current concepts in anesthesiology. N Engl J Med 1980;302:564–566.

46. Neuberger J, Williams R. Halothane hepatitis. Dig Dis 1988;6:52–64.

47. Greene NM. Halothane anesthesia and hepatitis in a high-rise population. N Engl J Med 1973;289:304–307.

48. Klotz U, Avant GR, Hoyumpa A, et al. The effects of age and liver disease on the disposition and elimination of diazepam in adult men. J Clin Invest 1975;55:347–359.

49. Morgan DD, Robinson JD, Mendengall CL. Clinical pharmacokinetics of chlordiazepoxide in patients with alcoholic hepatitis. Eur J Clin Pharmacol 1981;19:279–285.

50. Kraus JW, Desmond PV, Marshall JP, et al. Effects of ageing and liver disease on disposition of lorazepam. Clin Pharmacol Ther 1987;24:411–409.

51. Shull HJ, Wilkinson GR, Johnson R, et al. Normal disposition of oxazepam in acute viral hepatitis and cirrhosis. Ann Intern Med 1976;84:420–425.

52. Aranha GV, Sontag SJ, Greenlee HB. Cholecystectomy in cirrhotic patients: a formidable operation. Am J Surg 1982;143:55–60.

CHAPTER

18

Medical Management of the Surgical Patient, Third Edition,
edited by Michael F. Lubin, H. Kenneth Walker, and Robert B. Smith III.
J.B. Lippincott Company, Philadelphia, PA © 1995.

INFLAMMATORY BOWEL DISEASE

Suzy L. Kim
Steve Goldschmid

Crohn's disease and ulcerative colitis are two nonspecific inflammatory disorders of the gastrointestinal tract that are often referred to jointly as inflammatory bowel disease.[1] No definitive cause for either of these disorders has ever been identified; however, many theories exist that incorporate environmental and immunologic factors, genetic susceptibility, and transmissible agents.[2–6] Both disorders frequently require surgical therapy for numerous indications.

Initial differentiation of these diseases is of utmost importance because their medical and surgical treatment differ greatly. Crohn's disease and ulcerative colitis are diagnosed on the basis of characteristic clinical, radiologic, endoscopic, and histologic findings, although about 10% to 15% of patients have indeterminate diagnoses.[7] These patients are treated medically at first, depending on the location of active disease and the response to therapy. This approach is used because of the potential for recurrence if a diagnosis of Crohn's disease is confirmed.

CROHN'S DISEASE

Crohn's disease can affect any portion of the gastrointestinal tract from the mouth to the anus. Ileocolonic disease, or disease involving the terminal ileum and proximal colon, is most common, affecting about 55% of all patients. As many as 30% of patients have only small bowel disease.[8,9] When the disease affects the terminal ileum, other portions of the small intestine, the upper gastrointestinal tract, or the perianal region, the diagnosis is reasonably certain.

Crohn's disease is characterized by transmural inflammation, fistulas, strictures, and areas free of disease interspersed between areas of active disease (skip lesions). Frequently, deep linear ulcers (fissures) and small linear erosions or ulcerations (aphthous lesions) are found on the mucosa. Noncaseated granulomas are seen histologically but are found in only 15% to 30% of endoscopic biopsy samples and 70% of surgical specimens.[10,11] The rectum is uncommonly involved in Crohn's colitis, even when other portions of the colon are affected.[9] Patients usually complain of nonbloody diarrhea and abdominal pain but the clinical presentation varies with the distribution and extent of the Crohn's disease.[8] Patients with distal colonic Crohn's disease may have signs and symptoms similar to those seen in ulcerative colitis.

When disease is confined to the large intestine, distinguishing Crohn's disease from ulcerative colitis can be more difficult. The presence of skip lesions, fistulas, rectal sparing, and strictures favors a diagnosis of Crohn's disease. Fistulas may form between bowel and perineum, skin, or any visceral organ (including other parts of the bowel, bladder, or vagina). Perianal involvement is rare in ulcerative colitis and its presence markedly favors the diagnosis of Crohn's disease. The finding of noncaseated granulomas substantiates the diagnosis of Crohn's disease. If these distinguishing features are not present, patients should be asked whether they have oral ulcerations similar in description to aphthous lesions. This finding raises the suspicion of Crohn's disease when the other described manifestations make the distinction from ulcerative colitis difficult.

ULCERATIVE COLITIS

Ulcerative colitis is a nonspecific inflammatory disorder of the large intestine. In contrast to Crohn's disease, it affects only the mucosa. The rectum is involved in virtually all patients, and as many as 20% have pancolitis. The disease starts from the anal verge and involves the colon more proximally in a contiguous fashion (ie, without skip areas).[1] Endoscopic features include granularity, friability, and small ulcerations; however, fissures as seen in Crohn's disease are uncommon in ulcerative colitis. There is no pathognomonic histologic finding in ulcerative colitis. Findings of colonic crypt distortion, crypt abscesses, and plasma cell infiltration in the lamina propria extending to the mucosal base are suggestive of inflammatory bowel disease but do not differentiate ulcerative colitis from Crohn's disease.[13] The absence of these findings makes the diagnosis of ulcerative colitis equivocal. Previous therapy for inflammatory bowel disease, especially local rectal preparations given as enemas, may confuse the diagnosis because the rectum may appear to be spared. In this instance, skip areas may also be found. Painless bloody diarrhea, tenesmus, and rectal pain are characteristic complaints of patients with ulcerative colitis.

Again, the distinction between ulcerative colitis and Crohn's disease is not evident in 10% to 15% of patients. If surgery is elective, pathologic examination of removed colon often distinguishes between the two disorders. If it does not, or if surgery is urgent or emergent, patients should be approached conservatively, as though they have Crohn's disease, because of the likelihood of recurrence and its possible sequelae.

INDICATIONS FOR SURGERY

Operations for inflammatory bowel disease are usually elective because most patients have at least a partial response to medical therapy.[14,15] On occasion, however, emergency surgery is performed for some of the major complications of these two disorders. Indications for emergency surgery include free perforation, hemorrhage, and toxic megacolon.

Although hematochezia is found in one fourth of patients with Crohn's disease and in nearly all of those with ulcerative colitis, severe bleeding affects only 1% to 5%. Significant bleeding is usually seen in severe ulcerative colitis and ileocolonic Crohn's disease.[16] Hemorrhage is the most common complication requiring emergency surgery. Although many patients stop bleeding spontaneously, the outcome may be better if operation is performed early.[17]

Free perforation may be seen in up to 4% of patients with ulcerative colitis and in even fewer of those with Crohn's disease, although there are data suggesting that the percentage of patients with ulcerative colitis who have perforation is decreasing.[18] Free perforation requires immediate surgical intervention.[19–21] At highest risk are patients with ulcerative colitis who have pancolitis and patients with Crohn's disease who have small bowel involvement. Clinicians must remember that steroids may mask symptoms, and that perforation in patients who are receiving steroids may cause subtle signs and symptoms.

Toxic megacolon, an acute dilation of the colon, may be seen in as many as 8% of patients with ulcerative colitis and fewer of those with Crohn's disease.[12] Findings of increased amounts of small bowel gas and metabolic alkalosis may identify a group of patients with severe ulcerative colitis who are at higher risk for the development of toxic megacolon.[22] Toxic megacolon sometimes responds to medical therapy, which includes broad-spectrum antibiotics, intravenous corticosteroids, and bowel rest. Nearly 30% of patients, however, have recurrence of toxic megacolon or fulminant colitis during follow-up.[23] The decision to perform emergent operation is based on the condition of the patient. Medical therapy can be used in patients whose clinical condition permits waiting. If medical therapy is undertaken and no response is seen within 24 to 48 hours, urgent surgery to prevent free perforation is indicated.[21] Regardless, the mortality for emergency surgery in patients with toxic megacolon is as high as 30%, with higher rates in those patients who have associated colonic perforation.[24,25] Emergent colectomy carries significantly greater morbidity and mortality than does elective surgery. If emergent resection must be performed, the procedure should be limited to an abdominal colectomy without removal of the rectum. This minimizes the incidence of complications and helps lower the mortality rate.[26]

Indications for elective surgery in ulcerative colitis and Crohn's disease are similar[21]: disease unresponsive to medical therapy, colonic dysplasia or cancer, complications of medical therapy, stricture formation, bowel obstruction, and growth failure. When consideration is being given to elective surgery in patients with inflammatory bowel disease, there is a substantial difference between Crohn's disease and ulcerative colitis.

About 70% to 90% of patients with Crohn's disease require surgery.[27] The indications for surgery may vary depending on whether patients have colonic, small bowel, ileocolonic, or perirectal involvement.[28] Postoperative recurrence of symptoms is seen in 50% by 4 years, and recurrence of disease requiring reoperation is seen in 20% by 5 years and in 34% by 10 years.[29,30] Patients with ileocolonic disease seem to be at higher risk for recurrence. For these reasons, distinguishing Crohn's disease from ulcerative colitis is important before elective surgery is contemplated. Surgery in Crohn's disease should be as conservative as possible, with resection confined to areas of gross involvement.[31] In a select group of patients with Crohn's disease who have short fibrotic strictures and inactive disease, stricturoplasty may be appropriate because it minimizes the amount of bowel resected and has an outcome similar to that of conventional small bowel resection.[32,33]

Patients with ulcerative colitis who have pancolitis are more likely to undergo surgery within the first 3 years for medical failure.[1] In addition, the finding of high-grade dysplasia in patients with ulcerative colitis is an indication for surgery because of the increased risk of colon cancer. Some authors contend that the finding of a dysplasia-associated lesion or mass carries a significant risk of cancer and is also an indication for surgery.[34] In patients with ulcerative colitis, proctocolectomy is curative. Once the entire colon is removed, patients remain free of disease. In the past, permanent ileostomy was required. Psychologic, social, and appliance-related problems were frequent deterrents to a lifelong ileostomy. In 1947, abdominal colectomy, mucosal proctectomy, and ileoanal pull-through was proposed.[35] This initially was unsuccessful because of a high incidence of complications. The outcome of ileoanal pull-through has improved remarkably, however, with advances in ileal pouch configurations, although several late complications such as "pouchitis" and obstruction are being identified.[36-38] The availability of an ostomy-sparing operation that is curative and eliminates the possibility of colon cancer has induced patients to submit to operation more often than in the past. Finally, with patient education and participation in decision making, quality of life after surgery can be excellent, regardless of the type of surgery performed.[39]

PREOPERATIVE CARE

Several issues should be kept in mind during the evaluation of patients with inflammatory bowel disease. First, the diagnosis of ulcerative colitis or Crohn's disease must be confirmed. Next, the extent and distribution of the disease should be determined. This may entail reviewing previous radiographic, endoscopic, histologic, and surgical notes. Patients' symptom complexes and any existing complications, such as refractory symptoms, bleeding, infection, obstruction, and neoplasia, are important to know. The severity of disease can be evaluated by patients' general appearances; histories of fevers, weight loss, clinical bleeding, anemia, and hypoalbuminemia; and perceptions of pain. The indications for surgery should be clarified and the type of surgery to be performed planned well ahead.

It is most important that clinicians establish rapport with their patients, who may require one or several operations. Early in the course of the disease, patients should be educated as thoroughly as possible. Sufficient time should be allocated to allow patients' questions to be answered. This greatly assists patients in preparing psychologically for surgery, should it become necessary. We encourage our patients to become active in the Crohn's and Colitis Foundation of America, which has chapters throughout the country. Involving surgeons early in the course of the disease allows patients to establish good relationships with their other physicians and decreases some of the anxiety and emotional stress that accompanies these procedures. In our experience, however, educated patients are prepared to undergo operation when this becomes necessary. Patients can only benefit from psychologic preparation for surgery and medical therapy related to their disease. This can be accomplished in several ways. Even if formal counseling is used, this important aspect of care should not be neglected.

Emergent operation in patients with inflammatory bowel disease usually is necessitated by one of the severe complications mentioned earlier. Patient care in these situations is similar to that in virtually all emergent operations. Good intravenous access should be maintained, preferably with a central line. Fluid status should be monitored and losses replaced as they occur. Placement of a Foley catheter to monitor urine output is helpful. If major blood loss occurs, platelets, clotting factors, and acid–base balance can all be affected. Therefore, these also must be monitored and corrected as abnormalities arise. Blood should be replaced with packed red blood cells.

Once the decision is made to perform elective or emergent surgery, the administration of 5-aminosalicylic acid agents or corticosteroids serves no purpose. 5-Aminosalicylic acid agents are used primarily for mild to moderate inflammatory bowel disease and have no role in patients with moderate to severe disease requiring surgery.

If patients have not taken corticosteroids and surgery is contemplated, corticosteroids should not be used. If surgery is to be delayed and treatment with corticosteroids is appropriate, therapy with these agents should be instituted. There is no evidence in the literature that patients with inflammatory bowel disease who undergo surgery while they are receiving usual doses of corticosteroids have inferior outcomes. Therefore, patients should be treated appropriately, even if this means administering corticosteroids before surgery.[40]

Long-term corticosteroid therapy, even in small doses, depresses the response of the adrenocortical axis to stress.[41] Because this response can remain depressed for long periods, the potential for relative adrenal insufficiency is present even in patients who have not taken corticosteroids for some time. There are general guidelines regarding the preoperative and perioperative management of patients who are receiving or have previously received corticosteroid therapy.

If patients receiving long-term corticosteroid therapy show no clinical improvement, use of the drugs can be tapered slowly and possibly discontinued. Necessary surgery should not be delayed, however, simply to wean patients from corticosteroids. Tapering of the corticosteroid dose may be initiated after elective surgery has been performed.

If patients have not received corticosteroids for the past 1 to 2 years, then perioperative stress doses of corticosteroids to prevent an adrenal crisis are not needed. Any uncertainty regarding patients' adrenal responses to stress may be addressed with a cosyntropin (Cortrosyn) stimulation test. If corticosteroid treatment has been used in the past 12 months, or if adequate adrenal function cannot be confirmed with a cosyntropin stimulation test, the safest approach is to treat patients with corticosteroids immediately before, during, and after surgery.

INTRAOPERATIVE CARE

A dose of 300 mg of hydrocortisone per day is equivalent to the amount of steroid produced by the adrenal gland under stress and should prevent problems related to adrenal insufficiency. Patients are given 100 mg of hydrocortisone phosphate immediately before the operation. During the operation, 100 mg is administered by continuous intravenous infusion and another 100 mg is given immediately after the operation. This should be continued for 2 or 3 days after surgery. At that time, the steroid dosage can be tapered rapidly unless patients have received long-term corticosteroid therapy. Once patients' gastrointestinal tracts begin functioning, intravenous doses of hydrocortisone can be changed to the equivalent doses of prednisone (Table 18-1). Prednisone can be considered to have four times the strength of hydrocortisone.[42] Once the hydrocortisone dose is 200 mg/d, patients can be given 40 mg of prednisone daily as soon as the gastrointestinal tract is functioning.

POSTOPERATIVE CARE

Patients with ulcerative colitis who undergo colectomy are cured of their disease. Therefore, postoperative care revolves around recovery from major abdominal surgery. Patients who undergo surgery for Crohn's disease can be opti-mistic about being free of disease for a significant interval; some patients require much less medication and some need no medication at all.

Patients who have received the equivalent of 40 mg of prednisone for more than 2 weeks must have their corticosteroid therapy tapered. This can usually be accomplished within a few weeks.

The steroid dosage should be tapered more slowly in patients who have received prolonged corticosteroid therapy. Patients are instructed to reduce their dose of prednisone by 2.5 to 5 mg every 1 to 2 weeks. Once the dose is down to 20 mg, the drug can be taken every other day. The dose continues to be tapered by 2.5 to 5 mg every 1 to 2 weeks.[43] We see patients every 2 to 3 weeks and ask them to call us regarding any problems during the tapering period.

As long as diseased bowel has been removed, the use of other medications for inflammatory bowel disease is unnecessary. If diseased bowel has not been removed, patients must continue to receive therapy. Because the gastrointestinal tract does not function immediately after surgery, intravenous corticosteroids are usually administered. Once patients can tolerate oral medications, oral prednisone can be given.

Knowledge of patients' postoperative bowel anatomy, particularly any loss of continuity of the gastrointestinal tract, is important in determining which medications will be useful. Oral sulfasalazine or mesalamine preparations are not useful in treating the isolated segment of distal colon that is seen with a Hartmann's pouch. Disease of the Hartmann's pouch must be treated with oral corticosteroids or, if a reasonably short length of bowel is left, with topical enema preparations of corticosteroids or mesalamine. Sulfasalazine (Azulfidine) and osalazine (Dipentum) require colonic bacteria to cleave the diazo bond. Therefore, these preparations are not effective in patients with ileostomies or colectomies and are more appropriate in those with colonic disease. Agents that do not require cleavage by colonic bacteria, such as Pentasa or Asacol, are released in the small intestine and may be used in patients with ileostomies.

Wound dehiscence, incisional hernia, postoperative adhesions, sepsis, and wound-related problems can all occur in patients undergoing operation for Crohn's disease or ulcerative colitis.[29] Complications can be expected to be greatest when contamination occurs during surgery. Patients with preexisting infections are also at greater risk for the development of postoperative complications.[44] Nutritional markers, the type of surgery performed, and the timing of the surgery (elective versus emergent) do not help predict which patients will develop postoperative problems. No studies have implicated steroid use as an important factor in the rate of postoperative complications.[40] The appropriate use of corticosteroids in patients with inflammatory bowel disease should not influence decisions regarding the timing of surgery or the type of surgical procedure required.

TABLE 18–1. Equivalent Doses of Steroid Preparations

Agent	Relative Antiinflammatory Potency
Hydrocortisone	1
Prednisone	4
Methylprednisolone	5
Dexamethasone	25

REFERENCES

1. Podolsky DK. Inflammatory bowel disease (first of two parts). N Engl J Med 1991;325:928–937.
2. Biemond I, Burnham WR, D'Amaro J, Langman MJS. HLA-A and -B antigens in inflammatory bowel disease. Gut 1986; 27:934–941.
3. Ekbom A, Helmick C, Zack M, Adami HO. The epidemiology of inflammatory bowel disease: a large, population-based study in Sweden. Gastroenterology 1991;100:350–358.
4. Fiocchi C, Roche JK, Michener WM. High prevalence of antibodies to intestinal epithelial antigens in patients with inflammatory bowel disease and their relatives. Ann Intern Med 1989;110:786–794.
5. Gitnick G. Etiology: where have we been? where are we going? In: Gitnick G, ed. Inflammatory bowel disease: diagnosis and treatment. New York, Igaku-Shoin, 1991:29–33.
6. Orholm M, Munkhom P, Langholz E, et al. Familial occurrence of inflammatory bowel disease. N Engl J Med 1991; 324:84–88.
7. Lee KS, Medline A, Shockey S. Indeterminate colitis in the spectrum of inflammatory bowel disease. Arch Pathol Lab Med 1979;103:173–176.
8. Farmer RG, Hawk WA, Turnbull RB Jr. Clinical patterns in Crohn's disease: a statistical study of 615 cases. Gastroenterology 1975;68:627–635.
9. Mekhjian HS, Switz DM, Melnyk CS, et al. Clinical features and natural history of Crohn's disease. Gastroenterology 1979;77: 898–906.
10. Chambers TJ, Morson BC. The granuloma in Crohn's disease. Gut 1979;20:269–274.
11. Haggitt RC. Differential diagnosis of colitis. In: Goldman H, Appelman HD, Kaufman N, eds. Gastrointestinal pathology. Baltimore, Williams & Wilkins, 1988:325–355.
12. Purrmann J, Strohmeyer G. Pathogenesis and management of ulcerative colitis. Hepatogastroenterology 1989;36:209–212.
13. Nostrant TT, Kumar NB, Appelman HD. Histopathology differentiates acute self-limited colitis from ulcerative colitis. Gastroenterology 1987;92:318–328.
14. Geier DL, Miner PB Jr. New therapeutic agents in the treatment of inflammatory bowel disease. Am J Med 1992;93:199–208.
15. Peppercorn MA. Advances in drug therapy for inflammatory bowel disease. Ann Intern Med 1990;112:50–60.
16. Farmer RG. Lower gastrointestinal bleeding in inflammatory bowel disease. Gastroenterol Jpn 1991;26(Suppl 3):93–100.
17. Robert JR, Sachar DB, Greenstein AJ. Severe gastrointestinal hemorrhage in Crohn's disease. Ann Surg 1991;213:207–211.
18. Softley A, Clamp SE, Bouchier IA, et al. Perforation of the intestine in inflammatory bowel disease: an OMGE survey. Scand J Gastroenterol Suppl 1988;144:24–26.
19. Greenstein AJ, Sachar DB, Mann D, et al. Spontaneous free perforation and perforated abscess in 30 patients with Crohn's disease. Ann Surg 1987;205:72–76.
20. Greenstein AJ, Mann D, Sachar DB, Aufses AH Jr. Free perforation in Crohn's disease. I. A survey of 99 cases. Am J Gastroenterol 1985;80:682–689.
21. Zenilman ME, Becker JM. Emergencies in inflammatory bowel disease. Gastroenterol Clin North Am 1988;17:387–408.
22. Caprilli R, Vernia P, Latella G, Torsoli A. Early recognition of toxic megacolon. J Clin Gastroenterol 1987;9:160–164.
23. Grant CS, Dozios RR. Toxic megacolon: ultimate outcome in 38 patients after successful medical management. Am J Surg 1984;147:106–110.
24. Block GE, Moosa AR, Siminowitz D, Hassan SZ. Emergency colectomy for inflammatory bowel disease. Surgery 1977;82: 531–536.
25. Greenstein AJ, Sachar DB, Gibas A, et al. Outcome of toxic dilatation in ulcerative and Crohn's colitis. J Clin Gastroenterol 1985;7:137–143.
26. Telander TI, Smith SL, Marcinek HM, et al. Surgical treatment of ulcerative colitis in children. Surgery 1981;90:787–794.
27. Shorb PE Jr. Surgical therapy for Crohn's disease. Gastroenterol Clin North Am 1989;18:111–128.
28. Farmer RG, Hawk WA, Turnbull RB. Indications for surgery in Crohn's disease: analysis of 500 cases. Gastroenterology 1976; 71:245–250.
29. Michelassi F, Balestracci T, Chappell R, Block GE. Primary and recurrent Crohn's disease. Ann Surg 1991;213:230–240.
30. Sachar DB. The problem of postoperative recurrence of Crohn's disease. Med Clin North Am 1990;74:183–188.
31. Speranza V, Simi M, Leardi S, Del Papa M. Recurrence of Crohn's disease after resection: are there any risk factors? J Clin Gastroenterol 1986;8:640–646.
32. Fazio VW, Galandiuk S, Jagelman DG, Lavery IC. Strictureplasty in Crohn's disease. Ann Surg 1989;210:621–625.
33. Sayfran J, Wilson DA, Allan A, et al. Recurrence after strictureplasty or resection for Crohn's disease. Br J Surg 1989;76:335–338.
34. Blackstone MO, Riddell RH, Rogers BH, Levin B. Dysplasia-associated lesion or mass (DALM) detected by colonoscopy in longstanding ulcerative colitis: an indicator for colectomy. Gastroenterology 1981;80:366–374.
35. Ravitch MM, Sabiston DC. Anal ileostomy with preservation of the sphincter. Surg Gynecol Obstet 1947;84:1095–1099.
36. Becker JM, Parodi JE. Total colectomy with preservation of the anal sphincter. In: Nyhus M, ed. Surgery annual. Norwalk, CT, Appleton & Lange, 1989:263–302.
37. Mortensen N. Progress with the pouch-restorative proctocolectomy for ulcerative colitis. Gut 1988;29:561–565.
38. Santos MC, Thompson JS. Late complications of the ileal pouch-anal anastomosis. Am J Gastroenterol 1993;88:3–10.
39. McLeod RS, Churchill DN, Lock AM, et al. Quality of life of patients with ulcerative colitis preoperatively and postoperatively. Gastroenterology 1991;101:1307–1313.
40. Felder JB, Adler DJ, Korelitz BI. The safety of corticosteroid therapy in Crohn's disease with an abdominal mass. Am J Gastroenterol 1991;86:1450–1455.
41. Bondy PK. Disorders of the adrenal gland. In: Wilson JD, Foster DW, eds. Textbook of endocrinology, ed 7. Philadelphia, WB Saunders, 1985:816–890.
42. Hayes Jr RC, Murad F. Adrenocorticotropic hormone: adrenocortical steroids and their synthetic analogs: inhibitors of adrenocortical steroid biosynthesis. In: Gilman AG, Goodman LS, Gilman A, eds. Goodman and Gilman's the pharmacological basis of therapeutics, ed 6. New York, MacMillan, 1980:1466–1496.
43. Byyny RL. Withdrawal from glucocorticoid therapy. N Engl J Med 1976;295:30–32.
44. Hulten L. Surgical treatment of Crohn's disease of the small bowel or ileocecum. World J Surg 1988;12:180–185.

Medical Management of the Surgical Patient, Third Edition,
edited by Michael F. Lubin, H. Kenneth Walker, and Robert B. Smith III.
J.B. Lippincott Company, Philadelphia, PA © 1995.

CHAPTER

19

POSTOPERATIVE GASTROINTESTINAL COMPLICATIONS

J. Patrick Waring

Postoperative gastrointestinal (GI) bleeding is an uncommon but potentially serious problem.[1] Although 10% to 15% of patients who are scheduled for elective major surgery are found to have upper GI tract lesions on endoscopy,[2] significant bleeding occurs in only 0.5% to 1% of those who undergo cardiac, central nervous system, or transplantation procedures.[3–7] Major causes of postoperative GI bleeding include the following:

Upper Gastrointestinal Tract Bleeding
Preexisting lesion (peptic ulcer)
Stress ulceration
Anastomotic breakdown
Lower Gastrointestinal Tract Bleeding
Preexisting lesion
Ischemic colitis
Anastomotic breakdown
Remote Gastrointestinal Bleeding
Marginal ulceration
Aortoenteric fistula

Stress ulceration of the stomach and duodenum historically has been the most common cause of postoperative upper GI tract bleeding.[8] The incidence of stress ulceration and its complications appears to have been decreasing over the past few decades, however, probably as a result of better supportive measures in intensive care units and increased knowledge of stress ulcer prophylaxis.[9,10] Preexisting peptic

ulcer disease may now be the most common cause of postoperative GI bleeding.[3,11] In one study, six of seven patients with severe postoperative bleeding appeared to have preexisting peptic ulcers rather than postoperative stress ulcers.[11] Ulcer symptoms may not be present before surgery and only develop during the postoperative period. They are frequently associated with the use of nonsteroidal antiinflammatory drugs.[11] Patients with histories of peptic ulcer disease or peptic ulcer symptoms probably should be given H_2 blockers during the perioperative period. It is reasonable to discontinue the use of nonsteroidal antiinflammatory drugs for 7 to 10 days in patients who are scheduled for elective surgery.[12]

Another major cause of postoperative GI bleeding are problems related to the surgery itself, particularly if a GI anastomosis is involved.[13] The overall management of GI bleeding after surgery is similar to that under other circumstances. There may be a tendency to rely on a radiographic means of diagnosis and therapy in these cases, especially in patients with GI anastomoses.[14,15]

Lower GI tract bleeding in the postoperative period usually occurs from preexisting lesions (ie, diverticula or cancers), anastomotic problems, or ischemic colitis. Ischemic colitis is more common after intraabdominal vascular surgery and in elderly patients.

Remote GI bleeding related to surgical procedures may result from marginal ulceration after partial gastrectomy and the formation of an aortoenteric fistula.

STRESS ULCERATION

Cushing and Curling ulcers in patients with central nervous system trauma and burns, respectively, probably represent the first descriptions of stress ulceration.[16] These shallow ulcers can be found in the stomach or duodenum and may present with GI bleeding. Placebo-controlled studies suggest that about 15% of affected patients develop upper GI tract bleeding.[3,17–19] A smaller percentage require blood transfusions.[20] Mortality from stress ulcer bleeding has greatly decreased in the past few years and is usually related to the underlying illness.[16]

Stress ulceration probably develops in response to a combination of factors. Acid and pepsin are necessary to the process, although gastric acid hypersecretion is not always seen. Impaired blood flow to the stomach and duodenum is likely to be a contributory factor,[21] and postoperative stress ulceration is uncommon in the absence of prolonged hypotension, sepsis, or multiple organ failure.[22] The following situations put patients at risk for the development of stress ulceration with significant bleeding:

- Burns over 35% of the body
- Central nervous system trauma
- Sepsis
- Multiple organ system failure
- Prolonged ventilatory support
- Prolonged hypotension from any cause

The best therapy for stress ulceration is prevention. Supportive care during episodes of hypotension, shock, sepsis, or other medical illnesses is of crucial importance. The advances made in intensive care over the past few decades have probably had the most significant effect in decreasing the incidence of serious bleeding. Patients at risk for the development of stress ulcers should receive treatment designed to decrease gastric acid production.[23,24] Numerous therapies are available and have similar efficacy. Antacids have been shown to be superior to placebo and intermittent intravenous cimetidine in several studies.[17,25] These agents must be given on a regular basis to maintain the gastric pH level above 3.5. Frequent medication administration (often hourly) and gastric acid titration requires considerable nursing time and the placement of a nasogastric tube. Cimetidine should be given by continuous intravenous infusion.[26] Ranitidine and famotidine suppress gastric acid production with intermittent bolus infusion.[27] To achieve satisfactory gastric acid suppression in most patients, total daily dosages of cimetidine, ranitidine, and famotidine should be about 1200 mg, 300 mg, and 40 mg, respectively.[16] At these dosages, H_2 blockers are as effective as antacids in preventing serious complications of stress ulceration and are easier to use.[16,28] Sucralfate has been shown to produce results at least as good as those achieved with H_2 blockers.[28–30] Sucralfate is usually given in a crushed form and delivered through a nasogastric tube. The total daily dose is 4 to 6 g. Some studies suggest that sucralfate may be preferable for stress ulcer prophylaxis because it is associated with a lower incidence of pneumonia.[29,30] Gastric acid suppression may lead to bacterial colonization of the stomach and lower pharynx. Because sucralfate does not alkalinize the stomach, it does not alter these barriers to infection. Combination therapy with several medications is probably not necessary.

If stress ulcers develop despite prophylaxis, they should be treated similarly to standard peptic ulcers. Gastric acid production should be adequately suppressed. Patients with GI bleeding should be stabilized hemodynamically with intravenous fluids and blood.[31] When patients are stable, upper GI tract endoscopy can be performed safely to identify the source of bleeding. Endoscopic treatment using a heater probe, multipolar electrocoagulation, or injection therapy is often successful in patients with active bleeding or visible vessels.[32–34] No studies have specifically evaluated patients with stress ulceration. There is some evidence suggesting that patients who develop peptic ulcer bleeding during hospitalization have a significantly greater incidence of recurrent bleeding and death.[32,35] If endoscopic treatment is unsuccessful, radiographic attempts can be made to control bleeding. The results of surgery in this setting usually are extremely poor.

POSTOPERATIVE PEPTIC (MARGINAL) ULCER

The formation of ulcers after ulcer surgery is uncommon, occurring in about 4% of patients. There may be many causes, including retained antrum, Zollinger-Ellison syndrome, gastric cancer, bile reflux, *Helicobacter pylori* infection, and salicylate abuse.[36] The most common cause, however, is incomplete vagotomy. Serum gastrin levels and salicylate levels should be measured and gastric acid analyzed. Endoscopy with biopsy to exclude *H pylori* infection or malignancy may be performed in patients who develop marginal ulcers.[37] GI bleeding is common in these patients and is managed the same as in patients without previous ulcer surgery.[38] Their conditions are stabilized with fluid and blood products, and endoscopy is performed. All necessary coagulation techniques may be used to control bleeding. Treatment should be directed at the underlying cause if one has been identified. Eighty percent to 90% of marginal ulcers heal with standard medical therapy.[39] Recurrence is a major problem, however, and many patients require reoperation.

AORTOENTERIC FISTULA

Aortoenteric fistula formation is an uncommon but devastating complication after abdominal vascular surgery.[40] It occurs in 1% to 2% of patients, usually in the first 3 to 5 postoperative years. Three fourths of these fistulas occur in the area of the duodenum. Most patients have evidence of infection at the site of the fistula. An elevated white blood cell count and fever may be present. Patients usually are seen initially with a minor episode of bleeding, the so-called "herald bleed." The next bleeding episode may occur within hours to months and be so severe as to cause exsanguination. Patients with suspected aortoenteric fistulas should undergo endoscopy to search for another site of bleeding. If no other lesion is found, the presence of an aortoenteric fistula should be presumed. Computed tomographic scans, magnetic resonance imaging scans, and angiography may show the fistula but are insensitive methods of detecting this lethal problem.[41] If aortoenteric fistula is strongly suspected, patients should undergo exploratory laparotomy. Only one in three aortoenteric fistulas is demonstrated before surgery. Removal of the infected graft and reconstruction of the vascular anastomosis is usually successful.[42]

ISCHEMIC COLITIS

Numerous vascular diseases may affect the GI tract:

Acute
Superior mesenteric artery embolus
Superior mesenteric artery thrombosis
Nonocclusive mesenteric ischemia
Mesenteric venous thrombosis

Chronic
Chronic mesenteric ischemia
Chronic mesenteric thrombosis

The most common postoperative vascular complication is ischemic colitis. The condition is usually nonocclusive and results from hypoperfusion of the colon during the perioperative period. It may be seen after any surgery and is more common in elderly patients. Ischemic colitis occurs in only 1% to 7% of patients who have undergone elective aortic surgery but in as many as 60% of those who have had ruptured aortic aneurysms.[43] Depending on the degree of injury, symptoms may range from mild (diarrhea, bleeding) to severe (severe diarrhea, bleeding, stricture formation with obstructive symptoms, or gangrenous bowel).[44,45] Endoscopy is safe and diagnostic.[46] Hyperemia, pallor, and petechiae may be seen in the acute phase, followed by ulcer-

ation and exudation. Strictures may occur in the chronic phase of ischemic colitis. Angiography is rarely helpful and treatment is largely supportive. Most patients improve spontaneously in a few days to months. The administration of systemic corticosteroids, antibiotics, and vasodilators is not effective, although there have been anecdotal reports of some success with steroid enema preparations.[43] Patients with progressive abdominal tenderness, leukocytosis, fever, ileus, obstructive symptoms, or bleeding may benefit from resection of the affected area.

POSTOPERATIVE NAUSEA AND VOMITING

Early postoperative nausea and vomiting may be related to individual patient characteristics, the surgery itself, anesthetic agents, or postoperative medications.[47] Patients with underlying gastroparesis, histories of motion sickness, high anxiety, and obesity are more likely to be affected. The incidence of postoperative nausea and vomiting is much higher in women than in men. Patients undergoing abdominal or laparoscopic surgery also have a higher incidence of this complication. Longer operations are associated with an increased possibility of postoperative nausea and vomiting. Factors such as abdominal pain, dizziness, early refeeding, and ambulation after surgery can contribute to the incidence, as can medications such as narcotics.

The treatment of early postoperative nausea and vomiting is largely supportive.[48] If possible, the cause should be identified and corrected. Controlling the sensation of nausea with antiemetics such as chlorpromazine or prochlorperazine is important. Serotonin antagonists such as ondansetron may be helpful in more severe cases.[49] Early postoperative nausea and vomiting is usually self-limited and associated with little morbidity and mortality.

Remote postoperative nausea and vomiting may be a manifestation of intestinal obstruction, which is most commonly caused by adhesions after abdominal surgery. There also may be an obstruction at the site of an intestinal anastomosis.[13] It should be possible to locate the obstruction using endoscopic or barium studies. Surgery is often required, although there have been reports of successful balloon dilation of intestinal anastomotic strictures.[14]

Patients without obstruction may have nausea and vomiting related to medications, particularly narcotics, anticholinergics, digoxin, and theophylline preparations. Patients who have undergone gastric surgery may have gastroparesis associated with vagotomy. Many of these patients, especially those operated on for gastric outlet obstruction, may have had gastroparesis before operation. The cause of remote postoperative nausea and vomiting should be identified if possible and eliminated. The use of antiemetics may be helpful. Prokinetic agents such as metoclopramide, cisapride, or domperidone may provide additional benefits in patients with evidence of gastroparesis.[50]

POSTOPERATIVE DIARRHEA

Early postoperative diarrhea is usually associated with the following medications:

* Antacids containing magnesium
* Elixirs containing sorbitol, mannitol, or xylitol
* Colchicine
* Lactulose
* Diuretics
* Anticholinergics
* Quinidine
* Misoprostol

Patients with prolonged hospitalizations and impaired ambulation may have fecal impaction presenting as diarrhea.[51] Enteral feeding has been associated commonly with diarrhea. The factors responsible for this are controversial.[52–54] Antibiotic-associated diarrhea, particularly that caused by *Clostridium difficile* infection, may present within the first few weeks after surgery.

Remote postoperative diarrhea may be seen after vagotomy in 20% to 30% of patients. Again, the pathophysiology is controversial.[55–57] It may be related to disordered gastric emptying with the presentation of hyperosmolar loads to the proximal intestine, rapid transit through the intestinal tract, or an increase in the concentration of bile acids or fatty acids allowed to reach the colon. Patients with ileal resection may have bile salt malabsorption that leads to bile acid–induced diarrhea.[58] Bile acids that are not absorbed in the small bowel reach the colon and can stimulate colonic fluid secretion. Diarrhea may also be seen after cholecystectomy, although the pathogenesis of this is unknown.[59,60] Therapy for remote postoperative diarrhea involves identifying and treating the underlying cause if possible. Opiates such as codeine, diphenoxylate hydrochloride and atropine (Lomotil), or loperamide; cholestyramine to bind bile acids; and, in severe cases, anticholinergics such as atropine or hyoscyamine may provide symptomatic relief. Surgery is rarely beneficial.[55,57]

REFERENCES

1. Flint LM. Early postoperative acute abdominal complications. Surg Clin North Am 1988;68:445–455.
2. Rypins EB, Safeh IJ, Collins-Irby D, et al. Asymptomatic peptic disease in patients undergoing major elective operations: a prospective endoscopic study. Am J Gastroenterol 1988;83:927–929.
3. Rosen HR, Vlahakes GJ, Rattner DW. Fulminant peptic ulcer disease in cardiac surgical patients: pathogenesis, prevention, and management. Crit Care Med 1992;20:354–359.
4. Chan KH, Mann KS, Lai ECS, et al. Factors influencing the development of gastrointestinal complications after neurosurgery: results of multivariate analysis. Neurosurgery 1989;25:378–382.
5. Konno H, Sakaguchi S, Hachiya T. Bleeding peptic ulcer after abdominal aortic aneurysm surgery. Arch Surg 1991;126:894–897.
6. Lebovics E, Lee SS, Dworkin BM, et al. Upper gastrointestinal bleeding following open heart surgery: predominant finding of aggressive duodenal ulcer disease. Dig Dis Sci 1991;36:757–760.
7. Egleston CV, Wood AE, Gorey TF, McGovern EM. Gastrointestinal complications after cardiac surgery. Ann R Coll Surg Engl 1993;75:52–56.
8. Schiessel R, Feil W, Wenzl E. Mechanisms of stress ulceration and implications for treatment. Gastroenterol Clin North Am 1990;19:101–120.
9. Schuster DP, Rowley H, Feinstein S, et al. Prospective evaluation of the risk of upper gastrointestinal bleeding after admission to a medical intensive care unit. Am J Med 1984;76:623–630.
10. Reusser P, Gyr K, Scheidegger D, et al. Prospective endoscopic study of stress erosions and ulcers in critically ill neurosurgical patients. Crit Care Med 1990;18:270–274.
11. Matthews JB, Tortella BJ, Silen W. Gastroduodenal hemorrhage and perforation in the postoperative period. Surg Gynecol Obstet 1988;167:389–392.
12. Connelly CS, Panush RS. Should nonsteroidal anti-inflammatory drugs be stopped before elective surgery? Arch Intern Med 1991;151:1963–1966.
13. Jex RK, van Heerden JA, Wolff BG, et al. Gastrointestinal anastomoses: factors affecting early complications. Ann Surg 1987;206:138–141.
14. Nag D, Rogers CE, Nolan DJ. Early abdominal complications of intestinal surgery: the radiologist's role in management. Br J Hosp Med 1989;42:214–222.
15. Ng BL, Thompson JN, Adam A, et al. Selective visceral angiography in obscure postoperative gastrointestinal bleeding. Ann R Coll Surg Engl 1987;69:237–240.
16. Soll AH. Gastric, duodenal and stress ulcer. In: Sleisenger MH, Fordtran JS, eds. Gastrointestinal disease. Philadelphia, WB Saunders, 1993:580–678.
17. Hastings PR, Skillman JJ, Bushnell LS, Silen W. Antacid titration in the prevention of acute gastrointestinal bleeding: a controlled, randomized trial in 100 critically ill patients. N Engl J Med 1978;298:1041–1045.
18. Shuman RB, Schuster DP, Zuckerman GR. Prophylactic therapy for stress ulcer bleeding: a reappraisal. Ann Intern Med 1987;106:562–567.
19. Tryba M, May B. Conservative treatment of stress ulcer bleeding: a new approach. Scand J Gastroenterol 1992;191:16–24.
20. Kingsley AN. Prophylaxis for acute stress ulcers. Am Surg 1985;51:545–547.
21. Hinder RA, Pace E, Fimmel CJ, et al. Is there a relationship be-

tween gastric mucosal blood flow and stress lesions in hemorrhagic shock? Digestion 1987;38:74–82.

22. Bumaschny E, Doglio G, Pusajo J, et al. Postoperative acute gastrointestinal tract hemorrhage and multiple organ failure. Arch Surg 1988;123:722–726.

23. Zuckerman GR, Shuman R. Therapeutic goals and treatment options for prevention of stress ulcer syndrome. Am J Med 1987;83(Suppl 6A):29–35.

24. Peura DA. Prophylactic therapy of stress-related mucosal damage: why, which, who, and so what? Am J Gastroenterol 1990; 85:935–937.

25. Priebe HJ, Skillman JJ, Bushnell LS, et al. Antacid versus cimetidine in preventing acute gastrointestinal bleeding. N Engl J Med 1980;302:426–430.

26. Ostro MJ, Russell JA, Soldin SJ, et al. Control of gastric pH with cimetidine boluses versus primed infusions. Gastroenterology 1985;89:532–537.

27. Miller TA, Tornwall MS, Moody FG. Stress erosive gastritis. Curr Probl Surg 1991;28:453–509.

28. Tryba M. Prophylaxis of stress ulcer bleeding. J Clin Gastroenterol 1991;13:S44–S55.

29. Cannon LA, Heiselman D, Gardner W, Jones J. Prophylaxis of upper gastrointestinal tract bleeding in mechanically ventilated patients. Arch Intern Med 1987;147:2101–2106.

30. Eddleston JM, Vohra A, Scott P, et al. A comparison of the frequency of stress ulceration and secondary pneumonia in sucralfate or ranitidine-treated intensive care unit patients. Crit Care Med 1991;19:1491–1496.

31. Gogel HK, Tandberg D. Emergency management of upper gastrointestinal hemorrhage. Am J Emerg Med 1986;4:150–162.

32. Waring JP, Sanowski RA, Sawyer RL, et al. A randomized comparison of multipolar electrocoagulation and injection sclerosis for the treatment of bleeding peptic ulcer. Gastrointest Endosc 1991;37:295–298.

33. Laine L. Multipolar electrocoagulation in the treatment of peptic ulcers with nonbleeding visible vessels: a prospective, controlled trial. Ann Intern Med 1989;110:510–514.

34. Jensen DM. Heat probe for hemostasis of bleeding peptic ulcers: technique and results of randomized controlled trials. Gastrointest Endosc 1990;36(Suppl 5):S42–S49.

35. Jensen DM, Kovacs TOG, Randall GM, et al. Prospective study of patients who developed severe ulcer bleeding as inpatients compared to outpatients. (Abstract) Gastrointest Endosc 1992; 38:A235.

36. Matthews JB, Silen W. Operations for peptic ulcer disease and early postoperative complications. In: Sleisenger MH, Fordtran JS, eds. Gastrointestinal disease. Philadelphia, WB Saunders, 1993:713–730.

37. Hirschowitz BL, Lanas A. Intractable and recurrent postsurgical peptic ulceration is due to aspirin (ASA) abuse, much of it surreptitious. (Abstract) Gastroenterology 1992;102:A84.

38. Schirmer BD, Meyers WC, Hanks JB, et al. Marginal ulcer: a difficult surgical problem. Ann Surg 1982;195:653–661.

39. Festen HPM, Lamers CBH, Driessen WMM, van Tongeren JHM. Cimetidine in anastomotic ulceration after partial gastrectomy. 1979;83:83–85.

40. Peterson WL, Laine L. Gastrointestinal bleeding. In: Sleisenger MH, Fordtran JS, eds. Gastrointestinal disease. Philadelphia, WB Saunders, 1993:162–192.

41. Goldstone J, Cunningham CC. Diagnosis, treatment, and prevention of aorto-enteric fistulas. Acta Chir Scand Suppl 1990; 555:165–172.

42. Peck JJ, Eidemiller LR. Aortoenteric fistulas. Arch Surg 1992; 127:1191–1193.

43. Brandt LJ, Boley SJ. Ischemic and vascular lesions of the bowel. In: Sleisenger MH, Fordtran JS, eds. Gastrointestinal disease. Philadelphia, WB Saunders, 1993:1927–1962.

44. Robert JH, Mentha G, Rohner A. Ischaemic colitis: two distinct patterns of severity. Gut 1993;34:4–6.

45. Longo WE, Ballantyne GH, Gusberg RJ. Ischemic colitis: patterns and prognosis. Dis Colon Rectum 1992;35:726–730.

46. Scowcroft CW, Sanowski RA, Kozarek RA. Colonoscopy in ischemic colitis. Gastrointest Endosc 1981;27:156–161.

47. Watcha MF, White PF. Postoperative nausea and vomiting: its etiology, treatment, and prevention. Anesthesiology 1992;77: 162–184.

48. Rowbotham DJ. Current management of postoperative nausea and vomiting. Br J Anaesth 1992;69:46S–59S.

49. Russell D, Kenny GN. 5-HT3 antagonists in postoperative nausea and vomiting. Br J Anaesth 1992;69:63S–68S.

50. Ouyang A. Approach to the patient with nausea and vomiting. In: Yamada T, ed. Gastroenterology. Philadelphia, JB Lippincott, 1991:647–659.

51. Powell DW. Approach to the patient with diarrhea. In: Yamada T, ed. Gastroenterology. Philadelphia, JB Lippincott, 1991:732–778.

52. Edes TE, Walk BE, Austin JL. Diarrhea in tube-fed patients: feeding formula not necessarily the cause. Am J Med 1990; 88:91–93.

53. Heimburger DC. Diarrhea with enteral feeding: will the real cause please stand up? Am J Med 1990;88:89–90.

54. Kelly TWJ, Patrick MR, Hillman KM. Study of diarrhea in critically ill patients. Crit Care Med 1983;11:7–9.

55. Cuschieri A. Surgical management of severe intractable postvagotomy diarrhea. Br J Surg 1986;73:981–984.

56. Raimes SA, Smirniotis V, Wheldon EJ, et al. Postvagotomy diarrhea put into perspective. Lancet 1986;2:851–853.

57. Cuschieri A. Postvagotomy diarrhea: is there a place for surgical management? Gut 1990;31:245–246.

58. Hardison WGM, Rosenberg IH. Bile-salt deficiency in the steatorrhea following resection of the ileum and proximal colon. N Engl J Med 1967;277:337–342.

59. Fromm H, Tunuguntla AK, Malavolti M, et al. Absence of significant role of bile acids in diarrhea of a heterogeneous group of postcholecystectomy patients. Dig Dis Sci 1987;32:33–44.

60. Arlow FL, Dekovich AA, Priest RJ, Beher WT. Bile acid-mediated postcholecystectomy diarrhea. Arch Intern Med 1987;147: 1327–1329.

SECTION

VIII

HEMATOLOGY

Medical Management of the Surgical Patient, Third Edition,
edited by Michael F. Lubin, H. Kenneth Walker, and Robert B. Smith III.
J.B. Lippincott Company, Philadelphia, PA © 1995.

CHAPTER

DISORDERS OF RED BLOOD CELLS

20

James R. Eckman

The primary consideration in the medical management of red blood cell disorders during surgery is ensuring an optimal hemoglobin concentration to provide for adequate oxygen delivery to tissues. Blood hemoglobin concentration is a primary direct and indirect determinant of tissue oxygenation. Blood oxygen content increases directly as hemoglobin concentration rises. Tissue oxygen delivery is a complex function of hemoglobin level, cardiac output, hemoglobin oxygen affinity, and tissue oxygen content. As the hemoglobin level (more correctly, the number of red blood cells) increases, cardiac output decreases; therefore, there is an optimal range of hemoglobin concentration that provides maximal tissue oxygen delivery. The goal of preoperative and postoperative management is to maintain this optimal level at reasonable cost. Unfortunately, this level is poorly defined in most clinical settings, varies between patients and within individual patients over time, and, even if it is well defined, at times cannot be maintained without unacceptable monetary costs or complication rates. Perioperative management involves considering the optimal hemoglobin level for each clinical setting based on an informal cost-benefit analysis that usually is supported by incomplete outcome data.

An initial assessment should be done to determine whether the hemoglobin level is too high or too low for specific patients or surgical procedures. Alterations in the hemoglobin level may also suggest the presence of a clinical condition that may compromise surgical outcome if it is not properly diagnosed and treated. Anemia may require partial correction to prevent cardiovascular complications during surgery and may be a manifestation of nutritional problems that will lead to impaired healing, hemoglobinopathies that require specific therapy, or autoimmune diseases that may complicate blood transfusion. Polycythemia may require correction before surgery and could be a sign of acute or chronic volume depletion that requires specific therapy or of chronic diseases associated with hypoxemia, thrombosis, or excessive operative bleeding.

ANEMIA

Anemia is generally defined as a hemoglobin concentration of less than 14 g/dL in males and 12.3 g/dL in females. Corresponding lower limits of normal for the hematocrit are 42% in males and 36% in females.

DIAGNOSTIC CONSIDERATIONS

Evaluation of anemias with decreased production of red blood cells may reveal nutritional deficiencies that can be treated to maintain a maximal hemoglobin level and improve healing. Many microcytic and macrocytic anemias result from specific deficiencies that cause correctable anemia

189

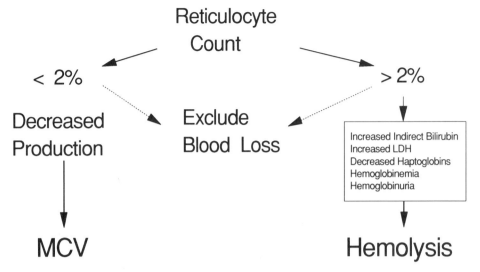

Reticulocyte Count

< 2%   > 2%

Decreased Production   Exclude Blood Loss

Increased Indirect Bilirubin
Increased LDH
Decreased Haptoglobins
Hemoglobinemia
Hemoglobinuria

MCV   Hemolysis

FIG. 20-1. Evaluation of anemia is initiated by obtaining a reticulocyte count to determine if there is decreased production or increased loss of erythrocytes as a primary cause of anemia. Blood loss must always be excluded. The mean corpuscular hemoglobin concentration (MCV) is the next step in determining the cause of anemia when the reticulocyte count is low. Tests are done to establish hemolysis when the reticulocyte count is elevated. LDH, lactic dehydrogenase.

and may delay healing and predispose to infection. Normocytic anemias may indicate the presence of underlying medical disease or define patients with marginal marrow reserve. Evaluation of hemolytic anemias must exclude hemoglobinopathies that may require special operative management, immune hemolysis that may complicate blood transfusion, and enzyme deficiencies that may influence the selection of medications.

Algorithms for the evaluation of anemias are presented in Figures 20-1 through 20-3. Blood loss always must be excluded because it is a common cause of anemia in surgical patients. Studies used to initiate diagnostic testing for most common anemias are presented in Figure 20-1. This approach uses the reticulocyte count as the first test to determine whether the primary cause of the anemia is related to decreased production or increased loss of red blood cells. The first step in characterizing anemias resulting from decreased red blood cell production with low or normal reticulocyte counts is to measure the mean corpuscular volume. The diagnostic tests outlined in Figure 20-2 establish the cause of most common anemias when the reticulocyte count is low. Tests indicated by the algorithm should be performed before surgery or transfusion in all but the most urgent surgical emergencies. When the reticulocyte count is high, the presence of a hemolytic anemia is first confirmed by excluding blood loss and detecting isolated increased in-

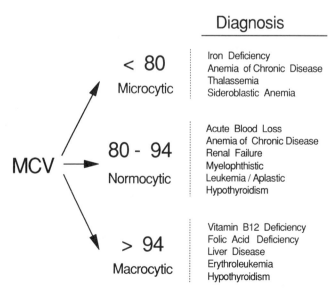

	Diagnosis	Diagnostic Test
< 80 Microcytic	Iron Deficiency Anemia of Chronic Disease Thalassemia Sideroblastic Anemia	Serum Ferritin Iron, TIBC Red Count, Hb ELP, DNA Bone Marrow Iron Stain
80 - 94 Normocytic	Acute Blood Loss Anemia of Chronic Disease Renal Failure Myelophthistic Leukemia / Aplastic Hypothyroidism	Exclude Bleeding Iron , TIBC BUN, Creatinine Bone Marrow Biopsy Bone Marrow with Biopsy TSH, T4, T3
> 94 Macrocytic	Vitamin B12 Deficiency Folic Acid Deficiency Liver Disease Erythroleukemia Hypothyroidism	Serum B12 Levels Serum, RBC Folate Blood Smear, Liver Profile Bone Marrow with Biopsy TSH, T4, T3

MCV

FIG. 20-2. The MCV is most useful in evaluating anemias with decreased red cell production. The most common diagnostic considerations for microcytic, normocytic, and macrocytic anemias are presented with the most useful confirmatory tests.

FIG. 20-3. Hemolytic anemias are best evaluated using the patient's history, the direct Coombs' test, and examination of the peripheral blood smear. The history divides hemolysis into acquired disorders where the red cell environment is the cause of increased destruction from inherited disorders where red cell abnormalities shorten survival. The Coombs' test and smear are most useful for acquired disorders while the smear alone initiates evaluation of inherited disorders.

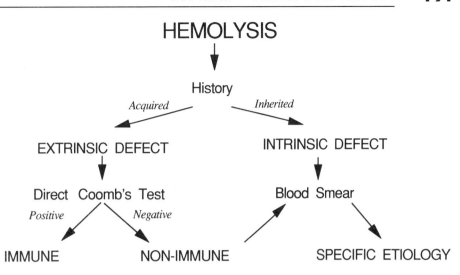

direct bilirubin, lactic dehydrogenase, decreased haptoglobin, or free hemoglobin in plasma or urine (see Fig. 20-1). Once hemolysis is confirmed, preoperative diagnosis of the cause of the hemolytic anemia is particularly important because many diseases that require special management during surgery present with hemolysis. A careful past medical and family history, a direct Coombs' test, and examination of the peripheral blood smear in combination with a few appropriate confirmatory tests usually results in a diagnosis (see Fig. 20-3).

MANAGEMENT CONSIDERATIONS

The perioperative management of anemia is not difficult because treatment by transfusion of red blood cells is readily available. Too often, to the potential detriment of patients, the transfusion of red blood cells is substituted for thoughtful clinical evaluation and optimal medical therapy. Diagnosis and treatment of the cause of the anemia is preferred over transfusion before elective surgery if the cause is treatable and time permits. If the anemia cannot be corrected or large losses are anticipated, careful planning can allow for surgery without transfusion or provide patients' own blood for transfusion, minimizing complications. In emergency situations, it is usually best to draw blood for appropriate diagnostic laboratory tests and proceed with transfusion and surgery before the cause of anemia is certain. There are no absolute criteria for the management of anemia in the perioperative period but several useful guidelines have been developed.

Anemia places increased physiologic demands on patients who are undergoing surgery. There is no evidence showing that mild to moderate anemia slows healing, increases the incidence of infection, or causes bleeding. The approach to preoperative transfusion must be individualized and there is no ideal hemoglobin level for surgery in all patients. Patients without underlying cardiovascular or respiratory problems have considerable physiologic adaptive capacity and can tolerate significant anemia without increased surgical morbidity or mortality. Patients with underlying medical problems, those with acute anemia, and those experiencing excessive blood loss, however, may be at risk for increased morbidity and mortality and require more aggressive treatment of anemia.

Factors in addition to hemoglobin level that affect tissue oxygen delivery include cardiac output, vascular volume, blood viscosity, hemoglobin oxygen affinity, and blood oxygen saturation. With chronic anemia, many of these factors are modified to provide optimal oxygen delivery to tissues in spite of the anemia. The "magic" hemoglobin level of 10 g/dL was challenged recently at a National Institutes of Health consensus conference. Studies also show no increase in mortality among patients with hemoglobin levels higher than 8 g/dL who lose less than 500 mL of blood during surgery. Because there is no evidence that mild to moderate anemia increases surgical morbidity or mortality, indications for perioperative transfusion must be based on careful assessment of coexisting diseases that may reduce tolerance for anemia, patients' physiologic adjustments to anemia, the stress of the surgical procedure, an estimate of potential operative blood loss based on the nature of the procedure and the skill of the surgeon, and plans for intraoperative procedures to reduce net blood loss such as hemodilution and intraoperative blood salvage.

Before transfusion is performed in the perioperative period, informed consent for homologous transfusions must be obtained that documents the risks of infection, alloimmunization, volume overload, and immediate and delayed transfusion reactions. Patients' religious and cultural beliefs must also be recognized and taken into account. The risks of direct complications from transfusion are not readily quantifiable and are changing because of evolving blood banking techniques. Reasonable rate estimates are presented in Table 20-1. Alternatives to homologous transfusion should be presented to patients who are undergoing elective surgical procedures in which blood administration is likely to be required. There is considerable evidence that autologous transfusion of blood with or without the administration of erythropoietin is a practical, safe, and underused approach to perioperative transfusion. These programs not only provide the safest transfusion for patients, they also diminish the need for donation by reducing homologous transfusion and providing unused units for others. Patients must be informed about autologous donation when the decision for elective surgery is made to allow sufficient time to collect the required blood. In patients with concurrent medical problems, medical consultants should supervise blood collection to prevent complications from donation and ensure optimal blood collection. Because liquid blood can be stored as long as 42 days, most surgical needs can be met as liquid units, reducing cost. Red blood cells can be frozen for more than 10 years to meet greater needs; however, this increases costs significantly.

Intraoperative approaches such as autotransfusion or hemodilution may be advocated by medical consultants but must be implemented by surgeons and anesthesiologists. Intraoperative blood salvage involves aspirating blood lost in the operative site and centrifuging or washing the cells for reinfusion. Numerous devices make this a practical, although somewhat expensive, approach when the loss of large amounts of blood is anticipated. Air embolus is a possible complication and this approach is contraindicated if the operative site is grossly contaminated by microorganisms or tumor cells. Intraoperative hemodilution involves removing blood after the induction of anesthesia and replacing it with colloid or crystalloid solutions to create acute normovolemic anemia. This allows the blood to be salvaged for reinfusion, decreases surgical loss of red blood cells from bleeding, and reduces blood viscosity, which may result in increased blood flow. Careful monitoring for volume overload during the infusion of salvaged units and accurate identification and labeling of units are critical to ensure safe reinfusion.

In patients with chronic anemia, preoperative transfusion must be planned with the understanding that total blood volume is probably increased. Necessary transfusion must be started well in advance of elective surgery and given slowly to prevent acute volume overload and to allow physiologic adaptation to the change in volume status. The transfusion of packed cells causes minimal volume overload but increases the total blood volume by an amount equal to the total volume of the unit, and this may persist for 24 hours or longer. In general, volume overload can be kept to a minimum by reducing the amount of cells transfused to 250 mL at one time, decreasing the rate of infusion to 1 mL/kg/h, and minimizing right atrial pressure by placing patients in sitting or semiupright positions.

Rapid transfusion with diuresis or partial exchange should be reserved for urgent or emergent surgery. Patients with heart failure or renal failure and volume overload who require rapid transfusion can be given 20 mg of furosemide by intravenous push before the transfusion is begun. Additional doses of furosemide can be given by separate intravenous injection based on the urine output and volume of cells infused. Partial-exchange transfusion can be used to raise the hemoglobin level acutely in patients with severe anemia and volume overload who require emergent transfusion. One approach is to remove whole blood from one vein as an approximately equal volume of packed red blood cells is infused through another vein. Severe anemia can be corrected rapidly by infusing a volume of 1000 to 1500 mL of packed red blood cells while 1200 to 1700 mL of whole blood is being removed from another large vein.

The transfused blood should be prewarmed to 37°C before large volumes are infused rapidly.

In patients with chronic anemia, surgical preparation requires individualized use of transfusion based on the presence of coexisting diseases, chronic hemoglobin levels, and estimated operative blood losses. If transfusion is required, careful planning may allow use of autologous donation. Preoperative transfusion in patients with chronic anemia should be done well in advance of surgery to allow physiologic adaptation to the changes in volume and blood viscosity.

ANEMIAS REQUIRING SPECIAL CONSIDERATION

Hematologic diseases that require special perioperative management include sickle hemoglobinopathies and immune hemolytic anemias. These disorders may be over-

TABLE 20–1. Approximate Complication Rates for Homologous Red Blood Cell Transfusion

Immune Reaction	
Alloimmunization	1 in 100 to 1 in 5
Hemolytic transfusion reaction	1 in 6000
Fatal transfusion reaction	1 in 100,000
Febrile reaction	1 in 100 to 1 in 50
Infection	
Human immunodeficiency virus	1 in 10^6 to 1 in 40,000
Hepatitis B	1 in 300 to 1 in 200
Hepatitis C (non-A, non-B)	<1 in 100

looked because anemia is not invariably present. Preoperative screening with a complete blood count, reticulocyte count, and blood typing and crossmatching identifies most patients with these disorders. Using the algorithm outlined in Figure 20-3, a definitive diagnosis should be obtained before surgery in all but the most emergent situations.

Sickle Cell Syndromes

Patients with sickle cell anemia are at significantly increased risk for complications during most operative procedures. Patients who are compound heterozygotes for hemoglobin S–thalassemia and hemoglobin C–thalassemia or for hemoglobin S–thalassemia and β-thalassemia may also be at increased risk; however, the perioperative complication rates are not well defined. Carriers of the sickle gene (hemoglobin AS) probably are not at increased risk for complications unless they experience profound hypoxia or undergo prolonged, complicated cardiovascular surgery. Even in these extreme situations, the risks have not been defined by appropriate controlled studies.

The optimal perioperative management of patients with sickle cell syndromes is not clear. It is generally agreed that the hemoglobin concentration should be corrected by the transfusion of packed red blood cells to a level of 9 to 10 g/dL for all but the most simple procedures. Transfusion above this level should not be done unless the hemoglobin S level is less than 50% from previous transfusion. The level of hemoglobin S can be monitored in the laboratory by performing standard hemoglobin electrophoresis and using a protein densitometry scanner to measure the amount of hemoglobin A and hemoglobin S on the membrane. This indicates the approximate percentage of erythrocytes with hemoglobin A and hemoglobin S after the transfusion of hemoglobin A–containing erythrocytes. For major surgery, many experts advocate transfusion or exchange transfusion to reduce the hemoglobin S level to less than 30% or 50% while maintaining the hemoglobin level between 8 and 10 g/dL. Even lower percentages of hemoglobin S are advocated for cardiovascular bypass surgery, retinal or eye surgery, and major neurosurgery. Whether simple transfusion to a hemoglobin level of 10 g/dL is better than exchange transfusion to reduce the hemoglobin S level to less than 30% is in the final stages of study in a multicenter collaborative trial.

Several other considerations are important in planning for transfusion or exchange transfusion in patients with sickle cell syndromes. The first is the extremely high rate of alloimmunization that accompanies transfusion in these patients. Because alloimmunization develops in as many as 20%, some experts advocate transfusion with red blood cells matched by phenotype for antigens commonly associated with delayed transfusion reactions in this population. Patients who have one alloantibody definitely should be considered for transfusion with phenotype-matched blood because of the high probability that they will develop multiple alloantibodies and the more remote possibility that they will develop autoantibodies. This is especially important with exchange transfusions because of the potential increased severity of a delayed transfusion reaction in this setting.

Patients can also be prepared electively with multiple transfusions over the weeks before surgery. The hemoglobin concentration should be determined before each transfusion to prevent hyperviscosity associated with transfusion to levels greater than 10 g/dL. Repeated hemoglobin electrophoresis with densitometry scanning can be used to document the desired percentage of hemoglobin S. If there is insufficient time to achieve the desired hemoglobin S percentage by simple transfusion, exchange transfusion is best accomplished by red blood cell pheresis using an automated cell separator. Manual exchange transfusion using published protocols can achieve the same result but is inefficient and labor-intensive in adults and older children.

Preliminary results of the multicenter transfusion study in sickle cell anemia indicate that complications still occur, even with extensive exchange transfusion. Transfusion or exchange transfusion cannot be substituted for excellent perioperative management to prevent hypoxia, hypothermia, excessive sedation, fluid overload, and acidosis. Acute chest syndrome, acute pain episodes, fever or infection, new alloantibodies, and delayed transfusion reactions appear to be among the most common complications. Predisposing factors for these complications are under investigation.

Recommendations for the perioperative management of patients with sickle cell syndromes are outlined in Table 20-2. Data support the need for transfusion to a hemoglobin level

TABLE 20–2. Perioperative Management of Sickle Syndromes

- Preoperative transfusion to a hemoglobin level of 10 g/dL using simple transfusion or exchange to obtain a hemoglobin S <50%.
- Preoperative evaluation to exclude pulmonary, renal, hepatic, or central nervous system complications.
- Prevention of hypoxia using careful anesthetic and postoperative respiratory management.
- Hydration with hypotonic intravenous solutions while withholding oral fluids to prevent increased viscosity, cellular dehydration, hypoperfusion, or acidosis.
- Careful maintenance of body temperature during and after surgery.
- Early ambulation and intensive respiratory care.
- Postoperative vigilance and aggressive evaluation and treatment of fever or infection.

of 10 g/dL in all patients. Until data from the multicenter trial are available, the choice of simple or exchange transfusion to reduce the percentage of hemoglobin S–containing cells remains a personal one. Careful preoperative evaluation and optimal preparation of pulmonary, renal, and hepatic function is important, especially in older patients in whom end-organ damage may have developed. Intravenous hydration must be adequate to prevent intravascular and intracellular dehydration during the period of restricted oral intake. This is made most important by the almost universal renal tubular defect that increases obligatory free water loss through the kidneys. Care must also be taken to prevent volume overload in these patients with expanded plasma volumes from chronic anemia. Hypoxia and acidosis should be prevented because of their direct effect on the rate of sickling. Decreases in temperature can increase peripheral resistance, reducing local blood flow in certain areas and predisposing to pain episodes. Early ambulation and intensive respiratory care are important in preventing acute chest syndrome and other pulmonary complications. Finally, because postoperative complications appear to be more common in these patients, diligent assessment of fevers and prompt diagnosis and treatment of infections are important in the postoperative period. Close collaboration between surgeons, anesthesiologists, and hematologists helps to improve the operative outcome in these patients with high rates of surgical complications.

Autoimmune Hemolytic Anemia

The care of patients with immune hemolysis entails several special considerations. Immune hemolytic anemias are mediated by antibodies directed against components of the red blood cell membrane or drugs that interact with the red blood cell membrane. In general, patients should be treated and the immune hemolytic anemia should be controlled before surgery is undertaken. With drug-related immune hemolytic anemias, this usually can be accomplished by discontinuing use of the drug and delaying surgery until the anemia corrects itself. Autoimmune hemolytic anemias pose a more difficult problem. These disorders usually are recognized by diagnosing hemolysis with the studies outlined in Figure 20-1 and documenting positive results on a direct Coombs' test.

Autoimmune hemolytic anemias may be idiopathic but are also commonly associated with autoimmune diseases, lymphomas, chronic lymphocytic leukemia, human immunodeficiency virus infection, other infections, and multiple myeloma. Warm antibody hemolytic anemias are caused by IgG antibodies and usually are associated with positive results on a direct Coombs' test for IgG, complement, or both. Initial treatment is with prednisone, 1 to 2 mg/kg/d. Therapeutic failures are usually treated with splenectomy or immunosuppressant drugs such as cyclophosphamide or azathioprine. Preparation for splenectomy may include the administration of intravenous immunoglobulin, which has been reported to have some activity in controlling immune hemolysis.

Cold-reacting autoantibodies are usually IgM antibodies that are associated with positive results on a complement Coombs' test and with high-titer cold agglutinin levels. These antibodies are more commonly caused by infections such as *Mycoplasma pneumoniae*, viruses, or lymphoproliferative disease. Management is difficult if the primary disease cannot be treated. Steroids and splenectomy are not effective and immunosuppressant drugs are often required for severe, refractory cases. Avoiding the use of transfusion and providing supportive care, including hydration, warmth, and infusions of fluids with temperatures higher than 37°C, are the mainstays of therapy.

Autoimmune hemolytic anemias create problems in patients who require surgery because the anemia may be profound and transfusions of red blood cells can precipitate serious complications. The autoantibody may cause accelerated destruction of the transfused cells, resulting in renal, coagulation, or pulmonary complications. This is particularly true with cold antibodies, in which endogenous circulating red blood cells may be protected from hemolysis by processed complement components on the membrane. The autoantibody almost always causes difficulties in finding compatible blood for transfusion because typing and crossmatching may be difficult or impossible. Autoantibodies can prevent the detection of alloantibodies that may precipitate immediate or delayed transfusion reactions and increase hemolysis caused by the autoimmune process.

Autoantibodies are uncommon, however, and infrequently present preoperative management problems. When present, they require coordinated management by experienced teams that include hematologists, clinical pathologists, and anesthesiologists who understand and will coordinate the special management issues. Elective surgery should be delayed if possible and the autoimmune hemolysis controlled with therapy. If the autoimmune process is resistant to therapy or the surgery is emergent, the blood bank should be given sufficient time to use special techniques to detect alloantibodies. In emergent situations, patients often are given the least incompatible blood. Patients with uncontrolled autoimmune hemolytic anemia require careful monitoring and transfusion of the fewest units possible. The initiation of high-dose steroid therapy is indicated for warm antibodies. Some advocate increasing steroid doses or administering high-dose intravenous immunoglobulin before transfusion in patients with poorly controlled autoimmune hemolysis.

With cold antibodies, patients must be kept warm so that the blood temperature exceeds 37°C throughout the body. All fluids and blood products must be warmed to 37°C before infusion. This may require maintenance of the entire operating suite at 37°C for patients with high-titer cold antibodies. Plasmapheresis is technically difficult because of the need to keep the fluids, blood, and patients warm, but is effective for the acute removal of these IgM antibodies and may be considered as emergency treatment before surgery in patients with significant, uncontrolled cold-antibody immune hemolysis.

POLYCYTHEMIA

Elevated hemoglobin or hematocrit levels require preoperative evaluation to exclude conditions that may increase perioperative complications. The upper limits of normal for hemoglobin and hematocrit levels, respectively, are 16.5 g/dL and 50% in males and 15.3 g/dL and 45% in females. Polycythemia or erythrocytosis is defined as elevation above these levels. The elevation may reflect a true polycy-

themia (erythrocytosis) with an increase in red blood cell mass or a relative increase in hemoglobin and hematocrit levels caused by a reduction in plasma volume. Relative polycythemia should be defined and corrected because the low plasma volume is usually associated with a reduced total blood volume. This may predispose to hypotension during the induction of anesthesia or performance of surgery. True polycythemia may be caused by polycythemia vera, which must be well controlled before surgery to minimize the high incidence of hemorrhagic and thrombotic complications. Relative polycythemia may result from physiologic processes that predispose to cardiovascular complications in the perioperative period.

DIAGNOSTIC CONSIDERATIONS

An algorithm for the evaluation of elevated hemoglobin levels in patients undergoing surgery is outlined in Figure 20-4. The most common cause of elevated hemoglobin lev-

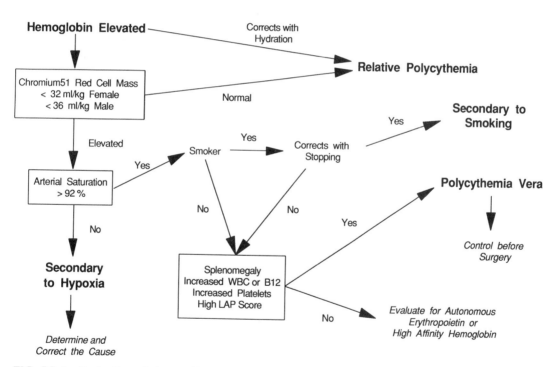

FIG. 20-4. Evaluation of elevated hemoglobin levels is important preoperatively because untreated polycythemia vera is associated with high morbidity and mortality. Evaluation is initiated if hydration does not normalize the hemoglobin level. Determination of red cell mass separates true elevation of the red cell mass from relative elevation caused by low plasma volume. True polycythemia is most commonly secondary to hypoxia or smoking, so blood gases and determining the response to cessation of smoking are important first steps. Splenomegaly or a combination of two of the other manifestations of polycythemia vera establish that diagnosis in true polycythemia without hypoxia. Other less common causes must be sought if these are not present.

els is relative polycythemia caused by reduced plasma volume. This may occur acutely from dehydration or be a chronic state associated with hypertension, adrenergic excess, and increased cardiovascular risk (eg, stress erythrocytosis, Gaisböck's syndrome). If hydration does not return the hemoglobin concentration to normal, a red blood cell mass should be determined to confirm the presence of true polycythemia. Blood gas analysis is used to document chronic hypoxia. Exercise-induced hypoxia and sleep apnea should also be considered as a cause of polycythemia because both may increase surgical complications. If patients smoke, they should stop smoking and undergo observation if time permits to see whether the hemoglobin level returns to normal. Determination of carbon monoxide levels may be helpful if surgery is urgent because these levels are usually elevated in smokers with erythrocytosis.

After these more common clinical conditions have been excluded, a careful evaluation to rule out polycythemia vera is indicated. Splenomegaly is a cardinal feature of polycythemia vera; spleen scanning is necessary if the spleen is not palpable because the presence of splenomegaly with true primary erythrocytosis establishes the diagnosis of polycythemia vera. If the spleen is normal, the presence of two other indicators of a myeloproliferative syndrome, such as an increased leukocyte or platelet count, an elevated white blood cell mass reflected in an increased vitamin B_{12} level, or a high leukocyte alkaline phosphatase score, establishes the diagnosis of polycythemia vera. Measurement of the erythropoietin level and performance of intravenous pyelography, sonography, or computerized tomography should be considered to search for occult kidney disease or tumors of other organs if the rest of the work-up for true polycythemia produces negative results.

MANAGEMENT CONSIDERATIONS

Polycythemia rubra vera should be treated to reduce the hemoglobin level to normal before surgery because of the high incidence of thrombotic and hemorrhagic perioperative complications in patients with uncontrolled or poorly controlled disease. To ensure minimal morbidity and mortality, the general recommendation is that the disease should be well controlled for 4 months before purely elective surgery is undertaken. Before more urgent surgery, patients should be treated to achieve normal hemoglobin levels. Phlebotomy alone can rapidly control the hemoglobin level in patients with primary elevations. Phlebotomy in combination with hydroxyurea administration should probably be used in patients with elevated hemoglobin levels and platelet counts or in those with systemic symptoms such as itching. Hemoglobin levels should be less than 15 g/dL in males and less than 14 g/dL in females because of evidence that cerebral blood flow is reduced at higher levels. Phlebotomy

can be accomplished rapidly in young patients by removing 250 to 500 mL of blood every other day. Patients who develop acute orthostatic symptoms may benefit from less frequent phlebotomy or concurrent hydration with an equal volume of normal saline solution. In older patients or those with underlying cardiovascular disease, slower phlebotomy is prudent, removing 200 to 500 mL twice a week. Again, the concurrent administration of normal saline solution may prevent acute orthostatic symptoms.

Reduction of the platelet count to less than 500,000 is advocated, although there are no data indicating that such treatment decreases thrombotic complications. Drugs that interfere with platelet function should not be used because platelets are often functionally abnormal and bleeding complications are increased.

Patients with polycythemia vera are at higher risk for serious perioperative complications, including stroke, myocardial infarction, pulmonary embolus, thrombophlebitis, splenic infarction, and portal or hepatic venous thrombosis. There is also an increased incidence of gastrointestinal and surgical hemorrhage. Alternatives to surgery should be considered. If surgery is necessary, however, the management plan should be formulated well in advance. Patients require close monitoring for common complications in the perioperative period. For emergency surgery, the hemoglobin level should be returned to normal rapidly by the removal of whole blood and infusion of colloid solution to maintain blood volume. Anticoagulation is indicated for thrombotic complications but generally is not recommended at full therapeutic levels for prophylaxis because of the increased risk of hemorrhage.

Recent publications suggest that patients with relative and secondary polycythemia do not have an increased rate of perioperative complications. It does seem prudent to define the cause of the polycythemia and to identify and correct the underlying pathology if possible. Relative polycythemia may indicate acute dehydration, which may predispose to hypotension during anesthesia or surgery. Chronic spurious polycythemia is often associated with hypertension, and control of the blood pressure with antihypertensive agents may correct the elevated hemoglobin level. Smokers with polycythemia should stop smoking in advance of elective surgery to reduce pulmonary complications. If this is done early, it may also lead to normalization of the hemoglobin concentration.

Although secondary polycythemia probably does not increase complications, evaluation of this condition may uncover underlying disease that requires special management in the perioperative period. Hypoxia resulting from pulmonary or cardiac disease is a common cause of secondary polycythemia. Certain types of renal disease that cause ischemia in the juxtaglomerular cells increase erythropoietin, resulting in secondary polycythemia. Several tumors, including renal cell tumors, hepatomas, cerebellar hemangioblastomas, uterine fibroids, and ovarian carcinomas, may cause polycythemia by increasing erythropoietin. Pheochromocytoma and adrenocortical carcinoma are important rare causes of polycythemia that are important to consider because of the management implications of these tumors during anesthesia and surgery.

If treatment of the underlying condition is impossible or does not correct the polycythemia, phlebotomy to normalize blood viscosity can be considered. Experimental data show that blood flow is decreased with any true elevation of hemoglobin levels. There is no compelling evidence that phlebotomy is beneficial for either relative or secondary polycythemia at lower levels. Evidence does suggest that reduction of the hematocrit level may be beneficial if it exceeds 60%, even if the elevation is the result of hypoxia caused by severe pulmonary disease or cyanotic heart disease.

BIBLIOGRAPHY

Anemia: General

Allen JB, Allen BA. The minimum acceptable level of hemoglobin. Int Anesthesiol Clin 1982;20:1–22.

Carson JL, Poses RM, Spence RK, Bonavita G. Severity of anaemia and operative mortality and morbidity. Lancet 1988;2:727–729.

Consensus Conference. Perioperative red blood cell transfusion. JAMA 1988;260:2700–2703.

Council on Scientific Affairs. Autologous blood transfusions. JAMA 1986;256:2378–2380.

Goodnough LT, Rudnick E, Price TH, et al. Increased preoperative collection of autologous blood with recombinant human erythropoietin therapy. N Engl J Med 1989;321:1163–1168.

Health and Public Policy Committee, American College of Physicians. Practice strategies for elective red blood cell transfusion. Ann Intern Med 1992;116:403–406.

Irving GA. Continuing medical education. Perioperative blood and blood component therapy. Can J Anaesth 1992;39:1105–1115.

Leone BJ, Spahn DR. Anemia, hemodilution, and oxygen delivery. Anesth Analg 1992;75:651–653.

Toy PTCY, Strauss RG, Stehling LC, et al. Predeposited autologous blood for elective surgery: a national multicenter study. N Engl J Med 1987;316:517–520.

Walker RH, ed. Technical manual. Arlington, Virginia, American Association of Blood Banks, 1990:341–448.

Welch HG, Meehan KR, Goodnough LT. Prudent strategies for elective red blood cell transfusion. Ann Intern Med 1992;116:393–402.

Anemia: Sickle Syndromes

Adu-Gyamfi Y, Sankarakutty M, Marwa S. Use of a tourniquet in patients with sickle-cell disease. Can J Anaesth 1993;40:24–27.

Bischoff RJ, Williamson II A, Dalali MJ, et al. Assessment of the use of transfusion therapy perioperatively in patients with sickle cell hemoglobinopathies. Ann Surg 1988;207:434–438.

Burrington JD, Smith MD. Elective and emergency surgery in children with sickle cell disease. Surg Clin North Am 1976;56:55–71.

Esseltine DW, Baxter MRN, Bevan JC. Sickle cell states and the anaesthetist. Can J Anaesth 1988;35:385–403.

Forrester K. Anesthetic implications in sickle cell anemia. J Assoc Nurs Anesth 1986;54:314–324.

Fullerton MW, Philippart AI, Sarnaik S, Lusher JM. Preoperative exchange transfusion in sickle cell anemia. J Pediatr Surg 1981;16:297–300.

Gibson JR. Anesthesia for the sickle cell diseases and other hemoglobinopathies. Semin Anesth 1987;6:27–35.

Janik J, Seeler RA. Perioperative management of children with sickle hemoglobinopathy. J Pediatr Surg 1980;15:117–120.

Morrison JC, Whybrew WD, Bucovaz ET. Use of partial exchange transfusion preoperatively in patients with sickle cell hemoglobinopathies. Am J Obstet Gynecol 1978;132:59–63.

Oduro KA, Searle JR. Anaesthesia in sickle-cell states: a plea for simplicity. Br Med J 1972;4:596–598.

Schlanger M, Cunningham AJ. Intraoperative hypoxemia complicating laparoscopic cholecystectomy in a patient with sickle hemoglobinopathy. Anesth Analg 1992;75:838–843.

Vichinsky EP, Earles A, Johnson RA, et al. Alloimmunization in sickle cell anemia and transfusion of racially unmatched blood. N Engl J Med 1990;322:1617–1621.

Polycythemia

Berk PD, Goldberg JD, Donovan PB, Fruchtman SM, Berlin NI, Wasserman LR. Therapeutic recommendations in polycythemia vera based on polycythemia vera study group protocols. Semin Hematol 1986;23:132–143.

Fitts WT, Erde A, Peskin GW, Frost JW. Surgical implications of polycythemia vera. Ann Surg 1960;152:548–558.

Kaplan ME, Mack K, Goldberg JD, Donovan PB, Berk PD, Wasserman LR. Long-term management of polycythemia vera with hydroxyurea: a progress report. Semin Hematol 1986;23:167–171.

Lubarsky DA, Gallagher CJ, Berend JL. Secondary polycythemia does not increase the risk of perioperative hemorrhagic or thrombotic complications. J Clin Anesth 1991;3:99–103.

Tartaglia AP, Goldberg JD, Berk PD, Wasserman LR. Adverse effects of antiaggregating platelet therapy in the treatment of polycythemia vera. Semin Hematol 1986;23:172–176.

Wallis PJW, Skehan JD, Newland AC, et al. Effects of erythropheresis on pulmonary haemodynamics and oxygen transport in patients with secondary polycythaemia and cor pulmonale. Clin Sci 1986;70:91–98.

Ware R, Filston HC, Schultz WH, Kinney TR. Elective cholecystectomy in children with sickle hemoglobinopathies. Ann Surg 1988;208:17–22.

Wasserman LR. The treatment of polycythemia vera. Semin Hematol 1976;13:57–78.

Wasserman LR, Gilbert HS. Surgery in polycythemia vera. N Engl J Med 1963;269:1226–1230.

Medical Management of the Surgical Patient, Third Edition,
edited by Michael F. Lubin, H. Kenneth Walker, and Robert B. Smith III.
J.B. Lippincott Company, Philadelphia, PA © 1995.

CHAPTER

21

ABNORMAL BLEEDING

Sidney F. Stein
Bruce L. Evatt

NORMAL HEMOSTASIS

The potential for abnormal bleeding is always a concern in patients who are about to undergo surgery. To understand how to predict the likelihood of bleeding, prevent it from happening, or treat it properly when it occurs, physicians must have some understanding of normal hemostatic mechanisms.

The maintenance of normal hemostasis depends on several factors, including platelets, the vessel wall, and several coagulation and fibrinolytic factors. Vasoconstriction plays an important role in achieving hemostasis in small vessels. When a vessel is damaged, endothelium is lost and platelets adhere to the denuded vascular surface. Once platelets become adherent, they release many potent mediators into the microenvironment. The most important of these is thromboxane A_2, although adenosine diphosphate, epinephrine, and serotonin also appear to have a functional role in producing vasoconstriction and recruiting other platelets to form a platelet plug. When platelets are activated, platelet surface glycoproteins undergo a conformational change and become exposed on the platelet surface. These newly exposed glycoproteins bind to plasma proteins (fibrinogen in the case of glycoprotein IIb/IIIa and von Willebrand's factor in the case of glycoprotein Ib). The binding of these plasma proteins is important for both the adhesion of platelets to the denuded vascular surface (von

Willebrand's factor) and the aggregation of platelets to form a platelet plug (fibrinogen). When platelets aggregate, platelet factor 3, a platelet phospholipid, also undergoes a conformational change, gains better surface exposure, and accelerates thrombin formation through both the intrinsic and extrinsic pathways of the coagulation system (Fig. 21-1).

PREOPERATIVE EVALUATION OF SURGICAL PATIENTS

HISTORY

When patients are being evaluated for the potential of abnormal bleeding before surgery, consulting physicians should obtain bleeding histories, perform physical examinations, and order selected laboratory tests. In assessing whether patients may develop bleeding problems, it is important to review carefully the bleeding histories of both patients and their family members to detect the presence of either congenital or acquired abnormalities. Patients may complain of easy bruising, report excessive bleeding (eg, longer than 24 hours or requiring transfusions) after dental extractions, or describe heavy menstrual bleeding (often with clots). There may be histories of hematuria, hematochezia, melena, hemarthroses, or muscle hematomas. Pa-

Coagulation Pathways

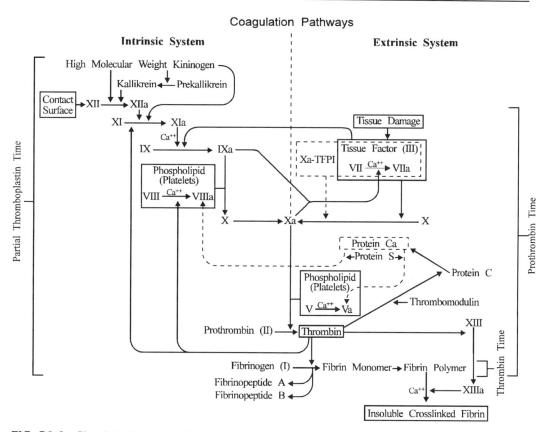

FIG. 21-1. Blood clotting starts through the extrinsic system when tissue factor, released as a result of tissue damage, activates factor VII to VIIa. Factor VIIa then either directly activates factors X to Xa or activates factors IX to IXa, which then proceed to activate factor X through the intrinsic system. The presence of a lipoprotein inhibitor called the tissue factor pathway inhibitor prevents further activation of factor X through the extrinsic pathway, thus making the intrinsic pathway the primary in vivo vehicle for coagulation once the process has started. Factor Xa converts prothrombin to thrombin. Thrombin then acts on fibrinogen to form a fibrin clot, which also contains the fibrinolytic precursor protein, plasminogen. As normal tissue repair proceeds, tissue plasminogen activator is released from surrounding endothelium and permeates the clot; it activates the zymogen plasminogen to the active fibrinolytic enzyme plasmin, which dissolves the fibrin clot. Ultimately, when remodeling is complete, vascular integrity is restored. (© Emory University. Used by permission.)

tients should be questioned about frequent nose bleeds, prolonged bleeding after minor scratches, bleeding that recurs long after the original insult to the blood vessel, and poor wound healing. Whenever histories are obtained, it is important to determine what medications patients use. Patients should be questioned about any of the stigmata of liver disease because impaired liver function frequently compromises the hemostatic system. Aspirin and oral anticoagulants are some of the more obvious drugs that can induce abnormal bleeding.

PHYSICAL EXAMINATION

When performing physical examinations, physicians should search for petechiae, purpura, ecchymoses, and mucosal bleeding. Deformed joints, hemarthroses, and muscle hematomas should be fairly obvious. The presence of pallor may be a sign of remote bleeding. Hepatomegaly or splenomegaly, jaundice, or spider angiomas may indicate previously undetected liver disease.

LABORATORY SCREENING

We believe that a substantial panel of preoperative tests should be obtained on all patients. A complete blood count, including a platelet count, is essential. A battery of chemistry tests should be ordered to detect hyperbilirubinemia and elevated liver enzyme levels. A screening prothrombin time and partial thromboplastin time should also be obtained. If patients have significant bleeding histories or physical findings suggestive of bleeding problems, an expanded laboratory evaluation may be necessary. Additional testing may include specific clotting factor assays or tests of platelet function. Although it may be useful to determine the bleeding time in patients with histories that point to congenital platelet abnormalities, the test as performed in many hospital settings may produce false-positive results in patients without histories suggestive of bleeding disorders.

POTENTIAL HEMOSTATIC DISORDERS IDENTIFIED BEFORE SURGERY

PLATELET DISORDERS

Platelet disorders can be divided into those that are quantitative and those that are qualitative. Thrombocytopenia is the most common quantitative abnormality that leads to abnormal bleeding. Normally, platelets remain in the circulation for almost 10 days and about one third of circulating platelets are sequestered in the spleen. Thus, thrombocytopenia may result from decreased or ineffective platelet production (eg, aplastic anemia or vitamin B_{12} deficiency, respectively); increased destruction (eg, immune thrombocytopenia or disseminated intravascular coagulation [DIC]); or abnormal distribution (eg, increased splenic sequestration with splenomegaly).

Quantitative Platelet Disorders

Thrombocytopenia. By far the most common cause of significant thrombocytopenia (a platelet count less than $100,000/\mu L$) is immune thrombocytopenia, in which platelet destruction is accelerated because of the presence of a platelet autoantibody. Patients with immune thrombocytopenia may have other associated autoimmune disorders, including autoimmune hemolytic anemia and systemic lupus erythematosus. Immune thrombocytopenia may also be associated with human immunodeficiency virus (HIV) infection and lymphoproliferative disorders such as chronic lymphocytic leukemia. The diagnosis of immune thrombocytopenia is made largely on clinical grounds after other specific causes of thrombocytopenia have been excluded. Typically, patients have thrombocytopenia in the face of bone marrow aspirates or biopsies that show increased numbers of megakaryocytes. It is generally possible to demonstrate increased binding of IgG to the circulating platelets of patients with immune thrombocytopenia, although this test is nonspecific and generally not necessary to make a clinical diagnosis. Heparin may occasionally cause an immune-mediated thrombocytopenia associated with in vivo platelet aggregation and platelet thrombus formation. Medications such as quinine, quinidine, or sulfa drugs may also be associated with immune thrombocytopenia. Most patients with immune thrombocytopenia, however, have autoantibodies.

Accelerated destruction may also occur by mechanisms that do not involve a platelet autoantibody. Examples of disorders that cause nonimmunologic accelerated platelet destruction include DIC (with or without sepsis) vasculitis, malfunctioning prosthetic heart valves, and conditions that result in vascular damage (eg, thrombotic thrombocytopenia purpura).

The second most common cause of thrombocytopenia is decreased platelet production. This is frequently associated with a bone marrow aspirate or biopsy showing a decreased number of megakaryocytes. Patients may relate histories of the use of several pharmacologic agents that are known to cause thrombocytopenia as a side effect; chloramphenicol, phenylbutazone, parenteral gold, alcohol, thiazide diuretics, and other sulfa drugs have all been reported to suppress megakaryocyte proliferation. Cytotoxic chemotherapy and radiotherapy are powerful suppressants of megakaryocyte formation. Infections such as hepatitis and a few less common viral infections also suppress platelet production. In addition, platelet production may be reduced because the bone marrow is replaced by leukemic or lymphomatous infiltrates, fibrosis, granulomas, or metastatic cancer.

Platelet production may also be decreased without a diminished number of megakaryocytes in the bone marrow. This may occur when patients have either vitamin B_{12} or folic acid deficiency causing a megaloblastic anemia. There are a few rare familial thrombocytopenias such as the May-Hegglin anomaly or the Wiskott-Aldrich syndrome that also have a kinetic profile consistent with ineffective thrombopoiesis. These disorders have characteristic morphologic platelet size abnormalities.

The last major cause of thrombocytopenia is distributional in nature. When patients have splenomegaly, more than the normal one-third proportion of circulating platelets is sequestered in the spleen. With massive splenomegaly, 80% to 90% of the intravascular platelet mass can be found in the spleen. Typically, patients with splenomegaly have no more than moderate thrombocytopenia because of the bone marrow's capacity to increase platelet production. If the bone marrow is incapable of increasing platelet production, thrombocytopenia associated with splenomegaly may become more significant.

Thrombocytosis. Thrombocytosis is seen much less frequently than is thrombocytopenia. There are two kinds of thrombocytosis. Essential thrombocythemia is a primary disorder of the bone marrow. Patients with this disorder generally have platelet counts in excess of 1 million/μL. The platelets appear large and abnormal on a peripheral blood smear. Essential thrombocythemia is often characterized by abnormal platelet aggregation and a prolonged bleeding time. A bone marrow examination reveals large numbers of abnormal-appearing megakaryocytes. This disorder may be associated with both thrombotic and hemorrhagic problems.

Secondary thrombocytosis is a much more common cause of thrombocytosis than is essential thrombocythemia. Patients with secondary thrombocytosis typically have platelet counts of less than 1 million/μL. Platelet morphology tends to be normal on blood smear. Although bone marrow examination reveals increased numbers of megakaryocytes, megakaryocyte morphology is usually normal. Secondary thrombocytosis is generally seen in association with acute and chronic inflammatory disorders, iron-deficiency anemia, hemorrhage, hemolytic anemias, and neoplasms. Thrombotic complications of this disorder are unusual.

Qualitative Platelet Disorders

Platelet dysfunction may be diagnosed when patients have prolonged template bleeding times and normal platelet counts.

Platelet dysfunction may also occur in association with thrombocytopenia and should be suspected when the bleeding time is prolonged out of proportion to the degree of thrombocytopenia.

Acquired forms of platelet dysfunction. The most common forms of platelet dysfunction are acquired. Many drugs can interfere with platelet function. Drugs such as ticlopidine are specifically used to inhibit platelet function. Aspirin is the most notorious inhibitor of platelet function because of its widespread use and ability to irreversibly interfere with the function of platelets in the circulation. It does so by inactivating the enzyme cyclooxygenase, which performs a primary role in prostaglandin synthesis. All the nonsteroidal antiinflammatory drugs impair platelet function to some extent by reversibly interfering with the same pathway. Plasma expanders such as dextran and hydroxyethyl starch interfere with platelet function by coating the platelet surface. High doses of penicillin analogues also in-

terfere with platelet function. A few other classes of drugs, including phenothiazines, tricyclic antidepressants, and some anesthetics, can interfere with platelet function. Uremia and dysproteinemias such as Waldenström's macroglobulinemia are also associated with platelet dysfunction. Finally, abnormal platelet function has been described in patients with myeloproliferative disorders.

Hereditary forms of platelet dysfunction. Hereditary forms of platelet dysfunction are less common than are acquired forms. Von Willebrand's disease is an autosomal dominant disorder associated with a defect in platelet adhesion. The Bernard-Soulier syndrome is a recessive disorder characterized by an abnormality in platelet glycoprotein Ib. As a result of this defect, the platelets do not properly bind the von Willebrand's factor required for normal platelet adhesion. Thrombasthenia is a recessive disorder associated with a global defect in platelet aggregation. Patients with this disorder have an abnormal receptor (glycoprotein IIb/IIIa) for fibrinogen on the platelet surface; without the binding of fibrinogen, platelets do not properly aggregate. Several disorders of platelet function have been described that are associated with the absence or abnormality of either the dense granules or the alpha granules of platelets. A heterogeneous group of hereditary platelet disorders has also been described in which platelets behave as if they had been exposed to aspirin; patients with this abnormality typically have a defect in the pathway of prostaglandin synthesis.

COAGULATION DISORDERS

Inherited Coagulation Abnormalities

Hemophilia and related coagulation disorders. Most adults with inherited coagulation disorders have already been identified because of abnormal bleeding during their childhoods. Hemarthroses and muscle hematomas generally identify patients with inherited coagulation disorders unless bleeding problems are detected immediately after birth as a result of circumcision. By far the most common inherited clotting factor defect is hemophilia A, or factor VIII deficiency, which occurs in about 1 in 5000 to 7500 male births; hemophilia B, or factor IX deficiency, is about one fifth as frequent as hemophilia A. Both these disorders have an X-linked pattern of inheritance and, therefore, are restricted primarily to males. Inherited defects in other clotting factors are rare and transmitted as autosomal traits. Patients with hemophilia have prolonged partial thromboplastin times. If their plasma is mixed with normal plasma at a ratio of 1:1, the partial thromboplastin times should correct to normal levels. This correction indicates that patients have a clotting factor deficiency rather than inhibitors interfering with the clotting process. Once it has been ascertained that patients have clotting factor deficiencies, specific factor assays should be performed to determine the type of abnormalities. In a similar fashion, a prolonged prothrombin time can lead to the diagnosis of factor VII deficiency. A classification of clotting factor deficiencies is found in Table 21-1.

Von Willebrand's disease. Von Willebrand's disease is an inherited hemorrhagic disorder that is most often transmitted in an autosomal dominant manner. The clinical presentation is highly variable and may range from a severe bleeding disorder to a mere laboratory abnormality. It is probably the most prevalent inherited bleeding disorder; some estimates range as high as 1:200 of the general population. Patients with von Willebrand's disease have a defect in platelet adhesion resulting from low levels or abnormal functioning of von Willebrand's factor. Von Willebrand's factor is a protein that binds to platelet glycoprotein Ib and bridges the gap between the platelet and collagen and other subendothelial surface proteins.

The defect in platelet adhesion can frequently be detected by an abnormal template bleeding time. The activity of von Willebrand's factor is most commonly measured by the ristocetin cofactor assay; ristocetin, which was originally developed as an antibiotic, agglutinates platelets as long as functional von Willebrand's factor is present. Because von Willebrand's factor circulates in the blood bound to factor VIII, and because factor VIII is quickly removed from the circulation if it is not protected by its association with von Willebrand's factor, patients with von Willebrand's disease frequently have low levels of factor VIII activity. The clinical hallmark of von Willebrand's disease is mucosal bleeding (eg, epistaxis, bruising, and gastrointestinal bleeding). Hemarthroses and muscle hematomas may occur (particularly in patients with extremely low factor VIII levels) but are much less common. Women with von Willebrand's disease may have very heavy menses.

Von Willebrand's factor is synthesized in endothelial cells and megakaryocytes. It exists in the circulation in a series of multimeric forms ranging in molecular weight from 1 million to 20 million daltons. The multimers with the highest molecular weights have the greatest ability to function in the platelet-subendothelium interaction. Abnormalities in the multimeric pattern of von Willebrand's disease have been used to classify the various forms of this disorder. Type I is by far the most common. Patients with type I disease have a normal multimeric pattern but appear to have a defect in the secretion of protein from the endothelium. Type IIa von Willebrand's disease is associated with a relative reduction in the multimers with higher molecular weights, those that are most important for normal platelet function. Type IIb von Willebrand's disease is characterized by an abnormal von Willebrand's factor that has an increased binding affinity for platelets. Patients with IIb dis-

ease may have occasional thrombocytopenia because of in vivo platelet agglutination. Platelets from patients with IIb disease agglutinate in vitro with lower than normal concentrations of ristocetin. Patients with type III disease have a near absence of all multimers of von Willebrand's factor in the circulation; this condition may represent a doubly heterozygous state. There is a rare type of von Willebrand's disease called platelet type or pseudo von Willebrand's disease. Clinically, it appears to be similar in phenotype to type IIb disease and is inherited in an autosomal dominant manner. Although patients with this disorder have normal von Willebrand's factor, they have a modified platelet receptor that has an abnormally high binding affinity for von Willebrand's factor. Patients with this disorder may also develop episodic thrombocytopenia as a result of in vivo platelet agglutination.

Acquired Coagulation Abnormalities

Most of the coagulation problems that internists are called to see are acquired rather than congenital.

Liver disease. Of the acquired defects, liver disease is the most common. Patients who have acquired coagulation abnormalities generally show stigmata of liver disease; they may have jaundice, ascites, hepatosplenomegaly, or spider angiomas. The albumin level is almost always decreased and the bilirubin and liver enzyme levels may be elevated. Because the liver is the site of production for most clotting factors, patients with liver damage or impaired function may have multiple clotting factor deficiencies that could place them at risk during surgery or be associated with spontaneous bleeding. Because of the multiple clotting deficiencies that are present, the fibrinogen level may be low and the prothrombin time, partial thromboplastin time, and thrombin time may be prolonged. The coagulopathy of liver disease may occasionally be confused with chronic DIC (see later). Patients with liver disease, in contrast to those with DIC, tend to have normal or high factor VIII levels. Protein C and protein S levels may also be low but hemostatic abnormalities remain the predominant clinical problem.

Vitamin K deficiency. Patients with vitamin K_1 deficiency may have hemorrhagic disorders. The activity of factors II, VII, IX, and X is depressed in patients with vitamin K deficiency. Vitamin K is required for the posttranslational addition of carboxyl groups to glutamic acid residues on the N-terminal end of these vitamin K–dependent zymogens. Without this modification, these enzymes do not function properly because they are unable to bind the calcium required for normal clotting. There are two sources of vitamin K. Vitamin K_1 is derived from food and vitamin K_2 is pro-

TABLE 21–1. Clotting Factor Deficiencies and Their Treatment

Clinical Deficiency	Inheritance	Incidence	Production Site in Body	Sex Affected	Therapy	Half-Life of Infused Factor (hours)
Factor I (fibrinogen)	Autosomal recessive	Rare	Liver	Both sexes	Cryoprecipitate, fresh frozen plasma	96–144
Factor II (prothrombin)	Autosomal recessive	Rare	Liver (vitamin K–dependent)	Both sexes	Prothrombin complex concentrate, fresh frozen plasma	50–80
Factor V (proaccelerin)	Autosomal recessive	Rare	Liver	Both sexes	Fresh frozen plasma	24
Factor VII (proconvertin)	Autosomal recessive	1 in 500,000	Liver (vitamin K–dependent)	Both sexes	Prothrombin complex concentrate, plasma	4–6
Hemophilia A						
Factor VIII (antihemophilic factor)	Sex-linked recessive	1 in 5000, males only	?Throughout reticuloendothelial system, ? liver, spleen, kidneys	Males (female carrier)	Factor VIII concentrate, cryoprecipitate	12
Hemophilia B						
Factor IX (plasma thromboplastin component)	Sex-linked recessive	1 in 25,000, males only	Liver (vitamin K–dependent)	Males (female carrier)	Factor IX concentrate, prothrombin complex concentrate, plasma	20–30
Factor X (Stuart-Prower)	Autosomal recessive	<1 in 500,000	Liver (vitamin K–dependent)	Both sexes	Prothrombin complex concentrate, plasma	25–60
Factor XI (plasma thromboplastin antecedent	Autosomal dominant	Rare	Unknown	Both sexes	Plasma	40–84
Factor XII (Hageman)	Autosomal recessive	Rare	Unknown	Both sexes	Treatment unnecessary	50
Factor XIII (fibrin-stabilizing factor)	Autosomal recessive?	Rare	Unknown	Both sexes	Plasma	150
von Willebrand's factor	Autosomal dominant	Unknown	Endothelial cells	Both sexes	Deamino D-arginine vasopressin, cryoprecipitate, certain factor VIII concentrates	24

(Modified from Evatt BL, Gibbs WN, Lewis SM, et al. Fundamental diagnostic hematology, ed 2. Atlanta, US Department of Health and Human Services, 1992)

duced by intestinal bacteria. A diet free of vitamin K does not necessarily lead to vitamin K deficiency unless the intestinal flora are affected by antibiotics. Vitamin K deficiency may also occur with malabsorption syndromes. The deficiency can be induced iatrogenically by the administration of oral anticoagulants such as warfarin, which interfere with the regeneration of reduced vitamin K after the carboxylation event takes place. Patients with clinically significant vitamin K deficiency show prolongation of both the prothrombin time and the partial thromboplastin time, with the prothrombin time being the most sensitive indicator. This sensitivity is related to the short half-life of factor VII and the inability of the liver to produce sufficient amounts of carboxylated factor VII with low levels of vitamin K.

Disseminated intravascular coagulation. Disseminated intravascular coagulation is characterized by the accelerated consumption of platelets and multiple clotting factors. This pathologic process has been associated with many disorders, including gram-negative sepsis and other bacteremias; viral and other infections; several complications of pregnancy (eg, toxemia, abruption, amniotic fluid embolism, retained dead fetus); metastatic cancer; leukemia; tissue damage (eg, from shock, burns, heat stroke); venomous snake bites; and hemolytic transfusion reactions. Patients with DIC typically bleed from multiple sites and often have thrombocytopenia, hypofibrinogenemia, and elevated fibrin degradation products (d-dimer). Regardless of what triggers DIC, the final common pathway leads to the activation of thrombin and subsequent consumption of fibrinogen and platelets. Fibrinolysis follows clot formation in a secondary fashion. The rapid consumption of clotting factors overwhelms the ability of the reticuloendothelial system to clear activated factors, further promoting clotting. The rapidly generated fibrin degradation products interfere with platelet function and fibrin stabilization.

Acquired circulating anticoagulants. Patients with hemophilia occasionally may develop an alloantibody to the normal factor they are lacking. Other patients, including those with systemic lupus erythematosus and other autoimmune disorders, postpartum women, and the elderly, may develop autoantibodies against normal clotting factors. These spontaneously occurring antibodies are termed *circulating anticoagulants* and are associated with prolongation of either the prothrombin time or the partial thromboplastin time. The presence of these inhibitors is characterized by the inability of a 1:1 mixture of patient plasma and normal plasma to correct the abnormal clotting time.

Patients sometimes are detected who have prolongation of either the prothrombin time or the partial thromboplastin time that cannot be corrected as described earlier, yet who appear to lack inhibitors directed against specific clotting factors. Patients with this problem are said to have a lupus-like anticoagulant; they usually have an antibody directed against phospholipid that interferes with the in vitro coagulation test. They may also have false-positive test results for syphilis and detectable anticardiolipin antibodies as a result of this abnormality. Several more sensitive clotting tests have been developed to detect this phenomenon, such as the tissue thromboplastin inhibition test and Russell's viper venom test. Generally, patients with the lupus-like anticoagulant do not have bleeding problems; paradoxically, they may have an increased frequency of thrombotic events.

Patients with massive transfusions. Massively transfused patients have thrombocytopenia and multiple clotting factor deficiencies. These patients are easily recognized and require special care.

PREPARATION FOR SURGERY

Once the potential for abnormal bleeding during surgery has been identified, consulting physicians must design plans to prepare patients for surgery and to care for them during and after the procedure. The management of each disorder is unique but general principles often can be applied in designing patient care for groups of disorders that fall within common categories.

PATIENTS WITH THROMBOCYTOPENIA

Patients with thrombocytopenia who have platelet counts of 60,000 to 100,000/μL or greater generally have no difficulty with most surgical procedures if massive blood loss does not substantially reduce the platelet count. Neurosurgical procedures are more comfortably performed with platelet counts toward the upper end of this range. Patients with platelet counts of less than 50,000 to 60,000/μL on a nonimmune basis require special attention in preparation for surgery. This is discussed below.

Thrombocytopenia Caused by Increased Platelet Destruction

The most common disorder associated with accelerated platelet destruction is immune thrombocytopenia. The single most effective therapy for patients with chronic immune thrombocytopenia is splenectomy. Thus, medical consultants frequently are called on for advice regarding the care of patients with immune thrombocytopenia who are scheduled for surgery. Patients with immune thrombocytopenia initially should be given either corticosteroids or intravenous immunoglobulin. Most adult patients respond only transiently to a course of intravenous immunoglobulin or short-term corticosteroid therapy. Although acceptable platelet counts can be maintained in many patients with long-term steroid administration, the side effects of such therapy reduces its practicality. Thus, splenectomy is a frequent choice for the treatment of chronic immune thrombocytopenia. Platelet transfusions are of little use in preparing patients with immune thrombocytopenia for surgery because platelet survival is extremely short. In the past, patients with severe immune thrombocytopenia have undergone splenectomy without any attempt to raise the platelet count before surgery because of the observation that the platelets in immune thrombocytopenia are hyperfunctional and that the platelet count generally rises to hemostatic levels immediately after the spleen is removed. Today, most clinicians prefer to raise the platelet count by administering a short course of intravenous immunoglobulin in the few days before surgery. Patients typically are treated with a course of intravenous immunoglobulin, 2 g/kg of body weight, total dose, administered by slow intravenous infusion over 2 to 5 days. Most patients require no further therapy after surgery. Occasionally, patients may benefit from the administration of supplemental intravenous immunoglobulin or low-dose steroids in the immediate postoperative period; intravenous immunoglobulin is preferred over steroids because of the tendency of the latter to impair wound healing.

Accelerated platelet destruction is also seen in patients with DIC. The care of patients with DIC is discussed later.

Other Causes of Thrombocytopenia

Patients with significant nonimmune thrombocytopenia require higher platelet counts to undergo surgery safely. Most patients who require platelet supplementation have bone marrow that does not release sufficient numbers of platelets into the circulation to maintain adequate platelet counts. Somewhat fewer patients have thrombocytopenia because of splenic sequestration resulting from splenomegaly. All these patients should benefit from platelet transfusions if they have not become alloimmune through multiple previous transfusions. Platelet concentrates for transfusion are generally prepared from whole blood. A typical platelet concentrate has a volume of 50 mL and recovers 60% to 80% of the platelets in a unit of whole blood. A single platelet concentrate usually yields an incremental rise in platelets of $10,000/\mu L/m^2$. Thus, a platelet increase of 5000 to $7500/\mu L$ generally is achieved with a single platelet concentrate. Once physicians have determined target preoperative platelet counts, the number of units of platelets that must be administered before surgery is easy to estimate. A platelet count should be obtained 1 hour after transfusion to confirm the estimate. Patients whose histories suggest that they

may be alloimmunized may require several serial platelet counts after transfusion to determine whether platelet survival will be sufficiently long to sustain them during the surgical procedure and immediate postoperative period. Patients who are alloimmunized require special preparation and consideration. They may need special platelet donors who are either HLA-compatible or appear to be nonreactive in a platelet crossmatch procedure. Compatible donors can donate platelets by pheresis; a typical single donor preparation is equal to about six units of random donor platelet concentrates. Patients with splenomegaly generally experience a lower than predicted incremental platelet rise because of increased splenic sequestration. These patients require additional platelet transfusions to compensate for their distributional problems.

PATIENTS WITH THROMBOCYTOSIS

Patients with secondary thrombocytosis generally have no hemostatic defects and do not require special preparation for surgery. Once their conditions have been properly diagnosed, surgery can be performed without increased risk of thrombotic complications.

Patients with essential thrombocythemia or other myeloproliferative disorders associated with high platelet counts require special preparation for surgery. These patients are prone to both thrombotic and hemorrhagic complications. If surgery is elective, patients should be treated with hydroxyurea, alkylating agents (eg, busulfan [Myleran], chlorambucil), or ^{32}P for 1 to 2 months before the operation. A new drug, anagrelide, can reduce the platelet count without suppressing other bone marrow cell lines. If emergency surgery is required, plateletpheresis should be performed to reduce the risk of thrombotic or hemorrhagic complications. It may be useful to monitor the bleeding times of these patients because their platelets frequently function poorly. Platelet transfusion may be necessary to maintain adequate hemostasis.

PATIENTS WITH ABNORMAL PLATELET FUNCTION

Of all patients with abnormal platelet function, those with acquired disorders are by far the most common. Measurement of the bleeding time helps in assessing the degree of platelet dysfunction. Aspirin and other nonsteroidal anti-inflammatory compounds may cause platelet dysfunction but generally do not pose a major problem for patients who are about to undergo surgery. Patients with uremia may have a substantial deficit of platelet function. They may respond to an infusion of deamino D-arginine vasopressin (DDAVP), 0.3 µg/kg in 50 mL of normal saline solution given over 30 minutes. Patients whose defects in platelet function are the result of dysproteinemias should be considered candidates for either chemotherapy or pheresis before surgery. Generally, patients with extrinsic causes of acquired platelet dysfunction benefit little from platelet transfusions; normal transfused platelets soon acquire the defect of the patients' platelets.

Consulting physicians encounter fewer patients with hereditary platelet dysfunction. Von Willebrand's disease is probably the most common inherited defect of platelet function but the defect results from the deficiency or abnormality of a plasma protein and is discussed later. Many inherited defects of platelet function are so mild that little special care is required during surgery. Some inherited defects, such as thrombasthenia, are associated with a severe functional deficit. Severe defects in platelet function require platelet transfusions to sustain patients throughout surgery and the postoperative period. Multiply transfused patients with hereditary defects in platelet function can be difficult to maintain if they have become alloimmunized. Raising the platelet count by at least 50,000/μL should provide adequate hemostasis for most patients with severe congenital platelet defects who are undergoing surgery.

PATIENTS WITH INHERITED COAGULATION ABNORMALITIES

Although there are numerous inherited disorders of blood clotting, this section focuses on the treatment of the three most common disorders: factor VIII deficiency, factor IX deficiency, and von Willebrand's disease. The treatment of most patients with factor VIII or factor IX deficiency is well defined today. Highly purified factor VIII and factor IX products are available that provide a high degree of safety from infection with HIV and hepatitis. Many formulas are available for computing the preoperative and postoperative doses of factor VIII and factor IX. In general, the circulating level of factor VIII in patients with severe factor VIII deficiency should be raised to 100% by the administration of a highly purified factor VIII concentrate at a dose of 50 U/kg After the initial loading dose, 25 U/kg can be given every 12 hours by slow intravenous push, with the goal of maintaining a minimum factor VIII level of 30%. Most surgical patients require hemostatic levels of factor VIII for 10 days. Some patients undergoing orthopedic or neurosurgical procedures need a few more days of therapy. Patients with mild hemophilia A sometimes may be successfully treated for surgery with DDAVP, which raises the level of factor VIII. If patients have shown the capacity to raise factor VIII to hemostatic levels in response to an infusion of DDAVP (0.3 μg/kg in 50 mL of saline solution administered over 30 minutes), this non–plasma-based product can be used for surgery. Patients with mild hemophilia frequently require twice daily infusions and may become refractory to

DDAVP, necessitating the use of supplemental factor VIII. Whenever DDAVP is used, patients should be observed for the development of hyponatremia.

Patients with factor IX deficiency who are undergoing surgery should be treated with the new, pure coagulation factor IX products rather than with prothrombin complex concentrates that also contain therapeutic amounts of factor IX. These prothrombin complex concentrates contain small amounts of activated clotting factors that carry the risk of DIC and both arterial and venous thrombosis when they are used in high doses for sustained intervals. Now that pure coagulation factor IX products are available, physicians can safely use higher levels of factor IX without risking thrombotic complications from factor treatment. The factor IX level should be elevated to the range of 80% to 100% in patients with severe factor IX deficiency by the administration of factor IX at a dosage of 100 U/kg. After the initial loading dose has been delivered, patients can be treated with 25 U/kg every 12 hours or with 50 U/kg once daily by slow intravenous push to maintain a minimum factor IX level of 25% to 30%. Patients with factor IX deficiency who are undergoing surgery should be treated for the same duration as are patients with factor VIII deficiency.

About 15% of patients with factor VIII deficiency and a smaller percentage of those with factor IX deficiency may exhibit a circulating inhibitor to the infused clotting factor. These inhibitors can usually be detected before surgery with an inhibitor screening test. In some patients, the inhibitor can only be demonstrated by a shortened survival of infused factor concentrate. The criteria for performing surgery on patients with inhibitors and the care of these patients during surgery is complicated and beyond the scope of this chapter.

During surgery, most patients with mild von Willebrand's disease respond well to therapeutic agents. Evaluating the response to therapy, however, requires monitoring levels of both factor VIII and von Willebrand's factor as well as monitoring patients for the occurrence of bleeding. It often is not possible to obtain serial measurements of von Willebrand's factor and clinical observation becomes more important. The appropriate therapy for patients with von Willebrand's disease depends on the type of disease they have. Patients who have the most common form of von Willebrand's disease, type I, can usually be treated with DDAVP at a dosage of 0.3 μg/kg infused over 30 minutes. A single daily infusion frequently is sufficient, although occasional patients require more frequent therapy. As in patients with mild factor VIII deficiency, tachyphylaxis to the drug as well as hyponatremia can develop. Some patients with type IIa von Willebrand's disease respond to DDAVP.

Patients with most other forms of von Willebrand's disease, including those with type IIb, platelet type, and type III disease, usually require replacement with a plasma-derived von Willebrand's factor. In the past, cryoprecipitate has been used as a source of this factor. Currently available cryoprecipitate preparations are not safe from hepatitis, although a solvent-detergent cryoprecipitate that does not contain infectious hepatitis B or C may soon be available. Humate-P (Armour Pharmaceutical, Collegeville, PA), a factor VIII concentrate that is rich in von Willebrand's factor, is the preferred source of replacement for von Willebrand's factor. Patients should be treated with an initial dose of 50 factor VIII units per kilogram. Repeated treatment is necessary at intervals of 12 to 24 hours with 50% to 100% of the initial dose. Some patients who have platelets deficient in von Willebrand's factor may also require platelet transfusions to maintain hemostasis. Because of the difficulty in monitoring the response to therapy, patients should be observed closely for abnormal bleeding.

PATIENTS WITH LIVER DISEASE

Preparing patients with significant liver disease for surgery can be challenging. If the preoperative prothrombin time exceeds 15 seconds, the likelihood of significant bleeding is great. These patients frequently have substantially reduced levels of almost all clotting factors. Their fibrinogen levels may be low or their fibrinogen may function abnormally; either problem may substantially impair their ability to form clots. These patients also often have thrombocytopenia, compounding the hemostatic defect. In addition, some of these patients show some evidence of modest consumption of clotting factors.

Preoperative therapy for patients with liver disease must be individualized to correct each patient's coagulation abnormalities. Because of the risk of hypervolemia, hypofibrinogenemia is best treated with cryoprecipitate, which is rich in fibrinogen. Fifteen bags of cryoprecipitate should be given as an initial dose and further therapy should be adjusted to achieve fibrinogen levels in excess of 100 mg/dL. To supply other clotting factors, fresh frozen plasma is required. Three to 10 units of fresh frozen plasma may be necessary to normalize the prothrombin time and the partial thromboplastin time. This correction may last only a few hours and nearly continuous infusion of fresh frozen plasma may be required, necessitating careful observation and management of the volume status. Thrombocytopenia should be treated as described earlier given the fact that many of these patients have splenomegaly resulting from portal hypertension.

PATIENTS WITH VITAMIN K DEFICIENCY

Several techniques are available for treating vitamin K deficiency in patients who are being prepared for surgery. The approach used depends on the urgency of the surgery. If patients require urgent surgery because of bleeding or other life-threatening problems, replacement with functional vitamin K–dependent clotting factors must be accomplished promptly. Patients may be infused with prothrombin complex concentrate that contains factors II, VII, IX, and X; its potency is typically expressed in units of factor IX. This product is appropriately treated to inactivate HIV and hepatitis viruses. Patients should receive between 50 and 70 factor IX units per kilogram. This dose quickly corrects abnormal bleeding caused by vitamin K deficiency. This strategy is accompanied on rare occasions by unexpected thrombosis or DIC. This treatment does not resolve the underlying vitamin K deficiency, and patients must be given supplemental vitamin K. An alternative to prothrombin complex concentrate is fresh frozen plasma. Generally, a minimum of four units of fresh frozen plasma are required to achieve hemostasis. Although fresh frozen plasma does not carry the thrombotic risk of prothrombin complex concentrate, it still may transmit infectious agents such as hepatitis or HIV, may produce volume overload, and may require more time for intravenous administration.

If surgery is not imminent, supplementing the diet of patients who do not have vitamin K malabsorption can restore adequate tissue concentrations in about 1 week. Using an oral supplement may not be reliable, however, and most physicians prefer to treat vitamin K deficiency with a parenteral preparation. Generally, 10 to 15 mg of vitamin K_1 is infused intravenously; this must be done cautiously because anaphylactic reactions have been reported with intravenous use of this preparation. Intramuscular injections usually are not used in patients with vitamin K deficiency because of the risk of intramuscular hematomas. Once patients have been treated with parenteral vitamin K, the prothrombin time should normalize within 24 hours.

Patients who have vitamin K deficiency caused by the use of oral anticoagulants such as warfarin should be treated with modified regimens. Usually, patients who are being treated with oral anticoagulants should be switched to heparin therapy for the surgical procedure. If surgery will not performed for several days, warfarin administration can be discontinued while patients are receiving heparin and begun again in the postoperative period. If surgery must be performed a day after the cessation of warfarin therapy, heparinized patients can be given 1 to 2 mg of intravenous vitamin K_1 to restore hemostatic levels of vitamin K–dependent factors. If immediate surgery is necessary, warfarin therapy should be stopped and patients should be heparinized and treated with prothrombin complex concentrate or fresh frozen plasma as described earlier.

PATIENTS WITH DISSEMINATED INTRAVASCULAR COAGULATION

Patients with active DIC are inherently unstable and are not candidates for surgery unless an operative procedure is required to resolve the process initiating the consumption of clotting factors. Draining a large abscess and removing a dead fetus are examples of necessary surgical intervention in patients with DIC. In the absence of these exceptions, DIC must be treated methodically and patients must be stabilized before any surgical procedure is attempted. The treatment of DIC should be directed toward correction of the underlying pathologic process. For example, if the DIC is caused by sepsis, appropriate antibiotic therapy should be administered. If the DIC is secondary to shock, the circulatory status must be normalized. Patients with DIC accompanied by bleeding require hemostatic support until the primary problem can be corrected. Bleeding in this setting may result from severe thrombocytopenia, coagulation factor deficiencies, or a combination of these. Initial therapy for the thrombocytopenia may include 8 to 10 units of platelets. If patients have hypofibrinogenemia, treatment with 15 bags of cryoprecipitate may be used in an attempt to raise the fibrinogen to hemostatic levels. Other clotting factor deficiencies should be treated with the infusion of multiple units of fresh frozen plasma. Prothrombin complex concentrate is contraindicated for the treatment of clotting factor deficiency in DIC because it contains low levels of activated clotting factors that may worsen the consumptive process. Heparin is generally not indicated for the treatment of DIC because it usually aggravates the bleeding. It may be used cautiously in patients who have evidence of thrombosis along with the consumptive process.

PATIENTS WITH ACQUIRED CIRCULATING ANTICOAGULANTS

Patients with certain types of circulating anticoagulants usually are not candidates for elective surgery. There are a few approaches that consultants can use to treat such patients who must undergo surgery. Some patients with inhibitors to factor VIII have been treated with activated prothrombin complex concentrates such as FEIBA or Autoplex. No simple laboratory method is available for monitoring the response to such therapy, however, and most clinicians have been reluctant to use these preparations. Patients who possess low antibody titers to factor VIII may respond to porcine factor VIII. This preparation has the advantages of allowing the measurement of porcine factor VIII levels and correcting the partial thromboplastin time. Some patients have had reactions to this product, however, and others have developed antibodies to it, with resultant loss of therapeutic effectiveness. Patients with low factor VIII antibody titers (eg, less than 4 Bethesda units) can frequently be treated with large doses of factor VIII concentrate. Continuous infusion has been shown to increase the effectiveness of the therapeutic regimen. Patients with antibodies who require surgery at a future date can undergo programs of immune tolerance. Many different programs are available for

the induction of immune tolerance. All require the infusion of large daily doses of the factors to which patients have antibodies, and several use other immune-modulating techniques such as chemotherapy, pheresis, and intravenous administration of immunoglobulin. Patients with hemophilia in whom tolerance has been successfully induced can be treated with normal amounts of replacement factor for surgery. In theory, recombinant activated factor VII can be used to treat most patients with acquired inhibitors, either alloantibodies or autoantibodies. It is unlikely to be useful in the treatment of the rare inhibitor of a step in the common pathway. This product is available for investigational use only but may prove to be a useful therapy for patients with inhibitors who require surgery. Managing patients with inhibitors during surgical procedures is challenging and should be undertaken only by those who are experienced in such situations. Patients with lupus-like anticoagulants usually do not have unusual bleeding problems during surgery. If anything, they should receive prophylactic therapy to prevent the development of venous thrombosis.

PATIENTS WHO HAVE RECEIVED MASSIVE TRANSFUSIONS

Rapidly bleeding patients who receive at least 10 units of blood in a short period are considered to meet the criteria for massive transfusion. The principal defect of their hemostatic system is thrombocytopenia. Such patients who develop generalized bleeding from this "dilutional" thrombocytopenia are best treated with 10 units of platelets. Most clotting factors are not abnormal in this group of patients but factors V and VIII disappear rapidly from stored blood and may become depressed. If patients are treated with packed red blood cells, fresh frozen plasma can be given to supplement volume and supply diminished clotting factors. Alternatively, if patients are transfused with whole blood, the administration of 1 unit of fresh whole blood for every 4 units of banked or stored whole blood should be sufficient to maintain adequate concentrations of factors V and VIII. Some rapidly bleeding patients have concomitant DIC. These patients may also require the infusion of cryoprecipitate as described earlier to treat the hypofibrinogenemia.

PATIENTS WHOSE SURGERY REQUIRES CARDIOPULMONARY BYPASS

The bleeding diathesis associated with cardiopulmonary bypass is complex and probably involves an acquired abnormality in platelet function, clotting factor consumption, and activation of the fibrinolytic system. In the past few years, many studies have demonstrated that administration of the serine protease inhibitor, aprotinin, during surgery diminishes perioperative and postoperative bleeding. This agent is available only for investigational use in the United States but may come to market in the next few years.

THE TREATMENT OF UNANTICIPATED POSTOPERATIVE BLEEDING

Inadequate surgical technique is the most common cause of postoperative bleeding. Such bleeding can be corrected by surgical intervention and this must be considered, especially when bleeding is localized to the area of the surgical procedure. Generalized bleeding, however, suggests a systemic problem and a defect in the coagulation system. Nonsurgical postoperative bleeding may occur in spite of the fact that patients lack histories or physical findings of underlying hemorrhagic diatheses. Preoperative laboratory testing may also fail to detect patients who will bleed excessively after an operation. Mild hemophilia, von Willebrand's disease, and factor XIII deficiency are examples of disorders that fall into this category. If surgical bleeding has been excluded, a methodical search for a systemic hemostatic abnormality must be undertaken.

DIAGNOSTIC PROCESS

Patients' medical histories should be reexamined in light of their current bleeding problems to search for previously missed clues to the existence of underlying bleeding disorders. For example, a history of delayed bleeding or poor wound healing may indicate the presence of factor XIII deficiency. Reassessment of the initial physical examination is less useful but the current physical examination may be of help in distinguishing surgical from nonsurgical bleeding problems. If the bleeding is not related to surgery, the examination may indicate whether patients have platelet or coagulation abnormalities. Once surgical bleeding has been excluded as a likely possibility, a rapid laboratory evaluation should be conducted. The most frequently performed tests are a platelet count, prothrombin time, partial thromboplastin time, fibrinogen level, and determination of fibrin split products (often d-dimers). The results of these tests may reveal a specific problem such as thrombocytopenia or clotting factor deficiency, or a combined disorder such as DIC. Following the diagnostic approach outlined at the beginning of this chapter, consultants should be able to identify the problem in most cases. If the results of all screening studies are normal, it may be necessary to reconsider the possibility of surgical bleeding or one of the entities mentioned earlier. The possibility of platelet dysfunction should also be considered if patients appear to have patterns of bleeding suggestive of platelet abnormalities associated with normal platelet counts.

DEVELOPMENT OF A DEFECT IN PLATELET FUNCTION

When patients appear to have developed isolated defects in platelet function after surgery, the differential diagnosis should focus on the common causes of acquired abnormal platelet function. Particular attention should be given to the use of cyclooxygenase inhibitors and plasma expanders such as dextran and high-dose semisynthetic penicillin derivatives. DDAVP at a dosage of 0.3 µg/kg is beneficial in some patients and platelet transfusions are useful in others. If an extrinsic agent such as dextran or another drug is causing the defect in platelet function, however, platelet transfusions will not be beneficial and consideration should be given to discontinuing use of the offending agent.

Patients with previously undiagnosed mild von Willebrand's disease may also have platelet dysfunction. Most of these patients can be appropriately characterized by the measurement of ristocetin cofactor activity. Factor VIII coagulant activity frequently is low, although the meaning of a low factor VIII level may be clouded by the complexity of the postoperative setting. Virtually all patients with von Willebrand's disease that is mild enough to have escaped diagnosis before an operation have type I disease, which is generally responsive to DDAVP at a dosage of 0.3 µg/kg. If DDAVP is used in a surgical setting, physicians must watch for the development of hyponatremia. If patients become refractory to DDAVP therapy, they should be treated with Humate-P.

DEVELOPMENT OF ISOLATED THROMBOCYTOPENIA

The development of isolated thrombocytopenia during the postoperative period is relatively uncommon. Most patients who develop thrombocytopenia after surgery have either DIC or massive blood loss (discussed later).

The occurrence of heparin-associated thrombocytopenia within a few days of surgery, however, is being recognized with increasing frequency in patients with histories of previous heparin exposure. In its most fulminant form, heparin-associated thrombocytopenia is manifested by in vivo platelet aggregation, white thrombus formation, and vascular occlusion. Because the laboratory tests used to identify heparin-associated thrombocytopenia are specialized and not well standardized, the diagnosis must often be made on clinical grounds alone. A sudden drop of 50% in the platelet count, even in the absence of thrombocytopenia, may provide a clue to the presence of this entity. Accompanying vascular occlusion makes the diagnosis virtually certain. Fortunately, only a few patients develop heparin-associated thrombocytopenia; those who do should discontinue use of the drug immediately. Patients can be treated with the defibrinating agent ancrod, which is a viper venom, while they are receiving careful anticoagulant therapy with warfarin (Coumadin). There are unconfirmed reports that intravenous immunoglobulin may be of benefit in treating patients with heparin-associated thrombocytopenia. Newer classes of systemic anticoagulants such as the heparinoids (but not the low-molecular-weight heparin formulations) may not be associated with the development of thrombocytopenia.

Several medications have been associated with the development of immune thrombocytopenia, including quinine, quinidine, and sulfa drugs. Therapy with these agents should be discontinued if they are suspected to be the cause of thrombocytopenia. Thrombocytopenia resulting from the use of these drugs is of short duration if bone marrow production is normal. Platelet transfusions are of little use in these patients because of the shortened platelet survival associated with the peripheral platelet destruction. Many drugs have been associated with the suppression of thrombopoiesis. If patients are sensitive to these agents and have been taking them on a long-term basis, thrombocytopenia most likely will have been noticed before surgery. For some patients, however, the hemostatic stress of surgery may uncover minimally compromised bone marrow. A drug-related hypoproliferative thrombocytopenia can be treated with platelet transfusions using the criteria discussed earlier.

DEVELOPMENT OF A COAGULATION ABNORMALITY

Several coagulation defects may be manifested for the first time in the postoperative period. Mild von Willebrand's disease with its associated low factor VIII level is one such disorder. Because of the extensive use of antibiotics, acquired vitamin K deficiency must be considered in the differential diagnosis of bleeding in postoperative patients, especially those whose diets have not included foods rich in vitamin K. These patients have prolonged prothrombin times and partial thromboplastin times, with normal or elevated fibrinogen levels and normal or minimally elevated fibrin degradation products. Platelet counts are generally normal in this setting. Treatment with vitamin K_1 should quickly reverse the coagulation abnormality.

Patients with mild factor VIII deficiency occasionally have normal partial thromboplastin times because of the in-

sensitivity of this screening test. Mild factor IX deficiency is missed in this fashion less frequently. If patients appear to have bleeding problems despite normal results on screening tests, specific factor assays should be performed in an attempt to uncover mild hemophilia.

Because the usual battery of screening tests cannot uncover factor XIII deficiency, this factor should be measured when patients with normal results on screening studies have delayed bleeding or abnormal wound healing. Factor XIII deficiency can be treated with a simple infusion of fresh frozen plasma; a factor XIII concentrate has also become available.

DISSEMINATED INTRAVASCULAR COAGULATION

Sepsis associated with DIC may appear for the first time early in the postoperative period. It is usually diagnosed with little difficulty and may be associated with thrombocytopenia, hypofibrinogenemia, elevated fibrin split products (d-dimers), and low factor VIII levels. If sepsis does not appear to be the cause of DIC, other etiologies, including incompatible blood transfusion, should be considered. The treatment of DIC has been discussed extensively.

ABNORMAL HEMOSTASIS ASSOCIATED WITH MASSIVE TRANSFUSIONS

Postoperative bleeding may become so severe that massive transfusion support is required. The transfusions themselves lead to coagulation abnormalities. The treatment of massively transfused patients may require platelet transfusions and fresh frozen plasma; the details of such therapy were discussed earlier.

CARING FOR PATIENTS DURING THE DIAGNOSTIC EVALUATION

The screening studies recommended help to differentiate most nonsurgical hemostatic problems and can be performed relatively quickly. Until the results become available, critically bleeding patients should be treated with both platelet transfusions and fresh frozen plasma unless the nature of the procedure performed, additionally elicited history, or physical findings suggest a specific problem that can be treated more narrowly.

Medical Management of the Surgical Patient, Third Edition,
edited by Michael F. Lubin, H. Kenneth Walker, and Robert B. Smith III.
J.B. Lippincott Company, Philadelphia, PA © 1995.

CHAPTER

PROPHYLAXIS FOR DEEP VENOUS THROMBOSIS AND PULMONARY EMBOLISM IN SURGERY

22

Geno J. Merli

Venous thrombosis is a major cause of disability and death in all patient populations. Autopsy studies of hospitalized patients have demonstrated that massive pulmonary embolism (PE) is the cause of death in 5% to 10% of all hospital deaths and have suggested that two thirds of all clinically important venous emboli are never recognized during life.[1,2] In a population-based study, Anderson and colleagues[3] estimated that 170,000 patients are treated for a clinically recognized initial episode of venous thromboembolism in US hospitals each year and that 90,000 patients are treated for recurrent disease. In addition, venous thromboembolism has been well documented as a common, serious, and, in some cases, fatal complication in the postoperative period. Despite the plethora of articles, books, and courses on the prevention of this complication, physicians continue to underuse prophylactic regimens to prevent thromboembolic disease. Anderson and colleagues[4] showed that 44% of university hospitals use prophylaxis compared to 19% of community hospitals. More striking was the fact that only 32% of the patients in this study who were at high risk for deep venous thrombosis (DVT) or PE received prophylaxis.

PATHOPHYSIOLOGY

The pathophysiologic changes of stasis, intimal injury, and hypercoagulability predispose surgical patients to the development of DVT or PE. The supine position on the operat-

ing room table, the anatomic position of the extremities for some surgical procedures, and the effect of anesthesia all contribute to stasis during surgery. Venographic contrast studies have shown that the supine position on the operating table decreases venous return.[5,6] In orthopedic, gynecologic, and urologic surgeries, the anatomic position of the extremities that provides the best surgical access to the joint impairs adequate venous drainage during the procedure.[7] For example, in total hip replacement and hip fracture repair, the flexion and adduction of the hip that is required for better anatomic access to the surgical field has been shown to impair venous return.[7] Anesthesia causes peripheral venous vasodilation, which results in increased venous capacitance and decreased venous return during the operative procedure.[8–10]

Intimal injury may be caused by anatomic positioning and the excessive vasodilation that results from anesthesia. Flexion and adduction of the hip during surgery has been shown to compress the femoral vein. Three intraoperative venographic studies provided clear evidence of distortion of the femoral vein during certain phases of total hip replacement.[11–13] The use of a tourniquet on the proximal thigh and flexion of the knee during total knee replacement also compresses the underlying venous structures. These types of prolonged positions may damage the delicate venous endothelium. Anesthesia also contributes to injury by causing excess vasodilation and endothelial damage.[14–17] Comerota and associates[14] demonstrated in dogs that the endothelial lesions occurred as multiple tears around the junction of small side branches with the major receiving

211

veins (jugular and femoral veins).[14] These tears extended through the endothelium and through the basement membrane, exposing subendothelial collagen, which is highly thrombogenic. On electron microscopic evaluation, the lesions were infiltrated with leukocytes, platelets, and red blood cells.[15] Limited studies have demonstrated the presence of biologically active substances such as histamine, complement fragment C3a, and leukotrienes, which may contribute to venous vasodilation and endothelial damage.[16] These may be the factors that contribute to thrombus formation at sites distant from the surgical procedure. All these mechanisms produce endothelial cell damage, creating a nidus for clot formation.

The third factor contributing to the development of postoperative DVT is hypercoagulability. Assessing this state has proved challenging. The current approach focuses on either coagulation cascade modulators or impairment of the fibrinolytic system. Levels of antithrombin III (AT-III) have been shown to be decreased for 3 to 5 days after total hip and knee surgery.[18] This results in impaired modulation of the clotting cascade at factors Xa and IIa, with an increased propensity toward thrombus formation. The fibrinolytic system also has been evaluated by the measurement of tissue plasminogen activator and plasminogen activator inhibitor-1 levels before and after operation.[19] Several surgical studies have demonstrated a shutdown of the fibrinolytic system as evidenced by reductions in these levels.[20] An increased level of plasminogen activator inhibitor-1 before operation appears to indicate an increased risk for the de-velopment of thrombosis in patients undergoing orthopedic surgery.[21] Another marker of an activated fibrinolytic system is the presence of α_2-antiplasmin, the primary function of which is to inactivate plasmin. Increased levels of plasmin–α_2-antiplasmin complexes are indicative of active fibrinolysis, which is an indirect measure of active thrombus formation.[21] This radioimmunoassay requires further study as a predictor of postoperative DVT. Coupled with stasis and intimal injury, however, it seems to suggest an increased risk for DVT or PE.

As Virchow postulated in 1856, the three factors described increase the risk for the development of DVT and, in some cases, PE. Our responsibility as consultants is to ameliorate these risk factors wherever possible.

RISK FACTOR CLASSIFICATION

In assessing the risk for DVT or PE before surgery, patient age, length and type of procedure, previous DVT or PE, and secondary risk factors must be documented. Secondary risk factors include prolonged immobilization, paralysis, malignancy, obesity, varicose veins, and estrogen therapy.[1,22] Using these criteria, patients are classified as being at low, moderate, or high risk for the development of DVT or PE[23] (Table 22-1).

Patients at low risk are younger than 40 years, have no secondary risk factors, and are undergoing minor, elective abdominal or thoracic surgery under general anesthesia for

TABLE 22–1. Classification of Risk for Postoperative Deep Venous Thrombosis (DVT) or Pulmonary Embolus (PE)

Risk Categories	Calf DVT	Proximal DVT	PE
High Risk	40%–80%	10%–20%	1%–5%
Age >40 y			
Surgery >30 min			
Orthopedic surgery			
Pelvic or abdominal cancer surgery			
Previous DVT or PE			
Secondary risk factors*			
Moderate Risk	10%–40%	2%–10%	0.1%–0.7%
Age >40 y			
Surgery >30 min			
Secondary risk factors*			
Low Risk	<10%	<1%	<0.01%
Age <40			
Surgery minor <30 min			
No secondary risk factors			

*Obesity, immobilization, malignancy, varicose veins, estrogen use, paralysis.
(Modified from Hull R, Raskob G, Hirsh J. Prophylaxis of venous thromboembolism: an overview. Chest 1986;85:379)

less than 30 minutes. In this group of patients, the risk of calf DVT is less than 10%, the risk of proximal vein DVT is less than 1%, and the risk of fatal PE is less than 0.01% if prophylaxis is not used.

Patients at moderate risk are older than 40 years, have one or more secondary risk factors, and are undergoing surgery under general anesthesia for more than 30 minutes. Without prophylaxis, this group has a 10% to 40% risk of developing calf vein thrombosis, a 2% to 10% risk of developing proximal vein clotting, and a 0.1% to 0.7% risk of developing fatal PE.

The high-risk group includes patients older than 40 years who either are undergoing surgery for malignancy or an orthopedic procedure of the lower extremities lasting longer than 30 minutes, have hereditary or acquired coagulopathies (eg, proteins C and S, AT-III, anticardiolipin antibodies), or have secondary risk factors. This group has a 40% to 80% risk of calf vein thrombosis, a 10% to 20% risk of proximal vein thrombosis, and a 1% to 5% risk of fatal PE if prophylaxis is not used.

Although this classification may appear to be artificial, it identifies high-risk patients who must be given some form of prophylaxis for surgery. It also serves as a guide for documenting risk factors in the history and physical examination that affect perioperative prophylactic therapy.

DURATION OF RISK FOR DEEP VENOUS THROMBOSIS OR PULMONARY EMBOLISM

The length of time during which patients are at risk for the development of DVT after surgery has become an important issue because of dramatic reductions in the duration of hospitalization after procedures. The publications reviewed for this chapter focused on a defined period of prophylaxis during the hospital stay and did not assess the risk of thrombosis after discharge from the hospital. All the research subjects underwent evaluation for thrombosis before they were discharged. Importantly, the recommended prophylactic regimens do not eliminate the incidence of thrombosis. In practice, venous imaging or venography cannot be performed before hospital discharge on all patients to detect the small percentage who will develop thrombosis despite prophylaxis. Determining the incidence of clinically significant thromboembolic disease after discharge and the risk-benefit ratio of prophylaxis is of critical importance.

In a study by Scurr,[24,25] 51 patients who underwent major abdominal surgery for benign and malignant disease were followed up for 6 weeks after discharge from the hospital. All patients underwent ^{125}I fibrinogen scanning and plethysmography studies. Thirteen of the 51 patients (25%) developed DVT during the 6-week study period. Only patients with positive results on noninvasive studies underwent venography. The highest incidence of DVT occurred during days 4 through 10 after discharge from the hospital. In a study by Paiement and coworkers,[26] 268 patients undergoing elective total hip replacement were evaluated. All patients received warfarin prophylaxis during their hospitalization and for 6 months after discharge. No standard noninvasive or invasive testing for DVT or PE was performed. Patients were assessed clinically on an outpatient basis. No fatal PE occurred during the study period and no known PE occurred after the patients were discharged from the hospital. Lausen and colleagues[27] assessed 89 general surgery patients. All received postoperative prophylaxis with low-molecular-weight heparin (LMWH; Logiparin). At the time of hospital discharge, 45 patients were given no extended prophylaxis and 44 were given LMWH for 3 weeks. The patients were followed up and DVT was assessed by venous imaging. None of the patients in the group that received LMWH developed DVT compared to 15.6% of the group that did not receive prophylaxis. DVT occurred predominantly in the calf between days 15 and 29 after discharge. Nationally, orthopedic surgeons are the primary group advocating the use of extended prophylaxis after hospital discharge. Six weeks is the accepted duration of prophylaxis with warfarin. The study by Paiement and colleagues involved a longer duration of therapy, with added costs and an increased risk of bleeding. The reports from the groups of Scurr and Lausen are the most provocative because patients were monitored intensely with ^{125}I fibrinogen scanning or venous imaging after abdominal surgery. All types of clots were discovered in these patients, many of which may not have been clinically significant, despite the potential implications drawn by Paiement's group.

This subject requires further study. For the present, I recommend that prophylaxis with warfarin be given for 6 weeks after discharge only to patients who have undergone orthopedic surgery. I do not recommend the use of extended prophylaxis in patients who have undergone abdominal surgical procedures for malignant or benign conditions. Studies are under way to assess this risk period and provide future direction regarding the optimal duration and risk-benefit ratio of extended prophylaxis.

TECHNIQUES OF PROPHYLAXIS

Seven techniques are used for the prophylaxis of DVT and PE in patients undergoing surgery. Each approach is reviewed with respect to dosage, administration, and length of therapy.

TABLE 22–2. Adjusted Low-Dose Heparin Prophylaxis

3500 U subcutaneously 2 h before surgery
3500 U subcutaneously q8h after surgery
Begin adjusting* the dosage 6 h after the morning dose on post-operative days 1 and 2; thereafter, adjust the dosage every second day
After 2 or 3 adjustments, either begin warfarin therapy (prothrombin time, INR 2–3) or maintain patients on the last total daily adjusted dose of heparin subcutaneously q12h until discharge

*<36 s = + 1000 U; 36–40 s = +500 U; 41–45 s = no additional heparin; 46–50 s = − 500 U; >50 s = + 1000 U.

HEPARIN

Heparin is administered at an initial dose of 5000 U given subcutaneously 2 hours before surgery. After surgery, 5000 U is given subcutaneously every 8 to 12 hours until patients are fully ambulatory or discharged from the hospital. In double-blind trials, the incidence of major hemorrhagic events using this regimen was 1.8% compared to 0.8% in the control group.[28] This difference is not statistically significant. The incidence of minor bleeding such as injection site and wound hematomas, however, was significant with heparin prophylaxis (6.3% compared to 4.1% in the control group). Rare complications of low-dose heparin therapy include skin necrosis, thrombocytopenia, and hyperkalemia.[29–32]

Adjusted low-dose heparin therapy was devised for use in patients undergoing total hip replacement. In the original description by Leyvraz and associates,[33] prophylaxis with heparin was begun at a dose of 3500 U given subcutaneously every 8 hours for 2 days before surgery. Adjustments were made on a sliding scale to maintain the partial thromboplastin time at the highest normal value of the laboratory. The practice of admitting patients on the same day as surgery or the evening before makes this regimen impractical. We administer 3500 U of heparin subcutaneously 2 hours before surgery, followed by 3500 U every 8 hours beginning the evening of the procedure (Table 22-2). The heparin dose is adjusted based on the activated partial thromboplastin time 6 hours after the postoperative afternoon dose. The next adjustment is based on the activated partial thromboplastin time 6 hours after the morning dose on the first postoperative day. Subsequent adjustments are made every other day. The heparin dose is derived from a sliding scale schedule of 4 seconds plus or minus the highest normal activated partial thromboplastin time value of the laboratory. The object is to maintain the activated partial thromboplastin time within 4 seconds of the highest normal value of the laboratory. The dose of heparin is adjusted for 7 to 10 days after surgery, at which point warfarin or the last total daily adjusted dose of heparin is given every 12 hours until discharge. Two studies using this method reported no increase in the risk of bleeding.[33,34]

WARFARIN

Three protocols have been devised for the use of warfarin prophylaxis (Table 22-3). The first involves the administration of 10 mg of warfarin the night before surgery, followed by 5 mg the evening of surgery.[35] The daily dose is determined by the prothrombin time (PT), which should be kept at 16 to 18 seconds. If oral intake is not possible, warfarin can be administered through a nasogastric tube. The second method involves the initiation of warfarin therapy 10 to 14 days before surgery.[36] The dose is adjusted to maintain the PT at 1.5 to 3 seconds longer than the laboratory control value before surgery. On the first postoperative day, the dose of warfarin is regulated to maintain a PT of 16 to 18 seconds. The third protocol begins with the administration of 10 mg of warfarin on the evening after surgery.[37] No warfarin is given on the first postoperative day. On the second postoperative day, the dose of warfarin is regulated to maintain a PT of 16 to 18 seconds. This therapy is continued until discharge. Prophylaxis for DVT after hospital discharge has been recommended as a management strategy for patients who have undergone total hip replacement.[38] Warfarin therapy is continued to maintain the PT at 16 to 18 seconds for a total of 6 weeks.[23] Further studies are necessary to support this clinical approach. The incidence of major postoperative bleeding with warfarin therapy has varied from 5% to 10%. The rare complication of warfarin, skin necrosis, has never been reported in studies using this agent as prophylaxis for DVT or PE.

TABLE 22–3. Warfarin Prophylaxis

Method 1
10 mg orally the evening before surgery
5 mg orally the evening of surgery
Adjust dose daily based on a prothrombin time of INR 2–3
Continue warfarin therapy until hospital discharge*

Method 2
Begin warfarin administration at home 1–14 d before hospital admission
Maintain the prothrombin time at 1.5–3 s above the control value
Postoperative day 1, begin adjusting the dose to maintain a prothrombin time of INR 2–3
Continue warfarin therapy until hospital discharge*

Method 3
10 mg orally the evening of surgery
No warfarin postoperative day 1
Postoperative day 2, begin warfarin administration to adjust the prothrombin time of INR 2–3
Continue warfarin therapy until hospital discharge*

*Warfarin therapy may be continued for 4–6 wk after discharge at a prothrombin time of INR 2–3

DEXTRAN

Dextran 40 or 70 has been used in numerous dosages and dosage intervals as prophylaxis for total hip replacement surgery.[39,40] Two dosing schedules are used, one based on a fixed dose and the other on milliliters per kilogram of body weight. The fixed-dose schedule is begun by administering 500 mL of dextran at the initiation of surgery and continuing it during the procedure. After operation, a second 500 mL of dextran 40 or 70 is infused over 8 to 12 hours. For 3 to 5 days after surgery, 500 mL of dextran is given over each 24-hour period. The second regimen is similar to the first except that dextran is given at a dose of 10 mL/kg of body weight during the surgery and 7.5 mL/kg of body weight afterward. This form of prophylaxis is not used as frequently as are the other techniques.

ANTITHROMBIN III

Antithrombin III has been approved for use in the United States for congenital and acquired AT-III deficiency. It is derived from purified human plasma. There have not been any reported cases of viral transmission with its use. A postoperative decrease in AT-III has been reported after orthopedic surgery.[18] This decrease has been cited as one of the factors contributing to the increased incidence of DVT. A combination of AT-III and heparin has been evaluated for use as DVT prophylaxis in patients undergoing total hip replacement.[41] Fifteen hundred units of AT-III and 5000 U of subcutaneous heparin were given 2 hours before surgery, followed by 1000 U of intravenous AT-III each day and 5000 U of subcutaneous heparin every 12 hours for 5 days. Two of 41 patients (5%) who received this therapy had documented thrombosis, compared with 12 of 42 patients (40%) who received dextran.

MECHANICAL METHODS

External pneumatic compression (EPC) sleeves are mechanical methods of improving venous return from the lower extremities.[42] They reduce stasis in the gastrocnemius-soleus pump and may increase fibrinolysis as a concomitant mechanism. These devices are placed on patients the morning of surgery. They are worn throughout the surgical procedure and for 3 to 5 days afterward. When patients resume ambulation, the sleeves can be removed and warfarin or heparin therapy initiated, depending on the surgical procedure that was performed. In patients who do not resume ambulation quickly, the sleeves should be kept in place. These patients may not tolerate the sleeves, however, because of increased warmth, sweating, or sleep disturbance. Warfarin or heparin therapy can be substituted until patients resume ambu-

lation or are discharged from the hospital. The sleeves may be removed temporarily from bedridden patients for skin care, bathing, physical therapy, or bedside commode use. Each manufacturer (eg, Kendall, Venodyne, Jobst, Baxter, Huntleight) provides specifications regarding the operation and cycle time of its device, but no statistically significant difference in the incidence of DVT has been demonstrated. If patients have been bedridden or immobilized for more than 72 hours without any form of prophylaxis, the placement of pneumatic sleeves is not recommended because of the possibility of disturbing newly formed clot. The lower extremity should be evaluated through noninvasive testing.

Calf-length gradient elastic stockings are worn during surgery and until discharge from the hospital. The stockings can be removed for skin care and bathing.

PROPHYLAXIS FOR SPECIFIC SURGERY

Table 22-4 outlines the incidence and prophylaxis of DVT in various surgical procedures.

ORTHOPEDIC SURGERY

The number of orthopedic joint replacement procedures performed has increased over the past 10 years commensurate with the aging of the population. The incidence of DVT has been documented at 40% to 50% in total hip replacement, 45% to 50% in hip fracture, and 72% in total knee replacement. The incidence of fatal PE is about 1% to 5% for all these procedures.[43,44] The high incidence of thrombotic complications in the absence of prophylaxis is a pressing concern. The prophylactic interventions that have been shown to be effective in reducing the incidence of DVT and PE in this high-risk population are reviewed here.

Venography is the gold standard for assessing the efficacy of DVT prophylaxis in orthopedic surgery. Thrombosis in this type of surgery can occur in an isolated proximal, proximal and distal, or isolated distal pattern. The noninvasive studies of venous imaging and impedance plethysmography are more sensitive and specific for proximal vein thrombosis and overlook distal vein thrombosis. The studies presented in this section focus on prophylactic techniques that have venographically demonstrated efficacy in reducing postoperative clot formation.

Total Hip Replacement

The incidence of DVT and fatal PE in total hip replacement surgery varies from 40% to 60% and from 1% to 3%, respectively.[34,45,46] In an attempt to reduce these rates, several

TABLE 22–4. Incidence and Prophylaxis of Deep Venous Thrombosis (DVT) in Surgery

Procedure	DVT Incidence	Recommended Prophylaxis
Orthopedic Surgery		
Total hip replacement	40%–60%	Warfarin
		LMW heparin* (Lovenox, 30 mg SC q12h)
		EPC sleeves
		Adjusted low-dose heparin
		Dextran
Fractured hip repair	40%–50%	Warfarin
		Adjusted low-dose heparin
Total knee replacement	40%–84%	Warfarin
		EPC sleeves
		LMW heparin* (Lovenox, 30 mg SC q12h)
General Surgery	20%–30%	Low-dose heparin (5000 U SC q8–12h)
		EPC sleeves
Neurosurgery		
Craniotomy	19%–40%	EPC sleeves
		Low-dose heparin (5000 U SC q8–12h)
Spinal surgery	4%–60%	EPC sleeves
		EPC sleeves plus low-dose heparin
Gynecologic Surgery		
Not related to malignancy		
Abdominal hysterectomy	12%–15%	Low-dose heparin (5000 U SC q8–12h)
Vaginal hysterectomy	6%–7%	Low-dose heparin (5000 U SC q8–12h)
Related to malignancy	35%–38%	Low-dose heparin (5000 U SC q8–12h)
		EPC sleeves
Urologic Surgery		
Transurethral resection of the prostate	7%–10%	EPC sleeves
		Low-dose heparin (5000 U SC q8–12h)
		Gradient elastic stockings
Open prostatectomy for malignancy	21%–51%	EPC sleeves
		Low-dose heparin (5000 U SC q8–12h)

EPC, external pneumatic compression; LMW, low-molecular-weight.
*The LMW heparins will soon become the drug of choice.

pharmacologic and mechanical approaches to the prevention of thrombosis have been advocated.

Warfarin is the pharmacologic agent of choice for total hip replacement surgery and may be administered as outlined earlier.[43] The use of warfarin prophylaxis has decreased the incidence of DVT from 40% to 60% to 17% to 30%, with a marked reduction in proximal vein thrombosis. The efficacy of fixed-dose heparin therapy was not supported by the National Institutes of Health Consensus Conference for orthopedic surgery.[43] In a metaanalysis of the literature, Collins and coworkers[45] reported that fixed-dose heparin therapy was associated with a lower incidence of proximal thrombosis and fatal PE in orthopedic surgery but with the same overall number of thrombi. Levine and colleagues[47] demonstrated a 23% incidence of DVT using 7500 U of subcutaneous heparin every 12 hours compared to a 19% incidence of DVT in an experimental group that received LMWH. In a study by Planes and associates,[48] fixed-dose heparin reduced the incidence of DVT in total hip replacement surgery to 25%.

Leyvraz and colleagues[33] adapted an adjusted low-dose heparin regimen that proved to be effective in reducing the incidence of DVT. This regimen has not been readily accepted, however, because of the necessity of frequent dose adjustment. Dextran 40 or 70 is another single pharmacologic agent that has been successful in DVT prophylaxis, but its use has declined because of the risk of fluid overload, the occurrence of hypersensitivity reactions, and the availability of more effective techniques. Finally, the replacement of AT-III levels depleted by surgery combined with the delivery of low-dose subcutaneous heparin therapy at a dose of 5000 U every 12 hours has been studied by Francis and coworkers.[41] DVT was identified in 5% of the patients who received AT-III plus low-dose heparin and in 40% of those who received dextran 40. Although it is effective, AT-III is expensive and exposes patients to the risks inherent in the use of human blood products.

The use of mechanical techniques to prevent DVT has been increasing in orthopedic surgery. Several studies have evaluated the use of calf-length or thigh-length EPC sleeves alone or in combination with a pharmacologic agent. The overall incidence of DVT was reduced significantly by this approach (from 40% to 60% to 6% to 35%).[46,49–52] Although these devices have been successful in reducing the incidence of calf vein DVT, they have not been as effective in decreasing proximal vein thrombosis. In these studies, the sleeve on the operated extremity was activated immediately after surgery, whereas the contralateral extremity was compressed throughout the procedure. The sleeves should be worn for 7 days and removed only for bathroom use and physical therapy. No studies have compared different types of sleeves (ie, calf-length versus thigh-length sleeves or sequential versus single-chamber compression devices).

These studies in total hip replacement indicate that the possible methods of prophylaxis for this group of patients are varied. Warfarin, EPC, adjusted-dose heparin, and dextran are the primary agents used (see Table 22-4). More studies are needed to assess the additive effect of EPC plus a single pharmacologic agent. The use of AT-III, although highly effective, has not been accepted nationally. LMWH preparations may soon prove to be the most effective agents.

Hip Fracture

The incidence of DVT in patients who undergo surgery for hip fracture without prophylaxis varies from 40% to 50%.[53–55] This increased risk results from the immobilization that is caused by both the fracture and the surgical procedure. Several prophylactic regimens have been evaluated in these patients but no consensus has been reached regarding the most effective approach.

An early study by Bergqvist and coworkers[53] evaluated the use of dicumarol and dextran as prophylaxis for DVT in patients with fractured hips. The incidence of DVT was about 30% with both agents. Taberner and associates[55] assessed the effectiveness of heparin as a prophylactic intervention in this population. In a small cohort study, adjusted-dose heparin reduced the incidence of DVT from 14% in patients receiving fixed doses to 7% in those receiving the adjusted regimen. This was a small study of 28 patients but the trend in outcome appears to be real. Powers and colleagues[54] compared three methods of prophylaxis in patients with hip fractures: placebo, warfarin, and aspirin. DVT was documented in 46% of the placebo group, 40.9% of the aspirin group, and 20% of the warfarin group. This was a significant reduction in the incidence of thrombosis.

Based on these few studies with venography as their end point, the use of warfarin or adjusted-dose heparin is recommended for prophylaxis (see Table 22-4). Extrapolating from the data obtained in patients undergoing total hip replacement, compression sleeves and dextran also seem to be reasonable alternative approaches.

Total Knee Replacement

The incidence of DVT in patients undergoing total knee replacement surgery without prophylaxis is 40% to 84% for isolated calf vein thrombosis and 3% to 20% for proximal vein thrombosis.[56–59] The high incidence of proximal thrombosis is significant because PE has been reported in about 1.7% of patients.[58,59] Despite this high incidence, the best method of prophylaxis in patients undergoing total knee replacement remains controversial.

No large-scale studies have evaluated pharmacologic agents as prophylaxis for DVT in total knee replacement. As part of a larger study of total hip replacement, Francis and colleagues[36] compared dextran 40 with two-step warfarin therapy in a few patients undergoing total knee replacement. All 8 patients who were given dextran 40 developed DVT compared to 3 of the 14 patients who were given warfarin (21%). A much larger, nonrandomized and nonblinded study by Stulberg and associates[59] evaluated 638 patients undergoing unilateral (338 patients), bilateral (121 patients), and unilateral revision (58 patients) knee replacement surgery. The overall incidence of calf thrombosis was 46.1% and the incidence of proximal vein thrombosis was 10.7%. In a small pilot study, Francis and coworkers[41] used AT-III replacement in two different doses with subcutaneous heparin as prophylaxis in patients undergoing total knee replacement. Fifty percent of those who received low-dose AT-III and 27% of those who received high-dose AT-III developed DVT. The results of these studies indicate that a significant, large-scale, controlled trial of single pharmacologic regimens as prophylaxis in total knee replacement has yet to be performed.

Three studies have evaluated the use of mechanical methods of prophylaxis either alone or in combination with pharmacologic agents.[46,57,60] Hull and colleagues[44] compared the use of calf-length EPC sleeves plus acetylsalicylic acid to the use of acetylsalicylic acid alone. The incidence of DVT was 6.3% in the former group and 65.5% in the latter group. All the thrombi occurred in the calf vein in patients who received EPC plus acetylsalicylic acid, whereas 36.8% of the thrombi extended from the calf into the popliteal and femoral veins in the control group. The EPC sleeves in this study were worn an average of 12 days. These devices had a 20-second, 50-mmHg compression cycle with a 60-second relaxation phase. Two problems with this study are the fact that different knee surgeries were performed and acetylsalicylic acid use was not randomized. Despite these inadequacies, the data regarding the efficacy of EPC are significant.

In another study, bilateral and unilateral total knee replacement were evaluated using the prophylactic regimen outlined earlier.[60] The incidence of DVT in patients who underwent bilateral total knee replacement was 48% in those who were treated with EPC and 68% in those who were treated with acetylsalicylic acid. Among patients who underwent unilateral total knee replacement, 22% of those in the EPC group developed DVT compared to 47% of those in the acetylsalicylic acid group. All the thrombi occurred in the calf vein in patients who underwent unilateral total knee replacement. The thrombi extended into the popliteal veins in 16.6% of patients who underwent bilateral total knee replacement compared to only 6.6% of those who received acetylsalicylic acid. The EPC sleeves were thigh-length, sequential compression devices. They had an 11-second inflation time at a pressure of 35 to 55 mmHg followed by a 60-second venting cycle. The EPC sleeves were worn for 5 to 7 days. An unexpected finding in this study was a higher incidence of highly suggestive results on lung scans among asymptomatic patients treated with EPC sleeves who had undergone single or bilateral knee replacement. The lung scan results were not confirmed by angiography.

The final mechanical intervention evaluated was continuous passive motion plus acetylsalicylic acid versus acetylsalicylic acid with active range of motion exercises.[57] A Kinetec 3080 provided the continuous range of motion for an average of 10 hours daily for 5 to 7 days. DVT was not significantly reduced in these two groups, being 45.3% in the former and 37.3% in the latter. The rates of proximal extension of thrombosis were 10.7% and 14.7%, respectively. This form of mechanical prophylaxis is not as effective as EPC for the reduction of both distal and proximal vein thrombosis.

After reviewing these studies, we recommend the use of warfarin or EPC for DVT prophylaxis in patients who undergo total knee replacement (see Table 22-4). A LMWH (enoxaparin) preparation has been approved for use in the United States. Because of their efficacy and safety, these new forms of heparin appear to be ideal for reducing the incidence of DVT in this high-risk group.

GENERAL SURGERY

The variety of procedures performed in general surgery make it difficult to accurately assess the incidence of DVT in this patient population. When reviewing studies, it is impossible to segregate patients according to the procedure they underwent. Individual surgical procedures are included in the next sections under their appropriate specialty heading.

Five trials were reviewed to document the incidence of DVT in general surgery.[61-65] These studies used ^{125}I fibrinogen scanning as the test of therapeutic efficacy. Only one study confirmed the accuracy of all positive ^{125}I fibrinogen scans by venography.[64] The incidence of thrombosis varied from 20% to 30%. A review by Clagett and coworkers[28] reported an incidence of 25%. Calf vein thrombosis has been the predominant type of thrombosis in these studies.

The approach to prophylaxis in general surgery has been directed toward single pharmacologic agents. Five studies used low-dose subcutaneous heparin, 5000 U given 2 hours before surgery followed by 5000 U every 8 to 12 hours after surgery until patients were ambulatory or discharged from the hospital. The incidence of postoperative DVT was reduced by 4% to 17% in the general surgery population studied. Clagett and associates[28] performed a metaanalysis of trials that were controlled, uncontrolled, or involved the comparison of heparin and other prophylactic methods. There appeared to be a trend toward a lower incidence of DVT when prophylactic heparin was administered on an 8-hour rather than a 12-hour schedule. Other methods of prophylaxis have been evaluated in general surgery, including dextran and dihydroergotamine plus heparin. Dextran did not prove to be effective in this population but dihydroergotamine plus heparin was beneficial.[61,65] This combination was withdrawn from the American market, however, because of adverse reports related to dihydroergotamine. EPC sleeves have been adopted as a mechanical means of preventing postoperative DVT. These devices have been studied primarily in orthopedic, urologic, neurologic, and gynecologic surgery, and not in general surgery.

Low-dose heparin administered every 8 or 12 hours is the primary method of prophylaxis for DVT in patients undergoing general surgery (see Table 22-4). If this approach is contraindicated, the use of EPC sleeves during surgery and for at least 48 to 72 hours afterward followed by low-dose heparin therapy until patients resume ambulation or are discharged from the hospital is acceptable.

NEUROSURGERY

The incidence and prevention of DVT in neurosurgical procedures have varied in the literature. This stems from the premise that all neurosurgical procedures carry the same risk for postoperative DVT. Studies using ^{125}I fibrinogen scanning or venous Doppler with or without venographic confirmation were evaluated to assess the incidence of DVT in neurosurgery. In six studies, patients underwent craniotomy for either tumor or vascular injury (eg, subdural hematoma, ruptured aneurysm).[66-71] The largest study that separated supratentorial and infratentorial procedures for tumors was conducted by Valladares and colleagues[71] and did not show a difference in DVT. Constantini and associates[72] did demonstrate a difference in thrombotic events in supratentorial compared to infratentorial surgery, but the study was not included in this assessment because only patients with a suspicion of DVT were evaluated by noninvasive or invasive testing. The remaining five studies documented a 19% to 40% incidence of thrombosis occurring within the first 7 days after surgery, with calf veins predominantly involved.

Turpie and coworkers[66] and Black and associates[70] were the only authors who addressed the issue of duration of risk for DVT in patients undergoing intracranial procedures. In the study by Turpie's group, the intervention portion lasted for 5 days.[66] After that time, patients continued to be monitored for DVT without being given prophylaxis. Seven of 52 patients (13.4%) in the initial treatment group developed thrombosis between postoperative days 6 and 14. Five of the 7 patients were not ambulatory and had paralyzed extremities. Black and colleagues[70] maintained prophylaxis until patients became ambulatory, were discharged from the hospital, or died. Among their patients, who underwent surgery for subarachnoid hemorrhage, DVT developed at a mean of 27 days in those who received no prophylaxis compared to 24 days in those who received prophylaxis.

The incidence of DVT is not as well defined in spinal surgery as in craniotomy studies. To assess the former group, three studies with mixed neurosurgical procedures were reviewed and the patients undergoing spinal surgery were abstracted for evaluation.[68–71] These patient groups were small and the spinal surgeries were performed for a variety of conditions, including tumors, disk disease, and undefined problems. The reported incidence of DVT varied from 4% to 60%. Rossi and colleagues[73] and Merli and associates[74] studied patients with spinal cord injuries who were undergoing fusion or stabilization procedures. Venographically confirmed thrombosis developed in 72% of patients in the former study and in 47% of patients in the latter study within the first 14 days after surgery.

In assessing the efficacy of prophylactic interventions, only those studies that used an accurate measure of DVT were chosen. Approaches to preventing DVT in this surgical population have been tempered by the risk of bleeding into such vulnerable tissues as the brain and spinal cord. Despite this potential risk, Cerroto and associates[67] showed that low-dose heparin reduced the incidence of DVT from 34% in control subjects to 6% in the treated group. Heparin (5000 U) was administered subcutaneously every 8 hours. A safe prophylactic dose was achieved by evaluating a plasma heparin concentration obtained 3 hours after the initial dose was given. A heparin level of less than 0.18 U/mL was desired. If a level higher than 0.18 U/mL was obtained, the heparin dose was decreased and the level was reassessed. Once the desired level was achieved, heparin was administered at that dose every 8 hours for 7 days. The risk of bleeding was not increased with this regimen.

An alternative approach to the prevention of postoperative DVT in neurosurgical patients is the use of mechanical devices to reduce stasis and hypercoagulability. Two studies using single-chamber, calf-length EPC sleeves demonstrated a decrease in the incidence of DVT from 18% to 19% in the control group to 1.9% to 5.5% in the treated patients.[66,70] The EPC sleeves were used for an extended period by Black and colleagues[70] (until patients resumed ambulation, were discharged from the hospital, or died) but were only applied for 5 days after the surgical procedure by Turpie and associates.[66] The extended treatment period used by Black was related to the longer postoperative recovery period after craniotomy for subarachnoid hemorrhage.[70] Zelikovski and associates[75] and Turpie and coworkers[76] used thigh-length sequential compression sleeves. Zelikovski and associates used a four-chamber, thigh-length device and noted a reduction in the incidence of DVT from 50% to 4.3%. Turpie and coworkers selected a thigh-length, six-chamber sequential compression sleeve with and without gradient elastic stockings.[76] This device reduced the incidence of thrombosis from 19.8% to 9%. The use of electrical calf stimulation plus dextran 70 was compared to the use of heparin (5000 U given subcutaneously every 12 hours) by Bostrom and colleagues.[77] DVT occurred in 13% of patients treated with the former approach and in 10% of those treated with the latter approach.

Patients undergoing spinal surgery have not been evaluated with respect to the indication for their procedures. Skillman and coworkers[69] compared calf-length EPC sleeves to placebo in patients undergoing cervical, thoracic, or lumbar laminectomies. No difference in the number of thrombi could be documented. In patients undergoing spinal surgery for traumatic injury with paralysis, both Green and associates[78] and Merli and colleagues[74,79] demonstrated a significant reduction in the incidence of DVT using VPC and low-dose heparin. Green and associates[78] compared prophylaxis with EPC sleeves to prophylaxis with EPC sleeves plus aspirin and dipyridamole. It was believed that mechanical methods plus antiplatelet therapy would be ideal for this patient population. The results were compared to historical controls and showed a reduction in the incidence of thrombosis. In their initial work, Merli and colleagues demonstrated a significant reduction in DVT using electrical stimulation plus low dose-heparin versus low-dose heparin alone. All patients had bilateral lower extremity venography as the end point of the study. In a second study, EPC sleeves were combined with gradient elastic stockings and low-dose heparin.[79] Again, a significant reduction in DVT was documented. In all the studies of spinal cord injury, the risk for the development of DVT was highest in the first 2 weeks after injury.

Medical consultants evaluating patients before neurosurgery must consider the type of surgery planned and the underlying indication for surgery in selecting appropriate prophylaxis for DVT (see Table 22-4). Their responsibility does not end with their initial recommendations; prophylactic therapy must be reassessed in the postoperative period in light of the degree of neurologic deficit. If neurologic impairment persists, prophylaxis should be maintained until patients are fully functional.

GYNECOLOGIC SURGERY

The incidence of DVT in gynecologic surgery varies according to the type of procedure performed and whether the disease process is malignant or benign. Numerous approaches to prophylaxis have been evaluated and have substantially reduced the incidence of DVT. Studies using ^{125}I fibrinogen scanning, impedance plethysmography, or venography have been selected to define the incidence of DVT and evaluate appropriate prophylactic interventions.

Four studies examined the incidence of DVT demonstrated on ^{125}I fibrinogen scanning in patients undergoing gynecologic surgery for benign indications.[80–83] Both Bonnar and coworkers[80] and Walsh and associates[81] separated their study populations according to abdominal or vaginal hysterectomy and reported the incidence of thrombosis in each group. Thrombosis was documented in 12% to 15% of patients undergoing abdominal hysterectomy and in 6% to 7% of those undergoing vaginal hysterectomy. Taberner and colleagues[82] and Walsh and associates[81] evaluated mixed gynecologic procedures, including both vaginal and abdominal hysterectomy, and documented thrombosis in 20% to 29% of patients. The discrepancy between these results and those of the other studies is most likely related to variation in the procedures included in the populations studied.

Gynecologic surgery for malignancy is associated with a much higher incidence of postoperative thrombotic events. Seven studies were reviewed.[81–88] Walsh,[81] Clarke-Pearson, and Crandon[85] demonstrated a 35% to 38% incidence of DVT in patients undergoing major pelvic procedures for malignancy. In contrast, the remaining four studies documented rates of DVT between 12% and 23%.[82,83,86,87] The surgical procedures performed were similar, as were the methods used to assess thrombosis. The reason for the differences in results is not known.

In assessing the efficacy of prophylactic interventions, the studies reviewed are divided according to whether they used pharmacologic interventions or mechanical devices and whether they involved surgery for malignant or benign conditions. This separation demonstrates the dual clinical approach used throughout the country.

Seven studies were evaluated.[82–84,86,88,89] Bonnar and colleagues[80] compared dextran to a control group in patients undergoing vaginal or abdominal hysterectomy. The dextran was administered during and shortly after the proce-

dure. The incidence of thrombosis was reduced from 15% to 0% in patients undergoing abdominal hysterectomy and from 6% to 1% in those undergoing vaginal hysterectomy. Taberner and coworkers[82] assessed the efficacy of low-dose heparin, warfarin, and placebo. Both low-dose heparin and warfarin reduced the incidence of DVT from 23% in the placebo group to 6% in the treated groups. The prothrombin ratios were maintained between 2 and 2.5 for the study. Ballard and associates[83] compared low-dose heparin with a control group and found that the incidence of DVT was decreased from 29% to 3.6%. Based on the results of these studies, the use of low-dose heparin or dextran alone is recommended as prophylaxis for DVT in patients undergoing gynecologic surgery for benign conditions. Because so few studies have been done on warfarin, I would not use this agent in this patient population unless no other alternative was available.

The efficacy of low-dose heparin for DVT prophylaxis in gynecologic surgery for malignancy has been assessed in three studies. In a study of 185 patients, Clarke-Pearson and colleagues[84] reported no difference in the incidence of DVT between patients who received low-dose heparin (14.8%) and a control group (12.4%). The same authors completed a second study comparing three protocols: the administration of a placebo, the administration of low-dose heparin only after surgery, and the administration of low-dose heparin both 2 or 3 days before surgery and after surgery.[88] The 18.4% incidence of DVT was reduced to 8% with postoperative administration of low-dose heparin and to 4.1% with additional preoperative administration of low-dose heparin. More recently, a third study by Clarke-Pearson comparing the administration of low-dose heparin (5000 U subcutaneously 2 hours before surgery and every 8 hours after surgery) to the use of EPC sleeves demonstrated heparin's effectiveness in reducing the incidence of DVT. Based on these results, we recommend low-dose heparin as a single pharmacologic agent of choice.

Prophylaxis may also be accomplished with mechanical devices. Two studies of such techniques have been completed using single-chamber calf compression devices for 5 days after surgery. The first study compared EPC sleeves to a control and documented DVT rates of 12.7% and 34.6%, respectively.[86] The second study compared EPC sleeves to low-dose heparin (5000 U given subcutaneously every 8 hours) and demonstrated no statistical difference in DVT incidence (1.9% versus 4.6%).[89] The patients who received low-dose heparin in this study required more blood transfusions after surgery and had an increased volume of retroperitoneal drainage. Mechanical methods are an effective alternative to pharmacologic therapy in this high-risk population.

These studies indicate the necessity of DVT prophylaxis in patients who are undergoing gynecologic surgery (see Table 22-4). Those who are being operated on for malignant conditions are at especially high risk and must be given DVT prophylaxis to reduce the incidence of thrombosis.

UROLOGIC SURGERY

It is difficult to evaluate the incidence of DVT in patients undergoing urologic surgery because of the lack of uniform study procedures and the variety of surgical procedures evaluated. All published studies in patients undergoing urologic surgery were reviewed. Those studies that had defined cohorts and objective end points for DVT are discussed here.

Transurethral resection of the prostate is a frequently performed surgical procedure in the United States. Two small studies have shown the incidence of DVT in patients undergoing this procedure to be 7% to 10% using ^{125}I fibrinogen scanning as the thrombosis end point.[90,91] Because of this low incidence, few studies of prophylaxis have been performed in these patients. In an uncontrolled randomized trial, Van Arsdalen and coworkers[92] compared EPC and gradient elastic stockings as prophylactic interventions. They reported DVT rates of 7.6% with EPC and 6.2% with gradient elastic stockings. This difference was not statistically significant. The low incidence of thrombosis in transurethral resection of the prostate requires a large cohort of patients to demonstrate the clinical benefit of a prophylactic intervention. The present recommendation for DVT prophylaxis in transurethral resection of the prostate is the use of EPC, low-dose heparin, or gradient elastic stockings.

Open prostatectomy is the primary surgical approach for the treatment of patients with prostate cancer. Seven studies using either ^{125}I fibrinogen scanning or venography have documented the incidence of DVT after this procedure to vary between 16% and 51%.[90,91,93–97] Two of the studies by Becker and colleagues[93,94] used venography at varying times after surgery. This approach did not provide an accurate natural history of the development of thrombosis after open prostatectomy. Even if these two studies are not included, the incidence of DVT remains high at 21% to 51%.

Preventing this postoperative complication is of major significance in urologic surgery. Six studies using several methods of prophylaxis for thrombosis have been completed.[96–101] The study populations in these protocols underwent a variety of urologic procedures, with open prostatectomy predominating. In four of the studies, EPC sleeves reduced the incidence of DVT significantly to about 6% to 12% compared to the control rate of 25% to 34%. Vandendris and associates[102] reported a reduction in the incidence of DVT from 39% in the control group to 10% in the patients who received low-dose heparin. Chandhoke and colleagues[101] used low-dose warfarin and reported no case of DVT by duplex scanning in 53 patients studied. No fatal PE occurred in any of these studies.

Patients undergoing prostatectomy or other radical urologic procedures require specific DVT prophylaxis (see Table 22-4). Additional studies are necessary to assess other prophylactic approaches.

NEW METHODS OF PROPHYLAXIS FOR DEEP VENOUS THROMBOSIS

PHARMACOLOGIC AGENTS

Low-molecular-weight heparin preparations are likely to become the primary agents for the prevention of postoperative DVT in orthopedic surgery. LMWH have been observed to have a more significant inhibitory effect on factor Xa than on factor IIa, as well as a lower bleeding risk than standard heparin.[103] Five LMWH preparations are approved for use in Europe; in the United States, one preparation has been approved for orthopedic surgery and two are nearing approval. Each of these LMWH preparations has a different molecular weight, anti-Xa to anti-IIa activity, rate of plasma clearance, and recommended dosage regimen.[104]

Six LMWH preparations have been developed (Table 22-5). They are fragments of commercial-grade standard heparin prepared by either chemical or enzymatic depolymerization. The resulting LMWH contains the pentasaccharide required for specific binding to AT-III.[104–106] This binding in-

TABLE 22–5. Low-Molecular-Weight Heparins

Drug	Molecular Weight (daltons)	Xa/IIa	Half-Life (hours)
PK 10169 (Enoxaparin)	4500	2.7:1	2–3
CY 216 (Fraxiparin)	4500	3.2:1	$2-2\frac{3}{4}$
KABI 2165 (Fragmin)	5000	2:1	$2-2\frac{1}{2}$
Novo LMWH (Logiparin)	4500	1.9:1	2
Org 10172 (Lomoparin)	6500	20:1	18
RD 11885 (Normiflo)	5000	2:1	$3-3\frac{1}{2}$

hibits Xa and IIa without forming the complex that occurs when standard heparin binds with these factors. Heparin molecules with fewer than 18 saccharides (molecular weight less than 5400 daltons) are unable to bind thrombin and AT-III but retain their ability to catalyze the inhibition of factor Xa by AT-III.[104–106]

LMWH formulations are not bound to plasma proteins (histidine-rich glycoprotein, platelet factor 4, vitronectin, fibronectin, and von Willebrand's factor), endothelial cells, or macrophages as is standard heparin.[104,105] This lower affinity contributes to a longer plasma half-life, more complete plasma recovery at all concentrations, and clearance that is independent of dose and plasma concentration.

In comparing the potential for hemorrhagic complications with standard heparin and LMWH, three factors must be considered. Standard heparin inhibits both collagen-induced and von Willebrand's factor–dependent platelet aggregation and increases vascular permeability.[104] These three qualities result in a higher bleeding potential with standard heparin than with LMWH, which does not have these effects.

In reviewing the literature regarding the safety and efficacy of LMWH preparations for the prevention of postoperative DVT, it must be remembered that these agents are distinct compounds with unique properties and different dosage regimens. Only one LMWH has been approved for use in orthopedic surgery in the United States, although several others are awaiting approval.

Four studies using ^{125}I fibrinogen scanning as an end point for thrombosis and a basis for comparing LMWH to low-dose heparin were reviewed[107–111] (Table 22-6). A large study multicenter[107] showed a significant reduction in the incidence of DVT. The remaining studies did not demonstrate any change. Only one study by Bergqvist and coworkers[108] recorded a lower bleeding risk in patients treated with LMWH. A recent metaanalysis of LMWH studies in Europe did not reveal any advantage with these agents.[111]

The largest number of studies have been conducted in patients undergoing elective total hip replacement (Table 22-7). Turpie and associates[112] compared placebo with enoxaparin and demonstrated a reduction in the incidence of DVT from 51.3% to 10.8%. Hoek and colleagues[113] evaluated 196 patients who were randomly assigned to receive either lomoparan or placebo. The incidence of DVT was 57% in the placebo group and 10% in the lomoparin group. Planes and coworkers[48] randomly assigned 237 patients to receive either enoxaparin or standard heparin after hip surgery. The incidence of DVT was reduced from 25% with standard heparin to 12.5% with LMWH. A fourth study by Levine and associates[47] compared LMWH with heparin (7500 U given subcutaneously every 12 hours). There was no difference in the incidence of DVT in either group but there was a lower incidence of bleeding in the LMWH-treated patients.

Le Clerc and colleagues[114] performed a randomized study of 111 patients undergoing total knee arthroplasty who were given either placebo or enoxaparin (see Table 22-7). The incidence of DVT was reduced from 65% in the placebo group to 20% in the enoxaparin group. Two other studies have been performed comparing LMWH to warfarin therapy in patients undergoing total knee replacement surgery (see Table 22-7).[115,116] Only two studies have been performed in patients with hip fractures (see Table 22-7).

TABLE 22–6. Deep Venous Thrombosis (DVT) Prophylaxis in General Surgery with Low-Molecular-Weight Heparins (LMWH)*

Author	Number of Patients	LMWH	DVT	Bleeding
Encke[†]	960	Fraxiparin	27 (2.8%)	47 (4.9%)
	936	LDH (q8h)	42 (4.5%)	42 (4.5%)
Bergqvist[‡]	505	Fragmin	28 (5.5%)	30 (6%)
	497	LDH (q12h)	41 (8.3%)	15 (3%)
Leizorovicz[§]	430	Logiparin	16 (3.7%)	13 (3%)
	429	LDH (q12h)	18 (4.2%)	14 (3.3%)
Samama[¶]	159	Enoxaparin	6 (3.8%)	4 (2.5%)
	188	LDH (q8h)	12 (7.6%)	4 (2.5%)

LDH, low-dose heparin.
*All patients screened with ^{125}I fibrinogen scanning.
[†]Fraxiparin, 7500 ICU SC qd.
[‡]Fragmin, 5000 U 2 h before surgery, then 5000 U SC qd.
[§]Logiparin, 3500 U SC qd.
[¶]Enoxaparin, 1600 U SC qd.

TABLE 22–7. Prophylaxis of Deep Venous Thrombosis (DVT) With Low Molecular-Weight Heparin in Various Orthopedic Procedures*

Study	Number of Patients	Prophylaxis	All DVT	Proximal DVT	Bleeding
Total Hip Replacement					
Turpie	50	Placebo	20 (51%)	9 (45%)	2 (4%)
	50	Enoxaparin, 30 mg SC q12h	4 (11%)	2 (50%)	2 (4%)
Planes	113	Heparin, 5000 U SC q8h	27 (25%)	20 (19%)	2 (2%)
	124	Enoxaparin, 40 mg SC qd	15 (12%)	9 (8%)	3 (2%)
Hoeck	99	Placebo	56 (57%)	25 (25%)	0 (0%)
	97	Lomoparin, 750 U SC q12h	15 (15%)	8 (8%)	6 (6%)
Levine	263	Heparin, 7500 U SC q12h	61 (23%)	17 (7%)	31 (9%)
	258	Enoxaparin, 30 mg SC q12h	50 (19%)	14 (5%)	17 (5%)
Total Knee Replacement					
Le Clerc	54	Placebo	8 (19%)	11 (20%)	5 (8%)
	41	Enoxaparin, 30 mg SC q12h	35 (65%)	0 (0%)	4 (6%)
Hull	317	Logiparin, 75 IU/kg qd	116 (37%)	20 (7%)	14 (4%)
	324	Warfarin, INR 2–3	154 (48%)	34 (11%)	8 (2%)
RD heparin	150	RD heparin, 50 IU/kg SC q12h	37 (25%)	9 (6%)	10 (6%)
	149	RD heparin, 90 IU/kg SC qd	41 (28%)	7 (5%)	11 (6%)
	147	Warfarin, INR 1.2–1.5	60 (41%)	15 (10%)	10 (6%)
Fractured Hip Repair					
Gerhart	131	Warfarin to maintain the prothrombin time at 1.5 times the control value after surgery	28 (21%)	7 (5%)	3 (2%)
	132	Lomoparin, 750 U SC q12h	9 (7%)	3 (2%)	5 (4%)
Bergqvist	146	Dextran, 50 mL IV qod before surgery, then 500 mL IV q24 h for 2 d	3 (29%)	10 (7%)	2 (1%)
	143	Lomoparin, 750 U SC q12h	14 (10%)	5 (4%)	5 (4%)

*All DVT confirmed by venography.

Bergqvist and coworkers[117] randomly assigned 289 patients to receive either lomoparin or dextran. The incidence of thrombosis was 10% in the lomoparin group and 29% in the dextran group. Interestingly, the dextran group required a significantly higher volume of transfused blood. Gerhart and associates[118] compared lomoparan with warfarin. Twenty-one percent of the patients in the warfarin group developed DVT compared to 7% of those in the lomoparan group.

In each of these studies, a significant reduction in the overall incidence of DVT and proximal thrombosis was demonstrated with LMWH prophylaxis (see Table 22-7). In addition, no increase in the incidence of bleeding was reported with these new agents.

NEW MECHANICAL DEVICES

Several mechanical devices used to prevent postoperative DVT have been reviewed in this chapter. These techniques are effective in reducing the incidence of thrombosis when they are applied appropriately and worn throughout the high-risk period. A new mechanical device has come under study for DVT prophylaxis in total hip replacement and total knee replacement.

In 1984, Gardner and colleagues[119] described a previously unrecognized physiologic pump mechanism in the sole of the foot that is activated by the flattening of the plantar arch that occurs with weight bearing. The arteriovenous impulse system foot pump (A-V Impulse System) was developed to perform this function. Fordyce and coworkers[120] randomly assigned 84 patients to treatment with either placebo or the A-V Impulse System. The incidence of DVT was 40% in the control group and 10% in the treated group. In a nonrandomized study of patients undergoing total knee arthroplasty, Wilson and associates[121] reported the incidence of DVT to be 50% in patients treated with the A-V Impulse System compared to 68.5% in those who received placebo therapy. Although it was not statistically significant, the incidence of proximal vein thrombosis was 17.8% in the treatment group versus 59.4% in the control group.

This new, easy to use mechanical device may prove to be effective in high-risk surgical fields such as orthopedics. Large-scale studies are necessary to assess its usefulness.

REFERENCES

1. Carter C, Gent M. The epidemiology of venous thrombosis. In: Colman R, Hirsh J, Marder V, Salzman E, eds. Hemostasis and thrombosis. Philadelphia, JB Lippincott, 1982:805–819.
2. Dismuke S, Wagner E. Pulmonary embolism as a cause of death: the changing mortality in hospitalized patients. JAMA 1986;255:2039–2042.
3. Anderson F, Wheeler H, Goldberg R, et al. A population based perspective of the hospital incidence and case fatality rate of deep vein thrombosis and pulmonary embolism: the Worchester DVT study. Arch Intern Med 1991;151:933–938.
4. Anderson F, Wheeler H, Goldberg R, et al. Physician practice in the prevention of venous thromboembolism. Ann Intern Med 1991;115:591–595.
5. Nicolaides A, Kakkar V, Renney J. Soleal sinuses and stasis. Br J Surg 1970;57:307.
6. Nicolaides A, Kakkar V, Field E, et al. Venous stasis and deep vein thrombosis. Br J Surg 1972;59:713–716.
7. Stamatakis J, Kakkar V, Sagar S, et al. Femoral vein thrombosis and total hip replacement. Br Med J 1977;112:223–225.
8. Clark C, Cotton L. Blood flow in deep veins of the legs: recording technique and evaluation of method to increase flow during operation. Br J Surg 1968;55:211–214.
9. Lindstrom B, Ahlman H, Jonsson O, et al. Blood flow in the calves during surgery. Acta Chir Scand 1977;143:335–339.
10. Linstrom B, Ahlman H, Jonsson O, et al. Influence of anesthesia on blood flow to the calves during surgery. Acta Anaesthesiol Scand 1984;28:201–203.
11. Johnson R, Carmichael J, Almond H, et al. Deep vein thrombosis following charneley arthroplasty. Clin Orthop 1978;132: 24–30.
12. Planes A, Vochelle N, Fagola M. Total hip replacement and deep vein thrombosis: a venographic and necropsy study. J Bone Joint Surg 1990;72B:9–13.
13. Stamatakis J, Kakkar V, Sagar S, et al. Femoral vein thrombosis and total hip replacement. Br Med J 1977;2:223–225.
14. Comerota A, Stewart G, Alburger P, et al. Operative venodilation: a previously unsuspected factor in the cause of postoperative deep vein thrombosis. Surgery 1989;106:301–309.
15. Schaub P, Lynch P, Stewart G. The response of canine veins to three types of abdominal surgery: a scanning and transmission electron microscope study. Surgery 1978;83:411–422.
16. Stewart G, Schaub R, Niewiarowske S. Products of tissue injury: their induction of venous endothelial damage and blood cell adhesion in the dog. Arch Pathol Lab Med 1980;104: 409–413.
17. Stewart G, Alburger P, Stone E, et al. Total hip replacement induces injury to remote veins in a canine model. J Bone Joint Surg 1983;65A:97–102.
18. Gitel S, Salvanti E, Wessler S, et al. The effect of total hip replacement and general surgery on antithrombin III in relation to venous thrombosis. J Bone Joint Surg 1979;61A:653–656.
19. Eriksson B, Eriksson E, Wessler S, et al. Thrombosis after hip replacement: relationship to the fibrinolytic system. Acta Orthop Scand 1989;60:159–163.
20. Kluft C, Verheijen J, Jie A, et al. The postoperative fibrinolytic shutdown: a rapidly reverting acute phase pattern for the fast acting inhibitor of tissue type plasminogen activator after trauma. Scand J Clin Lab Invest 1985;45:605–610.
21. D'Angelo A, Kluft C, Verheijen J, et al. Fibrinolytic shut down after surgery: impairment of the balance between tissue plasminogen activator and its specific inhibitors. Eur J Clin Invest 1985;15:308–312.
22. Salzman E, Hirsh J. Prevention of venous thromboembolism. In: Colman R, Hirsh J, Marder V, et al, eds. Hemostasis and thrombosis: basic principles of clinical practice. Philadelphia, JB Lippincott, 1987:986–999.
23. Hull R, Raskob G, Hirsh J. Prophylaxis of venous thromboembolism: an overview. Chest 1986;85:379–383.
24. Scurr J. How long after surgery does the risk of thromboembolism persist? Acta Chir Scand 1990;556:22–24.
25. Scurr J, Coleridge-Smith P, Hasty J. Deep vein thrombosis: a continuing problem. Br Med J 1988;297:28.
26. Paiement G, Wessinger S, Hughes R, et al. Routine use of adjusted low dose warfarin to prevent venous thromboembolism after hip replacement. J Bone Joint Surg 1993;75A: 893–898.
27. Lausen I, Jorgensen L, Jorgensen P, et al. Late occurring deep vein thrombosis following general surgery: incidence and prevention. Thromb Haemost 1993;69:1210.
28. Clagett G, Reisch J. Prevention of venous thromboembolism in general surgical patients: results of meta-analysis. Ann Surg 1988;208:227–239.
29. Hall J, McConahay D, Gibson D, et al. Heparin necrosis: an anticoagulation syndrome. JAMA 1980;244:1831–1832.
30. White P, Sadd J, Nensel R. Thrombotic complications of heparin therapy. Ann Surg 1979;190:595–608.
31. Hrushesky W. Subcutaneous heparin-induced thrombocytopenia. Arch Intern Med 1978;138:1489–1491.
32. Edes T, Edeste, Sunderrajan E. Heparin induced hyperkalemia. Arch Intern Med 1985;145:1070–1072.
33. Leyvraz P, Richard J, Bachmann F, et al. Adjusted versus fixed dose subcutaneous heparin in the prevention of DVT after total hip replacement. N Engl J Med 1983;309:954–958.
34. Leyvraz P, Bachman F, Vuilleumier B, et al. Adjusted subcutaneous heparin versus heparin plus dihydroergotamine in prevention of deep vein thrombosis after total hip arthroplasty. J Arthroplasty 1988;3:81–86.
35. Harris W, Salzman E, Athanasoulis C. Comparison of warfarin, low molecular weight dextran, aspirin, and subcutaneous heparin in prevention of venous thromboembolism following total hip replacement. J Bone Joint Surg 1974;56A:155–1562.
36. Francis C, Marder V, Evart C, et al. Two-step warfarin therapy: prevention of postoperative venous thrombosis without excessive bleeding. JAMA 1983;249:374–378.
37. Amstutz H, Friscia D, Dorey F, et al. Warfarin prophylaxis to prevent mortality from pulmonary embolism after total hip replacement. J Bone Joint Surg 1989;71A:321–326.
38. Goldhaber S, Morpurgo M, for the WHO/ISFC Task Force on

Pulmonary Embolism. Diagnosis, treatment, and prevention of pulmonary embolism. JAMA 1992;268:1727–1733.

39. Harris W, Athanasoulis C, Waltman A, et al. Dextran and external pneumatic compression compared with 1.2 or 0.3 gm of aspirin daily. J Bone Joint Surg 1985;67:57–62.

40. Kline A, Hughes L, Campbell H, et al. Dextran 70 in prophylaxis of thromboembolic disease after surgery: a clinically oriented randomized double blind trial. Br Med J 1975;2:109–112.

41. Francis C, Pellegrini V, Marder V, et al. Prevention of venous thrombosis after total hip arthroplasty: antithrombin III and low dose heparin compared with dextran 40. J Bone Joint Surg 1989;71A:327–335.

42. Caprini J, Scurr J, Hasty J. Role of compression modalities in a prophylactic program for deep vein thrombosis. Semin Thromb Hemost 1988;14:77–87.

43. Consensus Conference. Prevention of venous thrombosis and pulmonary embolism. JAMA 1986;256:744–749.

44. Hull R, Delmore J, Hirsh M, et al. Effectiveness of intermittent pulsatile elastic stockings for the prevention of calf and thigh vein thrombosis in patients undergoing elective knee surgery. Thromb Res 1979;16:37–45.

45. Collins R, Scrimogeour A, Yusuf S, et al. Reduction in fatal pulmonary embolism and venous thrombosis by perioperative administration of subcutaneous heparin: overview of results of randomized trials in general, orthopedic, and urologic surgery. N Engl J Med 1988;318:1162–1173.

46. Hull R, Raskob G, McLoughlin D, et al. Effectiveness of intermittent pneumatic leg compression for preventing deep vein thrombosis after total hip replacement. JAMA 1990;263:2313–2317.

47. Levine M, Hirsh J, Gent M, et al. Prevention of deep vein thrombosis after elective hip surgery: a randomized trial comparing low molecular weight heparin with standard unfractionated heparin. Ann Intern Med 1991;114:545–551.

48. Planes A, Vochelle N, Mazas F, et al. Prevention of postoperative venous thrombosis: a randomized trial comparing unfractionated heparin with low molecular weight heparin in patients undergoing total hip replacement. Thromb Haemost 1988;60:407–410.

49. Bailey J, Kruger M, Salano F, et al. Prospective randomized trial of sequential compression devices vs low-dose warfarin for deep venous thrombosis prophylaxis in total hip arthroplasty. J Arthroplasty 1991;6:S29–S35.

50. Francis C, Pellegrini V, Marder V, et al. Comparison of warfarin and external pneumatic compression in prevention of venous thrombosis after total hip replacement. JAMA 1992;267:2911–2915.

51. Gallus A, Raman K, Darby T. Venous thrombosis after elective hip replacement: the influence of preventive intermittent calf compression and of surgical technique. Br J Surg 1983;70:17–19.

52. Paiement G, Wessinger S, Waltman A, et al. Low dose warfarin versus external pneumatic compression against venous thromboembolism following total hip replacement. J Arthroplasty 1987;2:23–26.

53. Bergqvist E, Bergqvist D, Bronge A. An evaluation of early thrombosis prophylaxis following fracture of the femoral neck: a comparison between dextran and dicoumarol. Acta Chir Scand 1972;138:689.

54. Powers P, Bent M, Jay R, et al. A randomized trial of less intense postoperative warfarin or aspirin therapy in the prevention of venous thromboembolism after surgery for fractured hip. Arch Intern Med 1989;149:771–774.

55. Taberner D, Poller L, Thomson J, et al. Randomized study of adjusted versus fixed low dose heparin prophylaxis of deep vein thrombosis in hip surgery. Br J Surg 1989;76:933–935.

56. Cohen S, Ehrlich G, Kauffman M, et al. Thrombophlebitis following knee surgery. J Bone Joint Surg 1973;55A:106–112.

57. Lynch A, Bourne R, Rorabeck C, et al. Deep vein thrombosis and continuous passive motion after total knee arthroplasty. J Bone Joint Surg 1988;70A:11–14.

58. Stringer M, Steadman C, Hedges A, et al. Deep vein thrombosis after elective knee surgery: an incidence study in 312 patients. J Bone Joint Surg 1989;71B:492–497.

59. Stulberg B, Insall J, William G, et al. Deep vein thrombosis following total knee replacement: an analysis of six hundred and thirty-eight arthroplasties. J Bone Joint Surg 1984;66A:194–201.

60. Haas S, Insall J, Scuderi G, et al. Pneumatic sequential compression boots compared with aspirin prophylaxis of deep vein thrombosis after total knee arthroplasty. J Bone Joint Surg 1990;72A:27–31.

61. A multi-unit controlled trial. Heparin versus dextran in the prevention of deep vein thrombosis. Lancet 1974;11:118.

62. An international multi-center study. Prevention of fatal postoperative pulmonary embolism by low doses of heparin. Lancet 1975;11:45.

63. Gallus A, Hirsh J, O'Brien S, et al. Prevention of venous thrombosis with small subcutaneous doses of heparin. JAMA 1976;235:1980.

64. Groote-Schuur Hospital Thromboembolism Study Group. Failure of low dose heparin to prevent significant thromboembolic complications in high risk surgical patients: interim report of a prospective trial. Br Med J 1979;1:1447.

65. Multi-Center Trial Committee. DHE/heparin prophylaxis of postoperative DVT. JAMA 1984;251:2960–2966.

66. Turpie A, Gallus A, Beatties W, et al. Prevention of venous thrombosis in patients with intracranial disease by intermittent pneumatic compression of the calf. Neurology 1977;27:435–438.

67. Cerroto D, Ariano C, Fiacchino F. Deep vein thrombosis and low-dose heparin prophylaxis in neurosurgical patients. J Neurosurg 1978;49:378–381.

68. Joffe S. Incidence of postoperative deep vein thrombosis in neurosurgical patients. J Neurosurg 1975;42:201–203.

69. Skillman J, Collins R, Coe N, et al. Prevention of deep vein thrombosis in neurosurgical patients: a controlled, randomized trial of external pneumatic compression boots. Surgery 1978;83:354–358.

70. Black P, Crowell R, Abbott W. External pneumatic calf compression reduces deep venous thrombosis in patients with ruptured intracranial aneurysms. Neurosurgery 1986;18:25–28.

71. Valladares J, Hankinson J. Incidence of lower extremity deep vein thrombosis in neurosurgical patients. Neurosurgery 1980;6:138–141.

72. Constantini S, Kornowski R, Pomeranz S, et al. Thromboembolic phenomena in neurosurgical patients operated upon for

primary and metastatic brain tumors. Acta Neurochir (Wien) 1991;109:93–97.

73. Rossi E, Green D, Rosen J, et al. Sequential changes in factor VIII and platelets preceding deep vein thrombosis in patients with spinal cord injury. Br J Haematol 1980;45:143–151.

74. Merli G, Herbison G, Ditunno J, et al. Deep vein thrombosis: prophylaxis in acute spinal cord injured patients. Arch Phys Med Rehabil 1988;69:661–664.

75. Zelikovski A, Zucker G, Eliashiv A, et al. A new sequential pneumatic device for the prevention of deep vein thrombosis. J Neurosurg 1981;54:652–654.

76. Turpie A, Hirsh J, Gent M, et al. Prevention of deep vein thrombosis in potential neurosurgical patients: a randomized trial comparing graduated compression stockings alone or graduated compression stockings plus intermittent pneumatic compression with control. Arch Intern Med 1989;149: 679–681.

77. Bostrom S, Holmgren E, Jonsson O, et al. Post-operative thromboembolism in neurosurgery: a study on the prophylactic effect of calf muscle stimulation plus dextran compared to low dose heparin. Acta Neurochir (Wien) 1986;80:83–89.

78. Green D, Rossi E, Yao J, et al. Deep vein thrombosis in spinal cord injury: effects of prophylaxis with calf compression, aspirin, and dipyridamole. Paraplegia 1982;20:227–234.

79. Merli G, Crabbe S, Doyle L, et al. Mechanical plus pharmacological prophylaxis for deep vein thrombosis in acute spinal cord injury. Paraplegia 1992;30:558–562.

80. Bonnar J, Walsh J. Prevention of thrombosis after pelvic surgery by British dextran 70. Lancet 1972;1:614.

81. Walsh J, Bonnar J, Wright F. A study of pulmonary embolism and deep leg vein thrombosis after major gynecologic surgery using labelled fibrinogen-phlebography and lung scanning. J Obstet Gynaecol Br Comm 1974;81:311.

82. Taberner D, Poller L, Burslem R, et al. Oral anticoagulants controlled by the British comparative thromboplastin versus low heparin prophylaxis of DVT. Br Med J 1978;1:272.

83. Ballard R, Bradley-Watson P, Johnstone F, et al. Low doses of subcutaneous heparin in the prevention of DVT after gynecologic surgery. J Obstet Gynaecol Br Comm 1973;80:469.

84. Clarke-Pearson D, Colman R, Synan I, et al. Venous thromboembolism prophylaxis in gynecologic oncology: a prospective, controlled trial of low-dose heparin. Am J Obstet Gynecol 1983;145:606–613.

85. Crandon A, Koutts J. Incidence of postoperative deep vein thrombosis in gynecological oncology. Aust N Z J Obstet Gynaecol 1983;23:216–219.

86. Clarke-Pearson D, Creasman W, Colman R, et al. Perioperative external pneumatic compression as thromboembolism prophylaxis in gynecologic oncology. Gynecol Oncol 1984;18: 226–232.

87. Clarke-Pearson D, Synan I, Colman R, et al. The natural history of postoperative venous thrombolus in gynecologic oncology: a prospective study of 382 patients. Am J Obstet Gynecol 1984;148:1051–1054.

88. Clarke-Pearson D, DeLong E, Synan I, et al. A controlled trial of two low dose heparin regimens for the prevention of postoperative DVT. Obstet Gynecol 1990;75:684–689.

89. Clarke-Pearson D, Synan I, Dodge R, et al. A randomized trial of low dose heparin and intermittent pneumatic compression for the prevention of deep venous thrombosis after gynecologic oncology surgery. Am J Obstet Gynecol 1993;168: 1146–1154.

90. Mayo M, Hall T, Browse N. The incidence of deep vein thrombosis after prostatectomy. Br J Urol 1971;43:739–742.

91. Nicolaides A, Field E, Kakkar V, et al. Prostatectomy and deep vein thrombosis. Br J Surg 1972;50:487.

92. Van Arsdalen K, Barnes R, Clarke G, et al. Deep vein thrombosis and prostatectomy. Urology 1983;21:461–463.

93. Becker J, Borgstrom S, Salzman C. Occurrence and course of thrombosis following prostatectomy: a phlebographic investigation. Acta Radiol Diagn 1970;10:513.

94. Becker J, Borgstrom S. Incidence of thrombosis associated with epsilon-aminocaproic acid administration and with combined epsilon-aminocaproic acid and subcutaneous heparin therapy. Acta Chir Scand 1968;134:343.

95. Gordon-Smith I, Hickman J, Masri S. The effects of the fibrinolytic inhibitors epsilon-aminocaproic acid on the incidence of deep vein thrombosis after prostatectomy. Br J Surg 1972;59: 522–524.

96. Nicolaides A, Fernandes J, Pollock A. Intermittent sequential pneumatic compression of the legs in the prevention of venous stasis and postoperative deep vein thrombosis. Surgery 1980;87: 69–76.

97. Rosenberg I, Evans M, Pollock A. Prophylaxis of postoperative leg vein thrombosis by low dose subcutaneous heparin or preoperative calf muscle stimulation: a controlled clinical trial. Br Med J 1975;1:649.

98. Coe N, Collins R, Klein L, et al. Prevention of deep vein thrombosis in urological patients: a controlled, randomized trial of low dose heparin and external pneumatic compression boots. Surgery 1978;83:230–234.

99. Salzman E, Ploetz J, Bettmann M, et al. Intra-operative external pneumatic calf compression to afford longer term prophylaxis against deep vein thrombosis in urologic surgery. Surgery 1980;87:239–242.

100. Hansberry K, Thompson I, Bauman J, et al. A prospective comparison of thromboembolic stockings, external sequential pneumatic compression stockings and heparin sodium/dihydroergotamine mesylate for the prevention of thromboembolic complications in urological surgery. J Urol 1991;145:1205–1208.

101. Chandhoke P, Gooding G, Narayan P. Prospective randomized trial of warfarin and intermittent pneumatic leg compression as prophylaxis for postoperative deep venous thrombosis in major urological surgery. J Urol 1992;147:1056–1059.

102. Vandendris M, Kutnowski M, Futeral B. Prevention of postoperative deep vein thrombosis by low-dose heparin in open prostatectomy. Urol Res 1980;8:219–222.

103. Carter C, Kelton J, Hirsh J, et al. The relationship between the hemorrhagic and antithrombotic properties of low molecular weight heparins and heparin. Blood 1982;59:1239.

104. Hirsh J, Levine M. Low molecular weight heparin. Blood 1992;79:1–17.

105. Rosenberg R. The heparin-antithrombin system: a natural anticoagulant mechanism. In: Colman R, Hirsh J, Marder V, Salzman E, eds. Hemostasis and thrombosis: basic principles and clinical practice, ed 2. Philadelphia, JB Lippincott, 1987: 1373.

106. Lane D. Heparin binding and neutralizing protein. In: Lane D, Lindahl U, eds. Heparin, chemical and biological properties, clinical applications. London, Edward Arnold, 1989:363.

107. European Fraxiparin Study Group. A comparison of a low molecular weight heparin and unfractionated heparin for the prevention of deep vein thrombosis in patients undergoing abdominal surgery. Br J Surg 1988;75:1058.

108. Bergqvist D, Matzsch T, Burmark U, et al. Low molecular weight heparin given the evening before surgery compared with conventional low dose heparin in prevention of thrombosis. Br J Surg 1988;75:885.

109. Leizorovicz A, Picolet H, Peyrieux J. Prevention of postoperative deep vein thrombosis in general surgery: a multi-center double-blind study comparing two doses of logiparin and standard heparin. Br J Surg 1991;78:412.

110. Samama M, Bernard P, Bonnardot J, et al. Low molecular weight heparin compared with unfractionated heparin in prevention of postoperative thrombosis. Br J Surg 1988;75:128.

111. Nurmohamed M, Rosendaal F, Buller H, et al. Low molecular heparin versus standard heparin in general and orthopedic surgery: a meta-analysis. Lancet 1992;340:152–156.

112. Turpie A, Levine M, Hirsh J, et al. A randomized controlled trial of a low molecular weight heparin (enoxaparin) to prevent deep vein thrombosis in patients undergoing elective hip surgery. N Engl J Med 1986;315:925.

113. Hoek J, Nurmohamed M, ten Cate H, et al. Prevention of deep vein thrombosis following total hip replacement by a low molecular weight heparinoid. Thromb Haemost 1989;62: 1637.

114. Le Clerc J, Desjardins L, Geerds W, et al. A randomized trial of enoxaparin for the prevention of deep vein thrombosis after major knee surgery. Thromb Haemost 1991;65:753.

115. Hull R, Raskob G, Pineo G, et al. Low molecular weight heparin compared with less intense warfarin prophylaxis against venous thromboembolism following total knee replacement. Blood 1992;Suppl 1:167a.

116. The RD Heparin Arthroplasty Group. RD heparin versus warfarin in the prevention of venous thromboembolic disease following total hip or knee arthroplasty. Blood 1991;78(Suppl): 187a.

117. Bergqvist D, Kettunen K, Fredin H, et al. Thromboprophylaxis in hip fracture patients: a prospective comparative study between ORG 10172 and dextran. Surgery 1991;109:617.

118. Gerhart T, Yett H, Robertson L, et al. Low molecular weight heparinoid compared with warfarin for prophylaxis of deep vein thrombosis in patients who are operated on for fracture of the hip. J Bone Joint Surg 1991;73A:494–502.

119. Gardner A, Fox R. The venous pump of the human foot: a preliminary report. Bristol Med Chir J 1983;98:109–114.

120. Fordyce M, Ling R. A venous foot pump reduces thrombosis after total hip replacement. J Bone Joint Surg 1992;74B:45–49.

121. Wilson N, Das S, Kakkar V, et al. Thrombo-embolic prophylaxis in total knee replacement: evaluation of the A-V impulse system. J Bone Joint Surg 1992;74B:50–52.

Medical Management of the Surgical Patient, Third Edition,
edited by Michael F. Lubin, H. Kenneth Walker, and Robert B. Smith III.
J.B. Lippincott Company, Philadelphia, PA © 1995.

CHAPTER

23

HEMATOLOGIC MALIGNANCIES

John R. Wingard
Thomas E. Seay
Steven M. Devine

The hematologic malignancies are a heterogeneous group of malignant disorders that affect cells originating from bone marrow or lymphatic tissue.[1] The leukemias and multiple myeloma are systemic diseases and surgery plays only a minor role in their diagnosis, staging, and therapy (Tables 23-1 and 23-2). Biopsy of localized masses is occasionally required for diagnostic purposes. Chemotherapy is the mainstay of treatment. Measures such as surgical excision or radiotherapy are reserved for control of local complications. Splenectomy is occasionally performed to treat hypersplenism and is one therapeutic option for hairy-cell leukemia.

Hodgkin's disease and non-Hodgkin's lymphomas initially spread through the lymphatic system before becoming systemic. An excisional lymph node biopsy is the keystone for establishing the diagnosis in these conditions. Historically, staging laparotomy has been crucial in delineating the spread of lymphomas. Laparotomy is less commonly used today; however, appropriate management decisions depend on adequate surgical staging in selected patients with Hodgkin's disease.

Rarely, a hematologic malignancy may present with common surgical problems such as appendicitis; cholecystitis; or bowel, ureteral, or prostatic obstruction. These result from infiltration of the respective organ by malignant cells, creating obstruction followed by localized infection. These local infectious events can rapidly progress to generalized sepsis if patients have concomitant neutropenia from involved, dysfunctional bone marrow.

GENERAL ASPECTS OF THE DISEASES

ACUTE MYELOGENOUS LEUKEMIA

Leukemia is a malignant disease of the hematopoietic system in which a somatic mutation occurs in a bone marrow progenitor cell, followed by unrestrained clonal proliferation of the progeny of that altered cell. Leukemia constitutes about 10% of all cancers in adults. The leukemias are broadly divided into acute leukemias, which can progress if they are not treated and cause death in a matter of weeks to several months, and chronic leukemias, which have a more indolent course, with survival extending from months to years.

The myeloid leukemias originate in early progenitors at some point along the pathway of differentiation into not only myeloid, but also monocytoid, megakaryocytic, and, occasionally, erythroid cells. Although acute myelogenous leukemia is seen in all decades of life, its incidence increases in persons older than 40 years and it is the most common form of acute leukemia in adults. Classification of acute my-

TABLE 23–1. Role of Surgery in the Evaluation of Hematologic Malignancies

Purpose	Procedure	Disease
Diagnosis	Excisional lymph node biopsy	Hodgkin's disease, non-Hodgkin's lymphoma
	Biopsy of mass of uncertain etiology	Chloromas (acute myelogenous leukemia)
		Plasmacytomas (multiple myeloma)
Staging evaluation	Laparotomy	Hodgkin's disease
Evaluation of treatment response	Biopsy of lymph nodes or residual masses	Hodgkin's disease, non-Hodgkin's lymphona

elogenous leukemia is based on the differentiation stage of the progenitor cell in which the malignant change has occurred, and the French-American-British (FAB) system is used most commonly, according to morphology and differentiation of the leukemic blasts.[2]

The clinical manifestations at presentation often are non-specific and constitutional in nature, although symptoms attributable to anemia, thrombocytopenia, and infection are also common. Physical findings may include pallor, petechiae, and splenomegaly in about 40% of cases; gum hypertrophy in some cases; chloromas (localized tumors of leukemic blasts that can occur in the skin and, rarely, other organs) in occasional cases; and involvement of the leptomeninges in a few cases.

Diagnostic procedures include a complete blood count with differential and examination of the blood smear. A bone marrow aspirate and biopsy are essential for the diagnosis. Cytogenetic and immunophenotypic testing and his-

tochemical staining are necessary to confirm the type of leukemic blasts and classify the disease. A lumbar puncture with cytologic examination of the cerebrospinal fluid is performed to determine whether leptomeningeal involvement is present. Biochemical assessment is important because hyperuricemia, hypokalemia, hyperkalemia, lactic acidosis, and, occasionally, other electrolyte abnormalities may occur.[3] The electrolyte disturbances may become exaggerated once therapy is begun, as leukemic cells are destroyed and their contents are released into the circulation. Some subclasses of acute nonlymphocytic leukemia (FAB M4, M5) are noted for resulting in extreme potassium wasting because of lysozymal damage to the proximal tubule of the kidney,[4] but the potassium level may also be increased because of massive cellular breakdown and preexisting or concurrent renal damage. Spurious laboratory abnormalities may be seen occasionally with large numbers of circulating leukemic blasts (eg, hypoglycemia, hyperkalemia,

TABLE 23–2. Role of Surgery in the Management of Hematologic Malignancies

Purpose	Procedure	Disease
Treatment	Splenectomy	Hypersplenism, HCL
	Gastric or intestinal resection	NHL primary to the gastrointestinal tract
Venous access	Insertion of central venous catheter	Various
Management of complications		
Typhlitis, bowel infarction	Intestinal resection	AML, ALL during aplasia
Spinal cord compression	Laminectomy	Epidural mass from HD, NHL, MM, or vertebral collapse
Pathologic bone fracture	Orthopedic pinning and stabilization	MM
Bone marrow transplantation	Bone marrow harvest	AML, ALL, CML, MM, HD, NHL, MDS

HD, Hodgkin's disease; NHL, non-Hodgkin's lymphoma; HCL, hairy-cell leukemia; AML, acute myelogenous leukemia; ALL, acute lymphocytic leukemia; MM, multiple myeloma; CML, chronic myelogenous leukemia; MDS, myelodysplastic syndrome.

and hypoxemia may result from ex vivo metabolic activity of the blasts if there is a delay between the time of collection of blood specimens and their laboratory testing).[5,6]

Coagulation parameters should be assessed because disseminated intravascular coagulopathy (DIC) can occur to some degree in either acute or chronic forms in most patients with leukemia.[7,8] The release of coagulation activation agents contained in myelogenous leukemic blasts is thought to cause DIC in acute leukemia. Various activators are reported, such as urokinase-type or tissue-type plasminogen activators,[9,10] elastase-type proteolytic enzymes that have direct fibrinolytic or plasminogen activator activity,[11] direct procoagulant enzymes,[12,13] and lymphokines that mediate coagulation through endothelial cells.[14] DIC is frequently associated with promyelocytic leukemia (FAB class M3) and less commonly accompanies other classes of leukemia, especially myelomonocytic leukemia (FAB class M4). DIC should be evaluated at the time of diagnosis and before any planned procedure is undertaken. Replacement of coagulation factors, use of low-dose heparin, or administration of antithrombin III should be considered to return coagulation parameters to normal before an invasive procedure is attempted. Elective surgical procedures should be postponed until coagulation parameters have returned to normal, and emergent procedures should be done with the assistance of a specialist familiar with the management of coagulopathies. Cytoreductive therapy for leukemia is likely to exacerbate any preexisting DIC, or may precipitate acute DIC.[15]

When the number of circulating blasts is high (exceeding 50,000 cells/μL), leukostasis can result from the occlusion of small blood vessels by aggregations of blasts and from the infiltration of tissues; this can lead to alterations in cerebral function or hypoxemia with rapid deterioration if it is not treated promptly. Acute intracranial hemorrhage may result from cerebral leukostasis, and rarely may be a presenting problem to the neurosurgery service. Intracranial bleeding can be exacerbated by preexisting DIC, and widespread thrombosis and DIC may result from the release of tissue factors from damaged brain tissue.[16] The prognosis in such cases is extremely grim.

Vascular access is a critical issue before the institution of therapy. Multiple lines are required to administer chemotherapy, antibiotics, and other medications, as well as blood products, all of which are vital supportive care components. An external catheter such as a double-lumen or triple-lumen Hickman catheter is greatly preferred over an implantable injection port such as a Port-A-Cath because continuous access is usually necessary.

Treatment should be initiated promptly as soon as the diagnosis is confirmed. Hyperuricemia may be precipitated by therapy because of lysis of leukemic blasts; thus, allopurinol administration, hydration, and vigorous diuresis should be initiated before chemotherapy. Agents that are particularly useful for induction cytoreductive therapy include an antimetabolite, especially cytarabine, in combination with an anthracycline, such as daunorubicin, doxorubicin, idarubicin, or mitoxantrone. Chemotherapy causes marrow aplasia, and antibiotics and transfusion support therapy are necessary until normal marrow function is recovered, typically after several weeks. Once remission is achieved, one to three additional intensive chemotherapy courses usually are given, or patients are offered bone marrow transplantation to provide an optimal chance for converting the remission into a cure.[17]

ACUTE LYMPHOBLASTIC LEUKEMIA

Acute lymphoblastic leukemia is the most common malignancy in children, as well as the most common form of acute leukemia in children. It is much less common in adults, representing about 25% of the leukemias in adults. As with acute myelogenous leukemia, the clinical presentation is frequently nonspecific and includes fatigue, malaise, and symptoms associated with anemia, thrombocytopenia, or infection. Physical findings may include pallor, petechiae, hepatosplenomegaly, and lymphadenopathy. Involvement of the leptomeninges is more common than with acute myelogenous leukemia.

Evaluation should include complete blood count determination, examination of the blood smear, bone marrow aspiration and biopsy, and immunophenotypic and cytogenetic analyses. Histochemical stains are a useful adjunct to distinguish lymphoblasts from myeloblasts. Metabolic abnormalities, especially hyperuricemia, are noted occasionally. Untreated, patients develop life-threatening complications from the accumulation of excess leukemic blasts, replacement of normal tissues, and failure of bone marrow.

After evaluation, chemotherapy should be initiated promptly. Prednisone, vincristine, L-asparaginase, doxorubicin, methotrexate and 6-mercaptopurine, cytarabine, and cyclophosphamide are used frequently in various combinations and schedules. Allopurinol administration and adequate hydration with forced diuresis should be initiated before chemotherapy to prevent exacerbation of hyperuricemia. If the number of circulating blasts is high, a tumor lysis syndrome can occur, resulting in hyperphosphatemia, hyperuricemia, hyperkalemia, hypomagnesemia, hypocalcemia, and acidosis; these electrolyte disturbances can lead to life-threatening cardiac arrhythmias or acute renal failure. Careful monitoring of the metabolic status is important, with prompt correction of any electrolyte disturbances that develop. If acute renal failure occurs, early dialysis may be necessary until the tumor lysis syndrome and resulting renal damage resolves. After complete remission is achieved, generally within 4 to 6 weeks after the initiation of therapy, multiple courses of consolidation and maintenance therapy are given and bone marrow transplantation is considered to provide optimal long-term control.

CHRONIC MYELOGENOUS LEUKEMIA

Chronic myelogenous leukemia is uncommon in children. In adults, it increases in frequency with age and peaks at 50 to 60 years. The diagnosis frequently is made incidentally when a complete blood count is obtained for other reasons, and patients may be asymptomatic at the time of diagnosis or have only vague constitutional symptoms. The disease typically presents in a chronic phase and has an indolent course, but about 20% of cases progress to an accelerated phase within the first year after diagnosis and 15% accelerate during each subsequent year. Thus, the average survival is 3 to 4 years. The accelerated phase or blast crisis is similar in nature to the manifestations and tempo of progression of acute leukemia. On physical examination, splenomegaly is noted frequently. Hepatomegaly and lymphadenopathy are less common.

Diagnostic evaluation should include complete blood count determination, examination of the peripheral blood smear, bone marrow aspiration and biopsy, cytogenetic examination, and assessment of the leukocyte alkaline phosphatase (which typically is markedly reduced). The Philadelphia chromosome (a translocation between chromosomes 9 and 22) is diagnostic and present in about 90% of patients.

Treatment of the chronic phase is directed toward control of leukocytosis or symptomatic splenomegaly and can generally be effected with hydroxyurea, busulfan, or α-interferon. Once the accelerated phase or blast crisis occurs, more aggressive chemotherapy can be offered, although it frequently fails to reestablish the chronic phase. Splenectomy has not been shown to appreciably alter the prognosis and should not be routinely performed. If discomfort, infarction, or hypersplenism occurs, however, and cannot be controlled by medical measures, splenectomy can provide effective palliation. Allogeneic bone marrow transplantation should be considered early after diagnosis because it offers the only chance for cure.[18]

CHRONIC LYMPHOCYTIC LEUKEMIA

Chronic lymphocytic leukemia, like chronic myelogenous leukemia, is rare in children but increases in frequency with successive decades in adults. The condition is often detected incidentally through a complete blood count performed at a time when patients are asymptomatic. Symptoms initially tend to be constitutional and nonspecific. Infections, especially pneumonia, can be initial presenting events. Lymphadenopathy and splenomegaly are the most frequent physical findings. Nodular skin infiltrates can occur occasionally, especially in T-cell types of chronic lymphocytic leukemia.

The diagnosis is made through evaluation of the complete blood count, examination of the peripheral blood smear, aspiration of bone marrow, and assessment of biopsy samples. Hypogammaglobulinemia can occur; patients occasionally may have monoclonal immunoglobulins (which are detected by serum protein electrophoresis). Red blood cell autoantibodies sometimes are present, producing positive results on a Coombs' test, with a resultant hemolytic anemia. Autoimmune thrombocytopenia can also occur on occasion.

Staging takes into consideration the absence or presence of lymphadenopathy or splenomegaly (early to intermediate stages) or anemia or thrombocytopenia (advanced stages).[19] The course is generally indolent, with survival of 10 to 12 years in patients with early stage disease but only 2 to 4 years in those with advanced disease.[20] Treatment is directed toward controlling leukocytosis, symptomatic lymphadenopathy, splenomegaly, or bone marrow displacement. Agents such as chlorambucil, cyclophosphamide, and corticosteroids are used most commonly. Occasionally, radiotherapy delivered to localized masses of lymphoid tissue may be useful. Splenectomy may be helpful if autoimmune thrombocytopenia or hemolytic anemia is not controlled by medical measures.

HAIRY-CELL LEUKEMIA

Hairy-cell leukemia is an uncommon form of leukemia that is manifest most often by pancytopenia and splenomegaly. The diagnosis is confirmed by the identification of cells with villous cytoplasmic projections, so-called hairy cells. These cells have a tartrate-resistant acid phosphate isoenzyme; its presence is demonstrated by histochemical staining and confirms the diagnosis. The disease has a prolonged, indolent course. In the past, splenectomy was commonly used to control cytopenias (by correcting hypersplenism). Over the last few years, however, several agents, such as α-interferon, pentostatin, and especially 2-chlorodeoxyadenosine, have been used and appear to be highly effective. Thus, splenectomy may soon be relegated to a salvage therapeutic option when medical measures fail. Patients who derive greatest benefit from splenectomy are those whose bone marrow cellularity is under 85% and whose platelet count is 60,000/μL or higher.[21] Patients with marrow cellularity exceeding 85% should not be considered for splenectomy as initial therapy.

MYELODYSPLASTIC SYNDROME

Myelodysplastic syndrome, sometimes referred to as *preleukemia,* includes several entities characterized by cytopenias, especially anemia, which often terminate after months to years in acute myeloblastic leukemia.[22] The clinical manifestations include constitutional symptoms or symptoms related to anemia or other cytopenias. The diagnosis sometimes is made in asymptomatic patients by abnormalities noted incidentally in complete blood counts performed for other indications. Generally, treatment is directed toward control of infection or transfusion support if necessary. The role of growth factors such as erythropoietin and granulocyte-macrophage colony-stimulating factor is being investigated. The development of progressive cytopenias, trilineage involvement, the presence of excessive numbers of blasts, and the presence of certain cytogenetic abnormalities confer a grave prognosis.[23] Patients with adverse prognostic factors should be considered for bone marrow transplantation, which can be curative in some cases.

MULTIPLE MYELOMA

Multiple myeloma is a malignant proliferation of plasma cells. It occurs almost exclusively in adults, with more than 90% of cases occurring in patients older than 40 years. Its most common presenting manifestation is bone pain, especially in the lower back, caused by osteopenia, lytic bone lesions, or vertebral fractures. Pathologic bone fractures can occur in many sites but are especially common in the vertebral column. A hypoplastic anemia leading to fatigue is often present at diagnosis. Repeated infections, especially from pneumococci; hypercalcemia; coagulopathy; or carpal tunnel syndrome from deposition of amyloid may also occur and be presenting features.

Evaluation should include assessment of the complete blood count; serum and urinary protein electrophoresis; determination of serum calcium, uric acid, and creatinine levels; bone marrow aspiration and biopsy; and radiographic survey of the skeleton. Serum protein electrophoresis frequently reveals a monoclonal paraprotein that can be better characterized by immunoelectrophoresis. Paraproteins can also be excreted in the urine. Urinary excretion of light chains only results in the occurrence of Bence Jones proteinuria. Azotemia related to pyelonephritis, hypercalcemia, amyloidosis, or hyperuricemia can occur. Occasionally, localized infiltration of plasma cells can lead to plasmacytomas in soft tissues. Hyperviscosity resulting from a marked increase in paraprotein can occur and lead to "sludging" in capillaries, with purpura, retinal hemorrhages, papilledema, coronary ischemia, confusion, seizures, or vertigo. Interaction of the paraprotein with clotting factors can cause coagulopathy by several mechanisms.[24]

The diagnosis is confirmed in most cases by the results of bone marrow aspiration and biopsy, the detection of osteolytic lesions or osteopenia on radiographic bone survey, and the presence of a monoclonal paraprotein in the serum or urine on protein electrophoresis or immunofixation. Intravenous pyelography should not be used because it may precipitate renal failure, especially in association with dehydration.

Chemotherapy is generally used in patients with progressive disease or symptoms. Chemotherapy is not curative but can offer effective palliation of symptoms for prolonged intervals. Average survival ranges from 2 to 4 years but may be longer in some cases. Alkylating agents (eg, melphalan or cyclophosphamide) given alone or in combination with prednisone are used frequently.[25] Radiotherapy is used occasionally to relieve bone pain or prevent fractures from localized disease. Vigilant monitoring for infections, especially those caused by pneumococci, staphylococci, or streptococci, is important. Hypercalcemia should be vigorously managed with hydration, diuretics, or corticosteroids. Pathologic fractures may necessitate orthopedic pinning for restoration of limb function and symptomatic relief. Preoperative evaluation for coagulopathies and thrombotic potential is essential. Allogeneic bone marrow transplantation is curative in some patients when it is performed early during the course of the disease.[26]

HODGKIN'S DISEASE

Hodgkin's disease has a bimodal distribution of incidence, with peaks in early adulthood and later adulthood. The initial presentation typically is characterized by painless lymphadenopathy, especially in the cervical lymph nodes. Supradiaphragmatic lymph node involvement is present in about 90% of patients, with a subdiaphragmatic presentation being uncommon. Night sweats, pruritus, or weight loss (so-called "B" symptoms) may also accompany lymph node involvement. These symptoms represent adverse prognostic factors.

The diagnosis is made by excisional biopsy of a lymph node. Needle biopsy has limited value and should not be used. The largest, most central node in a group of enlarged nodes should generally be selected for biopsy. If multiple lymph node groups are enlarged, biopsy of cervical nodes is preferable to inguinal or axillary nodes because of lower morbidity and less chance of finding only nondiagnostic reactive changes.

The extent of disease involvement suggests the prognosis and guides appropriate therapy.[27–33] Stages I and II indicate the involvement of one or two lymph node groups, respectively, on the same side of the diaphragm. Stage III indicates the involvement of lymphatic tissue on both sides of the diaphragm. Stage IV indicates the involvement of other, nonlymphatic tissue such as bone marrow, liver, or other organs. After the diagnosis is made, additional tests should be performed, including computed tomographic (CT) scans of the chest, abdomen, and pelvis, as well as lymphangiography.[32] Bilateral bone marrow biopsies should be performed to look for marrow involvement.

Lymphangiography assesses the internal architecture of lymph nodes within the abdomen and is an important tool for detecting occult infradiaphragmatic involvement. It demonstrates retroperitoneal adenopathy in as many as 30% of patients with clinical stage I disease, 31% of those with clinical stage IIA disease, and 88% of those with clinical stage IIB disease. About 20% of these results prove to be false-negative at laparotomy.[33,34] Lymphangiography does not visualize certain lymph node groups well, such as high celiac, splenic, portal, and mesenteric lymph nodes. The CT scan can detect enlarged intraabdominal and intrapelvic nodes, which are considered to be suspicious if they exceed 1 cm in diameter and to be abnormal if they exceed 2 cm. Lymphangiography and CT scanning can provide complementary information. The CT scan can delineate lymph node groups that are poorly assessed by lymphangiography, and lymphangiography can detect abnormalities of normal-sized lymph nodes whose internal architecture is distorted by involvement by Hodgkin's disease. Compared to lymphangiography, however, CT scanning is less sensitive (80%), produces more false-positive results, and is more costly.[35]

Staging laparotomy used to be routinely advocated for all patients except those with stage IV disease detected on less invasive testing. Now, however, staging laparotomy is only routinely recommended in selected patients with clinical stage I, II, and IIIA disease, in whom treatment would be altered if the disease were up-staged.[36–39] Clinically normal spleens are pathologically involved in one third of cases. About 20% to 25% of patients with clinical stage IA disease are found to have occult intraabdominal disease at staging laparotomy. About 23% to 31% of patients with clinical stage IIA disease are found to have disease below the abdomen at staging laparotomy.[33] Conversely, 10% of patients are down-staged at laparotomy.[36]

Therapeutic approaches have evolved over the last two decades. In general, patients with stage I or II disease undergo surgical staging with laparotomy followed by extended-field radiotherapy. This results in a relapse-free survival rate of 70% to 80%. Several factors, such as systemic symptoms, bulky mediastinal disease, and contiguous extralymphatic extension, worsen the prognosis, and combined radiotherapy with chemotherapy is often advocated in these cases.[36,40] Patients with advanced Hodgkin's disease (stages III and IV) usually receive combination chemotherapy and have a relapse-free survival rate of about 50% at 10 years. The most commonly used regimens are ABVD (doxorubicin, bleomycin, vinblastine, and dicarbazine); MOPP (mechlorethamine, vincristine, prednisone, and procarbazine); or a hybrid of these. These regimens are administered cyclically over about 6 months.

If relapse occurs, salvage chemotherapy is often successful, producing a second remission. Cure can often be achieved in patients who have had a relapse after radiotherapy alone and in those who have undergone initial chemotherapy but had a first remission lasting longer than 12 months. For those with shorter remissions after chemotherapy, intensive salvage chemotherapy followed by bone marrow transplantation can lead to high rates of durable relapse-free survival.

Residual masses sometimes remain after initial radiotherapy or chemotherapy. In most instances, these represent scar rather than active disease.[41] Patients with residual masses do not need immediate biopsy but should be monitored closely over time (see later).

NON-HODGKIN'S LYMPHOMA

The peak incidence is later for non-Hodgkin's lymphoma than for Hodgkin's disease. The incidence climbs steadily from childhood to the age of 80 years. The signs and symptoms of non-Hodgkin's lymphoma are similar to those of Hodgkin's disease. Most patients seek medical attention because of lymphadenopathy. About 20% of patients experience constitutional symptoms.

Many histologic classifications have been proposed but the most widely used analysis is the working formulation.[42] This classification uses both the morphology of the lymphoma cells and the pattern of involvement in the lymph node (follicular or diffuse). There are three broad, general categories: low-grade, intermediate, and high-grade. These categories carry prognostic significance in that their prognosis for untreated disease often is years, months, and weeks, respectively.

The diagnosis of non-Hodgkin's lymphoma is made by excisional lymph node biopsy. Because histologic transformation can occur from the low-grade lymphomas to the intermediate lymphomas in about one third of instances, repeated biopsies are sometimes indicated, especially if the clinical picture changes.[43] In addition to a complete physical examination, a complete blood count; bone marrow biopsy; CT scans of the chest, abdomen, and pelvis; lumbar puncture; and, occasionally, lymphangiography should be performed.

The staging system is the same as that used in Hodgkin's disease. Laparotomy for staging purposes has not proved to be helpful and is not recommended. Involvement of extralymphatic tissue is more common in non-Hodgkin's lymphoma than in Hodgkin's disease and needle biopsy can be helpful in certain situations. The surgeon should collaborate closely with the pathologist to ensure that optimal samples are obtained for diagnostic purposes.

Therapy for the low-grade lymphomas should be tailored to the clinical course, with an emphasis on controlling manifestations of the disease. Because the median survival is about 8 years and the disease is not curable with aggressive therapy, the main goal of treatment is to control symptomatic disease. Radiotherapy to symptomatic lymphatic masses can provide effective local control. Single chemotherapeutic agents (eg, chlorambucil, fludarabine, pentastatin) or combination chemotherapy (eg, cyclophosphamide, vincristine, doxorubicin, prednisone) can be used to control more extensive lymph node involvement. Lymphoma primary to the gastrointestinal tract occasionally occurs; surgical resection can be useful to prevent or control perforation or bleeding.[44] Chemotherapy or radiotherapy often is provided as adjunctive therapy.

For intermediate and high-grade lymphomas, radiotherapy can be curative in patients with early stage disease.[45] In patients with more advanced disease, combination chemotherapy is the treatment of choice and cures can be effected in 30% to 50% of cases.[46–49] Several multiagent chemotherapy regimens are effective; CHOP (cyclophosphamide, doxorubicin, vincristine, and prednisone) is one commonly used regimen. Supportive measures before treatment include allopurinol administration and adequate hydration. Monitoring of biochemical parameters in patients with high-grade lymphomas is important because rapid tumor lysis can occur similar to that in acute leukemia therapy.[50]

Bone marrow transplantation can be curative as salvage therapy for relapsed intermediate or high-grade lymphomas. Its use is being investigated in low-grade lymphomas and as part of the initial treatment of certain intermediate and high-grade lymphomas with adverse prognostic factors.

PREOPERATIVE EVALUATION AND PERIOPERATIVE MANAGEMENT

In addition to the usual preoperative assessment, several unique features in patients with hematologic malignancies require consideration (Table 23-3).

The complete blood count requires close scrutiny because it is so commonly altered as part of the pathophysiology of hematologic malignancies. Anemia should be corrected to a hematocrit level of about 30%; typing and crossmatching should be performed before surgery whenever there is a possibility of blood loss during the operative procedure.

Neutropenia (a neutrophil count of less than 500/μL) places patients at risk for life-threatening infections, especially by gram-negative bacteria, *Candida,* and *Aspergillus* pathogens. Bacteremia or fungemia can be life-threatening and all patients with neutropenia should be monitored carefully for infection. Because the usual manifestations of infection are frequently masked by the body's inability to mount an inflammatory response, fevers in patients with neutropenia should be regarded as signs of infection until proven otherwise. Empiric antibiotic therapy is an important part of therapy for patients with fevers and neutropenia. Guidelines have been formulated for the treatment of such patients.[51]

Prompt initiation of intravenous antibiotic therapy at maximal therapeutic doses forms the cornerstone of empiric therapy for patients with neutropenia. Many antibiotics are available and have been used effectively in empiric regimens. In general, such coverage should provide a broad spectrum of activity against both gram-negative organisms such as *Pseudomonas aeruginosa* and gram-positive pathogens. No specific antibiotic or combination regimen is considered to be ideal. Before empiric therapy is initiated, patients must undergo prompt and thorough evaluations. Often, evidence of an inflammatory response to infection is absent. Nevertheless, a careful review of historical information and a complete physical examination is required. Particular attention should be paid to sites that are frequently infected or that serve as foci for the dissemination of infection, including the oropharyngeal mucosa (often damaged by chemotherapy), lungs, esophagus, paranasal sinuses, perirectal site, nail beds, and vascular access sites. Two sites of blood cultures, including one from a vascular access catheter if present, as well as cultures from the throat, urine, and stool should be obtained before antibiotics are administered. Chest radiography should be performed initially, in addition to CT studies of the paranasal sinuses or other sites that are suspected to harbor infection after a thorough review. The initial regimen may include single agents with broad-spectrum coverage, such as ceftazidime or imipenem, or combinations of aminoglycosides and antipseudomonal penicillins.[51–53] Such regimens may be equally efficacious, with response rates ranging from 65% to 88%. With the increased use of indwelling venous catheters, infections with gram-positive organisms that are resistant to methicillin have become prevalent and warrant consideration of the use of vancomycin in any initial empiric regimen.[54]

Fever may persist despite the use of appropriate broad-spectrum antibiotics. If patients continue to experience profound neutropenia (as commonly occurs after high-dose chemotherapy or bone marrow transplantation), the risk of fungal infection increases, as does the risk of infection by a bacterial pathogen that is resistant to the initial empiric regimen. Continued close evaluation to detect signs of occult infection and periodic repetition of the blood culture are important. Modification of the initial antibiotic regimen may be necessary to provide coverage for suspected gram-negative bacteria; knowledge of institution-specific antibiotic resistance patterns should be used to guide the choice of antibiotics. In patients with persistent or recurrent fevers, fungal species such as *Candida* and *Aspergillus* are the most common pathogens. Thus, fevers in patients with neutropenia that persist after 96 hours of therapy with broad-spectrum antibacterial regimens warrant the institution of antifungal therapy with amphotericin B. After a test dose, amphotericin B is administered at 0.5 mg/kg/d unless an invasive fungal infection such as *Aspergillus* has been documented that requires a higher dosage.

TABLE 23–3. Preoperative Evaluation: Special Considerations in Patient's With Hematologic Malignancies

Parameter	Concern	Intervention
Leukocyte count	Leukostasis (>50,000/μL)	Leukopheresis or chemotherapy
Neutrophil count	Infection if low (<500/μL)	Prophylactic/empiric antibiotic therapy
Hematocrit	Anemia	Transfusion to a hematocrit of 30% or more
Platelet count	Hemorrhage if low (<50,000/μL)	Platelet transfusion (preferably single-donor, irradiated)
Coagulation factors	Hemorrhage if disturbed (AML, MM)	
Prothrombin time	Prolonged (DIC or factor-deficient states)	Fresh frozen plasma, vitamin K, or specific factor deficiencies
Partial thromboplastin time	Prolonged (DIC or factor-deficient states)	Fresh frozen plasma, vitamin K, or specific factor deficiencies
Fibrinogen	↓ (DIC)	Cryoprecipitate
Fibrin split products	↑ (DIC)	Factor replacement, low-dose heparin, antithrombin III replacement
Hypercoagulable state	Thrombosis	May require heparin, thrombolytic therapy, or vena cava filter
Electrolyte balance	Disturbances with tumor lysis syndrome	
Potassium	↓ (Renal wasting)—arrhythmias	Replacement needed, quantities may be large
Potassium	↑ (Tumor lysis syndrome)—arrhythmias	Diuretics, hydration, dialysis*
Phosphate	↑ (Tumor lysis syndrome)	Amphojel, dialysis*
Calcium	↑ (Myeloma)—lethargy, nausea	Fluids, furosemide, calcitonin, diphosphonates, prednisone
Calcium	↓ (Tumor lysis syndrome)—tetany	Replacement
Magnesium	↓ (Renal tubular defect)	Replacement
Uric acid	Increased by disease (AML, ALL, MM) or its treatment (tumor lysis syndrome)	Allopurinol, hydration, vigorous diuresis
Hyperglycemia	Induced by corticosteroids	Insulin
Renal function and urine output	Impaired by tumor lysis syndrome, MM, hyperuricemia, or certain chemotherapeutic agents (eg, cisplatin, nitrosoureas)	Hydration, dialysis*
Thyroid function	Impaired after mantle irridation for HD	Thyroid hormone replacement*
Size of mediastinal mass	Anesthesia risk if massive; superior vena cava syndrome	Tumor reduction by chemotherapy or radiotherapy*
Pulmonary function	Certain chemotherapeutic agents (eg, bleomycin, busulfan) or irradiation to the thorax	*
Cardiac function	Certain chemotherapeutic agents (eg, anthracyclines)	*

*Requires appropriate subspecialty evaluation and treatment.
AML, acute myelogenous leukemia; MM, multiple myeloma; DIC, disseminated intravascular coagulopathy; ALL, acute lymphocytic leukemia; HD, Hodgkin's disease

The ultimate duration of antibiotic therapy depends on several factors, including the resolution of neutropenia, the resolution of all sites of infection, the eradication of any potential pathogen that may have been isolated, and the absence of any significant signs or symptoms suggesting infection.

Surgery should not be performed during episodes of neutropenia because of a high risk of infection and poor wound healing. Typhlitis, an infection of the intestinal mucosa, frequently by gram-negative or anaerobic bacteria, can be life-threatening and endanger viability of the bowel. Manifestations can include dilation of the ascending colon, guarding, rebound, and ileus. Pseudomembranous colitis is a rare complication of antibiotic therapy but also should be treated conservatively, even in the presence of toxic megacolon, if neutropenia and refractory thrombocytopenia are present. Surgical intervention in both these situations should be avoided if at all possible unless definite bowel infarction or perforation occurs.

Thrombocytopenia can place patients at risk for excessive blood loss during surgery. Generally, transfusions should be used to bring the platelet count up to at least 40,000 to 50,000/µL. The use of certain agents (eg, aspirin, some of the semisynthetic penicillins, nonsteroidal antiinflammatory agents) should be avoided to prevent impairment of platelet function.

DIC can occur de novo with some of the myeloid leukemias and be exacerbated by chemotherapy. Acquired hemostatic defects are frequently associated with dysproteinemias (eg, multiple myeloma, amyloidosis, and isolated gammopathies) and involve both coagulation proteins and platelets.[24] Prolonged bleeding and coagulopathy may occur through several mechanisms, including platelet dysfunction[55]; inhibition of fibrin polymerization[56]; direct inhibition of von Willebrand's factor and factor VIII[57]; accelerated clearance of coagulation proteins (factors V, VII, VIII, and X, prothrombin, protein C, and fibrinogen)[24]; direct binding of factor X[58]; production of heparin-like anticoagulants[59]; and pathologically excessive fibrinolysis.[60] Surgery should be postponed if possible until these complications are controlled.

Electrolyte disturbances are common in patients with hematologic malignancies and many of the chemotherapeutic regimens used exacerbate them. Tumor lysis syndrome can be precipitated by chemotherapy for rapidly proliferative malignancies, which can lead to life-threatening electrolyte disturbances and acute renal failure. Correction of electrolyte imbalances and maintenance of adequate urinary flow are important prerequisites for surgery. Hypercalcemia is an infrequent accompaniment of multiple myeloma and can be corrected by the administration of saline solution, furosemide, corticosteroids, calcitonin, and diphosphonates. Renal dysfunction is often encountered in multiple myeloma as a result of amyloidosis, pyelonephritis, hyperuricemia, or a combination of factors. Intravenous pyelography should not be performed because the dye can worsen marginal renal function, especially in patients who are dehydrated. Hyperuricemia or the tumor lysis syndrome can be precipitated by chemotherapy for acute leukemia.

Endocrine disturbances are possible. Corticosteroids can induce hyperglycemia. Hypothyroidism can be a late occurrence after mantle irradiation for Hodgkin's disease or non-Hodgkin's lymphoma. Because this can develop years later, evaluation of the thyroid status should be considered before surgery in patients who have previously received mantle irradiation.

Bulky mediastinal adenopathy can pose a risk to patients who are undergoing laparotomy because of difficulties in extubation, atelectasis, and pneumonia after operation.[61] Shrinkage of a bulky mass by chemotherapy or irradiation before surgery can be useful to reduce the hazard. Bulky retroperitoneal adenopathy can lead to ureteral obstruction, hydronephrosis, and acute renal failure. The placement of ureteral stents or performance of nephrostomy may be necessary in some cases to reestablish urinary flow until cytoreduction is accomplished.

Previous irradiation can impair small vessel integrity and vascularization of tissue may be compromised during surgery. Mantle or other thoracic irradiation can lead to pulmonary fibrosis and reduction in the ventilatory capacity. The use of pulmonary function tests should be considered in such patients. Reduced exercise tolerance resulting from impaired cardiac function and accelerated coronary atherosclerosis can occur years after patients undergo mantle irradiation. Therefore, evaluation of the ejection fraction can be useful in assessing cardiac function.

Numerous chemotherapeutic agents can impair organ function either briefly or permanently.[62] The anthracyclines (including doxorubicin and daunorubicin) have cumulative cardiac toxicity and can result in a cardiomyopathy. The risk correlates with the cumulative dose over time. Thus, ejection fractions should be evaluated in patients who have had previous anthracycline therapy. Bleomycin and high doses of busulfan and cyclophosphamide have cumulative pulmonary toxicities, resulting in a restrictive ventilatory pattern and reduced diffusion capacity. The risk is dose dependent. Assessment of the vital capacity, forced expiratory volume at 1 second, and diffusion capacity are useful guides to ventilatory impairment. Renal function can be impaired by agents such as cisplatin and the nitrosoureas. Neurologic function, especially of the peripheral nerves, can be impaired by vincristine. Severe vincristine toxicity can lead to a visceral neuropathy with functional ileus, which can mimic an acute intraabdominal crisis. This generally resolves over time with supportive care without surgical intervention.

SPECIAL SITUATIONS

AUTOLOGOUS BLOOD DONATION

The practice of donating one or more units of autologous red blood cells in anticipation of elective surgery has increased in recent years. Consideration of preoperative autologous donation should be an important part of preoperative planning. Such donation prevents transfusion reactions; avoids the transmission of infectious pathogens such as hepatitis, cytomegalovirus, and human immunodeficiency virus; and conserves the community blood supply. Because impairment of hemopoiesis is a common feature of hematologic malignancies, many patients have antecedent anemia caused by the disease process and cannot make donations; however, this should be considered in those who are candidates.[63,64] The procedure is safe in most patients, even those with other medical illnesses.[64] In one randomized, placebo-controlled trial, the administration of recombinant human erythropoietin was shown to increase the ability to donate blood in patients who were about to undergo elective surgery.[65] Erythropoietin was safe and prevented the development of anemia while it increased the volume of red blood cells that were collected before surgery. Even if preoperative blood donation is not possible, blood that is lost during surgery may be salvaged; technologic advances have improved the success of this technique.[63]

INDWELLING CENTRAL VENOUS CATHETERS

The placement of indwelling central venous catheters has made the treatment of patients with hematologic malignancies much easier in the last decade.[66] The need for frequent blood testing and multiple transfusions; the administration of repetitive doses of chemotherapeutic agents, many of which can sclerose peripheral blood vessels and surrounding tissues; the use of prolonged courses of parenteral antibiotics; and the need for parenteral nutritional support are some of the reasons these catheters are used. Many types of catheters are available. Some are implanted beneath the skin (eg, Port-A-Cath; Infuse-A-Port) and are particularly desirable because they require minimal care by patients.[67] This is particularly valuable in patients who are receiving relatively nonintensive but repetitive courses of chemotherapy for such conditions as Hodgkin's disease, non-Hodgkin's lymphoma, and multiple myeloma. Patients who are undergoing more intensive treatment, in whom neutropenia is profound or prolonged and frequent catheter access is necessary, require catheters with external ports (eg, Hickman or Groshong catheters). Such patients include those with acute leukemia and those who are undergoing bone marrow transplantation.

The catheter should be placed by an experienced clinician to reduce the risk of complications.[68] Platelet transfusions should be given to patients who have thrombocytopenia. After surgery, pressure dressings can be applied to minimize hemorrhage at the exit site or a hematoma within the catheter tunnel. Standard maintenance procedures are important to reduce complications.[69]

Complications of catheter placement can include pneumothorax, hemothorax, thrombosis, tunnel bleeding, incorrect placement of the catheter, and inadvertent arterial puncture.[68] Delayed complications can include infection (both at the entry site as well as bacteremia, especially by coagulase-negative staphylococci) and thrombosis of the superior vena cava or other central veins.[70] It is desirable to place an indwelling catheter promptly in patients with newly diagnosed acute leukemia so that one will be ready to manage vigorous fluid and electrolyte support and provide necessary transfusions. To minimize complications, however, catheters should not be placed during active systemic infections or while patients are in hypercoagulable states.

BONE MARROW HARVEST

Bone marrow transplantation has emerged as a major therapy for hematologic malignancies that cannot be controlled by conventional treatment regimens or for which prognostic factors indicate a high likelihood of failure with less intensive treatment regimens. An autologous unit of blood is collected 1 to 3 weeks before the procedure. Bone marrow stem cells are obtained by multiple needle punctures from the posterior iliac crest and occasionally from the anterior iliac crest and sternum.[71] The procedure is performed with the donor in the prone position using either general or epidural anesthesia. The number of cells obtained is generally between 2 and 5×10^8 per kilogram of ideal body weight. The volume of bone marrow mixed with blood that is removed usually ranges between 0.5 and 2 L. Although the blood volume can be substantial, the proportion of the total content of bone marrow stem cells removed is less than 10% of 1 day's normal production, and because of self-renewal, there are no permanent effects. After the cells are removed, they are filtered through fine wire meshes to remove bony spicules and fat globules that otherwise may lead to fat embolism. Then the cells are counted. If the donor and patient are ABO blood group incompatible, additional processing must be done to remove the red blood cells and plasma so that a blood transfusion reaction is not precipitated when the cells are administered. In the case of autologous bone marrow transplantation, the bone marrow frequently is treated ex vivo with either pharmacologic or immunologic maneuvers to try to reduce the number of contaminating tumor cells that may be present. The bone marrow progenitor cells are then cryopreserved for later use.

Bone marrow harvest is generally well tolerated; major risks are rare. Most patients experience discomfort at the puncture sites that lasts for several days to several weeks. There is a small risk of infection or hemorrhage at the needle puncture sites but these are minor complications and easily controlled with either pressure or antibiotics.[72]

STAGING LAPAROTOMY

Staging laparotomy should be performed by surgeons who are experienced in the procedure and should include careful attention to and sampling of multiple lymph node groups from paraaortic, iliac, celiac, mesenteric, portal, and splenic hilar nodes; biopsy of both lobes of the liver (wedge and needle); splenectomy; biopsy of any suspicious lymph nodes detected on lymphangiography and CT scanning; biopsy of the bilateral iliac crest bone marrow; placement of radiopaque markers at the splenic pedicle; biopsy of nodal sites and at margins of tumor masses; and oophoropexy in women of childbearing potential.

Staging laparotomy is generally well tolerated in young adults.[73–75] Perioperative mortality is about 0.5%. The morbidity is comparable to that encountered with other intraabdominal surgery. Small bowel obstruction is the most common major complication, occurring in under 1% of cases. Other major complications include pneumonia, pulmonary embolus, and wound dehiscence. Minor complications occur in 10% to 15% of patients and include wound infection, urinary tract infection, atelectasis, division of the lateral femoral cutaneous nerve, prolonged ileus, and pancreatitis. Laparotomy should not be performed in patients with bulky mediastinal masses because of excessive risk from airway obstruction during or after anesthesia.[61] Long-term complications include pneumococcal sepsis after splenectomy, the incidence of which approaches 10%.[76–78]

SPLENECTOMY

Complications of splenectomy include deep venous thrombosis, fever, pulmonary infection, pulmonary embolism, and ileus.[79] The removal of a massively enlarged spleen has been shown to be associated with higher rates of pneumonia, wound infection, and thromboembolism in some series but not in others.[80] Generally, significant morbidity is under 15% and mortality is under 5%.[81] Postoperative hemorrhage and pleural effusion are occasional complications.

In patients in whom splenectomy is planned, consideration should be given to the preoperative administration of pneumococcal vaccine because of the high risk for postoperative sepsis.[76–78] If possible, the vaccine should be administered at least 10 days before splenectomy to provide for optimal development of protective immunity.[78] If vaccination is not possible or fails to induce immunity, penicillin should be administered prophylactically.

EMERGENT SURGICAL INTERVENTION

The rare patients who require both immediate cytoreduction (eg, patients with impending leukostasis) and emergent surgical intervention present a special challenge. Preoperative pharmacologic cytoreduction may significantly increase the intraoperative and postoperative complications and complicate anesthetic management by worsening electrolyte abnormalities, renal function, or bleeding through the precipitation of acute tumor lysis syndrome or DIC. An alternate temporizing approach, mechanical cytoreduction by leukapheresis, can be performed rapidly in most major medical centers and facilitates the reduction of high blast counts with few complications, allowing patients to proceed to surgery in a timely fashion. Multiple sessions of leukopheresis can be performed in hemodynamically stable postoperative patients to allow some time for wound healing and recovery. Patients then may be given more definitive pharmacologic cytoreductive therapy once they are completely stable after operation.

RESIDUAL MASSES AFTER TREATMENT

About half of all patients with Hodgkin's disease have mediastinal adenopathy. After treatment, 64% to 88% of these patients have some residual mediastinal abnormality on radiographic examination. In nearly half this group, the remaining abnormality is substantial. With serial follow-up, most of these abnormalities return to normal without further intervention. Relapse rates do not appear to be any greater in the subset of patients with large residual masses. Most investigators suggest close observation in these cases; needle biopsy is not recommended because most biopsy specimens reveal only fibrosis. If gallium scanning reveals continued uptake within the mass, however, biopsy should be strongly considered because the likelihood of residual active disease is higher.[82,83]

Abdominal masses are detected in 30% to 50% of patients with aggressive non-Hodgkin's lymphoma. In as many as 40% of such cases, residual abdominal masses can be detected on CT scanning even after the administration of full-dose combination chemotherapy. The presence of residual abdominal masses in patients in whom all other evidence of disease has disappeared represents a substantial treatment dilemma for oncologists.[84] Repeated staging laparotomy or needle aspiration of such lesions is often considered to detect the persistence of active disease. Data from the National Cancer Institute, however, suggest that neither laparotomy nor needle biopsy is likely to detect residual disease in such instances. It is recommended that such masses be observed closely with radiography and that surgical exploration be deferred unless there is evidence that the lesion is enlarging.

PERIRECTAL INFECTIONS

Perirectal infections occur in about 4% to 10% of patients who undergo therapy for acute leukemia. Before the development of improved supportive care measures, such lesions were associated with high mortality rates, ranging from 45% to 78%. Physicians are frequently reluctant to drain these lesions because they are often nonfluctuant and may hemorrhage or heal poorly. Perirectal infections are characterized by perianal tenderness, edema, induration, and redness. Many patients have a previous history of rectal problems such as hemorrhoids or rectal fissures. Most lesions become clinically manifest within a week to 10 days after the onset of neutropenia, and are often preceded by fever and perirectal pain. Point tenderness and poorly delineated induration are the earliest signs, followed by erythema, increased tenderness, and widening induration. Many patients develop significant tissue necrosis, producing blue-black discoloration. If the problem progresses, further complications include fascial extension to involvement of the external genitalia and peritoneum. Some patients develop signs of peritonitis.

Blood culture results are positive in most patients with neutropenic perirectal infections and the presence of multiple organisms is common. *Escherichia coli* and *P aeruginosa* are the most commonly recovered organisms, although other enteric gram-negative bacilli and group D streptococci may be recovered.

Initial treatment is conservative and involves the administration of broad-spectrum antibiotics and analgesics as well as the use of local measures such as frequent sitz baths and warm compresses. Although spontaneous drainage often occurs within a week of the onset of infection, some patients develop increased induration and swelling. This is usually associated with persistent fever and breakthrough bacteremia in spite of the administration of antibiotics to which the organisms are susceptible. In these patients, surgical incision and débridement is justified and typically results in the resolution of symptoms within 4 to 7 days.[85] Diverting colostomy may be required only in those patients in whom persistent fecal soilage from rectal incontinence prevents wound healing.

Resolution of neutropenia is important to proper wound healing. If necessary, colony-stimulating factors can be administered to speed neutrophil recovery or granulocyte transfusions can be given if the infection does not respond to antimicrobial agents.

REFERENCES

1. Holleb AI, Fink DJ, Murphy GP. Textbook of clinical oncology, ed 1. Atlanta, American Cancer Society, 1991.
2. Bennett JM, Catovsky D, Daniel MT, et al. Proposed revised criteria for the classification of acute myeloid leukemia. Ann Intern Med 1985;103:620–629.
3. O'Regan S, Arson S, Chesney RW, et al. Electrolyte and acid-base disturbances in the management of leukemia. Blood 1977;49:345–354.
4. Osserman E, Lawlor D. Serum and urinary lysozyme (muramidase) in monocytic and monomyelocytic leukemia. J Exp Med 1966;124:921.
5. Hess CE, Nichols AB, Hunt WB, et al. Pseudohypoxemia secondary to leukemia and thrombocytosis. N Engl J Med 1979;301:361–363.
6. Salomon J. Spurious hypoglycemia and hyperkalemia in myelomonocytic leukemia. Am J Med Sci 1974;267:359–363.
7. Williams EC, Mosher DF. Disseminated intravascular coagulation. In: Hoffman R, Benz E, Shantil S, et al, eds. Hematology: basic principles and practice. New York, Churchill Livingstone, 1991:1394–1405.
8. Myers T, Rickles F, Bbarb C, Cronlund M. Fibrinopeptide A in acute leukemia: relationship of activation of blood coagulation to disease activity. Blood 1981;57:518.
9. Wilson EL, Jacobs P, Dowdle E. The secretion of plasminogen activators by human myeloid leukemic cells in vitro. Blood 1983;61:568.
10. Bennett B, Booth N, Croll A, Dawson A. The bleeding disorder in acute promyelocytic leukemia: fibrinolysis due to u-PA rather than defibrination. Br J Haematol 1988;71:511.
11. Eckhardt T, Koch M. Fibrinogen-proteolysis in acute myelogenous leukemia. Blut 1986;53:39.
12. Andoh K, Kubota T, Takada M, et al. Tissue factor activity in leukemic cells: special reference to disseminated intravascular coagulation. Cancer 1987;59:748.
13. Falanga A, Alessio M, Donati M, Barbui T. A new procoagulant in acute leukemia. Blood 1988;71:870.
14. Cozzolino F, Torcia M, Miliani A, et al. Potential role of interleukin-1 as the trigger for diffuse intravascular coagulation in acute nonlymphoblastic leukemia. Am J Med 1988;84:240.
15. Goldberg M. Is heparin administration necessary during induction chemotherapy for patients with acute promyelocytic leukemia? Blood 1987;69:187–191.
16. Drake T, Morrissey J, Edgington T. Selective cellular expression of tissue factor in human tissues: implications for disorders of hemostasis and thrombosis. Am J Pathol 1989;134:1087.
17. Champlin R. Bone marrow transplantation for acute leukemia: recent advances and comparison with alternative therapies. Semin Hematol 1987;24:55–67.

18. Thomas ED. Indications for marrow transplantation in chronic myelogenous leukemia. Blood 1989;73:861–864.

19. Binet J. Chronic lymphocytic leukemia: proposals for a revised prognostic staging system. Br J Haematol 1981;48:356–367.

20. Binet J. Effectiveness of "CHOP" regimen in advanced untreated chronic lymphocytic leukemia. Lancet 1986;1:1346–1349.

21. Ratain MJ, Vordman JW, Barker CM, et al. Prognostic variables in hairy cell leukemia after splenectomy as initial therapy. Cancer 1988;62:2420–2424.

22. Vallespie T, Torrabadella M, Julia A, et al. Myelodysplastic syndromes: a study of 101 cases according to the FAB classification. Br J Haematol 1985;61:83.

23. Kerhofs H, Hermans J, Haak HL, Leeksma CHW. Utility of the FAB classification for myelodysplastic syndromes: investigation of prognostic factors in 237 cases. Br J Haematol 1987;65:73.

24. Leibman H. Hemostatic defects associated with dysproteinemias. In: Hoffman R, Benz E, Shantil S, et al, eds. Hematology: basic principles and practice. New York, Churchill Livingstone, 1991:1406–1409.

25. Camba L, Durie BGM. Multiple myeloma: new treatment options. Drugs 1992;44:170–181.

26. Gahrton G, Tura S, Ljungman P, et al. Allogeneic bone marrow transplantation in multiple myeloma. N Engl J Med 1991;325:1267.

27. Lister TA, Crowther D, Sutcliffe SB, et al. Report of a committee convened to discuss the evaluation and staging of patients with Hodgkin's disease. J Clin Oncol 1989;7:1630.

28. Carbone PP, Kaplan HS, Mushoff K, et al. Report of the Committee on Hodgkin's Disease Staging Classification. Cancer Res 1971;31:1860–1861.

29. Jones SE. Importance of staging in Hodgkin's disease. Semin Oncol 1980;7:126–135.

30. Bennett JM, ed. Lymphomas I. Boston, Martinus Nijhoff, 1981.

31. Jones SE. Importance of staging in Hodgkin's disease. Semin Oncol 1980;7:126–135.

32. Lister TA, Crowther D, Sutcliffe SB, et al. Report of a committee convened to discuss the evaluation and staging of patients with Hodgkin's disease: Cotswolds meeting. J Clin Oncol 1989;7:1630–1636.

33. Moormeir JA, Williams SF, Golomb HM. The staging of Hodgkin's disease. Hematol Oncol Clin North Am 1989;3:237.

34. DeLaney TF, Glatstein E. The role of the staging laparotomy in the management of Hodgkin's disease. In: DeVita VT Jr, Hellman S, Rosenberg SA, eds. Cancer: principles and practice of oncology, ed 2, vol 1. Philadelphia, JB Lippincott, 1987:1.

35. Clouse ME, Harrison DA, Grassi CJ, et al. Lymphangiography, ultrasonography, and computed tomography in Hodgkin's disease and non-Hodgkin's lymphomas. J Comput Assist Tomogr 1985;9:1–8.

36. Rosenberg SA, Kaplan HS, eds. Malignant lymphomas: etiology, immunology, pathology, treatment: Bristol-Myers Cancer Symposia, vol 3. San Diego, Academic Press, 1982.

37. Mauch P, Larson D, Osteen R, et al. Prognostic factors for positive surgical staging in patients with Hodgkin's disease. J Clin Oncol 1990;8:257–265.

38. Leibenhaut MH, Hoppe T, Efron B, et al. Prognostic indicators of laparotomy findings in clinical stage I–II supradiaphragmatic Hodgkin's disease. J Clin Oncol 1989;7:81–91.

39. Taylor MA, Kaplan HS, Nelsen TS. Staging laparotomy with splenectomy for Hodgkin's disease: the Stanford experience. World J Surg 1985;9:449.

40. Dutcher JP, Wiernick PH. Combined modality treatment of Hodgkin's disease confined to lymph nodes: results 14 years later. In: Calvelli F, Bonadonna G, Rozencweig M, eds. Malignant lymphomas and Hodgkin's disease: experimental and therapeutic advances. Boston, Martinus Nijhoff, 1985:317.

41. Radford JA, Cowan RA, Flanagan M, et al. The significance of residual mediastinal abnormality on the chest radiograph following treatment for Hodgkin's disease. J Clin Oncol 1988;6:940.

42. Rosenberg SA. National Cancer Institute sponsored study of classification of non-Hodgkin's lymphomas. Cancer 1982;49:2112.

43. Cullen MH, Lister TA, Brearly RL, et al. Histological transformation of non-Hodgkin's lymphomas: a prospective study. Cancer 1979;44:645.

44. Weingrad DN, Decosse JJ, Sherlock P, et al. Primary gastrointestinal lymphoma: a 30-year review. Cancer 1982;49:1258–1265.

45. Hoppe RT. Role of radiation treatment in the management of NHL. Cancer 1985;55:2176–2183.

46. Schein PS, DeVita VT Jr, Hubbard S, et al. Bleomycin, adriamycin, cyclophosphamide, vincristine, and prednisone (BACOP) combination chemotherapy in the treatment of advanced diffuse histiocytic lymphoma. Ann Intern Med 1976;85:417–422.

47. Connors JM, Klimo P. Updated clinical experience with MACOP-B. Semin Hematol 1987;24(Suppl 1):26.

48. Coltman CA, Dahlberg S, Jones SE, et al. CHOP is curative in thirty percent of patients with large cell lymphoma: a twelve year Southwest Oncology Group follow up. (Abstract) Proc Am Soc Clin Oncol 1986;5:197.

49. DeVita VT Jr, Hubbard SM, Young RC, et al. The role of chemotherapy in diffuse aggressive lymphomas. Semin Hematol 1988;25:2–10.

50. Tsokos G, Balow J, Spiegel E, et al. Renal and metabolic complications of undifferentiated and lymphoblastic lymphoma. Medicine (Baltimore) 1981;60:218.

51. Hughes WT, Armstrong D, Bodey GP, et al. Guidelines for the use of antimicrobial agents in neutropenic patients with unexplained fever. J Infect Dis 1990;161:381–396.

52. Pizzo PA, Hathorn JW, Hiemenz J, et al. A randomized trial comparing ceftazidime alone with combination antibiotic therapy in cancer patients with fever and neutropenia. N Engl J Med 1986;315:552.

53. Bodey GP, Alvarez ME, Jons GP, et al. Imipenem–cilastatin as initial therapy for febrile cancer patients. Antimicrob Agents Chemother 1986;30:211.

54. Karp JE, Hick SD, Angelopulos C, et al. Empiric use of vancomycin during prolonged treatment-induced granulocytopenia. Am J Med 1986;81:237.

55. Cohen I, Amir J, Ben-Shaul Y, et al. Plasma cell myeloma associated with an unusual myeloma protein causing impairment of fibrin aggregation and platelet function in a patient with multiple malignancy. Am J Med 1970;48:766.

56. Wisloff F, Micahelsen TE, Godal HC. Inhibition or acceleration of fibrin polymerization by monoclonal immunoglobulins and immunoglobulin fragments. Thromb Res 1984;35:81.

57. Glueck HI, Coots MC, Benson M, et al. A monoclonal immuno-

globulin A (K) factor VIII: C inhibitor associated with primary amyloidosis: identification and characterization. J Lab Clin Med 1989;113:267.

58. Furie B, Voo L, McAdam KPW, Furie BC. Mechanism of factor X deficiency is systemic amyloidosis. N Engl J Med 1981;304:817.

59. Kaufman PA, Glockerman JP, Greenberg CS. Production of a novel anticoagulant by neoplastic plasma cells: report of a case and review of the literature. Am J Med 1989;86:612.

60. Sane DC, Pizzo SV, Greenberg CS. Elevated urokinase-type plasminogen activator level and bleeding in amyloidosis: case report and literature review. Am J Hematol 1989;31:53.

61. Piro AJ, Weiss D, Hellman S. Mediastinal Hodgkin's disease: a possible danger for intubation anaesthesia. Int J Radiat Oncol Biol Phys 1976;1:415–419.

62. Selvin BL. Cancer chemotherapy: implications for the anesthesiologist. Anesth Analg 1981;60:425–434.

63. AuBuchon JP. Autologous transfusion and directed donations: current controversies and future directions. Transfus Med Rev 1989;3:290–306.

64. Sandler SG, Sacher RA. Preoperative autologous blood donations by high-risk patients. Transfusion 1992;32:1–2.

65. Goodnough LT, Rudnick S, Price TH, et al. Increased preoperative collection of autologous blood with recombinant human erythropoietin therapy. N Engl J Med 1989;321:1163–1168.

66. Stacey R, Filshie J. Venous access. In: Treleaven J, Barrett J, eds. Bone marrow transplantation in practice. New York, Churchill Livingstone, 1992:207–218.

67. Stanislav GV, Fitzgibbons RJ, Bailey RT, et al. Reliability of implantable central venous access devices in patients with cancer. Arch Surg 1987;122:1280–1283.

68. Wagman LD, Kirkemo A, Johnston R. Venous access: a prospective, randomized study of the Hickman catheter. Surgery 1984;95:303–308.

69. Pritchard AP, David JA, eds. Royal Marsden Hospital manual of clinical nursing procedures, ed 2. London, Harper & Row, 1988:89–93.

70. Press OW, Ramsey PG, Larson EB, Fefer A. Hickman catheter infections in patients with malignancies. Medicine (Baltimore) 1984;63:189–200.

71. Patterson K. Bone marrow harvesting and preparation of harvested marrow. In: Treleaven J, Barrett J, eds. Bone marrow transplantation in practice. New York, Churchill Livingstone, 1992:219–226.

72. Buckner CD, Clift RA, Sanders JE, et al. Marrow harvesting from normal donors. Blood 1984;64:630–634.

73. Slavin R, Nelsen TS. Complications from staging laparotomy for Hodgkin's disease. Natl Cancer Inst Monogr 1973;36:457–459.

74. Kinsella TJ, Glatstein E. Staging laparotomy and splenectomy for Hodgkin's disease: current status. Cancer Invest 1983;1:87–91.

75. Slavin R, Nelsen TS. Complications from staging laparotomy for Hodgkin's disease. Natl Cancer Inst Monogr 1973;36:457–459.

76. Holdsworth RJ, Irving AD, Cuschieri A. Postsplenectomy sepsis and its mortality rate: actual versus perceived risks. Br J Surg 1991;78:1031–1038.

77. Shaw JHF, Print CG. Postsplenectomy sepsis. Br J Surg 1989;76:1074–1081.

78. Leonard AS, Giebink GS, Baesl TJ, et al. The overwhelming postsplenectomy sepsis problem. World J Surg 1980;4:423–432.

79. Gill PG, Souter RG, Morris PJ. Splenectomy for hypersplenism in malignant lymphomas. Br J Surg 1981;68:29–33.

80. Coon WW. Splenectomy for massive splenomegaly. Surg Gynecol Obstet 1989;169:235–237.

81. Wilhelm MC, Jones RE, McGehee R, et al. Splenectomy in hematologic disorders: the ever-changing indications. Ann Surg 1988;207:581–589.

82. Jochelson M, Muach P, Balikian J, et al. The significance of the residual mediastinal mass in treated Hodgkin's disease. J Clin Oncol 1985;3:637–640.

83. Radford JA, Cowan RA, Flanagan M, et al. The significance of residual mediastinal abnormality on the chest radiograph following treatment for Hodgkin's disease. J Clin Oncol 1988;6:940–946.

84. Subone A, Longo DL, DeVita VT, et al. Residual abdominal masses in aggressive non-Hodgkin's lymphoma after combination chemotherapy: significance and management. J Clin Oncol 1986;4:306–310.

85. Barnes SG, Sattler FR, Ballard JO. Perirectal infections in acute leukemia: improved survival after incision and debridement. Ann Intern Med 1984;100:515–518.

Medical Management of the Surgical Patient, Third Edition,
edited by Michael F. Lubin, H. Kenneth Walker, and Robert B. Smith III.
J.B. Lippincott Company, Philadelphia, PA © 1995.

CHAPTER

24

BLOOD TRANSFUSION

Carolyn F. Whitsett

Preoperative consultations usually focus on the ability of patients to tolerate the stress of surgery and on the management of preexisting medical conditions during surgery and the immediate postoperative period. Hematologic consultations present the opportunity to ensure optimal transfusion therapy and to prevent some types of transfusion reactions. Postoperative hematologic consultations usually are requested to determine whether signs and symptoms are caused by an adverse reaction to transfusion or by some other pathologic event. When the symptoms are clearly related to transfusion, consultants are expected to make recommendations regarding treatment and product selection for subsequent transfusions.

THE PREOPERATIVE CONSULTATION

The transfusion history characteristically addresses previous episodes of transfusion and any adverse reactions that may have accompanied them. Other sources of immunization should also be included. A history of bone grafting, organ and tissue transplantation, and past or current pregnancy may be relevant factors in transfusion recommendations. Patients' immune systems may be compromised by chemotherapy or other immunosuppressive medications, in which case the use of irradiated blood products may be

warranted. Patients who are pregnant or infected with the human immunodeficiency virus (HIV) and who have not been infected with cytomegalovirus (CMV) should receive CMV-seronegative blood products. Leukocyte-depleted blood products should be considered for patients with medical conditions that may be treated by allogeneic transplantation as well as for those with histories of recurrent febrile reactions. Patients with histories of severe allergic reactions to blood products should be evaluated for possible IgA deficiency.

The use of autologous blood precludes many of the hazards of blood transfusion. The preoperative consultation should specifically indicate whether patients' medical conditions safely permit autologous donation. Some high-risk patients who would not tolerate routine phlebotomy do well with isovolumic donations in which most of the blood volume removed is replaced with crystalloid solutions during or immediately after the phlebotomy. This procedure can be repeated with each donation. Iron supplements or erythropoietin may be needed to permit collection of all the autologous units required. Regional blood centers also collect and freeze autologous plasma for use in surgery, and perform plateletpheresis procedures to obtain autologous platelets. If the time before surgery is too short to permit preoperative donation, intraoperative salvage or phlebotomy with hemodilution in the immediate preoperative period remain as alternatives.

NEW INDICATIONS FOR COMPONENTS

The blood components that are regularly available for patient use are described in Table 24-1. Most of the units of whole blood that are collected are converted into components, although some regional blood centers collect whole blood for use in trauma centers. The addition of adenine to preservative solutions for red blood cells helps maintain intracellular adenosine triphosphate, extending the shelf life of red cells from 35 to 42 days. Platelet products have an expiration time of 5 days and are stored at 20° to 24°C. During the past 5 years, single-donor platelets obtained by apheresis have become more widely available. This single-donor product is the equivalent of six to eight units of platelet concentrate. Single-donor platelets have become the product of choice for many physicians because they are less immunogenic. Patients are exposed to only one donor for each transfusion, and the lymphocyte count is lower in platelet products obtained by apheresis than in those obtained by the centrifugation methods used for routine component preparation.

The basic components available for use remain unchanged. Three types of components are being used more frequently, however. First, the production and use of components from CMV-seronegative donors has increased substantially. In addition, the indications for leukocyte-depleted red cells and platelets have expanded. Finally, the observation of graft-versus-host disease in immunologically normal patients as well as in some patients receiving chemotherapy who were thought to have only moderate immunosuppression has increased the number of patients receiving irradiated blood products. The indications for these products are discussed in the following sections.

CYTOMEGALOVIRUS-SERONEGATIVE PRODUCTS

The indications for CMV-seronegative blood components were recently reviewed.[1] CMV-seronegative blood should be used in the following categories of CMV-seronegative patients: premature infants born to CMV-seronegative mothers, pregnant women, recipients of bone marrow transplants, patients with the acquired immunodeficiency syndrome (AIDS), and other HIV-positive patients. A larger group of patients who may also benefit from the use of CMV-seronegative blood has been identified. Among these are CMV-seronegative patients who are receiving tissue and organ transplants from CMV-seronegative donors and CMV-seronegative patients who have undergone splenectomy. In some areas, the request for CMV-seronegative blood products has exceeded the supply. Because the virus is found in peripheral blood mononuclear cells, leukocyte-depleted blood components have a lower risk of CMV transmission. Fresh frozen plasma is not associated with an increased risk of CMV transmission.[2]

LEUKOCYTE-DEPLETED BLOOD PRODUCTS

Leukocyte-depleted blood products are indicated primarily for the prevention of febrile nonhemolytic transfusion reactions caused by antileukocyte antibodies. The transfusion of leukocyte-depleted products may also prevent or delay immunization to HLA antigens.[3] Leukocyte-depleted red cells and platelets are being used increasingly in patients who are candidates for solid organ and bone marrow transplantation. Patients with cardiac disease who currently are being treated with surgery may become candidates for cardiac transplantation in the future. Blood transfusions given during a surgical procedure for an unrelated condition may seriously jeopardize a patient's ability to receive a transplant if immunization to HLA antigens occurs.

The degree of leukocyte depletion needed to prevent a febrile nonhemolytic reaction is generally less than that needed to prevent immunization to HLA antigens. Procedures that reduce the leukocyte count of the component below 5×10^8 cells/unit are adequate for preventing transfusion reactions but the number of contaminating leukocytes must be reduced below 5×10^6 cells/unit to prevent immunization to HLA antigens. Washed red cells may be used to prevent febrile transfusion reactions but are not suitable for preventing immunization to HLA antigens. Frozen deglycerolized red cells prepared by some methods may be used to prevent immunization to HLA antigens. Platelet products are contaminated with lymphocytes. Platelets prepared with apheresis techniques generally contain fewer lymphocytes than do platelet concentrates prepared from whole blood, and may eliminate febrile reactions in some patients. Only platelets prepared with high-efficiency leukocyte-depletion filters, however, have a low enough leukocyte count to prevent immunization to HLA antigens.

IRRADIATED BLOOD PRODUCTS

Irradiation of blood components prevents graft-versus-host disease. The minimum recommended dose of irradiation is 2500 cGy.[4,5] This dose limits the ability of contaminating lymphocytes to proliferate but does not harm the other cellular elements. During storage, irradiated red cells release more potassium than do untreated cells. The extra potassium does not usually cause problems in adults but may do so if large volumes of blood are needed and renal insufficiency is present. Washing the red cells eliminates the extra potassium.

TABLE 24–1. Blood and Blood Components

Component	Approximate Volume (mL)	Composition	Storage Period	Indications	Comments
Whole blood	500	200 mL red cells 250 mL plasma 63 mL anticoagulant	35 d (CPD-A1)	Simultaneous replacement of volume and red cell mass	Hematocrit ≃ 40% Not a reliable source of platelets, granulocytes, or labile coagulation factors V and VIII Variable availability depending on local need for component production
Red cells	250	200 mL red cells 50 mL plasma	35 d closed system (CPD-A1); 24 h open system	Replacement of red cell mass	Hematocrit 70%–80% Cannot be infused as rapidly as whole blood because of viscosity
Red cells (adenine saline added)	330	200 mL red cells 30 mL plasma 100 mL adenine saline solution*	42 d	Replacement of red cell mass	Hematocrit ≃ 60% Red cell product most commonly available Has flow characteristics similar to whole blood
Leukocyte-depleted red cells†: Washed red cells	200	180 mL red cells 20 mL isotonic saline (0.9%)	24 h	Increase red cell mass; prevent allergic and febrile reactions	Washing removes all of plasma and 70%–80% of leukocytes
Frozen deglycerolized‡ red cells	200	180 mL red cells 20 mL isotonic saline/ dextrose solution	24 h	Increase red cell mass; prevent allergic and febrile reactions	Freezing usually reserved for blood with rare phenotype Frozen red cells may be stored 10 years Plasma and ≃90% of leukocytes removed
Red cells depleted by leukocyte adhesion filters‡	200	160 mL red cells 40 mL plasma	35 d closed system; 24 h open system	Prevent febrile reactions; prevent immunization to HLA antigens	95%–99% of leukocytes removed
Platelet concentrate	50	≥ 5.5 × 10¹⁰ platelets; contains plasma, and variable number of red and white cells	5 d	Bleeding from decreased or abnormal platelet function	Average adult dose 8–10 units of concentrate May be pooled for infusion White cells can be removed with special leukocyte adhesion filter

(continued)

TABLE 24–1. (Continued)

Component	Approximate Volume (mL)	Composition	Storage Period	Indications	Comments
Platelet apheresis (single donor platelets)	300	$\geq 3 \times 10^{11}$ platelets/U; plasma, and variable number of red and white cells	24 h open system; 5 d closed system	Bleeding from decreased or abnormal platelet function	Equivalent to 6 units of concentrate Decreases number of donors to which patient is exposed Generally contains fewer lymphocytes than equivalent dose of platelet concentrate May minimize febrile reactions and delay onset of immunization to HLA antigen Form in which HLA-matched products provided. Equivalent in cost to 6–8 platelet concentrates in some places
Granulocytes (apheresis)	200–300	$\geq 1.0 \times 10^{10}$ granulocytes; contains platelets ($\approx 2 \times 10^{11}$); some red cells, plasma	24 h	Documented sepsis in patients with neutropenia or neutrophil dysfunction when response to antibiotics is unsatisfactory	Should be transfused as soon as possible Function deteriorates with storage Never given prophylactically May be replaced by treatment with granulocyte-macrophage colony-stimulating factor or granulocyte colony-stimulating factor in some patients
Fresh frozen plasma	220	Contains all coagulation factors	24 h after thawing if maintained at 1°–6°C; 12 mo frozen	Correction of coagulation deficiencies; partial replacement in exchange transfusions	Not for volume expansion only
Cryoprecipitated antihemophilia factor	15	Factor VIIIc ≥ 80/U factor VIII vWF; ≈ 250 mg fibrinogen; factor XIII	6 h after thawing; 12 mo frozen	Symptomatic deficiencies of factor VIIIc, factor VIII vWF, fibrinogen, or factor XIII; preparation of fibrin glue for use in surgery	Used primarily to treat von Willebrand's disease, congenital hypofibrinogenemia, and acquired coagulation disorders with deficiencies of fibrinogen or factor VIII Dose variable May be pooled for ease of transfusion In acquired deficiencies, therapy often initiated with 8–10 units

*Contains additional additives to improve red cell survival.
†Cannot be used to prevent graft-versus-host disease.
‡Considered cytomegalovirus-safe if cytomegalovirus-seronegative blood is unavailable.

Until recently, irradiated blood was routinely recommended only for patients with congenital immunodeficiency syndromes and those receiving bone marrow transplants. Fetuses, neonates undergoing exchange transfusions, and premature neonates should receive irradiated blood. In addition, patients who develop immunosuppression after intensive chemotherapy for hematologic diseases and some solid tumors are at risk. It is also recognized that immunologically competent patients may develop transfusion-induced graft-versus-host disease when they are transfused with blood from persons with similar HLA types. In the United States, blood donations from blood relatives are thought to pose the greatest risk, and these products are routinely irradiated by blood centers. In ethnically homogeneous populations such as the Japanese, however, blood from unrelated donors may pose some risk as well.

ADVERSE EFFECTS OF TRANSFUSION

HEMOLYTIC REACTIONS

Acute Hemolytic Reactions

Acute hemolytic reactions are rare, with a reported frequency of 1 in 8300 to 1 in 33,500 transfusions.[6] The antibodies involved invariably bind complement and cause intravascular destruction of red cells. Intravascular red cell destruction is usually associated with numerous signs and symptoms. Fever and fever with chills are the most common signs of a hemolytic transfusion reaction. Other manifestations include pain in the back or chest, dyspnea, flushing, nausea, vomiting, agitation, a feeling of impending doom, and pain in the infusing arm. Hypotension, disseminated intravascular coagulation (DIC), and renal failure may also occur. In a patient who is under anesthesia, unexplained hypotension, an unexplained bleeding diathesis, or hemoglobinuria without other signs may be the only indication that a transfusion reaction has occurred.

When a hemolytic transfusion reaction is suspected, blood and urine samples taken after the transfusion and the crossmatch tag and unit of blood implicated in the reaction (or the blood bag if the entire unit has been transfused) should be sent to the blood bank. A clerical check is performed first to determine whether an error occurred in patient identification when the blood transfusion was administered. Then the urine and serum samples that were obtained after the transfusion are inspected for hemolysis. Direct antiglobulin testing is performed to determine whether there is evidence of immunologic destruction. In most instances of immunologic destruction, the results of this test are positive. When the antibody causing red cell destruction binds complement, as in the case of anti-A and

anti-B, all incompatible cells may have been destroyed and the results of the direct antiglobulin test could be negative. If the results are positive, an eluate is performed to identify the antibody. The blood type, antibody screening test, and crossmatches are performed again with serum obtained before and after the transfusion. The typical hemolytic reaction involves the destruction of transfused cells, although passively administered antibody may occasionally cause hemolysis of patients' cells.

Most severe hemolytic transfusion reactions involve ABO incompatibility. Errors in patient or sample identification are usually responsible. Other blood group antibodies that may bind complement and cause acute intravascular hemolysis include anti-JK[a], anti-K (Kell), and anti-Fy[a]. Occasionally, clinical and laboratory data suggest that an acute hemolytic reaction has occurred but antibody is not demonstrable. Under these circumstances, consultation with a specialist in transfusion medicine is advisable.

If the serologic evaluation does not support a diagnosis of immune hemolysis, an evaluation for nonimmune hemolysis should be performed. Bacterial contamination of blood can cause in vitro hemolysis, with the contamination of the unit being recognized only after transfusion. The blood component implicated in a hemolytic transfusion reaction should be cultured. A faulty in-line blood warmer may result in heat damage to red cells. Mechanical hemolysis can be caused by excessive vacuum or inadequate washing during intraoperative salvage procedures, or by roller pumps used during cardiac bypass surgery. Inadequate deglycerolization of frozen red cells and the infusion of blood with hypotonic intravenous solutions are other possible causes of nonimmune hemolysis. Finally, diseases must be considered in which patients' red cells, but not transfused cells, may have hemolyzed. Paroxysmal nocturnal hemoglobinuria, glucose-6-phosphate dehydrogenase deficiency, and sickle cell anemia are examples.

The constellation of signs and symptoms that characterize the acute hemolytic transfusion reaction are caused primarily by activation of the complement system and coagulation cascade.[7] Immune complexes activate complement, generating C3a and C5a, which are anaphylatoxins. Immune complexes also activate Hageman factor and platelets; activated Hageman factor (XIIa) acts on the kinin system to produce bradykinin and activated platelets release histamine and serotonin. Hypotension results from the release of these vasoactive substances, and norepinephrine and other catecholamines are released into the circulation to counteract this hypotension. These catecholamines cause vasoconstriction in the renal, splanchnic, pulmonary, and cutaneous capillary beds. Until recently, the hypotension, renal failure, and bleeding diathesis characteristic of the acute hemolytic transfusion reaction was thought to be related to these mechanisms alone. An in vitro model of ABO red cell incompatibility has now demonstrated that interleukin-8 (IL-8) is released during hemolysis.[8] IL-8 is a cytokine with chemotactic and activating properties for neutrophils. It is produced by several kinds of cells, including monocytes and endothelial cells. The observed association between immune hemolysis and IL-8 production suggests that neutrophils may play a role in mediating the organ damage and DIC that is observed in acute hemolytic transfusion reactions.

The transfusion should be discontinued as soon as a reaction is suspected. In general, the severity of the reaction is proportional to the amount of blood transfused. Intravenous access should be maintained to permit adequate hydration and administration of medications. Hydration should be adjusted to maintain blood pressure and sustain a urine output of 100 mL/h. Diuretics such as furosemide (80 to 120 mg intravenously) or mannitol may be helpful in maintaining urine output. Vasopressors such as dopamine, which maintain blood pressure without impairing renal perfusion, should be used if hydration alone does not maintain an adequate blood pressure. If oliguria occurs despite these measures, fluid administration should be adjusted so that volume overload is prevented. Coagulation studies should be obtained to determine whether there is evidence of DIC. The management of DIC in this setting is controversial. Prophylactic heparinization has been recommended when the volume of incompatible blood transfused is large (more than 200 mL).[9] When coagulation abnormalities are present but patients are asymptomatic, supportive treatment with platelets, fresh frozen plasma, and cryoprecipitate is considered appropriate by some, whereas others recommend heparinization. Symptomatic DIC may require the administration of heparin as well as support with platelets, cryoprecipitate, and fresh frozen plasma.

Delayed Hemolytic Reactions

Delayed hemolytic transfusion reactions typically occur 2 to 10 days after a transfusion.[10] Often, the blood bank detects positive results on direct antiglobulin tests in asymptomatic patients during routine compatibility testing. The symptoms of a delayed hemolytic reaction are frequently mild because red cell destruction is usually extravascular and slower than with acute hemolysis. Patients may have fevers, elevated bilirubin levels, or unexplained anemia. Hemoglobinuria, hemoglobinemia, and renal failure are rare but may occur. The results of the direct antiglobulin test are usually positive and new antibodies are present in patients' sera. The positive results decrease in strength as the incompatible cells are destroyed and may be negative if patients are seen late in the course of the reaction.

Delayed hemolytic reactions usually occur because patients have been immunized by previous transfusions or pregnancies. Red cell antibodies fall below the level that can be detected through routine techniques. Occasionally, a technical error occurs and the blood bank fails to detect the presence of an antibody.

Compatibility testing has changed dramatically within the last decade. ABO and Rh typing and antibody screening tests are performed on patients' blood. If the results of the antibody screening tests are negative and patients are not known to be previously immunized to red cell antigens, compatibility testing with donor cells is confined to the immediate spin phase, which detects primarily ABO incompatibility. Only patients with demonstrable alloantibodies or histories of immunization have compatibility testing routinely carried through the antiglobulin phase. This abbreviated compatibility testing procedure for nonsensitized patients has proven to be safe and cost-effective. A technical error in antibody screening may not be detected in the compatibility testing, however, if only the immediate spin phase of testing is performed. Many hospitals provide immunized patients with a wallet card that lists the red cell antigens to which they are immunized. This procedure helps to ensure that patients receive truly compatible blood.

Most delayed hemolytic transfusion reactions do not require specific treatment. Additional blood transfusions may be needed in patients with symptomatic anemia when the incompatible cells are destroyed. Recognition that signs and symptoms result from a delayed transfusion reaction eliminates costly medical evaluation.

NONHEMOLYTIC REACTIONS

Febrile Reactions

A febrile transfusion reaction is defined as an increase in temperature of at least 1°C during or within several hours after transfusion. The most common cause of febrile reactions is immunization to HLA antigens and other antigens expressed on leukocytes and platelets. Every febrile reaction involving a red cell transfusion must be investigated as a possible hemolytic reaction because fever is the most common sign of hemolysis. Bacterial contamination of blood components may also cause febrile reactions. Recent studies on platelets revealed that IL-1, IL-6, and tumor necrosis factor are increased in the plasma of stored platelets.[11] These cytokines are thought to be synthesized or released by contaminating monocytes and lymphocytes. Because these cytokines can cause fever, febrile reactions caused by platelet reactions may not always be the result of bacterial contamination or immunization to HLA antigens.

In patients who have received multiple transfusions or women who have been pregnant, a presumptive diagnosis of febrile nonhemolytic reaction can be made if there is no evidence of red cell incompatibility and the blood is not contaminated. The presence of antibodies to leukocytes can be documented with several tests. Lymphocytotoxicity assays are sensitive for the detection of HLA antibodies. Antiplatelet antibody tests detect HLA and platelet-specific antibodies. Leukoagglutination assays and indirect fluorescence techniques may be needed to demonstrate other antibodies. Unless a hospital has an organ transplantation program, these assays may not be available; however, regional blood centers usually perform these tests.

The first episode of a febrile nonhemolytic reaction that is not accompanied by any other symptoms (ie, respiratory distress or hypotension) may be treated by the administration of acetaminophen. Although aspirin is also effective, it should not be used in the perioperative setting because of its effect on platelet function. Preventive measures should be taken if patients have repeated reactions. Premedication with antipyretics is often the first approach. Numerous leukocyte-poor red cell products are available to support patients who do not respond to premedication with antipyretics or who have more serious symptoms associated with febrile reactions. The least expensive product is leukocyte-poor red cells prepared by inverted centrifugation. This procedure removes 70% to 80% of leukocytes but has 20% to 25% fewer red cells than does a standard unit of packed red cells. This product also is not available in all areas. The most efficient way to deplete whole blood or red cells of leukocytes is with the third-generation leukocyte-depletion filters, which remove 95% to 99% of contaminating leukocytes. Washed red cells and frozen deglycerolized red cells are also considered to be leukocyte-depleted products. Platelets prepared by apheresis contain fewer lymphocytes than does an equivalent volume of platelet concentrate and may be suitable for use in some patients. Platelet products can be depleted of leukocytes only with special leukocyte-depletion filters designed for platelet products.

Transfusion-Related Acute Lung Injury

Patients who experience febrile reactions may also have chest pain, severe respiratory distress, and hypotension. The respiratory distress is associated with hypoxemia and a chest radiograph shows typical pulmonary edema, although the objective signs of heart failure are absent.[12] The pulmonary capillary wedge pressure is normal. This syndrome of noncardiac pulmonary edema is called transfusion-related lung injury and is associated with the presence of antibodies in donor plasma that react with patients' granulocytes. Clinical and experimental studies suggest that activation and agglutination of granulocytes in the lung is responsible for this syndrome.[13,14] Both HLA antibodies and antigranulocyte antibodies have been demonstrated in donor plasma.

The respiratory distress may begin shortly after transfusion is initiated or occur the next day. Typically, patients de-velop symptoms several hours after transfusion. Although the symptoms are extremely severe initially, they usually subside within 48 hours. Treatment is supportive. Some patients require mechanical ventilatory support. Treatment with high-dose corticosteroids appears to be helpful.

Blood products are not screened routinely for the presence of anti-HLA and antigranulocyte antibodies. Any donor product implicated in such a reaction should be reported to the blood-collecting facility.

Allergic Reactions

The manifestations of allergic reactions are usually mild and consist of hives, itching, and erythema of the skin. More severe symptoms are encountered occasionally. Bronchospasm is not unusual. On rare occasions, allergic reactions progress to anaphylaxis. Immunization to donor plasma proteins is the most common cause of allergic reactions. With severe reactions, patients are frequently found to have class-specific antibodies to IgA. These patients are usually IgA-deficient and serum IgA levels should be measured to help establish the diagnosis. Tests to detect and measure antibodies to IgA are available in some blood center reference laboratories but are not performed in most hospital laboratories. A presumptive diagnosis can be made based on failure to detect serum IgA.

Mild allergic reactions can be treated with antihistamines. If patients have recurrent allergic reactions and premedication with antihistamines does not completely prevent these reactions, washed or frozen deglycerolized cells should be administered. Platelet products may also be washed to remove plasma.

Patients who have severe reactions caused by immunization to IgA usually respond to therapy with epinephrine, antihistamines, and corticosteroids. Once antibodies to IgA have been documented as the cause of a severe allergic reaction, patients must be given products that lack IgA. Frozen deglycerolized red cells and red cells washed twice with an automated washer may be used. Platelet products and plasma products must come from IgA-deficient donors. Regional blood centers maintain lists of IgA-deficient donors who can provide blood components for IgA-deficient patients. Fresh frozen plasma from IgA-deficient donors is also available in some blood centers. Plasma protein fraction and albumin solutions may contain trace amounts of IgA and may also pose a risk for these patients.

EFFECTS OF MASSIVE TRANSFUSION

Certain adverse effects of blood transfusion develop in the setting of massive transfusion. The most common of these may be the bleeding diathesis that is associated with the transfusion of large volumes of red cells and crystalloid or colloid solutions, resulting in a dilutional coagulopathy. Laboratory studies should be performed in patients who receive one or more total blood volumes to evaluate the extent of the dilutional effect. There usually is a predictable fall in blood platelets and in most coagulation factors, except for factor VIII, which is an acute-phase reactant and may be normal or elevated. This dilutional coagulopathy may be asymptomatic or may present as unexplained oozing or excessive bleeding during surgery. When intraoperative blood salvage is used, the physicians caring for patients may not recognize that the entire blood volume has been replaced because banked blood may not have been required. Symptomatic dilutional coagulopathy may be more likely to develop in this setting.

The transfusion of large volumes of banked blood is also associated with the development of metabolic abnormalities. The rapid infusion of large volumes of blood may cause hypothermia. The use of a blood warming device prevents this problem. The development of other metabolic problems is related to the composition of stored blood. Blood is anticoagulated with citrate, which exerts its anticoagulant effect by complexing calcium ions. The infusion of large volumes, especially in a central line, may produce symptomatic hypocalcemia and cardiac arrhythmias. Although the pH of blood is between 7.2 and 6.7 (depending on the average length of storage), massive transfusion usually produces metabolic alkalosis rather than metabolic acidosis because the citrate is metabolized to bicarbonate. During storage, potassium also leaks from the red cells and ammonia accumulates in the supernatant plasma. The older the unit of blood, the higher is its load of potassium and ammonia. Massive transfusion usually produces hypokalemia because the metabolic alkalosis produced by the metabolism of citrate causes potassium to move into the cells. Patients with hepatic or renal insufficiency, however, may be at risk for hypocalcemia, acidosis, or hyperkalemia.

Microaggregates composed of leukocytes and platelets develop during storage. For patients receiving several units of blood, these microaggregates do not pose problems. A syndrome of pulmonary dysfunction that occurs after massive transfusion, however, is believed to result from lodging of these microaggregates in the pulmonary vasculature. Patients who undergo cardiovascular surgery that requires cardiopulmonary bypass have similar problems that are thought to be related to systemic embolization of these microaggregates. Microaggregate filters with a pore size of 40 μm have been developed to prevent this syndrome. The use of microaggregate filters is routine during cardiac surgery requiring bypass. Some microaggregate filters also remove leukocytes that are not in microaggregates and can be used to provide leukocyte-depleted red cells if a standard leukocyte-depletion filter is unavailable.

IMMUNOLOGIC EFFECTS

Immunization to antigens on blood cells and plasma proteins is one of the expected complications of blood transfusion. Preventing immunization to HLA antigens is desirable for patients who may require solid organ or bone marrow transplantation. In addition, some experts believe that matching blood transfusions for common red cell antigens may decrease the frequency of delayed transfusion reactions and facilitate the identification of compatible blood in patients with hemoglobinopathies such as sickle cell anemia.

Posttransfusion purpura is a rare syndrome in which immunization to platelet-specific antigens causes severe thrombocytopenia 2 to 10 days after transfusion. This form of thrombocytopenia usually develops in patients who are PLA-1–negative (a platelet-specific antigen) and who are transfused with blood products from a PLA-1–positive donor.[15] In the course of the immune response, the antibodies developed by the patients react with the patients' own PLA-1–negative platelets as well as with PLA-1–positive platelets. This syndrome usually develops in women who have been immunized by a previous pregnancy. Although thrombocytopenias associated with the administration of heparin and other medications are more common after surgery, this syndrome must be considered in the differential diagnosis. A hematologist or specialist in transfusion medicine should be consulted in the treatment of these patients.

Blood transfusion has been demonstrated to cause immunosuppression in all recipients. This immunosuppression may be manifest as an increased number of infections in surgical patients and may be associated with increased recurrence and decreased survival in patients with cancer.[16,17] Recent studies of blood transfusion in patients with AIDS have indicated an increased frequency of infectious complications and viral production associated with transfusion.[18,19] It is too soon to determine the ultimate clinical implications of these observations.

Graft-versus-host disease, a rare complication of transfusion, is caused by viable T lymphocytes that are present in cellular blood components and plasma that has not been frozen. Usually, patients develop symptoms 1 to 2 weeks after transfusion. The clinical presentation is similar to that after bone marrow transplantation. Skin rashes, fever, hepatic dysfunction, and diarrhea develop. Marrow aplasia is invariably present in the transfusion-induced form of the disorder. Treatment is ineffective and the disease is usually fatal.[20]

Patients at greatest risk for this disease are fetuses, premature newborns, infants undergoing exchange transfusions, patients with congenital immunodeficiency syndromes, and patients undergoing bone marrow transplants or intensive chemotherapy for Hodgkin's disease and other hematologic malignancies. Immunologically competent patients can also develop transfusion-induced graft-versus-host disease if the donor lymphocytes have similar HLA antigens. In ethnically heterogeneous societies, this is most likely to occur when donors are related to patients. In more homogeneous societies, it may also occur with unrelated persons.

The irradiation of blood products prevents graft-versus-host disease. The recommended minimal dose is 2500 cGy. The disease has been reported after the transfusion of leukocyte-depleted blood components, and the irradiation of blood components is the only effective preventive method.[21]

INFECTIOUS COMPLICATIONS

Numerous infections can be transmitted by transfusion. The most frequent infectious complication is posttransfusion hepatitis and the most feared is transfusion-transmitted AIDS. Several blood donor screening procedures have been implemented to make the blood supply safer. These include obtaining a past and current medical history, performing a limited physical examination, testing donor blood for numerous infectious agents, offering donors an opportunity to confidentially exclude their donations from use, and instructing donors to notify the blood center if they become ill after donating. Donated blood is tested for syphilis, alanine aminotransferase level, hepatitis B surface antigen (HBsAg), and antibodies to HIV-1, HIV-2, human T-cell lymphotrophic virus (HTLV-I and HTLV-II), hepatitis B core antigen (HBcAg), and hepatitis C virus (HCV). In addition, a donor deferral registry is consulted to determine whether donors have been permanently deferred after being evaluated during a previous donation. Some of the infections for which specific serologic testing is available have a window period (ie, a period in which blood donors are asymptomatically infected and have not developed specific antibodies). Both primary syphilis and AIDS have window periods. Other infections may go undetected because patients' antibodies have disappeared or are below the sensitivity level of the test being used. Donors with HCV infections may not have had clinical signs or symptoms, and their antibodies may have disappeared or fallen below detectable levels. Occasionally, donors also provide inaccurate histories, leading to the donation of units of blood that would not normally be accepted. This is especially likely with an infection such as malaria. In the United States, the only screening done for malaria is to obtain a medical and travel history. These potential problems associated with the donor screening procedure should be kept in mind when patients are evaluated for infections that can be transmitted by transfusion.

HEPATITIS VIRUSES

Hepatitis C Virus

HCV is a single positive-stranded RNA virus of about 10 kilobases. It is the most common cause of posttransfusion hepatitis, accounting for 90% of posttransfusion cases of non-A, non-B hepatitis. The serologic tests that are used to exclude potentially infected donors are an elevated serum alanine aminotransferase level, the presence of antibody to HCV, and antibody to HBc (a surrogate marker for non-A, non-B hepatitis in epidemiologic studies). Routine screening of blood donors for antibody to HCV using an enzyme immunoassay was first introduced in the summer of 1990. An improved second-generation test was marketed in 1992.

The average incubation period for HCV is 50 days but shorter and longer incubation periods have been observed. Seventy-five percent of cases are anicteric, with the most common presenting symptoms being fatigue, fever, and anorexia. The average time from the onset of clinical illness until the development of antibody to HCV is 15 weeks.[22] Antibody titers fluctuate and may disappear in some patients. A reverse transcriptase polymerase chain reaction test has been developed to detect the virus in clinical circumstances where establishment of the diagnosis is important and antibodies are not detectable. HCV progresses to chronic hepatitis in about 50% of patients.

Hepatitis B Virus

The hepatitis B virus is a double-shelled, partially double-stranded DNA virus. There is an inner protein core (HBcAg) surrounding the circular DNA and an outer coat consisting of HBsAg. Hepatitis B accounts for 5% to 10% of all cases of posttransfusion hepatitis. The serologic studies performed on donor blood to prevent hepatitis B include antibody to HBsAg and antibody to HBcAg. Both IgG and IgM antibodies to HBc are detected with the screening test. Antibody to HBc usually persists for many years after infection.

The average incubation period for hepatitis B is 90 days, with a range of 15 to 180 days. The incubation period overlaps that of hepatitis C, and only serologic studies can be used to distinguish between them. Chronic hepatitis develops in only 5% to 10% of all patients who are infected with hepatitis B virus.

Other Hepatitis Viruses

Transmission of the hepatitis A virus through transfusion has been documented.[23] This form of hepatitis is rarely transmitted, however, because it causes symptoms and does not have a carrier state. The virus may be present in serum for as long as 2 weeks before an infected person develops symptoms. During this period, it is possible for the virus to be transmitted through donated blood.

Delta agent is a defective RNA virus that depends on hepatitis B virus for survival.[24] Hepatitis B virus and hepatitis B delta may infect patients simultaneously, or hepatitis delta virus infection may develop in patients who are already infected with hepatitis B virus. Although the risk of infection from blood found to be HBsAg-negative is small, patients who have received multiple transfusions and those who have received other derivatives are at greatest risk.

Hepatitis E virus is responsible for an epidemic form of enteric hepatitis. It is not considered an important transfusion risk in developed countries.

TRANSFUSION-ASSOCIATED ACQUIRED IMMUNODEFICIENCY SYNDROME

The first case of transfusion-associated AIDS was reported to the US Centers for Disease Control and Prevention (CDC) in 1982. The first test to detect antibody to HIV-1 was licensed in 1983. Serologic testing was expected to eliminate transfusion-transmitted AIDS but the first reports of HIV-1 transmitted by seronegative blood were published in 1988.[25,26] Estimates used to determine the risk of HIV infection from screened blood have been summarized.[27] Statistical models based on the incidence and prevalence of HIV infection in blood estimate the risk of HIV infection per unit transfused to range from 1 in 38,000 to 1 in 153,000. Using the look-back model, which involves tracing seronegative donations from donors who subsequently became seropositive, the estimates suggest that between 1 in 68,000 and 1 in 225,000 screened blood transfusions transmit HIV. Prospective studies estimate the risk at 1 in 40,315 to 1 in 88,561. The antibody to HIV enzyme immunoassay tests that are currently in use are more sensitive than the ones that were originally introduced. The current assay is a sandwich assay using p24/41 antigen produced with recombinant DNA techniques. The earlier assays used whole virus lysates. When paired serum and cell samples from prospectively followed members of high-risk groups are analyzed with polymerase chain reaction and enzyme immunoassays, the window period for HIV with current tests is 33 to 40 days.

Infection with HIV-2 also causes a syndrome of immunodeficiency and opportunistic infections. Although the virus is endemic in West Africa, infection with HIV-2 is rare in the United States. The CDC estimates that less than three units per 10 million screened donations are positive for HIV-2. Nonetheless, the current licensed immunoassays are designed to detect HIV-1 and HIV-2.

HUMAN T-CELL LEUKEMIA/LYMPHOMA VIRUSES

The role of HTLV-I and HTLV-II in transfusion medicine was recently reviewed.[28] HTLV-I is the etiologic agent of adult T-cell leukemia and tropical spastic paraparesis/HTLV-I–associated myelopathy. The virus is endemic in Japan and in the Caribbean. Studies by the Japanese demonstrated that HTLV-I could be transmitted by blood transfusion, and the first kits to detect HTLV-I were licensed in late November of 1988. The risk of transmitting HTLV-I infection in screened blood is estimated to be 1 in 62,500 units.[27] Before the introduction of testing, the risk was estimated to be 1 in 5000 units. The incubation period for adult T-cell leukemia is long and transfusion-transmitted cases have not been confirmed. The development of tropical spastic paresis/HTLV-I–associated myelopathy after transfusion has been documented, however. HTLV-I is a cell-associated virus, and any procedure that would reduce the leukocyte content of blood would be expected to reduce or eliminate the risk of HTLV-I infection. Therefore, it is interesting to note that HTLV-I seroconversion occurred in an infant who received washed irradiated red cells.[29] The transfusion was administered before the introduction of serologic testing and the recipient was identified through a look-back study.

HTLV-II has not been convincingly demonstrated to cause disease.[28] Infection is endemic in Guyami Indians in Panama and has been identified in a few Native American and Hispanic blood donors in the United States. Infection with HTLV-II is common among intravenous drug users. HTLV-I and HTLV-II are similar, and the immunoassay for HTLV-I also detects HTLV-II.

CYTOMEGALOVIRUS

Cytomegalovirus is a member of the herpesvirus family. It is a double-stranded enveloped virus that, like other herpesviruses, remains in a latent state after primary infection. The transmission of CMV by blood transfusion was first documented in the 1960s. In adults, the frequency of seropositivity for CMV varies from 30% to 90%. Infection acquired in the community and by transfusion is usually subclinical and documented only by the development of antibodies to CMV. A syndrome similar to infectious mononucleosis, however, is occasionally seen in immunologically competent adults after transfusion. In infants and immunologically compromised adults, transfusion-transmitted CMV may be associated with severe morbidity and mortality.[30] Routine blood transfusions are not screened for CMV, although cellular blood components prepared from CMV-seronegative donors are provided for use in patient populations at risk. Fresh frozen plasma does not need to be obtained from CMV-seronegative donors because the virus is carried in blood mononuclear cells.[31]

OTHER INFECTIONS

Bacterial Infections

Bacterial contamination of blood products is extremely rare because of improvements in blood collection procedures. Sepsis related to blood transfusion is observed occasionally, however. Reports of fatal transfusion reactions to the US Food and Drug Administration indicated that 12 of 99 deaths occurring from 1991 to 1992 were related to bacterial contamination.[32] In 11 of the 12 cases, platelet products were implicated. Asymptomatic bacteremia in blood donors infected with *Yersinia enterocolitica* has also caused transfusion-transmitted sepsis. *Pseudomonas* and *Serratia* species believed to have been introduced through breaks in technique have also been cultured from red cell products that have caused sepsis.[33]

The transfusion of bacteria-contaminated blood components can produce a spectrum of symptoms. Mild bacterial contamination may provoke only a febrile reaction, whereas heavy contamination produces sepsis and shock. Bacterial contamination should be suspected in these cases and parenteral therapy with broad-spectrum antibiotics must be instituted immediately. Mortality is high, even with prompt diagnosis and treatment.

Strict adherence to guidelines regarding proper storage and infusion of blood components helps reduce the risk of bacterial contamination. Components prepared with an open system are more likely to become contaminated than are those prepared with closed systems. Blood components implicated in severe febrile reactions, hypotensive reactions, and hemolytic reactions should be sent for culture.

Syphilis may be transmitted by transfusion but such an event has not been reported recently in the United States. Red cell products are refrigerated between 1° and 6°C, and the spirochete does not survive more than 120 hours at this temperature. Platelet products, however, are not refrigerated. A platelet donor with primary syphilis in the window period could potentially transmit the disease. Blood donations from patients who have been treated for syphilis or gonorrhea are deferred for 12 months after the completion of therapy.

Parasitic Infections

Of the many parasitic diseases that can be transmitted by transfusion, malaria, babesiosis, and Chagas' disease are considered to be of importance in the United States. The CDC estimates that 1 case of transfusion-transmitted ma-

laria is reported for each 4 million units of blood collected.[34] Babesiosis appears to be symptomatic only in the immunocompromised transfusion recipient, because most affected patients have undergone splenectomy. Both malaria and babesiosis present as febrile hemolytic diseases occurring late after transfusion. Chagas' disease is of concern because of the many Latin American immigrants that are entering the United States. Chagas' disease presents as antibiotic-resistant fever accompanied by hepatosplenomegaly, myocarditis, and pericardial effusion. Transfusion-transmitted Chagas' disease has been documented in North America but the blood donors were from Central and South America, areas that are endemic for Chagas' disease. Donors with histories of babesiosis or Chagas' disease are permanently deferred but some donors have asymptomatic infection. Clinical studies are being conducted at a blood center in Los Angeles to determine whether a two-part screening system involving questions related to travel history followed by serologic testing will be useful in identifying donors who are capable of transmitting the disease.[35]

REFERENCES

1. Sayers MH, Anderson KC, Goodnough LT, et al. Reducing the risk for transfusion-transmitted cytomegalovirus infection. Ann Intern Med 1992;116:55–62.
2. Bowden RA, Meyers JD. Prophylaxis of cytomegalovirus infection. Semin Hematol 1990;27(Suppl 1):17–21.
3. Sniecinski I, O'Donnell MR, Nowicki B, et al. Prevention of refractoriness and HLA-alloimmunization using filtered blood products. Blood 1988;71:1402–1407.
4. American Association of Blood Banks. Standards for blood banks and transfusion services, ed 15. Arlington, VA, American Association of Blood Banks, 1993:30–31.
5. Anderson KC, Goodnough LT, Sayers MH, et al. Variation in blood component irradiation practice: implications for prevention of transfusion-associated graft-versus-host disease. Blood 1991;77:2096–2102.
6. Schroeder ML, Rayner HL. Transfusion of blood and blood components. In: Lee GR, Bithell TC, Foerster J, et al, eds. Wintrobe's clinical hematology, ed 9. Malvern, PA, Lea & Febiger, 1993:651–700.
7. Greenwalt TJ. Pathogenesis and management of hemolytic transfusion reactions. Semin Hematol 1981;18:84–94.
8. Davenport RD, Streiter RM, Standiford TJ, et al. Interleukin-8 production in red blood cell incompatibility. Blood 1990;76:2439–2442.
9. Rock RC, Bove JR, Nemerson Y. Heparin treatment of intravascular coagulation accompanying hemolytic transfusion reactions. Transfusion 1969;9:57–67.
10. Pineda AA. Delayed hemolytic transfusion reaction: an immunological hazard of blood transfusion. Transfusion 1978;18:1–7.
11. Muylle L, Joos M, Wouters E, et al. Increased tumor necrosis factor α (TNFα), interleukin 1 (IL-1), and interleukin 6 (IL-6)

levels in the plasma of stored platelet concentrates: relationship between TNFα and IL-6 levels and febrile transfusion reactions. Transfusion 1993;33:195–199.

12. Popovsky MA, Moore SB. Diagnostic and pathogenetic considerations in transfusion-related acute lung injury. Transfusion 1985;25:573–577.

13. Seeger W, Schneider U, Kreusler B, et al. Reproduction of transfusion-related acute lung injury in an *ex vivo* lung model. Blood 1990;76:1438–1444.

14. Gans ROB, Duurkens VAM, van Zundert AA, et al. Transfusion-related acute lung injury. Intensive Care Med 1988;14:754–757.

15. Mueller-Eckhardt C, Lechner K, Heinrich D, et al. Post-transfusion thrombocytopenic purpura: immunological and clinical studies in two cases and review of the literature. Blut 1980;40:249–257.

16. Tartter PI, Quintero S, Barren DM. Perioperative blood transfusion associated with infectious complications after colorectal cancer operations. Am J Surg 1986;152:479–482.

17. Van Aken WG. Does perioperative blood transfusion promote tumor growth? Transfus Med Rev 1989;3:243–252.

18. Sloand E, Kumar P, Klein HG, et al. Transfusion of blood components to persons infected with human immunodeficiency virus type I: relationship to opportunistic infection. Transfusion 1994;34:48–53.

19. Busch MP, Tzong-Hae L, Herman J. Allogeneic leukocytes but not therapeutic blood elements induce reactivation and dissemination of latent human immunodeficiency virus type I infection: implications for transfusion support of infected patients. Blood 1992;80:2128–2135.

20. Linden JV, Pisciotto PT. Transfusion-associated graft-versus-host disease and blood irradiation. Transfus Med Rev 1992;6:116–123.

21. Akahoshi M, Takanashi M, Masuda M. A case of transfusion-associated graft-versus-host disease not prevented by leukocyte depletion filters. Transfusion 1992;32:169–172.

22. Alter HJ, Purcell RH, Shih JW, et al. Detection of antibody to hepatitis C virus in prospectively followed transfusion recipients with acute and chronic non-A, non-B hepatitis. N Engl J Med 1989;321:1494–1500.

23. Sherertz RJ, Russell BA, Reuman PD. Transmission of hepatitis A by transfusion of blood products. Arch Intern Med 1984;144:1579–1580.

24. Rosina F, Saracco G, Rizzetto M. Risk of post-transfusion infection with the hepatitis delta virus: a multicenter study. N Engl J Med 1985;312:1488–1491.

25. Ward JW, Holmberg SD, Allen JR, et al. Transmission of human immunodeficiency virus (HIV) by blood transfusions screened as negative for HIV antibody. N Engl J Med 1988;318:473–478.

26. Cohen ND, Munoz A, Reitz BA, et al. Transmission of retroviruses by transfusion of screened blood in patients undergoing cardiac surgery. N Engl J Med 1989;320:1172–1176.

27. Busch MP. Retroviruses and blood transfusions: the lessons learned and the challenge yet ahead. In: Nance SJ, ed. Blood safety: current challenges. Bethesda, MD, American Association of Blood Banks, 1993:1–44.

28. Sandler GS, Fang CT, Williams A. Human t-cell lymphotropic virus type I and II in transfusion medicine. Transfus Med Rev 1991;5:93–107.

29. DePalma L, Luban NLC. Transmission of human T-lymphotropic virus type I infection to a neonatal infant by transfusion of washed and irradiated red cells. Transfusion 1993;33:582–584.

30. Zaia JA. Epidemiology and pathogenesis of cytomegalovirus disease. Semin Hematol 1990;27(Suppl 1):5–10.

31. Bowden R, Sayers M. The risk of transmitting cytomegalovirus infection by fresh frozen plasma. Transfusion 1990;30:762–763.

32. Regulatory affairs: fatality statistics. Am Assoc Blood Banks News Briefs 1992;August:14B-2.

33. Goldman M, Blajchman MA. Blood product-associated bacterial sepsis. Transfus Med Rev 1991;5:73–83.

34. Nahlen BL, Lobel HO, Cannon SE, et al. Reassessment of blood donor selection criteria for United States travelers to malarious areas. Transfusion 1991;31:798–804.

35. Kerndt PR, Waskin HA, Kirchhoff LV, et al. Prevalence of antibody to *Trypanosoma cruzi* among blood donors in Los Angeles, California. Transfusion 1991;31:814–818.

SECTION

INFECTIOUS DISEASE

Medical Management of the Surgical Patient, Third Edition,
edited by Michael F. Lubin, H. Kenneth Walker, and Robert B. Smith III.
J.B. Lippincott Company, Philadelphia, PA © 1995.

CHAPTER

25

PREVENTIVE ANTIBIOTICS IN SURGERY

John E. McGowan, Jr.

PREVENTION OF SURGICAL INFECTION

The preventive use of antibiotics, or surgical prophylaxis, is defined here as the administration of antimicrobial drugs during surgery to patients without evidence of established infection in anticipation of preventing infection.[1] Such use swiftly followed the development of the first antibiotics; studies of this indication have appeared for more than 50 years.[2] Antibiotic prophylaxis accounts for as much as 25% of all hospital antimicrobial drug use in the United States, representing a total expenditure of several hundred million dollars each year.[3] Excluded from consideration is the treatment of a preexisting infection that the procedure is designed to correct.[4]

For many years, this practice was based on a theoretical potential for averting infection: it seemed that it should be helpful. In the past decade, many studies (largely conducted by surgeons) have provided fresh data to identify when antimicrobial agents given at surgery do and do not benefit patients.[5–8] As a result, internists who must offer advice on whether to use prophylactic antimicrobials for a given procedure or which drugs to use for specific patients now have objective information to guide these decisions. This section provides prophylaxis guidelines for several surgical procedures and considers settings in which internists may wish to modify the usual regimens.

SURGICAL INFECTIONS AND THEIR CONSEQUENCES

Infections accompanying surgical procedures contribute significantly to surgical morbidity and mortality. A national survey from 1987 to 1990 by the Centers for Disease Control and Prevention (CDC) reported surgical wound infections in 2376 of 84,691 operations (2.8%).[9] If this study is extrapolated to the United States as a whole, postoperative wound infections afflict up to 1 million of the 23 million patients who undergo surgery each year.[2]

In the CDC study, the rate markedly increased when pus or a perforated viscus was found at operation. The infection rate for clean surgery (in which no infection was encountered, no hollow muscular organ was opened, and no break in aseptic technique occurred) was 2.1%, whereas that for clean-contaminated procedures (those in which a hollow muscular organ was opened but minimal spillage occurred) was 3.3%. After contaminated procedures (those involving acute inflammation without pus, gross spillage from a hollow viscus, a major break in aseptic technique during the operation, or acute trauma of less than 4 hours), the infection rate was 6.4%. When pus was encountered at operation or when traumatic wounds had existed for more than 4 hours (so-called dirty cases), the infection rate was 7.1%. Further analysis of surgical patients in the same CDC study from January 1986 to June 1992 found that wound infection was the most frequent type of infection and that a causal relationship between wound infection and death existed in 89% of patients in whom both factors were present.[10]

A similar survey in a Canadian hospital published in 1981 found wound infection rates after operations in these four classes to be 1.5%, 7.7%, 15.2%, and 40%, respectively.[11] Thus, rates were higher in the last three groups in the older survey but lower for clean procedures. These data support the observation of Condon, who noted in 1991 that some infection rates have not diminished in recent years and actually appear to have been increasing.[12]

In 1992, Ulualp and Condon[13] summarized infection rates after scheduled operations performed without antibiotic prophylaxis. Rates ranged from 5% to 56% for all except clean procedures, which had an infection rate of under 3%. Farber and Wenzel[14] determined the occurrence of wound infection in association with specific procedures in hospitals throughout Virginia. Rates ranged from under 1% for meniscectomy and thyroidectomy to 26% for removal of a ruptured appendix. Similar differences by site of operation were noted in a large study from Minneapolis.[15] Infection is the most common cause of death in injured patients who survive severe trauma.[16]

The presence of a wound infection has economic as well as medical consequences.[7] Wenzel[2] estimates the total direct cost of longer hospital stays associated with surgical wound infection to be well over $1.5 billion per year. In a study by the CDC, the average cost to a hospital of surgical wound infection was estimated at $2700 (in 1985 dollars), and the best-case estimate of the increase in reimbursement to the hospital was $233. Thus, the hospital's net loss would be in the range of $2500.[17] Wound infection added 12.2 days to the average stay of cardiac surgical patients in Freiburg, Germany, compared with matched patients without infection.[18] Finally, a study from the United Kingdom showed that an outbreak of wound infections in orthopedics produced an average increased hospital stay of 17 days and an additional cost of about $3400 (£2220).[19]

CURRENT PATTERNS OF PROPHYLACTIC ANTIBIOTIC USE

Surgical prophylaxis accounted for about one third of all antimicrobial drug use in one statewide survey in the 1970s.[20] Antimicrobial use for prophylaxis made up about the same proportion of total antibiotic costs at St. Thomas Hospital in Nashville in 1988.[21] In a random survey of short-stay hospitals in middle Tennessee from 1989 to 1990, perioperative prophylaxis was used in 48% of 905 surveyed surgical procedures.[22] The financial investment can be sizable; one study estimated that five orthopedic surgical procedures per week using a standard cefamandole prophylaxis regimen would entail drug acquisition and administration costs of $40,872 per year.[23] When these figures are extrapolated to all the surgery performed in the country, prophylaxis for surgery requires an aggregate expenditure of several hundred million dollars per year in the United States.[24]

Britt and colleagues[25] investigated antimicrobial use in surgical patients throughout Utah. Of 2782 patients, 42% received prophylactic antimicrobials, including 58% who had clean surgery involving the implantation of prostheses, 27% who underwent other clean surgery, 54% whose procedures were clean-contaminated, and 86% whose wounds were contaminated. Preventive antimicrobial therapy was begun within 6 hours of surgery and stopped within 48 hours afterward in only 9% of patients. Drug administration was initiated after the operation in 34% of patients and continued for more than 48 hours in 57%. In this study, cephalosporins were used most commonly. Gardner and associates[26] reviewed the use of preventive antimicrobials in 300 consecutive surgical patients in their hospital. Preventive drugs were used in 41% of the patients in this study. The authors evaluated the therapy in all patients and judged the indications for prophylaxis to be appropriate in about half of them. Major problems recorded were beginning therapy after the operation was completed (23 cases), administering prophylaxis for too long (9 cases) or too short (5 cases) a period, or having an insufficient indication for antibiotic coverage (39 cases). The authors also called attention to patients in whom the omission of prophylaxis represented what they considered to be inappropriate prescribing. These included three patients receiving metal orthopedic implants and one undergoing elective bowel resection.

Prophylaxis also produces substantial economic benefits.[2,27] The prevention of postoperative infections has an economic effect because these infections are expensive to treat when they occur. Costs are disproportionate to rates of occurrence; surgical wound infections constitute only about 25% of all nosocomial infections but account for about 50% of extra costs and additional hospital days for such infections.[28,29] These costs make postoperative infection one of the three most expensive types of nosocomial infection, along with pneumonia and bacteremia.[30]

CAN PERIOPERATIVE ANTIBIOTIC USE BE IMPROVED?

The use of perioperative prophylaxis, to Ehrenkranz, "may account for a substantial portion of hospital pharmacy antibiotic use that is regarded as inappropriate."[31] At the community hospitals surveyed by him, the mean duration of intravenous antimicrobial use in uninfected patients after elective large bowel operations was 4 days, longer than many studies would suggest as appropriate.[32] Several studies performed a decade or more ago demonstrated problems with indications for use, dose, and duration of administration.[20,25,26,33] More recent reports exist as well. In a survey of community hospitals in South Florida, the use of prophylaxis was determined to be justified in 366 of 486 operations.[34] Prophylaxis was used in all 366 of these cases but therapy was given in inadequate dosage in 32%, was started after operation in 24%, and was used for a longer period than studies suggest in 23%. Per surveyed operation, the authors identified an excess cost for prophylaxis of $26.93; $13.24 was wasted because of incorrect, inadequate, or prolonged use, and $9.26 for the use of more expensive drugs than were needed. For a hospital at which 1250 such operations are done per year, this could total more than $45,000 in resources wasted in the process of prophylaxis. These authors also noted that a lawsuit risk existed in situations where prophylaxis was indicated but was given in inadequate dosage or started after operation. They provided no estimate of the financial magnitude of this liability risk, however.[34] A survey in middle Tennessee from 1989 to 1990 showed that 60% of patients who underwent surgery for which there is a published indication actually received prophylaxis and that 41% of those who had a procedure for which prophylaxis is not usually recommended received prophylaxis as well.[22] This study also showed problems with the timing and duration of drug administration.

When attention has been given to improving the use of prophylaxis, the dollar impact has been dramatic. At Hartford Hospital in Connecticut, a program to emphasize the use of single rather than multiple doses of cefazolin for prophylaxis in obstetric and gynecologic surgical procedures cost $1733 to implement and led to a savings of $19.79 per patient, or about $14,000 annually.[35] Everitt[36] and coworkers found that an educational program for obstetricians produced improved prescribing practices and savings of more than $26,000 per year without an adverse effect on the infection rate.

Recent studies have focused on ways to produce better habits in the prescription of perioperative prophylaxis. One group has used computer-generated messages. In a Salt Lake City hospital, reminders about perioperative antibiotic use were placed in patients' records before surgery and the rate of postoperative wound infections declined by half.[37]

FACTORS MODIFYING USUAL RECOMMENDATIONS

Guidelines provided for prophylaxis in specific operations are for "usual" procedures. Internists must determine whether special circumstances require modification of the standard practices. Many factors must be considered in the consultation process. Nichols[38] noted that the most critical factors in the prevention of postoperative wound infection are the operative technique and judgment of the surgical staff and the patient's general health and disease stage. Each of these is considered in turn, as are organisms, drugs, and cost/benefit ratios.

Surgeon and Environmental Factors

As DiPiro and associates[39] suggested, the surgical techniques used and postoperative care provided have a greater influence on infection risks than does the prophylactic antimicrobial agent selected. The surgeon's skill in removing dead tissue, preventing hematoma, and providing adequate drainage is vital.[2] His or her ability to use newer mechanical techniques, such as zipper closure, also may affect infection rates. In addition, the rate of infection varies somewhat with the number of surgical procedures performed.[40,41] As a result, some surgeons may achieve acceptably low infection rates without prophylaxis in circumstances in which others have found prophylaxis to be effective or essential. Alternatively, some surgeons may have an inordinate number of infectious complications even with the use of prophylactic antibiotics.[42] Consulting internists must consider the track record of surgeons and other operative team members in deciding whether to recommend antimicrobial prophylaxis.

In the classifications of risk developed by Culver and associates[9] and by Garibaldi and colleagues,[6] long duration of surgery was a significant predictor of subsequent infection. Thus, the speed of performance as well as the relative complexity of the procedure must be considered in the decision regarding prophylaxis.

The operating room environment and other features of preoperative and postoperative care also are crucial to controlling the occurrence of postoperative wound infection.[43] Kaiser[44] noted that virtually all operative fields are contaminated with microorganisms by the end of surgical procedure, despite vigorous aseptic techniques. Garibaldi and colleagues[6] found that a positive intraoperative culture was an independent predictor of subsequent wound infection; this may relate in part to environmental contamination. The ward setting also can be important. Outbreaks have demonstrated that wounds closed in a primary fashion are still at risk for contamination and infection after the surgical procedure itself has been completed.[44] Weaknesses of the hospital setting must be known to consulting internists and may necessitate the use of antimicrobials when they usually would not be required.

About half the surgical procedures performed in the United States are done in outpatient facilities, and patient outcomes have not been studied as well in this setting as they have in the hospital.[2] It is assumed that risks associated with this environment are similar to those of the hospital but this remains to be confirmed.

Patient Factors

Numerous patient-specific factors that are independent of the antimicrobial drugs used and the types of surgery performed affect the occurrence of infection.[45–47] Burke[48] pointed out that host defenses ordinarily handle invading microorganisms without difficulty. In some patients, however, these defenses can be inhibited by primary diseases (eg, malignancy) or their therapy (eg, steroids or immunosuppression), or by procedures or equipment (eg, the insertion of foreign-body prostheses or the use of a heart–lung machine). Thus, investigators such as Ulualp and Condon consider that use of a prosthesis results in a procedure that is clean-contaminated rather than clean.[13]

Measuring a patient's inherent risk of infection is crucial in making decisions regarding prophylaxis.[49] Haley and colleagues[50] developed a risk index to predict a patient's likelihood of developing surgical wound infection. In this scheme, the most significant predictors were operations on the abdomen, operations classified as contaminated or dirty, and operations lasting more than 2 hours. After controlling for these factors, however, patients with more than three diagnoses (which the authors considered to be a measure of the complexity of the patient's underlying condition distinct from the surgery) were still at markedly higher risk for infection. In the CDC study of 1987 to 1990,[9] the risk of wound infection was best predicted by combining two non-patient factors, the type of procedure performed (eg, clean, clean-contaminated), and the length of the operation with an index (ASA score) constructed by the American Society of Anesthesiologists to assess patients' overall physical status. Garibaldi and colleagues[6] similarly found the ASA score to be one of four risk factors that were independent of each other in predicting likely wound infection. Including the ASA score is a practical way to assess risk because it is used almost universally in anesthesia practice.

Results of these risk assessments show that, for certain types of operations, the rate may be five or more times higher in particular groups of high-risk patients.[2] Higher wound infection rates are consistently found in obese patients, presumably because adipose tissue is poorly vascularized. Older age is associated with wound sepsis after some operations but this appears to relate to other specific factors (eg, diabetes) that are more often present in the elderly rather than to age in general.[51] For example, the high frequency of infection after colonic surgery in the elderly probably results from the greater concentration of bacteria usually found in their colons. Similarly, the use of prophy-

laxis in children must take into account differences in the procedures performed, the response of the host, and the altered pharmacology of many antimicrobials in this population.[52,53] The presence of infection at another site at the time of operation also increases the risk of infection.[10]

The advisability of using these patient risk classifications as a guide to prophylaxis is emphasized by Page and colleagues,[1] who point out that the presence of two or more of the risk factors used in the CDC study predict a high risk of postoperative infection regardless of the type of surgery performed. Patients in this risk group experience infection rates of 8% to 15% after clean surgery, which qualifies them for prophylaxis in most evaluations. Thus, these authors conclude that risk categories are an appropriate guide for determining the usefulness of prophylaxis.

Studies of patient risk usually have excluded several groups from evaluation, including pregnant women, children, and patients who have recently received therapeutic drugs. Thus, guidelines for prophylaxis are less clear for such patients.[4]

If possible, it is important to try to improve these defenses; the preservation and enhancement of host defenses is the oldest but the most neglected of preventive measures.[54] This can be done by enhancing nutrition, tissue perfusion, and oxygenation as alternatives to chemoprophylaxis. Immunoprophylaxis as an aid to improving defenses (eg, *Pseudomonas* vaccine for patients with burns) is still being evaluated. Appropriate preoperative care (eg, ensuring optimal nutrition, giving baths) also can modify the risk of postoperative infection.[55]

Organism Factors

It is imperative that prophylactic antibiotics be selected on the basis of those organisms that are most likely to cause infection, which vary dramatically with operative site.[56] More important, they also vary with previous antimicrobial therapy and depend on the local patterns of organism prevalence and resistance in a given area. Length of hospitalization before surgery also can affect the likelihood of infection with resistant organisms because changes in microbial flora can occur quickly after hospitalization.[56]

CORRECT DRUG USE

What Drug Characteristics Are Important?

The drug used should be effective against the pathogens that are most likely to cause infection. It does not necessarily have to kill all the organisms present but must inhibit their interactions. Regimens directed at only some microbial flora have been successful in some instances.[1] Drugs that are not effective for therapy may work for prophylaxis.[32] Therefore, benefit does not necessarily result from a better in vitro spectrum of activity for a new drug.[57]

Their absorption and duration of action are thought to be important features of prophylactic antimicrobial agents.[58] After drug blood levels decline, some groups of antimicrobials (eg, aminoglycosides) continue to have a residual antibacterial effect, whereas others (eg, β-lactams) have little or none.[32] The clinical effect of this pharmacologic interaction is not clear, especially because one member of the β-lactam family, cefazolin, has been shown to be effective in several studies over many years. In addition, improved pharmacokinetics and greater tissue penetration have not necessarily produced better clinical results.[4]

The potential for adverse reactions always should be considered in choosing a prophylactic regimen. According to Ehrenkranz,[31] given a large number of patients, routine use of an antimicrobial, however brief, will result in measurable side effects in some. For example, infusion-related adverse events of prophylaxis occurred in 3% and 4.9% of cases in two different studies summarized by Eisenberg and colleagues.[59] Each drug given also increases the chance for possible adverse drug interactions. Moreover, Bryan and colleagues[23] emphasize that "the extent to which we should base our choice of agents on reports of rare (however serious) side effects becomes a cost-effective issue with ethical overtones."

For some drugs and some types of surgery, the emergence of resistance is a fairly common occurrence. For example, low-level colonization of hospitalized patients with methicillin-resistant coagulase-negative staphylococci progressed to higher organism concentrations at the same sites after prophylaxis was administered for cardiac surgery.[60] The emergence of resistance potentially poses a problem both for the patients being treated and for other patients.[61] The use of agents with a broader spectrum of activity for prophylaxis increases the chance of superinfection with naturally resistant organisms such as *Clostridium difficile*.[32] Assigning a financial equivalent to ecologic costs is difficult, however.[61–64]

A final consideration is whether a drug otherwise may be useful for treating a postoperative infection. Page and associates[1] conclude that inappropriate use of valuable therapeutic agents may be one of the most serious errors made in the provision of prophylaxis.

Which Drug Should Be Used?

Kaiser[21] found that prophylactic antibiotics are more effective than placebos but differ little in effectiveness from one another. The true value of one antiinfective regimen over another has become difficult to assess because of the potency of available drugs.[46] The antimicrobials used for many studies have been selected because the manufacturer has supported the study. It is unclear in many instances whether other drugs would have had equal or greater effectiveness. Recent trials have compared the third-generation cephalosporins with earlier cephalosporins. Yet, the *Medical Letter* states emphatically that third-generation cephalosporins should not be used for surgical prophylaxis: "They are expensive, their activity against staphylococci is often less than that of cefazolin, their spectrum of activity against aerobic gram-negative bacilli includes organisms rarely encountered in elective surgery, and their widespread use for prophylaxis promotes emergence of resistance to these potentially valuable drugs."[65]

The most common pathogens and their antimicrobial resistance vary among hospitals and even over time at a particular hospital. Thus, a regimen that is successful at one hospital may prove relatively ineffective at another time at the same hospital or at a different institution. Medical consultants must know the local pattern of susceptibility before recommending prophylaxis.

Antiseptic and Topical Agents

Fitzgerald[66] has noted that local antiseptics are one of the most controversial topics in surgery. Sanderson[56] found good evidence that appropriate, locally administered prophylactic agents (eg, abdominal lavage, gentamicin cement) reduce the occurrence of postoperative infection. Finding the right setting for their use, however, has proven to be a problem. For example, the use of povidone-iodine solution as an irrigation agent in abdominal surgery has produced conflicting results.[67] In view of studies suggesting their potential for toxicity, iodophors should be used with caution.[68] Topical or local antibiotics also can contribute to the emergence of resistance. The value of these agents remains to be determined.[38]

When Should Prophylaxis Be Started?

Animal studies and other experiments suggest that antimicrobials are most likely to prevent colonization of a wound when they are given while the number of organisms is low, the organisms are multiplying rapidly, and the site is not yet deprived of its blood supply.[13] Thus, to prevent postoperative infection, antibiotics must be administered before or at the start of surgery; it appears that drugs must have an adequate concentration at the site of expected infection once bacteria are introduced into a wound.

Even though experimental studies suggest a golden period of 3 hours after incision during which antimicrobials have some preventive effect,[48,65] most clinical investigators agree that tissue levels of antibiotics should be present at the first incision and that initiating prophylaxis after patients have returned to regular hospital floors is useless.[67] In a study of 2847 patients undergoing elective clean or clean-contaminated surgery, those who were given postoperative antibiotics had a 5.8 times greater incidence of wound infection than did those who received perioperative antibiotics.[69] After intravenous administration, peak tissue levels usually appear within about 1 or 2 hours. Rates of infection also were increased if the drug was given more than 2 hours before the procedure. Moreover, administration too soon before the procedure can lead to the emergence of resistant organisms, whose introduction into the wound at surgery could make the treatment of subsequent infections difficult.[61]

As a result, parenteral antibiotics for surgical prophylaxis usually are begun 20 to 30 minutes before initial incision, depending on the pharmacology of the drug. Giving the drug in the operating room facilitates this timing, instead of giving it "on call," which may occur hours before the actual surgery.[38] For some kinds of abdominal surgery, a regimen of oral antimicrobials combined with mechanical bowel cleaning must be administered during the 24 hours before the operative procedure is begun.[13,38]

How Long Should Prophylaxis Be Continued?

According to Ehrenkranz,[32] prophylaxis ideally should be given immediately before or during operation and only for the shortest period of proven efficacy. He cites abundant data indicating that postoperative doses of antimicrobials do not provide an additional prophylactic benefit. Three to 4 hours after the incision, antimicrobials are no longer beneficial against possible subsequent infection,[38,48] so surgical prophylaxis is needed only for a short time.[4,55]

Page and coworkers[1] concluded that, in most instances, the course of antibiotic administration should be limited to intraoperative coverage, which they deemed a significant change from the usual 24- to 48-hour coverage. Support for this position has come from numerous studies. In operations involving the gastrointestinal tract, orthopedic operations, and cesarean section and gynecologic procedures, intraoperative prophylaxis was found to be at least as effective as longer courses of therapy.[1] There is far more danger of both drug reactions and the emergence of antibiotic-resistant bacteria with prolonged administration. Studies are being performed to define the minimum time needed for prophylaxis in various procedures. In many operations, the total duration of prophylaxis may be shortened to as little as one dose of parenteral drug without adverse effect.[13] Sanderson[56] suggests that an optimal regimen for many procedures may include the administration of one dose just before the first incision and a second dose as the incision is being closed.

A single dose, however, is not always successful. Maintaining effective levels throughout a surgical procedure appears to be a critical part of preventive care.[32] More than one dose may be needed when patients have been hemorrhaging or when the duration of surgery is prolonged. Ulualp and Condon[13] recommend that the dose be administered every 2 hours during the operation when the half-life of the drug is less than 1 hour. A few special situations may arise in which patients are at risk for more extended periods (eg, the presence of drains, trauma before operation), and these must be taken into account when defining the period of risk. For most of these, a regimen extending no longer than 2 days after surgery appears satisfactory. A longer period of prophylaxis sometimes is advocated for heavily contaminated wounds. These cases are managed better by delayed wound closure, however, than by reliance on antimicrobial agents to chance primary closure.[1,32]

Shortening the duration of prophylaxis can markedly affect expenditures for laboratory monitoring, potential adverse effects, selection of resistant bacteria, and other factors.[3] In a comparison of 5 days versus 1 day of prophylaxis with penicillin in elective neurosurgical procedures, no difference in infection rates was shown. This finding had important cost implications for the institutions at which the study was performed.[70]

COST/BENEFIT ASSESSMENT

Financial aspects of prophylactic therapy have become even more important since the institution of prospective payment systems for hospitals. The cost of postoperative infection must be measured by considering the frequency with which it occurs and its economic and medical consequences.[3] The ability of the antimicrobial agent to decrease this cost by reducing the risk of infection must be balanced against its potential harmful effects, such as toxic or allergic reactions and the selection of resistant organisms. Although the likelihood of the former is fairly well known, the potential for the emergence of resistant microorganisms in the patient or the environment is less readily measured or recognized.[61] Among *otherwise equal* antibiotics, the least expensive should be selected, with cost assessment including the expense of laboratory monitoring, drug procurement, drug administration, adverse effects, and infections.[1]

Based on cost/benefit studies, a general assessment of indications has been provided by Ulualp and Condon[13]: prophylaxis is generally used for clean-contaminated or contaminated operations and for operations that involve the insertion of a prosthesis. These authors define "less well-accepted indications" as clean operations in patients with impaired host defenses or operations in which the consequences of infection would be extremely severe (eg, neurosurgery, cardiac surgery, ophthalmology). Prophylaxis is not usually recommended for clean surgery that does not involve the implantation of prostheses.[65] The Antimicrobial Agents Committee of the Surgical Infection Society, however, recommends its use in clean surgery when patients have multiple risk factors for infection that classify them as being at high risk.[1]

This general guide has several applications:

1. In some operative settings (eg, carotid endarterectomy and cholecystectomy in patients at low risk), prophylaxis may be effective but infections develop only infrequently and are seldom life-threatening. For other operations (eg, hysterectomy), the infections being prevented are rarely life-threatening and are easily treated.[71] Infections in either of these settings may cost more to try to prevent than to treat.[72] These considerations may apply for certain operations that are classified as clean surgery.[32]

2. In procedures involving the placement of prostheses (eg, cardiac valves, vascular grafts, artificial joints), infection is difficult to eradicate if it occurs. Thus, although infection is unlikely, its occurrence is so detrimental that antimicrobial prophylaxis is often justified.[13]

3. In other than clean surgery, antimicrobial prophylaxis may be useful in an attempt to reduce levels of contaminating organisms, whether they originate in the endogenous flora or in the outside environment.[32]

4. Patients are at risk for hospital-acquired infections at other sites (eg, lungs, urinary tract) during the postoperative period.[73] These infections also can contribute to increased costs of hospitalization. In surgical patients, prolongation of the hospital stay as a result of infection varies markedly by site. In one survey, the average hospital stay was prolonged 5.1 days by urinary tract infection, 12.9 days by wound infection, 8 days by postoperative fever, and 18 days by multiple infections compared with uninfected matched control subjects.[74] In contrast, some studies have found little or no effect of postoperative urinary tract infections on the length of the hospital stay or the duration of postoperative fever.[75] Thus, equal economic benefit cannot be ascribed to the prevention of wound infections and the prevention of other postoperative infections without measuring the average cost of infection at each site. If prophylaxis decreases the occurrence of infection at these sites as well, the economic benefit can increase greatly and the overall cost/benefit comparison may change. Infections at some sites (eg, bronchitis, atelectasis) are unlikely to prolong the hospital stay, whereas those at other sites (eg, pneumonia, bacteremia, symptomatic urinary

tract infection) lead to extended hospitalization because they require significant treatment and patient care.[28,76] Greco and colleagues[77] noted a 39% decrease in the rate of postoperative pneumonia after the institution of a standardized approach to prophylaxis and other perioperative procedures.

5. All reoperations performed through fresh or healing wounds after clean procedures should be considered clean-contaminated surgery and the decision for prophylaxis made on this basis.[32]

6. As new procedures are developed and old ones are improved, acceptable infection rates will decrease. As this occurs, prophylaxis that is acceptable today may not be cost-effective tomorrow.[56]

METHODS OF SURGICAL PROPHYLAXIS

This chapter presents the usual guidelines for specific types of operations. Factors listed earlier may make it necessary to modify the recommendations given here for specific patients.

PREVENTING RECURRENCE OF RHEUMATIC FEVER AFTER SURGERY

Antibiotics have long been used against recurrent episodes of rheumatic fever to prevent pharyngitis caused by group A streptococcus. Although such therapy is usually given for many years, the optimal duration of prophylaxis remains unknown.[78] Patients who have undergone valve surgery must avoid recurrent streptococcal infection, and prophylaxis is often continued longer in these patients than in patients who have not undergone valve surgery. Recommended drugs are benzathine penicillin G, 1.2 million units intramuscularly every 4 weeks; penicillin V, 125 to 250 mg orally twice daily; or sulfadiazine, 1 g orally daily for adults. Erythromycin, 250 mg orally twice daily, may be used if patients are allergic to both penicillin and sulfonamides.

Patients who have had rheumatic fever but have no evidence of rheumatic heart disease do not need endocarditis prophylaxis.

PATIENTS WITH VALVULAR HEART DISEASE WHO ARE UNDERGOING SURGICAL OR OTHER PROCEDURES

Before surgical, dental, and invasive diagnostic procedures are performed, antimicrobial agents usually are given to patients with congenital, rheumatic, or other valvular diseases of the heart.[79] This therapy is provided in an attempt to reduce the incidence or intensity of the associated transient bacteremia and decrease the likelihood of colonization of the valve. The risk of valvular infection depends on the age of the patient, the organisms that are likely to enter the bloodstream, and the type of cardiac disease that is present.[80]

No controlled studies of the efficacy of prophylaxis have been conducted because the large numbers of patients needed to demonstrate differences between regimens are impractical.[81] The recommendations in Tables 25-1 and 25-2 apply to adults and children weighing more than 27 kg and are adapted from the American Heart Association guidelines.[79] Some experts question the need to provide prophylaxis to patients with prosthetic joint replacements who are undergoing routine dental procedures but administer prophylaxis when more extensive periodontal disease or dental infection is involved.[82]

Head and Neck, and Ear, Nose, and Throat Surgery

Antimicrobial prophylaxis may be useful when the dura is entered, when areas contaminated with oropharyngeal flora are opened, or when implant material is being used.[65] These include orthognathic procedures, craniofacial revisions, maxillofacial fracture corrections, and major resections and reconstructions that involve the mucous membranes and deep tissue.[1] Antibiotics do not seem to be useful in clean otologic and oncologic operations of the head and neck, including the ear, in minor nasopharyngeal procedures, and for laryngectomy in patients with normal host defenses.[65,84] Further trials are needed to determine whether short-course prophylaxis is effective in tonsillectomy.[84] Gentamicin ear drops may decrease the occurrence of otorrhea after tympanostomy tube insertion.[65]

No clearcut choice of antimicrobial agent has emerged for use in these situations. Shapiro[84] believes that the use of

TABLE 25–1. Recommendations for Prophylactic Antimicrobial Agents for Preventing Endocarditis in Adults and Children Over 27 kg

Procedure	Drugs and Administration
DENTAL SURGERY: All dental procedures likely to induce gingival bleeding (including routine professional cleaning but not simple adjustment of orthodontic appliances or shedding of deciduous teeth), oral surgery, and upper respiratory procedures in patients who are at risk* Standard therapy: regimen A Amoxicillin- or penicillin-allergic patients: regimen B Patients allergic to both amoxicillin or penicillin and erythromycin: regimen C Patients unable to take oral medications: regimen D Amoxicillin- or penicillin-allergic patients unable to take oral medications: regimen E Alternate regimen for patients at highest risk† whose physicians prefer parenteral prophylaxis: regimen F Alternate regimen for patients at highest risk who are allergic to amoxicillin or penicillin: regimen G *GENITOURINARY AND GASTROINTESTINAL PROCEDURES* Standard therapy: regimen F Amoxicillin- or penicillin-allergic patients: regimen H Alternate for low-risk patients (those without prosthetic heart valves or histories of endocarditis): regimen A	*Regimen A:* Amoxicillin, 3 g orally 1 hour before the procedure, then 1.5 g 6 hours after the initial dose *Regimen B:* Erythromycin ethylsuccinate, 800 mg (or erythromycin stearate, 1 g) orally 2 hours before the procedure, then half the dose 6 hours after the initial dose *Regimen C:* Clindamycin, 300 mg orally 1 hour before the procedure and 150 mg orally 6 hours after the initial dose *Regimen D:* Ampicillin, 2 g IM or IV 30 minutes before the procedure, then 1 g IV 6 hours after the initial dose (can substitute amoxicillin 1.5 g orally for this second dose) *Regimen E:* Clindamycin, 300 mg IV 30 minutes before the procedure, then 150 mg IV or orally 6 hours after the initial dose *Regimen F:* Ampicillin, 2 g IV or IM, plus gentamicin, 1.5 mg/kg (not to exceed 80 mg), 30 minutes before the procedure; follow-up with amoxicillin, 1.5 g orally 6 hours after the initial dose (or repeat parenteral ampicillin and gentamicin 8 hours after the initial dose) *Regimen G:* Vancomycin, 1 g IV slowly over 1 hour, starting 1 hour before the procedure *Regimen H:* Vancomycin, 1 g IV slowly over 1 hour, starting 1 hour before the procedure, plus gentamicin 1.5 mg/kg IV or IM (not to exceed 80 mg) 1 hour before the procedure; this regimen may be repeated once 8 hours after the initial dose

*Patients with prosthetic cardiac valves, including bioprosthetic and homograft; previous bacterial endocarditis; most congenital cardiac malformations; rheumatic and other acquired valvular dysfunction (even after valve surgery); hypertrophic cardiomyopathy; mitral valve prolapse with valvular regurgitation.
†Patients with prosthetic heart valves or a previous history of endocarditis, or surgically constructed systemic-pulmonary shunts or conduits.
(Adapted from Dajani AS, Bisno AL, Chung KJ, et al. Prevention of bacterial endocarditis: recommendations by the American Heart Association. JAMA 1990;264:2919)

TABLE 25–2. Recommendations for Drug Choice in Selected Situations for Prevention of Surgical Wound Infection in Adults and Children Over 27 kg*

Procedure

Major head and neck procedures (incision of oral or pharyngeal mucosa or implant): regimen A or B

Eye surgery: regimen C

Cardiac operations with sternotomy or cardiopulmonary bypass: regimen D

Noncardiac vascular operations involving aorta, abdomen, or lower extremities; vascular prosthesis placement; or lower extremity amputation: regimen D

Noncardiac chest surgery involving thoracotomy: regimen A

Esophageal surgery: regimen A

Percutaneous endoscopic gastrostomy or gastric bypass for obesity: regimen A

Gastroduodenal surgery in high-risk patients (see text): regimen A

Biliary tract infection in high-risk patients (see text): regimen A

Colorectal elective surgery: regimen E or F (regimen F especially when urgency of surgery precludes use of oral therapy with regimen E)

Appendectomy: regimen G

Abdominal hernia repair: regimen A

Penetrating abdominal wound, treated immediately: regimen F or (for high-risk patients) H

Face or chest trauma with minimal contamination: regimen A

Cardiac trauma: regimen I

Orthopedic operations with implanted devices or prostheses: regimen I

Closed fractures treated with open reduction and internal fixation: regimen I

Open extremity fracture treated surgically within 6 hours of occurrence: regimen I

Clean neurosurgical procedures other than shunt insertion or revision: regimen A

Prostatectomy: treat bacteriuria if present before operation, according to organism susceptibilities

Transrectal biopsy of the prostate, stone removal, or renal trauma treated operatively: regimen I

Penile prosthesis insertion: regimen J

Hysterectomy or reconstructive fallopian tube surgery on previously infected tissues: regimen A

Laparoscopy with hydrotubation or hysterosalpingography: regimen K

First-trimester abortion in high-risk patients (see text): regimen L

Cesarean section in high-risk patients (see text): regimen A, given after umbilical cord is clamped

Elective breast surgery: regimen A

Drugs and Administration

Regimen A: Cefazolin, 1–2 g IV preoperatively, repeated every 4 hours during operative procedure, or if massive hemorrhage occurs. For patients allergic to cephalosporins: vancomycin or clindamycin. If methicillin-resistant staphylococci are frequent: vancomycin, 15 mg/kg IV slowly and in a dilute solution (no IV push) over 1 hour started 1 hour preoperatively.

Regimen B: Clindamycin, 600 mg IV, with or without gentamicin, 1.5 mg/kg IV, preoperatively and every 8 hours for a total of 3 doses.

Regimen C: Gentamicin drops topically over 2 to 24 hours *or* neomycin-gramicidin-polymyxin B drops topically over 2 to 24 hours *or* cefazolin, 100 mg subconjunctivally, at end of procedure.

Regimen D: Cefazolin, 1–2 g IV preoperatively, 2 g IV after completion of bypass and 2 g IV 8 hours later (some suggest another dose 8 hours later). If the patient is allergic to cephalosporins: vancomycin, 15 mg/kg IV given slowly and in a dilute solution over 1 hour (no IV push) preoperatively and 10 mg/kg IV given slowly in the same fashion after completion of bypass. Omit second dose if renal function is compromised. In some cases, a topical agent may suffice (see text).

Regimen E: Gastrointestinal lavage followed by erythromycin base, 1 g orally, and neomycin, 1 g orally, at 1 PM, 2 PM, and 11 PM on the day before surgery.

Regimen F: Cefoxitin, cefotetan, or cefmetazole, 2 g IV preoperatively and every 3 hours during surgery or if massive hemorrhage occurs.

Regimen G: Cefoxitin, cefotetan, or cefmetazole, 2 g IV preoperatively and every 3 hours during surgery or if massive hemorrhage occurs. (Alternative: add 1 dose of intravenous metronidazole at time of first dose of cephalosporin.)

Regimen H: Cefotaxime, 2 g preoperatively and every 8 hours, combined with metronidazole, 1 g IV preoperatively and every 12 hours. Alternative: clindamycin, 900 mg IV preoperatively and every 8 hours, plus gentamicin, 1.5 mg/kg IV at the same intervals.

Regimen I: Cefazolin 2 g IV preoperatively and every 8 hours for a total of 3 doses.

Regimen J: Cefazolin, 1 g IV, with gentamicin, 1.5 mg/kg IV, preoperatively, followed by 2 doses of the same 2 drugs at 8-hour intervals for a total of 24 hours of therapy.

Regimen K: Doxycycline, 200 mg orally before the procedure.

Regimen L: Aqueous penicillin G, 1 million units IV. Alternative: doxycycline, 100 mg orally 1 hour before the procedure and 200 mg orally 30 minutes after the procedure.

*See text for additional recommendations and cautions.
(Data from references 1, 13, 32, and 65)

a drug directed against oral anaerobes is essential. Cephalosporins (primarily cefazolin), penicillin, clindamycin, and amoxicillin/clavulanic acid in short perioperative courses have been used.[65,84,85] Short perioperative courses appear to be as effective as prolonged therapy.[86]

Ocular Surgery

Infection after intraocular lens implantation or other ophthalmologic procedures occurs infrequently but can be severe. The analogy to hip prostheses suggests that prophylaxis is reasonable. Antimicrobial eye drops and subconjuctival injection at the end of the procedure are widely prescribed.[65] Poor tissue penetration of most antimicrobials has discouraged the use of systemic antibiotic prophylaxis, however.[87]

Cardiovascular Surgery

Cardiac operations with sternotomy or cardiopulmonary bypass. The use of prophylactic antibiotics can decrease the incidence of infection after open heart surgery on valves and after coronary artery bypass grafting.[65] Single doses may be as effective as more prolonged therapy but this is not as clear for this type of surgery as for many others.[1] Because *Staphylococcus aureus* and coagulase-negative staphylococci are the most frequent causes of these infections, cefazolin or similar drugs are usually used for preventive therapy.[65] In hospitals where methicillin resistance is common among the staphylococci, vancomycin may be required. Tissue levels of short-acting cephalosporins in the heart decrease quickly after an intravenous or intramuscular dose, so another dose of a drug such as cefazolin may be needed during long surgical procedures. A dose of cefazolin or a similar drug should be given at the end of cardiopulmonary bypass because an adequate serum drug level is necessary at the time that electrocautery is performed and the sternum is closed.[88] For coronary artery bypass, a narrow-spectrum cephalosporin with a long half-life, used for no more than 1 day, appears to be a reasonable regimen.[88,89]

Cardiac catheterization and angioplasty. Although data are scanty, the use of prophylactic antimicrobials does not appear to be necessary in cardiac catheterization or angioplasty.[88,90]

Pacemaker insertion. Authors disagree on the value of prophylaxis in pacemaker insertion. Most now suggest that prophylactic antimicrobials are not needed.[65,88] Institutions with a high incidence of infection, however, may choose to use prophylaxis.[65]

Vascular surgery. Antimicrobial prophylaxis is commonly used in patients who are receiving vascular grafts because postoperative graft infections are difficult to treat. Antimicrobial prophylaxis is suggested for all vascular grafts of the aorta and for grafts of the lower extremities in which groin incisions are performed.[13,65] Kaiser and associates,[91] however, found that the infection rate after carotid or brachial artery surgery that did not involve prosthetic materials was so low (1 in 400 patients) that it did not outweigh the risk of drug administration. Any vascular procedure that involves the insertion of a prosthesis, including grafts for vascular access in hemodialysis, probably should include prophylaxis.[65]

Cephalosporins usually are used. Single doses or short periods (24 hours or less) of therapy are recommended. One study suggested that an intraoperative topical agent was as effective as parenteral administration.[92] Similarly, the topical use of mupirocin ointment has been found to be an effective prophylactic measure for the insertion of vascular shunts for hemodialysis access.[88]

Lower extremity amputation. The perioperative administration of a cephalosporin can decrease the incidence of infection after lower extremity amputation.[65]

Varicose vein surgery. The value of prophylactic antimicrobials in varicose vein surgery is unclear.[93]

Chest and Thoracic Surgery

The administration of a first-generation cephalosporin such as cefazolin for 24 hours is recommended by Malangoni and Jacobs[16] for emergency thoracotomy, regardless of whether lung resection is performed. In contrast, the same authors suggest that no perioperative prophylaxis be used for patients with pulmonary contusion.

A prospective randomized trial of cefazolin versus placebo for patients with chest tubes after stab wounds showed a definite benefit associated with antibiotic use.[94] The subject remains controversial, however[9]; some recommend brief periods of prophylaxis and others suggest that there are insufficient data to support prescription.[65]

Bowel Surgery

Patients who are undergoing operations associated with significant contamination of the peritoneal cavity should receive prophylaxis because it is well demonstrated to decrease the likelihood of intraabdominal sepsis. Well-controlled, prospective, blind studies are available to assist in prescribing decisions.[1]

Esophageal surgery. The potential for mediastinal contamination after operations on the esophagus is relatively great because the organ has a poor blood supply and motility is impaired after the operation. The risk is particularly increased when obstruction is present. Thus, a single dose or brief course of a first-generation cephalosporin is recommended.[13]

Percutaneous endoscopic gastrostomy. Antimicrobial prophylaxis with a single dose of cefazolin has been shown to be effective in patients undergoing percutaneous endoscopic gastrostomy.[65,95]

Gastroduodenal surgery. After surgery for nonobstructing duodenal ulcer, infection is infrequent and prophylaxis probably is not warranted.[87] In contrast, in patients with upper gastrointestinal tract bleeding, benign gastric ulcer, gastric tumor, obstruction, or other causes of decreased motility or lessened acidity of the stomach (eg, cimetidine therapy), infection is more likely and its occurrence is reduced by antimicrobial perioperative prophylaxis.[87] In addition, cephalosporins can decrease infectious complications in gastric bypass surgery for obesity.[65]

Mouth aerobes and anaerobes as well as the aerobes of the mid-bowel are often present in these patients. First-generation cephalosporins (primarily cefazolin or cefoxitin) have been used in most studies but their superiority over other drugs for this indication is unclear because few comparative trials have been performed. A single dose of a first-generation cephalosporin is probably adequate. Discontinuing therapy with agents that block or neutralize acid secretion for 1 or 2 days before operation also is important.[13]

Biliary surgery. Prophylaxis with antibiotics is not considered to be useful for gallbladder surgery in general but is useful for patients with certain risk factors that place them at higher than average risk for infection.[3] The high-risk category includes older patients (arbitrarily set at more than 60 years) and those with acute cholecystitis in the past 30 days, previous biliary tract surgery, obstructive jaundice, empyema of the gallbladder, chills or fever within 1 week of operation, or stones or stricture in the common bile duct.[13] Many of these categories represent the presence of established infection, so antibiotic use can be viewed as therapy rather than prophylaxis. Prophylaxis is unnecessary for patients who are not in these high risk-categories. If it is unclear whether common duct exploration will be needed, however, patients may be given a single perioperative dose of a systemic antibiotic.

First-generation cephalosporins have been used frequently in clinical trials. Biliary excretion of a drug has not correlated with prophylactic efficacy.[96] No evidence indicates that rates of infection are reduced when newer cephalosporins are used instead of first-generation drugs. This is

a setting in which a single dose of cephalosporin seems to be as beneficial as a long course of therapy.[13] As an alternative, intraoperative irrigation with topical polymyxin and neomycin is recommended by some.[55]

Colorectal surgery. Several regimens have been found to be effective in reducing the occurrence of infection and decreasing mortality in colorectal surgery.[97] It remains unclear whether the perioperative administration of parenteral antibiotics is superior or inferior to a regimen of preoperative oral antimicrobials; both approaches have been successful in reducing infection rates compared with placebo or mechanical cleaning of the bowel alone.

Currently recommended parenteral regimens include a second-generation cephalosporin (cefoxitin, cefotetan, or cefmetazole) alone; doxycycline alone; or metronidazole and clindamycin plus an aminoglycoside. First-generation cephalosporins should not be used.[13] The use of third-generation cephalosporins instead of drugs with a more narrow spectrum has not reduced infection rates[61] and these agents should not be used.[65] All these parenteral regimens should be instituted just before surgery.

One commonly used oral regimen includes erythromycin base plus neomycin base in conjunction with polyethylene glycol–electrolyte solution for mechanical cleaning of the bowel.[13] When prophylaxis is accomplished with such orally administered antibiotics, the agents should be given only during the 24 hours before the operation. Longer periods of therapy are not effective and have been associated with the isolation of resistant organisms within the colonic flora.[38] Oral regimens should not be used for emergency surgery or when gastrointestinal function is unreliable. It is not clear whether combining parenteral antibiotic therapy with a regimen of oral antibiotics and mechanical cleaning adds to the effectiveness of either approach alone.[13,65] In a survey of surgeons, however, combining an oral regimen with a short course (1 to 3 doses) of cefoxitin or cefotetan was a frequent practice.[97]

Studies examining the value of instilling antibiotics or antiseptics into the operative site at surgery have produced conflicting results.[24] Local or topical antimicrobials or antiseptics deliver activity directly to the wound edges at the time of closure but studies have not controlled for the confounding effects of systemic or oral antimicrobials administered concurrently.

Appendectomy. Infection rates in acute appendectomy can be low if the appendix has not perforated but rates as high as 90% result when perforation is present. As is true in abdominal trauma, antibiotics for appendiceal perforation represent therapy rather than prophylaxis.

In cases of perforation, wound infection rates have been reduced with the use of several parenteral and topical agents and with the rectal administration of metronidazole.[97] Drugs with activity against both aerobes and anaerobes (especially *Bacteroides*) are preferred.[13] Thus, first-generation cephalosporins such as cefazolin are not recommended for this indication. A short course of antibiotics (1 to 3 doses) appears to be sufficient.[4] In most instances, a single dose of a second-generation cephalosporin such as cefoxitin, with or without one dose of intravenous metronidazole, can be effective.[13,65] If patients subsequently are found to have diffuse peritonitis or abscess formation, continuing the regimen for an additional 4 or 5 days may be useful but this represents therapy, not prophylaxis.[4]

Abdominal hernia repair. A large controlled study suggested that prophylactic antimicrobials were useful in reducing the rate of infection after elective repair of abdominal hernias.[98] Infection rates (4%) in patients receiving placebo were higher than would be expected nationally, however, so it is not clear how applicable these findings are to other institutions.[88] A further study in several centers showed fewer wound infections in patients receiving prophylaxis, even after adjusting for duration of surgery and type of procedure.[99] Surgeons in these studies administered prophylaxis preferentially to patients at higher risk. These data suggest that prophylaxis should be seriously considered for hernia repair; oral therapy for this elective procedure may be more cost-efficient.[100] A study that compared the local injection of cefamandole into the operative wound to placebo showed a reduction of the infection rate in the group that received the antibiotic.[101] This study requires confirmation before the practice is widely adopted.

Lymph Node Dissection

Prophylaxis with cefazolin made little difference in infection rates after inguinal lymph node dissection, although it may have a role in the dissection of axillary nodes.[102]

Trauma Surgery

Antimicrobials are frequently used in surgery of traumatic wounds, which by definition are classified as contaminated or dirty.[9] This is properly defined as therapeutic use rather than prophylaxis.[4] Therapy is often directed against gastrointestinal or skin flora. As a result, parenteral penicillinase-resistant penicillins are commonly used in surgery for trauma above the waist and cephalosporins are used in penetrating abdominal trauma.[103] Antibiotic therapy seems to be especially important in surgery of soft tissue injuries of the hand or human bites. Drugs effective against mouth flora are needed for the latter situation.

For abdominal trauma, many regimens have included an aminoglycoside (for aerobic gram-negative bacilli) combined with one of numerous agents effective against *Bacteroides fragilis* and other anaerobes (some parenteral cephalosporins, metronidazole, and carbenicillin-like drugs).[9,104] Other successful therapy has included cefotaxime and antibiotic combinations containing β-lactamase inhibitors.[104] Cefazolin was compared with cefotaxime for abdominal infections other than colon surgery and in patients with peritonitis at the time of operation. Both drugs were better than placebo in reducing both the overall infection rate and the total amount of postoperative antibiotics given but no difference in these factors was noted for one drug compared with the other.[105] Single-drug therapy with cefoxitin was recommended for this situation in one recent review.[9] The duration of therapy can be as short as one or two doses.

In chest trauma, prophylaxis is suggested for thoracic esophageal injury resulting from penetrating trauma, especially when repair has been delayed for more than 12 hours.[9] A single day of cefazolin administration is recommended for patients with little or no contamination. The duration of therapy for more extensive mediastinal spillage of organisms is usually longer, although the optimal course is unclear.

Prophylaxis usually is given in cardiac trauma because of the risk of sternal wound infection and subsequent mediastinitis. A first-generation cephalosporin administered for 24 hours or less is a frequent choice.[9]

Head and neck fractures usually are contaminated with oral flora, and with skin flora when fractures communicate with the skin. A first-generation cephalosporin often is used for prophylaxis, although penicillin can be given when fractures communicate with skin and not with the oral cavity. Therapy is continued until the fracture is repaired.

The rate of infection after basilar skull fracture has not been reduced by prophylaxis, even in subsets of patients with cerebrospinal rhinorrhea or otorrhea.[9]

Burn Surgery

Both topical and systemic drugs have been used as antimicrobial prophylactic agents for patients with burns.[106] Systemic drugs can help limit spread to other tissues but are slow to cross the interface between eschar and underlying tissue. Topical drugs such as silver nitrate, mafenide acetate, chlorhexidine, and silver sulfadiazine delay colonization in moderate burns (under 50% of body surface area) but neither topical nor systemic antimicrobials prevent colonization in major burns (over 50% of body surface area). Penicillin and penicillin-like drugs are usually given for the first 3 to 5 hospital days to prevent group A streptococcal infection and are effective if the blood supply can deliver the drug to the injured area. Prophylactic therapy in this situation must be brief because of the increased risk of colonization with resistant strains of gram-negative rods and staphylococci.[106] Antimicrobials appear to be of little benefit in the outpatient treatment of burns.[107]

Orthopedic Surgery

Systemic drugs. Because of the severe consequences of infection after joint replacement (with both bone and metal grafts), perioperative prophylaxis with a parenteral drug usually is undertaken even though infection rates are low.[65,82] Many drugs have been used successfully. Cefazolin appears to be reasonable because of its low cost.[82] Institutions with a high prevalence of methicillin-resistant staphylococci must consider the use of vancomycin. One day of therapy with cefazolin appears to be as effective as 3 or 7 days; some authorities recommend a 24-hour course.[65,82] If the surgeon wishes to obtain cultures of the site where a replacement joint prosthesis is being inserted, prophylaxis may be withheld until the cultures are obtained, then given immediately, and always sooner than 60 minutes after the procedure is begun.[88] Controlled trials are necessary to determine whether patients with prosthetic joints should receive prophylactic antibiotics during dental, genitourinary, or gastrointestinal procedures (as do patients with prosthetic heart valves).[65,82,88] The organisms recovered from prosthetic joint infections are not typical mouth organisms, so the use of antibiotics at the time of dental work does not seem reasonable.

When closed hip fractures are treated by open reduction with internal fixation by nail, screw, wire, or plate, prophylaxis is effective.[65,82] In contrast, prophylaxis is not indicated for fractures that are treated with open reduction alone.[9]

Systemic antibiotics are important in the treatment of open fractures that have been managed surgically within a few hours of the trauma. This represents therapy (not prophylaxis) and usually involves the administration of first-generation cephalosporin drugs for a brief period.[1,9] When surgical therapy is not possible within a few hours of injury, treatment with the same drugs usually is continued for a week.[88,104] No superiority of the second-generation or third-generation cephalosporins has been demonstrated in comparison with the first-generation drugs.

Antibiotic-containing cement. A different approach to prophylaxis has been the inclusion of an antibiotic (usually gentamicin) in the cement that is used to secure a hip or other prosthesis, or in beads.[108] Some studies have shown antibiotic-impregnated cement to be as effective as systemic antibiotics in the prevention of early postoperative infection after total joint replacement.[82] However, prospective randomized trials with longer follow-up still are needed to determine the role of this approach used alone rather than combined with parenteral therapy.[4,9]

Neurosurgery

Data are scanty to confirm or refute a benefit of antibiotic prophylaxis in neurosurgery, regardless of the procedure being considered.[84] An exception may be craniotomy, in which antistaphylococcal antibiotics may decrease infection rates.[65] As a result, there is no consensus in recent reviews regarding appropriate indications for this therapy. Many authors advise against the use of prophylactic antibiotics in clean procedures that do not involve a prosthesis[88,109] but Shapiro[84] suggests that, except in institutions with very low infection rates (0.1%), the use of prophylaxis is documented as beneficial in clean and clean-contaminated procedures. Regimens that have been suggested are vancomycin alone, vancomycin plus gentamicin, vancomycin plus antistaphylococcal penicillins, or gentamicin and cefazolin.

No consistent data show the efficacy of antibiotic prophylaxis for ventricular shunt operations or dural fistula repairs.[88,109] One author strongly recommends the use of prophylaxis in shunt surgery when institutions experience shunt infection rates exceeding 15%.[110] Prophylaxis is not indicated in an attempt to prevent central nervous system infection after routine intracranial monitor use.[9]

Genitourinary Surgery

Patients with positive results on urine cultures at the time of prostatic surgery or other elective surgical exploration of the urinary tract receive some benefit from antimicrobial therapy directed at the organisms present.[88] The optimal duration of prophylaxis for prostate surgery is unclear because the length of time that the catheter was in place varied among studies, confounding analysis. Conte and colleagues,[93] however, suggest that short-term antibiotic regimens are inexpensive, produce fewer antibiotic-resistant organisms, and are associated with fewer adverse effects.

Studies suggest a benefit of antimicrobial coverage for patients with positive results on urine cultures during transrectal biopsy of the prostate.[1] Antibiotics are usually unnecessary for ureterolithotomy, pyelolithotomy, nephrectomy, and cystotomy when patients have sterile urine.[111] Some recommend prophylaxis with cefazolin or ampicillin for stone removal, especially if patients have had urinary tract infections or are immunocompromised.[55]

Most blunt renal injuries can be treated without operation, whereas about half of all renal stab wounds and most renal gunshot wounds require surgery. A brief (less than 1-day) course of a first-generation cephalosporin appears to be suitable prophylaxis.[9]

Postoperative irrigation of the bladder with antiseptic solutions appears to provide no benefit other than that provided by saline solutions alone.[93]

The insertion of penile prostheses is a procedure involving heavy contamination with groin flora in which perioperative prophylaxis has been found to be effective.[112] One author suggests preoperative doses of cefazolin and gentamicin followed by two doses of the same two drugs at 8-hour intervals after the surgery.[88]

Gynecologic Surgery

The value of short perioperative courses of antibiotics for transvaginal hysterectomy, especially in premenopausal women or after cervical cone procedures, is established and has been shown to reduce net health care costs.[65,113] The risk of infection associated with abdominal hysterectomy (whether routine or radical) is lower and it is not as clear that antibiotic prophylaxis is beneficial in routine cases. It is likely that a benefit exists, however, and patients should receive prophylaxis before this operation as well.[65,114] First-generation cephalosporins have been as effective as other drugs and are much less expensive.[65] Therapy probably should consist of a single dose of 1 to 2 g of cefazolin given intravenously in the operating room after intravenous line placement and before the induction of anesthesia.[114] When the operation lasts for more than 3 hours, an additional dose should be given if a shorter-acting antimicrobial (eg, cefazolin) is being used.

In infertility surgery, no advantage has been noted for antimicrobial prophylaxis.[115] Some recommend the use of prophylaxis for reconstructive fallopian tube surgery on previously infected tissues (one dose of cefazolin, 1 to 2 g intravenously) or for laparoscopy with hydrotubation (one dose of doxycycline, 200 mg orally) but not for other infertility procedures.[114]

Hysterosalpingography infrequently results in acute pelvic infection but such infections can be tragic for patients whose procedures are performed to investigate infertility. The oral administration of 200 mg of doxycycline has been recommended in at least one review.[114] Prophylaxis for the insertion of an intrauterine contraceptive device resulted in a decrease in unscheduled repeated visits for infection. The oral administration of 200 mg of doxycycline is recommended before these devices are inserted.

For first-trimester abortion procedures, antimicrobials should be given only to high-risk patients (eg, women with previous pelvic inflammatory disease, previous gonorrhea, or multiple sex partners).[65] The use of prophylaxis in all cases is better established in second-trimester abortions.[55] Intravenous penicillin or doxycycline are the suggested drugs and should be given just before surgery and continued for no more than 24 hours.[65,116] One suggested regimen is doxycycline, 200 mg orally before the procedure and 100 mg orally 12 hours later.[114]

In pelvic surgery for cancer, studies have reported benefit from the prophylactic use of cefamandole and doxycy-

cline.[115] Other studies are needed to confirm or refute these findings. Antimicrobials are routinely used in pelvic exenteration procedures because they involve colorectal surgery, in which the value of prophylaxis is clear.

Obstetric Surgery

Antimicrobial prophylaxis in cesarean section is recommended for patients who are at moderate or high risk for postoperative infection (eg, those with onset of labor before operation, those with rupture of membranes).[65] Such prophylaxis is clearly cost-effective.[113] Single-dose regimens are as effective as regimens lasting as long as 48 hours.[114] Penicillin, ampicillin, or first-generation cephalosporins are used commonly but there is little evidence to suggest that one is better than the others. A reasonable regimen is 2 g of cefazolin or ampicillin administered intravenously after clamping and cutting of the umbilical cord.[114]

Data are conflicting in regard to the value of prophylaxis in surgery for ectopic pregnancy, and a controlled trial is needed. Prophylaxis also may be indicated for cervical cerclage procedures in some patients but a high-risk group has not been defined.[114]

Breast Surgery

No controlled data are available regarding the value of prophylaxis with antibiotics in the insertion of breast implants but the higher rates of infection observed in patients who have previously undergone subcutaneous mastectomy suggest a benefit.[117] One dose of a first-generation cephalosporin has been recommended. A large controlled study suggested that prophylactic antimicrobials were useful in reducing the occurrence of infection after elective breast surgery.[98] A metaanalysis of 2587 breast surgeries, which included excisional biopsy, lumpectomy, mastectomy, reduction mammoplasty, and axillary node dissection, found that prophylaxis significantly reduced the risk of postoperative infection.[118] Infection rates were higher (12%) in those receiving placebo than would be expected nationally, however, so it is not clear how applicable these findings are to other institutions.[88] Another multicenter study has also obtained evidence that prophylaxis is likely to be worthwhile for elective breast surgery.[99]

Transplant Surgery

Few controlled studies are available that evaluate the effect of antimicrobial prophylaxis during transplant surgery. Antimicrobial agents are usually given because infection is common after transplantation.[119] It is difficult, however, to separate the confounding effects of the patient's immuno-suppressive and other nonantibiotic therapies (eg, "prophylactic" granulocytes) from the contribution of antimicrobial prophylaxis.[120]

Many renal transplant centers use perioperative prophylactic regimens but there are few controlled studies examining their value. No overall difference in the incidence of infection was seen after the use of tobramycin and cefamandole for prophylaxis in renal transplantation, although the frequency of urinary tract infection during the first postoperative week was diminished in the treatment group.[121] Ulualp and Condon[13] recommend the use of a second-generation cephalosporin in renal transplantation procedures.

In bone marrow transplantation, both bacterial and non-bacterial infections are major postoperative threats. Perioperative prophylaxis often involves multiple antibacterial and antifungal agents. According to van der Meer and colleagues, there is as yet no best method of infection prevention; the regimens vary, sometimes greatly, from one bone marrow transplant center to another.[122] Comparative trials are needed.

Patients undergoing heart transplantation should receive the usual antimicrobial prophylaxis given to other patients having open heart surgery. Again, no comparative trials are available to suggest which regimen is optimal.

Ulualp and Condon[13] recommend that hepatic and pancreatic transplant recipients be given a broad-spectrum cephalosporin but the data to support this practice are minimal.

CONCLUSION

Kunin[123] has noted that preoperative and postoperative prophylaxis is an area of considerable, but correctable, overuse in most facilities. The incidence of surgical wound infection has decreased in US hospitals during the past decade. This is the only site of nosocomial infection for which a consistent reduction was seen during this period. One explanation is the use of prophylaxis. Liss and Batchelor[124] concluded that for many uses of prophylaxis, "the reduction in real-dollar terms in the amount of illness and disability resulting from the use of developed and marketed antibiotics far outweighs costs of adverse effects, including resistance."

The major focus for future studies in this area should not be whether perioperative prophylactic antibiotics in general are worth their cost but whether the ways in which they are used can be made more efficient and cost-effective.[124] Many of the easy studies in this area already have been done. Further work must deal with surgical procedures that have not been evaluated. These represent more difficult questions for

which data will be both difficult and expensive to obtain. The answers to these questions are likely to be extremely valuable in improving the care of surgical patients, however.

Problems with prophylaxis are being attacked primarily by surgeons, who are performing clinical trials using methods that permit evaluation of efficacy. Educational programs designed to disseminate these data among both medical and surgical practitioners are proving effective. Even though gaps remain, recent advances in our knowledge about and use of surgical prophylaxis are impressive. This is now an area in which consulting internists can be confident that most recommendations are based on the comforting bedrock of objective data.

REFERENCES

1. Page CP, Bohnen JMA, Fletcher JR, et al. Antimicrobial prophylaxis for surgical wounds: guidelines for clinical care. Arch Surg 1993;128:79–88.
2. Wenzel RP. Preoperative prophylactic antibiotics: brief historical note. Infect Control Hosp Epidemiol 1993;14:121–122.
3. McGowan JE Jr. Cost and benefit of perioperative antimicrobial prophylaxis: methods for economic analysis. Rev Infect Dis 1991;13(Suppl 10):S879–889.
4. Gorbach SL, Condon RE, Conte JE Jr, et al. Evaluation of new anti-infective drugs for surgical prophylaxis. Clin Infect Dis 1992;15(Suppl 1):S313–338.
5. Platt R. Methodologic aspects of clinical studies of perioperative antibiotic prophylaxis. Rev Infect Dis 1991;13(Suppl 10):S810–814.
6. Garibaldi RA, Cushing D, Lerer T. Risk factors for postoperative infection. Am J Med 1991;91(Suppl 3B):158S–163S.
7. McGowan JE Jr. Improving antibiotic use has become essential: can surgery lead the way? Infect Control Hosp Epidemiol 1990;11:575–577.
8. American Society of Hospital Pharmacy Commission on Therapeutics. ASHP therapeutic guidelines on antimicrobial prophylaxis in surgery. Clin Pharm 1992;11:483–513.
9. Culver DH, Horan TC, Gaynes RP, et al. Surgical wound infection rates by wound class, operative procedure, and patient risk index. Am J Med 1991;91(Suppl 3B):152S–157S.
10. Horan TC, Culver DH, Gaynes RP, et al. Nosocomial infections in surgical patients in the United States, January 1986–June 1992. Infect Control Hosp Epidemiol 1993;14:73–80.
11. Cruse P. Wound infection surveillance. Rev Infect Dis 1981;3:734–737.
12. Condon RE. Retrospect and prospect: ruminations after the first decade of the Surgical Infection Society. Arch Surg 1991;126:19–22.
13. Ulualp K, Condon RE. Antibiotic prophylaxis for scheduled operative procedures. Infect Dis Clin North Am 1992;6:613–625.
14. Farber BF, Wenzel RP. Postoperative wound infection rates:

results of prospective statewide surveillance. Am J Surg 1980;140:343–346.

15. Olson M, O'Connor M, Schwartz ML. Surgical wound infections: a 5-year prospective study of 20,193 wounds at the Minneapolis VA Medical Center. Ann Surg 1984;199:253–259.

16. Malangoni MA, Jacobs DG. Antibiotic prophylaxis for injured patients. Infect Dis Clin North Am 1993;6:627–630.

17. Haley RW, White JW, Culver DH, et al. The financial incentive for hospitals to prevent nosocomial infections under the prospective payment system: an empiric determination from a nationally representative sample. JAMA 1987;257:1611–1614.

18. Kappstein I, Schulgen G, Fraedrich G, et al. Added hospital stay due to wound infections following cardiac surgery. Thorac Cardiovasc Surg 1992;40:148–151.

19. O'Donoghue MA, Allen KD. Costs of an outbreak of wound infections in an orthopedic ward. J Hosp Infect 1992;22:73–79.

20. Shapiro M, Townsend T, Rosner B, et al. Use of antimicrobial drugs in general hospitals: patterns of prophylaxis. N Engl J Med 1979;301:351–355.

21. Kaiser AB. Overview of cephalosporin prophylaxis. Am J Surg 1988;155(Suppl 5A):52–55.

22. Currier JS, Campbell H, Platt R, et al. Perioperative antimicrobial prophylaxis in middle Tennessee, 1989–1990. Rev Infect Dis 1991;13(Suppl 10):S874–878.

23. Bryan CS, Ervin FR, John JF Jr, et al. Cost-effective antimicrobial therapy: an approach for physicians and community hospitals. J S Car Med Assoc 1986;82:121–248.

24. Platt R. Antibiotic prophylaxis in surgery. Rev Infect Dis 1984;6(Suppl 4):S880–S886.

25. Britt MR, Goodell N, Turner R, et al. A 1979 statewide study on the "non-usage" of perioperative antibiotics in surgical prophylaxis: a continuing problem. Clin Res 1980;28:43A.

26. Gardner FT, Jones CE, Polk HC Jr. Further definition of antibiotic use and abuse in the surgical setting. Arch Surg 1979;114:883–886.

27. Davey PG, Parker SE, Malek MM. Pharmacoeconomics of antimicrobial prophylaxis. J Antimicrob Chemother 1993;31(Suppl B):107–118.

28. Pinner RW, Haley RW, Blumenstein BA, et al. High cost nosocomial infections. Infect Control 1982;3:143–149.

29. Haley RW. Managing hospital infection for cost-effectiveness: a strategy for reducing infectious complications. Chicago, American Hospital Association, 1986:91.

30. Daschner F. Cost-effectiveness in hospital infection control: lessons for the 1990's. J Hosp Infect 1989;13:325–336.

31. Ehrenkranz NJ. Containing costs of antimicrobials in the hospital: a critical evaluation. Am J Infect Control 1989;17:300–310.

32. Ehrenkranz NJ. Antimicrobial prophylaxis in surgery: mechanisms, misconceptions, and mischief. Infect Control Hosp Epidemiol 1993;14:99–106.

33. Crossley K, Gardner LC, Task Force on Prophylactic Antibiotics in Surgery. Antimicrobial prophylaxis in surgical patients. JAMA 1981;245:722–726.

34. Fiore P, DiNunzio A, Ehrenkranz NJ. Antibiotic prophylaxis in community hospitals: patterns and costs of incorrect use. Am J Infect Control 1984;12:245.

35. Smith K, Quercia RA, Chow MSS, et al. Multidisciplinary program for promoting single prophylactic doses of cefazolin in obstetrical and gynecological surgical procedures. Am J Hosp Pharm 1988;45:1338–1342.

36. Everitt DE, Soumerai SB, Avorn J, et al. Changing surgical antimicrobial prophylaxis practices through education targeted at senior department leaders. Infect Control Hosp Epidemiol 1990;11:578–583.

37. Larsen RA, Evans RS, Burke JP, et al. Improved perioperative antibiotic use and reduced surgical wound infections through use of computer decision analysis. Infect Control Hosp Epidemiol 1989;10:316–320.

38. Nichols RL. Surgical wound infection. Am J Med 1991;91(Suppl 3B):54S–64S.

39. DiPiro JT, Bowden TA, Hooks VH III. The prophylactic use of cephalosporins for surgery. JAMA 1985;253:3399–3400.

40. Farber BF, Kaiser DL, Wenzel RP. Relation between surgical volume and incidence of postoperative wound infections. N Engl J Med 1981;305:200–204.

41. Garnick DW, Luft HS, McPhee SJ, et al. Surgeon volume vs. hospital volume: which matters more? JAMA 1989;262:547–548.

42. Hirschmann JV, Inui TS. Antimicrobial prophylaxis: a critique of recent trials. Rev Infect Dis 1980;2:1–23.

43. Ayliffe GAJ. Role of the environment of the operating suite in surgical wound infection. Rev Infect Dis 1991;13(Suppl 10):S800–804.

44. Kaiser AB. Surgical-wound infection. N Engl J Med 1991;324:123–124.

45. Nichols RL. Classification of the surgical wound: a time for reassessment and simplification. Infect Control Hosp Epidemiol 1993;14:253–254.

46. Bohnen JMA, Solomkin JS, Dellinger EP, et al. Guidelines for clinical care: anti-infective agents for intra-abdominal infection: a Surgical Infection Society policy statement. Arch Surg 1992;127:83–89.

47. Guillou PJ. Biological variation in the development of sepsis after surgery or trauma. Lancet 1993;342:217–220.

48. Burke JF. Preventing bacterial infection by coordination of antibiotic and host activity: a time-dependent relationship. South Med J 1977;70(Suppl 1):24–26.

49. Haley RW. Nosocomial infections in surgical patients: developing valid measures of intrinsic patient risk. Am J Med 1991;91(Suppl 3B):145S.

50. Haley RW, Culver DH, Morgan WM, et al. Identifying patients at high risk of surgical wound infection: a simple multivariate index of patient susceptibility and wound contamination. Am J Epidemiol 1985;121:206–215.

51. Ehrenkranz NJ. Surgical wound infection occurrence in clean operations: risk stratification for interhospital comparison. Am J Med 1981;70:909–914.

52. Chang JHT. The use of antibiotics in pediatric abdominal surgery. Pediatr Infect Dis J 1984;3:195–198.

53. Committee on Infectious Diseases, Pediatrics AAO. Antimicrobial prophylaxis in pediatric surgical patients. Pediatrics 1984;74:437–439.

54. Hunt TK. Surgical wound infections: an overview. Am J Med 1981;70:348–351.

55. Paluzzi RG. Antimicrobial prophylaxis for surgery. Med Clin North Am 1993;77:427–441.

56. Sanderson PJ. Antimicrobial prophylaxis in surgery: microbiological factors. J Antimicrob Chemother 1993;31(Suppl B): 1–9.

57. Sahm DA, Neuman MA, Thornsberry C, et al. Cumitech 25: current concepts and approaches to antimicrobial agent susceptibility testing. Washington, DC, American Society for Microbiology, 1988:1–17.

58. Redington J, Ebert SC, Craig WA. Role of antimicrobial pharmacokinetics and pharmacodynamics in surgical prophylaxis. Rev Infect Dis 1991;13(Suppl 10):S790–799.

59. Eisenberg JM, Koffer H, Finkler SA. Economic analysis of a new drug: potential savings in hospital operating costs from the use of a once-daily regimen of a parenteral cephalosporin. Rev Infect Dis 1984;6(Suppl 4):S909–S923.

60. Kernodle DS, Barg NL, Kaiser AB. Low-level colonization of hospitalized patients with methicillin-resistant coagulase-negative staphylococci and emergence of the organisms during surgical antimicrobial prophylaxis. Antimicrob Agents Chemother 1988;32:202–208.

61. McGowan JE Jr. Is antimicrobial resistance in hospital microorganisms related to antibiotic use? Bull N Y Acad Med 1987;63:253–268.

62. Holmberg SD, Solomon SL, Blake PA. Health and economic impacts of antimicrobial resistance. Rev Infect Dis 1987;9: 1065–1078.

63. McGowan JE Jr, Hall EC, Parrott PL. Antimicrobial susceptibility in gram-negative bacteremia: are nosocomial isolates really more resistant? Antimicrob Agents Chemother 1989;33: 1855–1859.

64. Liss RH, Batchelor FR. Economic evaluations of antibiotic use and resistance: a perspective: report of Task Force 6. Rev Infect Dis 1987;9(Suppl 3):S297–S312.

65. Antimicrobial prophylaxis in surgery. Med Lett Drugs Ther 1992;34:5–8.

66. Fitzgerald RH Jr. Postoperative surgical skin infection. JAMA 1980;242:2889.

67. Pollock AV. Surgical wound sepsis. Lancet 1979;1:1283–1286.

68. Lineaweaver W, Howard R, Soucy D, et al. Topical antimicrobial toxicity. Arch Surg 1985;120:267–270.

69. Classen DC, Evans RS, Pestotnik SL, et al. The timing of prophylactic administration of antibiotics and the risk of surgical-wound infection. N Engl J Med 1992;326:281–286.

70. Cartmill TDI, Al Zahawi MF, Sisson PR, et al. Five days versus one day of penicillin as prophylaxis in elective neurosurgical operations. J Hosp Infect 1989;14:63–68.

71. Shapiro M, Schoenbaum SC, Tager IB, et al. Benefit-cost analysis of antimicrobial prophylaxis in abdominal and vaginal hysterectomy. JAMA 1983;249:1290–1294.

72. Kaiser AB. Antimicrobial prophylaxis in surgery. N Engl J Med 1986;315:1129–1138.

73. Garibaldi RA. Postoperative pneumonia and urinary tract infection: epidemiology and prevention. J Hosp Infect 1988;11 (Suppl A):265–272.

74. Rubenstein E, Green M, Modan M, et al. The effects of nosocomial infections on the length and costs of hospital stay. J Antimicrob Chemother 1982;9(Suppl A):93–100.

75. Egarter C, Fitz R, Brehm R, et al. Prophylactic perioperative use of clindamycin and metronidazole in vaginal hysterectomy without pelvic floor repair. Arch Gynecol Obstet 1988;244:53–57.

76. Penin GB, Ehrenkranz NJ. Priorities for surveillance and cost-effective control of postoperative infection. Arch Surg 1988;123:1305–1308.

77. Greco D, Moro ML, Tozzi AE, et al. Effectiveness of an intervention program in reducing postoperative infections. Am J Med 1991;91(Suppl 3B):164S–169S.

78. Shulman ST, Amren DP, Bisno AL, et al. A statement for health professionals by the Committee on Rheumatic Fever. Circulation 1984;70:1118A–1122A.

79. Dajani AS, Bisno AL, Chung KJ, et al. Prevention of bacterial endocarditis: recommendations by the American Heart Association. JAMA 1990;264:2919–2922.

80. Durack DT. Current issues in prevention of infective endocarditis. Am J Med 1985;78(Suppl 6B):149–156.

81. Chemoprophylaxis for infective endocarditis: faith, hope and charity challenged. Lancet 1992;339:525–526.

82. Norden CW. Antibiotic prophylaxis in orthopedic surgery. Rev Infect Dis 1991;13(Suppl 10):S842–846.

84. Shapiro M. Prophylaxis in otolaryngologic surgery and neurosurgery: a critical review. Rev Infect Dis 1991;13(Suppl 10):S858–868.

85. Johnson JT, Wagner RL, Schuller DE, et al. Prophylactic antibiotics for head and neck surgery with flap reconstruction. Arch Otolaryngol Head Neck Surg 1992;118:488–490.

86. Fee WE Jr, Glenn M, Handen C, et al. One day vs. two days of prophylactic antibiotics in patients undergoing major head and neck surgery. Laryngoscope 1984;94:612–614.

87. Gilbert DN. Current status of antibiotic prophylaxis in surgical patients. Bull N Y Acad Med 1984;60:340–357.

88. Ehrenkranz NJ. Antimicrobial prophylaxis in surgery: mechanisms, misconceptions, and mischief. Infect Control Hosp Epidemiol 1993;14:99–106.

89. Ariano RE, Zhanel GE. Antimicrobial prophylaxis in coronary bypass surgery: a critical appraisal. Drug Intell Clin Pharm 1991;25:478–484.

90. Heupler FA Jr, Heisler M, Keys TF, et al. Infection prevention guidelines for cardiac catheterization laboratories: Society for Cardiac Angiography and Interventions Laboratory Performance Standards Committee. Cathet Cardiovasc Diagn 1992; 25:260–263.

91. Kaiser AB, Clayson KR, Mulherin JL Jr, et al. Antibiotic prophylaxis in vascular surgery. Ann Surg 1978;192:356–364.

92. Pitt HA, Postier RG, MacGowan AW, et al. Prophylactic antibiotics in vascular surgery. Ann Surg 1980;192:356–364.

93. Conte JE Jr, Jacobs LS, Polk HC Jr. Antibiotic prophylaxis in surgery: a comprehensive review. Philadelphia, JB Lippincott, 1984.

94. Cant PJ, Smyth S, Smart DO. Antibiotic prophylaxis is indicated for chest stab wounds requiring closed tube thoracostomy. Br J Surg 1993;80:464–466.

95. Jain NK, Larson DE, Schroeder KW, et al. Antibiotic prophylaxis for percutaneous endoscopic gastrostomy. Ann Intern Med 1987;107:824–828.

96. DiPiro JT, Bivins BA, Record KE, et al. The prophylactic use of antimicrobials in surgery. Curr Probl Surg 1983;20:76–132.

97. Gorbach SL. Antimicrobial prophylaxis for appendectomy and colorectal surgery. Rev Infect Dis 1991;13(Suppl 10):S815–819.

98. Platt R, Zaleznik DF, Hopkins CC, et al. Perioperative antibi-

otic prophylaxis for herniorrhaphy and breast surgery. N Engl J Med 1990;322:153–160.

99. Platt R, Zucker JR, Zaleznik DF, et al. Prophylaxis against wound infection following herniorrhaphy or breast surgery. J Infect Dis 1992;166:556–560.

100. Ranaboldo CJ, Kerran SE, Bailey IS, et al. Antimicrobial prophylaxis in "clean" surgery: hernia repair. J Antimicrob Chemother 1993;31(Suppl B):35–41.

101. Lazorthes F, Chiotasso P, Massip P, et al. Local antibiotic prophylaxis in inguinal hernia repair. Surg Gynecol Obstet 1992;175:569–570.

102. Coit DG, Peters M, Brennan MF. A prospective randomized trial of perioperative cefazolin treatment in axillary and groin dissection. Arch Surg 1991;126:1366–1372.

103. Nichols RL, Smith JW, Robertson GD, et al. Prospective alterations in therapy for penetrating abdominal trauma. Arch Surg 1993;128:55–64.

104. Dellinger EP. Antibiotic prophylaxis in trauma. Rev Infect Dis 1991;13(Suppl 10):S847–857.

105. Rotman N, Hay J, Lacaine F, et al. Prophylactic antibiotherapy in abdominal surgery. Arch Surg 1989;124:323–327.

106. American College of Surgeons, Committee on Surgical Infections. Manual on control of infection in surgical patients, ed 2. Philadelphia, JB Lippincott, 1984.

107. Boss WK, Brand DA, Acampora D, et al. Effectiveness of prophylactic antibiotics in the outpatient treatment of burns. J Trauma 1985;25:224–227.

108. Strachan CJL. Antibiotic prophylaxis in peripheral vascular and orthopaedic prosthetic surgery. J Antimicrob Chemother 1993;31(Suppl B):65–78.

109. Brown EM. Antimicrobial prophylaxis in neurosurgery. J Antimicrob Chemother 1993;31(Suppl B):49–63.

110. Haines SJ. Antibiotic prophylaxis in neurosurgery: the controlled trials. Neurosurg Clin N Am 1992;3:355–358.

111. Childs SJ. Genitourinary surgical prophylaxis. Infect Surg 1983;2:701–710.

112. Blum MD. Infections of genitourinary prostheses. Infect Dis Clin North Am 1989;3:259–274.

113. Shapiro M, Schoenbaum SC, Tager IB, et al. Benefit-cost analysis of antimicrobial prophylaxis in abdominal and vaginal hysterectomy. JAMA 1983;249:1290–1294.

114. Hemsell DL. Prophylactic antibiotics in gynecologic and obstetric surgery. Rev Infect Dis 1991;13(Suppl 10):S821–841.

115. Hirsch HA. Prophylactic antibiotics in obstetrics and gynecology. Am J Med 1985;78(Suppl 6B):170–176.

116. Grimes DA, Schulz KF, Cates W Jr. Prophylactic antibiotics for curettage abortion. Am J Obstet Gynecol 1984;150:689–694.

117. LeRoy J, Given KS. Wound infection in breast augmentation: the role of prophylactic perioperative antibiotics. Aesthetic Plast Surg 1991;15:303–305.

118. Platt R, Zucker JR, Zaleznik DF, et al. Perioperative antibiotic prophylaxis and wound infection following breast surgery. J Antimicrob Chemother 1993;31(Suppl B):43–48.

119. Garibaldi RA. Infections in organ transplant recipients. Infect Control 1983;4:460–464.

120. Navari RM, Buckner CD, Clift RA, et al. Prophylaxis of infection in patients with aplastic anemia receiving allogenic marrow transplants. Am J Med 1984;76:564–572.

121. Townsend TR, Rudolf LE, Westervelt FB Jr, et al. Prophylactic antibiotic therapy with cefamandole and tobramycin for patients undergoing renal transplantation. Infect Control 1980;1: 93–96.

122. van der Meer JWM, Guiot HFL, van den Brooek PJ, et al. Infections in bone marrow transplant recipients. Semin Hematol 1984;21:123–140.

123. Kunin CM. Resistance to antimicrobial drugs: a worldwide calamity. Ann Intern Med 1993;118:557–561.

124. Liss RH, Batchelor FR. Economic evaluations of antibiotic use and resistance. Rev Infect Dis 1987;9(Suppl 3):S297–S312.

Medical Management of the Surgical Patient, Third Edition,
edited by Michael F. Lubin, H. Kenneth Walker, and Robert B. Smith III.
J.B. Lippincott Company, Philadelphia, PA © 1995.

CHAPTER

26

HUMAN IMMUNODEFICIENCY VIRUS INFECTION IN THE SURGICAL PATIENT AND HEALTH CARE WORKER

Sumner E. Thompson III

The human immunodeficiency virus-1 (HIV-1) that causes HIV infection and its more severe later form, acquired immunodeficiency syndrome (AIDS), is transmitted in virtually the same manner as is the hepatitis B virus: (1) through direct injection of blood into the bloodstream by reuse of contaminated syringes and needles, blood transfusion, or use of contaminated blood products, or by the accidental injection of blood through needles and sharp surgical equipment; (2) through sexual intercourse, primarily rectal homosexual or heterosexual intercourse and heterosexual vaginal intercourse; or (3) from mothers to infants either in utero, during the perinatal period with vaginal delivery, or through breastfeeding. Bizarre routes of transmission such as through skin abrasions or bites have been suggested but rarely proved.

After infection, HIV-1 replicates in lymph node tissue for several weeks and then disseminates hematogenously to most tissues of the body. At that time, patients may experience the symptoms of primary or acute HIV-1 infection, which consist of a transient influenza-like syndrome accompanied by a skin rash. Roughly 6 weeks into the infection, antibodies to many HIV-1 antigens become detectible. In some cases, antibodies may not be produced for as long as 6 months, although this is the exception. This "window" (ie, the interval between actual infection and the time when antibodies can be detected) has important implications for testing and screening programs (see later).

Before antibodies can be detected in serum, virus may be grown from blood, and p24 antigen, a surface marker de-

noting the presence of virus, may be detected. The p24 antigen test, or the polymerase chain reaction, which detects viral DNA and is even more sensitive, may reveal the presence of infection before detectable antibodies appear. The HIV-1 polymerase chain reaction may soon be the test of choice. Virus then enters several types of cells, such as lymphocytes, dendritic cells of the skin, glial brain cells, and splenic cells. It merges with host DNA to produce chronically infected cells that are capable of living in a latent state, dividing to produce more infected cells, or, by accelerating viral proliferation, killing the host cell and releasing new infectious virions.

As antibodies appear, most of the circulating virus and p24 antigen disappear from the circulation. It had been thought that the virus, under the influence of an intact immune system, underwent a long period of latency. It is now believed that virus continues to proliferate in spleen and lymph node tissue, even during the height of the immune response, and that the bloodstream is probably never entirely free of circulating virus, even when the disease appears to be nonprogressive, as it usually does during the first few years after infection.

Most patients suffer inevitable damage to the immune system over time, with selective loss of CD4+ cells. Because CD4 lymphocytes are central to the regulation of the immune system, advancing HIV infection is accompanied by increasing dysregulation of the entire immune system, including cell-mediated immune responses, antibody production, and mucosal immunity. Eventually, virus production accelerates and the disease progresses rapidly, with death resulting from the opportunistic infections or tumors that cannot be controlled by the destroyed immune system. The time from initial infection to death may average 10 to 15 years. During most of this period, patients may experience good health and lead productive lives.

TRANSMISSION OF HUMAN IMMUNODEFICIENCY VIRUS IN THE CLINICAL SETTING

Of primary concern to surgeons and other operating room personnel is the possibility that they may contract HIV infection from infected patients during surgery and, to a lesser extent, that they may transmit HIV infection to uninfected patients.

TRANSMISSION OF HUMAN IMMUNODEFICIENCY VIRUS TO PATIENTS

HIV can be transmitted from infected health care workers to patients. Most surgeons routinely describe cuts and scratches from needles, scalpels, and other instruments during operations. Direct inoculation is possible if injured health care workers bleed directly into wounds or reuse instruments that they have contaminated. No case of infection from such contact during surgery has been reported, however. In one important 13-year look-back study of an infected orthopedic surgeon, none of the 1174 former patients who underwent invasive procedures and were tested for HIV were found to be seropositive.[1] In a study of 15,795 patients cared for by 32 HIV-infected health care workers, no case of HIV transmission was documented.[2]

Many articles document the transmission of HIV to patients through the transplantation of organs such as the heart,[3] lungs,[4] liver,[5] skin,[6] cornea,[7] kidney,[8–10] and bone,[11] as well as through semen.[12]

The first report of transplantation-related AIDS occurred in a woman who received an infected bone allograft. The US Centers for Disease Control and Prevention has since developed guidelines for bone transplantation.[14] They recommend using bone autografts whenever possible, evaluating all donors of tissue and organ allografts for risks associated with HIV infection, and performing tests for HIV antibody. Furthermore, because bone can be stored, living donors should be tested again for antibody at least 90 days after procurement. Donation is refused from persons with histories of sepsis, intravenous drug use, neoplasia, hepatitis, syphilis, slow virus infection, AIDS, HIV infection, or perceived high risk for these conditions. High-risk patients singled out by the US Public Health Service include those with

clinical or laboratory evidence of HIV infection, men who have had sex with other men since 1977, past or present intravenous drug abusers, persons immigrating since 1977 from countries where heterosexual activity is thought to play a major role in the transmission of HIV, persons with hemophilia who have received clotting factor concentrates, sexual partners of any of the above, and men and women who have engaged in prostitution since 1977 and persons who have been their heterosexual partners within the past 6 months.

With the institution of such guidelines and care in testing potential donors, the rate of infection in recipients is now low. Because of the window phase of infection, however, it will not reach zero. The addition of a rapid polymerase chain reaction test to the armamentarium may help reduce infection rates further.

Some physicians who perform transplants fear that the course of HIV infection may be more severe in patients who contract the virus through organ transplantation. Data from a study by Dummer and colleagues[15] indicate that the course is no more severe in patients who receive cyclosporine than in other hosts. A study by Tzakis and associates[16] from the same center, however, concludes that transplantation and immunosuppression appears to shorten the AIDS-free interval in patients who become HIV-positive through transplantation compared with patients with hemophilia who are HIV-positive and with transfusion control groups. Because many of these patients were infected before transplantation, the two studies are not comparable, however.

HIV is transmitted through blood transfusion with high efficiency (over 90%). Screening of all blood by HIV testing has reduced this rate to less than 1 in 60,000 U. This is probably a minimum. Blood testing with p24 antigen and polymerase chain reaction has not substantially decreased these figures further.

Adequate history taking coupled with HIV testing of donated blood has resulted in an extremely low risk for HIV infection in recipients of blood, organs, and other types of grafts. The introduction of new tests may lead to small additional decreases but will not reduce the incidence to zero.

TRANSMISSION OF HUMAN IMMUNODEFICIENCY VIRUS TO HEALTH CARE WORKERS

In a 6-year study of 179 percutaneous needlesticks from HIV-positive patients, Henderson and coworkers[17] found one case of seroconversion. In several other studies in which both the numerator (number converting) and the denominator (number exposed)[18–20] are known and transmission can be calculated directly, the average rate of nosocomial HIV transmission after parenteral exposure was 0.32%

and the risk from mucous membrane contact with HIV-infected blood or body fluids was zero.

Blood always has been found to be the vehicle of transmission. Other fluids contain viral particles but probably at such low titer that transmission is difficult. About 45 cases of occupational HIV transmission from needlestick exposure or more major exposure to blood have occurred since 1981.[20] Aerosols of infected blood or saliva can occur in the operative or dental suite. No case of HIV transmission by aerosol through surgical masks has been described.

The risk of transmission probably is increased primarily by the size of the blood inoculum (ie, the amount of virus in the inoculum); deep penetration with a hollow-bore needle (also related to the size of the inoculum); and the duration of contact with the inoculum.[21] Less clear, but possibly important, is the stage of disease in the patient. In general, viral burden is highest during the early, asymptomatic stage of disease (the first few months after infection) and again during the late stages of symptomatic AIDS. The cumulative risk from repeated exposure to HIV has not been well studied but it appears logical that dentists, surgeons, nurses, persons who work in proximity to patients in trauma centers, and obstetric labor and delivery personnel would be at higher risk. The prevalence of HIV infection in the population encountered in the workplace is also an important factor. In one inner city emergency department, the prevalence of HIV infection in unselected patients presenting for care was 5%.[22] Given all these factors, the risk of acquiring HIV infection from working with HIV-infected patients is not zero but the degree of risk is small.

The fear of acquisition of HIV infection among health care workers should be put into proper perspective by assuming all patients to be infected and working to decrease the risk of parenteral exposure. It is almost never possible to avoid all contact with HIV-infected patients; attempting to do so creates an illusion of safety that may actually increase the possibility of transmission from patients who are not considered to be infected to clinicians who do not feel the need to practice stringent infection control. Frank communication between providers and patients in discussing possible infection and risks is preferable to an atmosphere of mistrust and ignorance. Physicians should be willing to openly discuss the risk status of patients and to request testing, and equally prepared to honestly answer the same questions posed to them by patients.

PREVENTION OF PARENTERAL EXPOSURE

Preventing needlesticks and other parenteral exposure is the mainstay of risk reduction. Although blood has been the only fluid implicated in HIV transmission, prevention of exposure to all infected fluids should be the goal. The US Cen-

ters for Disease Control and Prevention has recommended universal precautions for all patients, regardless of diagnosis, for the prevention of transmission of blood-borne pathogens.[23,24] These precautions consist of using gloves for any procedure involving contact with blood or any other potentially infected fluid, using masks and protective eyewear when spatters of such fluids are expected, and wearing gowns when wider soilage of clothing is anticipated. Proper management of needles and other sharp instruments during surgery and their disposal afterward is also an important part of infection control.

Exercising total control of sharp instruments during surgery is becoming common practice (ie, placing instruments on intermediate tables rather than passing them from nurses to surgeons, directly visualizing instruments before using them, and blunting sharp scalpel tips). It is now well recognized that using the index finger of the nondominant hand to blindly palpate the needle during suturing accounts for more than half of all intraoperative injuries.[25] The use of more stab-resistant gloves is also spreading but will not completely solve the problem. Wearing two pairs of gloves decreases the rate at which the inner glove is perforated by 60% to 80%.[26] In a survey of two cities, however, 50% of surgeons did not recommend universal precautions and only 24% routinely used two pairs of gloves.[27] Finally, refraining from recapping needles and disposing of them immediately after use in containers that cannot be reopened can markedly reduce the incidence of needlestick injuries.

PROPHYLAXIS WITH ANTIRETROVIRAL AGENTS AFTER EXPOSURE

Zidovudine (AZT, Retrovir) and the other two similar antiretroviral agents (ddC—Zalcitabine and ddI—Hivid) can prevent the replication of HIV within infected cells. Thus, there is a theoretic possibility that they could prevent initial HIV infection if they were administered soon enough after initial HIV exposure. There are no studies available to prove this point and, given the low rate of seroconversion after parenteral exposure (0.3%), no study is likely to obtain a sample size that could convincingly demonstrate an effect. Failure of prophylaxis has been demonstrated in at least three patients.[28,29] Large blood inocula and delay in instituting prophylaxis may have contributed to these failures but the efficacy is definitely not 100%.

Despite the lack of data regarding its efficacy, many institutions have developed guidelines for zidovudine prophylaxis. Many centers have a person or a team that can be called on at any time to discuss and assess an exposure. All such guidelines are experimental and they should be offered with that understanding. Informed consent should be obtained before zidovudine or other antiretroviral agents are administered whenever possible.

The general approach taken by most institutions is that the decision to use zidovudine depends on the severity of the exposure and the time elapsed since the exposure.[30] Treatment priority increases with the size of the inoculum and the speed with which the drug can be administered. Thus, with a massive exposure such as a transfusion, zidovudine is highly recommended if it can be given within several hours. With a definite injection of blood, but a small amount, the use of zidovudine is still recommended. For lesser injuries, use of the drug is permitted but discouraged, and for splashes without breaks in the skin or mucosa, the drug should not be offered. Most authorities believe that drug administration should be started within minutes to no longer than 1 hour after the injury to maximize efficacy but this is conjectural. The optimal dose and length of prophylaxis has not been established either. The average recommended dose is 1000 mg/d in divided doses for 2 to 6 weeks, although no consensus exists. Serious adverse reactions are rare with the 2-week regimen. It is reasonable to monitor the hemoglobin and hematocrit levels and the white blood cell count at least once during therapy if the 6-week course is given.

SURGICAL INTERVENTION IN PATIENTS WHO ARE INFECTED WITH THE HUMAN IMMUNODEFICIENCY VIRUS

Concise information gleaned from the surgical literature regarding surgical intervention in patients with HIV infection or AIDS is presented in this section. It is not intended to be an extensive review of the literature.

CARDIOTHORACIC SURGERY

Cardiac disease appears to be common in patients with HIV infection or AIDS, with an incidence as high as 60% in one autopsy study. Most of these conditions do not require surgery, however.[31] No study has shown an increase in mortality associated with cardiac surgery in patients with HIV, and no study directly addresses which patients most benefit from surgery and which should be deferred. One study did not show an influence of cardiopulmonary bypass on the progression to AIDS but the sample was small and follow-up was short.[32] Another retrospective study showed no increased progression to AIDS among these patients.[33] Valve replacement should be done when necessary in patients with AIDS and does not seem to accelerate disease progression.[34]

PULMONARY PROCEDURES

Open lung biopsy is occasionally indicated for patients with AIDS, usually in the setting of nondiagnostic bronchoscopy or transbronchial biopsy. In a series of patients meeting these criteria, a diagnosis was established in 84% and therapy was changed in 60%; however, there was a complication rate of 56% (pneumothorax, persistent air leak, and difficulty with extubation).[35]

Most authorities agree that bronchoscopy should be the initial diagnostic approach in patients with AIDS who have pulmonary disease.[35] Determining how much a diagnosis will benefit a patient is more important than deciding how the diagnosis should be made. We suggest that open lung biopsy be used as follows[36]:

1. Nondiagnostic bronchoscopy, with or without deteriorating clinical status
2. Diagnostic bronchoscopy with failure to respond to medical therapy, with or without deteriorating clinical status
3. Nondiagnostic bronchoscopy with empiric therapy based on radiologic survey with deteriorating clinical status
4. Failure to yield a pathogen after repeated bronchoscopy or failure of radiologic improvement for any of the above
5. Respiratory failure or mechanical ventilation are contraindications to open lung biopsy

CENTRAL NERVOUS SYSTEM SURGERY

Central nervous system involvement with AIDS is relatively common, occurring in up to half of patients. Computed tomography and magnetic resonance imaging, even with gadolinium contrast, cannot distinguish with assurance between cerebral toxoplasmosis, central nervous system lymphoma, and some cases of progressive multifocal leukoencephalopathy. Most of the papers reviewed suggest that computed tomography–guided stereotactic biopsy is a safe and effective means of establishing a diagnosis in most cases.[37,38]

ABDOMINAL SURGERY

In a study from the University of California, Los Angeles, School of Medicine involving 36 major abdominal operations, 22 were elective (usually for a mass) and the rest were performed for emergencies such as perforated viscus or bleeding. Non-Hodgkin's lymphoma was the most common malignant condition. Gloomy predictions of "great difficulty" in operating on patients with AIDS was not borne out in this study for elective operations but the mortality was extremely high for emergency surgery.[39] In a report 2 years earlier from the same institution, even elective surgery was associated with a high mortality rate (43%), a finding that the authors attributed to the progression of opportunistic infections or malignant diseases.[40] Changes in surgical indications and types of presentations may account for some of the improvement.

For patients with immune thrombocytopenia, a common manifestation of HIV infection, splenectomy can usually be accomplished without increased morbidity.[41] Other authors also conclude that splenectomy is safe and effective treatment in HIV-infected patients with severe thrombocytopenic purpura that is resistant to medical therapy.[42]

DENTAL PROCEDURES

Delayed healing has been included as an oral manifestation of HIV infection. In a large HIV-dedicated dental clinic, a 26-month retrospective study did not show any difference in healing between HIV-positive and HIV-negative men in regard to complications such as dry socket (3% versus 4.3%). The authors concluded that prophylactic antimicrobial agents were not necessary for extractions in these patients.[43] Others have obtained essentially identical results.[44]

Virtually all the current literature now suggests that elective surgery is safe in HIV-infected patients and should be offered when it provides some advantage. Ferguson[45] concludes that the presentation of surgical complications is similar in both HIV-infected and noninfected patients, except that leukocytosis is often absent in the former. He states that, "most important, the management of the surgical problem follows standard surgical principles regardless of the state of HIV infection."

REFERENCES

1. von Reyn CF, Gibert TT, Shaw FE, et al. Absence of HIV transmission from an infected orthopedic surgeon: a 13 year look-back study. JAMA 1993;264:1807–1811.
2. Centers for Disease Control and Prevention. Update: investigation of patients who have been treated by HIV-infected health care workers. MMWR 1992;41:344–346.
3. Rubin RH, Tolkoff-Rubin NE. The problem of human immunodeficiency virus (HIV) infection and transplantation. Transpl Int 1988;1:36–42.
4. Tzakis AG, Cooper MG, Dummer JS, et al. Transplantation in HIV (patients). Transplantation 1990;49:354–358.
5. Erice A, Rhame FA, Heussner RC, et al. Human immunodeficiency virus infection in patients with solid organ transplants: report of five cases and a review. Rev Infect Dis 1991;13:537–547.
6. Clarke JA. HIV transmission and skin grafts. (Letter) Lancet 1987;1:983.
7. Prepose JS, McRae S, Quinn TC, et al. Serologic markers after transplantation of corneas from donors infected with human immunodeficiency virus. Am J Ophthalmol 1987;103:798–804.
8. Carbone L, Cohen D, Hardy M, et al. Determination of acquired immunodeficiency syndrome (AIDS) after renal transplantation. Am J Kidney Dis 1988;11:378–392.
9. Kumar P, Pearson JE, Martin JH, et al. Transmission of human immunodeficiency virus (HIV) by transplantation of a renal allograft with development of the acquired immunodeficiency syndrome. Ann Intern Med 1987;106:244–245.
10. Bowen PA, Lobel SA, Caruana RJ, et al. Transmission of human immunodeficiency virus (HIV) by transplantation: clinical aspects and time course analysis of viral antigenemia and production. Ann Intern Med 1988;108:46–48.
11. Buck BE, Resnick L, Shah SM, et al. Bone transplantation and human immunodeficiency virus: an estimate of risk of acquired immunodeficiency virus syndrome (AIDS). Clin Orthop 1990;251:249–253.
12. Semen banking, organ and tissue transplantation and HIV antibody testing. MMWR 1988;37:57–58.
14. Transmission of HIV through bone transplantation: case report and public health recommendations. MMWR 1988;37:597–599.
15. Dummer JS, Erb S, Breinig MK, et al. Infection with human immunodeficiency virus in the Pittsburgh transplant population: a study of 538 donors and 1043 recipients, 1981, 1986. Transplantation 1989;47:134–140.
16. Tzakis AG, Cooper MH, Dummer JS, et al. Transplantation of HIV (+) patients. Transplantation 1990;49:354–358.
17. Henderson DK, Fahey BJ, Willy M, et al. Risk for occupation transmission of human immunodeficiency virus type-1 (HIV-1) associated with clinical exposure: a prospective evaluation. Ann Intern Med 1990;113:740–746.
18. The risk for occupational/nosocomial transmission of human immunodeficiency in health care workers. (Abstract) Programs and abstracts of the 28th ICAAC, Washington, DC, 1988.
19. Kuhls JL, Vikers S, Paris NB, et al. Occupational risk of HIV, HBV and HSV-2 infections in health care personnel caring for AIDS patients. Am J Public Health 1987;77:1306–1309.
20. Centers for Disease Control and Prevention. Update: investigation of patients who have been treated by HIV-infected healthcare workers. MMWR 1992;41:344–346.
21. Mast S, Gerberding JL. Factors predicting needlestick infectivity following exposure to HIV: an in vitro model. Clin Res 1991;39:58A.
22. Kelen GD, Fritz S, Quaqish B, et al. Unrecognized human immunodeficiency virus infection in emergency department patients. N Engl J Med 1988;318:1645–1650.
23. Recommendation for prevention of HIV transmission in health care settings. MMWR 1987;36(Suppl B):1817.
24. Recommendations for preventing transmission of HIV invasive and hepatitis B virus to patients during exposure-prone procedures. MMWR 1991;40:1–9.
25. Wilson SE, Williams RA, Robinson G. Operating on HIV-positive patients: what are the risks to healthcare workers? to patients? Postgrad Med 1990;88:193–201.
26. Gerberding JL, Schechter WP. Surgery and AIDS: reducing the risk. JAMA 1991;265:1572–1573.

27. Mandelbrot DA, Smythe WR, Normal SA, et al. A survey of exposures, practices and recommendations of surgeons in the care of patients with human immunodeficiency virus. Surg Gynecol Obstet 1990;171:99–106.

28. Lange JMA, Boucher CAB, Hollak CEM, et al. Failure of zidovudine prophylaxis after accidental exposure to HIV. N Engl J Med 1990;322:1375–1377.

29. Looke DRM, Grove DI. Failed prophylactic zidovudine after needlestick injury. (Letter) Lancet 1990;335:1280.

30. Henderson DK, Gerberding JL. Prophylactic zidovudine after occupational exposure to the human immunodeficiency virus: an interim analysis. J Infect Dis 1989;160:321.

31. Roldan EO, Moskowitz L, Genley GT. Pathology of the heart in acquired immunodeficiency syndrome. Arch Pathol Lab Med 1987;111:943.

32. Lemma M, Vanelip P, Meretta L, et al. Cardiac surgery in HIV-positive intravenous drug addicts: influence of cardiopulmonary bypass on the progression to AIDS. Thorac Cardiovasc Surg 1992;40:279–282.

33. Aris A, Pomar JL, Saura E. Cardiopulmonary bypass in HIV-positive patients. Soc Thorac Surg 1993;55:1104–1107.

34. Brau N, Esposito RA, Simberkoff MS. Cardiac valve replacement in patients infected with the immunodeficiency virus. Soc Thorac Surg 1992;54:552–554.

35. Bonfils-Roberts EA, Nickodem A, Nealon TF. Retrospective analysis of the efficacy of open lung biopsy in acquired immunodeficiency syndrome. Ann Thorac Surg 1990;49:115–117.

36. Trachiotis GD, Hafner GH, Hix WR, Aaron BL. Role of open lung biopsy in diagnosis of pulmonary complications of AIDS. Soc Thorac Surg 1992;54:898–902.

37. Pell MF, Thomas DGT, Whittle IR. Stereotactic biopsy of cerebral lesions in patients with AIDS. Br J Neurosurg 1991;5:585–589.

38. Levy RM, Russel E, Yungbluth M, et al. Efficacy of image guided stereotaxic brain biopsy in neurologically symptomatic AIDS patients. J Neurosurg 1992;30:186–190.

39. Wilson SE, Robinson G, Williams RA, et al. Acquired immune deficiency syndrome (AIDS): indications for abdominal surgery, pathology and outcome. Ann Surg 1989;210:428–434.

40. Robinson G, Wilson SE, Williams RA. Surgery in patients with the acquired immunodeficiency syndrome. Arch Surg 1987;122:170–174.

41. Ravikumar TS, Allen JD, Bothe A, Stelle G. Splenectomy: the treatment of choice for human immunodeficiency virus-related immune thrombocytopenia? Arch Surg 1989;124:625–627.

42. Alonso M, Gossot D, Borstyn E, et al. Splenectomy in human immunodeficiency virus-related thrombocytopenia. Br J Surg 1993;80:330–333.

43. Robinson PG, Cooper H, Hatt J. Healing after dental extractions in men with HIV infection. Oral Surg Oral Med Oral Pathol 1992;74:426–430.

44. Porter SR, Scully C, Luker J. Complications of dental surgery in persons with HIV disease. Oral Surg Oral Med Oral Pathol 1993;75:165–167.

45. Ferguson CM. Surgical complications of HIV infections. N Y State J Med 1991;91:383–384.

Medical Management of the Surgical Patient, Third Edition,
edited by Michael F. Lubin, H. Kenneth Walker, and Robert B. Smith III.
J.B. Lippincott Company, Philadelphia, PA © 1995.

CHAPTER

Postoperative Fever and Infection

James P. Steinberg

Fever is common in the postoperative period, and its causes are diverse (Table 27-1). Fever may result from a benign process such as the release of pyrogens from traumatized tissue and have no bearing on the clinical outcome. Alternatively, fever may be an early sign of a potentially life-threatening infection. The clinician's challenge is to distinguish those fevers that are significant from the large pool of "routine" fevers while avoiding the excessive use of diagnostic resources and therapeutic interventions such as antibiotics.

Evaluation of a febrile surgical patient begins with a careful history and review of the medical record. The presence of symptoms or signs of infection before the operative procedure or underlying medical problems that increase the likelihood of postoperative complications are valuable clues. The type of surgical procedure performed, the operative findings, and the temporal relationship between the operation and the onset of fever are also important. Although prolonged endotracheal intubation, indwelling bladder catheters, and intravascular catheters may be important components of patient care, they violate normal host defenses and increase the likelihood of postoperative infection. When a patient has a significant infection, symptoms and signs in addition to fever usually are present. Thus, a careful physical examination is essential. Laboratory and radiographic studies should be directed by the relevant clinical data and not obtained by an undirected "shotgun" approach.

The incidence of postoperative fever varies widely depending on the surgical procedure performed and the defi-

nition of fever. There is no consensus regarding what constitutes fever in the postoperative setting. Investigators have used temperatures ranging from 37.5° to 38.5°C to define fever, with 38°C being the most popular cutoff point. In addition, some investigators require that the temperature be elevated on consecutive measurements to meet their definition of fever, whereas others require that the temperature be elevated for 2 consecutive days. Thus, it is not surprising that the reported incidence of postoperative fever ranges from 13.7% after general surgery to nearly 100% after cardiac surgery.[1,2] Even among studies that involve only abdominal operations, there still is considerable variation in the reported incidence of fever (Table 27-2).

Postoperative fever can be divided into two broad categories—infectious and noninfectious. The reported proportion of febrile episodes attributed to bacterial infection also varies widely. In general, high fevers are more likely caused by infection, although considerable overlap exists.

TEMPORAL ASPECTS OF POSTOPERATIVE FEVER

The time of onset of postoperative fever is a helpful clue that can suggest a particular cause. Fever that develops within 24 hours after surgery usually is not caused by infection (Fig. 27-1). The time-honored dogma that atelectasis causes most early postoperative fever may be inaccurate,

TABLE 27–1. Causes of Postoperative Fever

Noninfectious
Adrenal insufficiency
Alcohol withdrawal
Atelectasis
Blood (hematoma or in cerebrospinal fluid)
Dehydration
Drug fever (including anesthetics)
Factitious
Malignant hyperthermia
Myocardial infarction
Neoplasms
Pancreatitis
Pheochromocytoma
Pulmonary embolism
Thrombophlebitis
Thyrotoxicosis
Tissue trauma
Transfusion reaction

Infectious
Abscess
Bloodstream infection
Cholecystitis
Clostridium difficile colitis
Endocarditis
Intravascular device infection
Parotitis
Peritonitis
Pneumonia
Surgical site infections
    Superficial incisional
    Deep incisional
    Organ/space
Transfusion-related (cytomegalovirus, hepatitis)
Urinary tract infection

however.[3–5] Garibaldi and colleagues[5] found that unexplained (and presumed noninfectious) early postoperative fever did not occur more frequently after thoracic and upper abdominal surgeries, procedures that predispose to atelectasis and pneumonia. In addition, Roberts and associates[6] did not find a high correlation between early fever (48 hours or less) after abdominal surgery and radiographic evidence of atelectasis. Tissue trauma during surgery with systemic release of pyrogenic substances may be the major cause of early postoperative fever, although definitive evidence is lacking. Other noninfectious causes of early postoperative fever include drug hypersensitivity reactions (including anesthetic agents) and transfusion reactions, which may cause hemolysis. Malignant hyperthermia usually manifests with high fever (39° to 44°C) beginning within 30 minutes of the administration of an anesthetic agent. Rarely, the fever associated with malignant hyperthermia is delayed and develops several hours after operation.

On occasion, infection does occur within 1 or 2 days after surgery. *Streptococcus pyogenes* and *Clostridium perfringens* infections, although rare, are the classic causes of early postoperative wound infections and can produce high fever within 24 hours of surgery. With streptococcal infections, erythema around the surgical site develops early and spreads rapidly. Clostridial wound infections typically occur after biliary tract or intestinal surgery. Severe pain is present and tense edema develops at the surgical site. A bronze or violaceous hue may develop, followed by hemorrhagic bullae and the formation of tissue gas. Toxic shock syndrome also produces high fever early in the postoperative period. Hypotension, diffuse erythematous rash, confusion, and other signs of toxemia often are present. In contrast to other wound infections, signs of local inflammation are absent, even though the surgical site harbors the toxige-

TABLE 27–2. Incidence of Fever and Infection Causing Fever After Abdominal Surgery

Procedure	Definition of Fever	Number of Patients	Percentage With Fever	Percentage of Those Febrile With Infection
Major abdominal[20]	≥38.5°C (rectally) on 2 consecutive measurements during first 6 postoperative days	464	15	27*
Cholecystectomy[21]	≥38.4°C or ≥38.0°C (orally) on consecutive measurements 4 hours apart	176	16	7†
Abdominal[22]	≥38.1°C during first 7 postoperative days	434	38	16†
Intraabdominal, duration >1 hour[23]	≥38.0°C (rectally) on 2 measurements >1 hour apart	608	43	36
	Group A: 38°–38.4°C; group B: ≥38.5°C		A: 15 B: 27	A: 19 B: 45

*Required culture confirmation.
†Uses CDC definition of infection; 8 other patients had infection but were afebrile.

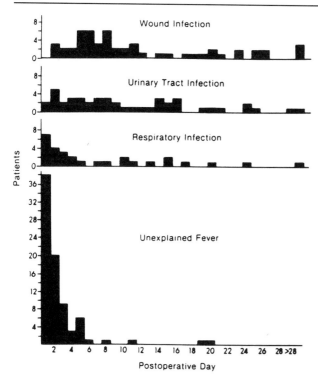

FIG. 27-1. Days of onset for postoperative infections and unexplained fever. (Garibaldi RA, Brodine S, Matsumiya S, Coleman M. Evidence for the noninfectious etiology of early postoperative fever. Infect Control 1985:6;274)

pear later. Bacterial pneumonias are often precipitated by perioperative aspiration or early postoperative atelectasis and, consequently, tend to occur within the first week after surgery. UTIs can appear at any time; the major risk factors for UTI development are instrumentation of the urinary tract and indwelling urinary catheter placement. The probability of bacterial colonization in the bladder increases with the duration of catheterization. Bloodstream infections may result from any of these infections but are most commonly caused by intravascular devices. The risk of bloodstream infection increases with the duration of intravascular access.

Thrombophlebitis, pulmonary embolism, and pulmonary infarction are important causes of postoperative fever that can occur early or late in the postoperative period, depending on the clinical situation. Diagnosis can be difficult and a high index of suspicion is necessary. Hematomas can produce occult fevers or mimic intraabdominal abscesses. The possibility of a hematoma should be considered when the hematocrit continues to decline after the operation in the absence of other explanations, such as gastrointesti-

nic *Staphylococcus aureus*. If significant aspiration of oropharyngeal or gastric contents occurred during the induction of anesthesia, a postoperative pneumonia may manifest within 1 or 2 days of surgery. If the surgery is prompted by infection, such as peritonitis after a ruptured viscus, fever can antedate or occur shortly after the procedure. On occasion, an unrelated infection is incubating at the time of surgery and produces early fever. Accurate diagnosis can be difficult, especially when patients are intubated or sedated after operation and are unable to relate their history.

Fever that develops 72 hours or more after operation suggests the presence of infection. Rates of infection vary considerably with the type of operation performed (Fig. 27-2), ranging from 2% after herniorrhaphy to 20.8% after gastric surgery. Although the causes of postoperative infection are numerous (see Table 27-1), surgical site infections, bloodstream infections, pneumonia, and urinary tract infections (UTIs) account for 80% to 90% of all cases. Wound infections are most common overall but the distribution of infections depends on the type of operation performed (Table 27-3). Wound infections typically manifest 5 to 10 days after operation, although deep organ space abscesses may ap-

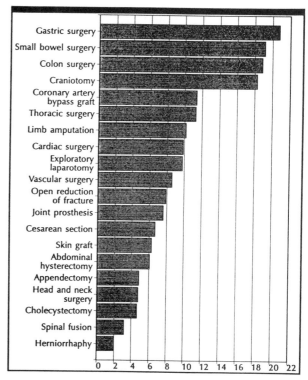

FIG. 27-2. Overall infection rates by type of operation (number of nosocomial infections at all sites per 100 operations). (Horan TC, Culver DH, Gaynes RP, Jarvis WR, Edwards JR, Reid CR. Nosocomial infections in surgical patients in the United States, January 1986–June 1992. Infect Control Hosp Epidemiol 1993;14:75)

TABLE 27–3. Distribution of Nosocomial Infections in Surgical Patients by Site for Operations With 750 Infections or More Reported

Operation	Number of Infections	Incisional Surgical Site Infection (%)	Organ/Space Surgical Site Infection (%)	Urinary Tract Infection (%)	Pneumonia (%)	Primary Bloodstream Infection (%)	Other (%)
Coronary artery bypass graft	4559	25	8	19	21	8	19
Thoracic surgery	1418	11	6	18	34	11	21
Cardiac surgery	1586	14	8	18	21	15	24
Open reduction of fracture	3507	18	4	48	14	4	12
Joint prosthesis	2742	21	7	52	9	2	9
Spinal fusion	1789	29	5	42	10	4	10
Limb amputation	1493	36	1	29	11	6	17
Cesarean section	4908	19	5.5	12	3	2	9
Abdominal hysterectomy	2491	22	24	37	6	2	9
Colon surgery	5312	26	12	26	15	8	12
Exploratory laparotomy	4024	25	8	23	18	10	16
Cholecystectomy	2245	24	9	26	19	7	15
Gastric surgery	2127	20	12	19	22	10	16
Small bowel surgery	1209	27	13	18	16	10	16
Appendectomy	817	51	24	6	8	2	9
Herniorrhaphy	787	46	4	21	15	4	10
Vascular surgery	4057	29	4	23	20	8	16
Craniotomy	2297	5	3	39	25	9	19
Skin graft	925	31	1	22	11	7	28
Head and neck surgery	789	37	4	14	25	7	13

*National Nosocomial Infection Surveillance System, January 1986 to June 1992.
(Horan TC, Culver DH, Gaynes RP, et al. Nosocomial infections in surgical patients in the United States, January 1986–June 1992. Infect Control Hosp Epidemiol 1993;14:73)

nal blood loss. Resorption of clotted blood can produce hyperbilirubinemia and an elevated lactate dehydrogenase level. Hematomas also can become secondarily infected, further complicating the clinical picture. Medications are an important cause of postoperative fever. Drug fever caused by antibacterial agents classically develops 7 to 10 days after administration of the agent is begun.[7] Misconceptions abound regarding drug fever; rash, eosinophilia, and other signs of drug allergy are frequently absent. In addition, drug fever can produce a hectic fever curve.

Late fever, developing more than 2 weeks after surgery, usually occurs in patients with underlying medical problems or complicated hospital courses. Prolonged intravenous access, bladder catheterization, and endotracheal intubation present ongoing risks for infection. Transient bacteremias can lead to metastatic foci of infection that declare themselves in the late postoperative period. Drug fevers can occur several weeks or longer after a new medication is introduced. Transfusion-related infections, partic-

ularly cytomegalovirus infection, can produce fever weeks to months after the receipt of blood products. Screening of blood products for human immunodeficiency virus and hepatitis B and C has reduced transfusion-associated infection to extremely low levels. *Clostridium difficile* diarrhea occurs days to several weeks after antibiotics are administered. Single-dose antibiotic prophylaxis before surgery rarely induces this infection.

SURGICAL SITE INFECTIONS

In 1992, the Centers for Disease Control and Prevention (CDC) modified the definition of surgical wound infections.[8] The term *surgical site infection* replaced *surgical wound infection*. Surgical site infections are categorized as incisional or organ/space infections. An organ/space surgical site infection involves any part of the anatomy beyond the incision opened or manipulated during the procedure. In addition, incisional surgical site infections are subdivided into superficial incisional and deep incisional infections. This semantic change should eliminate confusion in that the surgical "wound" in standard parlance extends from the skin to the deep soft tissues and not to the organ space. Thus, the term *deep wound infection,* referring to infections at or deep to the fascial layers, was ambiguous. The distinction between incisional and organ/space infections also has relevance because certain procedures (eg, cesarean section) are more likely to lead to organ/space infection, whereas other procedures (eg, herniorrhaphy, appendectomy, exploratory laparotomy) are complicated more often by incisional infections (see Table 27-3).

The standard classification of surgical wound infections has four categories—clean, clean-contaminated, contaminated, and infected—based on the degree of bacterial contamination at the time of the procedure. Although it is helpful, this system has limited capability to stratify the risk of surgical site infections[9] (Table 27-4). Host factors such as age, obesity, and underlying medical illnesses also contribute to the risk of postoperative infection.[10] Other factors related to the operation, such as duration, independently predict risk of infection. To account for these other risk factors, the Surgical Wound Infection Task Force recommended a composite risk index for stratifying the risk of surgical site infection.[10] This index incorporates three elements: (1) the standard wound classification, (2) a severity of illness marker such as the American Society of Anesthesiologists class, and (3) the duration of operation. This index greatly

TABLE 27–4. Surgical Site Infection Rates Among 84,691 Operations Stratified by Wound Classification and Risk Index*

Risk Factor	Surgical Site Infection Rate: Infections per 100 Operations
Wound Classification	
Clean	2.1
Clean-contaminated	3.3
Contaminated	6.4
Dirty-infected	7.1
Risk Index	
0	1.5
1	2.9
2	6.8
3	13.0

*Risk index determined by giving 1 point for each risk factor present: (1) American Society of Anesthesiologists score of 3, 4, or 5; (2) operation classified as contaminated or dirty-infected; (3) prolonged duration of surgery with time cutoff depending on the type of procedure.
(Adapted from Culver DH, Horan TC, Gaynes RP, et al. Surgical wound infection rates by wound class, operative procedure, and patient risk index: National Nosocomial Infections Surveillance System, Am J Med 1991;91:1525)

enhances the ability to stratify the risk of infection (see Table 27-4). When confronting patients with postoperative fever, clinicians can use the index to estimate the probability of a surgical site infection.

Superficial incisional infections are heralded by pain at the surgical site disproportionate to usual postoperative pain. Edema, tenderness, erythema, and purulent drainage are frequently evident on inspection of the wound. The wound should be examined closely for areas of fluctuance. Occasionally, crepitus is present and suggests the involvement of anaerobic organisms. Deep incisional infections may not show the typical local signs and diagnosis may be delayed. Fever and leukocytosis are usually present but are not invariable.

Effective wound drainage, which usually includes suture removal, is the cornerstone of therapy for incisional infections. Purulent drainage should be sent to the microbiology laboratory for Gram stain and culture. If cellulitis and systemic signs of infection are absent, drainage is usually curative and the use of systemic antibiotics can be avoided. Antibiotic selection should be based on Gram stain results, if these are available. Staphylococci and streptococci are the major causes of superficial incisional infections. The emergence of methicillin-resistant *S aureus* as a significant nosocomial pathogen complicates empiric antibiotic coverage. The need to consider vancomycin as part of empiric therapy depends on the prevalence of methicillin-resistant *S aureus* at the particular institution, the severity of the infection, the duration of hospitalization, and previous antibiotic administration.

Organ/space infections involving the peritoneal cavity or the pelvis are frequently polymicrobial, and empiric antibiotics should have activity against gram-negative and anaerobic pathogens. Peritonitis typically occurs after procedures that enter contaminated areas such as the bowel or the biliary tract. Procedures that include anastomoses of the gastrointestinal tract pose an increased risk of peritonitis. Anastomotic leaks usually occur between the third and fifth postoperative days, when edema of the suture line begins to resolve. The diagnosis of peritonitis in the postoperative period is usually straightforward. Signs of peritoneal irritation are often heralded by fever, tachycardia, and abdominal pain. Intraabdominal or pelvic abscesses occurring after gastrointestinal or gynecologic surgery can have a subtle presentation. Abdominal pain and other localizing signs may or may not be present. Persistent or recurrent fever and leukocytosis may be early clues. Computed tomography is invaluable, both for diagnosis and for percutaneous drainage of abscesses. On average, computed tomographic scans are obtained 1 week after the initial surgery if abscess is suspected. During this interval, some of the expected inflammatory changes in the operative area should resolve, whereas any infection that is present may evolve into a discrete abscess.

Infection after median sternotomy may be superficial, involve the sternum, or result in mediastinitis. After the procedure, the sternum is contiguous with the deeper mediastinal structures and the pericardium. Thus, differentiating superficial from deep infection may be difficult. When mediastinitis is present, patients are often critically ill with accompanying bacteremia. On occasion, fever and systemic signs of infection develop before other clinical signs of wound infection, such as purulent drainage. *S aureus* and coagulase-negative staphylococci are common causes of sternal wound infections. In some institutions, gram-negative bacteria predominate. Therapy involves the prolonged administration of intravenous antibiotics and aggressive surgical débridement. Prolonged surgery, reoperation, underlying diseases such as diabetes mellitus, cigarette smoking, obesity, and the use of internal mammary arteries are risk factors for the development of sternal wound infections.

BLOODSTREAM INFECTIONS

Bloodstream infections in the postoperative setting can result from localized processes such as surgical site infections, pneumonia, or UTIs. The rate of secondary bloodstream infection varies considerably depending on the operative procedure performed. Rates of bacteremia accompanying incisional and organ/space infections are highest (13.2% and 39.7%, respectively) after cardiac surgery.[11] Postoperative pneumonia is more likely to lead to secondary bacteremia in patients who are mechanically ventilated than in those who are not.

Primary bloodstream infections, usually a consequence of intravascular access devices, are more common than secondary bloodstream infections and account for 7% of nosocomial infections in surgical patients.[11] These infections are unfortunate, not only because of the significant attendant mortality but because they are largely preventable. Although any device can serve as the source of a bacteremia or fungemia, most device-related bloodstream infections in the postoperative setting are caused by central venous catheters. Several studies of percutaneously inserted subclavian or internal jugular vein catheters have found a septicemia rate of 3% to 5%.[12] Cutaneous colonization of the insertion site by bacteria, increased duration of placement, frequent manipulation, and poor line care are risk factors for central venous catheter–related infection. The risk of infection with internal jugular vein catheters is higher than with subclavian catheters, probably because the former are more difficult to secure and are located close to oropharyngeal secretions. Swan-Ganz catheters inserted with maximal barrier precautions (ie, surgical gowns, masks, sterile gloves, and a large sterile sheet drape) are less prone to infection than are catheters inserted in the operating room under less stringent conditions.[13] With short-term catheters (versus cuffed tunneled lines such as Hickman catheters), most bloodstream infections are caused by bacteria that colonize the skin site and then gain access to the bloodstream from the insertion wound (ie, outside the lumen). With increased manipulation of the catheter, the hub may become colonized and serve as the source of bacteremia. Contaminated infusates are uncommon but can be the source of epidemic nosocomial bacteremias. The insertion site may show erythema or purulence, although these findings are often absent with catheter-associated bacteremia, especially if the catheter hub or infusate is the source of infection.

Peripheral catheters can be the source of phlebitis and bloodstream infection. Phlebitis, or inflammation of the vein, manifests with pain, erythema, tenderness, and an indurated thrombosed vein. Phlebitis is a reaction to the catheter material or the infusate and does not imply the presence of infection. The inflammation associated with phlebitis can produce fever. There is a significant correlation between phlebitis and the development of catheter-related infection. Consequently, the presence of phlebitis mandates catheter removal. The absence of phlebitis, however, does not exclude a catheter-related bloodstream infection. With routine replacement every 72 hours, peripheral venous catheters rarely cause bloodstream infection. An erythematous or indurated catheter site should be assessed for signs of suppurative phlebitis, which include fluctuance over the course of the vein and purulence that can be expressed from the insertion site by milking the vein. Suppurative phlebitis is the cause of a sustained bacteremia; patients frequently appear septic with high, spiking fevers. Excision of the involved vein is often necessary.

In the assessment of febrile postoperative patients, any intravascular catheter should be considered a potential source of infection, especially if no other site is apparent. If catheter-associated infection is suspected, the device should be removed and the tip sent for quantitative cultures. Two sets of blood cultures should be obtained by separate peripheral venipunctures. *Candida* species and *Torulopsis glabrata*, the most common causes of fungemia, grow on routine media, so it is not necessary to order fungal blood cultures in most situations. Blood cultures obtained through the device are more likely to be contaminated. The practice of obtaining one culture through a central catheter and one culture through a peripheral vein should be discouraged unless peripheral access is poor or quantitative blood cultures are performed. On quantitative culturing, a greater concentration of organisms from the device culture compared with a peripheral culture supports the diagnosis of catheter-associated bacteremia. Most hospital laboratories, however, do not perform quantitative blood cultures routinely.

If catheter-related bacteremia is suspected, empiric antibiotic therapy is warranted. Coagulase-negative staphylococci and *S aureus* are the most common pathogens but many types of bacteria and fungi have been associated with infusion-related infections. Prolonged antibiotic therapy, hyperalimentation, underlying medical problems such as diabetes mellitus, central venous access, and previous surgery are risk factors for catheter-related fungemia. If patients with central venous catheter–related bacteremia remain febrile despite the administration of appropriate antibiotics, and if follow-up blood cultures show sustained bacteremia, an infected thrombus should be suspected. Unlike septic phlebitis of peripheral veins, there are few clues on the physical examination to suggest septic thrombosis of a central vein. Endocarditis is also a cause of sustained bacteremia but is less common in the postoperative setting.

PNEUMONIA

Pneumonia and other pulmonary sources of postoperative fever are discussed in Chapter 15.

URINARY TRACT INFECTIONS

According to CDC data, UTIs account for 27% of all postoperative infections.[11] Although they are the second most common infection in surgical patients, UTIs cause less morbidity and mortality than do pneumonias, bloodstream infections, or surgical site infections. UTIs occur almost exclusively in patients with bladder catheterization or previous urinary tract manipulation. The risk of bacteriuria increases with the duration of catheterization. The microbiology of nosocomial UTIs is much broader than that of community-acquired UTIs, with *Escherichia coli* accounting for only about 30%. The intensive use of broad-spectrum antibiotics, including third-generation cephalosporins, in the postoperative setting has contributed to the increase in the number of UTIs caused by enterococci, resistant gram-negative bacilli, and yeast. Removal of the bladder catheter as soon as feasible is the best means of minimizing the risk of UTI.

Seventy to 80% of patients with catheter-associated bacteriuria are asymptomatic. Pyuria is common, even when symptoms are absent. The presence of the bladder catheter obscures the symptoms of lower tract infection. Signs of upper tract infection, including fever and flank pain, are rare; secondary bacteremia occurs in about 1% of patients with bacteriuria. Because bacteriuria is common and the course usually is benign, other sources of infection should be considered in febrile postoperative patients who have pyuria and positive results on urine cultures.

After the removal of short-term urinary catheters, symptomatic lower UTIs developed in 7 of 42 patients (17%) with catheter-associated bacteriuria.[14] Consequently, it is prudent to treat patients with asymptomatic bacteriuria after catheter removal. Single-dose antibiotic therapy is usually effective in women.[14] The best approach for patients with funguria is unknown.[15]

OTHER INFECTIONS

Ten to 20% of infections in surgical patients are from other sources. The diagnosis may be cryptic, especially in critically ill patients in intensive care units. Physical examination, although difficult to perform, is nonetheless essential. Maxillary sinusitis, often staphylococcal, occurs in patients with nasotracheal intubation or nasogastric tubes. Sinus tenderness may be present, even in obtunded patients. A boggy, tender, and enlarged parotid gland suggests parotitis, an uncommon complication seen in sick patients with volume depletion. A careful funduscopic examination should be performed to search for evidence of fungal endophthalmitis, especially in patients with risk factors for candidemia. Acute cholecystitis can occur after surgery remote to the gallbladder. Right upper quadrant pain is usually present but recognition can be delayed in sedated and paralyzed patients. Calculi may be absent on imaging studies. Without prompt diagnosis and surgical intervention, perforation, peritonitis, and sepsis can develop. Diarrhea is sometimes absent or mild with *C difficile* colitis; this diagnosis should be considered in postoperative patients who have fevers and abdominal tenderness.

ANTIBIOTIC USE IN THE PERIOPERATIVE AND POSTOPERATIVE SETTING

Perioperative prophylactic antibiotics effectively reduce the rates of postoperative infection after many operative procedures.[16,17] Timing of the preoperative dose is critical; infection rates are higher if the antibiotic is administered more than 2 hours before surgery or after the incision is made.[18] One preincisional dose is usually sufficient, although a second dose administered during procedures that last more than 3 to 4 hours is advised. Some authorities recommend the continued administration of prophylactic antibiotics for 24 hours after surgery.[17] Antibiotics given beyond this time should be considered therapeutic and not prophylactic. Prolonging therapy longer than 48 hours in the absence of established infection should be avoided because of increased cost and the increased likelihood of colonization and infection with antibiotic-resistant bacteria. The use of broad-spectrum agents also exerts selective pressure on the microbiologic flora. These agents, especially third-generation cephalosporins, have no role in perioperative prophylaxis. There is a temptation to continue the administration of perioperative antibiotics because of early postoperative fever. This temptation should be balanced by the realization that fever on the first postoperative day is rarely caused by infection and by knowledge of the hazards of prolonged antibiotic coverage. Recent data from the CDC show an increase in wound and other nosocomial infections caused by antibiotic-resistant pathogens, including methicillin-resistant *S aureus,* enterococci, coagulase-negative staphylococci, *Enterobacter* species, and *Candida albicans.*[19] The intensive use of antibiotics has played a major role in the selection of these and other resistant organisms. In choosing an antibiotic regimen for a postoperative infection, the clinician must be cognizant not only of the likely pathogens but also of previous antibiotics administered to the patients and resistance trends in the hospital.

REFERENCES

1. Galicier C, Richet H. A prospective study of postoperative fever in a general surgery department. Infect Control 1985;6:487.
2. Livelli FD Jr, Johnson RA, McEnany MT, et al. Unexplained in-hospital fever following cardiac surgery. Circulation 1978; 57:968.
3. Hiyama DT, Zinner MJ. Surgical complications. In: Schwartz SI, ed. Principles of surgery, ed 6. New York, McGraw-Hill, 1994:455.
4. Fry DE. Postoperative fever. In: Mackowiak PA, ed. Fever: basic mechanisms and management. New York, Raven Press, 1991:243.
5. Garibaldi RA, Brodine S, Matsumiya S, Coleman M. Evidence for the non-infectious etiology of early postoperative Fever. Infect Control 1985;6:273.
6. Roberts J, Barnes W, Pennock M, Browne G. Diagnostic accuracy of fever as a measure of postoperative pulmonary complications. Heart Lung 1988;17:166.
7. Mackowiak PA. Drug fever. In: Mackowiak PA, ed. Fever: basic mechanisms and management. New York, Raven Press, 1991:255.
8. Horan TC, Gaynes RP, Martone WJ, et al. CDC definitions of nosocomial surgical site infections, 1992: a modification of CDC definitions of surgical wound infections. Infect Control Hosp Epidemiol 1992;13:606.
9. Culver DH, Horan TC, Gaynes RP, et al. Surgical wound infection rates by wound class, operative procedure, and patient risk index: National Nosocomial Infections Surveillance System. Am J Med 1991;91:152S.
10. The Society for Hospital Epidemiology of America, The Association for Practitioners in Infection Control, The Centers for Disease Control, The Surgical Infection Society. Consensus paper on the surveillance of surgical wound infections. Infect Control Hosp Epidemiol 1992;13:599.
11. Horan TC, Culver DH, Gaynes RP, et al. Nosocomial infections in surgical patients in the United States, January 1986–June 1992: National Nosocomial Infections Surveillance (NNIS) System. Infect Control Hosp Epidemiol 1993;14:73.
12. Maki DG. Infections due to infusion therapy. In: Bennett JV, Brachman PS, eds. Hospital infections, ed 3. Boston, Little, Brown, 1992:849.
13. Mermel LA, McCormick RD, Springman SR, Maki DG. The pathogenesis and epidemiology of catheter-related infection with pulmonary artery Swan-Ganz catheters: a prospective study utilizing molecular subtyping. Am J Med 1991;91(Suppl 3B):197S.
14. Harding GKM, Nicolle LE, Ronald AR, et al. How long should catheter-acquired urinary tract infections in women be treated? Ann Intern Med 1991;114:713.
15. Wong-Beringer A, Jacobs RA, Guglielmo J. Treatment of funguria. JAMA 1992;267:2780.
16. Page CP, Bohnen JMA, Fletcher JR, et al. Antimicrobial prophylaxis for surgical wounds. Arch Surg 1993;128:79.
17. Kaiser AB. Antimicrobial prophylaxis in surgery. N Engl J Med 1986;315:1129.
18. Classen DC, Evans RS, Pestotnik SL, et al. The timing of prophylactic administration of antibiotics and the risk of surgical-wound infection. N Engl J Med 1992;326:281.
19. Schaberg DR, Culver DH, Gaynes RP. Major trends in the microbial etiology of nosocomial infection. Am J Med 1991; 91:73S.
20. Freischlag J, Busuttil RW. The value of postoperative fever evaluation. Surgery 1983;94:358.
21. Giangobbe MJ, Rappaport WD, Stein B. The significance of fever following cholecystectomy. J Fam Pract 1992;34:437.
22. Mellors JW, Kelly JJ, Gusberg RJ, et al. A simple index to estimate the likelihood of bacterial infection in patients developing fever after abdominal surgery. Am Surg 1988;54:558.
23. Jorgensen FS, Sorensen CG, Kjaergaard J. Postoperative fever after major abdominal surgery. Ann Chir Gynaecol 1988;77:47.

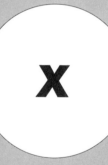
RENAL DISEASE

Medical Management of the Surgical Patient, Third Edition,
edited by Michael F. Lubin, H. Kenneth Walker, and Robert B. Smith III.
J.B. Lippincott Company, Philadelphia, PA © 1995.

CHAPTER

28

SURGERY IN THE PATIENT WITH RENAL DISEASE

Deepak Kikeri

End-stage renal disease (ESRD) develops in about 1.6 in 10,000 Americans each year and has a four times higher incidence in blacks than in whites.[1] Diabetes mellitus and hypertension are believed to be the major causes of chronic renal failure and ESRD but histologic evidence is lacking and the true incidence of ESRD associated with these disease processes is unknown.[1] More than 160,000 patients now participate in the ESRD Medicare program and this number is expected to continue to increase.[1]

Patients with ESRD can be treated by hemodialysis, peritoneal dialysis, or renal transplantation, and many are treated with more than one modality during their lifetime. For example, patients who have been undergoing peritoneal dialysis may receive renal transplants, then require hemodialysis years later when the transplants fail because of chronic rejection.

In hemodialysis, blood is drawn from an arteriovenous fistula (eg, Cimino-Brescia fistula, synthetic grafts). Clearance of uremic toxins and other substances (eg, potassium) from the blood occurs across a semipermeable membrane by diffusion into a dialysate. Blood "cleaned" by this method is then returned to the same arteriovenous access. To remove fluid (ultrafiltration), a pressure gradient is produced across the semipermeable membrane. To maintain homeostasis without excessive accumulation of waste products, patients with ESRD usually undergo hemodialysis three times a week.

To treat patients with peritoneal dialysis, dialysate is introduced into the peritoneal cavity through a pliable cathe-ter (usually a Tenckhoff catheter). Removal of waste products and ions from the blood (ie, clearance) occurs by diffusion from the capillaries in the peritoneal membrane into the dialysate. A high dextrose concentration in the dialysate provides an osmotic gradient that permits fluid removal (ie, ultrafiltration). Peritoneal dialysis may be performed continuously (eg, continuous ambulatory peritoneal dialysis, continuous cycler-assisted peritoneal dialysis) or intermittently (eg, intermittent peritoneal dialysis).

A transplanted kidney (from a cadaver or a living donor) is generally placed in the right or left lower quadrant in the extraperitoneal space. The blood vessels of the transplanted organ are usually anastomosed to the recipient's external iliac vessels and the ureter is anastomosed to the recipient's bladder. Immunosuppressive drugs, such as azathioprine, prednisone, and cyclosporine, are used in different combinations to prevent rejection of the renal transplant. These drugs have potentially serious side effects ranging from bone marrow suppression and infections to cyclosporine-induced renal damage. Consequently, the treatment of these patients is complex and beyond the scope of this chapter.

The incidence of heart disease is high in patients who are undergoing dialysis and in transplant recipients. Cardiac-related deaths accounted for over 40% of all deaths in the European Dialysis and Transplant Registry.[2] Therefore, patients must be carefully evaluated for evidence of heart disease and measures taken to ensure optimal cardiac function before any surgical procedure is performed.

291

PREOPERATIVE EVALUATION AND TREATMENT

Patients with advanced renal failure (particularly those receiving dialysis) and patients with renal transplants should undergo preoperative evaluation by nephrologists if possible. One of the many reasons for this is that the timing of surgery must be closely coordinated with the hemodialysis schedule. This simple practice minimizes the risk of fluid overload with associated hypertension and pulmonary edema, as well as electrolyte disturbances such as hyperkalemia and acidosis.

EXTRACELLULAR VOLUME STATUS

It is imperative that excess extracellular fluid be removed by diuretics in patients with renal failure who are in the predialysis stage of disease, or by progressive ultrafiltration in those who are receiving dialysis, otherwise, fluid administration during surgery and in the perioperative period can cause hypertension and pulmonary edema. Excessive removal of fluid before surgery is also undesirable, however, because it can cause hypotension in the perioperative period. As a general rule, enough fluid is removed so that patients return to their "dry weights" within 24 hours of the planned surgery. During surgery and in the perioperative period, fluid, salt, and potassium intake should be minimized.

Extracellular Fluid Overload

Extracellular fluid overload in patients with renal failure can be recognized as hypertension, edema, or increased jugular venous pressure. Severe fluid overload causes pulmonary edema, which requires emergent treatment. In patients with pulmonary edema, it is important to distinguish whether heart failure (eg, after a myocardial infarction) or fluid overload is the primary cause because the former may require specific therapy. Fluid overload occurs when salt and fluid intake exceed losses through urination or dialysis. Restricting dietary salt and fluid intake, avoiding unnecessary blood products (see later), and accomplishing adequate diuresis (in patients with predialysis disease) or dialysis can prevent the development of volume overload.

In patients with renal failure and predialysis renal disease, diuretics plus a low-salt diet are used to treat extracellular volume (ECV) overload. For patients with severely compromised renal function, a high dosage of furosemide (eg, 140 to 200 mg) or bumetanide (eg, 6 to 8 mg) may be necessary. Although high dosages of loop diuretics such as furosemide can cause ototoxicity and even permanent deafness, this is unusual and mainly associated with the con-

comitant administration of another ototoxic drug (eg, an aminoglycoside) or the bolus intravenous administration of furosemide.[3] Excessive diuresis, however, can result in ECV depletion, reduced renal perfusion, and worsening renal function. Other complications of diuretic use include hypokalemia, metabolic alkalosis, hyperuricemia, and hypomagnesemia.

In patients who are undergoing dialysis, the key to treating fluid overload is restricting salt and fluid intake while the excess fluid is removed during dialysis. Unfortunately, the rapid removal of large volumes of fluid during dialysis may result in cramping and hypotension. In addition, blood glucose levels should be monitored carefully in these patients, especially those who have diabetes, because severe hyperglycemia can develop when high dialysate dextrose concentrations are used to enhance fluid removal.

Extracellular Fluid Depletion

Intravascular volume depletion can result from direct losses of ECV (ie, hemorrhage, diarrhea, excessive diuresis or ultrafiltration) or from the movement of fluid from the intravascular to the extravascular space (ie, third-space losses from such causes as pancreatitis, intestinal sequestration of fluid, and crush injuries). This can cause hypotension in all patients and worsening renal function in those with predialysis disease. Treatment involves volume expansion, usually with isotonic fluids such as normal saline solution, although excessive volume administration to patients with renal failure may result in pulmonary edema. Monitoring the intravascular volume through a pulmonary artery catheter may be exceedingly helpful in critically ill patients. Potassium supplements should not be used unless significant hypokalemia is present (see later).

ARTERIAL BLOOD PRESSURE STATUS

Hypertension

Hypertension in patients with renal failure is largely mediated by ECV expansion and by the renin–angiotensin axis.[4,5] The removal of excess extracellular fluid to achieve dry weight reduces blood pressure into the normal range in most patients with severe renal failure.[4] The excess ECV is removed by diuretics in patients who have not yet required dialysis or by ultrafiltration in those who have. In addition, the intake of salt and fluid must be restricted to maintain a nonexpanded ECV.

Antihypertensive agents such as angiotensin-converting enzyme (ACE) inhibitors, calcium channel blockers, and β-blockers are used to control hypertension if the removal of excess ECV fails to lower blood pressure into the desired range. If antihypertensive medications are used, they should not be administered before hemodialysis to prevent hypotension during the dialysis session. ACE inhibitors provide an attractive form of treatment in these patients, given the involvement of the renin system in hypertension in renal failure.[6] For patients with predialysis renal disease, ACE inhibitors can raise the serum potassium level by reducing the secretion of aldosterone. In addition, ACE inhibitors can cause a reduction in renal function when glomerular perfusion is reduced and, consequently, glomerular filtration becomes dependent on angiotensin II–induced efferent glomerular arteriolar constriction (eg, bilateral renal artery stenosis, ECV depletion). For these reasons, ACE inhibitors should be used cautiously in patients with renal failure who have predialysis renal disease, and the potassium and creatinine levels should be monitored closely.

Hypotension

Hypotension can be caused by many factors, including intravascular volume depletion (see earlier); sepsis with vasodilation; reduced cardiac function (eg, myocardial infarction, uremic pericarditis with tamponade); and antihypertensive medications. It is essential that the specific cause be determined and the hypotension be treated rationally. Excessive reliance on intravenous fluids results in pulmonary edema in patients with renal failure. Pulmonary artery catheterization may provide valuable information in making the diagnosis and monitoring therapy in selected patients with refractory disease.

ELECTROLYTE STATUS

Hyponatremia

Mild hyponatremia, and consequently hypoosmolality, is common in patients with renal failure because of excessive free water intake when renal clearance of water is impaired. In patients who are undergoing hemodialysis, this can be corrected easily by using a dialysate that contains a higher sodium concentration. It is also critical that the intake of free water be restricted. For patients who are receiving peritoneal dialysis and those who have predialysis renal disease, free water intake should be restricted only if the serum sodium concentration is below normal. There is no need to restrict water intake in patients who have edema alone; in these cases, sodium intake should be restricted.

Severe hypoosmolality resulting from hyponatremia causes cerebral edema and encephalopathy, especially when it occurs rapidly. Hypertonic saline is commonly used to treat severe symptomatic hyponatremia. The optimal rate and extent of correction of hyponatremia using

hypertonic saline is controversial because some studies suggest that overly aggressive correction may lead to demyelinating lesions, especially in the pons.[7–9] Risk factors for osmotic demyelination include greater than 25 mEq/L correction of the sodium concentration or correction to above 140 mEq/L within 48 hours, and the presence of hypoxic encephalopathy.[9–11] In the absence of symptoms, it has been suggested that the sodium concentration be increased at a rate of 0.5 mEq/L/h until a level of 120 mEq/L is reached.[9,11,12] A higher initial rate of correction (1 to 1.5 mEq/L/h until the sodium concentration increases by 5 to 10 mEq/L) may be advisable if severe symptoms attributable to hypoosmolality are present, such as altered mental status or seizures.[13]

The amount of sodium required to increase the serum sodium to 120 mEq/L can be estimated from the formula:

$$\text{Na deficit (mEq)} = 0.5 \text{ (lean body weight in kg) (120} - \text{serum Na)}$$

It should be emphasized, however, that this equation provides only an estimate of the sodium deficit; serial measurements of the serum sodium are mandatory to monitor the rate and extent of the correction of hyponatremia.

Hyponatremia is usually associated with reduced plasma osmolality (hypoosmolality). Occasionally, hyponatremia is caused by hyperosmolality (eg, mannitol administration, severe hyperglycemia) because of water movement from the intracellular to the extracellular space. Isoosmolar hyponatremia (pseudohyponatremia) occurs with severe hyperlipidemia and hyperproteinemia.

Hypernatremia

Hypernatremia is rare in patients with renal failure and occurs when losses of free water (eg, skin losses with fever, osmotic diuresis) exceed the intake of free water. Occasionally, the rapid administration of hypertonic solutions (eg, hypertonic saline, hypertonic sodium bicarbonate) can cause hypernatremia. It is not generally appreciated that potassium salts are osmotically active; the combination of isotonic saline plus potassium chloride results in a hypertonic solution. Severe hypernatremia and the consequent hyperosmolality leads to cerebral dehydration.

Hypernatremia can be corrected by giving patients free water. For patients with hypernatremia who are receiving hemodialysis, the sodium concentration in the dialysate can be set at a lower value than that in the blood. Rapid correction of hypernatremia, however, can cause cerebral edema.[14] It has been recommended that the plasma sodium concentration be reduced gradually to normal levels over 2 to 3 days.[13]

The water deficit can be estimated from the formula:

$$\text{Water deficit (L)} = 0.5 \text{ (lean body weight in kg) ([serum Na}/140] - 1)$$

This equation provides only an estimate of the water deficit; serial measurements of the serum sodium are mandatory to monitor the rate and extent of the correction of hypernatremia.

Hyperkalemia

Mild hyperkalemia occurs commonly in patients with renal failure because of reduced renal clearance of potassium in the diet. Hypoaldosteronism (eg, from ACE inhibitors, nonsteroidal antiinflammatory drugs [NSAIDs], or heparin); treatment with potassium-sparing diuretics; and volume depletion with the consequent reduction in delivery of sodium to the distal, potassium-secreting segments of the nephron can further reduce the renal excretion of potassium. Redistribution of potassium from cells to the extracellular space after tissue trauma (eg, rhabdomyolysis, hemolysis, hematomas) is another cause of hyperkalemia. A similar mechanism occurs with metabolic acidosis; insulin deficiency; hyperosmolality (eg, hyperglycemia, mannitol); drugs such as β-blockers and succinylcholine; and digitalis intoxication.

Trauma, bleeding, and blood transfusions are other factors that can worsen hyperkalemia in surgical patients. For these reasons, it is desirable to dialyze hemodialysis patients within 24 hours of the planned surgery so that excess potassium is removed. Potassium intake (oral and parenteral) must be restricted. Patients with hyperkalemia who are receiving peritoneal dialysis must restrict their potassium intake, and either the frequency of dialysis exchanges or the volume of the dialysate can be increased to enhance the removal of potassium.

In patients who have predialysis renal disease and asymptomatic mild hyperkalemia, potassium intake should be restricted, the use of medications contributing to the development of hyperkalemia should be discontinued, and, if possible, salt intake should be increased while diuretics are used. In addition, acidosis should be corrected and hyperglycemia should be treated with insulin. If these measures fail, cation-exchange resins can be used. A dose of Kayexalate, 15 to 60 g, is given orally or by retention enema and may be repeated as needed.

Therapy is dictated by the severity and physiologic consequences of hyperkalemia. Potassium levels above 7 to 8 mEq/L, severe muscle weakness, or marked electrocardiographic changes require immediate therapy. Treatment options include the administration of 10 mL of intravenous 10% calcium gluconate (with increased risks for metastatic calcification if the calcium × phosphorus product is high, and for the precipitation of digitalis toxicity in patients who

are taking digitalis preparations); sodium bicarbonate (45 mEq); insulin (1 U of regular insulin per 3 to 5 g of glucose) or glucose (50 mL of 50% solution [glucose should not be given if patients have marked hyperglycemia, and insulin may not be necessary in patients who do not have diabetes]); and β2-adrenergic agonists such as albuterol. Concomitantly, excess potassium must be removed from the body by diuretics, cation-exchange resins, or dialysis. Cation-exchange resins can be given by retention enemas if oral therapy is not possible (eg, because of nasogastric suction or ileus). Hemodialysis is more effective than peritoneal dialysis in the treatment of severe hyperkalemia.

Pseudohyperkalemia may be caused by hemolysis during or after the blood sample is drawn, severe leukocytosis or thrombocytosis, or repeated clenching of the fist after the tourniquet has been applied. Careful venipuncture and assessment of plasma potassium levels (instead of serum potassium levels) may be necessary to exclude pseudohyperkalemia.

Hypokalemia

Hypokalemia in patients with renal failure usually results from insufficient intake of potassium with continued excretion of potassium (eg, through dialysis, diuretics, or diarrhea). Redistribution of potassium from the extracellular fluid into cells occurs with alkalemia, hypothermia, insulin therapy, β2-adrenergic activity, and carbohydrate intake, and these factors can cause or aggravate hypokalemia. In patients with hypokalemia who are taking digitalis, or who have electrocardiographic changes or cardiac arrhythmias, it may be necessary to administer potassium. This can be dangerous in patients with renal failure. If potassium is given, the serum potassium level must be monitored carefully to prevent life-threatening hyperkalemia. In patients receiving dialysis, the potassium level in the dialysate should be increased to reduce dialysis-associated potassium losses and to help replenish body potassium stores.

Metabolic Acidosis

Patients with renal failure usually have mild metabolic acidosis because of the accumulation of nonvolatile acids resulting from the metabolism of food (about 1 mEq/kg/d). In most cases, the acidosis can easily be corrected by oral base supplementation (eg, sodium bicarbonate) or by dialysis. If stable patients with renal failure develop progressive acidosis, other causes should be vigorously investigated. These include lactic acidosis, ketoacidosis, intoxications (eg, ethylene glycol), and severe diarrhea.

The initial goal in severe metabolic acidosis (blood pH less than 7.2) is to rapidly (over several hours) give enough intravenous sodium bicarbonate to increase the blood pH to 7.2, a level at which abnormalities in cardiovascular function become less likely.[13] Rapid intravenous administration of bicarbonate can lead to fluid overload, however, worsening tissue oxygenation, hypokalemia, and cerebrospinal fluid acidosis (because the blood–brain barrier is more permeable to CO_2 than to bicarbonate).[15] To minimize these complications, intravenous bicarbonate therapy either should be halted or should proceed at a much slower pace once the blood pH has reached 7.2. Treating the underlying cause of metabolic acidosis is critical, especially with lactic acidosis and diabetic ketoacidosis. Administering sodium bicarbonate to patients with lactic acidosis is controversial[16,17]; in addition, accumulated lactate and keto-anions are metabolized to bicarbonate with successful therapy. In these two situations (ie, lactic acidosis and diabetic ketoacidosis), bicarbonate is usually not given unless the blood pH is less than 7.10 to 7.15. Bicarbonate therapy may be useful in diabetic ketoacidosis when the anion gap is relatively normal, however, because of the excretion of keto-anions in the urine.[17,18] Other complications of treatment with sodium bicarbonate include hypernatremia (if hypertonic bicarbonate solutions are used), hyponatremia (if hypotonic solutions are used), and metabolic alkalosis (if excessive bicarbonate is given).

The amount of sodium bicarbonate required to raise the serum bicarbonate to a desired level can be estimated from the formula:

$$HCO_3 \text{ deficit (mEq)} =$$
$$(HCO_3 \text{ space}) (\text{desired serum } HCO_3 - \text{serum } HCO_3)$$

The bicarbonate space can be variable, from 0.5 times lean body weight (in kilograms) in patients with mild metabolic acidosis to more than 0.7 times lean body weight in those with severe metabolic acidosis. In addition, it should be emphasized that this equation provides an estimate of the bicarbonate deficit; serial measurement of the blood pH and serum bicarbonate is mandatory to monitor the rate and extent of the correction of metabolic acidosis.

Metabolic Alkalosis

Metabolic alkalosis in patients with renal failure is usually caused by acid losses from vomiting, nasogastric suction, or diuretic use (in those with predialysis disease). The administration of excessive alkali (eg, sodium bicarbonate, citrate-anticoagulated blood transfusion) also results in metabolic alkalosis because the excretion of bicarbonate is markedly reduced in patients with renal failure. Treatment must be directed at the underlying cause. The administration of H_2 blockers may be useful when gastric acid loss causes alkalosis.[19] If patients are volume-contracted or hypokalemic, then careful volume expansion with isotonic saline or supplementation with potassium chloride is indicated. Hemodialysis or hydrochloric acid administration can be used to treat symptomatic or severe alkalosis.[20,21] When metabolic

alkalosis is treated with dialysis, it is necessary to reduce the concentration of base in the dialysate.[20] Alternatively, bicarbonate can be removed by isolated ultrafiltration (ie, fluid removal alone without dialysis) and replacement of the fluid that is removed with intravenous normal saline. If hydrochloric acid is used, it must be administered as an isotonic solution, slowly (over 12 to 24 hours) and through a central venous catheter.[21]

The amount of hydrochloric acid required to normalize the serum bicarbonate is equal to the bicarbonate excess, which can be estimated by the equation:

$$HCO_3 \text{ excess (mEq)} =$$
$$0.5 (\text{lean body weight in kg}) (\text{serum } HCO_3 - 24)$$

This equation provides an estimate of the bicarbonate excess; serial measurement of the blood pH and serum bicarbonate is mandatory to monitor the rate and extent of the correction of metabolic alkalosis.

Respiratory Acid–Base Disturbances

Patients who are receiving dialysis do not develop the usual metabolic compensations for either respiratory acidosis or alkalosis because there is little or no renal bicarbonate transport. Instead, the serum bicarbonate level is determined by the base concentration in the dialysate, the intensity of dialysis, and the rate of generation of nonvolatile acids.

ANEMIA

The major cause of chronic anemia in patients with renal failure is erythropoietin deficiency.[22,23] Even with recombinant erythropoietin administration, there can be resistance to the drug from "uremic toxins"; blood loss (eg, during hemodialysis or through the gastrointestinal tract as a result of ulcers, gastritis, or angiodysplasias); nutritional deficiencies (eg, iron deficiency); aluminum toxicity; hyperparathyroidism with marrow fibrosis; hemolysis; or inflammation.[23]

In the past, hematocrit levels of 15% to 25% were usual in patients undergoing dialysis, and many required repeated blood transfusions to treat symptoms of severe anemia. Recombinant erythropoietin therapy has revolutionized the treatment of anemia in renal failure and patients with ESRD commonly maintain hematocrits above 30%. The major cause of erythropoietin resistance is iron deficiency but this can be effectively treated with oral or parenteral iron. Folate is routinely administered to patients who are undergoing dialysis.

Blood transfusions should not be given solely to treat low hematocrit levels in patients with renal failure because the associated risks (eg, transfusion reactions, volume overload, hyperkalemia, hepatitis C infection, iron overload, transplant sensitization) may outweigh the potential benefits.[22,23] Fortunately, these patients often tolerate chronic anemia well. Blood transfusions should be given only if absolutely necessary, preferably during dialysis in patients who are undergoing hemodialysis and slowly in patients who are undergoing peritoneal dialysis and those with predialysis renal disease. To prevent fluid overload, higher concentrations of dextrose can be used during peritoneal dialysis and diuretics can be given during the predialysis phase. The serum potassium level must be monitored closely in patients with renal failure who are given blood transfusions.

UREMIC PLATELET DYSFUNCTION

The responses of platelets exposed to damaged endothelium are often abnormal in patients with severe renal failure. These abnormalities have been attributed to "uremic toxins," to anemia, and to abnormalities in both factor VIII/von Willebrand's factor complex activity and prostaglandin metabolism.[24-28] Evidence of abnormal platelet function is a prolonged bleeding time despite a normal platelet count. Treatment strategies that have been successful in reducing the abnormal bleeding time include vigorous dialysis, raising the hematocrit to more than 30%, administering deamino D-arginine vasopressin, 0.3 μg/kg intravenously, to release endothelial factor VIII/von Willebrand's factor complexes,[27] administering cryoprecipitate, 10 U, to increase circulating factor VIII/von Willebrand's factor complex activity,[28] and administering conjugated estrogens, 0.6 mg/kg/d intravenously for 5 days.[29] Conjugated estrogens should be given at least a week before surgery because the onset of the effect is delayed.

EFFECT OF HEPARIN DURING HEMODIALYSIS

Heparin is typically used during hemodialysis to prevent thrombosis of the extracorporeal dialysis circuit. The half-life of heparin is not changed in ESRD; it is about 1 hour but may vary considerably. Generally, we do not use heparin immediately before surgery. If hemodialysis is required just before surgery, heparin-free techniques, protamine reversal of heparinization, or citrate anticoagulation can be used with close follow-up of coagulation parameters as indicated.

PERIOPERATIVE CARE

Patients who are receiving hemodialysis should undergo dialysis within 24 hours of the planned surgery, and their fluid, potassium, and sodium intake should be restricted. Patients who are receiving peritoneal dialysis can be dia-

lyzed until the time of surgery, when the dialysate fluid is drained from the peritoneal cavity.

During surgery, care must be taken to avoid placing pressure on the arteriovenous dialysis fistula. Adherence to this simple rule prevents many incidents of thrombosis of dialysis fistulas. The consequences of fistula thrombosis (thrombectomy of the clotted arteriovenous access, placement of temporary dialysis catheters) increase morbidity and cost. The extremity containing the fistula must not be used for blood pressure measurements, intravenous fluid lines, or blood drawing.

Patients receiving peritoneal dialysis who are undergoing abdominal surgery may have their catheters left in place if they do not interfere with the surgical incision, if sterility of the peritoneal cavity can be maintained, and if peritoneal dialysis will be continued after surgery.[30] In general, these patients are treated by hemodialysis for a variable period after surgery to allow the peritoneal and abdominal wall incisions to heal.

A critical part of the perioperative care of patients with renal failure is minimizing the use of intravenous fluids. Intravenous fluids should be used judiciously to correct hypotension caused by volume depletion but their routine administration leads to fluid overload and pulmonary edema. In critically ill patients, a pulmonary arterial catheter can provide invaluable assistance in guiding fluid management. If fluids are needed, isotonic, potassium-free fluids such as normal saline should be used with close monitoring and, if necessary, measurement of the pulmonary capillary wedge pressure. Hypotonic fluids (eg, D_5W, D_5 half-normal saline) lead to hyponatremia, and potassium administration (eg, potassium chloride, lactated Ringer's solution) usually causes hyperkalemia. Blood transfusions between dialysis sessions often result in both fluid overload and hyperkalemia. Consequently, blood transfusions should not be given unless the anemia is severe enough to result in adverse complications and are preferably given during dialysis sessions in patients who are receiving hemodialysis. The precautions that must be observed when blood transfusions are given were discussed earlier.

MUSCLE RELAXANTS AND ANESTHETIC DRUGS

The half-life of certain neuromuscular agents, such as atracurium and vecuronium, is not increased in patients with renal failure. The half-life of other neuromuscular agents, such as alcuronium, pancuronium, metocurine, tubocurarine, and gallamine, is prolonged, however, and these drugs should not be used. Renal failure also changes the effects of other drugs. For example, the dosage of the depolarizing agent succinylcholine is not altered in patients with renal failure but it can cause hyperkalemia by redistributing potassium from the intracellular fluid to the extracellular fluid. The pharmacology of fentanyl, ketamine, halothane, and nitrous oxide is not altered by renal failure. Finally, anesthesia with methoxyflurane and enflurane has been associated with acute renal failure, and these agents should not be used in such patients.

POSTOPERATIVE CARE

In the immediate postoperative period, heparin should not be used during hemodialysis to decrease the risk of bleeding; otherwise, patients who have stable blood pressure and cardiovascular status can be dialyzed just after surgery. Likewise, peritoneal dialysis may be restarted immediately if patients have not undergone abdominal surgery. Patients receiving peritoneal dialysis who have undergone abdominal surgery are supported by hemodialysis using temporary vascular access until the peritoneal and abdominal wall incisions have healed.

Intravenous fluids, especially those that contain potassium, must be restricted to prevent volume overload and electrolyte imbalances. Sodium and potassium in the diet are usually restricted unless patients are sodium-depleted (ie, hypovolemic) or hypokalemic. The intake of phosphates is also restricted unless hypophosphatemia is present (see later). Besides waste products, dialysis removes water-soluble vitamins and amino acids, and with peritoneal dialysis there are significant losses of protein. To prevent deficiencies, water-soluble vitamins are routinely prescribed and a high-protein diet (more than 1 g/kg/d) is recommended for patients who are receiving dialysis. In contrast, protein intake should be restricted (to 0.6 to 0.8 g/kg of protein with high biologic value) in patients with renal failure who are not dialyzed to prevent excessive accumulation of nitrogen and high blood urea nitrogen (BUN) levels.

An increase in the BUN level in patients with renal failure may indicate excessive protein intake; reduced renal perfusion or function (in the predialysis phase of disease); excessive catabolism of body proteins (eg, steroids, tetracyclines, gastrointestinal bleeding); or inadequate dialysis. A reduced BUN level may be a sign of protein malnutrition rather than improved renal function.

During the predialysis phase of disease, an increase in the serum creatinine level may indicate reduced glomerular filtration or drug-induced inhibition of tubular creatinine secretion (eg, trimethoprim, cimetidine). Other factors that can increase the serum creatinine level include cooked meat intake and drugs or products that interfere with the assay of creatinine (eg, flucytosine, cefoxitin, acetoacetic acid). Reduced serum creatinine levels in patients with renal failure may signal the loss of muscle mass rather than improved renal function. Values of serum electrolytes (eg, sodium, potassium, bicarbonate, calcium) and some other com-

pounds (eg, BUN) should be interpreted in relation to the time of the last dialysis session. For example, the serum potassium levels of stable patients who are receiving hemodialysis may be between 2 and 3 mEq/L after dialysis against a low potassium dialysate. Subsequently, they increase rapidly and could exceed 5 mEq/L 2 days later. The low initial value should not be treated with supplemental potassium because life-threatening hyperkalemia may develop. Rarely, supplemental potassium is needed for a serious complication such as a cardiac arrhythmia with hypotension.

In addition, several rules should be followed:

1. Change the dosage of all medications in relation to the degree of renal dysfunction (see later discussion).
2. Do not use nephrotoxic drugs in patients with residual renal function (eg, aminoglycosides, radiographic contrast media, NSAIDs [including ketorolac]).
3. Do not use drugs that are converted to toxic metabolites that accumulate in patients with renal failure (eg, meperidine, propoxyphene).
4. Do not use medications that contain magnesium (eg, magnesium citrate, magnesium-based antacids, milk of magnesia), phosphate (eg, phosphate-containing laxatives or enemas), or potassium (eg, potassium salts of penicillin).

TREATMENT OF OTHER COMPLICATIONS

RENAL OSTEODYSTROPHY

Virtually all patients with ESRD have secondary hyperparathyroidism, which is caused by calcitriol deficiency and hypocalcemia. Phosphate retention, recognized clinically as an increased serum inorganic phosphorus level, plays a central role in the pathogenesis of secondary hyperparathyroidism. Phosphate intake directly suppresses the conversion of 25-hydroxyvitamin D to 1,25-dihydroxyvitamin D (calcitriol) in proximal renal tubule cells.[31] This effect, combined with the reduced functional nephron mass in renal failure, leads to reduced calcitriol formation. Both calcitriol deficiency (reduced calcium absorption from the intestine, skeletal resistance to parathyroid hormone) and hyperphosphatemia itself (precipitation of ionized calcium) contribute to the development of hypocalcemia, which directly stimulates the secretion of parathyroid hormone. Perhaps more important, the regulation of parathyroid hormone secretion by ionized calcium is altered in the presence of calcitriol deficiency so that parathyroid hormone secretion is greater for any given level of ionized calcium.[32,33] Thus, severe renal failure is almost invariably associated with hyperparathyroidism, and phosphate retention plays a major role in its pathogenesis.

Because the excretion of phosphate is markedly decreased in renal failure, dietary phosphates must be restricted (less than 800 mg/d) to reduce serum phosphorus levels. Phosphate binders, given with meals, are widely used to further reduce intestinal absorption of phosphates. Calcium-containing binders (eg, calcium carbonate) are preferable to aluminum-based binders because of the risk of aluminum-induced osteomalacia, anemia, and encephalopathy. The most serious side effect of calcium-based binders is hypercalcemia, and when the calcium times phosphorus product exceeds 60 mg^2/dL^2, there is an enhanced risk of metastatic calcification. As a result, it may be preferable to temporarily use aluminum-based binders when either severe hyperphosphatemia or a high calcium times phosphorus product is present. After the serum phosphorus level is reduced through the ingestion of a low-phosphate diet and the administration of phosphate binders, calcitriol is given if secondary hyperparathyroidism or hypocalcemia persists. Parathyroidectomy is used to treat hyperparathyroidism that is resistant to medical therapy.

Osteomalacia is the second major type of bone disease observed in patients with renal failure. Aluminum accumulation in the bone is believed to play a major role in its pathogenesis.[34,35] Although both a high level of circulating aluminum[36] and a significant increase in the circulating aluminum level after the administration of the chelator, deferoxamine,[37] indicate the presence of aluminum intoxication, the definitive diagnosis of aluminum-induced osteomalacia is made only by bone biopsy. Treatment strategies include avoidance of aluminum and chelation of aluminum with deferoxamine.

ABNORMALITIES IN SERUM INORGANIC PHOSPHORUS LEVELS

Hyperphosphatemia

Hyperphosphatemia is common in patients with renal failure and is caused by increased phosphate intake in the presence of reduced renal phosphorus excretion. Other causes include increased intestinal phosphate absorption with vitamin D treatment; tissue breakdown (rhabdomyolysis, tumor lysis); and medications (phosphate-containing laxatives and enemas). Hyperphosphatemia plays a significant role in the development of secondary hyperparathyroidism and hypocalcemia in patients with renal failure (see earlier discussion). The cornerstone of therapy for hyperphosphatemia in patients with renal failure is restricting dietary phosphate intake (less than 800 mg/d) and avoiding the use of phosphate-based laxatives and enemas. Generally, phosphate binders are used with meals to further decrease intestinal phosphate absorption (see earlier discussion).

Hypophosphatemia

Hypophosphatemia is unusual and occurs because of malnutrition, excessive use of oral phosphate binders, infusion of hyperalimentation fluids without phosphate, or intensive dialysis. Insulin treatment, respiratory alkalosis, and glucose can aggravate or cause hypophosphatemia by driving phosphate into cells. After parathyroidectomy, phosphate deposition in bone ("hungry bone syndrome") can cause hypophosphatemia.

Prolonged, severe hypophosphatemia can lead to cardiomyopathy, respiratory arrest, hemolysis, rhabdomyolysis, and osteomalacia. The use of oral phosphate binders should be discontinued if mild hypophosphatemia is present, and phosphate supplements (oral or parenteral) should be given for severe hypophosphatemia. The easiest method is to add milk to the diet. Serum phosphorus levels must be closely monitored because severe hyperphosphatemia, leading to hypocalcemia and metastatic calcification, can occur when excessive phosphates are given.

ABNORMALITIES IN SERUM CALCIUM LEVELS

Hypercalcemia

Hypercalcemia is less common than hypocalcemia in patients with renal failure. The use of calcium-based phosphate binders plus calcitriol to treat secondary hyperparathyroidism often causes hypercalcemia; therefore, serum calcium levels must be monitored closely in these patients. Although the secondary hyperparathyroidism of renal failure is usually associated with hypocalcemia, hypercalcemia can develop with severe secondary hyperparathyroidism. Aluminum-induced osteomalacia appears to predispose patients to the development of hypercalcemia. More unusual causes include immobilization, malignant tumors, sarcoidosis, and vitamin A intoxication.

Emergency treatment of severe hypercalcemia in patients with predialysis disease who have renal failure begins with saline volume expansion to induce a saline diuresis; the natriuresis is sustained by furosemide. Other therapies include glucocorticoids and calcitonin. Hemodialysis with a low-calcium dialysate should be used if conservative treatment does not succeed in these patients. Low-calcium hemodialysis is also the treatment of choice for severe hypercalcemia in patients who are receiving dialysis. Newer drugs include plicamycin and etidronate, which act by inhibiting bone resorption. The use of these drugs in patients with renal failure is uncertain, however, because plicamycin can aggravate renal failure and renal excretion provides the major route of elimination of etidronate.

Hypocalcemia

Hypocalcemia is common in patients with renal failure; both low levels of calcitriol and hyperphosphatemia play critical roles in its development (see earlier). Other causes include parathyroidectomy (hungry bone syndrome); pancreatitis; anticonvulsant medications (eg, phenytoin, phenobarbital); and malabsorption. If hyperphosphatemia is also present, mild hypocalcemia is initially treated by correcting the serum phosphorus level by restricting phosphate intake and using phosphate binders with meals (see earlier). Calcitriol is given if hypocalcemia persists after the serum phosphorus level is reduced. Calcium supplementation between meals may also be necessary. Intravenous calcium can be used to treat severe, symptomatic hypocalcemia but may cause metastatic calcification if the calcium × phosphorus product is high.

ABNORMALITIES IN SERUM MAGNESIUM LEVELS

Hypermagnesemia

Hypermagnesemia in patients with renal failure occurs most commonly because of the administration of magnesium-containing agents such as milk of magnesia, magnesium citrate, and magnesium-based antacids. It is treated by discontinuing the use of these drugs. Severe, symptomatic hypermagnesemia can be treated by intravenous calcium (with the risk of metastatic calcification), insulin and glucose, or dialysis.

Hypomagnesemia

Hypomagnesemia is rare in patients with renal failure and usually results from severe malnutrition, prolonged therapy with magnesium-free hyperalimentation fluids, diarrhea, or diuretics (in patients who have predialysis disease). Severe hypomagnesemia has been associated with tetany, cardiac arrhythmias, and hypocalcemia. The serum magnesium level should be monitored closely if magnesium supplements are given, to prevent severe hypermagnesemia.

HEMORRHAGE

The bleeding time should be determined in patients with renal failure who experience hemorrhage. Performing dialysis, raising the hematocrit to over 30%, and administering deamino D-arginine vasopressin, cryoprecipitate, or estrogens have been useful in treating the functional platelet abnormality of renal failure (see earlier). The risks of blood transfusion and the precautions that must be observed when blood transfusions are given already have been discussed.

INFECTION

Patients with renal failure exhibit impaired immunologic and inflammatory responses; for example, macrophage Fc receptor function and neutrophil chemotaxis are abnormal.[38,39] Therefore, these patients are predisposed to the development of infection. Common sources of infection are repeated puncture of dialysis fistulas leading to bacteremia and fistula infections; infections from the peritoneal dialysis catheter leading to peritonitis; subcutaneous "tunnel" infections and exit site infections; and urinary tract infections (even in anuric patients receiving dialysis), which can result in pyelonephritis or pyocystitis. The search for the origin of an infection should include blood cultures, urine culture, careful evaluation of the dialysis fistula, and peritoneal dialysate fluid cell counts and cultures plus evaluation of the exit site and subcutaneous tunnel of the peritoneal dialysis catheter. Bladder catheterization and lavage may be necessary in symptomatic patients with anuria to document the presence of bladder infections.

The incidence of bacterial endocarditis may be as high as 3% to 5% in patients receiving hemodialysis, possibly because of the high incidence of bacteremia combined with the high prevalence of calcific valvular heart disease.[40–43] The latter may be related to secondary hyperparathyroidism. A high index of suspicion, repeated blood cultures and physical examinations, and echocardiographic assessment are necessary to diagnose infective endocarditis.

Antibiotic dosages must be adjusted for the degree of renal failure, and nephrotoxic antibiotics should not be used in patients with significant residual renal function (see later discussion).

UREMIC PERICARDITIS

Since dialysis has become widely available, the incidence of symptomatic uremic pericarditis has decreased. Pericarditis does occur in dialyzed patients, however, possibly related to the inadequate removal of uremic toxins. Other causes include coincident diseases such as viral infections, tuberculosis, or systemic lupus erythematosus, and drugs such as minoxidil. When other causes have been excluded, the mainstay of therapy for dialysis-associated pericarditis is intensified dialysis (eg, daily hemodialysis). It is important to limit the use of heparin during dialysis to prevent pericardial hemorrhage.

Most patients with pericarditis have pericardial effusions, which can cause cardiac tamponade. An important clue to the presence of tamponade is the development of hypotension during dialysis, especially when patients are above their dry weights. About 15% to 20% of stable asymptomatic patients who are undergoing dialysis have small pericardial effusions.[44] It is unclear whether intensification of dialysis is beneficial in these patients but frequent evaluation of the size and hemodynamic significance is prudent. The treatment of large pericardial effusions with intensified dialysis may result in improvement but pericardiotomy or pericardiectomy is indicated if hemodynamic compromise occurs, or if the effusion shows no improvement with conservative therapy.

UREMIC ENCEPHALOPATHY

Symptoms and signs of uremic encephalopathy are nonspecific and include impaired mentation, asterixis, hyperreflexia, and an abnormal electroencephalogram. These findings should be reversible with dialysis. The differential diagnosis should include other causes of neurologic disease such as strokes, seizures, subdural hemorrhage, central nervous system infections, drug intoxications, and electrolyte disturbances. Intensive initiation of dialysis in patients with severe uremia may lead to cerebral edema and the "dysequilibrium syndrome," with confusion, headache, and seizures. Finally, aluminum deposition in the brain may result in dialysis dementia, a disorder that is characterized by progressive speech disturbances, impaired memory, seizures, and global dementia, and eventually leads to death.[45]

ACUTE RENAL FAILURE IN PATIENTS WITH CHRONIC RENAL FAILURE

Acute renal failure is defined as a rapid decrease in the glomerular filtration rate and it usually is recognized by a rising serum creatinine level. Factors that can increase the serum creatinine level in the absence of renal failure already have been discussed.

The causes of acute renal failure can be conveniently divided into prerenal causes, intrinsic renal causes, and postrenal causes. Prerenal acute renal failure occurs when there is reduced renal perfusion from intravascular volume depletion (eg, hemorrhage, diarrhea, excessive diuresis, burns, "third-spacing" with diseases such as intestinal obstruction); hypotension; heart failure; liver failure; or drugs such as NSAIDs or ACE inhibitors. Many intrinsic renal diseases can cause acute renal failure. For example, acute tubular necrosis can result from severe prerenal disease or from nephrotoxins such as aminoglycosides, radiocontrast media, cisplatin, or heme pigments (eg, myoglobin). In contrast, drugs such as the penicillins, cephalosporins, and NSAIDs can cause acute interstitial nephritis, and consequently acute renal failure. Another cause is precipitation of

poorly soluble compounds such as uric acid (eg, with tumor lysis), acyclovir, or methotrexate within the nephron lumen. Renal vascular disease can result in either ischemia or infarction of renal parenchyma. Finally, postrenal acute renal failure occurs with urinary tract obstruction.

The BUN and serum creatinine levels, urinary indices, and a careful urinalysis including microscopic examination are helpful in distinguishing prerenal disease from acute tubular necrosis. In typical prerenal disease, the ratio of BUN to serum creatinine is high (greater than 20:1), the urinary sodium concentration is low (less than 20 mEq/L), the fractional excretion of sodium is low (less than 1%), the urine osmolality is high (greater than 500 mOsm/kg), and the urinalysis is normal. In contrast, tubular damage in acute tubular necrosis results in a normal ratio of BUN to serum creatinine (10:1 to 15:1), a high urinary sodium concentration (greater than 40 mEq/L), a high fractional excretion of sodium (greater than 2%), a low urine osmolality (less than 350 mOsm/kg), and an abnormal urinalysis containing many "muddy brown" granular casts and renal tubular epithelial cells and casts. The urinalysis in acute interstitial nephritis is different and typically contains many white blood cells (especially eosinophils) with or without white blood cell casts. Renal ultrasonography is critical in evaluating for urinary tract obstruction.

Treatment depends on the cause of acute renal failure. For example, urinary tract obstruction should be relieved, volume depletion should be treated with volume expansion, and the use of nephrotoxic agents (eg, gentamicin) should be discontinued. Conservative treatment of acute renal failure includes maintaining a normal ECV, preventing and treating serum electrolyte disorders (see earlier), avoiding the use of all nephrotoxic agents, changing medication dosages based on the loss of renal function, and restricting protein intake (0.6 to 0.8 g/kg/d of protein with high biologic value) to reduce the rate at which the BUN increases. The indications for dialysis are discussed later.

INDICATIONS FOR DIALYSIS OR DIALYTIC TECHNIQUES

Absolute indications for dialysis are severe ECV expansion or pulmonary edema (unresponsive to diuretics in patients with predialysis disease), severe hyperkalemia (unresponsive to conservative therapy), severe metabolic acidemia (when bicarbonate cannot be given because of fluid overload), and uremic complications (eg, pericarditis, encephalopathy). Other indications include intoxications (eg, ethylene glycol), severe hypercalcemia, and severe hyperuricemia (eg, tumor lysis) when conservative therapy has failed or is not expected to succeed.

Hemodialysis is the treatment of choice when efficient clearance is required (eg, in patients with hypercatabolism or severe hyperkalemia). Peritoneal dialysis is often more appropriate in patients with unstable hemodynamics (eg, after myocardial infarction) because the removal of fluid and waste products is more gradual. Continuous arteriovenous hemofiltration, with or without dialysis, is used in hemodynamically unstable patients for whom volume removal is the major goal.

DRUG THERAPY

Renal failure affects the pharmacology of many drugs. Bioavailability may be reduced by the use of phosphate-binding antacids, by uremic vomiting, and by decreased small bowel absorptive capacity in patients with uremia.[46,47] In addition, the volume of distribution may be increased because of altered protein binding and the presence of significant edema. Reduced protein binding also increases the amount of drug that is available for action and degradation. Finally, decreased glomerular filtration and renal tubular secretion of drugs reduces the elimination of many drugs or their active metabolites. In this respect, "normal" serum creatinine levels in elderly patients or those with reduced muscle mass may not reveal substantial reductions in renal function.

Drugs that are nephrotoxic must be used with extreme caution and only if absolutely indicated because even small reductions in glomerular filtration in patients with severe renal failure (eg, a 5-mL/min decrement in glomerular filtration from 10 to 5 mL/min) can result in overt uremia.

A comprehensive discussion of the use of drugs in patients with renal failure is beyond the scope of this chapter. General principles regarding the use of some of the more common drugs in these patients are presented later. The use of muscle relaxants and anesthetics has already been discussed.

ANTIBIOTICS

Vancomycin

The half-life of vancomycin is prolonged in patients with renal failure and drug accumulation can result in ototoxicity. In patients undergoing dialysis, the half-life of vancomycin is about 200 hours, and the drug may only need to be given every 5 to 7 days.[48] Blood levels must be monitored closely.

Aminoglycosides

The aminoglycoside antibiotics have a narrow therapeutic range and are excreted almost exclusively by glomerular filtration. Drug accumulation can cause nephrotoxicity and ototoxicity. In patients with significant residual renal function, the use of other antibiotics should be strongly consid-

ered. The initial loading dose is the same as in patients with normal renal function but subsequent doses must be adjusted for the degree of renal failure. For example, in patients with renal function of 50 mL/min, either the dose should be reduced by 50% or the interval between doses should be doubled. Monitoring of renal function and blood levels of the aminoglycoside (especially in patients with predialysis renal disease) is mandatory when these drugs are used.

Cephalosporins

The dosages of most cephalosporins must be adjusted for the degree of renal failure. Cefoperazone and ceftriaxone may be used without dosage modifications, however. Cephalosporins can cause acute interstitial nephritis and acute renal failure. Cefoxitin may falsely increase the serum creatinine level by interfering with the assay.

Penicillins

The dosages of most penicillins must be adjusted in patients with renal failure; nafcillin, oxacillin, dicloxacillin, and cloxacillin may be used without dosage modifications. Penicillins can cause acute interstitial nephritis as well as serum sickness, and both these disease processes can cause acute renal failure. The accumulation of penicillins can result in seizures, especially when high dosages are used.

Miscellaneous Antibiotics

Tetracyclines are antianabolic, can raise the BUN and serum inorganic phosphorus levels, and may potentiate acidosis. The dosages of ciprofloxacin, aztreonam, erythromycin, imipenem, co-trimoxazole, sulfonamides, fluconazole, flucytosine, isoniazid, ethambutol, pentamidine, acyclovir, ganciclovir, and zidovudine need to be adjusted in patients with renal failure. Chloramphenicol, clindamycin, ketoconazole, and rifampin may be used without dosage modifications. Amphotericin is nephrotoxic, and can cause hypokalemia and renal tubular acidosis.

CARDIOVASCULAR DRUGS, ANTIHYPERTENSIVE AGENTS, AND DIURETICS

Digoxin

The loading dose of digoxin should be reduced by 50% in patients with ESRD because the volume of distribution is decreased. Maintenance dosages should also be reduced because the primary route of elimination is by renal excretion. In the absence of a loading dose, the time required to reach a steady state is markedly prolonged (eg, 2 to 3 weeks) because of the drug's extended half-life in patients with renal failure. Blood levels should be monitored when digitalis is used in these patients. Concomitant administration of quinidine and verapamil can result in digoxin toxicity. In patients who are receiving hemodialysis, consideration should be given to using 3 mEq/L of potassium in the dialysate instead of the more usual 2 mEq/L to prevent serious arrhythmias during dialysis. This practice requires rigid restriction of potassium intake between dialysis sessions to prevent the development of life-threatening hyperkalemia.

Procainamide

The half-life of procainamide and its active metabolite *N*-acetylprocainamide are prolonged in patients with renal failure, so maintenance dosages must be adjusted to prevent toxicity. Close monitoring of the levels of both procainamide and its metabolite is mandatory.

Nitroprusside

In the presence of renal failure, thiocyanate accumulates when nitroprusside is administered, and this can result in neurologic toxicity. Nitroprusside use should be restricted in patients with renal failure, and thiocyanate levels should be monitored.

Angiotensin-Converting Enzyme Inhibitors

The half-life of most ACE inhibitors is prolonged in patients with renal failure, so dosage reduction is necessary. In patients with predialysis disease, ACE inhibitors can cause both hyperkalemia, by reducing the secretion of aldosterone, and acute renal failure. ACE inhibitor–induced renal failure occurs when renal blood flow is reduced and glomerular filtration becomes dependent on angiotensin II (eg, severe volume depletion, severe bilateral renal artery stenosis). Captopril can cause bone marrow suppression, especially in patients with renal failure who have collagen vascular diseases. In addition, proteinuria can occur when captopril is administered either in high dosages or in the presence of renal disease.

Diuretics

Acetazolamide is an ineffective diuretic in patients with severe renal failure and may potentiate acidosis. Amiloride and other potassium-sparing diuretics can cause hyperkalemia in patients with renal failure and should not be used. In general, thiazide-type diuretics are ineffective in severe renal failure, although metolazone is effective in high dosages. Loop diuretics, such as furosemide, bumetanide, and ethacrynic acid, are effective in high dosages, even with severe renal failure, but can cause ototoxicity (see earlier). Mannitol administration to patients with renal failure may cause hyperosmolality, which can result in volume overload, hyponatremia, and hyperkalemia. In contrast, mannitol administration to patients with adequate renal function can result in osmotic diuresis, leading to hypernatremia and volume depletion.

Miscellaneous Cardiovascular Drugs

β-Blockers can cause hyperkalemia in patients with renal failure by reducing the cellular uptake of potassium. In general, calcium channel blockers do not need dosage adjustments in patients with renal failure. Dosages of bretylium, disopyramide, flecainide, and encainide must be reduced, whereas lidocaine can be used without adjustment.

PSYCHOACTIVE DRUGS

Psychiatric Drugs

Dosages of tricyclic antidepressants, phenothiazine agents, and haloperidol are unchanged in patients with renal failure. Tricyclics and phenothiazines can cause urinary retention and obstructive nephropathy, however.

The half-life of lithium is inconsistent and markedly prolonged in patients with renal failure. Moreover, lithium may cause renal interstitial fibrosis, nephrogenic diabetes insipidus, and renal tubular acidosis.

Sedatives

The benzodiazepines and barbiturates may cause excessive sedation and encephalopathy in patients with ESRD. In addition, barbiturates may exacerbate hypocalcemia and osteomalacia in these patients by interfering with the metabolism of vitamin D. The half-life of phenobarbital is prolonged in patients with renal failure and dosage modification is necessary. Chloral hydrate and ethchlorvynol should not be used because accumulation of these drug or their active metabolites may occur in patients with renal failure.

ANALGESICS

Narcotic Analgesics

Narcotic analgesics can cause profound sedation in patients with renal failure. In general, dosages of narcotic analgesics are reduced in these patients. Meperidine should not be used because normeperidine, one of its metabolites, accumulates in patients with renal failure and can reduce the seizure threshold. Propoxyphene should not be used in patients with ESRD because the metabolite, norpropoxyphene, accumulates.

Nonnarcotic Analgesics

Because of the qualitative platelet defect in patients with renal failure (see earlier), the use of aspirin and other NSAIDs should be limited. In patients with predialysis disease, NSAIDs have many undesired side effects. They can cause acute renal failure by reducing glomerular perfusion or causing acute interstitial nephritis, and can produce the nephrotic syndrome, hyperkalemia, and sodium retention.

MISCELLANEOUS DRUGS

Phenytoin

Because the binding of phenytoin to plasma proteins is abnormal in patients with renal failure, the concentration of unbound phenytoin is higher for any given total (bound plus unbound) phenytoin level. Hence, attempts to maintain the total phenytoin level in the "therapeutic" range may result in toxicity. Measurement of free phenytoin (Dilantin) levels may be useful. Generally, a standard dosage of 300 mg/d is used because this usually provides an adequate free drug level. Phenytoin can cause acute interstitial nephritis, and can aggravate hypocalcemia and osteomalacia by interfering with the metabolism of vitamin D.

H₂ Receptor Antagonists

H_2 receptor antagonists such as cimetidine, ranitidine, and famotidine should be administered in reduced dosages to patients with renal failure because the half-life of these drugs is prolonged.

Allopurinol

The half-life of allopurinol is prolonged in patients with renal failure. Moreover, the active metabolite, oxypurinol, accumulates in these patients and may cause exfoliative dermatitis and acute interstitial nephritis. Therefore, dosages must be reduced. In patients taking azathioprine (eg, renal transplant recipients), allopurinol can precipitate severe bone marrow toxicity because of its inhibition of the degradative pathway of azathioprine.

Antidiabetic Drugs

The hypoglycemic effects of certain antidiabetic agents, such as acetohexamide and chlorpropamide, are markedly prolonged in patients with renal failure and should not be used. The renal metabolism of insulin decreases with renal failure and, consequently, the dosage of insulin may need to be reduced.

Other Drugs

The half-life of clofibrate is prolonged in patients with renal failure and administration of the drug may result in myopathy. The dosage of metoclopramide should be reduced in these patients because extrapyramidal side effects are common.

REFERENCES

1. Excerpts from the United States renal data system 1991 annual data report. Am J Kidney Dis 1991;18:1–127.
2. Brynger H, Brunner FP, Chantler C, et al. Combined report on regular dialysis and transplantation in Europe, X, 1979. Proc Eur Dial Transplant Assoc 1980;17:2–87.
3. Gallagher KL, Jones JK. Furosemide-induced ototoxicity. Ann Intern Med 1979;91:744–745.
4. Vertes V, Cangiano JL, Berman LB, Gould A. Hypertension in end-stage renal disease. N Engl J Med 1969;280:978–981.
5. Weidmann P, Maxwell MH, Lupu AN, et al. Plasma renin activity and blood pressure in terminal renal failure. N Engl J Med 1971;285:757–762.
6. Vaughan Jr ED, Carey RM, Ayers CR, Peach MJ. Hemodialysis-resistant hypertension: control with an orally active inhibitor of angiotensin-converting enzyme. J Clin Endocrinol Metab 1979;48:869–871.
7. Sterns RH, Thomas DJ, Herndon RM. Brain dehydration and neurologic deterioration after rapid correction of hyponatremia. Kidney Int 1989;35:69–75.
8. Laureno R. Central pontine myelinolysis following rapid correction of hyponatremia. Ann Neurol 1983;13:232–242.
9. Ayus JC, Krothapalli RK, Arieff AI. Treatment of symptomatic hyponatremia and its relation to brain damage: a prospective study. N Engl J Med 1987;317:1190–1195.
10. Sterns RH, Riggs JE, Schochet Jr SS. Osmotic demyelination syndrome following correction of hyponatremia. N Engl J Med 1986;314:1535–1542.
11. Laureno R, Karp BI. Pontine and extrapontine myelinolysis following rapid correction of hyponatremia. Lancet 1988;1:1439–1440.
12. Narins RG. Therapy of hyponatremia: does haste make waste? N Engl J Med 1986;314:1573–1575.
13. Rose BD. Clinical physiology of acid-base and electrolyte disorders, ed 3. New York, McGraw-Hill, 1989.
14. Hogan GR, Dodge PR, Gill SR, et al. Pathogenesis of seizures occurring during restoration of plasma tonicity to normal in

animals previously chronically hypernatremic. Pediatrics 1969; 43:54–64.

15. Posner JB, Plum F. Spinal-fluid pH and neurological symptoms in systemic acidosis. N Engl J Med 1967;277:605–613.

16. Stacpoole PW. Lactic acidosis: the case against bicarbonate therapy. Ann Intern Med 1986;105:276–278.

17. Narins RG, Cohen JJ. Bicarbonate therapy for organic acidosis: the case for its continued use. Ann Intern Med 1987;106:615.

18. Adrogue HJ, Eknoyan G, Suki WK. Diabetic ketoacidosis: role of the kidney in the acid-base homeostasis re-evaluated. Kidney Int 1984;25:591–598.

19. Barton CH, Vaziri ND, Ness RL, et al. Cimetidine in the management of metabolic alkalosis induced by nasogastric drainage. Arch Surg 1979;114:70–74.

20. Swartz RD, Rubin JE, Brown RS, et al. Correction of postoperative metabolic alkalosis and renal failure by hemodialysis. Ann Intern Med 1977;86:52–55.

21. Abouna GM, Veazey PR, Terry Jr DB. Intravenous infusion of hydrochloric acid for treatment of severe metabolic alkalosis. Surgery 1974;75:194–202.

22. Eschbach JW, Egrie JC, Downing MR, et al. Correction of the anemia of end-stage renal disease with recombinant human erythropoietin: results of a combined phase I and II clinical trial. N Engl J Med 1987;316:73–78.

23. Eschbach JW, Adamson JW. Anemia of end-stage renal disease (ESRD). Kidney Int 1985;28:1–5.

24. Di Minno G, Martinez J, McKean M, et al. Platelet dysfunction in uremia: multifaceted defect partially corrected by dialysis. Am J Med 1985;79:552.

25. Remuzzi G, Benigni A, Dodesini P, et al. Reduced platelet thromboxane formation in uremia: evidence for a cyclooxygenase defect. J Clin Invest 1983;71:762–768.

26. Moia M, Vizzotto L, Cattaneo M, et al. Improvement in the haemostatic defect of uraemia after treatment with recombinant erythropoietin. Lancet 1987;2:1227–1229.

27. Mannucci PM, Remuzzi G, Pusoneri F, et al. Deamino-8-D-arginine vasopressin shortens the bleeding time in uremia. N Engl J Med 1983;308:8–12.

28. Janson PA, Jubelirer SJ, Weinstein MJ, Deykin D. Treatment of the bleeding tendency in uremia with cryoprecipitate. N Engl J Med 1980;303:1318–1322.

29. Livio M, Mannucci PM, Vigano G, et al. Conjugated estrogens for the management of bleeding associated with renal failure. N Engl J Med 1986;315:731–735.

30. Bansal VK, Vertuno LL. Surgery. In: Daugirdas JT, Ing TS, eds. Handbook of dialysis. Boston, Little, Brown, 1988:416–422.

31. Portale AA, Halloran BP, Murphy MM, Morris Jr RC. Oral intake of phosphorus can determine the serum concentration of 1,25-dihydroxyvitamin D by determining its production rate in humans. J Clin Invest 1986;77:7–12.

32. Delmez JA, Tindira C, Grooms P, et al. Parathyroid hormone suppression by intravenous 1,25-dihydroxyvitamin D: a role for increased sensitivity to calcium. J Clin Invest 1989;83:1349–1355.

33. Dunlay R, Rodriguez M, Felsenfeld AJ, Llach F. Direct effect of calcitriol on parathyroid function (sigmoidal curve) in dialysis. Kidney Int 1989;36:1093–1098.

34. Hodsman AB, Sherrard DJ, Alfrey AC, et al. Bone aluminum and histomorphometric features of renal osteodystrophy. J Clin Endocrinol Metab 1982;54:539.

35. Lee DBN, Goodman WG, Coburn JW. Renal osteodystrophy: some questions on an old disorder. Am J Kidney Dis 1988;11: 365–376.

36. Winney RJ, Cowie JF, Robson JS. Role of plasma aluminum in the detection and prevention of aluminum toxicity. Kidney Int 1986;29:S91–S95.

37. Nebeker HG, Andress DL, Milliner DS, et al. Indirect methods for the diagnosis of aluminum bone disease: plasma aluminum, the desferrioxamine infusion test, and serum iPTH. Kidney Int 1986;29:S96–S99.

38. Ruiz P, Gomez F, Schreiber AD. Impaired function of macrophage F_c receptors in end-stage renal disease. N Engl J Med 1990;322:717–722.

39. Clark RA, Hamory BH, Ford GH, Kimball HR. Chemotaxis in acute renal failure. J Infect Dis 1972;126:460–463.

40. Leonard A, Raij L, Shapiro FL. Bacterial endocarditis in regularly dialyzed patients. Kidney Int 1973;4:407–422.

41. Cross AS, Steigbigel RT. Infective endocarditis and access site infections in patients on hemodialysis. Medicine (Baltimore) 1976;55:453–466.

42. Nsouli KA, Lazarus JM, Schoenbaum SC, et al. Bacteremic infection in hemodialysis. Arch Intern Med 1979;139:1255–1258.

43. Forman MB, Virmani RV, Robertson RM, Stone WJ. Mitral annular calcification in chronic renal failure. Chest 1984;85:367–377.

44. Lazarus JM, Gottleib MN, Lowerie EG, et al. Echocardiographic findings in stable hemodialysis patients. Proc Clin Dial Transplant Forum 1976;6:53.

45. Alfrey AC, LeGendre GR, Kaehney WD. The dialysis encephalopathy syndrome: possible aluminum intoxication. N Engl J Med 1976;294:184.

46. Hurwitz A. Antacid therapy and drug kinetics. Clin Pharmacokinet 1977;2:269–280.

47. Craig RM, Murphy P, Gibson TP, et al. Kinetic analysis of D-xylose absorption in normal subjects and patients with chronic renal failure. J Lab Clin Med 1983;101:496.

48. Magera BE, Arroyo JC, Rosansky SJ, Postic B. Vancomycin pharmacokinetics in patients with peritonitis on peritoneal dialysis. Antimicrob Agents Chemother 1983;23:710–714.

Medical Management of the Surgical Patient, Third Edition,
edited by Michael F. Lubin, H. Kenneth Walker, and Robert B. Smith III.
J.B. Lippincott Company, Philadelphia, PA © 1995.

CHAPTER

29

POSTOPERATIVE ELECTROLYTE DISTURBANCES

Michael F. Lubin
Charles M. Ferguson
Roger Sherman

WATER AND ELECTROLYTE ABNORMALITIES

Surgical patients are at risk for the development of disorders of fluid balance, electrolyte composition, and acid–base balance. These occur because of fluid losses resulting from surgery and the body's physiologic response to surgical trauma. Before specific electrolyte disorders are addressed, a brief review of normal fluid balance is provided.

REVIEW OF NORMAL FLUID BALANCE

Water constitutes 50% to 70% of total body weight and is distributed among intracellular, interstitial, and intravascular compartments. Extracellular fluid volume (ie, interstitial and intravascular) is determined by total body sodium content. The distribution of extracellular fluid between intravascular and interstitial fluid compartments is determined by the hydrostatic and oncotic pressures of the two compartments. Osmolality of body fluids is precisely controlled through the release of antidiuretic hormone (ADH). Although the normal kidney has a large reserve capacity for concentration and dilution, abnormalities of fluid regulation are common after surgery, resulting in hypernatremia

and hyponatremia and, thus, hyperosmolality and hypoosmolality.

Under normal circumstances, the body loses about 1400 mL of water a day. This is made up of 500 mL of urine (at maximum concentrating capacity) and 300 mL of water through the lungs, 400 mL through the skin, and 200 mL in feces. The body obtains 200 to 400 mL of water a day through oxidation and, thus, requires a minimum of 1 L of water each day to stay in balance. After operation, these fluid needs are increased by fever, warm environment, and increased urinary solute load resulting from catabolism.

Complicating factors in postoperative fluid balance are the body's reaction to trauma and fluid losses resulting from surgery that can affect fluid volume, composition, and concentration. ADH is released after most injuries and persists for 3 to 5 days after operation, depending on the degree of trauma. This excess secretion of ADH predisposes to overhydration and hyponatremia. A spontaneous brisk diuresis often is observed on the third or fourth postoperative day, coincident with the reduction in ADH to normal levels. Fluid losses resulting from surgery or trauma are equally important in the management of fluid balance. These include such obvious losses as nasogastric or fistula drainage and more subtle losses such as the third-space losses of major retroperitoneal dissection or burns. Thus, the treatment of postoperative fluid and electrolyte disorders must

305

take into account patient status (eg, congestive heart failure, renal disease); preexisting disorders (eg, small bowel obstruction with dehydration); the operation (eg, major third-space losses); and patient response.

Abnormalities of fluid volume must be diagnosed largely by clinical means because no reliable laboratory methods exist for identifying acute changes in fluid volume. For the most part, examination of the pulse, blood pressure, neck veins, tissue turgor, and mucous membranes, and measurement of the urine output provide an indication of volume status. In confusing situations, however, measurement of the central venous pressure or pulmonary artery wedge pressure is necessary. Volume changes sometimes also involve alterations in composition or concentration. For example, loss of blood at operation causes a volume deficit but no change in electrolyte concentration or composition in the remaining bodily fluid. On the other hand, loss of electrolyte-rich gastric fluid through nasogastric suction depletes the body not only of volume but of potassium and chloride, resulting in hypokalemic alkalotic dehydration.

Volume deficit is the most common fluid disorder in patients undergoing surgery. Common causes of fluid loss include persistent vomiting, nasogastric suction, diarrhea, third-space sequestration from dissection, intestinal obstruction, burns, and bleeding at surgery. Although composition and concentration changes vary according to the particular fluid lost, the volume loss is the same regardless of the mechanism and is manifested in a similar fashion for all causes. Dehydrated patients may show changes in neurologic function (sleepiness, apathy, stupor); gastrointestinal function (anorexia, nausea, vomiting, ileus); metabolic function (hyperthermia); and cardiovascular function (tachycardia, collapsed veins, hypotension). Correction of these disorders requires replacement of the volume deficit. This can be done with isotonic solution (usually normal saline) while awaiting laboratory results that will define concentration and composition abnormalities. Once all the information is available, precise fluid replacement can be directed to the specific abnormality; however, volume deficit can be treated clinically before electrolytes are measured.

Excesses in extracellular fluid in surgical patients are generally iatrogenic in nature. Because patients who have undergone operation have higher than normal levels of ADH, overaggressive fluid administration can easily result in volume excess. Although renal insufficiency may lead to volume excess, it accounts for relatively few postoperative cases of this disorder. Volume excess is generally manifested in the cardiovascular system by elevated venous pressure with distended neck veins, gallops, and pulmonary edema, and in tissues by pitting edema and anasarca. As in volume deficit, treatment is based largely on clinical findings and consists of fluid restriction for mild overload and diuretic therapy for more severe cases.

Although the following sections deal in general terms with specific abnormalities, most patients have multiple abnormalities of fluid volumes and concentrations.

SODIUM

PSEUDOHYPONATREMIA

Pseudohyponatremia is uncommon in patients who have undergone operation but is included for completeness. In patients with severe hyperlipidemia, the portion of plasma that is aqueous is reduced by the nonaqueous lipids. Because sodium is limited to the aqueous portion of plasma but is measured as milliequivalents per milliliter of whole plasma, its concentration appears low because the aqueous portion of plasma is decreased.[1] Severe hyperglycemia decreases sodium concentration by its osmotic effect of drawing water into the vascular space because the glucose cannot get into cells. Hyperglycemia thus pulls fluid from cells and the sodium concentration falls.[2,3] In either case, the hyponatremia is corrected by correcting the underlying disorder (ie, hyperlipidemia or hyperglycemia).

HYPONATREMIA

True hyponatremia is generally the result of some impairment of diluting capacity (water-excreting deficit). In patients who have undergone operation, this is generally related to elevated levels of ADH, although renal insufficiency sometimes plays a part. Assessment of the volume status is of great importance in uncovering the cause of hyponatremia. Specific settings of hyponatremia—hypervolemic, normovolemic, and hypovolemic—are discussed separately. The manifestations of hyponatremia depend not only on the absolute level of sodium but also on its rate of change. Slow changes of great magnitude may cause no symptoms, whereas rapid changes of lesser magnitude may result in major problems. Neurologic manifestations of hyponatremia are of most concern and include restlessness, confusion, seizures, and coma.[4–6]

Hypervolemic Hyponatremia

Hyponatremia with volume expansion is common in patients who have undergone operation, particularly those with renal insufficiency, congestive heart failure, and severe liver disease. In patients with the last two conditions, the total body water and sodium are elevated, although there is often a decrease in effective intravascular volume, which activates the neurogenic and renal mechanism for sodium and water retention despite the total body excess.[7] In patients with chronic renal insufficiency, the water excretory deficit is intrinsic but the result is the same.

Regardless of the underlying cause, if hypervolemic hyponatremia is present, fluid restriction is the preferred therapy. If there are severe neurologic manifestations of hyponatremia (eg, altered mental status, seizures), saline or hypertonic saline should be administered, along with intravenous furosemide to correct the volume overload.

Normovolemic Hyponatremia

Normovolemic hyponatremia is the result of increased ADH activity. ADH levels normally rise in response to surgery and trauma, although the increase is usually mild and of little clinical significance.[8] In surgical patients with mild cardiac or renal dysfunction, however, the administration of hypotonic solutions (eg, D_5W, $D_{10}W$, $D_{5/0.45}NS$ or $D_{0.45}NS$) may produce normovolemic hyponatremia. Similarly, large volumes of hyponatremic solutions may produce normovolemic hyponatremia in normal persons. More important, many drugs used in anesthesia and surgery, including halothane, thiopental, nitrous oxide, morphine, and barbiturates, stimulate ADH release, thus predisposing to this problem.[9] The treatment of normovolemic hyponatremia in these settings is modest water restriction and avoidance of unnecessary drugs.

In some settings (brain tumor or abscess, subdural hemorrhage, skull fracture, carcinoma of the lung, carcinoma of the pancreas), there may be an inordinate outpouring of ADH, resulting in the syndrome of inappropriate ADH secretion (SIADH). The usual findings in this syndrome are normal fluid volumes, hyponatremia, hypoosmolality of the serum, inappropriately high urine osmolality, and high urinary sodium. Volume assessment is important to differentiate SIADH from hypervolemic hyponatremia and from dehydration that has been partially corrected with hypotonic solutions. Serum and urine osmolality help confirm the diagnosis. Serum osmolality should be below normal, often in the range of 220 to 260 mOsm/L, and, although urine osmolality is higher than is serum osmolality, it does not often reach the maximum concentration of 900 to 1110 mOsm/L. The urinary sodium level often is inappropriately elevated but is not particularly helpful in making a diagnosis.

The treatment of SIADH is fluid restriction. Although sodium replacement seems attractive for correction of the hyponatremia, it is virtually doomed to fail because the mechanism of the disorder is excessive retention of free water. Again, if severe neurologic manifestations exist, such

as confusion, seizures, or coma, the use of hypertonic saline therapy and furosemide is indicated.[10]

Hypovolemic Hyponatremia

Hypovolemic hyponatremia is relatively uncommon in surgical patients and is generally the result of insufficient sodium and water replacement. This can occur in patients with extrarenal volume losses from diarrhea, vomiting, or nasogastric suction. Another important cause is the overzealous use of diuretics. Hypovolemia prevents the formation of dilute urine through both direct and indirect (ADH-mediated) mechanisms. Volume depletion, be it from intravascular, renal, or third-space losses, causes water retention, predisposing to the development of hyponatremia if hypotonic fluids are administered. The treatment of hypovolemic hyponatremia involves replacement with isotonic sodium chloride.

HYPERNATREMIA

Hypernatremia is always associated with hyperosmolality and may result from dehydration after excessive depletion of free water or the administration of hypertonic solution. Clinically, hypernatremia is manifested by central nervous system depression ranging from lethargy to coma.[4] The severity of central nervous system depression is related not only to the degree of hypernatremia but also to its rate of development. Other manifestations of hypernatremia from dehydration are poor skin turgor, dry mucous membranes, and orthostatic hypotension. The blood urea nitrogen:creatinine ratio is elevated and the urinary sodium level is usually less than 10 mEq/L.

Insensible water losses are increased after operation and may predispose to hypernatremia if this is not accounted for in planning fluid management. In addition, any cause of excess renal water loss predisposes to hypernatremia. This is seen after neurosurgical operations in patients who develop diabetes insipidus, with the osmotic diuresis of uncontrolled diabetes, and with the osmotic diuresis that occurs after mannitol administration in patients who have undergone neurosurgery and vascular surgery. The result of this diuresis is greater loss of free water than of sodium, resulting in hypernatremia.[11] Occasionally, hypernatremia may occur from extrarenal losses such as extensive burns or massive diarrhea.

Hypernatremia with dehydration is treated with saline and water. Even though these patients have hypernatremia, their total body sodium is depleted and normal saline replacement is indicated until their volume depletion is corrected. The major concern during the correction of hypernatremia is to prevent too rapid a change in osmolality. A rapid decrease of plasma osmolality risks brain swelling and a worsened neurologic condition. It is better to attempt a gradual correction of hypernatremia over 24 to 48 hours.[12,13]

Less commonly, hypernatremia may be caused by the administration of hypertonic solution. This may result from the overzealous correction of hyponatremia, from the administration of sodium bicarbonate for cardiopulmonary resuscitation,[14] from absorption of the hypertonic saline used in saline abortion,[15] or, more rarely, from the transfusion of blood or blood products. These patients may have hypervolemia or hypovolemia, depending on the clinical situation. The hypernatremia is corrected with hypotonic saline and diuretics in patients with hypervolemia and with saline in patients with hypovolemia.

POTASSIUM

NORMAL POTASSIUM BALANCE

Potassium is largely an intracellular cation but is of great clinical significance because of the cardiovascular effects of hypokalemia or hyperkalemia in extracellular fluid. About 98% of potassium is intracellular and largely in muscle. The extracellular potassium concentration depends on total body potassium and the transcellular potassium flux. Insulin and aldosterone promote cellular uptake of potassium. Acidosis tends to increase extracellular fluid potassium, whereas chronic alkalosis leads to hypokalemia and total body potassium depletion by kaliuresis in exchange for hydrogen ion.

HYPERKALEMIA

Because of the kidney's ability to excrete large amounts of potassium (as much as 1000 mEq/d) independent of the glomerular filtration rate, hyperkalemia is uncommon in healthy patients who are undergoing elective surgery. Hyperkalemia may develop in patients with renal insufficiency, however, if careful attention is not given to potassium balance. Metabolic acidosis from diabetic ketoacidosis, shock, or ischemia of an organ or extremity may result in hyperkalemia through the exchange of potassium for hydrogen ion.[16] The release of potassium from cells that is associated with cellular necrosis in hemolysis, burns, rhabdomyolysis, or chemotherapy may result in hyperkalemia.[17] Similarly, succinylcholine inhibits cell membrane repolarization and potassium uptake. This can be of clinical significance in patients with severe trauma, burns, or preexisting neuromuscular disease; succinylcholine should not

be used in these patients.[18,19] In these causes of hyperkalemia, total body potassium may be normal, increased, or decreased but the extracellular potassium is increased and causes the problems. Unless there are changes in cardiac rhythm and conduction, therapy can be aimed at the underlying cause. The hyperkalemia associated with renal insufficiency results from lack of excretion, and total body potassium is increased. Thus, therapy in these patients must be aimed at removing potassium.

The usual step-by-step electrocardiographic changes of hyperkalemia are (1) tall, peaked T waves; (2) diminished P wave and prolonged PR interval; (3) disappearance of the P wave; (4) prolonged QRS complex; (5) slurred QRS complex; and (6) cardiac standstill. T-wave peaking and minor changes in the P wave are common and not life-threatening but disappearance of the P wave or a widened QRS complex indicate imminent danger of cardiac standstill, and therapy must be instituted immediately.

Immediate treatment of severe hyperkalemia begins with the administration of intravenous calcium chloride. Although calcium has no effect on extracellular fluid potassium or total body potassium, it directly antagonizes the effect of potassium on cardiac muscle electrical activity. This effect lasts for about 30 minutes, and repeated doses are limited by hypercalcemia. Sodium bicarbonate can be used because it directly antagonizes potassium's effects on cardiac muscle and also increases blood pH, increasing the exchange of extracellular potassium for intracellular hydrogen ion and, thus, decreasing extracellular fluid potassium while not affecting total body stores. Its onset of action is 15 to 20 minutes and its duration is several hours. Sodium bicarbonate is particularly effective in the presence of acidosis. Repeated dosing is limited by increased extracellular fluid volume, hypernatremia, and alkalosis. Intravenous glucose and insulin decrease the serum potassium level by redistributing potassium into cells. Again, there is no change in total body potassium. The onset and duration of action are similar to those of sodium bicarbonate. Doses may be administered frequently if blood sugar is monitored carefully. The administration of 50 g of glucose with 25 U of regular insulin is a reasonable schedule.

When total body stores are believed to be elevated (as in renal failure), potassium may be removed through the gastrointestinal tract or by dialysis. Kayexalate (20 to 50 g with a cathartic such as sorbitol, 30 mL) every 6 hours orally or rectally binds potassium and causes enteral loss. The onset of action is slow (several hours) and the duration of action varies (as long as 6 hours). Long-term use is somewhat limited by gastrointestinal intolerance. Diuresis is effective in depleting total body potassium and may be instituted by saline infusion if there is good cardiac reserve or by small doses of furosemide if the kidneys are not severely diseased and are able to respond to the volume or furosemide challenge. The serum potassium level drops fairly quickly after the onset of diuresis. The duration of action is generally several hours, depending on the degree of hyperkalemia and the increase in total body potassium.

Finally, dialysis may be used to decrease extracellular and total body potassium. Hemodialysis is much quicker in onset than is peritoneal dialysis, although both methods may maintain normal potassium levels for several days. Because of the technical difficulties of dialysis and the other available treatment methods, dialysis is usually reserved for patients with anuria and renal failure.

HYPOKALEMIA

Hypokalemia is very common in surgical patients, particularly those who have been taking loop diuretics or who have prolonged upper gastrointestinal tract fluid losses from vomiting or nasogastric suction. Loop diuretics increase potassium excretion along with natriuresis. In patients with persistent nasogastric losses, the alkalosis resulting from the loss of hydrochloric acid causes increased potassium loss by exchange of potassium for hydrogen ion in the distal tubule.[20] This potassium loss continues as long as chloride deficiency and metabolic alkalosis persist.

Hypokalemia is usually first manifested by its effects on cardiac muscle conduction. The electrocardiogram shows a flattened T wave and, at times, a new U wave. In addition, there may be arrhythmias such as numerous or multifocal premature ventricular contractions or paroxysmal atrial tachycardia with block, particularly in the presence of digoxin. More severe depletion of total body potassium may induce skeletal muscle weakness, ileus, and even respiratory muscle paralysis.[21] Rarely, severe hypokalemia can cause rhabdomyolysis with acute renal failure.[22]

Treatment of hypokalemia is replacement. Because most potassium in the body is intracellular, equilibration between intracellular and extracellular levels takes time. Only an approximation of the amount of potassium needed to correct the hypokalemia is possible because there is no good correlation between the serum potassium level and total body potassium stores. An attempt at rapid correction of hypokalemia may turn a benign laboratory abnormality into a life-threatening arrhythmia of hyperkalemia. Thus, correction with oral agents over several days is preferred if possible. If the intravenous route is used, the rate of infusion should not exceed 20 mEq/h in concentrations of 50 mEq/L.

ACID–BASE DISTURBANCES

Blood pH is carefully maintained between 7.38 and 7.42. The principal buffer system in the extracellular fluid is the carbonic acid–bicarbonate system, which is represented in the following equation:

$$H^+ + HCO_3^- \rightleftharpoons H_2CO_3 \rightleftharpoons CO_2 + H_2O$$

The relationship of bicarbonate concentration and partial pressure of CO_2 is expressed in the Henderson-Hasselbalch equation as follows:

$$pH = 6.1 + \log \frac{HCO_3^-}{0.03 \times Pa_{CO_2}}$$

Thus, blood pH depends on metabolic mechanisms (controlling bicarbonate concentration) and respiratory mechanisms (controlling CO_2 concentration). A rise in pH above 7.42 is alkalosis; a fall in pH below 7.38 is acidosis. If the change in pH results from a change in bicarbonate concentration, it is metabolic. If it results from a change in CO_2 concentration, it is respiratory. It is apparent that one system can compensate for the other. Thus, if a metabolic acidosis occurs, a decrease in CO_2 concentration by respiratory compensation tends to correct the pH.

Mild changes in pH are well tolerated by most patients but severe acidosis or alkalosis can have significant effects during the postoperative period. Severe acidosis (pH less than 7.2) reduces myocardial contractility and responsiveness of the myocardium to catecholamines.[23] Acidosis may increase cerebral blood flow but low cerebrospinal fluid pH may cause cerebral dysfunction, resulting in lethargy or even coma. Alkalosis has little effect on the myocardium except indirectly through hypokalemia (see earlier discussion) but does shift the hemoglobin dissociation curve to the left, limiting oxygen delivery in the tissues. Respiratory alkalosis also decreases cerebral blood flow and, thus, should be prevented.[24,25] Alkalosis can have a higher associated mortality rate than acidosis, depending on the underlying cause, and must be addressed quickly.

METABOLIC ACIDOSIS

Metabolic acidosis occurs when there is a reduction in the serum bicarbonate concentration. This can result from a loss of total body bicarbonate or buffering of a strong acid. The basic cause is generally determined by the anion gap, which is the difference between the serum sodium concentration and the sum of the serum chloride and carbon dioxide concentrations, with a normal value being 8 to 12 mEq/L, but it depends on the normal values of the testing laboratory. Metabolic acidoses are divided into two groups: normal anion gap and elevated anion gap.

In surgical patients, metabolic acidosis with a normal anion gap is usually the result of loss of bicarbonate from the gastrointestinal tract. This may occur in the setting of profuse diarrhea or high small bowel fistula in which there is loss of bicarbonate-rich fluid. It may also occur in patients with ureterosigmoidostomy as a result of exchange of bicarbonate for chloride in the sigmoid; this operation is infrequently performed today. The addition of hydrochloric acid can cause metabolic acidosis with a normal anion gap, and this is seen clinically with the administration of chloride salts of cationic amino acids in total parenteral nutrition.[26,27] Less common causes of metabolic acidosis with a normal anion gap in surgical patients are renal tubular acidosis (which is seen at times in patients with intrinsic renal disease, diabetes, or the acquired immunodeficiency syndrome) and the administration of carbonic anhydrase inhibitors such as acetazolamide.

Metabolic acidosis with an elevated anion gap results from the accumulation of unmeasured organic acids or failure of the kidneys to excrete normally produced acid (renal insufficiency). In surgical patients, lactic acidosis is by far the most common cause. Lactate is produced by anaerobic metabolism in ischemic tissues. Thus, patients with cardiopulmonary arrest, shock, or ischemic organs or extremities commonly develop this disorder.[28] Other causes of metabolic acidosis with an elevated anion gap in surgical patients are sepsis, diabetic ketoacidosis (acetoacetic and β-hydroxybutyric acids), and renal failure. Again, the clinical picture should elucidate the cause.

In general, therapy for metabolic acidosis involves treating the underlying cause. Loss of bicarbonate must be stopped by controlling losses from diarrhea or fistulas, or the production of lactate must be slowed by improving tissue perfusion. In patients with gastrointestinal tract losses, replacement can be given by the oral or intravenous route when the serum bicarbonate level falls below 15 mEq/L.

When the acidosis is severe (bicarbonate level less than 10 mEq/L) and the clinical situation is critical (respiratory or cardiovascular decompensation), bicarbonate replacement may be indicated for lactic acidosis. The amount of bicarbonate and rate at which it should be administered is difficult to estimate because of the variability in lactate production. Giving bicarbonate to patients who are not critically ill may actually increase the acidosis because it can contribute to the formation of lactate. Thus, frequent measurement of pH during replacement is often of more value than are the various formulas designed to calculate the required dosage and rate.

METABOLIC ALKALOSIS

Metabolic alkalosis occurs when there is an elevation in the plasma bicarbonate level. This can result from a loss of chloride (gastrointestinal or renal), an increase in bicarbonate resorption by the kidney, or the administration of exogenous alkali. Metabolic alkalosis is a very common disorder in surgical patients and usually is caused by gastrointestinal tract losses from either nasogastric suction or prolonged vomiting. Loss of hydrochloric acid from the stomach produces the metabolic alkalosis and, as a compensatory mechanism, the kidney wastes potassium to conserve hydrogen

ions and sodium, resulting in the accompanying hypokalemia. In a similar fashion, loop diuretics produce renal losses of chloride, alkalosis, and hypokalemia. Rarer causes for metabolic alkalosis in surgical patients are hyperaldosteronism and Cushing's syndrome, which cause increased bicarbonate resorption, and the exogenous administration of alkali.

Alkalosis is common during the postoperative period and generally of little clinical significance. In patients with severe metabolic alkalosis, however, there can be compensatory hypoventilation to a point that makes weaning from a ventilator difficult. For patients with typical mild postoperative alkalosis, therapy with intravenous sodium chloride and potassium chloride is adequate. Replacement of chloride is usually the most significant factor. In patients with severe metabolic alkalosis (serum bicarbonate 40 to 50 mEq/L), rapid correction can be achieved with hydrochloric acid or ammonium chloride. Hydrochloric acid can be administered in 0.1 N solution through a central venous catheter,[29] and ammonium chloride can be given as an isotonic (160 mEq/L) solution peripherally. As in the correction of acidosis, it is better to correct the pH slowly over 24 to 48 hours.

RESPIRATORY ACIDOSIS

Respiratory acidosis occurs when hypoventilation raises the concentration of CO_2 in the blood. Unless there is an increase in the inspired oxygen fraction, concomitant hypoxia is often the most important clinical abnormality. Symptoms of respiratory acidosis depend largely on how fast the disorder develops and are most severe in acute cases. Anxiety, disorientation, headaches, stupor, and even coma may be seen.

In the postoperative period, acute respiratory acidosis is most commonly a complication of the respiratory-depressant effects of anesthesia and narcotics. Other causes are pneumothorax; airway obstruction (foreign body, laryngospasm, severe bronchospasm); and ventilator malfunction. Chronic causes include obstructive pulmonary disease, respiratory nerve or muscle damage, and restrictive disorders of the thorax. Treatment of acute respiratory acidosis is adequate ventilation. In the case of respiratory depression, this may mean administering a narcotic antagonist (naloxone). Maintaining an adequate airway is critical and intubation and mechanical ventilation are often required.

RESPIRATORY ALKALOSIS

Respiratory alkalosis results from hyperventilation with a consequent decrease in Pco_2. Causes in the postoperative period include anxiety; early septicemia; pulmonary embolus; hypoxemia (from any cause); hepatic failure; central nervous system disease (cerebrovascular accident, trauma); and iatrogenic mechanical hyperventilation. Respiratory alkalosis usually does not cause symptoms but can produce a rapid rise in pH with paresthesias, tetany, and even seizures. Therapy must be directed at the underlying cause because treatment of the alkalosis is unrewarding. Thus, a careful history, physical, and evaluation of the clinical situation is necessary to arrive at the diagnosis and initiate therapy.

OLIGURIA

Decreased urine output is common after operation and has many causes. It is generally defined as a urine output of less than 25 mL/h for 2 consecutive hours. The clinical significance of oliguria is that it is a marker for other problems. Urine output is monitored for two reasons: as an index of intravascular volume and as a marker for the development of postoperative renal failure. In patients with relatively normal myocardial function, oliguria is among the first signs of intravascular volume depletion that develop subacutely. Thus, in patients who undergo operation with significant third-space losses, oliguria precedes the development of tachycardia and hypotension, and allows earlier intervention. Similarly, oliguria is commonly the first manifestation of postoperative renal failure. Although nonoliguric renal failure can develop in the postoperative period, oliguric renal failure is more common and has a much graver prognosis.[30] Again, early recognition of the problem allows early intervention.

In the evaluation of oliguria, it is helpful to consider the production of urine in three states: prerenal, renal, and postrenal. Prerenal factors are events that deliver blood to the kidneys to produce urine. Adequate intravascular volume must be delivered at sufficient pressure through open renal arteries for the production of urine. Renal factors involve glomerular and tubular function. Postrenal factors involve the drainage of urine from the kidney through the ureters to the bladder and its excretion from the bladder through the urethra. In evaluating patients with oliguria, this approach is helpful both diagnostically and therapeutically.

Anuria is uncommon in the postoperative period. Even with complete renal shutdown, a small amount of urine is usually produced. The common causes of anuria are mechanical, with bladder outlet obstruction being the most frequent. Although many medications, most notably narcotics, can cause difficulty in voiding, an enlarged prostate is the most common cause and is usually apparent on digital rectal examination. Therapy involves simple catheterization. If patients have been obstructed for some time or have a large amount of urine in the bladder, however, drainage should

be slow. There have been reports of arrhythmias and cardiovascular collapse occurring after the release of large volumes of urine from obstructed bladders. In addition, a vigorous postobstructive diuresis occasionally occurs after the release of urinary obstruction. The other postrenal cause of anuria or oliguria is bilateral ureteral obstruction. This is important to keep in mind when anuria is found after an operation that requires dissection in the area of both ureters (ie, hysterectomy). Because the kidneys are paired organs and can compensate for each other, however, the ligation of one ureter does not cause anuria or oliguria.

Prerenal and renal causes of oliguria are much more complex than are postrenal causes and require in-depth evaluation of the patient's volume status and risk for the development of renal failure. Because prerenal oliguria usually involves intravascular volume depletion, evaluation for this cause is the first area targeted for exploration by history, physical examination, and laboratory testing. First, the nature of the particular illness should be reviewed and the presence or absence of preoperative volume depletion determined. Major burns, small bowel obstruction, mesenteric infarction, and peritonitis all involve intravascular depletion from third-space losses as part of their pathophysiology. Next, intraoperative losses that can lead to such depletion should be considered. Examples are unreplaced major blood loss or third-space losses from major dissection or prolonged bowel exposure. Last, postoperative losses such as ongoing bleeding or third-space losses should be explored. Evaluation of the state of hydration by physical examination is the next step. Orthostatic changes in blood pressure and pulse are good indicators of intravascular dehydration.

Similarly, information relating to renal causes of oliguria should be collected. Risk factors for the development of postoperative renal failure include preexisting renal failure, exposure to radiographic contrast material (particularly in patients with diabetes),[31,32] exposure to aminoglycosides,[33] preoperative shock or relative hypotension, major soft tissue crush injuries, systemic sepsis, transfusion reactions, and preoperative intravascular depletion from dehydration. There is little to be found by physical examination in the diagnosis of intrinsic renal failure, although a clinical evaluation of volume status is necessary for treatment.

It is usually possible to determine by clinical evaluation whether postoperative oliguria is caused by prerenal or renal factors. In severely ill patients (particularly those with some degree of preexisting renal disease), however, this differentiation may be difficult or impossible. Examination of the urine sediment may reveal casts indicative of acute tubular necrosis. Also helpful are measurement of the urine sodium level, osmolality, and creatinine level. In prerenal oliguria, the kidney attempts to preserve intravascular volume. Thus, the urine is concentrated (osmolality greater than 500), with little sodium (less than 20). In patients with renal failure, the urine has an osmolality similar to that of serum because the tubules have lost their concentrating mechanisms. Thus, osmolality is less than 400 and the sodium level is greater than 40. Often, the values for osmolality and sodium are nondiagnostic in individual patients. Further tests for differentiation include the renal failure index and fractional excretion of sodium.[34] The renal failure index is computed by dividing the urine sodium concentration by the urine:plasma creatinine ratio and multiplying by 100. A value of less than 1 is consistent with prerenal azotemia and a value of greater than 2 usually indicates renal failure. Specimens for these tests must be drawn before therapy is instituted and, most important, before any diuretics are administered.

The treatment of prerenal azotemia involves the restoration of effective intravascular volume and cardiac output. This is accomplished through the administration of adequate intravenous saline solution to restore normal urinary output. In acutely ill patients, evaluation of intravascular volume may be difficult because of concomitant adult respiratory distress syndrome or congestive heart failure. In these patients, monitoring of cardiac output and pulmonary artery wedge pressure with a Swan-Ganz catheter helps to guide therapy. If the wedge pressure is low (less than 15 cm H_2O), additional intravascular volume may help. Therapy for renal causes of oliguria involves the treatment of renal failure and is addressed in Chapter 28. In the immediate postoperative period, however, the crucial factor is maintaining adequate intravascular volume. In complicated patients, pulmonary capillary wedge pressure monitoring with a Swan-Ganz catheter may be crucial.

REFERENCES

1. Steffes MV, Freier EF. A simple and precise method of determining true sodium, potassium, and chloride concentrations in hyperlipidemia. J Lab Clin Med 1976;88:683–688.
2. Katz MA. Hyperglycemia-induced hyponatremia: calculation of expected serum sodium depression. N Engl J Med 1973; 289:843–844.
3. Jenkins PG, Larmore C. Hyperglycemia-induced hyponatremia. N Engl J Med 1974;290:573.
4. Arieff AI, Guisado R. Effects on the central nervous system of hypernatremic and hyponatremic states. Kidney Int 1976;10: 104–116.
5. Arieff AI, Llach F, Massry SG. Neurological manifestations and morbidity of hyponatremia: correlation with brain water and electrolytes. Medicine (Baltimore) 1976;55:121–129.
6. Scott JC, Welch JS, Berman IB. Water intoxication and sodium depletion in surgical patients. Obstet Gynecol 1965;26: 168–175.
7. Berliner RW, Davidson DG. Production of hypertonic urine in the absence of antidiuretic hormone. J Clin Invest 1957; 36:1416.
8. Weitzman R, Kleeman CR. Water metabolism and the neurohypophyseal hormones. In: Maxwell MH, Kleeman CR, eds. Clinical disorders of fluid and electrolyte metabolism. New York, McGraw-Hill, 1980:531–645.
9. Miller M, Moses AM. Drug induced states of impaired water excretion. Kidney Int 1976;10:96–103.
10. Hantman D, Rossier B, Zohlman R, Schrier R. Rapid correction of hyponatremia in the syndrome of inappropriate secretion of antidiuretic hormone: an alternative treatment to hypertonic saline. Ann Intern Med 1973;78:870–875.
11. Epstein FM. Disturbances in renal concentrating ability. In: Andreoli TE, Grantham JJ, Rector FC, eds. Disturbances in body fluid osmolality. Bethesda, American Physiological Society, 1977:251–266.
12. Finberg L. Hypernatremic (hypertonic) dehydration in infants. N Engl J Med 1973;289:196–198.
13. Ross EJ, Christie SBM. Hypernatremia. Medicine (Baltimore) 1969;48:441–473.
14. Mattar JA, Weil MH, Shubin H, et al. Cardiac arrest in the critically ill. Am J Med 1974;56:162–168.
15. DeVillota ED, Cavanilles JM, Stein L, et al. Hyperosmolal crisis following infusion of hypertonic sodium chloride for purposes of therapeutic abortion. Am J Med 1973;55:116–122.
16. Cohen JJ, Kassirer JP. Acid base metabolism. In: Maxwell MH, Kleeman CR, eds. Clinical disorders of fluid and electrolyte metabolism. New York, McGraw-Hill, 1980:181–232.
17. Kunau RT, Stein JH. Disorders of hypo- and hyperkalemia. Clin Nephrol 1977;7:173–190.
18. Weintraub HD, Heisterkamp DV, Cooperman LH. Changes in plasma potassium concentration after depolarizing blockers in anesthetized man. Br J Anaesth 1969;41:1048–1052.
19. Cooperman LH. Succinylcholine-induced hyperkalemia in neuromuscular disease. JAMA 1970;213:1867–1871.
20. Seldin DW, Rector FC. The generation and maintenance of metabolic alkalosis. Kidney Int 1972;1:306–321.
21. Duggin GG, Price MA. Hypokalemic muscular paresis in migratory Papua/New Guineans. Lancet 1974;1:649–652.
22. Relman AS, Schwartz WB. The nephropathy of potassium depletion: clinical and pathological entity. N Engl J Med 1956;255: 195.
23. Mitchell JH, Wildenthal K, Johnson RL Jr. The effects of acid-base disturbances on cardiovascular and pulmonary function. Kidney Int 1972;1:375–389.
24. Betz E. Cerebral blood flow: its measurement and regulation. Physiol Rev 1972;52:595–630.
25. Shenkin HA, Bouzarth WF. Clinical methods of reducing intracranial pressure. N Engl J Med 1970;282:1465–1471.
26. Heird WC, Dell RB, Driscoll JM Jr, et al. Metabolic acidosis resulting from intravenous alimentation mixture containing synthetic amino acids. N Engl J Med 1972;287:943–948.
27. Fraley DS, Adler S, Bruns F, et al. Metabolic acidosis after hyperalimentation with casein hydrolysate. Ann Intern Med 1978;88:352–354.
28. Oliva PB. Lactic acidosis. Am J Med 1970;48:209–225.
29. Wagner CW, Nesbit RR, Mansberger RR. The use of intravenous hydrochloric acid in the treatment of 34 patients with metabolic alkalosis. Am Surg 1980;46:140–146.

30. Anderson RJ, Linas SL, Berns AS, et al. Nonoliguric acute renal failure. N Engl J Med 1977;296:1134–1138.

31. Alexander RD, Berkes SL, Abuelo G. Contrast media induced oliguric renal failure. Arch Intern Med 1978;138:381–384.

32. Swartz RD, Rubin JE, Leeming BW, et al. Renal failure following major angiography. Am J Med 1978;65:31–37.

33. Appel GB, Neu HC. The nephrotoxicity of antimicrobial agents. N Engl J Med 1977;296:663–670.

34. Miller TR, Anderson RJ, Linas SL, et al. Urinary diagnostic indices in acute renal failure: a prospective study. Ann Intern Med 1978;89:47–50.

ENDOCRINOLOGY

Medical Management of the Surgical Patient, Third Edition,
edited by Michael F. Lubin, H. Kenneth Walker, and Robert B. Smith III.
J.B. Lippincott Company, Philadelphia, PA © 1995.

CHAPTER

DIABETES MELLITUS

30

Ruth M. Lawrence
Robert M. Walter, Jr.

Surgery has major effects on carbohydrate metabolism and, thus, presents special risks for patients with diabetes. Surgical mortality rates for patients with diabetes have declined recently but the successful perioperative care of these patients requires close cooperation between surgeons, anesthesiologists, and primary physicians to prevent complications. More than 10 million people in the United States have diabetes and at least half of them will require surgery at some point in their lives. In addition to surgical conditions typical of the general population, patients with diabetes experience increased intervention for occlusive vascular disease; cholelithiasis; ophthalmic disease (ie, cataract extraction, vitrectomy); renal disease; and infection. Three of four patients with diabetes are older than 40 years and approaching a time of life when surgical indications increase. The presence of diabetes typically is known before operation, although a new diagnosis of diabetes is made in the perioperative period in as many as 20% of cases.

PATHOPHYSIOLOGY

The endocrine pancreas, which consists of the islets of Langerhans, accounts for less than 3% of the total pancreatic mass in adults. The islets are unevenly distributed through the pancreas and contain four cell types: A (α) cells, which secrete glucagon; B (β) cells, which secrete insulin; D (δ) cells, which secrete somatostatin; and F cells, which secrete pancreatic polypeptide. Insulin, the major secretory product, is synthesized as a precursor molecule, preproinsulin, in the endoplasmic reticulum and cleaved by microsomal enzymes to proinsulin. Proinsulin is then converted by proteolysis to insulin and an amino acid residue, connecting peptide, which has no known biologic function. After secretion into the portal venous system, insulin passes through the liver and the portion that is not extracted enters the peripheral circulation. There, it binds to specific cell-surface receptors, initiating multiple phosphorylations of receptor and intracellular proteins and the internalization of the insulin-receptor complex.

The normal basal production of insulin is about 1 U/h, with an additional 3 to 5 U produced after meals. The usual fasting serum insulin concentration is 10 µU/mL; peak postprandial values rarely exceed 100 µU/mL. Endogenous insulin, which has a half-life of less than 5 minutes in plasma, is metabolized by hepatic and renal insulinases. Its major function is to promote the storage of ingested nutrients in many tissues, especially the liver, muscle, and fat. The major biologic effects are outlined in Table 30-1. Deficiency or reduced effectiveness of insulin has profound consequences on metabolism.

Diabetes mellitus is classified as either type I (insulin-dependent) or type II (non–insulin-dependent). Occasional

TABLE 30–1. Major Biologic Effects of Insulin

Organ or System	Effect
Liver	Promotes glycogen synthesis and storage, inhibits glycogenolysis
	Promotes triglyceride, very low-density lipoprotein, and cholesterol synthesis
	Inhibits ketogenesis
	Promotes glycolysis, inhibits gluconeogenesis
Fat	Promotes triglyceride storage, inhibits lipolysis
Muscle	Promotes protein synthesis
	Promotes glycogen synthesis and storage
Vascular	Promotes lipoprotein lipase activity

patients have diabetes as a result of other conditions, including pregnancy (gestational diabetes); pancreatic disease; endocrine disorders (Cushing's syndrome, thyrotoxicosis, pheochromocytoma, acromegaly, glucagonoma, somatostatinoma); acanthosis nigricans (related to insulin receptor abnormalities); and other rare genetic diseases. In 1979, the criteria used to diagnose diabetes were redefined to prevent overdiagnosis. In the absence of acutely decompensated, symptomatic disease, two fasting glucose levels that exceed 140 mg/dL or a sustained level of more than 200 mg/dL after the administration of 75 g of oral glucose are diagnostic.

Patients with type I diabetes (10% to 20% of all patients with diabetes in the United States) typically have circulating antibodies to islet cells and insulin that precede the clinical manifestations of the disease and persist for a few years after the onset of illness. Type I diabetes has strong HLA–haplotype associations that vary among different racial groups. Viral infection has been implicated as the cause in some patients. Patients with type I diabetes secrete little insulin, are prone to ketosis, and require insulin for treatment. Patients with type II diabetes commonly are obese (85%), are not prone to ketosis, and demonstrate insulin resistance that precedes impaired insulin secretion.

EFFECTS OF DIABETES ON SURGERY

Surgical mortality rates for patients with diabetes have declined substantially over the years with improved perioperative care. Uncomplicated diabetes is no longer associated with an increased mortality rate after cholecystectomy or peripheral vascular surgery and is associated with only a slightly increased risk after coronary artery bypass grafting. Nonetheless, multiple anatomic and functional complications of the disease do introduce specific problems during surgery.

Infection is the most common postoperative complication in patients with diabetes. Both in vitro and in vivo studies demonstrate the deleterious effect of hyperglycemia on leukocyte function. Hyperglycemia impairs chemotaxis and decreases phagocytosis by polymorphonuclear leukocytes. An increased incidence of surgical wound infection has been noted in patients with diabetes and, in a retrospective study, a positive correlation between mean plasma glucose and subsequent development of wound infections was shown. Studies assessing the effect of hyperglycemia on wound healing have been done in animals. A 50% decrease in wound tensile strength and in tissue hydroxyproline has been noted in rats with streptozotocin-induced diabetes compared with control rats without diabetes. Intensive insulin therapy (in which the glucose level is constantly maintained at less than 200 mg/dL) prevents these differences. Depressed leukocyte function may contribute to impaired collagen synthesis. Epithelial wounds (ie, corneal) require little leukocyte infiltration and collagen synthesis; their repair is not slowed in patients with diabetes.

The chronic complications of diabetes may also complicate surgery. The presence of neuropathy, particularly autonomic neuropathy, places patients at increased risk for perioperative cardiac arrest. Resting tachycardia or little change in the pulse with deep inspiration or exercise are warning signs and should encourage close postoperative cardiac and respiratory monitoring. The presence of gastroparesis increases the risk of aspiration, and appropriate perioperative therapy with metoclopramide and H_2 blockers is indicated. Ileus and urinary retention are additional complications of autonomic neuropathy. Renal disease can complicate fluid and electrolyte management. Of critical importance is macrovascular disease affecting coronary, cerebral, and peripheral vessels. Cardiac morbidity and death are also predicted by preexisting congestive heart failure and valvular disease. Noncardiac vascular complications are best predicted by the presence of retinopathy, neuropathy, nephropathy, congestive heart failure, and peripheral vascular disease. Control of diabetes has not been shown to be predictive. There is evidence, however, that patients with diabetes who experience cerebral ischemia after cardiac arrest or stroke have poorer short-term and long-term outcomes if their mean glucose levels are greater than 250 mg/dL.

EFFECTS OF SURGERY (STRESS) ON DIABETES

It has been known for more than 50 years that patients who do not have diabetes can develop hyperglycemia during the stress of surgery. Marked elevations are reached in intraoperative and postoperative levels of the counterregulatory hormones (glucagon, catecholamines, cortisol, and growth hormone). Experimental data indicate that the effects of these hormones are synergistic. In diabetes, the effects of stress are magnified by limited insulin availability or effectiveness. Furthermore, insulin release is significantly depressed during surgery. The hormonal milieu fosters hyperglycemia, and the markedly increased ratio of glucagon to insulin can result in ketoacidosis. Hormonal effects induced specifically by the newer inhalational anesthetic agents or by spinal anesthesia are not of great significance.

CARE OF SURGICAL PATIENTS WITH DIABETES

A careful history, physical examination, and selected laboratory tests (eg, blood count, urinalysis, fasting blood glucose level, electrolyte levels, creatinine level, hemoglobin A_{1c}, electrocardiogram, home glucose monitoring records) provide information regarding specific risk factors and assist in the care of surgical patients with diabetes. When possible, optimal control of diabetes should be achieved before surgery, although early admission to the hospital for this purpose often is not possible because of diagnosis-related group regulations.

Surgery should be performed early in the day to limit the time that patients are without food and are not receiving their usual treatment regimens. The goal of diabetes management in the perioperative period is to prevent marked hyperglycemia, ketosis, postoperative infections, and impaired wound healing, while also preventing unrecognized and potentially fatal hypoglycemia. This requires an intense coordinated effort between the internist or endocrinologist, surgeon, anesthesiologist, and nursing staff. The capacities of this team in part dictate the glycemic goals of therapy because frequent and precise monitoring of the perioperative glucose level is the most important factor in achieving optimal control. Plasma glucose levels of 250 mg/dL or less are desirable. If the plasma glucose level can be monitored every 30 minutes, even tighter control (a glucose level of 150 mg/dL or less) is desirable.

PATIENTS WITH TYPE I DIABETES

Several methods of insulin administration have been implemented with few comparative studies reported. The traditional method of treatment is to give one third to one half the usual dose of intermediate-acting insulin on the morning of surgery along with an infusion of 5% dextrose in water. About 10 to 20 mEq of potassium chloride is infused with each liter of solution. The blood glucose level is monitored every 1 or 2 hours and supplemental regular insulin is given subcutaneously every 4 to 6 hours according to the sliding scale shown in Table 30-2. According to some surveys, this is the most commonly used method and, with monitoring, it provides satisfactory control, particularly for minor surgery in an ambulatory setting. The disadvantages of this method relate to the variable and somewhat unpredictable absorption of insulin. If surgery is delayed, the effects of the previously administered NPH or Lente insulin cannot be modified. Another approach for brief, minor elective surgery is to withhold insulin and glucose during the procedure; this method is not recommended. High intraoperative glucose levels can be anticipated, as well as increased fatty acid and ketone levels.

A newer method, the use of continuous intravenous insulin infusions (CIII), has improved intraoperative glucose control and is recommended for major surgical procedures that require prolonged general anesthesia. There are two basic regimens for administering insulin and glucose. The preferable approach is to infuse insulin by pump independent of the other intravenous solutions; this permits greater flexibility. For CIII to be successful, the infusion must be monitored closely and blood glucose levels measured every 30 to 60 minutes, which requires the availability of skilled personnel throughout the intraoperative and postoperative periods. If such staffing is not available, less rigorous control using the traditional method described earlier may be preferable. The infusion of 5% dextrose at a rate of 100 to 150 mL/h with 10 to 20 mEq of potassium chloride per liter is probably sufficient to prevent catabolism, although more research is needed to confirm this. The administration of 1 to 3 U of regular insulin per hour is usually sufficient. Increased insulin needs can be expected in the face of obesity, sepsis, and glucocorticoid therapy, as well as in coronary artery bypass surgery because of the use of sympathomimetic drugs, glucose-containing priming solutions, and

TABLE 30–2. Traditional Method of Insulin Administration for Type I Diabetes

On morning of surgery, give one third to one half the usual dose of intermediate-acting insulin.

Infuse dextrose 5% in water at 100–150 mL/h with 10–20 mEq of potassium chloride added to each liter.

Monitor blood glucose every 1–2 hours; supplement with subcutaneous regular insulin every 4–6 hours; A representative scale follows:

Blood Glucose (mg/dL)	Regular Insulin (U)
<180	0
180–240	4
241–300	6
301–400	8
>400	10 (monitor closely)

hypothermia. Until patients can resume their usual diets, CIII remains the optimal mode of therapy and should be continued, provided adequate monitoring is available. When using CIII, it must be remembered that the serum half-life of insulin is less than 5 minutes and the biologic half-life is about 20 minutes. Total discontinuation of the insulin drip is promptly associated with catabolism leading to hyperglycemia and subsequent ketosis. Thus, a dose of regular insulin should be given 20 to 30 minutes before the drip is stopped. Table 30-3 outlines a suggested method of continuous insulin infusion.

In the other method, insulin and glucose are infused in the same bottle at a preestimated individualized concentration. This is not recommended because the occurrence of either hyperglycemia or hypoglycemia requires that new solutions with different relative concentrations be made.

PATIENTS WITH TYPE II DIABETES

For minor surgery, most patients with diet-controlled type II diabetes do not require insulin treatment. Patients who are taking the shorter-acting sulfonylureas (tolbutamide, tolazamide, acetohexamide, and glipizide) should have the dose held on the day of surgery, whereas those who are taking the longer-acting agents (chlorpropamide and glyburide) should have the dose held on the day before surgery as well. Blood glucose levels should be checked every 6 hours. When perioperative insulin is required, it should be given using a sliding scale with intravenous 5% dextrose running at 100 mL/h. Patients with type II diabetes who normally use insulin can be treated in the perioperative period either by the traditional method using sliding-scale regular insulin (Table 30-4) or by CIII (see Table 30-3). Patients with type II diabetes can be expected to require more insulin than those with type I diabetes because of inherent insulin resistance. Patients with type II diabetes who are undergoing major surgery are best treated with continuous intravenous insulin infusion if adequate glucose monitoring is available.

POSTOPERATIVE CARE

In the postoperative period, all patients with diabetes must be closely monitored to prevent both hyperglycemia and hypoglycemia. As soon as possible, patients should resume their usual diets and regimens of insulin or oral hypoglycemic agents. Because of the increased risk of postoperative infection, wound care must be assiduous and devices such as Foley and vascular catheters should be removed as soon as possible. In patients at high risk for coronary events, postoperative electrocardiographic monitoring can be helpful to monitor for new changes. With careful glucose monitoring and insulin infusions as needed, patients with diabetes can safely undergo major surgical procedures.

TABLE 30–3. Continuous Intravenous Insulin Infusion (CIII) Method of Glucose Control

Prepare solution of 25 U of regular insulin in 250 mL of normal saline (1 U/10 mL).

Flush 50 mL of solution through line (insulin adsorbs to glass and tubing).

Piggyback solution to perioperative maintenance fluid, which should be 5% dextrose with 10–20 mEq of potassium chloride added to each liter, infused at 100–150 mL/h.

Monitor glucose every 30–60 minutes during intraoperative and postoperative periods.

Blood Glucose (mg/dL)	Insulin (U/h)
<80	0 (give dextrose, resume infusion)
81–100	0.5
101–140	1.0
141–180	1.5
181–220	2.0
221–260	2.5
261–300	3.0
301–400	4.0
>400	5.0

Give a subcutaneous dose of regular insulin 20–30 minutes before discontinuing CIII. This dose, which can vary substantially, depends on the original insulin requirement and the degree of insulin resistance.

TABLE 30–4. Traditional Method of Insulin Administration for Insulin-Requiring Type II Diabetes

On morning of surgery, give one half to one third the usual dose of intermediate-acting insulin.

Infuse dextrose 5% in water with 10–20 mEq of potassium chloride per liter at 100–150 mL/h.

Monitor blood glucose every 6 hours. Supplement with regular insulin. A representative scale follows:

Blood Glucose (mg/dL)	Regular Insulin (U) Subcutaneously q6h
<140	0
141–180	4
181–240	6
241–300	8
>300	10

REFERENCES

1. Gavin LA. Perioperative management of the diabetic patient. Endocrinol Metab Clin North Am 1992;21:457–475.
2. Hirsch IB, McGill JB. Role of insulin in management of surgical patients with diabetes mellitus. Diabetes Care 1990;13:980–991.
3. MacKenzie CR, Charlson ME. Assessment of perioperative risk in the patient with diabetes mellitus. Surg Gynecol Obstet 1988;167:293–299.
4. Pezzarossa A, Taddei F, Cimicchi MC, et al. Perioperative management of diabetic subjects. Diabetes Care 1988;11:52–58.
5. Schade DS. Surgery and diabetes. Med Clin North Am 1988;72:1531–1543.
6. Stagnero-Green A. Perioperative glucose control: does it really matter? Mt Sinai J Med 1991;58:299–304.

Medical Management of the Surgical Patient, Third Edition,
edited by Michael F. Lubin, H. Kenneth Walker, and Robert B. Smith III.
J.B. Lippincott Company, Philadelphia, PA © 1995.

CHAPTER

31

DISORDERS OF THE THYROID

Ruth M. Lawrence
Robert M. Walter, Jr.

Because thyroid hormones exert regulatory effects on multiple organ systems, thyroid function should be aggressively evaluated and abnormal function treated in patients who require surgery. Thyroid hormones also significantly affect the metabolism of many drugs, and dose adjustments may be required when function is abnormal. Medical consultants performing preoperative evaluations should always include clinical assessments of thyroid function and perform confirmatory tests when indicated.

The adult thyroid gland weighs 15 to 20 g, typically consists of two lobes connected by an isthmus, and is located just below the cricoid cartilage. A remnant of the thyroglossal duct, the pyramidal lobe may be noted arising superiorly from the isthmus or medial side of a lobe. Enlargement of the pyramidal lobe indicates a diffuse thyroidal abnormality. The thyroid gland consists of follicles, which are spheres lined by a single layer of cuboidal cells and filled with a colloid that is composed primarily of thyroglobulin. A rich capillary network surrounds the follicles, explaining why a bruit is sometimes heard over hyperactive, enlarged thyroid glands. Scattered throughout the thyroid are calcitonin-secreting perifollicular cells. Hyperplasia or malignant transformation of these cells does not result in abnormalities of thyroid function.

Inorganic iodide is actively transported from the blood into the follicular cells, immediately oxidized by peroxi-

dase, and rapidly incorporated into the tyrosine residues of thyroglobulin. These monoiodotyrosine and diiodotyrosine residues couple to form the iodothyronines thyroxine (T_4) and triiodothyronine (T_3), which are stored in the follicles. In response to thyroid-stimulating hormone (TSH), follicular cells extend pseudopods into the colloid and take it up by endocytosis. Subsequent hydrolysis of thyroglobulin in cellular lysosomes yields T_4 and, to a lesser extent, T_3, which are then secreted into the blood. Thyroid function is closely regulated by the hypothalamic-pituitary-thyroidal axis. Hypothalamic thyrotropin-releasing hormone (TRH) stimulates the synthesis and release of TSH. TSH secretion is modulated by negative feedback from T_3 produced in the pituitary by monodeiodination of T_4. The thyroid gland also exhibits autoregulation in response to iodine availability.

Only 0.03% of T_4 and 0.3% of T_3 circulates as free hormones. The remainder is bound to thyroid-binding globulin, T_4-binding prealbumin, and albumin. Virtually all circulating T_4 is secreted from the thyroid gland, whereas 85% of T_3 is derived from peripheral deiodination of T_4. Deiodination at the 5' and 5 positions on T_4 yields T_3 and the biologically inactive reverse T_3 (rT_3), respectively.

Although a wide range of tests is available for evaluating thyroid function, metabolic status can usually be evaluated economically. Tests may be classified as those that (1) measure products secreted by the thyroid, (2) evaluate the functional anatomy of the thyroid, (3) test the functional effects of thyroid hormones, (4) assess the hypothalamic-pituitary-thyroidal axis, and (5) measure antibodies to assist with pathologic diagnosis.

MEASURING THYROID PRODUCTS

The measurement of total T_4 by radioimmunoassay is an inexpensive, useful test. Because alterations in the concentration of thyroid-binding proteins affect total T_4, an indirect measurement of the free T_4 concentration, the in vitro T_3 resin uptake, is done at the same time. In this test, radiolabeled T_3 is added to the serum to be tested; the specimen is incubated briefly and an aliquot is then added to a thyroid hormone–binding resin. The fraction of the radiolabeled T_3 that is bound by the resin correlates inversely with the number of unbound sites on thyroid-binding proteins in the serum. A high T_3 resin uptake occurs in hyperthyroidism where thyroid binding proteins are saturated because of the secretion of more T_4, when binding sites are occupied by a competing substance such as salicylate, and when binding protein production is decreased (eg, cirrhosis, nephrotic syndrome, glucocorticoids, androgen therapy). A decrease in T_3 resin uptake is seen when less T_4 is secreted (hypothyroidism) and when the production of binding proteins is increased (eg, pregnancy, estrogen therapy, heroin abuse). Multiplication of the T_3 resin uptake by the total T_4 concentration provides an index of the free T_4. In recent years, direct measurement of the free T_4 by radioimmunoassay has been shown to reliably assess thyroid function and has replaced the free T_4 index in some laboratories. In severe nonthyroidal illness, problems of test interpretation exist with both methods and it may be necessary to perform both tests. The measurement of T_3 by radioimmunoassay is useful in those patients who appear to have hyperthyroidism but whose levels of total and free T_4 are normal (T_3 thyrotoxicosis). This test is less useful for the diagnosis of hypothyroidism because T_3 levels remain normal early in the course, and may be misleadingly low in acute or chronic nonthyroidal illness, trauma, and surgery because of inhibition of 5′-monodeiodinase. Measurement of rT_3 by radioimmunoassay is not often necessary but can help to differentiate severe nonthyroidal illness from hypothyroidism because levels are normal to increased in the former and decreased in the latter. Although thyroglobulin measured by radioimmunoassay is typically elevated in hyperthyroidism and subacute thyroiditis, this test is used mainly to monitor patients with thyroid cancer after total thyroidectomy; measurable levels in that situation suggest recurrent disease.

EVALUATING THYROID ANATOMY

Although the radioactive iodine uptake test is typically increased in hyperthyroidism and decreased in hypothyroidism, it is not commonly used for differentiation. A low radioactive iodine uptake test result accompanying hyperthyroidism suggests subacute thyroiditis, exogenous thyroid administration, resolving hyperthyroidism, struma ovarii, iodine-induced thyrotoxicosis, or functional thyroid cancer metastases after thyroidectomy. Radionuclide scanning with iodine or technetium isotopes provides information regarding the functional status of nodules and thyroid size but is not helpful with respect to metabolic status. Thyroid ultrasound does not give functional information but does define nodules to help determine whether they are cystic, mixed, or solid. Fine-needle aspiration of thyroid nodules has decreased the need for ultrasound and radionuclide scanning and is typically the first test performed in the evaluation of a thyroid nodule.

TESTING FUNCTIONAL EFFECTS OF THYROID HORMONES

Tests of biologic effects of thyroid hormone include the basal metabolic rate and photomotogram (measuring the speed of relaxation of the Achilles tendon reflex). Many nonthyroidal conditions affect the results and these tests are not commonly used. Increases in cholesterol, creatine phosphokinase, and lactic dehydrogenase may be seen in hypothyroidism, reflecting in part their prolonged plasma half-lives.

ASSESSING THE HYPOTHALAMIC-PITUITARY-THYROIDAL AXIS

The measurement of TSH by radioimmunoassay is of great utility in evaluating thyroid function. The new "supersensitive" assays distinguish hyperthyroidism as well as hypothyroidism from normal thyroid activity. A normal or low TSH accompanying hypothyroidism is evidence for hypothalamic or pituitary disease. The TRH stimulation test measuring the response of TSH assists in distinguishing hypothalamic from pituitary disease in such patients. In the past, the TRH stimulation test was used mainly to confirm the diagnosis of hyperthyroidism: a flat TSH response is seen in this condition. The supersensitive TSH assays have largely replaced the TRH test for this purpose.

MEASURING ANTIBODIES TO MAKE A PATHOLOGIC DIAGNOSIS

Marked elevations in serum antithyroglobulin and antimicrosomal antibodies suggest Hashimoto's thyroiditis and increase concern for hypothyroidism. The measurement of thyroid-stimulating immunoglobulins by cyclic adenosine monophosphate generation or TSH binding inhibition is helpful in the diagnosis and treatment of Graves' disease.

HYPERTHYROIDISM

Hyperthyroidism results from Graves' disease (the most common cause), toxic adenoma, toxic multinodular goiter, subacute thyroiditis, the hyperthyroid phase of Hashimoto's thyroiditis (reflecting overlap with Graves' disease), thyrotoxicosis factitia from exogenous hormone, and iodine-induced thyrotoxicosis. Rare causes include ovarian struma, hydatidiform mole, metastatic follicular carcinoma, and a TSH-producing adenoma. Measurement in serum of free T_4 or of the free T_4 index (total T_4 with T_3 resin uptake) plus a sensitive TSH should confirm the diagnosis. Serum T_3 is increased in hyperthyroidism but may be normal after iodine ingestion or when severe nonthyroidal illness is present. A flat TSH response to TRH is confirmatory when the TSH level is equivocal or sensitive measurements are not available. An increased serum thyroid-stimulating immunoglobulin level is seen with Graves' disease. In younger patients, the clinical presentation of hyperthyroidism is typically dramatic, with obvious signs of increased sympathetic activity. The diagnosis is often more subtle in elderly patients, who may be markedly apathetic, with weight loss, weakness, poor appetite, and congestive heart failure without tachyarrhythmias or goiter.

SURGERY IN PATIENTS WITH HYPERTHYROIDISM

The preoperative diagnosis and treatment of hyperthyroidism is of great importance to prevent tachyarrhythmias and life-threatening thyroid storm. If surgery is not emergent, patients should be rendered euthyroid. β-Adrenergic blockade provides prompt symptomatic relief but does not significantly affect thyroid hormone levels. Some β-blockers (eg, propranolol, alprenolol) block the peripheral conversion of T_4 to T_3 but the therapeutic importance of this is questionable and β-blockers without this action are equally effective. The risks and benefits of β-blockade must be weighed in patients with congestive heart failure or bronchospasm. Both propylthiouracil, 300 to 600 mg in three divided doses daily, and methimazole, 30 to 40 mg in two divided doses daily, are effective inhibitors of thyroid hormone synthesis. Propylthiouracil blocks peripheral conversion of T_4 to T_3 and is favored by some endocrinologists for this reason, but again, this effect may be of little clinical consequence. The decreased frequency of dosing required with methimazole may improve compliance. Propylthiouracil is preferred during pregnancy and nursing because it crosses the placenta one fourth as well as methimazole and enters breast milk one tenth as well. With adequate doses of antithyroid drugs, patients may be nearly euthyroid within 3 weeks. The clearance of β-blockers is increased in hyperthyroidism. Thus, dose reductions are needed as the euthyroid state is approached.

Emergent surgery in hyperthyroid patients requires a different approach. The antithyroid drugs that only block organification and thyroid hormone synthesis are ineffective because of their slow onset of action. β-Adrenergic blockade alone has been used successfully. If propranolol is selected, it should be given at the rate of 40 to 80 mg orally every 6 hours and continued after operation because fever, tachycardia, and thyroid storm can occur with inadequate dosing or too rapid discontinuation. Propranolol, 1 to 5 mg, can be given slowly by the intravenous route if time does not permit oral administration, and this should be continued every 6 hours as needed through the perioperative period.

Iodide should be used in conjunction with β-blockade in emergency preparation for surgery. Iodide acutely blocks the release of thyroid hormone from the gland as well as inhibits organification. A decline of T_4 levels to normal may be reached in a week using 10 drops of an oral saturated solution of potassium iodide or 1 g of intravenous sodium iodide daily. Recent experience with iodine-containing oral cholecystographic agents has shown them to be effective in treating hyperthyroidism. Sodium ipodate (Oragrafin) and iopanoic acid (Telepaque) have structural homology with T_4 and competitively inhibit 5'-monodeiodinase. A marked reduction in T_3 levels is seen with these agents in addition to the previously noted iodine effects. Future studies will better define their role in treatment.

Although they are not immediately effective, therapy with antithyroid drugs should be initiated in patients who are undergoing emergent surgery. The rectal route has been shown to provide adequate serum levels when oral administration is precluded. If patients develop signs of thyroid storm (eg, hyperthermia, vomiting, hypertension, tachycardia, altered mental state, impending vascular collapse), prompt treatment with β-blockers, iodide, antithyroid drugs, and glucocorticoids (hydrocortisone, 75 to 100 mg intravenously every 8 hours) is required. Glucocorticoids cover potential inadequate adrenal reserve as well as inhibit 5'-monodeiodinase, thereby lowering T_3 levels. Salicylates should not be used because they displace thyroid hormone from binding proteins, resulting in increased free levels. The diagnosis of thyroid storm is a clinical one. Thyroid hormone levels are not higher than those in hyperthyroidism without storm. Presumably, concomitant stress increases catecholamine levels, with a profound effect on the already increased β-adrenergic receptor activity characteristic of the hyperthyroid state.

HYPOTHYROIDISM

The clinical presentation of hypothyroidism ranges from mild symptoms of fatigue to myxedema coma. A higher index of suspicion of the disease is required in the elderly because many mild symptoms and signs of hypothyroidism may be attributed to the aging process per se. The diagnosis of hypothyroidism is made by measuring free T_4 or the free T_4 index and TSH. An increase in TSH precedes the decline in circulating thyroid hormone levels; a low TSH suggests a hypothalamic–pituitary cause. The most common cause of hypothyroidism, Hashimoto's thyroiditis, is associated with high levels of antimicrosomal and antithyroglobulin antibodies.

The results of thyroid hormone deficiency are varied and affect surgery. Cardiovascular manifestations include bradycardia, decreased cardiac output, atrioventricular conduction defects, and pericardial effusions. Respiratory effects include decreased alveolar ventilation because of blunted responsiveness to anoxia and hypercarbia, and pleural effusions. Decreased glomerular filtration and probable inappropriate release of antidiuretic hormone result in hyponatremia. Delayed gastric emptying and intestinal mobility can lead to abdominal distention and ileus. Women may have menorrhagia or amenorrhea. Decreased metabolism of administered drugs may lead to toxicity and trigger respiratory failure.

SURGERY IN PATIENTS WITH HYPOTHYROIDISM

When possible, surgery should be postponed until hypothyroidism can be corrected. Studies have shown a small increase in intraoperative hypotension and postoperative congestive heart failure, ileus, and confusion when patients were moderately hypothyroid. These studies support the need for close monitoring of respiratory status, attention to fluid balance, and cautious use of narcotics and sedatives. If surgical patients demonstrate signs of myxedema coma (eg, stupor, hypothermia, hypoventilation, hypoglycemia, hyponatremia, hypotension), emergency treatment is required. L-Thyroxine is given intravenously at a dosage of 400 µg. Glucocorticoids (hydrocortisone, 75 to 100 mg intravenously every 8 hours) are administered because relative adrenal insufficiency may be present (eg, hypopituitarism, coincident autoimmune Addison's disease). Because most patients with hypothyroidism do well in surgery, this vigorous treatment should not be routine. In young patients without evidence of cardiac disease, full replacement with L-thyroxine, 100 to 125 µg intravenously or orally per day, may be initiated and continued through the perioperative period. A 20% reduction in dose is appropriate when long-term parenteral administration is needed. When coronary artery disease is present, a starting dose of 25 µg/d is more appropriate; if angina or arrhythmias occur, the dose should be reduced. For patients undergoing coronary revascularization surgery, thyroid replacement is best not initiated. These patients do well with surgery and the replacement of thyroid hormone often increases angina and induces arrhythmias. If thyroid function tests are inconclusive or not available, and hypothyroidism is clinically suspected, it is prudent to treat patients with replacement doses of L-thyroxine and reevaluate when they are stable.

Patients who are euthyroid while receiving replacement therapy can be maintained on parenteral therapy through the perioperative period. Alternatively, interruption of thyroid replacement for as long as 1 week is not detrimental.

EFFECT OF SURGERY ON THYROID FUNCTION

Nonthyroidal surgery is associated with several changes in circulating thyroid hormone levels. Most profoundly, an abrupt decline in T_3 levels occurs within 24 hours as a result of inhibition of 5'-monodeiodinase. Reverse T_3 levels rise for the same reason. The effect on T_4 levels is less predictable but a decline is usually noted when the procedure is prolonged and associated with greater stress and extended fasting. Free T_4 and TSH levels are typically normal. These patients are considered to be euthyroid (the "euthyroid sick" syndrome) and should not be treated with thyroid hormone.

REFERENCES

1. Baeza A, Guayo J, Barria M, et al. Rapid preoperative preparation in hyperthyroidism. Clin Endocrinol (Oxf) 1991;35:439–442.
2. Geffner DL, Hershman JM. β-Adrenergic blockade for the treatment of hyperthyroidism. Am J Med 1992;93:61–68.
3. Hennessey JV, Evaul JE, Tseng Y, et al. L-thyroxine dosage: a

reevaluation of therapy with contemporary preparations. Ann Intern Med 1986;105:11–15.

4. Ladenson PW, Levin AA, Ridgeway EC, et al. Complications of surgery in hypothyroid patients. Am J Med 1984;77:261–266.

5. Robuschi G, Safran M, Braverman LE, et al. Hypothyroidism in the elderly. Endocrinol Rev 1987;8:142–153.

6. Walter RM, Bartle WR. Rectal administration of propylthiouracil in the treatment of Graves' disease. Am J Med 1990;88:69–70.

Medical Management of the Surgical Patient, Third Edition,
edited by Michael F. Lubin, H. Kenneth Walker, and Robert B. Smith III.
J.B. Lippincott Company, Philadelphia, PA © 1995.

CHAPTER

32

DISORDERS OF THE ADRENAL CORTEX

Ruth M. Lawrence
Robert M. Walter, Jr.

Serum cortisol levels rise within 30 minutes of the induction of anesthesia and remain elevated for hours to days in the face of postoperative stress. Because of cortisol's critical role in the successful handling of stress, a careful clinical assessment of adrenal function is necessary before surgery. Either deficiency or excess of cortisol can adversely affect surgical outcome. The physiology and metabolism of the adrenal cortex are briefly reviewed in this chapter to help clarify the appropriate selection of tests to verify a clinical diagnosis of an adrenal cortex disorder. The adrenal medulla is discussed in Chapter 33.

Human adult adrenal glands weigh 4 to 5 g each and reside in the retroperitoneal space superomedial to the kidneys. The cortex, of mesodermal origin, occupies the outer 90% of the gland. It consists of three concentric histologic zones, two of which have apparently identical function. The outermost zona glomerulosa produces aldosterone but, because it lacks 17α-hydroxylase activity, is unable to synthesize cortisol or androgens. The middle zona fasciculata is the largest area of the adrenal cortex, and the small innermost zona reticularis encircles the medulla. These two zonae produce cortisol, androgens, and small amounts of estrogen but lack the 18-hydroxysteroid dehydrogenase required for aldosterone synthesis. Histologic evidence suggests that the zona fasciculata responds to acute adrenocorticotropic hormone (ACTH) stimulation, whereas the zona reticularis responds to prolonged stimulation.

Adrenal steroid synthesis is controlled by the hypothalamic-pituitary-adrenal axis. Hypothalamic corticotropin-releasing hormone (CRH) is released in response to stress and induces the release of ACTH from the anterior pituitary. ACTH release is episodic and exhibits a circadian rhythm, with levels highest in the morning (peaking about 8 hours after the onset of sleep) and lowest in the afternoon. The synthesis of all steroid hormones, including glucocorticoids (eg, cortisol) and adrenal androgens (eg, androstenedione), begins with cholesterol. The rate-limiting step in both cortisol and adrenal androgen synthesis is the conversion of cholesterol to pregnenolone within the mitochondria, and it is here that ACTH exerts its main adrenal effects.

Cortisol synthesis proceeds through several microsomal enzymatic steps, the final being the hydroxylation in mitochondria of 11-deoxycortisol to cortisol. Feedback inhibition by cortisol of both CRH and ACTH is the final regulator of cortisol secretion. Cortisol is the most important glucocorticoid in humans. As a group, glucocorticoids are defined as those hormones that exert their effects by binding to glucocorticoid-specific cytosolic receptors. These receptors, which are present in most tissues, enter the nucleus after binding with the hormone and bind to specific areas in nuclear DNA to initiate the glucocorticoid response.

Glucocorticoids have multiple actions. They increase cardiac output and peripheral vascular tone. Deficiency can result in refractory shock in the stressed state, whereas excess can cause hypertension. Glucocorticoids stimulate hepatic gluconeogenesis, glycogen storage, lipolysis, and proteolysis—effects that protect against hypoglycemia in the fasted state. An excess of glucocorticoids can lead to hyperglycemia. All glucocorticoids increase glomerular filtration, and those with mineralocorticoid activity (eg, cortisol) cause sodium retention, hypokalemia, and hypertension. Excess glucocorticoids inhibit connective tissue and bone formation, decrease gastrointestinal absorption of calcium, and increase calciuria. Glucocorticoids increase intravascular polymorphonuclear leukocytes yet decrease circulating lymphocytes, monocytes, and eosinophils. Both excess and deficiency of glucocorticoids have major effects on the central nervous system.

The most important adrenal androgens are dehydroepiandrosterone (DHEA), DHEA sulfate, and androstenedione. Although DHEA and DHEA sulfate are present in larger amounts, androstenedione is of greater biologic significance because of its ready conversion to the potent androgen, testosterone. Adrenal androgen synthesis in adults is stimulated by ACTH; both DHEA and androstenedione exhibit diurnal variation with ACTH but the long plasma half-life of DHEA sulfate precludes this. The physiologic effects of adrenal androgens in adult men are inconsequential. In women, however, in whom the adrenals supply roughly 50% of premenopausal and all postmenopausal androgens, excess adrenal production results in acne, hirsutism, and virilization.

The production of aldosterone by the adrenal cortex is controlled primarily by the renin–angiotensin system and secondarily by ACTH. Acute increases in serum potassium, depletion of body sodium, and renin production by the kidneys are also potent stimulators of aldosterone production. Excess production is manifested by hypertension, hypokalemia, suppression of the renin system, and normal to low cortisol secretion.

ADRENAL INSUFFICIENCY

Because a patient's response to the stress associated with surgery requires adequate adrenal reserves, it is critical that adrenal insufficiency be diagnosed and treated before operation. Medical consultants should always inquire about any use of glucocorticoids in patients who are about to undergo surgery. Although the inhaled steroids used to treat obstructive pulmonary disease are usually not associated with adrenal suppression, high doses of these drugs can result in suppression that is sufficient to require the perioperative administration of systemic glucocorticoids.

In the United States, 80% of primary adrenocortical insufficiency (Addison's disease) is a result of autoimmune adrenalitis. This is often associated with other autoimmune disorders, including Hashimoto's thyroiditis, Graves' disease, type I diabetes mellitus, premature ovarian failure, hypoparathyroidism, and, rarely, testicular failure. Associated nonendocrine conditions include mucocutaneous candidiasis, vitiligo, alopecia, pernicious anemia, and chronic active hepatitis. Worldwide, tuberculosis remains the most common cause of Addison's disease; it is the second most common cause in the United States. Rare causes include hemorrhage (a risk of anticoagulant therapy), fungal infections, tumor metastases, surgical adrenalectomy, radiation, amyloidosis, sarcoidosis, hemochromatosis, congenital enzyme defects, and medications (eg, metyrapone, ketoconazole, aminoglutethimide, etopamide, mitotane).

The most common cause of secondary adrenal insufficiency is ACTH deficiency resulting from exogenous glucocorticoid therapy. The administration of replacement doses of glucocorticoids (ie, 5 mg of prednisone or 20 mg of hydrocortisone daily) for more than 2 weeks is sufficient to suppress the hypothalamic-pituitary-adrenal axis. Subnormal cortisol responses to stimuli can persist for as long as 1 year after the discontinuation of glucocorticoid therapy. Pituitary recovery precedes adrenal recovery by months. Endogenous secondary adrenal insufficiency is most commonly caused by pituitary or hypothalamic tumors.

Patients with primary adrenal insufficiency are weak and fatigued. Appetite is decreased despite increased taste and smell sensation; nausea, vomiting, and weight loss are common. Hyperpigmentation, hyponatremia, and fasting hypoglycemia (especially in children) can occur. Because of the associated mineralocorticoid deficiency, volume depletion with orthostatic hypotension, hyperkalemia, and acidosis occur. Acute adrenal crisis is characterized by fever, volume depletion with refractory hypotension, nausea, weakness, depressed mentation, and hypoglycemia. Patients with secondary adrenocortical insufficiency have most of the same symptoms but are not hyperpigmented because the production of ACTH and β-lipotropin is reduced. Because their aldosterone production is typically intact, they do not have volume depletion, hyperkalemia, or acidosis. Hyponatremia from impaired excretion of water does occur, and there is the potential for hypotension with a stress-induced crisis.

Primary adrenal insufficiency is best diagnosed with the ACTH stimulation test. A normal serum cortisol response (at least 18 μg/dL 30 to 60 minutes after a 250-μg dose of intravenous or intramuscular synthetic ACTH [cosyntropin]) excludes the diagnosis. To rule out the diagnosis of Addison's disease in patients who have been receiving glucocorticoids, several daily doses of synthetic ACTH or a 6-hour infusion of ACTH may be needed to achieve a normal cortisol response because of superimposed secondary adrenal insufficiency. Although it is not routinely measured, an aldosterone response to ACTH is evidence against primary adrenal insufficiency. Plasma ACTH and β-lipotropin levels are typically elevated in untreated primary adrenal insufficiency. In secondary adrenal insufficiency, the serum cortisol response to ACTH is frequently blunted but can be normal.

Hypothalamic-pituitary-adrenal axis function can be evaluated by the overnight metyrapone test. After bedtime administration of 30 mg/kg of oral metyrapone, an agent that blocks the conversion of 11-deoxycortisol to cortisol, blood levels of serum cortisol and 11-deoxycortisol are measured at 8:00 AM the next day. A cortisol level of less than 5 μg/dL indicates that the level of blockade was adequate, and a marked increase (80-fold) in 11-deoxycortisol confirms that the adrenal response was normal.

Alternatively, the hypothalamic-pituitary-adrenal axis can be tested with insulin-induced hypoglycemia. After the intravenous injection of 0.1 U/kg of regular insulin, a serum glucose nadir occurs in 20 to 30 minutes. The serum cortisol should increase to more than 18 μg/dL 30 to 60 minutes after the glucose nadir. Because of the potential morbidity of hypoglycemia, this test requires the presence of a physician and should not be performed in the elderly or in patients with significant cardiovascular or cerebrovascular disease. Measurement of plasma ACTH and serum cortisol after CRH administration has been disappointing in distinguishing between hypothalamic and pituitary disease. Predictably, the ACTH response to CRH is exaggerated in primary adrenal insufficiency.

Adrenal insufficiency is treated with steroid replacement. For primary adrenal insufficiency, maintenance doses are 20 to 30 mg/d of hydrocortisone in at least two divided doses or 5 to 7.5 mg/d of prednisone in a single or divided dose. Patients who are also receiving drugs such as rifampin, barbiturates, and phenytoin, which induce hepatic metabolism of glucocorticoids, may require modest increases in the glucocorticoid dosage. The necessity for mineralocorticoid replacement with Florinef (9α-fluorocortisol) at a dosage of 0.05 to 0.2 mg/d is determined by assessment of the blood pressure and serum potassium level. Patients are instructed to increase their dosages of glucocorticoids two- to four-fold when they are experiencing stress and to notify their physicians if symptoms persist. Surgery represents a major form of stress and patients should receive maximal stress doses (10 times the maintenance dose, or 300 mg of hydrocortisone per day) in the perioperative period. The first dose of 100 mg of hydrocortisone should be given at least 1 hour before the induction of anesthesia and the dose should be repeated every 8 hours for at least 24 hours (longer when major stress persists after operation). The intravenous route is preferable because intramuscular medication may be absorbed erratically. Daily doses of hydrocortisone exceeding 50 to 60 mg supply adequate mineralocorticoid replacement but comparable doses of methylprednisolone and dexamethasone do not share

this degree of mineralocorticoid activity. Blood pressure, electrolyte, and glucose measurements, as well as fluid status, must be carefully monitored. If patients develop any signs suggestive of acute adrenal crisis, intravenous hydrocortisone at a dosage of 300 mg/d (100 mg every 8 hours) plus glucose and saline infusions must be given emergently. Once the acute stress has passed, patients can be weaned over several days to maintenance doses. Patients with secondary adrenal insufficiency should also receive these doses of intravenous glucocorticoids perioperatively and be tapered to their usual oral dosages when possible. Table 32-1 outlines the perioperative management of adrenocortical insufficiency.

CUSHING'S SYNDROME

The most common cause of Cushing's syndrome (the term for any state characterized by increased glucocorticoid effect) is exogenous glucocorticoid administration, which results in pituitary adrenal suppression. Cushing's disease, adrenal hyperplasia resulting from excess pituitary production of ACTH, is the cause of 70% of all cases of endogenous Cushing's syndrome. A pituitary adenoma is identified in most cases. Autonomous adrenal hyperfunction resulting from an adrenal adenoma or carcinoma, and ectopic production of ACTH by tumors (especially small cell carcinomas of the lung) each account for about 15% of all cases of endogenous Cushing's syndrome. Common signs and symptoms include obesity, facial plethora, hirsutism, menstrual irregularities, hypertension, proximal muscle weakness, back pain, and skin striae. Psychologic symptoms (eg, euphoria, mania, psychosis) are probably underreported. Patients with ectopic ACTH production have fewer chronic signs of glucocorticoid excess but demonstrate more mineralocorticoid effect with hypertension and hypokalemia associated with weight loss. Adrenal carcinomas often

TABLE 32–1. Perioperative Management of Adrenal Insufficiency

Inquire about any preoperative use of glucocorticoids (systemic or inhaled) and symptoms suggestive of adrenal insufficiency.

Administer hydrocortisone (hemisuccinate or phosphate) 100 mg intravenously q8h. Give first dose at least 1 h before induction of anesthesia.

Once the patient is stable after operation, taper the hydrocortisone dose over 3–4 days to maintenance levels (30 mg/d in at least two divided doses) or to the patient's preoperative dose of glucocorticoid.

Prevent volume depletion and hypoglycemia with the use of intravenous saline and glucose.

are accompanied by signs of marked androgenicity as well as glucocorticoid effect.

The two screening tests for Cushing's syndrome are the 1-mg overnight dexamethasone suppression of serum cortisol and measurement of the 24-hour urinary free cortisol. Suppression of the morning serum cortisol level to less than 5 μg/dL after the administration of 1 mg of oral dexamethasone and the presence of normal secretion of urine cortisol both are strong evidence against abnormal cortisol secretion. High-dose dexamethasone (2 mg orally every 6 hours for 48 hours) suppresses serum cortisol in the face of Cushing's disease but not adrenal tumors. Serum ACTH levels are low with adrenal tumors, normal to slightly elevated in Cushing's disease, and often markedly elevated with ectopic production. Metyrapone and CRH administration each induce exaggerated ACTH responses in Cushing's disease but have little effect in other causes of Cushing's syndrome.

Therapy for Cushing's disease involves removal of the pituitary or adrenal tumor. Cure rates for pituitary microadenomas are very good and the transsphenoidal surgery itself has low morbidity and mortality. Transient postoperative diabetes insipidus can occur. Complications after the resection of cortisol-producing adrenal tumors are more frequent and include wound infection, bleeding, pulmonary embolism, and respiratory infections. After surgery, a period of secondary adrenal insufficiency ensues. Unfortunately, adrenal carcinoma is often widely metastatic at the time of presentation, and the prognosis is poor. When surgical resection is not possible, medical therapy with ketoconazole, metyrapone, aminoglutethimide, or mitotane may be useful to decrease cortisol levels.

Patients with Cushing's syndrome have an increased incidence of hypertension, cardiovascular disease, diabetes mellitus, thromboembolism, delayed wound healing, and increased susceptibility to infection. Despite this increased risk of operative complications, emergent surgery can usually be safely performed in the face of hypercortisolism. If surgery can be postponed, the carefully monitored use of one or more of the agents mentioned above to control hypercortisolism may be of benefit in reducing surgical complications. After operation, patients must be observed for evidence of steroid withdrawal symptoms, which may require replacement steroids that are then slowly tapered.

PRIMARY ALDOSTERONISM

Primary aldosteronism is manifested by hypertension, increased aldosterone levels, low plasma renin levels, metabolic alkalosis, and hypokalemia. In about two thirds of pa-

tients, it results from a unilateral adrenal adenoma; in the remainder, idiopathic hyperplasia is the usual cause. Adrenal carcinoma is an extremely rare cause. Adenomas are treated with adrenalectomy of the affected side, which cures about three fourths of patients. Before operation, sodium restriction and a potassium-sparing diuretic such as spironolactone are used to correct the electrolyte abnormalities and hypertension. It is preferable to treat medically for 1 to 2 months before surgery to reduce the incidence of postoperative complications. After surgery, electrolyte concentrations and blood pressure must be monitored. Recovery of the renin–aldosterone system may take many months but normal function is the usual outcome.

HYPOALDOSTERONISM

Aldosterone deficiency without concomitant glucocorticoid deficiency is usually hyporeninemic hypoaldosteronism and rarely results from a primary abnormality of the adrenal cortex. Diabetes mellitus and tubulointerstitial renal disease are disorders that can be associated with decreased renin secretion, leading to subsequent hypoangiotensinemia and low aldosterone levels. The mineralocorticoid deficiency is manifested by hyperkalemia, hyperchloremic metabolic acidosis, and occasional sodium depletion. Most patients with hyporeninemic hypoaldosteronism are asymptomatic but hyperkalemia can lead to arrhythmias. Treatment with furosemide, 40 to 120 mg/d, helps relieve hyperkalemia and metabolic acidosis, although hypotension may be induced. This is typically combined with Florinef, which increases renal potassium and hydrogen ion excretion and causes salt retention. Correction of hyporeninemic hypoaldosteronism is desirable before surgery to prevent potential complications.

REFERENCES

1. Angermeier KW, Montie JE. Perioperative complications of adrenal surgery. Urol Clin North Am 1989;16:597–606.
2. Blichert-Toft M, Christiansen V, Enquist A, et al. Influence of age on the endocrine-metabolic response to surgery. Ann Surg 1979;190:751–770.
3. Chin R. Adrenal crisis. Crit Care Clin 1991;7:23–42.
4. Cook DM. Safe use of glucocorticoids. Postgrad Med 1992;91:145–154.
5. Lindholm J, Kehlet H. Re-evaluation of the clinical value of the 30 minute ACTH test in assessing the hypothalamic-pituitary-adrenocortical function. Clin Endocrinol (Oxf) 1987;26:53–59.

6. Novick AC. Surgery for primary hyperaldosteronism. Urol Clin North Am 1989;16:535–545.

7. Oelkers W, Diederich S, Bahr V. Diagnosis and therapy surveillance in Addison's disease: rapid adrenocorticotrophin (ACTH) test and measurement of plasma ACTH, renin activity, and aldosterone. J Clin Endocrinol Metab 1992;75:259–263.

8. Wagner RL, White PF, Kan PB, et al. Inhibition of adrenal steroidogenesis by the anesthetic etomidate. N Engl J Med 1984; 310:1415–1421.

Medical Management of the Surgical Patient, Third Edition,
edited by Michael F. Lubin, H. Kenneth Walker, and Robert B. Smith III.
J.B. Lippincott Company, Philadelphia, PA © 1995.

CHAPTER

33

PHEOCHROMOCYTOMA

Ruth M. Lawrence
Robert M. Walter, Jr.

Although pheochromocytomas are not a common medical/surgical problem (they are estimated to cause only 0.1% to 0.5% of all cases of hypertension, and are operated on only once or twice per year in most centers), medical consultants are likely to be asked to evaluate and prepare for surgery patients with suspected pheochromocytomas at some time during their careers. Because catecholamines have major regulatory effects on many different body systems, it is vital that these be anticipated and properly managed in the perioperative period. Pheochromocytomas are associated with an increased risk of adverse reactions to many commonly prescribed drugs and clinicians must also be aware of this potential hazard.

PATHOPHYSIOLOGY

Pheochromocytomas arise from chromaffin cells of the neural crest that migrate to form the adult adrenal medulla and sympathetic ganglia. These cells synthesize catecholamines through a series of enzymatically controlled steps, starting with the conversion of tyrosine to dihydroxyphenylalanine (dopa) by tyrosine hydroxylase. This is the rate-limiting step in catecholamine synthesis. Dopa is then converted to dopamine, which is subsequently decarboxylated to norepinephrine. The methylation of norepinephrine to epinephrine is accomplished through the action of phenylethanolamine-N-methyl transferase, an enzyme that is induced by glucocorticoids that reach the adrenal medulla in high concentrations through the corticomedullary venous sinuses from the adrenal cortex. Norepinephrine and epinephrine are the major products of most pheochromocytomas. Epinephrine is produced mainly in the adrenal medulla; thus, a pheochromocytoma that produces epinephrine is nearly always located in the adrenal. Norepinephrine is produced and secreted in the central nervous system and the sympathetic postganglionic nerve endings as well as in the adrenal medulla. Dopamine is also produced and secreted by some pheochromocytomas. Once catecholamines reach the plasma, they have a half-life of only 1 to 2 minutes before they are taken up by cells or enzymatically degraded. Metanephrine, normetanephrine, and vanillylmandelic acid are the major metabolites.

Catecholamines bind to adrenergic and dopaminergic cell-surface receptors, which in turn induce second messengers. Norepinephrine is primarily an α-adrenergic agonist that causes vasoconstriction and hypertension with little metabolic activity. Epinephrine, a β-adrenergic agonist, has positive inotropic and chronotropic effects on the heart and causes vasodilation. Its metabolic effects include inhibition of insulin secretion and stimulation of glycogenolysis in the liver. Hypersecretion of catecholamines has many dramatic physiologic effects. In contrast, adrenal medullary hypofunction is not clinically significant because norepinephrine is available from other sources.

DIAGNOSIS

Nearly 90% of pheochromocytomas in adults occur in the adrenal medulla. Of those that occur outside the adrenal, 9% are found in the abdomen, 1% in the chest, and 1% in the urinary bladder. The incidence of pheochromocytoma is increased in neuroectodermal dysplasias such as tuberous sclerosis, Sturge-Weber syndrome; and von Recklinghausen's disease, and in multiple endocrine neoplasia type IIA (pheochromocytoma, medullary carcinoma of the thyroid, and hyperparathyroidism) and type IIB (pheochromocytoma, medullary carcinoma of the thyroid, and mucosal neuromas). In multiple endocrine neoplasia, the incidence of bilateral adrenal tumors increases. Because nearly all pheochromocytomas are functional and produce high levels of catecholamines, a wide variety of symptoms and signs can occur. Hypertension is the most common feature and, despite the emphasis usually placed on the intermittent nature of pheochromocytoma symptoms, is more likely to be sustained than intermittent. Only about half of all patients have the classic paroxysmal symptoms of headache, pallor, palpitations, and sweating associated with hypertension. Orthostasis is frequent. The sudden onset of hypertension in a previously normotensive person, especially occurring during the induction of anesthesia, should suggest the possibility of pheochromocytoma. Other reported symptoms include a sense of doom or apprehension, anxiety, trembling, mild abdominal pain, and constipation. Less common presentations include intestinal pseudoobstruction and ileus, cardiomyopathy, Prinzmetal's coronary spasm, and peripheral vascular spasm. In elderly patients, symptoms may be less marked because of the decline in sensitivity to catecholamines that occurs with advanced age. A serious complication of pheochromocytoma is myocarditis and subsequent congestive heart failure. Infiltrates of histiocytes, plasma cells, and other inflammatory cells are seen in the myocardium on postmortem studies.

Few physical findings suggest pheochromocytoma other than hypertension. In the associated endocrine neoplasias and neuroectodermal disorders, thyroid enlargement, neurofibromas, or café au lait spots may be present.

The diagnosis of pheochromocytoma is made by documenting the excess secretion of catecholamines. These can be measured in blood or urine. Plasma levels of norepinephrine and epinephrine must be obtained under carefully controlled conditions with patients in the supine position and as free of stress as possible because the venipuncture itself can cause levels to be falsely elevated. Urinary catecholamines are also prone to false-positive and false-nega-tive results from numerous interfering substances, including decongestants; several antibiotics (chloramphenicol, nalidixic acid, tetracycline, and erythromycin); antihypertensives (reserpine, guanethidine, and methyldopa); and amphetamines. The usual screening tests are 24-hour measurements of urinary metanephrines, vanillylmandelic acid, and catecholamines. Metanephrine levels are less likely to be elevated by psychic stress and other conditions. The failure of 0.3 mg of oral clonidine to reduce plasma levels of norepinephrine in patients with hypertension is suggestive of pheochromocytoma. Provocative tests for catecholamine release, such as histamine or glucagon stimulation, have high rates of morbidity and even mortality, and have largely been abandoned.

Once the diagnosis of pheochromocytoma is suspected, the tumor must be localized. The use of computed tomography or magnetic resonance imaging has supplanted angiography for this purpose. Computed tomography is extremely sensitive for lesions greater than 1.0 cm but is less helpful in distinguishing types of intraadrenal masses or localizing extraadrenal tumors. On magnetic resonance scanning, pheochromocytomas appear hyperintense on T2-weighted images, allowing them to be differentiated from nonfunctioning adenomas. Extraadrenal pheochromocytomas are easier to identify on magnetic resonance scanning. The radionuclides, ^{131}I-metaiodobenzylguanidine or ^{125}I-metaiodobenzylguanidine, are taken up by adrenergic granules and are useful in localizing intraadrenal and extraadrenal tumors.

PERIOPERATIVE MANAGEMENT

Surgery is the preferred therapy for pheochromocytoma but patients must be carefully prepared before operation to prevent severe hypertensive crises and arrhythmias induced by the procedure. Careful planning and cooperation among internists, anesthesiologists, and surgeons are essential. Because most tumors secrete norepinephrine, the most important aspect of preoperative therapy is α-adrenergic blockade to lower the blood pressure, prevent paroxysms of severe hypertension, and replace intravascular volume. Oral phenoxybenzamine or prazosin is usually given. Phenoxybenzamine has a half-life of 36 hours but prazosin has a shorter half-life and can be titrated more rapidly. Whenever possible, α-blockade should be started at least 2 weeks before surgery to allow normalization of the decreased intravascular volume. If acute α-blockade is necessary, intravenous phentolamine or nitroprusside can be used. β-Blockade is occasionally necessary to control tachyarrhythmias but should be used only after adequate α-blockade is established. Propranolol is preferred because it has a short half-life and can be given intravenously if necessary.

The goal of preoperative therapy is to control hypertension without causing symptomatic postural hypotension. Metyrosine (α-methyl p-tyrosine) is a catecholamine analogue that inhibits tyrosine hydroxylase and catecholamine synthesis. This can be administered before operation but has several severe side effects, including crystalluria, extrapyramidal symptoms, and dystonia. This agent is usually given only when symptoms and signs cannot be controlled with other medications. Table 33-1 outlines suggested regimens for perioperative management.

Meticulous intraoperative control of the blood pressure, heart rate, and fluid status is essential for a good outcome. Because complete adrenergic blockade is neither obtainable nor desirable, catecholamine release during the procedure must be anticipated and managed. Hemodynamic monitoring is done with an intraarterial catheter and a central venous line with a Swan-Ganz catheter. Volume management is critical. Thiopental, nitrous oxide, and enflurane or

TABLE 33–1. Suggested Regimens for Perioperative Management of a Patient with Pheochromocytoma

Preoperative Considerations
α-Adrenergic blockade
10–14 days before surgery, begin treatment
　Phenoxybenzamine, 10 mg twice a day; increase to maximum
　　of 40 mg once a day
　　　or
　Prazosin, 1 mg twice a day; increase to maximum of 5 mg
　　three times a day
β-Adrenergic blockade
After α-adrenergic blockade is established, if tachyarrhythmias
　occur, give propranolol, 10 mg three times a day; increase to
　maximum of 80 mg three times a day

Considerations for Intraoperative Monitoring and Management
Electrocardiogram
Arterial catheter
Central venous access using Swan-Ganz catheter
To control paroxysms of hypertension
　Intravenous phentolamine, 0.5- to 1-mg bolus every 3–5 minutes
　　as needed
　　　or
　Sodium nitroprusside, 250-μg bolus or 1–5 μg/kg/min
To reverse hypotension
　Volume expanders
　Norepinephrine infusion
For tachyarrhythmias
　Lidocaine infusion
　Propranolol by bolus or infusion if α-blockade established

Postoperative Complications to Be Anticipated
Hypotension
Hypoglycemia
Bronchospasm

TABLE 33–2. Drugs With Potential Hazard in Pheochromocytoma

Histamine-Induced Catecholamine Release
Antihistamines
Opiates
Plasma expanders

Potentiation of Pressor Effect of Catecholamines
Adrenal steroids
Atropine
β-Blockers
Bretylium
Monoamine oxidase inhibitors
Metoclopramide
Phenylpropanolamine and other decongestants
Tricyclic antidepressants

Potentiation of Arrhythmias
Inhalational anesthetics, such as cyclopropane and halothane
Digoxin (theoretic, avoid concomitant use)
Thyroid hormone (through increase in number of β-receptors)

Increase of Release of Catecholamines, Inhibition of Reuptake
Amphetamines
Cocaine
Marijuana

isoflurane are the usual anesthetic agents. If severe hypertension accompanies intubation or manipulation of the tumor, nitroprusside infusions or the administration of boluses of phentolamine may be required for blood pressure control. Once the tumor is removed, hypotension can occur, requiring liberal use of volume expanders.

After operation, close monitoring must be continued and all the complications of any large intraabdominal procedure anticipated. In addition, several problems unique to pheochromocytoma may occur. Severe hypotension requires the replacement of large volumes of intravenous fluids and, occasionally, intravenous norepinephrine for control; severe hypoglycemia requires intravenous glucose replacement. Bronchospasm can recur in patients with asthma who were asymptomatic before the surgical procedure, requiring the use of inhaled bronchodilators for relief. In experienced surgical hands, the outcome should be good, with a surgical mortality of under 2%.

Numerous drugs, some of which may be used in the perioperative period, can cause adverse effects because of increased release of catecholamines from the tumor or peripheral stores, interference with neuronal uptake of catecholamines, or increased sensitivity to catecholamine effects. Table 33-2 lists some of the drugs that have the potential to cause adverse reactions in the presence of pheochromocytoma.

Catecholamine levels fall quickly after surgery but may

not return to completely normal levels for 2 weeks or longer because of peripheral stores and postoperative stress. High levels after this time suggest residual tumor. Some patients may have continued hypertension, especially those who had long-standing blood pressure elevations before surgery. A search for other causes of hypertension should be undertaken because essential hypertension and renal vascular hypertension have been reported in patients with pheochromocytoma.

REFERENCES

1. Angermeir KW, Montie JE. Perioperative complications of adrenal surgery. Urol Clin North Am 1989;16:597–606.
2. Boutros AR, Bravo EL, Zanettin G, Straffon RA. Perioperative management of 63 patients with pheochromocytoma. Cleve Clin J Med 1990;57:613–617.
3. Bretan PN, Lorig R. Adrenal imaging: computed tomographic scanning and magnetic resonance scanning. Urol Clin North Am 1989;16:505–513.
4. Greene JP, Guay AT. New perspectives in pheochromocytoma. Urol Clin North Am 1989;16:487–503.
5. Malone MJ, Libertino JA, Tsapatsaris NP, Woods BO. Preoperative and surgical management of pheochromocytoma. Urol Clin North Am 1989;16:567–582.
6. Proye CAG, Carnaille BM, Flament JBE, et al. Intraoperative radionuclear ^{125}I-labeled metaiodobenzylguanidine scanning of pheochromocytomas and metastases. Surgery 1992;111:634–639.
7. Robertson D, Oates JA, Berman ML. Preoperative and anesthetic management of pheochromocytoma. In: Scott HW, ed. Surgery of the adrenal glands. Philadelphia, JB Lippincott, 1989:225–239.
8. Scott HW, Van Way CW, Gray GF, Sussman CR. Pheochromocytoma. In: Scott HW, ed. Surgery of the adrenal glands. Philadelphia, JB Lippincott, 1989:187–223.
9. Stoelting RK, Dierdorf SF. Endocrine disease. In: Anesthesia and co-existing disease, ed 3. New York, Churchill Livingstone, 1993:339–373.

Medical Management of the Surgical Patient, Third Edition,
edited by Michael F. Lubin, H. Kenneth Walker, and Robert B. Smith III.
J.B. Lippincott Company, Philadelphia, PA © 1995.

CHAPTER

34

DISORDERS OF CALCIUM METABOLISM

Ruth M. Lawrence
Robert M. Walter, Jr.

Both hypercalcemia and hypocalcemia may be associated with life-threatening cardiac arrhythmias as well as morbidity affecting other organ systems. Effective treatment is available and clinicians should be alert to abnormalities in serum calcium, which are present in more than 2% of hospitalized patients. Furthermore, both hypercalcemia and hypocalcemia suggest significant underlying pathology, and efforts to diagnose and treat these conditions should be instituted.

Adult humans contain more than 1 kg of calcium, of which over 99% is skeletal and dental and only 0.1% is in extracellular fluids. About half the calcium in serum is bound to protein, primarily albumin. Decreases in serum albumin are accompanied by decreases in calcium (a drop of 1 g/dL of albumin lowers the calcium by about 0.8 mg/dL). Several calcium determinations and measurement of ionized (physiologically active) calcium levels may be needed to accurately assess calcium status.

Serum ionized calcium levels are tightly controlled by the interplay of parathyroid hormone, calcitonin, and 1,25-dihydroxycholecalciferol (1,25-[OH]$_2$D$_3$). Parathyroid hormone is synthesized in the parathyroid glands and, after cleavage of precursor molecules, is released into the circulation as an 84–amino-acid polypeptide and smaller fragments.

The amino-terminal 1-34 amino acids compose the biologically active portion of the molecule. Highly specific immunoradiometric assays are available that measure the intact hormone, permitting accurate diagnosis. Parathyroid hormone release is primarily controlled by serum calcium levels, although modest hypomagnesemia also evokes a parathyroid hormone response, whereas severe hypomagnesemia impairs release. Parathyroid hormone increases serum calcium by increasing bone resorption, decreasing calciuria, and indirectly increasing gastrointestinal absorption of calcium by its effects on the production of 1,25-(OH)$_2$D$_3$ and stimulation of the vitamin D–dependent calcium pump. Calcitonin is synthesized in the thyroidal perifollicular cells in response to hypercalcemia. Calcitonin directly inhibits bone resorption and may indirectly increase calciuria. The physiologic importance of calcitonin in humans is questioned. The renal synthesis of 1,25-(OH)$_2$D$_3$ from 25-(OH)D$_3$ is regulated directly by serum levels of parathyroid hormone and phosphate and, at least indirectly, by serum calcium. This sterol hormone increases intestinal absorption of calcium and phosphorus and is critical for normal mineralization of osteoid.

HYPERCALCEMIA

Hypercalcemia affects the function of many organs. When it is severe, hypercalcemia can cause decreased cardiac automatism with resultant arrhythmias and heart block. Effects of digitalis are exaggerated. Gastrointestinal symptoms include anorexia, nausea, vomiting, constipation, and ileus. Prolonged hypercalcemia may be associated with peptic ulcer disease and pancreatitis. Affected patients may exhibit polyuria and polydipsia resulting from reversible nephrogenic diabetes insipidus. Acute and chronic renal failure with nephrolithiasis and nephrocalcinosis may occur. Neuropsychiatric symptoms include poor concentration and memory, weakness, lethargy, depression, coma, and, rarely, psychosis.

Causes of hypercalcemia are listed in Table 34-1. The most common cause is primary hyperparathyroidism. Prolonged duration of hypercalcemia, hypophosphatemia, and hyperchloremic acidosis suggest the diagnosis, which usually can be easily confirmed by measuring intact parathyroid hormone levels with specific immunoradiometric assays.

The next most common (and most common inpatient) cause is hypercalcemia associated with malignancy. This is believed to virtually always have a systemic or local osseous humoral cause. The most common cause of solid tumor hypercalcemia is excessive elaboration of parathyroid hormone–related protein. This protein, which is a product of many normal tissues, has substantial homology with the amino-terminal end of parathyroid hormone and binds to

the same receptor. It can be measured by specific assays that do not measure parathyroid hormone, permitting laboratory distinction between these two common causes of hypercalcemia. The hypercalcemia of malignancy may also be mediated by various cytokines, including lymphotoxin, interleukin-1, and tumor necrosis factor, and by tumorous production of $1,25\text{-}(OH)_2D_3$ or prostaglandins.

Familial hypocalciuric hypercalcemia may be difficult to discern from hyperparathyroidism. Parathyroid hormone levels are typically not elevated yet are not appropriately suppressed. Lack of tissue damage, onset in childhood, family history, and low urinary calcium levels should help with the diagnosis. Although parathyroidectomy is the usual therapy for primary hyperparathyroidism, it is neither required nor recommended for familial hypocalciuric hypercalcemia.

Granulomatous disease causes hypercalcemia in a few patients and this is typically mediated by $1,25\text{-}(OH)_2D_3$ hydroxylated in the granuloma. Vitamin D and vitamin A cause bone resorption. Thiazide diuretics, by decreasing calciuria, can cause a transient hypercalcemia; if this persists, a work-up to exclude another cause is appropriate. Lithium alters the set-point for calcium feedback of parathyroid hormone release, resulting in mild hypercalcemia without appropriate suppression of parathyroid hormone. Immobilization leads to hypercalcemia in states of increased bone turnover (adolescence, Paget's disease, hyperthyroidism) and aggravates hypercalcemia resulting from other causes. Other, less common, causes are listed.

Patients with hypercalcemia who need surgery require careful evaluation. The cardiac effects of significant hypercalcemia have been noted. Nephrogenic diabetes insipidus combined with nausea, vomiting, and decreased mentation can lead to significant volume depletion, which in turn can further raise the serum calcium concentration. Restoration of plasma volume with normal saline is essential. Saline induces a calciuresis and is a mainstay of treatment. After adequate volume has been restored, furosemide may be added to facilitate continued saline administration.

If further treatment is necessary, salmon calcitonin (4 to 12 MRC U/kg every 6 to 12 hours subcutaneously or intramuscularly) exhibits a hypocalcemic effect in 2 hours and can be used safely in the presence of hepatic and renal disease. Unfortunately, no more than a 1.5-mg/dL decline in serum calcium can be anticipated with this agent. Several more powerful inhibitors of bone resorption are available that lower calcium levels in 1 or 2 days, with the therapeutic effect persisting for 1 to 3 weeks. The bisphosphonate, pamidronate, is the newest agent available. When it is infused at a dosage of 60 to 90 mg over 24 hours (some European investigators have used 12-hour infusions), it results in nearly 100% efficacy, particularly at the higher dose. Slightly less effective are infusions of another bisphosphon-

TABLE 34–1. Causes of Hypercalcemia

Primary hyperparathyroidism
Familial hypocalciuric hypercalcemia
Malignancy (PTHrP, cytokines, prostaglandin E, $1,25\text{-}[OH]_2D_3$)
Granulomatous disease ($1,25\text{-}[OH]_2D_3$)
    Sarcoid
    Tuberculosis
    Fungal infections
    Leprosy
    Silicone
Hyperthyroidism
Hypothyroidism (rare)
Adrenal insufficiency
Pheochromocytoma (rare)
Acromegaly (rare)
Calcium ingestion
Vitamin D intoxication
Vitamin A intoxication
Thiazides
Lithium
Immobilization in association with:
    Adolescence
    Paget's disease
    Any state with increased bone resorption
Renal disease
    Diuretic phase of acute renal failure
    Renal transplantation
    Tertiary hyperparathyroidism

ate, etidronate disodium, which is given at a rate of 7.5 mg/kg daily for 3 days. Gallium nitrate is also effective when it is infused at a rate of 200 mg/m^2 over 5 days, although it has the potential for nephrotoxicity. Plicamycin, formerly mithramycin, in doses of 15 to 25 μg/kg, is effective but must be used extremely cautiously in patients with renal, hepatic, or platelet dysfunction. The bisphosphonates have decreased the need for these other therapies. Although intravenous phosphate is effective and more rapid in lowering serum calcium levels, it does so by causing precipitation of calcium and phosphorus in tissues. It should be used rarely and only given cautiously when critical hypercalcemia exists in patients with hypophosphatemia.

Glucocorticoids are only effective in treating those causes of hypercalcemia that result from increased 1,25-(OH)$_2$D$_3$ (ie, granulomatous disease and lymphoma) or those that are associated with the production of cytokines (ie, multiple myeloma). A therapeutic response may take days to weeks to achieve and high doses (5 to 8 times maintenance doses) are typically required. Nonsteroidal anti-inflammatory drugs are occasionally effective in the few patients who have malignancy and prostaglandin E–mediated hypercalcemia. Patients with hypercalcemia and thyrotoxicosis may show a hypocalcemic response to β-blockers, and postmenopausal women with hyperparathyroidism may have a beneficial response to estrogen replacement therapy. Selected patients with renal failure and hypercalcemia require dialysis. Weight-bearing exercise should be attempted in all patients.

HYPOCALCEMIA

Modest hypocalcemia commonly occurs in critically ill patients but is not clinically significant. When symptoms do occur, they involve multiple organs. Neuropsychiatric symptoms include tetany, muscle spasms, hyperreflexia, paresthesias (circumoral, extremities), weakness, irritability, depression, dementia, and, rarely, psychosis. The Chvostek's sign is mildly positive in as many as 20% of normocalcemic research subjects but Trousseau's sign is more specific. Cardiovascular manifestations include hypotension, bradycardia, arrhythmias, and digitalis and catecholamine insensitivity. Electrocardiographic QT intervals are prolonged. Laryngospasm and bronchospasm may occur as well.

Causes of hypocalcemia are listed in Table 34-2. Hypocalcemia results from a deficiency of parathyroid hormone, impaired parathyroid action, a deficiency of vitamin D, impaired vitamin D action, complexing or precipitation of calcium, increased osteoblastic activity, or drugs that inhibit bone resorption. Patients with hypoparathyroidism typically have hyperphosphatemia, whereas those with vi-

TABLE 34–2. Causes of Hypocalcemia

Hypoparathyroidism (subnormal parathyroid hormone release)
  Idiopathic (autoimmune)
  Postsurgical
  Infiltrative (metastatic cancer, hemochromatosis, amyloidosis, granulomatous disease, Wilson's disease)
  Irradiation
  Severe hypomagnesemia
Pseudohypoparathyroidism
Vitamin D deficiency
  Decreased absorption
  Decreased 25-(OH)D$_3$ (severe liver disease)
  Decreased 1,25-(OH)$_2$D$_3$ (renal failure, vitamin D–dependent rickets)
Hyperphosphatemia
  Tumor lysis
  Rhabdomyolysis
  Iatrogenic
Massive blood transfusion (citrate)
Osteoblastic metastases
Parathyroidectomy (hungry bones)
Drugs
  Anticalcemic agents (discussed in text)
  Asparaginase
  Cisplatin
  Cytosine arabinoside
  Foscarnet
  Ketoconazole

tamin D deficiency have low serum phosphorus levels. Measurement of serum parathyroid hormone levels distinguishes hypoparathyroidism from pseudohypoparathyroidism because levels are increased in the latter. Levels of 25-(OH)D$_3$ are a measure of vitamin D availability, whereas levels of 1,25-(OH)$_2$D$_3$ assess renal hydroxylation. Severe hypomagnesemia (less than 1 mg/dL) impairs both parathyroid hormone release and activity.

Surgical patients with hypocalcemia require treatment to prevent the cardiorespiratory and neurologic manifestations of this metabolic derangement. Ionized calcium determinations should be performed in patients with hypoalbuminemia, although the reliability of this measurement is variable. Patients with hyperphosphatemia should be treated with dietary restrictions and phosphate binders (aluminum hydroxide or aluminum carbonate) to lower their serum phosphate levels because vigorous administration of calcium may result in enhanced soft tissue precipitation. Patients with hypomagnesemia require normalization of their serum magnesium levels to achieve normal calcium levels. Symptomatic hypocalcemia should be treated emergently with intravenous calcium. A 100- to 200-mg bolus of elemental calcium, diluted to minimize venous irritation, should be given over a 10-minute period. Calcium chloride provides more elemental calcium per gram than does either calcium gluconate or calcium gluceptate but all are acceptable for therapy. Subsequent treatment varies according to the cause of the hypocalcemia. A continuous calcium infusion (100 to 200 mg of elemental calcium in 500 mL over 6 hours) may be adequate in the acute perioperative setting but oral calcium or the addition of vitamin D may be indicated for future long-term therapy. Patients who experience hypocalcemia after neck surgery, which could damage parathyroid tissue, should be treated with calcium and, if needed, with a short-acting vitamin D preparation such as $1,25\text{-}(OH)_2D_3$, but should be maintained at mildly hypocalcemic levels to stimulate the remaining parathyroid tissue to recover. Serum calcium levels should be monitored every few hours during treatment because

hypercalcemia, nausea, arrhythmias, bradycardia, and toxicity from digitalis, when this is used, may occur.

REFERENCES

1. Davis KD, Attie MF. Management of severe hypercalcemia. Crit Care Clin 1991;7:175–190.
2. Nussbaum SR. Pathophysiology and management of severe hypercalcemia. Endocrinol Metab Clin North Am 1993;22:343–362.
3. Tohme JF, Bilezkian JP. Hypocalcemic emergencies. Endocrinol Metab Clin North Am 1993;22:363–375.
4. Zaloga GF. Hypocalcemia crisis. Crit Care Clin 1991;7:191–199.

CHAPTER

35   PITUITARY INSUFFICIENCY

Medical Management of the Surgical Patient, Third Edition,
edited by Michael F. Lubin, H. Kenneth Walker, and Robert B. Smith III.
J.B. Lippincott Company, Philadelphia, PA © 1995.

Ruth M. Lawrence
Robert M. Walter, Jr.

The clinical onset of hypopituitarism may be protracted and subtle, and physicians evaluating preoperative patients should be alert to pertinent symptoms and signs. Failure to recognize pituitary insufficiency can result in morbidity or mortality caused by unrecognized secondary thyroid and adrenal hypofunction. These conditions are discussed in detail in Chapters 31 and 32. If hypothalamic disease is also present, diabetes insipidus can complicate fluid balance in the perioperative period. Deficiencies of gonadotropin, growth hormone, and prolactin provide clinical clues to the diagnosis of hypopituitarism but are not of critical perioperative importance.

CAUSES OF HYPOPITUITARISM

Hypopituitarism most commonly results from neoplastic involvement of the pituitary (secondary endocrine insufficiency) or the hypothalamus (tertiary endocrine insufficiency). Either functional or nonfunctional adenomas can result in hypopituitarism by gradually compressing normal tissue or by causing pituitary apoplexy with hemorrhage, acute swelling, and necrosis. Necrosis occurring after postpartum uterine hemorrhage and hypotension is known as Sheehan's syndrome. Craniopharyngioma, the most common hypothalamic neoplasm in childhood, typically im-

pairs hypothalamic function. Primary central nervous system tumors and metastatic cancer may also cause pituitary insufficiency. Infiltrative diseases (sarcoidosis, hemochromatosis, and the histiocytoses) can involve the hypothalamus and the pituitary, as can infections (tuberculosis, syphilis, fungal infections), trauma, surgery, radiation, and autoimmune disease (lymphocytic hypophysitis). Idiopathic deficiencies of isolated hypothalamic and pituitary hormones also occur.

CLINICAL PRESENTATION AND DIAGNOSIS

The first symptoms of hypopituitarism are most commonly those of hypogonadism (ie, loss of libido, impotence in men, amenorrhea in women, decreased secondary sexual characteristics in both sexes). The symptoms, signs, and laboratory presentation of thyroid and adrenal insufficiency are reviewed in Chapters 31 and 32. It is important to remember that patients with secondary or tertiary adrenal insufficiency have neither hyperpigmentation (adrenocorticotropic hormone is decreased) nor hyperkalemia (aldosterone is present). Those with secondary or tertiary hypothyroidism do not have goiters (thyroid-stimulating hormone is decreased). Although impaired growth hormone release is the most common abnormal laboratory finding in hypopituitarism, it is clinically silent in adults. Loss of postpartum lactation suggests prolactin deficiency. Combined deficiency of cortisol and thyroid can result in severe hyponatremia and hypoglycemia. In addition, low levels of gonadal hormones and gonadotropin may be seen. Patients with hypothalamic disease may have diabetes insipidus and hyperprolactinemia because vasopressin is synthesized in the hypothalamus and prolactin is primarily regulated by hypothalamic inhibition. Testing with the hypothalamic hormones, thyrotropin-releasing hormone, gonadotropin-releasing hormone, growth hormone–releasing hormone, and corticotropin-releasing hormone, may distinguish between hypothalamic and pituitary lesions. An increase in the corresponding pituitary hormone suggests hypothalamic disease; lack of response supports a pituitary lesion. Diabetes insipidus can be diagnosed with serial measurements of serum and urine osmolality during a carefully monitored water deprivation test. Measurement of plasma vasopressin and evaluation of the response to administered vasopressin confirm the diagnosis and distinguish central from nephrogenic diabetes insipidus. After clinical and laboratory evidence of hypothalamic or pituitary disease is established, magnetic resonance imaging is superb for identifying anatomic pathology.

The treatment of adrenal and thyroid insufficiency is discussed in Chapters 31 and 32. Patients with secondary and tertiary adrenal insufficiency do not require mineralocorticoid replacement because aldosterone levels are adequate. Thyroid-stimulating hormone levels cannot be used to monitor thyroxine replacement doses in patients with secondary or tertiary thyroid deficiency. Men with hypogonadism should be treated with testosterone given intramuscularly at intervals of 2 to 3 weeks. Premenopausal women should be treated with estrogen plus progesterone. For postmenopausal women, hormone replacement is administered on an individual basis. Growth hormone replacement is not recommended for adults, although research is being conducted in this field. Central diabetes insipidus is effectively treated with twice daily intranasal administration of desmopressin acetate, a synthetic analogue of vasopressin.

PERIOPERATIVE MANAGEMENT

The importance of glucocorticoid replacement during perioperative stress is discussed in Chapter 32. Intravenous glucocorticoid should be given at doses 8 to 10 times higher than maintenance levels (ie, 240 to 300 mg of hydrocortisone in three divided doses) on the day of surgery, then tapered to maintenance levels over the next 3 to 7 days as dictated by the patient's level of stress. Mineralocorticoids are not needed. Although patients with hypothyroidism should be rendered euthyroid before elective surgery, hypothyroidism should not delay emergent surgery. When myxedema coma is suspected, the intravenous administration of 400 µg of levothyroxine is immediately indicated, accompanied by stress doses of glucocorticoid. Patients with diabetes insipidus can have urine volumes as high as 400 mL/h, resulting in severe plasma hypertonicity when access to water is restricted. Parenteral treatment can be achieved with intravenous desmopressin at a dosage of 1 to 4 µg/d. Its duration of action is 12 to 24 hours. During treatment, electrolyte levels must be observed closely and intravenous fluids monitored carefully to prevent hyponatremia. Cardiovascular monitoring with Swan-Ganz catheters is indicated in surgical patients who have diabetes insipidus to prevent hypovolemia and hypervolemia. Patients with hypopituitarism can undergo major surgery successfully if necessary hormone replacement is given and fluid and electrolyte status are monitored closely.

REFERENCES

1. Abboud CF. Laboratory diagnosis of hypopituitarism. Mayo Clin Proc 1986;61:35–48.
2. Blondell RD. Hypopituitarism. Am Fam Physician 1991;43: 2029–2036.
3. Cobb WE, Spare S, Reichlin S. Neurogenic diabetes insipidus: management with DDAVP. Ann Intern Med 1978;88:183–188.
4. Post KD, McCormick PC, Bello JA. Differential diagnosis of pituitary tumors. Endocrinol Metab Clin North Am 1987;16:609–645.
5. Rolih CA, Ober KP. Pituitary apoplexy. Endocrinol Metab Clin North Am 1993;22:291–302.

SECTION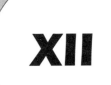

RHEUMATOLOGY

Medical Management of the Surgical Patient, Third Edition,
edited by Michael F. Lubin, H. Kenneth Walker, and Robert B. Smith III.
J.B. Lippincott Company, Philadelphia, PA © 1995.

CHAPTER

RHEUMATOLOGIC DISEASES

36

John O. Meyerhoff
Marc C. Hochberg

Arthritic disorders are estimated to affect about 15% of the adult population in the United States; based on 1989 census figures, this amounts to almost 37 million people.[1] Patients with arthritis, particularly osteoarthritis and rheumatoid arthritis (RA), undergo surgical procedures most often for comorbid conditions that are not necessarily related to their arthritis, although orthopedic procedures such as arthroscopy and total joint arthroplasty are also commonly performed. The perioperative evaluation and treatment of patients with arthritis focuses on documenting the extent and severity of arthritis and the use of medications, especially nonsteroidal antiinflammatory drugs (NSAIDs) and glucocorticoids.

The second major group of disorders are the connective tissue diseases, including systemic lupus erythematosus (SLE) and systemic sclerosis (scleroderma). These disorders are also referred to as autoimmune diseases and are characterized by multisystem involvement, with arthritis usually a minor component. Patients with autoimmune connective tissue diseases almost always undergo surgical procedures for complications of their specific disease and its treatment or for comorbid conditions. As in patients with arthritic conditions, perioperative evaluation and therapy focus on documenting the extent, activity, and severity of the con-

nective tissue disease and the need for medications, especially glucocorticoids and cytotoxic/immunosuppressive drugs.

ARTHRITIC CONDITIONS

OSTEOARTHRITIS

Osteoarthritis is the most common form of arthritis and typically affects middle-aged or elderly women. Although osteoarthritis may involve small as well as large joints in both the upper and lower extremities, the most common symptomatic sites are the knees, carpometacarpal joints at the base of the thumb, interphalangeal joints of the fingers, hips, and apophyseal joints of the cervical and lumbar spine.

The diagnosis of osteoarthritis is suggested by the presence of joint pain, which usually is worse with use of the joint and relieved by rest, and morning stiffness of less than 30 minutes' duration. Physical examination commonly reveals signs of bony enlargement or tenderness as well as crepitus on passive motion of the joint. The diagnosis is confirmed by finding evidence of osteophytes, often accompa-

345

nied by joint space narrowing and subchondral sclerosis, on radiographs of affected joints. The results of routine laboratory studies are usually normal. Systemic and extraarticular manifestations are not a feature of osteoarthritis.[2]

Surgical Considerations

Before surgery is performed, the major concern in the medical treatment of patients with osteoarthritis is their use of NSAIDs; issues regarding these agents are covered in a separate section of this chapter. Additional consideration must also be given to the evaluation and treatment of comorbid conditions, particularly obesity, hypertension, cardiovascular and renal diseases, and diabetes mellitus.

The major indications for orthopedic procedures in patients with osteoarthritis are pain that is unresponsive to medical therapy and functional limitation. The underlying distortion in the anatomy of the joint, weakness of the periarticular muscles, and the ability of patients to participate in postoperative rehabilitation programs also must be considered in the overall risk–benefit analysis. These issues as well as the types of orthopedic procedures that are available for treating osteoarthritis have been reviewed elsewhere.[3]

RHEUMATOID ARTHRITIS

The diagnosis of RA is based primarily on the presence of an inflammatory, symmetric, polyarthritis usually involving the small and large joints of the upper and lower extremities, most commonly the hands, wrists, knees, and feet.[4] Most patients are seropositive for rheumatoid factor, an IgM autoantibody to IgG. Radiographic changes such as juxtaarticular demineralization, joint space narrowing, erosions, and subluxation are present in varying degrees.

It is vital to ensure that patients in whom RA has been diagnosed actually have this disease. Seronegative RA should be confirmed by a rheumatologist because this diagnosis may be confused with polymyalgia rheumatica, erosive osteoarthritis, or gout. Moreover, the frequency of rheumatoid factor increases in older populations. Thus, as the frequency of false-positive results for rheumatoid factor rises in the elderly along with the frequency of symptomatic osteoarthritis, the potential exists for the incorrect diagnosis of RA in patients with osteoarthritis.

The articular system is involved most often. The hands and wrists are most frequently affected, followed by the feet, ankles, and knees. The shoulders and elbows are also commonly involved. Involvement of the cervical spine, temporomandibular joints, or cricoarytenoid joints is much less common but can lead to significant problems with anesthesia.

Extraarticular involvement usually occurs after the disease has been present and active for some time. Rheuma-

toid nodules are seen on extensor surfaces and bony prominences in about one fourth of patients but rarely affect surgery. Pleurisy and pericarditis are common on echocardiography and autopsy studies but less often detected clinically. Although they may cause symptoms, effusions that are large enough to result in pulmonary or cardiac compromise are extremely rare. Interstitial lung disease does occur but usually does not cause symptoms, with only bibasilar infiltrates seen on chest radiographs and a mild restrictive defect detected on spirometry. The disease may progress to produce symptoms.

Neurologic involvement of all types can occur. Patients often develop entrapment syndromes such as carpal tunnel syndrome when peripheral nerves are compressed by the swelling in peripheral joints, primarily the wrists and elbows. Many patients have stocking–glove paresthesia. Although this results from a small vessel vasculitis, it is benign and often resolves without treatment. Mononeuritis multiplex may be caused by vasculitis in a larger vessel and is a serious complication that is often associated with vasculitis of internal organs.

Sjögren's syndrome (keratoconjunctivitis sicca) occurs in almost one fourth of patients and is characterized by dryness of the eyes and mouth resulting from decreased tear and saliva production, respectively. Raynaud's phenomenon may be present in patients with RA. The temperature in an operating room may be cool enough to induce an episode of this disorder.

The skin of patients with RA may be affected by their medications, particularly corticosteroids, and may be thin and easily bruised. Bruising is often compounded by the almost universal use of NSAIDs, which interfere with platelet aggregation.

Surgical Considerations

Joint involvement. Cervical spine involvement and its attendant risks depend on the amount of laxity in the spine and the degree to which the dens (odontoid process) is intact. The production of collagenases and proteinases may lead to laxity and destruction of the joints and other structures in the cervical spine. If the dens is still intact, this excessive laxity allows the dens to "pith" the spinal cord on forward flexion. Alternatively, if the dens has been eroded by active disease, there may be a clunking sensation on flexion or extension as C-1 moves either forward or backward on C-2. With even more severe disease, the odontoid can subluxate vertically into the foramen magnum.[5] Patients may report this clunking sound or complain of paresthesias on movement of the neck. Bowel and bladder symptoms may also occur and are more chronic. Cranial neuropathies are suggestive of vertical subluxation.

Because cervical spine involvement does not occur in RA without peripheral involvement, patients with minimal joint changes (from mild disease) are unlikely to have spinal involvement. Those without neurologic symptoms are unlikely to have significant cord compression. Patients may have paresthesias, however, which have been attributed by them or their physicians to peripheral nerve entrapment or the benign neurovasculitis noted earlier. Women may assume that mild bladder dysfunction is the result of urinary tract infection. If any question exists, radiographic assessment is indicated.

The condition of the cervical spine can be assessed by simple flexion and extension views of the spine. Normal motion is 3 mm or less. The dens can be evaluated best by an open mouth view. If severe destruction of the upper cervical spine is seen or cranial neuropathies are reported, a magnetic resonance scan of the cervical spine is indicated. If excessive motion without neurologic symptoms is detected, patients should wear hard or Philadelphia collars at least until some time during the postoperative period. If neurologic symptoms are also present, neurosurgical consultation may be helpful to determine whether stabilization is possible and when it should be done in regard to any other scheduled surgery. In emergency surgery, particularly in unconscious patients, the presence of significant articular deformities in patients with RA should be assumed to indicate cervical spine disease, and hard collars should be placed to reduce cervical movement.

Although these concerns are less likely to be important in patients who are undergoing procedures that do not involve the use of general anesthesia, consideration should be given to obtaining radiographs if risk factors exist because of the unpredictable nature of emergencies.

Joint involvement in the head and neck may also lead to difficulty with intubation. Temporomandibular joint involvement may result in a small oral aperture. This is easily assessed by asking patients to open their mouths fully. Cricoarytenoid arthritis rarely is clinically apparent but as many as 30% of patients with RA report some hoarseness. This can lead to a small opening at the vocal cords. Patients with juvenile-onset RA may have micrognathia, which may also cause difficulty with intubation.

Joint contractures can develop in any involved joint. The position required for surgery should be reviewed as patients are examined to ensure that no problems exist.

Extraarticular manifestations. Pulmonary involvement is most likely to lead to operative problems, particularly with general anesthesia. Interstitial lung disease can be assessed by auscultating the lungs and obtaining a chest radiograph. Clinically significant involvement is unlikely in the absence of rales or abnormal radiographic results. The extent of involvement can be determined with pulmonary function tests. Significant pericardial and pleural effusions are rare, are preceded by clinical symptoms, and can be seen on chest radiographs.

The evaluation of Raynaud's phenomenon and Sjögren's syndrome are outlined later.

Disease activity. The level of RA activity is usually best determined by asking patients how active their arthritis is (patient global assessment). In addition, the number of painful or swollen joints can be noted on physical examination. Disease activity sometimes is accompanied by a mild anemia and an elevated erythrocyte sedimentation rate. Although the level of disease activity may not directly affect the timing or outcome of surgery, it forms the foundation for much of the preoperative and postoperative planning. Patients who are doing well may be able to quit taking some of their medications for a longer period if there is concern regarding side effects. Patients who have active disease are likely to develop joint contractures quickly if active joints are not exercised. If these patients are going to be inactive for more than several days, physical or occupational therapists should be asked to initiate passive range-of-motion exercises.

Medications. Patients with RA are often taking a combination of medications with different modes of action, therapeutic half-lives, and routes of delivery. This often enables them to undergo surgery without any significant interruption in their therapeutic regimen. For details concerning medications, see the section at the end of the chapter.

GOUT

Gout is an acute inflammatory arthritis provoked by monosodium urate crystals in the joint space. Untreated, acute episodes generally resolve over 1 to 2 weeks. Further episodes occur over subsequent months to years with increasing frequency and duration. This may lead to chronic arthritis, with deformities sometimes mimicking those of RA. In the past, it was thought that hyperuricemia and gout frequently led to renal insufficiency. The association resulted, however, from the fact that patients with hypertension and hypertensive renal disease often have secondary gout induced by thiazide diuretics.

With the medications currently available, virtually all patients who are compliant with their regimen can control gout. Acute episodes are usually treated with NSAIDs, particularly indomethacin, 200 mg/d in divided doses. Indomethacin remains the drug of choice because it reliably treats acute episodes in almost all patients. Colchicine is equally effective in preventing attacks when it is used prophylactically. Urate-lowering drugs (allopurinol and probenecid) can be used in those patients whose gout is not controlled with NSAIDs and colchicine.

Surgical Considerations

One third of patients with gout may have flares at the time of acute medical or surgical illness.[6] This propensity may also be exacerbated by the interruption of treatment at the time of surgery. Discontinuation of therapy with urate-lowering drugs can also induce an episode of gout. If medications cannot be given for several days, physicians should remain alert to the possibility of a flare. Early treatment may abort such an attack.

If acute episodes occur in the perioperative period, and patients can take oral medications, NSAIDs should be given if there are no contraindications. A dosage at the upper end of the approved dosage range should be used initially and then tapered as symptoms resolve. If NSAIDs are contraindicated, intramuscular adrenocorticotropic hormone, 40 to 80 IU, or intravenous methylprednisolone, 20 mg, may be effective at doses equivalent to 20 mg of prednisone daily. Last, if only a joint or two is involved, aspiration may be effective in reducing symptoms with or without the concurrent injection of corticosteroids. If there is concern that the joints may be infected, steroids should not be injected. Intravenous colchicine is usually not used because of its potential toxicity.

PSEUDOGOUT

Calcium pyrophosphate dihydrate crystals can cause several different patterns of arthritis that mimic other forms of arthritis. These include an acute monarticular inflammatory disease that usually involves the knee (pseudogout), a symmetric polyarthritis that resembles RA (pseudorheumatoid presentation), a noninflammatory process similar to osteoarthritis, and, particularly in patients with neurologic disease, a Charcot-like arthritis.

The diagnosis of pyrophosphate disease is confirmed by finding chondrocalcinosis on radiography and positively birefringent crystals in synovial fluid.

Surgical Considerations

Acute flares, particularly of pseudogout, can occur in the postoperative period, as can gout. Therapy is similar to that for acute gout.

SPONDYLOARTHROPATHIES

Ankylosing spondylitis (AS), psoriatic arthritis, arthritis associated with inflammatory bowel disease, and Reiter's syndrome are grouped together because of their similar clinical presentations and immunogenetics. AS has the fewest peripheral joint manifestations. In its most classic presentation, it begins as low back pain in the sacroiliac joints in a young man. The disease may then proceed up the spine, leading to fusion and deformity if NSAIDs and physical therapy are not used. In women and in younger children, the disease is more likely to have peripheral involvement and less likely to start in the sacroiliac joints and involve the lumbar spine. Inflammatory bowel disease arthritis, when it involves the spine, resembles AS. Reiter's syndrome and psoriatic arthritis are less symmetric than is AS.

The other common feature among these diseases is their association with HLA-B27. Almost 90% of patients with AS have HLA-B27, as do 75% of patients with Reiter's syndrome. In patients with psoriatic and inflammatory bowel disease arthritis, the presence of HLA-B27 increases the likelihood of spinal involvement. As is the case with many of the rheumatic diseases, the exact relationship between the immunogenetic or serologic findings and the disease manifestations is not known.

In all these diseases, joint contractures and ankylosis are frequent, particularly in the spine. This can lead to loss of motion and even complete fusion in the spine. Thoracic involvement may result in decreased range of motion in the chest with resultant restrictive lung disease. Patients with AS may also develop fibrotic changes in the upper lobes. Involvement of the aortic valve can lead to aortic insufficiency, although this rarely causes symptoms. Fibrosis around the aortic valve can extend into the aorta or into the conduction system, with subsequent arrhythmias occurring in 5% to 10% of patients.

All the spondyloarthropathies are treated initially with NSAIDs in doses adequate to control the symptoms. Physical therapy in the form of daily range-of-motion exercises should be used to minimize joint contractures. When NSAIDs are ineffective, sulfasalazine and methotrexate may be used.

Surgical Considerations

When surgery is being considered in these patients, the major concerns are the range of motion in the spine and cardiopulmonary function. Decreased cervical motion may make intubation difficult. Pulmonary evaluation with chest radiographs and pulmonary function tests should be considered in patients who have decreased range of motion in the thorax. Electrocardiograms and even echocardiograms should be considered in patients with severe AS, who are the most likely to have the cardiac abnormalities noted earlier. Positioning patients for surgery may also be difficult in the presence of spinal fusion. AS may involve the shoulders and hips, and all the other spondyloarthropathies can cause destruction and loss of motion of any other joints.

CONNECTIVE TISSUE DISEASES

SYSTEMIC LUPUS ERYTHEMATOSUS

Systemic lupus erythematosus is a multisystem disease characterized by the presence of autoantibodies to nuclear and cell-surface antigens.[7] Articular disease is the most common manifestation of SLE, although it is as deforming as RA in only 10% of patients. Cutaneous manifestations (butterfly rash, malar rash, photosensitivity, and alopecia) are the next most common signs. Pleuritic or pericardial symptoms occur in about half of all patients, as do cytopenias. The leukopenia is rarely sufficient to cause problems, although thrombocytopenia or hemolytic anemia can be clinically important. Similarly, about half of all patients have evidence of kidney involvement. This may range in severity from microscopic hematuria and mild proteinuria with normal renal function to end-stage renal disease requiring dialysis.

One third of patients have neuropsychiatric manifestations; an organic brain syndrome is the most common psychiatric manifestation and seizures are the most common neurologic finding. About one fifth of patients have nasal or oral ulcerations. Raynaud's phenomenon and Sjögren's syndrome can also occur in patients with SLE at the same frequency as in patients with RA.

Gastrointestinal involvement is unusual. In patients with active vasculitis, there may be involvement of the mesenteric arteries leading to bowel ischemia and perforation. Because these patients are often receiving corticosteroids and cytotoxic drugs, the degree of immunosuppression may cause the abdomen to be quiet on examination. It is not uncommon for patients with SLE to have months of abdominal symptoms before a major abdominal injury is discovered. At times, patients may have chronic abdominal pain, presumably caused by peritonitis; the results of all radiographic studies, including angiography, are normal.

Over 90% of patients with SLE have antinuclear antibodies but there are several different antigens in the nucleus that are typically the target antigens. Patients may make antibodies to cytoplasmic antigens and to nuclear antigens, including native DNA.

Awareness of the importance of antiphospholipid antibodies in patients with SLE is increasing.[8] These antibodies can give rise to a prolonged partial thromboplastin time, a false-positive RPR, or anticardiolipin antibodies. The presence of these antibodies, particularly in patients with SLE, is associated with venous and arterial thrombosis, cardiac valvular lesions, and frequent miscarriages.[8–10] IgG anticardiolipin antibodies, when they are present at a level greater than 5 SD above normal, may be the most significant of these antibodies.

Surgical Considerations

The three major surgical considerations are (1) the level of disease activity, (2) the organs currently involved, and (3) the medications being taken. Most of this information should be provided by patients' rheumatologists. All patients with SLE should be seen by consulting rheumatologists in the preoperative period if possible.

Disease activity. Numerous quantitative measures are being used by rheumatologists in clinical practice to provide a more reproducible and sensitive assessment of disease activity. Active SLE is associated with more surgical complications.[11] Wound complications, respiratory difficulties, infectious complications, deep venous thrombosis and pulmonary embolism, renal insufficiency, and urinary tract infections have all been reported to occur more frequently after surgery in patients with SLE when the disease is active.

Elective procedures should be performed when SLE is inactive or under control and surgery should be delayed until SLE is inactive, if possible. If not, even closer attention should be paid to prophylactic measures and surgical technique.

Organ involvement. The extent of organ involvement should be reviewed before surgery. Because active internal organ involvement may not be immediately obvious, a physical examination should be performed. The physical examination should focus on the skin for lesions of SLE; the joints for signs of inflammation; the heart for signs of intrinsic heart disease and pericarditis; the lungs for signs of consolidation, pleurisy, and pleural effusions; and the abdomen for abnormalities of the liver and splenomegaly.

A complete blood count (CBC) should be obtained. Leukopenia in SLE rarely results in fewer than 1000 granulocytes. Thrombocytopenia low enough to be of concern (fewer than 50,000 cells) occurs in under 10% of patients but, if necessary, can be treated acutely with platelet transfusions to raise the platelet count to an adequate level. Hemolytic anemia is much less common than are anemias of chronic disease or iron-deficiency anemia. The hemolysis can occur intermittently, causing stepwise reductions in the hemoglobin and hematocrit levels. If the hematocrit is more than 5% (absolute) below either normal or the patient's usual value, a hemolytic episode may have occurred for which the patient has not been able to compensate. This should be evaluated with a Coombs' test, serum lactic dehydrogenase level, and indirect bilirubin and urine hemosiderin measurements. Serologic studies (C3, C4, CH50, and anti–single- or double-stranded DNA antibody levels) may be helpful in assessing disease activity in patients with known patterns of disease exacerbation if changes are noted in their results.

Clotting studies should be obtained. If the partial thromboplastin time is prolonged, the patient's serum should be mixed 50:50 with normal serum. If the partial thromboplastin time continues to be prolonged, a lupus anticoagulant is present. In SLE, a circulating anticoagulant is associated with thrombosis, not excessive bleeding.[8] If an anticoagulant is present, care must be taken to prevent postoperative thrombosis using the appropriate deep venous thrombosis prophylaxis for the procedure being done.

The pulmonary manifestations of SLE are similar to those of RA, with pleurisy occurring commonly but significant effusions being rare. Interstitial disease presents initially with basilar rales and may progress to involve the entire lung. A chest radiograph usually is abnormal if there is clinically significant hypoxia; pulmonary function tests should be obtained if time permits in patients with abnormal physical findings.

Libman-Sacks endocarditis can occur in patients with SLE. These vegetations can be detected by echocardiography along with other clinically significant abnormalities of the valves (rigidity and thickening with stenosis or regurgitation) in as many as one fifth of all patients. Patients with anticardiolipin antibodies are more prone to these lesions. Prophylactic antibiotics should be given to all patients with SLE who have evidence of valvular heart disease.

The extent of renal disease should be assessed before surgery. The blood urea nitrogen or serum creatinine level may be normal, however, even in patients with some underlying renal involvement. A urinalysis, looking for hematuria, proteinuria, and other abnormalities in the sediment, is important. In patients with renal insufficiency, hypotension during surgery can cause worsening renal function.

Only 10% of patients with SLE have deforming arthritis similar to RA. Such patients, particularly those with neck involvement, should undergo radiographic evaluation of the neck as outlined earlier for RA.

SYSTEMIC SCLEROSIS (SCLERODERMA)

Systemic sclerosis is a disorder characterized by fibrosis that is manifest by the presence of thickened skin known as scleroderma. The two major forms of systemic sclerosis are generalized scleroderma and limited scleroderma; these are classified by the extent of skin involvement.[12] These two conditions were referred to previously as progressive systemic sclerosis and the CREST syndrome. The former name

was felt to be too pessimistic about the outcome and the latter name was misleading because all the features of the CREST syndrome (calcinosis, Raynaud's phenomenon, esophageal dysfunction, sclerodactyly, and telangiectasia) occur in patients with generalized skin involvement. In patients with limited scleroderma, the sclerodermatous skin changes are confined to the hands, face, and forearms, and do not involve the trunk.

Although many of the connective tissue diseases are inflammatory at both the microscopic and macroscopic level, scleroderma tends to be noninflammatory at the macroscopic level and often at the microscopic level. The cause of scleroderma is unknown but the fibroblast seems to be the most likely target organ because fibrosis is the most common finding in many organs. The lack of classic inflammatory changes led to uncertainty about an autoimmune cause. In the past decade, two autoantibodies have been discovered in patients with scleroderma. Systemic sclerosis is associated with an antibody to topoisomerase I (initially known as anti–Scl-70), whereas limited scleroderma produces anticentromere antibodies that are detected on Hep-2 cell lines during testing for antinuclear antibodies. Neither antibody test is sufficiently sensitive or specific for use in screening or definitive diagnosis. The tests are most helpful in patients with consistent histories or suspicious physical findings in the absence of definite sclerodermatous skin changes.

The characteristic finding in scleroderma is sclerodactyly (ie, thickened and bound-down skin over the fingers). Swelling in the fingers may occur early in the course, leading to a condition described as puffy fingers. As the disease progresses, there is loss of subcutaneous fat and the fingers become smaller than normal. The fibrosis can lead to severe loss of range of motion in the fingers with the development of a "clawlike" hand. Similarly, patients may develop a frozen shoulder if the skin in this area is involved. Interestingly, over a period of years, the skin may loosen and appear almost normal.

Raynaud's phenomenon occurs in 90% of patients with systemic sclerosis. Unlike patients with RA or SLE, patients with scleroderma are much more likely to develop digital tip ulcerations and subsequent infection. Raynaud's phenomenon can lead to gangrene of the involved digit.

Pulmonary involvement is common. The most frequent finding, particularly in patients with generalized scleroderma, is diffuse interstitial fibrosis that usually begins insidiously. There may be fine basilar rales and minimal reduction in exercise capacity. As the process continues, the symptoms and physical findings increase. Routine chest radiographs may appear normal until significant disease is present. Pulmonary function tests, including D$_{LCO}$, are the best way to monitor the development of the resulting restrictive lung disease and loss of diffusion capacity.

When limited scleroderma was called CREST syndrome,

pulmonary involvement was not believed to be part of the disease. It has become obvious that pulmonary hypertension can occur in these patients, however, and that it may cause death. This condition presents as shortness of breath in the absence of pulmonary findings and leads to cor pulmonale.

Symptomatic pericardial involvement is infrequent but echocardiography demonstrates effusions in many patients. Arrhythmias may occur because of fibrosis in the conduction system. Congestive heart failure may be seen if myocardial fibrosis develops and is resistant to therapy.

The renal involvement is a vasculopathy that usually develops suddenly, leading to malignant hypertension with the rapid onset of renal failure. Until minoxidil was introduced, aggressive therapy with antihypertensive agents was unsuccessful. With the use of minoxidil, angiotensin-converting enzyme inhibitors, and other agents, aggressive multiple drug treatment of renal crisis usually results in blood pressure control without loss of renal function.

Gastrointestinal involvement occurs frequently in patients with scleroderma. Esophageal involvement is extremely common, leading to dysphagia and reflux esophagitis. Dysmotility in the small intestine can lead to malabsorption because of bacterial overgrowth; this can sometimes be treated with antibiotics. When larger segments are involved with fibrosis, serious malabsorption can develop and surgery may be necessary to remove the diseased segments. This process can occur in multiple areas and some patients require total parenteral nutrition to maintain adequate nutrition. Patients may also develop pneumatosis intestinalis, or the presence of air in the bowel wall, which may appear to be free air in the peritoneum. In the colon (and occasionally the distal small bowel), pathognomonic wide-mouth diverticula may develop, usually along the antimesenteric border of the distal two thirds of the colon.

No specific treatment is available for scleroderma, although D-penicillamine may have some effect and is being tested in a prospective trial. Treatment of the specific manifestations of scleroderma often is effective in relieving symptoms.

Surgical Considerations

As in SLE, the level of disease activity should be determined and surgery delayed if possible until systemic sclerosis is under good control. The tightness of the skin in patients with scleroderma may be a problem in performing particular procedures. It may be more difficult to obtain the surgical exposure needed for a procedure or to position patients' limbs. Patients with facial involvement may have small oral apertures, which can make intubation difficult. Skin incisions will heal with appropriate care.

Patients should be questioned carefully before surgery regarding cardiopulmonary symptoms. Pulmonary symptoms in particular may develop slowly and patients may have adapted to these changes without being aware of them. All patients should undergo preoperative pulmonary function testing because of the high frequency of asymptomatic lung involvement. Esophageal dysfunction may also be long-standing and patients may not volunteer this information. After operation, blood pressure elevations should be monitored carefully and treated aggressively if they persist. Most potent antihypertensive agents are effective in these cases when they are used in adequate dosages.

RAYNAUD'S PHENOMENON

Raynaud's phenomenon is vasospasm of the peripheral arteries that is induced by anxiety or cold. In its full-blown form, a triphasic color change occurs in the affected digits. First, there is blanching as the vessel goes into spasm and blood flow is cut off. As the blood in the digit becomes more deoxygenated, it turns blue. With rewarming, there is reflex vasodilation and the digit becomes red with hyperemia. These events are often painful and may be accompanied by paresthesias that are usually described as a feeling of "pins and needles." All three phases may not occur in some patients, and the nose or external ear may also be involved. Depending on the size and number of vessels involved, the entire hand or foot may be affected or only half a digit supplied by one of the digital arteries may be affected. There also is evidence that the heart and lung may be affected by the same process, leading to microscopic infarction.

Raynaud's phenomenon may occur idiopathically, or after frostbite; the use of vibrating devices (eg, jackhammers, carving tools); trauma; or therapy with certain drugs (ergotamines, polyvinyl chloride, bleomycin, and vinblastine). It often affects patients with connective tissue disease (10% of those with RA, 30% of those with SLE, and 90% of those with scleroderma).

In most patients with Raynaud's phenomenon, the symptoms develop at varying temperatures during the year. Temperatures in the range of 50° to 60°F may induce an attack at the beginning of winter, whereas colder temperatures may be required later. Similarly, although an outdoor or indoor temperature of 70°F usually does not induce symptoms, walking into an air-conditioned room of that temperature in the middle of the summer may do so. Most patients suffer no obvious morbidity from Raynaud's phenomenon with the exception of pain. Patients with scleroderma, however, often develop digital tip infarctions and ulcerations from prolonged episodes.

Surgical Considerations

Patients who have Raynaud's phenomenon, particularly those with scleroderma or histories of digital tip infarctions or ulcerations, should be kept warm throughout the operative procedure and in the recovery room and intensive care unit. An attack can be induced with central cooling in some patients, not just peripheral cooling. Heated operating room tables are available and should be used routinely for patients who have significant morbidity from Raynaud's phenomenon.

Nifedipine may be helpful in some patients in preventing attacks or lowering the temperature at which attacks occur. Intravenous prostacyclin may have beneficial long-term effects in patients with Raynaud's phenomenon, and may be particularly helpful in those with poor symptom control if nifedipine is not effective. Other calcium channel blockers do not seem to be efficacious.

SJÖGREN'S SYNDROME

In 1933, Henrik Sjögren described a constellation of symptoms including keratoconjunctivitis sicca (dry eyes), xerostomia (dry mouth), and polyarthritis (although the first two manifestations had been described earlier). Today, the term *Sjögren's syndrome* is used to refer to three major groups of patients.

One group of patients with the triad of symptoms described by Sjögren have an autoimmune exocrinopathy. They have no other connective tissue diseases and are considered to have primary Sjögren's syndrome. These patients often have a photosensitive rash, decreased bronchial and vaginal secretions, and a high frequency of anti-Ro antibodies. Many patients with other connective tissue diseases have secondary Sjögren's syndrome, which is often asymptomatic.

Many elderly patients have dry eyes and mouths (along with symptomatic osteoarthritis), and abnormal results on Schirmer's tests. They do not have autoimmune diseases with abnormal serologies, however, but fibrosis of the exocrine glands. Thus, although these patients have Sjögren's syndrome, they have a different disease than do patients with primary and secondary Sjögren's syndrome.

The dry eyes and mouth of this condition result from decreased lacrimal and salivary gland function. The eyes may be so dry that severe corneal irritation occurs and the eyes become red. Many patients use artificial tears on a regular basis. In the mouth, the absence of saliva may lead to frequent caries and stomatitis. In the bronchial tree, the absence of secretions predisposes to frequent bronchial infections. Additional manifestations, depending on the organ system involved, include dry skin, dysphagia, type II renal tubular acidosis, and dyspareunia. Neurologic findings

similar to those of neuropsychiatric lupus have been reported but the frequency of such events varies dramatically from center to center.

Surgical Considerations

Patients with RA, SLE, or scleroderma should be questioned about symptoms of dryness, particularly in the eyes, mouth, and esophagus, as well as bronchial involvement. Artificial tears should be used in patients with dry eyes to prevent injury during surgery. Patients with dryness in the gastrointestinal tract may require additional care in intubation because of the dry surfaces. Those with histories of recurrent bronchitis and pneumonia require particular attention to pulmonary care.

POLYMYOSITIS AND DERMATOMYOSITIS

Polymyositis and dermatomyositis result from inflammation in the muscles and present with symptoms of loss of muscle function. Almost all patients have muscle weakness, elevated muscle enzyme levels, characteristic skin changes (in dermatomyositis), abnormal electromyograms, and abnormal results on muscle biopsy. Patients with the first two findings should undergo muscle biopsy to rule out infectious causes of muscle disease such as *Trichinella* and unusual conditions such as inclusion-body myositis, which generally is not as responsive to treatment. The cause of polymyositis and dermatomyositis is not known but many patients have antibodies to transfer RNA synthetases and signal recognition particles. These antibodies are associated with an increase in interstitial lung disease. The most common is called anti–Jo-1 antibody. The role of these autoantibodies in the development of polymyositis and dermatomyositis is unknown. The onset of the conditions in some patients is temporally associated with the diagnosis of a malignant tumor.

Patients with myositis develop muscle weakness gradually and may lose a significant amount of muscle function before they become aware of the problem. The most common symptoms are difficulty getting out of a chair or off of a toilet. Patients can develop pharyngeal weakness with dysphagia and aspiration, aspiration pneumonia (which may play a role in the development of the interstitial lung disease), and diaphragmatic weakness with respiratory insufficiency. Cardiac involvement may include myocarditis and rhythm disturbances.

Most patients respond well to the administration of corticosteroids, with muscle enzymes returning to normal levels over a period of 1 to 2 months. Once this has been achieved, the steroid dosage can be tapered and active physical therapy can be instituted to restore muscle strength. Many patients have disease flares as the steroid dosage is being tapered or are unable to discontinue steroid therapy completely. Azathioprine and methotrexate are sometimes used as steroid-sparing agents.

Surgical Considerations

Patients with well-controlled disease should have no problems undergoing surgery. Those who have active disease or have just begun treatment should be observed carefully for pharyngeal and diaphragmatic weakness. Neck flexor strength often correlates with pharyngeal weakness and may be used to estimate pharyngeal strength. Pulmonary function tests may be helpful in assessing weakness, the presence of restrictive disease, and diaphragmatic function.

VASCULITIC SYNDROMES

Vasculitis can occur as a primary syndrome or secondarily in association with most of the conditions discussed in this chapter: RA, SLE, scleroderma, Sjögren's syndrome, and polymyositis or dermatomyositis. No universally accepted classification system has been developed because pathologically similar diseases (eg, Takayasu's arteritis and temporal arteritis) may have dissimilar clinical pictures, and similar clinical findings (eg, palpable purpura) may occur in syndromes with differing pathology and outcomes. These disparities make it difficult to discuss every possible vasculitic syndrome. Moreover, once these conditions are diagnosed, the major surgical considerations revolve around the effects of the medications used in individual patients. These considerations are discussed here.

The American College of Rheumatology has developed classification criteria for seven of the primary vasculitides that were felt to be specific enough to allow differentiation: polyarteritis nodosa, Wegener's granulomatosis, Churg-Strauss syndrome, hypersensitivity vasculitis, Henoch-Schönlein purpura, giant cell arteritis, and Takayasu's arteritis.

The most common of the primary vasculitic syndromes is giant cell arteritis, which has an estimated prevalence in Olmstead County, Minnesota, of 223 per 100,000 population older than 50 years and an annual incidence of 17 cases per 100,000 patients of the same age. The common findings are headache, polymyalgia rheumatica, an abnormal temporal artery on examination, and an elevated sedimentation rate occurring in a person older than 50 years. This disease most commonly affects the large extracranial arteries or the ophthalmic artery and rarely results in ischemic damage other than in the eye. Giant cell arteritis responds to corticosteroid therapy, which is usually initiated at a dosage of 50 to 60 mg/d. immunosuppressive therapy is usually re-

quired only to prevent steroid side effects in patients who cannot discontinue the use of these agents.

Polyarteritis nodosa is the next most common condition, with an incidence of less than 1 per 100,000 in Olmstead County, Minnesota. This disease involves small to medium-sized vessels throughout the body and may lead to serious ischemic disease and infarctions. At least half of all patients have nonspecific symptoms: arthralgia, myalgia, malaise, and fever. A similar number have cutaneous manifestations, which are often suggestive of a vascular process (nodules, ulcers, or livedo reticularis) without being specific for any particular systemic vasculitis. Other patients may appear seriously ill, with obvious palpable purpura and ischemic digits, and clearly have a systemic vasculitis. The kidneys, lungs, and gastrointestinal tract are the most commonly involved organs. Particularly in elderly patients, gastrointestinal involvement may be relatively asymptomatic until a ruptured viscus occurs. Cholecystitis may be the presenting symptom.

Because of the toxicity of treatment, the diagnosis of giant cell arteritis, polyarteritis nodosa, or Wegener's granulomatosis should be based on positive biopsy results if possible. Characteristic radiographic changes may be found in patients with polyarteritis nodosa and Takayasu's arteritis. A specific diagnosis of polyarteritis nodosa may be difficult to confirm, and a clinical diagnosis of "systemic necrotizing vasculitis" may be sufficient to initiate treatment. Hypersensitivity angiitis and Henoch-Schönlein purpura may not require treatment; corticosteroids are almost always effective in giant cell arteritis. Takayasu's arteritis and Churg-Strauss syndrome are usually treated with steroids but occasionally require the administration of immunosuppressive agents. Cyclophosphamide is the treatment of choice for polyarteritis nodosa, Wegener's granulomatosis, and cases of unspecified necrotizing vasculitis.

Surgical Considerations

Patients with these conditions are generally receiving corticosteroids or immunosuppressive drugs with the expected side effects described in the next section. Biopsy of involved or presumably involved blood vessels rarely leads to complications, although meticulous wound care should be observed in those patients who are receiving immunosuppressive doses of drugs.

Patients with suspected or diagnosed polyarteritis or necrotizing vasculitis frequently have intestinal involvement. In older patients and those who are receiving immunosuppressive therapy, there may be significant organ involvement, including ischemic or necrotic changes in the gallbladder, mesentery, or intestine. Surgeons must be aware of these possibilities. Waiting for the classic findings of an acute abdomen to develop before increasing immunosuppressive treatment or performing exploratory surgery is associated with an extremely high mortality.[13]

DRUG THERAPY

The medications used to treat rheumatologic diseases can be classified in three major groups: NSAIDs, corticosteroids, and "remittive" drugs (including some that generally are not thought to be immunosuppressive in nature, such as gold, D-penicillamine, antimalarials, and sulfasalazine, and those that clearly are immunosuppressive, such as methotrexate, azathioprine, and cyclophosphamide).

Studies have shown that many of the drugs used in rheumatology have multiple effects on the immune system and inflammatory mediators. No one mechanism is sufficient to explain the action of these drugs.

NONSTEROIDAL ANTIINFLAMMATORY DRUGS

Mode of Action

Phospholipids in the cell wall are converted to arachidonic acid by phospholipases, which can be inhibited by corticosteroids. Arachidonic acid is converted by cyclooxygenase to prostaglandin G_2, which is quickly converted to prostaglandin H_2. This compound is then converted by isomerases to thromboxanes (in platelets), prostacyclin (in endothelial cells), and prostaglandins (prostaglandin G_2 and prostaglandin E_2 in various organs, including the kidney and stomach). Although the inhibition of cyclooxygenase may be the primary action of many NSAIDs, nonacetylated salicylates appear to have antiinflammatory activity based on inhibition of the isomerases rather than cyclooxygenase.

If this were the only action of NSAIDs, they all would have the same effects. Evidence suggests that their effects on white blood cells vary dramatically, however, and are not dependent on their ability to inhibit cyclooxygenase.

All these drugs have potentially equal efficacy and their selection is usually based on side effects and dosing frequency.

Surgical Considerations

Platelet effects. The most important effect of the NSAIDs in surgery is the inhibition of platelet aggregation. These drugs can be divided into three groups based on their effects on platelets: aspirin, nonacetylated salicylates, and other NSAIDs.

Aspirin causes irreversible acetylation of platelets for their life-span, which is 10 days. Therefore, aspirin use must be discontinued at least 10 days before surgery to ensure that all the platelets present at the time of surgery can aggregate. The number of normal platelets decreases by 10% each day if aspirin is discontinued for a shorter period.

Nonacetylated salicylates (choline magnesium trisalicylate and salsalate are used most commonly) have no effect on platelet aggregation and may be used up to the time of surgery.

The other NSAIDs cause reversible acetylation of platelets and exert their effects as long as they are present in the circulation. Because it takes about five half-lives for any drug to be eliminated from the circulation, these agents can be taken nearer to the time of surgery than can aspirin. Table 36-1 lists the NSAIDs and their half-lives.

Side effects. NSAIDs have their major side effects on the stomach and the kidney. It is impossible to screen for NSAID gastropathy except by endoscopy but the presence of NSAID nephropathy is quickly determined by measuring the blood urea nitrogen and creatinine levels.

In drug trials, about one third of all patients receiving NSAIDs have gastrointestinal side effects, and as many as 10% discontinue use of the drug for this reason. Adverse drug effects range from mild dyspepsia and heartburn to intolerable epigastric pain and severe diarrhea. The most serious side effect, gastric ulceration and bleeding, is unpredictable. Even among patients with the side effect of abdominal pain, only one fourth have ulcers, and the frequency of ulcers in unselected patients in unknown.

TABLE 36–1. Half-Lives of Nonsteroidal Antiinflammatory Agents

Generic Name	Half-Life (h)
Choline magnesium trisalicylate	9–17
Diclofenac	2
Diflunisal	8–12
Etodolac	7.3
Fenoprofen	3
Flurbiprofen	5.7
Ibuprofen	2
Indomethacin	4.5
Meclofenamate	0.8–21
Nabumetone	24
Naproxen	13
Piroxicam	50
Salsalate	3.5–16
Sulindac	16.4
Tolmetin	5

(Physician's desk reference, ed 47. Montvale, NJ, Medical Economic Data, 1993)

Risk factors for gastric ulcer formation include age greater than 50 years, concomitant corticosteroid use, RA, disability, and the presence of abdominal pain as a drug side effect.[14] Neither frequent stool guaiac examinations nor CBCs reveal the presence of an ulcer.[15] The higher the NSAID dosage used, the more likely is the development of gastric ulceration.[16] The nonacetylated salicylates and several of the newer NSAIDs (eg, etodolac and nabumetone) produce less gastric irritation as demonstrated on endoscopy but this may not translate into a lower risk of ulceration. Even very low-dose aspirin therapy (81 mg/d) may result in an increased risk of bleeding in older patients. Endoscopy is only indicated in patients with evidence of current gastrointestinal bleeding.

In patients with compromised renal perfusion or renal insufficiency, blood flow to the renal cortex is often maintained by the intrarenal production of prostaglandin E. When such patients are exposed to NSAIDs, there may be enough inhibition of prostaglandin production to result in shunting of blood away from the cortex with a resultant rise in blood urea nitrogen and creatinine levels. This effect is usually reversible with discontinuation of NSAID use. The likelihood of this effect does not increase with the duration of therapy. If the blood urea nitrogen and creatinine levels do not increase in the first 1 to 3 weeks after therapy is initiated, they are unlikely to do so unless renal hemodynamics are altered by other drugs or changes in patient health.

This effect develops more quickly with drugs that have shorter half-lives. The nonacetylated salicylates are less likely to cause this complication because they are only half as effective in reducing prostaglandin E production as are other NSAIDs. Sulindac may also be less likely to produce this effect because it circulates as a prodrug and may not be active in the kidney. Therapy with most of these drugs is discontinued preoperatively, so any adverse effect they have had on the kidneys will be reversed by the time of surgery.

Route of administration. Because NSAIDs traditionally have been given orally in pill form, patients have not been able to take them while their oral intake was restricted. Indomethacin is available as a rectal suppository, however, and ketorolac is available for intramuscular injection. Neither of these routes eliminates the side effects associated with NSAIDs. Naproxen and several of the nonacetylated salicylates are available as liquids for those patients who have nasogastric or percutaneous gastric feeding tubes in place.

Role of the nonsteroidal antiinflammatory drug. In general, the more antirheumatic drugs patients are taking, the less vital are NSAIDs in controlling symptoms. Surgeons may discontinue NSAID therapy sooner and reinstitute it

later in patients who are receiving more than one drug. Patients with RA, SLE, and other diseases who are taking corticosteroids are given extra steroids at the time of surgery (see later discussion). This often suppresses the disease symptoms that are being treated with the NSAID sufficiently so that discontinuation of NSAID therapy does not produce symptoms. Patients who have osteoarthritis can be given analgesic drugs, including acetaminophen (as much as 4000 mg/d), until their NSAIDs can be taken again.

NSAID therapy usually is discontinued before surgery because of concern regarding perioperative bleeding. Drug use should be discontinued at least five half-lives before surgery for most NSAIDs, 10 days (if possible) before surgery for aspirin, and the day before surgery for nonacetylated salicylates. Therapy can be reinitiated when the risk of bleeding has returned to baseline levels.

When the discontinuation of NSAID therapy results in a flare of disease before the drug can be given again, several options are available. Corticosteroids can be given intraarticularly for a flare in one or two joints and can be administered systemically for several days (generally, 20 mg/d of prednisone) for a more generalized flare of articular or serosal symptoms.

CORTICOSTEROIDS

Although corticosteroids have myriad effects on the human body and are of major importance in many rheumatologic diseases, they have few effects that relate to surgery. Because they can be administered parenterally, their use does not need to be discontinued at the time of surgery.

Wound healing may be affected by corticosteroids, and bruising after minimal trauma is common during therapy with these drugs. Patients should be given the lowest dose that controls their underlying disease before surgery.

A major concern in patients who are taking steroids is their ability to produce additional endogenous steroids at the time of surgery. The degree to which the hypothalamic-pituitary-adrenal axis can be suppressed by exogenous steroids and the rapidity of recovery vary between patients. Doses of prednisone exceeding 10 mg/d suppress the axis, and it may take as long as 1 year before it returns to normal. In patients who have taken more than 10 mg/d or have taken steroids for more than several weeks within the past year, either the expected steroid surge can be replaced or the hypothalamic-pituitary-adrenal axis can be tested before operation.

The maximal amount of corticosteroids produced in the stress situation of surgery is about equivalent to 300 mg of hydrocortisone or 60 mg of prednisone. Patients who are receiving dosages at least this high do not require supplemental steroids at the time of surgery and should continue to be given an equivalent parenteral dose until they are able to resume their preoperative steroid regimen. Those who are taking lower dosages can be given hydrocortisone (which has mineralocorticoid activity), 100 mg three times daily, or methylprednisolone (which does not have mineralocorticoid activity), 16 mg three times daily.[17]

To test the hypothalamic-pituitary-adrenal axis, 40 U of cosyntropin, a synthetic adrenocorticotropic hormone analogue, is given intravenously and plasma cortisol levels are drawn before and 45 minutes after the injection. If the baseline level doubles, rises more than 7 μg, or exceeds 18 μg at 45 minutes, the hypothalamic-pituitary-adrenal axis is intact and supplementation is unnecessary.

SECOND-LINE ANTIRHEUMATIC DRUGS

Second-line antirheumatic drugs are a broad class of agents that have gone by many names because it is not clear whether they are "remittive" or "disease-modifying" in RA. Some of these drugs are not thought to be immunosuppressive (eg, gold, D-penicillamine, hydroxychloroquine, azulfidine), whereas others are (eg, azathioprine, cyclophosphamide, methotrexate). The risk of postoperative infections is increased with the latter agents, but discontinuing their use before surgery to eliminate this risk is likely to result in a flare of the underlying disease. Therefore, the general recommendation is to continue to administer all these drugs until the time of surgery and to give them again as soon as possible afterward. Some controversy exists in regard to methotrexate, however.

Azathioprine

The mode of action of azathioprine is not precisely known. It is presumed to inhibit inflammation related to white blood cell activity by inhibiting DNA synthesis through its known effects on purine biosynthesis. It is given in a dosage of 100 to 250 mg/d and is most commonly used in patients with RA. It is also used in patients with SLE, myositis, or one of the vasculitides, primarily as a steroid-sparing agent. The most common serious acute side effect is leukopenia, which may require reduction in the dosage or temporary cessation of therapy. Some patients have reproducible reductions in their white blood cell counts at particular dosage levels.

Because of its effect on white blood cells, patients who are taking azathioprine are more likely to have immunosuppression and are more susceptible to all types of infection. This susceptibility may not be associated with the absolute white blood cell count. Prolonged discontinuation of therapy with the drug causes a flare of the underlying dis-

ease, so the drug-free interval before surgery should be as short as possible.

Cyclophosphamide

Cyclophosphamide is the most commonly used alkylating agent in the United States. By cross-linking with DNA, cyclophosphamide impairs cellular replication and leads to a diminution of the immune response. Cyclophosphamide is usually given either daily as an oral medication (2 to 3 mg/kg/d) or monthly or quarterly as an intravenous bolus. The dosage is usually adjusted to cause leukopenia, either chronically with the daily oral dose or 10 to 14 days later with the intravenous bolus. It is most frequently used in patients who have necrotizing vasculitis (eg, polyarteritis nodosa, Wegner's granulomatosis); SLE with acute renal or neurologic involvement; or RA with evidence of an acute large vessel vasculitis (usually a mononeuritis multiplex).

Because cyclophosphamide is given to induce leukopenia, the risk of infection is increased. Therefore, if patients are receiving the drug on a daily basis, extreme care must be taken to prevent postoperative infections by limiting urinary catheterization as much as possible and changing intravenous lines frequently and carefully. For patients who are receiving intermittent therapy, surgery should be scheduled between doses if possible.

Cyclophosphamide can interact with suxamethonium, prolonging recovery from anesthesia because of decreased plasma cholinesterase levels.

Gold

Intramuscular gold is one of the oldest therapies available for RA and is usually given as gold sodium thiomalate. More recently, an oral form of gold, auranofin, has become available. The mode of action of this therapy is not known, although these drugs have multiple effects in humans. Gold therapy is rarely used in any other rheumatic disease; it is sometimes used in psoriatic arthritis.

The major side effects of intramuscular gold are bone marrow depression and proteinuria. These usually develop after a period of drug therapy, and permanent effects can be largely prevented by checking the CBC and urinalysis each week before giving the injection, and reducing the dosage or increasing the dosing interval if changes occur. The usual dose is 50 mg intramuscularly per week, although patients who have taken gold for a long time and are in remission frequently receive monthly injections. Oral gold can cause the same effects, although they appear to occur less frequently. Diarrhea is its most common side effect. The usual dosage is 3 mg twice daily, with a maximum dosage of 3 mg three times daily.

These drugs do not appear to have any effects specific to patients who are undergoing surgery. Patients who are receiving intramuscular gold can continue this therapy as long as a CBC and urinalysis are performed weekly. Oral gold can be given as long as patients can take oral medications. If oral intake must be restricted for a prolonged period, intramuscular gold can be given weekly. When auranofin therapy is reinitiated, it should be given at a rate of one tablet a day for a while before increasing to the usual dosage to decrease the likelihood of diarrhea.

Hydroxychloroquine

Antimalarial drugs have been used to treat RA and SLE for many years. Hydroxychloroquine is more commonly used today than is chloroquine. The mode of action of these drugs is unknown and, in most patients, there is a period of weeks to months after therapy is instituted or discontinued before any change is observed in their condition. Hydroxychloroquine has no significant effects relating to surgery. The usual recommendation is that therapy with this drug be discontinued the night before surgery and reinitiated as soon as patients can take oral medications.

Methotrexate

Methotrexate is a folic acid analogue that interferes with thymidine synthesis, leading to the inhibition of DNA synthesis and cellular proliferation. Unlike cyclophosphamide, its efficacy does not seem to depend on the production of leukopenia. Over the past 10 years, it has assumed a much more important role in the treatment of rheumatic diseases, particularly RA.

Methotrexate has a much faster onset of action than do many of the other second-line drugs. In long-term studies, 50% to 60% of patients who begin methotrexate therapy continue to receive it 5 years later, compared with 20% to 30% of patients who begin therapy with all other remittive drugs. Methotrexate is effective in patients with RA and psoriatic arthritis, and is used in patients with other spondyloarthropathies and inflammatory muscle diseases. Dosages range from 5 to 15 mg orally once a week, although intramuscular dosing can be used.

The major concern with the use of methotrexate is the development of cirrhosis. When this drug was initially used for psoriasis, usually in dosages higher than those used for RA, the development of cirrhosis in the absence of liver test abnormalities was reported. As a result, it was recommended that patients receiving methotrexate undergo yearly liver biopsies. With the passage of time, it has become clear that methotrexate-induced cirrhosis (or even fibrosis) in RA is an extremely rare event, occurring in fewer

than 1 in 1000 patients who take the drug for at least 5 years.[18]

The other significant side effect is acute methotrexate lung toxicity, which is an idiosyncratic inflammatory response that usually responds to the discontinuation of methotrexate therapy and administration of corticosteroids. This complication has been reported to occur in as many as 8% of patients who take methotrexate but this has not been confirmed in other large studies.

Many patients receiving methotrexate have nausea, dyspepsia, and stomatitis. The frequency of these side effects appears to be decreased if 1 mg of folic acid is given daily. This does not appear to reduce the efficacy of methotrexate.

Surgical considerations. Several reports have been published regarding surgical risks in patients treated with methotrexate. These studies are retrospective reviews of the experiences of particular hospitals. It is difficult, therefore, to make definitive recommendations concerning how or when methotrexate should be discontinued before surgery.

Perhala and colleagues found no statistically significant increase in the incidence of infection in patients who had taken methotrexate within 4 weeks of surgery compared with those who had never taken this drug.[19] Patients who had last taken methotrexate more than 4 weeks before surgery were not evaluated.

West and Vogelgesang compared patients who were instructed to discontinue methotrexate therapy the week before, week of, and week after surgery with those who continued to take the drug.[20] No increase in the incidence of infection was noted in those patients who continued to receive methotrexate therapy. Nonetheless, we routinely advise patients to stop taking methotrexate for 3 weeks.

Bridges and associates compared patients who had discontinued methotrexate therapy more than 4 weeks before surgery to those who had taken methotrexate within 4 weeks of surgery (even if they had discontinued therapy for some shorter period).[21] These authors found an increase in complications in the group who took methotrexate within the month before surgery. Only four patients had complications: two had wound dehiscence (in the knee), one had infection (in the knee), and one had both (tendon transfer). It appears that most of the patients in both groups were told to reinitiate methotrexate therapy 4 to 6 weeks after operation. This study suggests that wound dehiscence may be as much of a problem as infection, particularly in patients undergoing knee replacement, in whom physical therapy can be vigorous.

None of the three studies found any evidence to implicate other medications or disease activity as contributing factors. We recommend withholding methotrexate therapy for the week before surgery, the week of surgery, and the week after surgery.

Penicillamine

Penicillamine is also known as D-penicillamine and shares a sulfhydryl group with intramuscular gold. As a result, it has a similar side effect profile, which must be monitored with frequent CBCs and urinalyses. The onset of action is very slow, and rapid increases in the dosage seem to increase the frequency of side effects. Dosing is begun at 125 or 250 mg/d and increased gradually by 125 to 250 mg every 1 to 2 months as indicated by clinical response until a dosage of 750 mg is reached. This drug is effective in patients with RA and may be effective in those with scleroderma. In a large retrospective study from the University of Pittsburgh, patients who were given D-penicillamine were less likely to develop involvement in new organ systems compared with patients who did not receive this agent. A prospective multicenter trial is in progress.

Poor wound healing has been reported in some patients taking D-penicillamine but the effect does not seem to be any greater than that seen with corticosteroids and there is no increase in the rate of wound infection or dehiscence.

Sulfasalazine

The mode of action of sulfasalazine is not known and administering either of its two components alone is not efficacious. It is used in patients with RA and in those with spondyloarthropathy. The usual dose is 500 to 1500 mg twice daily. Administration of this agent can be discontinued the night before surgery and restarted as soon as patients are able to tolerate oral intake.

REFERENCES

1. Lawrence RC, Hochberg MC, Kelsey JL, et al. Estimates of the prevalence of selected arthritic and musculoskeletal diseases in the United States. J Rheumatol 1989;16:867–884.
2. Hochberg MC. Osteoarthritis. In: Stobo JD, Hellmann DB, Traill TA, eds. The principles and practice of medicine, ed 23. Norwalk, CT, Appleton & Lange, in press.
3. Goldberg VM. Surgery in osteoarthritis: general considerations. In: Moskowitz RW, Howell DS, Goldberg VM, Mankin HJ, eds. Osteoarthritis: diagnosis and medical/surgical management, ed 2. Philadelphia, WB Saunders Co, 1992:535–544.
4. Arnett FC, Edworthy S, Bloch DA, et al. The American Rheumatism Association 1987 revised criteria for the classification of rheumatoid arthritis. Arthritis Rheum 1988;31:315–324.
5. Parish DC, Clark JA, Liebowitz SM, Hicks WC. Sudden death in rheumatoid arthritis from vertical subluxation of the odontoid process. J Natl Med Assoc 1990;82:297–304.
6. Wallace SI, Robinson H, Masi AT, et al. Selected data on primary gout. Bull Rheum Dis 1979;29:992–995.
7. Tan EM, Cohen AS, Fries JF, et al. The 1982 revised criteria for the classification of systemic lupus erythematosus. Arthritis Rheum 1982;25:1271–1277.
8. Petri M, Rheinschmidt M, Whiting-O'Keefe Q, et al. The frequency of lupus anticoagulant in systemic lupus erythematosus. Ann Intern Med 1987;106:524–531.
9. Asherson RA, Lubbe WF. Cerebral and valve lesions in SLE: association with antiphospholipid antibodies. J Rheumatol 1988;15:539–543.
10. Locksin MD, Druzin ML, Goei S, et al. Antibody to cardiolipin as a predictor of fetal distress or death in pregnant patients with systemic lupus erythematosus. N Engl J Med 1985;313:152–156.
11. Papa MZ, Shiloni E, Vetto JT, et al. Surgical morbidity in patients with systemic lupus erythematosus. Am J Surg 1989;157:295–298.
12. Masi AT, Rodnan GR, Medsger TA, et al. Preliminary criteria for the classification of systemic sclerosis (scleroderma). Bull Rheum Dis 1981;31:1–6.
13. Zizic TM, Classen JN, Stevens MB. Acute abdominal complications of systemic lupus erythematosus and polyarteritis nodosa. Am J Med 1982;73:525–531.
14. Fries JF, Williams CA, Bloch DA, Michel BA. Nonsteroidal antiinflammatory drug-associated gastropathy: incidence and risk factors. Am J Med 1991;91:213–222.
15. Bahrt KM, Korman LY, Nashel DJ. Significance of a positive test for occult blood in stools of patients taking anti-inflammatory drugs. Arch Intern Med 1984;144:2165–2166.
16. Griffin MR, Piper JM, Daugherty JR, et al. Nonsteroidal anti-inflammatory drug use and increased use risk for peptic ulcer disease in elderly patients. Ann Intern Med 1991;114:257–263.
17. Goldmann DR. Steroid use in surgical patients. Hosp Pract (Off Ed) 1991;26:54–61.
18. Walker AM, Funch D, Dreyer NA, et al. Determinants of serious liver disease among patients receiving low-dose methotrexate for rheumatoid arthritis. Arthritis Rheum 1993;36:329–335.
19. Perhala RS, Wilke WS, Clough JD, Segal AM. Local infectious complications following large joint replacement in rheumatoid arthritis patients treated with methotrexate versus those not treated with methotrexate. Arthritis Rheum 1991;34:146–152.
20. West SG, Vogelgesang SA. Methotrexate (MTX) and postoperative joint infection in rheumatoid arthritis patients undergoing total joint arthroplasty (TJA). Arthritis Rheum 1990;33:S61.
21. Bridges SL, Lopez-Mendez A, Han KC, et al. Should methotrexate be discontinued before elective orthopedic surgery in patients with rheumatoid arthritis? J Rheumatol 1991;18:984–988.

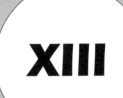

NEUROLOGY

Medical Management of the Surgical Patient, Third Edition,
edited by Michael F. Lubin, H. Kenneth Walker, and Robert B. Smith III.
J.B. Lippincott Company, Philadelphia, PA © 1995.

CHAPTER

DEMENTIA · 37

David A. Olson
Alexander P. Auchus
Robert C. Green

The demographic profile of our society is rapidly changing into one in which those older than 65 years will represent 13.9% of the American population by the year 2010,[1] and the rising number of older persons with dementia is now a major public health concern.[2,3] In this country, 188 new cases of dementia per 100,000 persons are recognized annually, and this figure increases dramatically to 1055 in 100,000 persons per year among those 80 years and older.[4] Many older persons live and function in the community with early or mild forms of dementia that often go unrecognized by physicians.[4-8] The prevalence of dementia among hospitalized patients is even higher and has been estimated at 12% to 20%.[9]

At the same time that these demographic changes have occurred, surgical procedures that were once considered too dangerous for older patients have become safer. For example, many studies have demonstrated the feasibility and efficacy of open heart surgery for the elderly.[10,11] Thus, patients with mild or moderate dementia, and perhaps more significantly, with unsuspected dementia, are increasingly becoming operative candidates.

This chapter explores the medical, legal, and ethical issues affecting the decision to operate on patients with known or suspected dementia. The term *dementia* is used here to describe age-associated, progressive decline in cognitive abilities, most often resulting from Alzheimer's disease or vascular causes. This chapter does not address issues concerning patients with static neurologic deficits (eg, cerebral palsy, mental retardation, traumatic brain injury); patients with dementia associated with progressive and fatal neurologic problems (eg, acquired immunodeficiency syndrome, malignant brain tumors); or patients with reduced cognitive capacity related purely to psychiatric disease.

On rare occasions, surgery is indicated as a diagnostic or therapeutic procedure for patients with dementia. For example, brain biopsies may be performed on some patients with potentially treatable dementias, and ventricular shunting procedures are indicated for patients with symptomatic hydrocephalus. These special cases typically come to surgery after extensive neurologic evaluation of the dementing condition. For most patients with known or suspected dementia, however, surgery is under consideration for an unrelated condition. Only some of these patients will have undergone a thorough diagnostic evaluation for their cognitive difficulties. Three critical questions must be asked in regard to all patients with dementia during the presurgical period: (1) What is the cause of the dementia? (2) How will the dementia affect the preoperative care of the patient? (3) How will the dementia affect the care and recovery of the patient after surgery?

CAUSES OF DEMENTING DISORDERS

Dementia is the final common pathway for many disease processes and may result from more than 50 neurologic, medical, and psychiatric causes.[12] Alzheimer's disease, either alone or in combination with another dementing illness, accounts for about 60% of cases and, depending on the population studied, vascular dementia may be responsible for another 20% of cases. Other disorders, such as Parkinson's disease and Huntington's disease, depression, metabolic and nutritional disorders, and infections, account for most of the remaining causes. "Reversible" dementias may be present in as many as 10% of all patients with dementia, and include the dementia syndrome of depression (sometimes called depressive "pseudodementia"), hypothyroidism, vitamin B_{12} deficiency, normal-pressure hydrocephalus, some chronic meningitides, and the long-term effects of medications, especially sedative and hypnotic agents (Table 37-1).

When surgery is being considered in patients with cognitive impairment, it is important that the cause of the deficit be determined before the decision to operate is made. A careful history obtained from family and close friends usually provides the most reliable data about patients' cognitive status.[13] Questions about how patients spend their days should elicit information regarding whether any previously independent tasks (eg, cooking, shopping, managing personal finances, driving) have been assumed by others. Consideration should also be given to complaints of anxiety, low mood, and vegetative signs suggestive of depression such as loss of appetite, loss of libido, and sleep disturbance.

Because medical syndromes have such an important effect on operative risk and can cause or exacerbate cognitive impairments, the preoperative medical examination, with subsequent optimization of any medication regimens, is of paramount importance. Careful neurologic and mental status examinations are also essential and may uncover findings that help to determine the cause of the cognitive deficits. For example, focal findings on the neurologic examination may suggest a vascular dementia, whereas extrapyramidal signs such as cogwheel rigidity or bradykinesia may reveal undiagnosed Parkinson's disease. Primitive signs, such as the grasp, palmomental, or snout reflexes, often occur in patients with dementia but do not add specific diagnostic information.[15]

A reasonable mental status examination can be performed in the office or at the bedside with little difficulty. Sensitivities over 80% and specificities over 90% have been demonstrated for the detection of Alzheimer's disease by both a simple delayed word recall task[16] and a bedside clock-drawing task.[17] For clinicians who are not accustomed to performing these tests as part of their regular patient evaluations, several brief, standardized mental status

TABLE 37–1. Drugs That Can Cause Delirium in Elderly Patients With Dementia

Sedatives	**Antihypertensives**
Benzodiazepines	β-Blockers
Diazepam (Valium)	Methyldopa
Flurazepam (Dalmane)	Clonidine
Others	**Anticonvulsants**
Barbiturates	Phenytoin (Dilantin)
Meprobamate (Miltown)	Phenobarbital
Ethanol	**Antiinflammatories**
Antihistamines	Indomethacin (Indocin)
Diphenhydramine	Prednisone
(Benadryl)	**Antimicrobials**
Cimetidine (Tagamet)	Cephalexin
Others	Isoniazid
Anticholinergics	Rifampin
Antiparkinsonian agents	Metronidazole
Benztropine (Cogentin)	**Cardioglycosides**
Trihexyphenidyl (Artane)	Digoxin
Others	Digitoxin
Antispasmodics	**Antiarrhythmics**
Phenothiazines	Quinidine
Chlorpromazine	Procainamide
(Thorazine)	Disopyramide
Thioridazine (Mellaril)	Mexiletine
Others	**Stimulants**
Scopolamine patches	Amphetamines
Tricyclic antidepressants	Methylphenidate
Amitriptyline (Elavil)	**Topicals**
Imipramine (Tofranil)	Pilocarpine eyedrops
Others	**Miscellaneous**
Dopaminergics	Seleqiline (Eldepryl)
Carbidopa/levodopa	Lithium
(Sinemet)	
Bromocriptine (Parlodel)	
Others	
Analgesics	
Salicylates	
Narcotics	
Meperidine (Demerol)	
Others	

examinations are available. The Mini Mental State Examination[18] takes about 10 minutes to administer and has reasonable sensitivity and specificity for detecting moderate dementia.[19] Unfortunately, it is less accurate in patients who are educationally disadvantaged or have only mild cognitive symptoms.[19–21] Other popular brief assessment instruments include the Short Portable Mental Status Questionnaire,[22] the Cognitive Capacity Screening Examination,[23] and the Dementia Rating Scale.[24]

Once cognitive impairment is documented by history and physical examination, the diagnostic evaluation should include a complete blood count, an electrolyte and metabolic panel, a thyroid-stimulating hormone level, vitamin B_{12} and folate levels, a *Treponema pallidum* microhemagglutination, and a human immunodeficiency virus antibody test (if clinically appropriate). A brain imaging study (computed tomography or magnetic resonance imaging) is also obtained to evaluate for the presence of mass lesions, hydrocephalus, or multiple infarctions. Any positive results from these diagnostic studies may have implications for surgery. For example, because patients with vascular dementia may have impaired autoregulation of cerebral blood flow, they may demonstrate improved cognition when their blood pressures are within a higher range than is customary. Special attention should be devoted to blood pressure management in the operative and perioperative periods in such patients.[25]

PREOPERATIVE CONSIDERATIONS

Even if only a mild dementia is present before general anesthesia is induced, the preoperative period is the best time to warn family members of the increased probability of postoperative delirium. Time devoted to educating the family in this regard before any surgical intervention is well spent and makes any occurrence of postoperative delirium less stressful for all involved parties.

Preoperative evaluation does not always include nutritional assessment but this may be extremely important in patients with dementia. Patients with even mild dementia may have poor nutrition, and protein-calorie malnutrition may be present in more than half the institutionalized elderly, among whom the prevalence of dementia is especially high.[26] Therefore, such patients may require a nutritional build-up period before elective procedures, and patients who need emergency surgery may require nutritional supplementation during their hospitalizations.

All but the most emergent surgical procedures require informed consent but the ability of patients to give informed consent or to make informed refusals hinges on their competency, which is a legal status determination based on subjective assessment of the ability to make informed judgments about specific treatment options and their attendant risks.[27] The extent to which patients with dementia have the capacity to make such informed decisions poses difficult, and sometimes irresolvable, questions. Decisions about antibiotic therapy and other low-risk health care procedures may require only that patients communicate simple choices, whereas decisions about experimental or high-risk procedures require substantially more cognitive capacity.[28] If mental competence is in question, a formal assessment by a psychiatrist or neurologist should be carried out. Family members or other patient advocates should be encouraged to seek legal recognition as surrogate decision makers in matters relating to both health care decisions and financial decisions.

Durable Power of Attorney is a written legal document signed by patients in which they specify the powers conferred.[29] This is frequently sought by patients' families because, unlike the traditional Power of Attorney, Durable Power of Attorney remains valid even after patients are incapacitated. Durable Power of Attorney can be used either for medical purposes (the Durable Power of Attorney for Health Care) or for financial purposes (the Durable Financial Power of Attorney). Formal guardianship may be necessary if patients are too incapacitated to participate meaningfully in decisions about the Power of Attorney but guardianship, even emergency guardianship, is time-consuming, expensive, and extremely burdensome.

Issues surrounding the use of advance directives have recently received considerable attention with regard to the use of long-term life support measures for patients with irreversible dementias and other incurable illnesses. Although, in actual practice, most situations involving decisions to restrict or terminate care are handled by quiet consensus between physicians and family members, an increasingly litigious climate has forced both individuals and institutions to follow more formal guidelines. In 1990, the Supreme Court ruled in *Cruzan v Director, Missouri Department of Health*, that the state could require "clear and convincing" evidence regarding patients' wishes for life-sustaining procedures, noting that affidavits produced by family members detailing patients' premorbid verbal directives are considered as supportive, but not definitive, evidence.[30] Thus, these policies vary depending on the state and the institution involved.

The regulatory confusion surrounding advance directives has been simplified in many states by the formal recognition of "living wills." These are popular advance directives that usually define the duration, degree of invasiveness, and type of health care that patients wish to receive in the event of a terminal illness. Arguing that the number and complexity of scenarios involving health care issues in the terminal phases of life may be limitless, Justice O'Connor, in her concurring opinion in *Cruzan*, recommended the premorbid appointment of a surrogate decision maker. Several states have even created a "springing" Durable Power of Attorney that may be enacted only if patients become incapable of making their own decisions.[29]

It has been argued that withdrawal and withholding of treatment are ethically synonymous. For patients and their families, however, these two courses often evoke different emotional responses.[31] Although the legal system generally supports these practices under defined circumstances, this varies from jurisdiction to jurisdiction, and it is strongly recommended that decisions regarding the withdrawal and withholding of treatment be addressed explicitly with both patients and their families.[32]

POSTOPERATIVE ISSUES

Patients who have severe cognitive or physical problems after major surgery frequently require institutionalization, even if they were previously independent.[33,34] Even when institutionalization is not necessary, the activities of patients with dementia may be more limited on discharge from the hospital. If the dementia was discovered at the time of the surgery, the treating physician may need to restrict such potentially dangerous activities as cooking and driving. Driving in particular is more dangerous in persons with dementia but it is such a symbol of independence in our society that restrictions are difficult to broach with patients.[35–37]

Transient cognitive impairment during the first postoperative week is common in the elderly, and is more likely after general than after regional anesthesia, unless the regional anesthesia includes intraoperative intravenous sedation with agents such as fentanyl, diazepam, or droperidol.[38,39] Some poorly controlled studies have suggested that permanent cognitive impairment results from general anesthesia[40–42] but several more recent reports have found no difference between large numbers of elderly patients undergoing regional and general anesthesia who were tested with several neuropsychologic measures before and several months after surgery.[43–45] General anesthesia, therefore, does not seem to produce lasting cognitive impairment. Most of these studies, however, deliberately excluded patients with demonstrable dementia. At times, the surgery or the anesthesia is inappropriately held responsible for the appearance of a dementia after an operative procedure. In our experience, it is far more likely that a postoperative delirium has developed, and this delirium represents the unmasking of an already present dementia.

The most common cognitive problem affecting both patients with dementia and normal elderly patients in the postoperative period is restlessness, confusion, and agitation, also known as delirium. Rates of postoperative delirium among the elderly vary widely depending on the patient population studied, the surgery performed, and the assessment techniques used. For example, although the prevalence of postoperative delirium has been reported as 7% in general surgical patients,[46] 44% of elderly patients undergoing repair of femoral neck fractures experienced postoperative delirium.[47] Delirium can be caused by sedating medications, medical complications, removal of ambient sensory input, and cerebral damage from microemboli.[48,49] Occult infection or organ failure are common in delirious patients but sometimes a specific cause of postoperative delirium cannot be identified.[46] In such situations, the correction of several mildly abnormal metabolic and pharmacologic parameters frequently produces improvement.[50] The impression that sensory and sleep deprivation can produce "intensive care unit psychosis" has been difficult to substantiate.[48,51–53]

Our clinical experience suggests that, when it is sought, postoperative delirium is far more common among elderly patients, even those without dementia, than is generally realized. Delirious patients may be quietly confused in a manner not readily noticed through casual conversation; therefore, more direct cognitive assessment should be a routine element of postoperative care.[54] Several predisposing factors for postoperative delirium in the elderly include decreased brain weight, reduced cerebral blood flow and metabolic rate, and decrements in brain neurotransmitter levels.[50] Such abnormalities in persons with preclinical or early dementing syndromes may diminish the "neurologic reserve" of elderly patients and thereby predispose them to postoperative delirium.[55] Patients with overt dementia have even less neurologic reserve and, consequently, are far more vulnerable to the development of delirium.[56] In light of this association, the risk of postoperative delirium should be discussed with the families of all patients who have dementia, and perhaps with all elderly patients before surgery.

Patients with dementia who have decreased neurologic reserve are often particularly vulnerable to cognitive dysfunction with even low doses of anticholinergic medications.[47,57] Typical doses of commonly prescribed medications that are not traditionally considered to be anticholinergic, such as ranitidine, codeine, nifedipine, and warfarin (Coumadin), recently have been shown to have potential anticholinergic effects.[58] Other common medications, including digitalis, benzodiazepines, barbiturates, catecholamine-depleting antihypertensives, and neuroleptics, can produce postoperative delirium.[50,59] Table 37-1 lists some drugs that can cause delirium in the elderly.

Elderly patients with dementia sometimes exhibit nocturnal agitation and an apparent cyclicity in their cognitive functioning. This is commonly referred to as "sundowning," a widely used term for a clinical phenomenon that is characterized by the onset or exacerbation of agitation, restlessness, panic, intensified disorientation, and verbal or physical outbursts in the afternoon or evening. Sundowning is probably not related to ambient lighting, as implied by older studies,[60] but may reflect a cyclical behavior pattern in some patients. A disorder of the sleep–wake cycle has been implicated,[61–64] and circadian behavior changes may increase in frequency and intensity as the season changes from longer light exposures (autumn) to shorter light exposures (winter).[65,66]

Depression in elderly patients with dementia is an important treatable cause of postoperative decline that is frequently overlooked. Elderly patients often deny affective symptoms or have atypical depression that lacks the prominent emotional features commonly recognized in younger patients.[67] Nonetheless, patients who have undergone an operation may be effectively treated for depression with antidepressant medication,[68,69] psychotherapy,[70] or electroconvulsive therapy.[71]

TREATMENT OF POSTOPERATIVE DELIRIUM AND AGITATION

Delirium in the postoperative period produces significant morbidity and can even be fatal. Effective treatment depends on the cause but some principles can be applied to almost any case (Table 37-2). The use of all nonessential medications should be discontinued. Centrally acting medications should be reevaluated and replaced with more peripherally acting equivalents. Metabolic derangements and other medical disorders should be sought for and corrected. Environmental adjustments to provide more soothing and simplified surroundings may help to reduce symptoms.[72] Restraints should be used as a last resort in markedly agitated patients to prevent falls and self-induced injuries.[73] Recommended guidelines for restraint orders include the reason for the restraint, the type of restraint to be applied, and the length of time the restraint should be used. "As needed" restraint orders are not appropriate. Attention should be paid to the correct application and monitoring of restraints because accidental self-strangulation can occur.[74]

Despite the tremendous frequency of postoperative delirium, the utility of pharmacologic therapies for this problem is not well validated.[75,76] Most clinicians treat delirium with low doses of neuroleptics[77,78] or benzodiazepines. Haloperidol is frequently chosen because of its relatively low anticholinergic side effect profile.[79] Age-related reductions in liver and kidney function, increased body fat proportions, and changes in brain receptors all make the elderly particularly sensitive to even small amounts of psychoactive medications, and dosages should be monitored carefully during the first days of treatment to achieve effective steady-state concentrations.[72,80] It is important to frequently assess patients clinically for signs of toxicity and oversedation, and for control of target symptoms.[72] Even with such precautions, however, dangerous side effects such as orthostatic hypotension and falls can occur.[81]

TABLE 37–2. The Treatment of Agitation in Elderly Patients With Dementia

---

Reexamine the patient for signs of infection, fecal impaction, painful injury, or new neurologic compromise.

Correct any demonstrable metabolic disturbances.

Eliminate or reduce all nonessential medications.

Simplify the patient's environment and provide bedside supervision (especially by available family members).

Consider chloral hydrate if sleep disturbance is severe.

Consider a short course of a low-dose neuroleptic.

Consider physical restraints to prevent accidental self-injury (with daily reevaluation of need for continued restraint).

Despite these cautions, pharmacologic control of behavioral problems in patients with dementia can be achieved. Coccaro and colleagues[77] found less agitation and improved self-care in 59 elderly patients with dementia who were treated with low doses of haloperidol, oxazepam, or diphenhydramine. A double-blinded study of a group of 56 elderly outpatients with abnormal mood and behavior found not only improvement in the psychiatric parameters after treatment with haloperidol or thioridazine but also significant improvement in the cognitive functioning of the patients who received haloperidol.[79]

We generally use oral or intramuscular haloperidol in dosages ranging from 0.5 mg every 24 hours to 1 mg every 8 hours as an initial pharmacologic step to control excessive agitation in hospitalized patients with dementia. Parkinsonism with poor gait function is a common side effect of haloperidol and should be looked for carefully. Benzodiazepines such as lorazepam (given orally or intramuscularly in dosages ranging from 0.5 mg every 12 hours to 1 mg every 8 hours) are sometimes recommended to control agitation. Impairment of balance and oversedation can develop easily, however. We try not to use benzodiazepines except when sedative or alcohol withdrawal is suspected. Chloral hydrate in a dosage of 250 to 1000 mg orally at bedtime may be used safely for sleep induction. It is critically important that the dosage of any psychoactive agents given to control postoperative delirium be tapered once the delirium has cleared.

Persistent behavioral problems after surgical procedures may sometimes be treated effectively with anticonvulsants (eg, carbamazepine or valproic acid), sedating antidepressants (eg, trazodone), or "atypical" neuroleptics (eg, clozapine); however, such treatment strategies are beyond the scope of this chapter.

SUMMARY

The aging of the US population, together with advances in surgical techniques, will make surgery in elderly patients with dementia increasingly common. Careful preoperative evaluation is essential to detect and correctly diagnose dementia in surgical candidates. Impaired cognition is a major risk factor for surgical morbidity and mortality among normal aged patients as well as among patients with dementia. Early communication with patients and their families is important to establish clear choices regarding any advance directives. Postoperative delirium and agitation are common and should be anticipated. The delirium is often reversible and a wide array of effective therapies are available for postoperative patients with confusion and agitation. Used wisely, these therapies may increase the number of elderly patients with dementia who can successfully tolerate surgical intervention.

REFERENCES

1. Bureau of the Census, Statistical Abstract of the United States, ed 119. Washington, DC, US Government Printing Office, 1990:16.
2. Weiler P. The public health impact of Alzheimer's disease. Am J Public Health 1987;77:1157–1158.
3. Sun R, Speers M. Mortality from Alzheimer disease: United States, 1979–1987. MMWR 1990;39:785–788.
4. Schoenberg B, Kokmen E, Okazaki H. Alzheimer's disease and other dementing illnesses in a defined United States community: incidence rates and clinical features. Ann Neurol 1987;22:724–729.
5. Rocca WA, Amaducci LA, Schoenberg BS. Epidemiology of clinically diagnosed Alzheimer's disease. Ann Neurol 1986;19:415–424.
6. Jorm AF, Korten AE, Henderson AS. The prevalence of dementia: a quantitative integration of the literature. Acta Psychiatr Scand 1987;76:465–479.
7. Katzman R, Aronson M, Fuld P, et al. Development of dementing illnesses in an 80-year-old volunteer cohort. Ann Neurol 1989;25:317–324.
8. Evans DA, Funkenstein HH, Albert MS, et al. Prevalence of Alzheimer's disease in a community population of older persons: higher than previously reported. JAMA 1989;262:2551–2556.
9. Erkinjuntti T, Autio L, Wikstrom J. Dementia in medical wards. J Clin Epidemiol 1988;41:123–126.
10. Knapp WS, Douglas JS Jr, Craver JM, et al. Efficacy of coronary artery bypass grafting in elderly patients with coronary artery disease. Am J Cardiol 1981;47:923–930.
11. Edmunds LH Jr, Stephenson LW, Edie RN, et al. Open-heart surgery in octogenarians. N Engl J Med 1988;319:131–136.
12. Cummings J, Benson D. Dementia: a clinical approach, ed 2. Boston, Butterworth-Heinemann, 1992:1–17.
13. Mayeux R, Foster NL, Rossor M, Whitehouse PJ. The clinical evaluation of patients with dementia. In: Whitehouse J, ed. Dementia. Philadelphia, FA Davis Company, 1993:92–129.
15. Basavaraju NG, Silverstone FA, Libow LS, et al. Primitive reflexes and perceptual sensory tests in the elderly: their usefulness in dementia. J Chronic Dis 1981;34:367–377.
16. Knopman DS, Ryberg S. A verbal memory test with high predictive accuracy for dementia of the Alzheimer type. Arch Neurol 1989;46:141–145.
17. Wolf-Klein GP, Silverstone FA, Levy AP, et al. Screening for Alzheimer's disease by clock drawing. J Am Geriatr Soc 1989;37:730–734.
18. Folstein M, Folstein S, McHugh P. "Mini-mental state": a practical method for grading the cognitive state of patients for the clinician. J Psychiatr Res 1975;12:189–198.
19. Anthony JC, LeResche L, Niaz U, et al. Limits of the "Mini-Mental State" as a screening test for dementia and delirium among hospital patients. Psychol Med 1982;12:397–408.
20. Faustman WO, Moses JA, Csernasnsky JG. Limitations of the Mini-Mental State Examination in predicting neuropsychological functioning in a psychiatric sample. Acta Psychiatr Scand 1990;81:126–131.
21. Berent S, Giordani B, Gilman S, et al. Neuropsychological changes in olivopontocerebellar atrophy. Arch Neurol 1990;997:1001.
22. Pfeiffer E. A short portable mental status questionnaire for the assessment of organic brain deficit in elderly patients. J Am Geriatr Soc 1975;23:433–441.
23. Jacobs JW, Bernhard MR, Delgado A, et al. Screening for organic mental syndromes in the medically ill. Ann Intern Med 1977;86:40–46.
24. Mattis S. Dementia Rating Scale professional manual. Odessa, FL, Psychological Assessment Resources, 1973.
25. Meyer JS, Judd BW, Tawaklna T, et al. Improved cognition after control of risk factors for multi-infarct dementia. JAMA 1986;256:2203–2209.
26. Rudman D, Fellar AG. Protein-calorie undernutrition in the nursing home. J Am Geriatr Soc 1989;37:173–183.
27. Beresford HR. Competency in the elderly and demented. New York, American Academy of Neurology, 1993:139–151.
28. Applebaum JC, Griss T. Assessing patient's capacities to consent to treatment. N Engl J Med 1988;319:1635–1638.
29. Hornbostel R. Legal and financial decision making in dementia care. In: Whitehouse PJ, ed. Dementia. Philadelphia, FA Davis Company, 1993:417–432.
30. Cruzan v. Director, Missouri Department of Health, 1990 US Lexicus 3301 (US June 25,1990).
31. Fairman RP. Lessons from Nancy Cruzan. Arch Intern Med 1992;15:25–27.
32. Printz LA. Terminal dehydration: a compassionate treatment. Arch Intern Med 1992;152:697–700.
33. Williams JH, Collin J. Surgical care of patients over eighty: a predictable crisis at hand. Br J Surg 1988;75:371–373.
34. Colenda CC, Schoedel K, Hamer R. The delivery of health services to demented patients at a university hospital: a pilot study. Gerontologist 1988;28:659–662.
35. Reuben DB, Silliman RA, Traines M. The aging driver: medicine, policy, and ethics. J Am Geriatr Soc 1988;36:1135–1142.
36. Parasuraman R, Nestor P. Attention and driving skills in aging and Alzheimer's disease. 1991;33:537–557.
37. Gilley DW, Wilson RS, Bennett DA, et al. Cessation of driving and unsafe motor vehicle operation by dementia patients. Arch Intern Med 1991;151:941–946.
38. Chung F, Meier R, Lautenschlager E, et al. General or spinal anesthesia: which is better in the elderly? Anesthesiology 1987;67:422–427.
39. Chung FF, Chung A, Meier RH, et al. Comparison of perioperative mental function after general anaesthesia and spinal anaesthesia with intravenous sedation. Can J Anaesth 1989;36:382–387.
40. Bedford PD. Adverse effects of anesthesia in the elderly. Lancet 1955;2:259–263.
41. Blundell E. A psychological study of the effects of surgery on eighty-six elderly patients. Br J Soc Psychol 1967;6:297–303.
42. Hole A, Terjesen T, Breivik H. Epidural versus general anesthesia for total hip arthroplasty in elderly patients. Acta Anaesthesiol Scand 1990;24:279–287.
43. Ghoneim MM, Hinrichs JV, OHara MW, et al. Comparison of psychologic and cognitive functions after general or regional anesthesia. Anesthesiology 1988;69:507–515.
44. Nielson WR, Gelb AW, Casey JE, et al. Long-term cognitive and social sequelae of general versus regional anesthesia during arthroplasty in the elderly. Anesthesiology 1990;73:1103–1109.

45. Jones MJ, Piggott SE, Vaughan RS, et al. Cognitive and functional competence after anaesthesia in patients aged over 60: controlled trial of general and regional anaesthesia for elective hip or knee replacement. BMJ 1990;300:1683–1687.

46. Seymour DG, Vaz FG. A prospective study of elderly general surgical patients: post-operative complications. Age Ageing 1989;18:316–326.

47. Berggren D, Gustafson Y, Eriksso B, et al. Postoperative confusion after anesthesia in elderly patients with femoral neck fractures. Anesth Analg 1987;66:497–504.

48. Schor JD, Levkoff SE, Lipsitz LA, et al. Risk factors for delirium in hospitalized elderly. JAMA 1992;267:827–831.

49. Barclay L. Evaluation of dementia. In: Barclay L, ed. Clinical geriatric neurology. Philadelphia, Lea & Febiger, 1993:53–69.

50. Blass JP, Plum F. Metabolic encephalopathies in older adults. In: Katzman R, Terry R, eds. The neurology of aging. Philadelphia, FA Davis Company, 1983:189–220.

51. Layne OL, Yudofsky SC. Postoperative psychosis in cardiotomy patients: the role of organic and psychiatric factors. N Engl J Med 1971;284:518–520.

52. Wilson LM. Intensive care delirium. Arch Intern Med 1972; 130:225–226.

53. Millar HTR. Psychiatric morbidity in elderly surgical patients. Br J Psychiatry 1981;138:17–20.

54. Lipowski ZJ. Delirium in the elderly patient. N Engl J Med 1989;283:1015–1020.

55. Satz P. Brain reserve capacity on symptom onset after brain injury: a formulation and review of evidence for threshold theory. Neuropsychology 1993;7:273–295.

56. Erkinjuntti T, Wikstrom J, Palo J, et al. Dementia among medical inpatients: evaluation of 2000 consecutive admissions. Arch Intern Med 1986;146:1923–1926.

57. Sunderland T, Tariot PN, Cohen RM, et al. Anticholinergic sensitivity in patients with dementia of the Alzheimer type and age-matched controls: a dose-response study. Arch Gen Psychiatry 1987;44:418–426.

58. Tune L, Carr S, Hoag E, et al. Anticholinergic effects of drugs commonly prescribed for the elderly: potential means for assessing risk of delirium. Am J Psychiatry 1992;149:1393–1394.

59. Risse SC, Lampe TH, Cubberley L. Very low-dose neuroleptic treatment in two patients with agitation associated with Alzheimer's disease. J Clin Psychiatry 1987;48:207–208.

60. Cameron D. Studies in senile nocturnal delirium. Psychiatr Q 1941;15:47–53.

61. Evans L. Sundown syndrome in institutionalized elderly. J Am Geriatr Soc 1987;35:101–108.

62. Gierz M, Campbell SS, Gillin JC. Sleep disturbances in various nonaffective psychiatric disorders. Psychiatr Clin North Am 1987;10:565–581.

63. Reynolds CF, Hoch CC, Stack J, et al. The nature and management of sleep/wake disturbance in Alzheimer's dementia. Psychopharmacol Bull 1988;24:43–48.

64. Cohen-Mansfield J. Does sundowning occur in residents of an Alzheimer's unit. Int J Geriatr Psychiatry 1989;4:293–298.

65. Bliwise DL, Lee K, Carroll JS, et al. A rating scale for assessing sundowning in nursing home patients. Sleep Res 1989; 18:111.

66. Bliwise DL, Carroll JS, Dement WC. Apparent seasonal variation in sundowning behavior in a skilled nursing facility. Sleep Res 1989;18:408.

67. Popkin MK, Mackenzie TB, Callies AL. Psychiatric consultation to geriatric medically ill inpatients in a university hospital. Arch Gen Psychiatry 1984;41:703–707.

68. Liston EH. Delirium in the aged. Psychiatr Clin North Am 1982;5:49–66.

69. Roccaforte WH, Burke WJ. Use of psychostimulants for the elderly. Hosp Community Psychiatry 1990;41:1330–1333.

70. Moberg PJ, Lazarus LW. Psychotherapy of depression in the elderly. Psychiatric Annals 1990;20:92–96.

71. Greenberg L, Fink M. Electroconvulsive therapy in the elderly. Psychiatric Annals 1990;20:99.

72. Knopman DS, Sawyer-DeMaris S. A practical approach to managing behavioral problems in dementia patients. Geriatrics 1990;45:27–35.

73. Scherer YK, Janelli LM, Wu YW, et al. Restrained patients: an important issue for critical care nursing. Heart Lung 1993;22:77–83.

74. Dube AH, Mitchell ER. Accidental strangulation from vest restraints. JAMA 1986;256:2725–2726.

75. Rader J, Doan J, Schwab M. How to decrease wandering, a form of agenda behavior. Geriatr Nurs 1985;July/Aug:196–197.

76. Hall GR, Buckwalter KC. A conceptual model for care of adults with Alzheimer's disease. Arch Psychiatr Nurs 1987;1:399–406.

77. Coccaro EF, Kramer E, Zemishlany Z, et al. Pharmacologic treatment of noncognitive behavioral disturbances in elderly demented patients. Am J Psychiatry 1990;147:1640–1645.

78. Schneider LS, Pollock VE, Lyness SA. A metaanalysis of controlled trials of neuroleptic treatment in dementia. J Am Geriatr Soc 1990;38:553–563.

79. Rosen HJ. Double-blind comparison of haloperidol and thioridazine in geriatric outpatients. J Clin Psychiatry 1979;40:17–20.

80. Maletta GJ. Management of behavior problems in elderly patients with Alzheimer's disease and other dementias. Clin Geriatr Med 1988;4:719–747.

81. Ray WA, Griffin MR, Schaffner W, et al. Psychotropic drug use and the risk of hip fracture. N Engl J Med 1987;316:363–369.

CHAPTER

38

NEUROMUSCULAR DISEASES

Medical Management of the Surgical Patient, Third Edition,
edited by Michael F. Lubin, H. Kenneth Walker, and Robert B. Smith III.
J.B. Lippincott Company, Philadelphia, PA © 1995.

David A. Krendel

MYASTHENIA GRAVIS

Of all the neuromuscular diseases, myasthenia gravis probably most often has significant implications for surgical patients.[1] It is caused by an autoimmune attack on the acetylcholine receptors of the postsynaptic (muscle) side of the neuromuscular junction. Characteristic clinical features include fluctuating weakness and fatigue, usually involving the extraocular muscles and eyelids (producing diplopia and ptosis). Weakness of the limbs can be severe, sometimes resulting in almost total paralysis. Sensation and deep tendon reflexes are normal. Respiratory muscle weakness is common and can be fatal. The introduction of practical mechanical ventilation has resulted in a dramatic decrease in the mortality rate.

Although the clinical features of myasthenia gravis are sufficiently characteristic in some cases, confirmatory tests are usually necessary.[2] The edrophonium test is often used. A specific weak muscle test should be performed before and after the intravenous administration of 8 mg of edrophonium. Atropine should be available in case significant bradycardia develops, and a test dose of 2 mg of edrophonium should always be given first. Electrodiagnostic studies are often useful, particularly in patients with cardiac disease or asthma, in whom edrophonium is relatively contraindicated. The characteristic finding on 2- to 3-Hz repetitive motor nerve stimulation is a progressive decrease in the amplitude of the response. The ace-

tylcholine receptor-antibody level is elevated in over 80% of patients with myasthenia gravis; positive test results are extremely specific for this disease.

Many effective therapies have been developed for myasthenia gravis.[3] Acetylcholine esterase inhibitors increase the concentration of acetylcholine near the impaired receptors. Pyridostigmine (Mestinon) is used most commonly and is generally given at a dosage of 60 mg every 3 to 6 hours, depending on patient response.

Immunosuppression with prednisone frequently is efficacious. Patients beginning prednisone therapy should be cautioned that weakness may increase during the first 10 to 14 days before its beneficial effect becomes apparent. Azathioprine has also been found to be effective and is often used in patients who have had no response to other treatments or are at increased risk for complications from prednisone.

Thymectomy is recommended for patients with generalized myasthenia, except at the extremes of age. About 10% of patients with myasthenia have a thymoma and their prognosis is worse, even if the tumor is removed. The incidence of thymoma increases with age and the tumor may develop at any time during the course of the illness. Chest computed tomography should be performed at the time of diagnosis. Thymectomy produces permanent remission in about 50% of patients, although remission may not occur for many months after surgery.

Hyperthyroidism is found in 5% of patients with myasthenia. Hypothyroidism also is more common in these patients than in the general population. Treatment of the thyroid abnormality usually improves muscle strength.

The term *myasthenic crisis* refers to progressive respiratory or bulbar weakness. Intubation usually should be done when the vital capacity falls to about 15 mL/kg. Causes of myasthenic crisis include infection, thyroid malfunction, and medications that adversely affect neuromuscular transmission. The most common pharmacologic offenders are aminoglycosides, quinine, quinidine, magnesium, and neuromuscular blocking agents. Many medications are reported to exacerbate myasthenia occasionally, including most antiarrhythmic agents. Hypokalemia is a common cause of increased weakness in patients with myasthenia, especially those who are taking prednisone. As a precautionary measure, potassium replacement is advisable in these patients. In addition to correcting any precipitating factor, the most effective treatment for myasthenic crisis is plasma exchange, which almost always has a dramatic effect over a few days. High-dose intravenous γ-globulin (400 mg/kg daily for 5 days) is also efficacious.[4]

ISSUES RELEVANT TO SURGICAL PATIENTS

Thymectomy is often performed in patients with myasthenia gravis to remove thymomas, if present, and attempt to induce remission. Patients should not undergo this surgery until medical management has been used to increase their strength, particularly in the respiratory muscles. If respiratory function remains significantly impaired (vital capacity 20 mL/kg or less) after maximal medical improvement, a course of intravenous γ-globulin (400 mg/kg daily for 5 days) should be given. Patients who undergo surgery with significant respiratory weakness are more likely to require prolonged postoperative mechanical ventilation. After sternotomy, accurate measurement of the vital capacity usually is not possible because of incisional pain. If the use of medications with neuromuscular blocking potential is avoided during surgery, a normal potassium level is maintained, and preoperative medication regimens are resumed, problems with extubation are unlikely. Intravenous pyridostigmine (Mestinon) can be given but the dosage used (1 to 4 mg) should be one thirtieth to one fifteenth the oral dosage (60 to 90 mg every 4 to 6 hours) because of first-pass hepatic metabolism. After surgery, remission may occur within a few weeks but can be delayed for several months. Medical therapy can gradually be withdrawn on an outpatient basis according to patients' clinical status. The prednisone dosage can often be tapered over 6 to 8 weeks. A dose of pyridostigmine can be omitted during the day to determine whether the drug is still needed.

Patients occasionally develop weakness as a result of unsuspected myasthenia gravis during hospitalization for a surgical procedure. This is most often related to the administration of a medication with neuromuscular blocking activity, although hypokalemia, hypermagnesemia, and infection are also capable of unmasking myasthenia gravis.[5] Intravenous magnesium should not be used in patients with myasthenia, except when life-threatening hypomagnesemia exists.[6] The use of aminoglycosides, quinine, quinidine, and intraoperative neuromuscular blocking agents also should be avoided. In addition, lincomycin, clindamycin, polymyxin, and colistin are capable of exacerbating myasthenia. Other antibiotics and antiarrhythmics have been implicated rarely but are not considered to be contraindicated. These include erythromycin, penicillins, sulfonamides, tetracyclines, ciprofloxacin, vancomycin, procainamide, calcium channel blockers, and β-blockers. There are anecdotal reports of numerous medications that have been associated with worsening of myasthenia, and it is prudent to suspect any newly added medication in this setting.

LAMBERT-EATON SYNDROME

Lambert-Eaton syndrome is a rare disorder of neuromuscular transmission caused by autoantibodies directed against calcium channels in the presynaptic terminal.[7] This impairs acetylcholine release. Patients have proximal muscle weakness but it differs from myasthenia gravis in that extraocular muscles are rarely involved and deep tendon reflexes are reduced. About half of patients are eventually found to have small cell carcinoma of the lung. Repetitive nerve stimulation is necessary to make the diagnosis and shows a characteristic increase in the potential recorded over a muscle after exercise or rapid repetitive stimulation.

Immunosuppressant agents that are useful in myasthenia gravis are also useful in Lambert-Eaton syndrome but pyridostigmine (Mestinon) is not as helpful. The response to treatment of small cell carcinoma is unpredictable. Medications that exacerbate myasthenia gravis may also exacerbate Lambert-Eaton syndrome.

PERIPHERAL NEUROPATHY

Peripheral neuropathy may be generalized (polyneuropathy), focal (mononeuropathy), or multifocal (multiple mononeuropathy). All three syndromes may cause clinically significant problems for surgical patients.

Mononeuropathies present as the dysfunction of an individual peripheral nerve and are common in patients undergoing surgical procedures. Compression neuropathies are probably the most frequent disorders. Patients with diabetes and other conditions associated with polyneuropathy are predisposed to their development. Patients who are undergoing general anesthesia are at risk because they may be positioned in such a way that continuous pressure is applied to a nerve. This is analogous to the well-known "Saturday night palsy," in which a person awakens from alcohol-induced anesthesia with a wristdrop.[8] The arm may have been draped over an object, resulting in damage to the radial nerve in the spiral groove of the humerus. Continuous pressure over the mid-humerus also can occur during surgery or be associated with impaired mobility before or after surgery. There is weakness of wrist extension and the brachioradialis with a normal triceps. Intrinsic hand muscles appear to be weak because they cannot be effectively activated without adequate wrist extension. There may be loss of sensation over the dorsum of the hand in the web space between the thumb and index finger. The prognosis is good, with recovery usually occurring over weeks to months. A splint should be used to keep the hand in a more functional position and prevent contracture.

Ulnar neuropathy resulting from compression at the elbow is a common problem.[9] Pressure over the medial elbow is the usual cause when this condition develops during surgery. There is numbness of the fifth and medial portion of the fourth digits and palm. In more severe cases, weakness of abduction and, sometimes, flexion of the ulnar digits may be seen. Recovery is usual when the condition is mild but some permanent disability is common in severe cases. Patients should be advised to avoid pressure over the elbow and prolonged elbow flexion (which stretches the nerve across the ulnar groove).

The other common pressure palsy involves the peroneal nerve as it passes behind the head of the fibula.[10] Pressure behind the knee, resulting from prolonged leg crossing or squatting, is the usual cause, and patients who have recently experienced significant weight loss are predisposed. This also can occur during surgery when pressure is applied to that area. There is weakness of ankle dorsiflexion and often eversion, without weakness of ankle inversion. There may be sensory loss in the web space between the first two toes and, sometimes, the anterolateral foot and leg. The prognosis is good, with most patients recovering in 3 to 8 weeks. A brace (ankle-foot orthosis) improves the ability to walk by relieving footdrop.

In addition to the pressure palsies, mononeuropathies related to the trauma of an invasive procedure are commonly encountered in surgical patients. The femoral nerve is often damaged after femoral artery catheterization.[11] This usually is related to pressure from a hematoma, although inaccurate needle placement also may be a potential cause. A hematoma may be evident on physical examination or it may lie proximal to the inguinal ligament and be hidden. Computed tomographic scanning or magnetic resonance imaging through the pelvis is necessary in this setting because evacuation of the hematoma can be beneficial. Femoral neuropathy is also a relatively common complication of

hysterectomy or other gynecologic surgery, probably because of traction on the nerve. Femoral neuropathy causes weakness of knee extension that often is not recognized until patients begin to ambulate. The knee jerk is reduced or absent and there may be loss of sensation over the anterior thigh and medial leg (the saphenous branch of the femoral nerve provides sensory innervation to the medial leg). When they are severe, these nerve injuries commonly result in prolonged or permanent disability, although significant recovery is possible even after 1 year.

Median, ulnar, and radial nerve injury may occur after an upper extremity arterial access procedure or placement of a shunt for hemodialysis. In both situations, hematoma is a possible cause, but ischemia is usually implicated. Among patients undergoing dialysis, ischemic nerve injury related to vascular diversion occurs almost exclusively in those who have diabetes. These patients are predisposed because of diabetic neuropathy and small vessel disease. Early recognition of this complication is important because patients may improve after prompt ligation.[12]

Damage to the spinal accessory nerve is a common complication of lymph node biopsy. An incision over the lateral neck puts this nerve at risk as it crosses the sternocleidomastoid muscle. Patients often develop insidious shoulder pain that increases with continued use of the shoulder joint. There is weakness of the trapezius, which causes scapular winging and instability of the shoulder joint. The winging is most evident when patients abduct the shoulders to 90 degrees. Testing for weakness of the shoulder shrug is rarely useful because this action is also served by muscles other than the trapezius. Depending on the level of injury, there may be weakness of the sternocleidomastoid muscle. This can be recognized by asking patients to turn their heads in the opposite direction against resistance. This injury commonly results in long-term disability because this slender nerve is usually severed and reanastomosis is difficult. Range-of-motion exercises prevent frozen shoulder but strenuous use of the joint should be avoided because it may hasten the development of degenerative arthritis.

POLYNEUROPATHY

Polyneuropathy occasionally requires diagnostic or therapeutic intervention in surgical patients. Typical clinical features include distal numbness, tingling, or burning; weakness of distal muscles; and reduced deep tendon reflexes. Numerous metabolic, toxic, inflammatory, and hereditary causes are known (Table 38-1). The most common are diabetes and alcoholism.

Neuropathies can be conveniently divided into two categories: (1) those in which peripheral axons are primarily damaged (axonal neuropathies), and (2) those in which peripheral myelin is the primary target (demyelinating neu-

TABLE 38–1. Peripheral Neuropathies

Axonal Sensory and Motor
Toxic
  Alcohol
  Vincristine
  Macrodantin
  Amiodarone
  Disulfiram
  Lead
  Arsenic
  Triorthocresyl phosphate (organophosphate)
  N-Hexane (glue sniffing)
  Acrylamide
  Ciguatera toxin
Nutritional deficiency
  Vitamin B_{12}
  Vitamin B_6
  Vitamin B_1
  Vitamin E
Metabolic
  Diabetes
  Uremia
  Hypothyroidism
  Acute intermittent porphyria
Vasculitis
  Polyarteritis nodosa
  Rheumatoid vasculitis
  Associated with human immunodeficiency virus
  Isolated
Malignancy-associated
  Remote effect
  Infiltrative (hematologic malignancy)
Granulomatous
  Leprosy
  Sarcoidosis
Associated with monoclonal gammopathy
Hereditary
Amyloidosis
  Hereditary
  Associated with monoclonal gammopathy

Demyelinating Sensory and Motor
Acute (Guillain-Barré syndrome)
Chronic inflammatory demyelinating polyradiculoneuropathy
  (chronic Guillain-Barré syndrome)
Hereditary
  Dominant (Charcot-Marie-Tooth disease)
  X-linked
  Recessive
    Déjérine-Sottas syndrome
    Refsum's syndrome
    Metachromatic leukodystrophy
    Krabbe's syndrome

Pure Sensory Neuropathies
Paraneoplastic (usually small cell)
Idiopathic
B_6
Cisplatin
Associated with Sjögren's syndrome

ropathies). Secondary damage to myelin or axons can occur in either type but they can often be differentiated with nerve conduction studies and electromyography. Demyelinating neuropathies show more slowing and blocking of conduction than do axonal neuropathies.

Virtually all toxic and metabolic neuropathies are axonal, as is the neuropathy caused by vasculitis. Demyelinating neuropathies are either inflammatory (Guillain-Barré syndrome in its acute or chronic form) or hereditary (most commonly the dominantly inherited Charcot-Marie-Tooth disease).

Guillain-Barré syndrome commonly occurs after an infection but may also develop during the postoperative period.[13] The reason for both these associations is unknown. Patients usually develop tingling or numbness in the feet and hands, followed by weakness of the lower and then the upper extremities, the respiratory muscles, and the facial muscles. Deep tendon reflexes are lost or reduced and mild distal sensory loss is common. There is frequently autonomic nerve involvement, causing fluctuations in blood pressure and pulse rate. Atypical clinical patterns are fairly common, with asymmetry, greater involvement of upper extremity or facial muscles, and a predilection for the proximal muscles occurring in individual cases. Muscle pain is common and the creatine kinase level is sometimes elevated (although usually less than 1000 U/L). This sometimes mimics polymyositis. The cerebrospinal fluid cell count is usually normal and the protein level elevated, although the latter is frequently normal during the first week of illness. Progression to maximum weakness usually occurs during the first few weeks but quadriplegia with respiratory paralysis may be seen as early as the first day of illness. Spontaneous recovery is the rule over several weeks to months, although a significant minority of patients retain some permanent disability.

Plasma exchange has been found to be beneficial, as has the less involved but equally expensive use of intravenous γ-globulin.[14,15] Some authorities believe that plasma exchange is still the treatment of choice because it has a longer track record. A study is being conducted to compare the two approaches.

Careful attention to respiratory function is probably the most important aspect of therapy for Guillain-Barré syndrome. In patients with actively progressing disease, respiratory function should be monitored at least twice a day. When the vital capacity reaches about 15 mL/kg, nonemergent intubation should usually be done. Inspiratory force can be estimated by asking patients to forcefully inhale through the nose (sniff) and vital capacity can be approximated by asking them to inhale and forcefully exhale. Patients should be instructed to cough to assess their ability to clear the airway and prevent aspiration. Patients with impending respiratory failure related to neuromuscular disease typically take rapid, shallow breaths and become diaphoretic. Blood gas analysis usually shows hyperventilation initially, with carbon dioxide retention being a late, preterminal finding.

MULTIPLE MONONEUROPATHY

Multiple mononeuropathy is occasionally encountered after surgery. It is most commonly associated with open heart surgery, and there is a predilection for involvement of the shoulder girdle and other upper extremity nerves. Traction on nerves during sternotomy may be responsible in some instances but the involvement of nerves distant from the incision suggests that embolic occlusion of small vessels with nerve ischemia also may be contributory.

Neuralgic amyotrophy (Parsonage-Turner syndrome) is a form of multiple mononeuropathy involving an upper extremity.[6] Pain in the shoulder region is followed after a few days by weakness resulting from multiple lesions in the brachial plexus or peripheral nerves. It has occurred after viral illness and immunization, and also is seen occasionally during the postoperative period. The prognosis for multiple mononeuropathies after surgery is good, with most patients recovering after several weeks or months.

MYOPATHIES

Primary myopathies rarely present clinical problems in patients undergoing surgical procedures, with the notable exception of malignant hyperthermia.[16] This causes life-threatening muscle rigidity and is precipitated by potent inhaled anesthetics and depolarizing neuromuscular blocking agents. Severe episodes are characterized by extreme hyperthermia, combined metabolic and respiratory acidosis (inability to ventilate because of rigidity), and myoglobinuria. This is usually an inherited disorder with a variable pattern of inheritance. The potential for this reaction should be anticipated in anyone with a personal or family history of malignant hyperthermia. Safe anesthetic agents for these patients include nitrous oxide, thiopental, opiates, droperidol, and pancuronium. Dantrolene is the specific pharmacologic agent used to treat an episode. It is given at a rate of 2 mg/kg every 5 minutes to a total dose of 10 mg/kg. There appears to be an increased incidence of malignant hyperthermia in patients with other myopathies, most notably central core disease (a congenital myopathy) and

Duchenne muscular dystrophy. Patients with myotonic dystrophy occasionally experience transient rigidity after the administration of succinylcholine but the mechanism for this is probably different and treatment usually is not required.

REFERENCES

1. Johns TR, Howard JF, eds. Myasthenia gravis. Semin Neurol 1982;2:193–280.
2. Phillips LH, Melnick PA. Diagnosis of myasthenia gravis in the 1990's. Semin Neurol 1990;10:62–69.
3. Finley JC, Pascuzzi RM. Rational therapy of myasthenia gravis. Semin Neurol 1990;10:70–82.
4. Arsura EL, Bick A, Brunuer NG, et al. High-dose intravenous immunoglobulin in the management of myasthenia gravis. Arch Intern Med 1986;146:1365–1368.
5. Howard JF. Adverse drug effects on neuromuscular transmission. Semin Neurol 1990;10:89–102.
6. Krendel D. Hypermagnesemia and neuromuscular transmission. Semin Neurol 1990;10:42–45.
7. Pascuzzi RM, Kim YI. Lambert-Eaton syndrome. Semin Neurol 1990;10:35–41.
8. Stewart JD. The radial nerve. In: Stewart JD, ed. Focal peripheral neuropathies. New York, Elsevier Science Publishing, 1987:194–210.
9. Stewart JD. The ulnar nerve. In: Stewart JD, ed. Focal peripheral neuropathies. New York, Elsevier Science Publishing, 1987:163–193.
10. Stewart JD. The common peroneal nerve. In: Stewart JD, ed. Focal peripheral neuropathies. New York, Elsevier Science Publishing, 1987:290–306.
11. Stewart JD. The femoral and saphenous nerves. In: Stewart JD, ed. Focal peripheral neuropathies. New York, Elsevier Science Publishing, 1987:322–332.
12. Riggs JE, Moss AH, Labosky DA, et al. Upper extremity ischemic monomelic neuropathy: a complication of vascular access procedures in ureanic diabetic patients. Neurology 1989;39:997–998.
13. Hughes RAC. Epidemiology. In Hughes RAC, ed. Guillain-Barré syndrome. London, Springer-Verlag, 1990:101–119.
14. Guillain-Barré Syndrome Study Group. Plasmapheresis and acute Guillain-Barré syndrome. Neurology 1985;35:1096–1104.
15. Van der Meché FGA, Schmitz PIM. A randomized trial comparing intravenous immune globulin and plasma exchange in Guillain-Barré syndrome. N Engl J Med 1992;326:1123–1129.
16. Gromert GA. Malignant hyperthermia. In: Engel AG, Banker BQ, eds. Myology. New York, McGraw-Hill, 1986:1763–1784.

Medical Management of the Surgical Patient, Third Edition,
edited by Michael F. Lubin, H. Kenneth Walker, and Robert B. Smith III.
J.B. Lippincott Company, Philadelphia, PA © 1995.

LARGE VESSEL OCCLUSIVE DISEASE

39

Bruce C. Mackay
Michael R. Frankel

Internists are often asked to assess cardiac risk in patients awaiting surgery. Similarly, neurologists are frequently asked to determine cerebrovascular risk in patients with previous transient ischemic attacks (TIAs) or strokes. Although Goldman[1] has well-established criteria to guide physicians in assessing cardiac risk, data about perioperative cerebrovascular risk are limited. This chapter addresses some of the important issues in surgical patients at risk for ischemic stroke. The discussion relates largely to stroke caused by atherosclerosis.

Stroke may result from ischemic or hemorrhagic causes. Cerebral infarction accounts for about 80% of all strokes.[2] Large vessel occlusive disease is responsible for as many as 50% of cerebral infarctions. Most of these are related to atherothromboembolic disease.

Atherosclerosis is a systemic disease that most prominently affects the aorta, the coronary arteries, the extracranial carotid and vertebral arteries, and the arteries to the extremities.[3] Atherosclerosis causes stroke by producing progressive stenosis, local thrombosis with occlusion, or distal embolization. The most common cause is a combination of all three mechanisms, making the term *atherothromboembolism* appropriate. Any one of these mechanisms, however, can be the primary cause. For example, progressive atherosclerotic occlusion can cause distal hypoperfusion severe enough to result in tissue ischemia and infarction. Mild or moderate atherosclerotic stenosis that does not cause distal hypoperfusion can be the site of thrombosis and cause intraarterial embolization, leading to occlusion of an intracerebral artery.

The relative significance of local thrombosis versus intraarterial embolization varies according to the site of atherosclerosis. Most strokes resulting from stenosis of the proximal internal carotid artery are caused by distal embolic occlusion of the middle cerebral artery, whereas infarction in the basilar artery usually results from occlusion of the small perforating vessels by local thrombosis.

MECHANISMS SPECIFIC TO SURGICAL INTERVENTION

Surgical intervention can cause or predispose to stroke in several different ways. The most straightforward cause is hypotension resulting from hemorrhage, fluid loss, or anesthesia. In patients who do not have hypertension or cerebrovascular disease, cerebral blood flow is maintained at a constant level until cerebral perfusion pressure reaches a mean of 60 mmHg.[4] This perfusion pressure is called the lower level of autoregulation. Chronic hypertension raises this lower limit so that decreases in cerebral blood flow occur at higher mean arterial blood pressures. Arterial occlusive disease also affects tolerance to hypotension. This effect is highly variable and depends on the adequacy of the collateral supply distal to the site of occlusion.[4] Flow across a region of stenosis varies directly with the pressure difference. Therefore, a decrease in pressure proximal to the stenosis requires a decrease in pressure distally to maintain the same perfusion pressure. This is accomplished by decreasing the resistance to flow distally by dilating resistance vessels. If resistance vessels are already maximally dilated, there is no means of decreasing resistance further and the pressure difference decreases, as does the flow.[5] This concept is called hemodynamic reserve. Although this can be evaluated before surgery by several methods, including xenon cerebral blood flow and transcranial Doppler, the usefulness of such data remains unclear.[6] The bottom line for most patients is that hypotension can cause stroke, especially in those who have no hemodynamic reserve.

Another straightforward mechanism involves dislodged thrombus or plaque causing distal embolization. This can occur during angiography or when arteries are manipulated (ie, during clamping of the carotid artery or aorta). Intraoperative ultrasound and transesophageal echocardiography have demonstrated extensive atherosclerosis and thrombus in the aortic arch, which likely serves as a source of embolism.[7,8] Aortic manipulation and crossclamping are probably a common cause of perioperative stroke and "can stir up recurrent bouts of embolization for days."[3] Marshall and colleagues[9] have suggested that intraoperative ultrasound of the aorta allows the surgeon to modify cannulation and operative techniques, and thereby reduce the risk of perioperative stroke.

Cardiopulmonary bypass plays a definite role in the postoperative encephalopathy that is frequently seen after coronary artery bypass grafting (CABG), although the mechanism is not well understood. This encephalopathy is a state of general mental slowing, particularly in frontal lobe functions of planning, concentration, shifting set, and choice reaction time. Microemboli consisting of gas bubbles and particulate matter generated from aortic cannulation appear to have a significant role in causing this disorder.[10] About 25% of patients undergoing CABG show a significant decrease in cognitive capacity after surgery with prospective testing.[11] Some of this decrement is long lasting. Advanced age also increases the risk for loss of cognitive function. The number of microemboli detected by transcranial Doppler during surgery appears to correlate with the neuropsychologic outcome.[12]

PERIOPERATIVE STROKE RISK

A few studies have examined the risk of stroke in patients undergoing major vascular[8,13–18] and minor nonvascular surgical procedures.[3] Most perioperative strokes that occur in patients undergoing cardiopulmonary bypass are aortoembolic or cardioembolic.[3] Hypotension also is a potential, although probably less common, cause of stroke.

Several studies have attempted to identify risk factors that contribute to perioperative stroke. Ropper and colleagues[19] performed a well-designed prospective study looking for the presence of carotid bruits as a marker for perioperative stroke risk in patients scheduled for elective surgery. They found bruits in 104 of 735 patients (14%) and noted no correlation with perioperative stroke. The overall stroke rate was 0.7% and all strokes occurred in patients undergoing CABG.[16] A separate retrospective study by Reed and colleagues[16] produced somewhat contradictory data indicating that there is a statistically significant, albeit small, increase in perioperative stroke in patients with carotid bruits who undergo CABG. They added that the small increase in risk was comparable to the reported risk of stroke from carotid endarterectomy and did not recommend routine carotid endarterectomy before CABG. A history of heart failure, mitral regurgitation, postoperative atrial fibrillation, cardiopulmonary bypass time greater than 120 minutes, and previous myocardial infarction also were significant factors contributing to the risk of perioperative stroke.

Four additional studies offer further support for the theory that perioperative stroke in patients undergoing CABG uncommonly results from carotid atherosclerosis. Furlan and Cracium[14] found that asymptomatic unilateral internal carotid artery stenosis less than 90%, or internal carotid artery occlusion, did not increase the risk of stroke during CABG. VonReutern and colleagues[18] monitored middle cerebral artery velocities with transcranial Doppler during CABG in patients with severe carotid stenosis or occlusion and found no change in velocities compared with patients without carotid stenosis. Three patients in this study developed postoperative encephalopathy, none of whom had evidence of reduced blood flow during cardiopulmonary bypass. Hise and colleagues[20] reviewed computed tomographic scans and angiographic results in patients who had strokes related to CABG and concluded that "the main mechanism of injury was cerebral embolization rather than cerebral hypoperfusion." A significant number of these patients had evidence of multiple emboli, suggesting a cardiac or aortic source. Last, Moody and colleagues[10] looked at neuropathologic material and found focal arteriolar and capillary dilation as well as evidence of birefringence suggesting the previous presence of air or fat emboli in four of five patients after CABG. Based on this evidence, there does not appear to be an indication for carotid endarterectomy in asymptomatic patients with carotid stenosis before cardiac surgery.

In a retrospective univariate analysis performed by Gardner and colleagues,[21] the following factors were found to correlate significantly with the risk of stroke: increased age, preexisting cerebrovascular disease, severe atherosclerosis of the ascending aorta, protracted cardiopulmonary bypass time, and severe perioperative hypotension. The last factor was defined as a systolic blood pressure of 40 mmHg or less for at least 5 minutes during normothermia. A separate prospective study by Breuer and colleagues[13] of 421 patients undergoing CABG found no correlation between age, pump time greater than 2 hours, and stroke. The use of an intraaortic balloon pump or pressor agents, however, was significantly correlated with prolonged encephalopathy. The reason for these different findings is not readily apparent.

A recent retrospective review of patients with histories of recent or remote strokes who underwent open heart surgery compared the incidence of perioperative stroke in these two groups.[17] A recent stroke was defined as one that occurred less than 3 months before open heart surgery. There was no significant difference in new stroke rates between patients with recent and remote strokes. There was a suggestion, however, that patients with recent strokes were more susceptible to perioperative hypotension.

CAROTID ENDARTERECTOMY

Carotid endarterectomy for patients with symptomatic (hemispheric transient ischemic attack or minor stroke) internal carotid artery stenosis of 70% to 99%, as measured by angiography, is indicated as long as the combined surgical mortality and morbidity is less than 6%.[22] These patients should undergo carotid endarterectomy before they have any other surgery, except in immediate life-threatening or urgent situations.[23] Table 39-1 summarizes the timing of carotid endarterectomy and CABG based on patient characteristics.

Prior to the clinical advisory released by the National Institutes of Health on September 28, 1994, regarding the early termination of the Asymptomatic Carotid Atherosclerosis Study (ACAS), only three randomized trials had tested the effectiveness of carotid endarterectomy in this setting. The Carotid Artery Stenosis With Asymptomatic Narrowing: Operation Versus Aspirin (CASANOVA) study found no significant difference between medical and surgical groups.[24] Unfortunately, they excluded the most severely affected patients (ie, those with over 90% stenosis). Therefore, the possibility remained that a subgroup of asymptomatic patients may benefit from carotid endarterectomy. The Mayo Clinic study ended early because of an excess of myocardial infarction in the surgical group, and no meaningful conclusions can be drawn from the limited data.[25] The Veterans Affairs Cooperative Study reported results on 444 asymptomatic randomized patients.[26] Using the end point of stroke, there was only a trend toward benefit only in the surgical group. Combining stroke and death as an end point revealed neither a significant difference nor a trend with surgery. The authors had to include TIA in their end point analysis to show statistical benefit. Given the obvious inability to blind such a study, the determination of the relevance of transient symptoms by patients and physicians should not be given as much weight as stroke and death. Therefore, TIA should not be part of the primary end point analysis of efficacy.[27] Because this was a relatively small study, it does not exclude the possibility that carotid endarterectomy may benefit patients with asymptomatic stenosis, particularly those with high-grade lesions. ACAS was a large randomized trial designed to compare endarterectomy with medical therapy in patients with asymptomatic internal carotid artery stenosis of more than 60% as measured by arteriography. The primary end point for the study was any stroke or death after randomization. On September 28, 1994, the National Institutes of Health announced the early termination of ACAS after an interim analysis revealed a significant difference between the two groups.[28] The information provided in the clinical advisory indicated a statistically significant benefit in favor of surgery, which reduced the relative risk of the primary end points by 55% ($P = .004$) over 5 years. To achieve similar results, surgeons should have documented perioperative morbidity and mortality rates of less than 3% when performing endarterectomy for asymptomatic carotid stenosis. In addition, all patients should receive aspirin and aggressive management of modifiable risk factors. Preliminary data suggest a greater benefit of surgery in men. Formal publication of these results is not available at this time.

TABLE 39–1. Recommendations for Combined Carotid and Coronary Disease*

Carotid Disease	Coronary Disease	Recommendation
Active, severe	Inactive	Carotid endarterectomy
Inactive	Active, severe	Coronary artery bypass grafting
Active, severe combined	Active, severe	Coronary artery bypass grafting and carotid endarterectomy

*Active carotid disease: ipsilateral hemispheric or retinal transient ischemic attacks or recent stroke and severe internal carotid artery stenosis (70%–99% stenosis). Active coronary disease: unstable angina, silent ischemia, or a recent myocardial infarction with severe surgically operable disease by coronary angiography.
(Caplan LR. Stroke, a clinical approach, ed 2. Boston, Butterworths-Heinemann, 1993)

PREVENTION OF PERIOPERATIVE STROKE

Patients should be screened before operation for histories of stroke and stroke risk factors such as hypertension, peripheral vascular disease, and coronary artery disease. Perioperative medical therapy does not differ substantially from good routine care except for extra care to prevent hypotension. Because atherosclerosis is a systemic disease, carotid atherosclerosis and coronary artery disease frequently coexist.[3] Myocardial infarction is the major cause of mortality in patients with stroke and all patients with histories of TIA or stroke should be screened before surgery with a thorough history and electrocardiogram looking for cardiac disease. The indications for carotid endarterectomy were outlined earlier.

The indications for anticoagulation in patients with cardioembolic stroke are relatively clear and an excellent review of the indications for antithrombotic therapy in cerebrovascular disease has been published.[29] The use of anticoagulants in patients with large vessel occlusive disease is less clear, however, and surgical considerations may take precedence when patients receiving anticoagulants require surgery.

Communication and mobility concerns need to be addressed in all patients. Range-of-motion exercises, splints, communication devices, and extra care to prevent bedsores all must be taken into consideration in patients with stroke.

The prevention of deep venous thrombosis and pulmonary embolus is an important concern after almost any major surgery. When patients are hemiplegic, the risk of embolic complications is even greater. Prophylaxis for deep venous thrombosis should be initiated in all patients with stroke who are not ambulatory. This usually consists of the administration of 5000 U of subcutaneous heparin every 12 hours, the application of compression stockings, and the institution of early mobilization for gait training.

Bowel and bladder continence play a major role in quality of life for patients with strokes. These concerns must be addressed during postoperative care. Timed voiding and elimination are the main tools for retraining. Medications should be chosen with their autonomic side effects in mind.

Seizures can occur in patients after stroke. In general, prophylaxis with antiepileptic medication is not used in patients with stroke. These drugs are given only to patients who have had at least one seizure. Patients with histories of seizures who are receiving antiepileptic medications must maintain adequate blood levels in the postoperative setting, when seizures could have serious consequences. Changes in kidney, liver, and heart function can affect the metabolism, protein binding, and volume of distribution of anticonvulsants. The use of various concomitant medications can also have an effect on the efficacy and toxicity of anticonvulsants during the perioperative period.

REFERENCES

1. Goldman L, Caldera DL, Nussbaum SR, et al. Multifactorial index of cardiac risk in non-cardiac surgical procedures. N Engl J Med 1977;297:845–850.
2. Caplan LR. Diagnosis and the clinical encounter. In: Stroke, a clinical approach, ed 2. Boston, Butterworth-Heinemann, 1993:67–98.
3. Caplan LR. Strokes, cerebrovascular disease, and surgery. In: Stroke, a clinical approach, ed 2. Boston, Butterworth-Heinemann, 1993:497–514.
4. Heiss WE. Experimental evidence of ischemic thresholds and functional recovery. Stroke 1992;23:1666–1672.
5. Bullock R, Mendelow AD, Bone I, et al. Cerebral blood flow and CO2 responsiveness as an indicator of collateral reserve capacity in patients with carotid arterial diseases. Br J Surg 1985;72:348–351.
6. Henriksen L, Hjaims E, Lindeburgh T. Brain hyperperfusion during cardiac operations: cerebral blood flow measured in man by intra-arterial injection of xenon 133—evidence suggestive of intraoperative microembolism. J Thorac Cardiovasc Surg 1983;86:202–208.
7. Karalis DG, Chandrasekaran K, Victor MF, et al. Recognition and embolic potential of intra-aortic atherosclerotic debris. J Am Coll Cardiol 1991;17:73–78.
8. Kartchner MM, McRae LP. Carotid occlusive disease as a risk factor in major cardiovascular surgery. Arch Surg 1992;117: 1086–1088.
9. Marshall WG, Barzilai B, Kouchoukos NT, et al. Intraoperative ultrasonic imaging of the ascending aorta. Ann Thorac Surg 1989;48:339–344.
10. Moody DM, Bell MA, Chaila VR, et al. Brain microemboli during cardiac surgery or aortography. Ann Neurol 1990;28:477–486.
11. Shaw PJ, Bates D, Cartidge NEF, et al. Neurologic and neuropsychological morbidity following major surgery: comparison of coronary artery bypass and peripheral vascular surgery. Stroke 1987;18:700–707.
12. Pugsley W, Klinger L, Paschalis C, et al. Microemboli and cerebral impairment during cardiac surgery. Vasc Surg 1990;24:34–43.
13. Breuer AC, Furian AJ, Hanson MR, et al. Central nervous system complications of coronary artery bypass graft surgery: prospective analysis of 421 patients. Stroke 1993;14: 682–687.
14. Furlan AJ, Cracium AR. Risk of stroke during coronary artery bypass graft surgery in patients with internal carotid artery disease documented by angiography. Stroke 1965;16: 797–798.
15. Kamik R, Valentin A, Bonner G, et al. Transcranial Doppler monitoring during percutaneous transluminal aortic valvuloplasty. Angiology 1990;41:106–111.
16. Reed GL, Singer DE, Picard E, DeSanctis RW. Stroke following coronary-artery bypass surgery: a case–control estimate of the risk from carotid bruits. N Engl J Med 1988;319:1246–1250.
17. Rorick MB, Furlan AJ. Risk of cardiac surgery in patients with prior stroke. Neurology 1990;40:835–837.
18. VonReutern GM, Hetzel A, Bimbaum D, Schlosser V. Transcranial doppler ultrasonography during cardiopulmonary by-

pass in patients with severe carotid stenosis or occlusion. Stroke 1988;19:674–680.

19. Ropper AH, Weschsier LR, Wilson LS. Carotid bruit and the risk of stroke in elective surgery. N Engl J Med 1992;25:1388–1390.

20. Hise JH, Nipper MN, Schnitker JC. Stroke associated with CABG. Am J Neuroradiol 1991;12:811–814.

21. Gardner TJ, Hornetter PJ, Manolio TA, et al. Stroke following CABG: a 10 year study. Ann Thorac Surg 1985;40:574–581.

22. North American Symptomatic Carotid Endarterectomy Trial Collaborators. Beneficial effect of carotid endarterectomy in symptomatic patients with high-grade carotid stenosis. N Engl J Med 1991;325:445–453.

23. Hertzer NR, Loop Fd, Beven EG, et al. Surgical staging for simultaneous coronary and carotid disease: a study including prospective randomization. J Vasc Surg 1988;9:455–463.

24. CASANOVA Study Group. Carotid surgery versus medical therapy in asymptomatic carotid stenosis. Stroke 1991;22:1229–1235.

25. Mayo Asymptomatic Carotid Endarterectomy Study Group. Effectiveness of carotid endarterectomy for asymptomatic carotid stenosis: design of a clinical trial. Mayo Clin Proc 1989;64:897–904.

26. Hobson RW, Weiss DG, Fields WS, et al. Efficacy of carotid endarterectomy for asymptomatic carotid stenosis. N Engl J Med 1993;328:221–227.

27. Barnett HJM, Haines SJ. Carotid endarterectomy for asymptomatic stenosis. (Editorial) N Engl J Med 1993;328:276–278.

28. National Institutes of Health. Clinical advisory: carotid endarterectomy for patients with asymptomatic carotid artery stenosis. September 28, 1994.

29. Sherman DG, Dyken ML, Fisher M, et al. Antithrombotic therapy for cerebrovascular disorders. Chest 1992;102:529S–537S.

Medical Management of the Surgical Patient, Third Edition,
edited by Michael F. Lubin, H. Kenneth Walker, and Robert B. Smith III.
J.B. Lippincott Company, Philadelphia, PA © 1995.

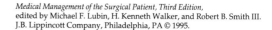

CHAPTER

40

DELIRIUM

Alan Stoudemire

Delirium (formerly referred to as acute organic brain syndrome) is the most common cause of altered mental status in surgical patients. The cardinal feature of delirium is an alteration in the level of consciousness that fluctuates over time—usually involving an alteration or clouding of consciousness. Multiple signs and symptoms may accompany delirium. Patients may be grossly psychotic with severe perceptual distortions that can include hallucinations (tactile, auditory, visual, olfactory); paranoia; and delusions; and have thought disorganization and language incoherence that can resemble schizophrenia. Signs of cognitive dysfunction such as disturbances in memory, attention, concentration, and orientation are usually the first to be recognized. Behavioral abnormalities such as agitation, impulsiveness, disinhibition, and combativeness may occur concurrently. Patients may become uncooperative, angry, irritable, frantic, aggressive, and hostile, and may exhibit a variety of bizarre behaviors. Often unrecognized or ignored, however, are confused patients who are quietly delirious and withdrawn but who demonstrate severe mental status abnormalities on formal examination.

The hallmark of delirium usually involves fluctuations in the level of consciousness that vary over time in a "sine wave" fashion and may be interspersed with periods of relative lucidity (the lucid interval). A clouding of consciousness is most common but patients can also show hyperalert, irritable, or agitated behavior similar to that seen in alcohol withdrawal delirium (or delirium tremens). The sleep-wake cycle can be, and generally is, markedly disrupted as well. Sleep is usually fragmented, shallow, and poor, with restlessness and agitation. Disturbances in psychomotor behavior may vary from hyperactivity to lethargy, stupor, obtundation, and catatonia. Tremor, asterixis, and other signs of neurologic dysfunction may be seen, such as in delirium caused by metabolic and hepatic encephalopathies or drug intoxication. Alcohol and sedative drug withdrawal states are particularly accompanied by irritability, anxiety, agitation, and insomnia.

Delirium by definition is usually acute in onset but may develop gradually over days or even weeks depending on the underlying cause. Most cases of delirium improve or resolve within 1 to 4 weeks if sufficient attention is given to correcting the underlying disorder causing the cerebral dysfunction.

Elderly patients are at high risk for the development of delirium, particularly those with preexisting cognitive impairment such as Alzheimer's disease or cerebrovascular dementia. Delirium tends to be common among the hospitalized elderly. One British study found that as many as 35% of patients older than 65 years had delirium at the time of admission or developed it during the course of hospitalization.[1] Other studies have shown prevalence rates for delirium for the hospitalized elderly to range from 16% to 25% in general medical wards[2,3] and from 10% to 15% in general surgical wards.[4]

Delirium may be a grave prognostic sign. One study reported that 33% of 4000 patients admitted to the hospital with a diagnosis of delirium died within a month.[5] Other studies have found a mortality rate of about 25%.[1,6]

DIAGNOSIS

The diagnosis of delirium is based on a combination of clinical observations and formal mental status changes. Nursing observations often provide the earliest and best sources for suspecting the diagnosis, especially for assessing the degree to which mental status fluctuates over a 24-hour period. The family's description of a patient's baseline mental status outside the hospital, especially regarding the use of prescription and nonprescription drugs and the use of alcohol, is extremely important. A past history of previous mental status changes during hospitalization or after surgery can help predict future episodes.

Although overt behavioral signs of delirium, such as agitation, insomnia, psychosis, and marked disorientation, are relatively easy to detect, subtle cognitive impairments in quiet, apathetic, and withdrawn patients require more rigorous testing. Several screening tests are available, including a short bedside mental status examination, the Folstein Mini-Mental State Examination, which can be completed in about 7 minutes[7] (Table 40-1). Any marked difficulties with this examination, and in particular a score below 24 (or scores that change over time), should lead to a presumptive diagnosis of delirium, especially in light of fluctuating mental status changes or alterations in level of consciousness. A normal examination does not necessarily exclude the diagnosis because patients can perform relatively well during lucid intervals. The examination may be repeated periodically every 24 to 48 hours.

FACTORS CAUSING DELIRIUM AND HIGH-RISK GROUPS

Psychotropic agents and other medications are probably the most common cause of delirium in hospitalized elderly patients, especially psychotropic and analgesic drugs that have sedative and anticholinergic effects.[8] Table 40-2 contains a partial list of drugs that cause delirium.

As reviewed by Lipowski,[8] the most common physical illnesses associated with delirium in the elderly include congestive heart failure, pneumonia, urinary tract infection, cancer, uremia, malnutrition, hypokalemia, dehydration, sodium depletion, and cerebrovascular accidents.[1,3,6,9–11] Systemic illnesses that result in cerebral dysfunction are more common causes of delirium than are primary illnesses of the central nervous system.

In addition to elderly patients, patients with alcoholism should be observed closely, particularly those with histories of recent heavy drinking in whom the possibility of a withdrawal syndrome exists. Delirium tremens (alcohol withdrawal delirium) carries its own morbidity and mortality, and the situation is made even more serious if withdrawal is superimposed on other medical or surgical conditions. A history of the use of other drugs that have significant withdrawal symptoms (eg, barbiturates, sedative-hypnotics, and benzodiazepines) warrants detoxification before surgery if possible. If emergent surgery is required, these drugs should not be withheld abruptly; instead, patients should be treated with a pharmacologic detoxification regimen after surgery (such as a barbiturate or benzodiazepine taper). Table 40-3 lists organic mental syndromes that are associated with psychoactive substances. See Chapter 47 for more information.

Injured patients, particularly those with head trauma, are at higher risk. Patients with sensory impairment (ie, those who are blind, deaf, undergoing cataract surgery, or facing extensive bandaging of the eyes and cephalic region) are prone to become confused because of sensory deprivation and require special efforts to promote orientation to the environment. Patients with preexisting cognitive impairment, mental retardation, or dementia have less ability to organize and adapt rapidly to the strangeness of the hospital and the stresses of surgery, and also may need special attention.

Differentiating between dementia and delirium is important. Dementia tends to be chronic, slowly progressive, and often insidious in onset; delirium usually is relatively dramatic in onset and fluctuating in nature. Dementia involves global impairments in intellect, cognition, personality, mood control, orientation, memory, judgment, and behavior, but alertness and level of consciousness are usually intact until the very late stages of illness. Although mental status does not usually fluctuate markedly during the day in dementia, when it does, exacerbations classically occur in the evening ("sundowning") when the orienting effects of patients' daily routines and sensory input decrease. Dementia has a gradual onset and does not remit unless an occult medical disorder is contributing to it. Most cases of dementia in patients older than 65 years are related to Alzheimer's disease, and most of the remainder result from cerebrovascular causes.[13] About 5% of patients with dementia have an underlying disorder that is potentially reversible (eg, meningioma).[14] Delirium may be superimposed on patients with underlying dementia, and patients with dementia are at higher risk for the development of delirium in the medical–surgical setting.

CAUSE

Delirium can arise from failure or dysfunction in any organ system (hepatic, pulmonary, renal, cardiovascular, endocrine, gastrointestinal) that causes secondary metabolic ab-

(text continues on page 383)

TABLE 40–1. The Mini-Metal State Examination and Instructions

Patient _____

Examiner _____

Date _____

MINI-MENTAL STATE EXAMINATION

Maximum
Score   Score

ORIENTATION

Max	Score	
5	( )	What is the (year) (season) (date) (day) (month)?
5	( )	Where are we: (state) (county) (town) (hospital) (floor)?

REGISTRATION

3   ( )   Name three objects: 1 second to say each. Then ask the patient all three after you have said them. Give 1 point for each correct answer. Then repeat them until he or she learns all three. Count trials and record.

Trials _____

ATTENTION AND CALCULATION

5   ( )   Serial 7's. 1 point for each correct. Stop after five answers. Alternatively spell *world* backward.

RECALL

3   ( )   Ask for the three objects repeated above. Give 1 point for each correct.

LANGUAGE

9   ( )   Name a watch and pencil. (2 points)
Repeat the following, "No ifs, ands or buts." (1 point)

Follow a 3-stage command:
  "Take a paper in your right hand, fold it in half, and put it on the floor." (3 points)
Read and obey the following:
  Close your eyes. (1 point)
  Write a sentence. (1 point)
  Copy design. (1 point)

TOTAL SCORE

Perfect Score = 30
Any score below 25 indicates the presence of significant cognitive dysfunction.

ASSESS level of consciousness along a continuum:
Alert   Drowsy   Stupor   Coma

(continued)

TABLE 40–1. (Continued)

INSTRUCTIONS FOR ADMINISTRATION
OF MINI-MENTAL STATE EXAMINATION

ORIENTATION

1. Ask for the date. Then ask specifically for parts omitted. For example, "Can you also tell me what season it is?" One point for each correct.

2. Ask in turn, "Can you tell me the name of this hospital?" (e.g, town, county). One point for each correct.

REGISTRATION

Ask the patient if you may test his or her memory. Then say the names of three unrelated objects, clearly and slowly, about one second for each. After you have said all three, ask him or her to repeat them. This first repetition determines his score (0 to 3), but keep saying them until the patient can repeat all three, up to six trials. If he or she does not eventually learn all three, recall cannot be meaningfully tested.

ATTENTION AND CALCULATION

Ask the patient to begin with 100 and count backward by 7. Stop after five subtractions (93, 86, 79, 72, 65). Score the total number of correct answers.

If the patient cannot or will not perform this task, ask him or her to spell the word *world* backward. The score is the number of letters in correct order. That is, dlrow = 5, dlorw = 3.

RECALL

Ask the patient if he can recall the three words you previously asked him or her to remember. Score 0 to 3.

LANGUAGE

Naming: Show the patient a wrist watch and ask him or her what it is. Repeat with a pencil. Score 0 to 2.

Repetition: Ask the patient to repeat the sentence after you. Allow only one trial. Score 0 or 1.

Three-stage command: Give the patient a piece of plain blank paper and repeat the command. Score 1 point for each part correctly executed.

Reading: On a blank piece of paper print the sentence "Close your eyes" in letters large enough for the patient to see clearly. Ask him or her to read it and do what it says. Score 1 point only if the patient actually closes his or her eyes.

Writing: Give the patient a blank piece of paper and ask him or her to write a sentence for you. Do not dictate a sentence, it is to be written spontaneously. It must contain a subject and verb and be sensible. Correct grammar and punctuation are not necessary.

Copying: On a clean piece of paper, draw intersecting pentagons, each side about 1 inch, and ask the patient to copy it exactly as is. All 10 angles must be present and 2 must intersect to score 1 point. Tremor and rotation are ignored.

Estimate the patient's level of sensorium along a continuum, from alert on the left to coma on the right.

(Folstein MF, Folstein SE, McHugh PR. Mini-Mental State: a practical method for grading the cognitive state of patients for the clinician. J Psychiatr Res 1975;12:189–198)

TABLE 40–2. Drugs That Cause Delirium (Partial Listing)

Antibiotics
Acyclovir (antiviral)
Amphotericin B (antifungal)
Cephalexin
Chloroquine (antimalarial)

Anticholinergics
Antihistamines
   Chlorpheniramine
   Diphenhydramine
Anticholinergics
   Benztropine
   Biperiden
Antispasmodics
Atropine/homatropine
Belladonna alkaloids
Phenothiazines (especially thioridazine)
Promethazine
Scopolamine
Tricyclic antidepressants (especially amitriptyline)
Trihexyphenidyl

Anticonvulsants
Phenobarbital
Phenytoin
Sodium valproate

Antiinflammatories
Adrenocorticotropic hormone
Corticosteroids
Ibuprofen
Indomethacin
Naproxen
Phenylbutazone

Antineoplastics
5-Fluorouracil

Antiparkinsonians
Amantadine
Carbidopa
Levodopa

Antituberculous Agents
Isoniazid
Rifampicin

Analgesics
Opiates
Salicylates
Synthetic narcotics

Cardiac Agents
β-Blockers (propranolol)
Clonidine
Digitalis
Disopyramide
Lidocaine
Mexiletine
Methyldopa
Quinidine
Procainamide

Drug Withdrawal
Alcohol
Barbiturates
Benzodiazepines

Sedative-Hypnotics
Barbiturates
Benzodiazepines
Glutethimide

Sympathomimetics
Amphetamines
Phenylephrine
Phenylpropanolamine

Miscellaneous
Aminophylline
Bromides
Chlorpropamide
Cimetidine
Disulfiram
Lithium
Metrizamide
Metronidazole
Ranitidine
Podphyllin by absorption
Propylthiouracil
Quinacrine
Theophylline
Timolol ophthalmic

Over-the-Counter Agents (Most Have Anticholinergic Effects)
Compoz
Sleep-Eze
Sominex

(Stoudemire A. Organic mental disorders. In: Clinical psychiatry for medical students. Philadelphia, JB Lippincott, 1990:99)

TABLE 40–3. Mental Syndromes Associated With Psychoactive Substances

Substance	Intoxication	Withdrawal	Delirium	Withdrawal Delirium	Delusional Disorder	Mood Disorder	Other Syndromes
Alcohol	X	X		X			*
Amphetamine and related substances	X	X	X		X		
Caffeine	X						
Cannabis	X				X		
Cocaine	X	X	X		X		
Hallucinogen	X (hallucinosis)				X	X	†
Inhalant	X						
Nicotine		X					
Opioid	X	X					
Phencyclidine (PCP) and related substances	X		X		X	X	‡
Sedative, hypnotic, or anxiolytic	X	X		X			§

*Alcohol idiosyncratic intoxication, alcohol hallucinosis, alcohol amnestic disorder, dementia associated with alcoholism.
†Posthallucinogen perception disorder.
‡Phencyclidine (PCP) or similarly acting arylcyclohexylamine mental disorder, nonspecific.
§Sedative, hypnotic, or anxiolytic amnestic disorder.
(Stoudemire A. Organic mental disorders. In: Clinical psychiatry for medical students. Philadelphia, JB Lippincott, 1990:78; and Diagnostic and statistical manual of mental disorders, ed 4. Washington, DC, American Psychiatric Association, 1994)

normalities (electrolyte imbalance, hypoglycemia, adrenal failure, hyperosmolarity or hypoosmolarity, uremia, hypoxemia, hypercarbia, hypercalcemia or hypocalcemia, severe hypertension). Decreases in cardiac output can lead to decreased cerebral perfusion with subsequent confusion. Peripheral as well as central nervous system infections can cause fever and sepsis, leading to altered mental status, as can meningeal infiltration in certain forms of leukemia.

Direct insults to the central nervous system from bacterial meningitis, viral encephalitis, cerebrovascular hemorrhage, subdural hematoma, strokes, and vasculitis associated with collagen vascular diseases can induce delirium. Gliomas and meningiomas may cause delirium, although the onset may be insidious if the tumor is growing slowly and may not be associated with focal neurologic findings in the early stages.

Medication side effects, particularly in the elderly and even in therapeutic doses, may cause mental status changes, especially when coexisting medical problems exist. Common offenders include narcotic analgesics, barbiturates, benzodiazepines, and other sedative-hypnotic medications. Antidepressants, particularly those with strong anticholinergic and sedating effects, such as amitriptyline (Elavil), can cause delirium that is referred to as *anticholinergic delirium*. Much attention has recently focused on triazolam (Halcion), an ultrashort-acting benzodiazepine that can cause amnesia, confusion, and disorientation, particularly in the elderly at doses greater than 0.125 mg/d.

Numerous nonpsychiatric medications cause symptoms of delirium even under physiologically normal conditions, almost always at toxic levels. These include antihistamines (sedative and anticholinergic effects); atropine-like drugs; H_2 blockers (cimetidine, ranitidine); phenytoin; phenobarbital; digitalis; procainamide; lidocaine; and L-dopa. Steroids, particularly when they are administered rapidly and in high doses (greater than the equivalent of 40 mg/d of prednisone), can cause steroid psychosis, which is more appropriately termed a delirium with psychotic features.

Mention should also be made of the intensive care unit syndrome, intensive care unit psychosis, and postcardiotomy syndrome. Although the behavioral abnormalities that have been described in patients in the intensive care unit often have been referred to as postoperative psychosis, most of these patients suffer from delirium with psychotic features. These delirious states are usually determined by multiple factors and may at least partially arise from the stresses inherent in the intensive care setting itself.[15] These stresses include the strange, technologically oriented environment; physical incapacitation; multiple monitors; intravenous lines; catheters; lack of privacy; and noise. Most patients in the intensive care unit are elderly, medically compromised, and receiving multiple medications. Sleep deprivation caused by pain and the stress of the intensive care unit also may contribute. A functional psychosis should be diagnosed only after metabolic causes have been ruled out.

Delirium also may occur after open heart surgery and is

TABLE 40–4. Differential Diagnosis of Delirium and Dementia

Feature	Delirium	Dementia
Onset	Acute, often at night	Insidious
Course	Fluctuating, with lucid intervals, during day; worse at night	Stable over course of day
Duration	Hours to weeks	Months or years
Awareness	Reduced	Clear
Alertness	Abnormally low or high	Usually normal
Attention	Lacks direction and selectivity, distractibility, fluctuates over course of day	Relatively unaffected
Orientation	Usually impaired for time, tendency to mistake unfamiliar for familiar place and persons	Often impaired
Memory	Immediate and recent impaired	Recent and remote impaired
Thinking	Disorganized	Impoverished
Perception	Illusions and hallucinations usually visual and common	Often absent
Speech	Incoherent, hesitant, slow or rapid	Difficulty in finding words
Sleep-wake cycle	Always disrupted	Fragmented sleep
Physical illness or drug toxicity	Either or both present	Often absent, especially in Alzheimer's disease

(Stoudemire A. Organic mental disorders. In: Clinical psychiatry for medical students. Philadelphia, JB Lippincott, 1990:97; and Lipowski ZJ. Delirium [acute confusional states]. JAMA 1987;258:1789–1792)

known as postcardiotomy delirium. The syndrome as classically described occurred after 3 or 4 days of lucidity and then was typified by progressive disorientation, confusion, and other features of delirium, often psychotic in nature. Several factors may contribute to the development of postcardiotomy delirium, including advanced age, extended duration of cardiopulmonary bypass, intraoperative hypotension, severity of illness, sleep deprivation, and sensory monotony.[16–20] Heller and associates[21] found that postcardiotomy delirium is also directly related to a low postoperative cardiac index, leading to a greater likelihood of impaired cerebral perfusion and oxygenation. As a result of advances in cardiopulmonary bypass procedures that have shortened the length of surgery, the incidence of postcardiotomy delirium appears to have markedly decreased. Table 40-4 presents the differential diagnosis for cognitive impairment in medical–surgical patients.

DIAGNOSTIC EVALUATION

The principal rule in assessing patients with delirium is to evaluate and correct the underlying disorder or disorders contributing to cerebral dysfunction. Appropriate treatment must be preceded by an extensive and in-depth search for the underlying cause of the brain syndrome. Although the differential diagnosis of delirium is extensive, the actual diagnostic work-up is relatively straightforward (Table 40-5).

A review of preoperative factors that may be contributing to the development of delirium may assist in more focally identifying its cause (ie, alcoholism, medication use, dementia) and in evaluating intraoperative factors that may have resulted in a central nervous system insult (ie, hypoxia, hemorrhage, hypotension, emboli). Because medications are always likely factors, the cumulative dose of medications received during the past week should be checked, as should blood levels when possible (eg, anticonvulsants, digoxin, theophylline, cyclosporine). Psychotropic, sedative- hypnotic, analgesic, and atropine-like drugs should be scrutinized especially closely.

Once the history, operative course, and medications have been reviewed, the vital signs should be evaluated and physical and neurologic examinations performed. Evaluations should be done on an organ-system basis, looking for evidence of cardiovascular (arterial blood gases, chest radiograph); pulmonary; renal (electrolyte imbalances, uremia); endocrine (thyroid panel, hypoglycemia, Ca^{2+}); hepatic (hepatic encephalopathy); and gastrointestinal (impaction, obstruction, ileus, hemorrhage, volvulus) disease. A search for infection (sepsis, occult abscess, meningitis) is crucial. The fundamental clinical principle is to detect and correct, to the greatest extent possible, the underlying ab-

TABLE 40–5. Comprehensive Evaluation of Dementia and Delirium

Physical examination, including thorough neurologic examination
Vital signs
Mental status examination
Mini-Mental State Examination
Review of medications and drug levels
Blood and urine screens for alcohol, drugs, and heavy metals*
Physiologic work-up
    Serum electrolytes/glucose/Ca^{2+}, Mg^+
    Liver and kidney function tests
    SMA-12 or equivalent serum chemistry profile
    Urinalysis
    Complete blood cell count with differential cell type count
    Thyroid function tests (including thyroid-stimulating hormone level)
    Rapid plasma reagin (serum screen)
    Fluorescent treponemal antibody absorption test (if central nervous system disease suspected)
    Serum B_{12} level
    Folate levels
    Urine corticosteroids*
    Erythrocyte sedimentation rate (Westergren)
    Antinuclear antibody* (ANA), C_3, C_4, anti-DS DNA*
    Arterial blood gases*
    Human immunodeficiency virus screen[†]
    Urine porphobilinogens*
Chest radiograph
Electrocardiogram
Neurologic work-up
    Computed tomographic or magnetic resonance scan of head*
    Lumbar puncture*
    Electroencephalogram*
Neuropsychologic testing[‡]

*If indicated by history and physical examination.
[†]Requires special consent and counseling.
[‡]May be useful in differentiating dementia from other neuropsychiatric syndromes if this cannot be done clinically.
(Stoudemire A. Organic mental disorders. In: Clinical psychiatry for medical students. Philadelphia, JB Lippincott, 1990:85)

normality causing the altered mental status. Among the elderly, a causative factor can be identified in 80% to 90% of patients.[8]

TREATMENT

Therapy for delirium primarily involves diagnosing and treating its underlying cause. Until this is accomplished or the delirium resolves, several environmental strategies can help to keep patients oriented. A window (properly secured to prevent jumping) through which patients can observe light and dark patterns can help provide orientation and correct sleep cycles. Family members or sitters can be allowed at the bedside to provide frequent orientation. Large calendars, clocks, familiar objects (such as family photographs), a radio, and a television also may help patients stay connected to the outside world. Providing night-lights and sensory input is helpful for patients who are heavily bandaged or in casts. Elderly patients undergoing cataract operations are at risk for delirium, and most of these procedures should be done on one eye at a time. Patients who are on ventilators or are unable to speak because of mechanical problems or tubes should be communicated with at frequent intervals and given the opportunity to respond through hand signals, writing, or lap computers.

PHARMACOLOGIC THERAPY

Antipsychotic medications have traditionally been used to control the severe behavioral symptoms of delirium, although they do nothing to correct the underlying structural or metabolic derangements causing the central nervous system dysfunction. These medications do suppress psychotic symptoms, control agitated and possibly dangerous behavior, and provide sedation. Antipsychotic agents have been preferred because other tranquilizing psychotropic drugs, such as the usual benzodiazepines, have a disinhibiting effect on behavior and usually exacerbate the symptoms of delirium. Some clinicians have advocated the use of lorazepam and midazolam in the intensive care unit setting for the treatment of delirium (see later discussion).

Antipsychotics can be roughly categorized as high-potency or low-potency agents. Chlorpromazine (Thorazine) and thioridazine (Mellaril) are relatively low-potency agents, whereas haloperidol (Haldol), thiothixene (Navane), fluphenazine (Prolixin), and trifluoperazine (Stelazine) are high-potency agents. High-potency agents such as haloperidol tend to be the drugs of choice in delirium, primarily because they are generally less sedating, have fewer anticholinergic effects, and have little propensity to cause hemodynamic effects. These higher potency agents, however, are more likely to cause extrapyramidal side effects, such as pseudoparkinsonism.

The side effects of antipsychotic drugs may be serious and are often more pronounced in elderly or physically compromised patients. These drugs must be used conservatively with frequent monitoring for side effects and periodic reevaluation for the necessity of continued treatment. The initiation of antipsychotic therapy should never delay the search to identify, stabilize, and correct the primary cause of the delirium.

The side effects of these drugs can be divided into six groups: anticholinergic, extrapyramidal, hypotensive, sedating, allergic, and neuroendocrine. The anticholinergic effects, which are most prominent with thioridazine and chlorpromazine, include dry mouth, blurred vision, urinary retention, nausea, constipation, tachycardia, decreased sweating, and confusion.

Extrapyramidal side effects, which are most prominent with higher potency drugs such as haloperidol, may be subdivided into (1) parkinsonian side effects (eg, resting tremor, masklike facies, bradykinesia, cogwheel rigidity, festinating gait, dysphagia, and drooling); (2) akathisia (eg, restless legs and agitation); (3) dystonic reactions (eg, oculogyric crises, opisthotonus, tonic contractions of muscle groups); and (4) tardive dyskinesia (eg, development of involuntary movements of the oral-buccal musculature, tongue, trunk, and extremities). Tardive dyskinesia may develop after only a few months of use in the elderly.

Orthostatic side effects result from α-adrenergic blockade and are most pronounced with chlorpromazine. Therefore, this drug should not be used in the elderly, patients with cardiovascular disease, or patients who have volume compromise or hypotension.

Sedating side effects are often desired but must be carefully monitored. Although these drugs do not have a great potential for respiratory depression, restriction of respiratory capacity may occur in higher doses or in patients with severe lung disease. Chlorpromazine and thioridazine tend to be more sedating on a dose-unit basis, and the sedative and confusional effects are compounded by their higher anticholinergic affinity. Sedative effects of these drugs are also related to antihistaminic effects.[22]

More rare reactions with these agents include agranulocytosis, cholestatic jaundice, dermatitis, lowering of seizure threshold, and galactorrhea.

One of the most overlooked causes of akathisia and extrapyramidal side effects is metoclopramide (Reglan). The drug has dopamine blocking properties similar to neuroleptics and may cause akathisia (restless legs), parkinsonian symptoms, and even tardive dyskinesia. Its dosage should be adjusted downward with decreased renal function and increased age.

A rare but highly lethal side effect of the higher potency neuroleptics (antipsychotic drugs) is the neuroleptic malignant syndrome.[23] This syndrome is primarily associated with haloperidol and fluphenazine and is characterized by the sudden onset of severe extrapyramidal symptoms (muscle rigidity, hyperthermia, and hyperadrenergic autonomic dysfunction). Patients may become stuporous and catatonic.[24] Because creatine kinase levels are almost always elevated, monitoring these levels is an excellent way to observe the course of the syndrome. Leukocytosis and elevated liver enzyme levels may also occur. If it is recognized early, this potentially lethal disorder is reported to respond to treatment with dantrolene sodium, 1.25 to 1.5 mg/kg by intravenous push, or bromocriptine, 5 mg orally three times daily. The crucial component of treatment, however, is rec-

ognizing that the hyperthermia is related to the central nervous system effect of the neuroleptics and discontinuing these agents if fever cannot be explained on other medical grounds.[25] Adequate hydration is critical to prevent renal shutdown caused by rhabdomyolysis.

CLINICAL USE OF NEUROLEPTICS IN DELIRIUM

Because the higher potency neuroleptics cause less orthostatic hypotension, they are usually the drugs of choice for medical–surgical patients, although patients should be monitored for extrapyramidal side effects. A typical initial dose is 2 to 5 mg of haloperidol given orally or intramuscularly. Because the peak action of intramuscular haloperidol occurs 30 minutes after administration, patients can be reevaluated within the first hour in emergencies and repeated doses can be given hourly if rapid tranquilizing is desired. Peak action after oral ingestion occurs within 2 to 4 hours. After patients are adequately sedated, doses can be given orally or intramuscularly every 4 to 6 hours. It is almost always preferable to administer these drugs orally, and giving them in elixir form hastens their onset of action.

The use of intravenous haloperidol and lorazepam in the treatment of delirium has increased markedly. Initial doses of haloperidol are usually 2 to 5 mg (given at a rate of 1 mg/min) and may be repeated every 30 to 60 minutes as outlined in Table 40-6.[26]

Some clinicians also advocate the simultaneous use of intravenous lorazepam (Ativan) with haloperidol, usually in doses of 1 to 2 mg with careful monitoring for respiratory depression. Some patients may exhibit extremely high tolerance of haloperidol, requiring doses in excess of 100 mg intravenously per day but such cases are the exception.

More detailed discussions of the use of intravenous haloperidol and lorazepam for the behavioral control of delirium are available.[27]

The need for continued medication use should be reevaluated every 24 hours. Most patients become stable within 72 hours if adequate attention is devoted to treating the underlying cause of the delirium. If treatment is necessary beyond a week or more, psychiatric consultation should be requested. In most instances, resolution of the delirium should be accompanied by a gradual tapering and discontinuation of the antipsychotic agent dosage as soon as possible.[28]

The extrapyramidal side effects of these drugs may be treated with diphenhydramine (Benadryl) at a dosage of 25 to 50 mg orally three times daily for 5 days, benztropine mesylate (Cogentin) at a dosage of 1 to 2 mg orally two or three times daily for 5 days, or trihexyphenidyl hydrochloride (Artane) at a dosage of 2 to 5 mg orally three times

TABLE 40–6. Treatment Guidelines for the Use of Intravenous Haloperidol in the Intensive Care Setting

Degree of Agitation	Starting Dose (mg)
Mild	0.5–2.0
Moderate–severe	2.0–10

Titration and Maintenance

Allow 20–30 minutes before the next dose.

If agitation is *unchanged*, administer double dose every 20–30 minutes until patient begins to calm.

If patient is calming down, repeat the last dose at next dosing interval.

Adjust dose and interval to patient's clinical course. Gradually increase the interval between doses until the interval is 8 hours, then begin to decrease dose.

Once stable for 24 hours, give doses on a regular schedule and supplement with as-needed doses.

Once stable for 36–48 hours, begin attempts to taper dose.

When agitation is very severe, very high boluses (up to 40 mg) may be required.

(Goldstein MG. Intensive care unit syndromes. In: Stoudemire A, Fogel BS, eds. Principles of medical psychiatry. Orlando, Grune & Stratton, 1987: 412)

daily for 5 days. In acute dystonic reactions (such as oculogyric crisis), diphenhydramine at a dosage of 25 to 50 mg intravenously, or benztropine mesylate at a dosage of 1 to 2 mg intramuscularly, can be given.

REFERENCES

1. Hodkinson HM. Mental impairment in the elderly. J R Coll Physicians Lond 1973;7:305–317.
2. Bergmann K, Eastham EJ. Psychogeriatric ascertainment and assessment for treatment in an acute medical ward setting. Age Ageing 1974;3:174–188.
3. Seymour DG, Henschke PJ, Cape RDT, et al. Acute confusional states and dementia in the elderly: the role of dehydration/volume depletion, physical illness and age. Age Ageing 1980;9:137–146.
4. Millar HR. Psychiatric morbidity in elderly surgical patients. Br J Psychiatry 1981;138:17–20.
5. Bedford PD. General medical aspects of confusional states in elderly people. BMJ 1959;2:185–188.
6. Simon A, Cahan RB. The acute brain syndrome in geriatric patients. Psychiatric Res Rep 1963;16:8–21.
7. Folstein MF, Folstein SE, McHugh PR. Mini-Mental State: a practical method for grading the cognitive state of patients for the clinician. J Psychiatr Res 1975;12:189–198.
8. Lipowski ZJ. Transient cognitive disorders (delirium, acute confusional states) in the elderly. Am J Psychiatry 1983;140:1426–1436.
9. Flint FJ, Richards SM. Organic basis of confusional states in the elderly. BMJ 1956;2:1537–1539.
10. Kay DWK, Roth M. Physical accompaniments of mental disorder in old age. Lancet 1955;2:740–745.
11. Roth M. The natural history of medical disorder in old age. J Ment Sci 1955;101:281–301.
12. Stoudemire A. Organic mental disorders. In: Stoudemire A, ed. Clinical psychiatry for medical students. Philadelphia, JB Lippincott, 1990:72–106.
13. Schneck MK, Reisberg B, Ferris SH. An overview of current concepts of Alzheimer's disease. Am J Psychiatry 1982;139:165–173.
14. Stoudemire A, Thompson TL. Recognizing and treating dementia. Geriatrics 1981;36:112–120.
15. Houpt JL, Stoudemire A. Diagnosis and treatment of delirium. In: Kortz WJ, Lamb PD, eds. Surgical intensive care. Chicago, Year Book Medical Publishers, 1984:283–292.
16. Heller SS, Frank KA, Malm JR, et al. Psychiatric complications of open-heart surgery: a reexamination. N Engl J Med 1970;283:1015–1020.
17. Kornfeld DS, Zimberg S, Malm JR. Psychiatric complications of open-heart surgery. N Engl J Med 1965;273:287–292.
18. Kornfeld DS, Heller SS, Frank KA, et al. Personality and psychological factors in postcardiotomy delirium. Arch Gen Psychiatry 1974;31:249–253.
19. Kornfeld DS, Heller SS, Frank KA, et al. Delirium after coronary artery bypass surgery. J Thorac Cardiovasc Surg 1978;76:93–96.
20. Tufo HM, Ostfeld AM, Shekelle R. Central nervous system dysfunction following open heart surgery. JAMA 1970;212:1333–1340.
21. Heller SS, Kornfeld DS, Frank KA, Hoar PF. Postcardiotomy delirium and cardiac output. Am J Psychiatry 1979;136:337–339.
22. Richelson E. Neuroleptic affinities for human brain receptors and their use in predicting adverse effects. J Clin Psychiatry 1984;45:331–336.
23. Stoudemire A, Luther JS. Neuroleptic malignant syndrome and neuroleptic-induced catatonia: differential diagnosis and treatment. Int J Psychiatry Med 1984;14:57–63.
24. Stoudemire A. The differential diagnosis of catatonic states. Psychosomatics 1982;23:245–252.
25. Harpe C, Stoudemire A. Aetiology and treatment of the neuroleptic malignant syndrome. Med Toxicol 1987;2:166–176.
26. Goldstein MG. Intensive care unit syndromes. In: Stoudemire A, Fogel BS, eds. Principles of medical psychiatry. Orlando, FL, Grune & Stratton, 1987:403–422.
27. Goldstein MG, Haltzman SD. Intensive care. In: Stoudemire A, Fogel BS, eds. Psychiatric care of the medical patient. New York, Oxford University Press, 1993:241–264.
28. Slaby AE, Erle SR. Delirium and dementia. In: Stoudemire A, Fogel BS, eds. Psychiatric care of the medical patient. New York, Oxford University Press, 1993:415–453.

Medical Management of the Surgical Patient, Third Edition,
edited by Michael F. Lubin, H. Kenneth Walker, and Robert B. Smith III.
J.B. Lippincott Company, Philadelphia, PA © 1995.

CHAPTER

41

PARKINSON'S DISEASE

Jorge L. Juncos

After a brief overview, this chapter focuses on clinical issues of importance to the perioperative care of patients with Parkinson's disease.

Parkinson's disease is an adult-onset neurodegenerative disorder characterized by progressive slowness of movement (bradykinesia), muscular rigidity, tremor, gait abnormalities, and varying degrees of cognitive impairment. It affects close to 1 million, mostly elderly, Americans with an annual incidence of 20 new cases per 100,000 and a prevalence of 130 cases per 100,000.[1,2] Its primary pathology is limited to the brain and consists of selective degeneration of the nigrostriatal dopaminergic pathway and the presence of Lewy bodies in surviving mesencephalic dopamine neurons.[3] Biochemically, this denervation results in striatal dopamine depletion, which is linked to the signs and symptoms of the illness.[4] The cause of selective neuronal death, and therefore the cause of Parkinson's disease, is unknown, although hereditary and environmental factors are thought to play a role.[5-7]

Symptomatic control of the illness depends on reestablishing dopamine transmission in the striatum. This strategy involves (1) enhancing the cerebral availability of levodopa, the precursor amino acid of dopamine; (2) using dopamine agonists (eg, bromocriptine, pergolide) to stimulate dopamine receptors directly; and (3) blocking the oxidative breakdown of dopamine with the selective monoamine oxidase (MAO) inhibitor, selegiline. Other MAO inhibitors and noncatechol-O-methyl transferase inhibitors

(which also block the breakdown of dopamine) should be available soon. Additional drugs that are useful in individual cases include anticholinergics (eg, trihexyphenidyl, benztropine), which reestablish the equilibrium between striatal cholinergic and dopaminergic transmission, and amantadine, which enhances cerebral dopamine transmission through still unclear mechanisms.

Special features of Parkinson's disease that may be important to its perioperative management include the presence of mild to moderate autonomic dysfunction, such as mild orthostatic hypotension or hypersensitivity to drugs that cause hypotension. Some patients exhibit nonspecific urinary difficulties (eg, urinary hesitancy not related to prostatism), vasomotor paroxysms with profuse unprovoked sweating, discoloration and mottling of the distal limbs, temperature sensitivity, and constipation. More severe forms of autonomic failure suggest a disorder other than Parkinson's disease (see later). A slowing of mental processes that parallels the slowing of motor processes may make some patients particularly sensitive to psychoactive drugs and anesthesia.[8] In addition, about 15% to 20% of patients with Parkinson's disease have or develop coexisting dementia.[9] The dementia is clinically and pathologically indistinguishable from senile dementia of the Alzheimer's type and is an important feature to identify before surgery.[9,10]

Drug-induced aggravation of parkinsonian signs and symptoms can be transient or chronic. It may involve the antiparkinsonian drugs, Parkinson–promoting drugs, or other drug interactions. Transient aggravation of symptoms is typified by motor fluctuations that result from the interaction between disease progression and the properties, long-term use, and schedule of antiparkinsonian therapy. Motor fluctuations range from the premature or sudden termination of drug effects ("off spells") to an excessive and aberrant sensitivity to therapy (ie, denervation hypersensitivity) that leads to dyskinesias and dystonias ("on" symptomatology). The fluctuations are mediated in part by the progressive loss of dopamine nerve end terminals, which destroys the ability of the striatum to buffer fluxes in dopamine availability.[11] In Parkinson's disease, the cerebral availability of dopamine is subject to fluctuations in plasma levodopa levels. These in turn reflect levodopa's short half-life (about 2 hours when it is given with carbidopa) and its intermittent oral administration. Because levodopa is absorbed primarily in the proximal small intestine, its availability is also subject to the vagaries of gastric emptying, which is a function of a myriad of factors, including the timing, quantity, and composition of meals.[12]

Chronic toxicity from antiparkinsonian drug therapy may also involve affective and cognitive functions. These include typical visual hallucinations, sleep disturbances (insomnia and hypersomnia), positive sleep phenomena such as vivid dreams (rapid eye movement–related behavioral disturbances such as screaming and ballistic movements during sleep), and nocturnal myoclonus (leg jerking). More subtle and insidious are personality changes that evolve over weeks to months. These consist of increasingly demanding and selfish attitudes, intolerance to any discomfort, and a seeming unawareness of impositions on other family members. It is important to recognize these early signs because their presence suggests that the threshold for postanesthetic delirium is low. In delirious patients with Parkinson's disease, motor symptoms respond poorly to drug therapy and increasing drug therapy only aggravates the delirium. Abrupt discontinuation of antiparkinsonian therapy also carries the risk of a potentially serious withdrawal reaction, as detailed later.

PREOPERATIVE CARE

GENERAL MEDICAL CONSIDERATIONS

The preoperative medical evaluation of patients with Parkinson's disease, regardless of their age, is similar to that of other elderly patients as outlined in Chapter 42. Areas that require special attention in Parkinson's disease are outlined here.

In Parkinson's disease, mild pharyngeal dysfunction leads to decreased spontaneous swallowing, accumulation of saliva in the posterior pharynx, and sialorrhea. With sedation, this otherwise minor dysfunction may worsen acutely and result in aspiration during the immediate postoperative period. To prevent this, frequent and extended suctioning is needed. Pharyngeal dysfunction may predispose patients with Parkinson's disease to severe laryngospasm if all antiparkinsonian therapy is removed abruptly, and the staff should be prepared to provide extra care if necessary.

The pulmonary status also requires special attention because pulmonary function tests often reveal restrictive deficits even in asymptomatic patients with Parkinson's disease. These abnormalities are partially relieved by levodopa therapy.[13] The restrictive findings are caused by the postural abnormalities (ie, stooping, scoliosis); the rigidity of the chest wall musculature; and the advanced spinal osteoarthritis that are often associated with the illness.[14–16] If patients are asymptomatic, they need only a routine preoperative evaluation consisting of a good history, chest examination, and chest radiograph. If pulmonary reserve is in doubt, the performance of abbreviated pulmonary function tests with arterial blood gases should be considered. Patients with Parkinson's disease do poorly once they develop pneumonia because of their easy fatigability, decreased respiratory capacity, and weak cough reflex.

The autonomic nervous system is of particular interest in Parkinson's disease. Although patients with Parkinson's disease technically do not have autonomic failure, they can have autonomic instability and special sensitivity to drugs that may cause hypotension, including antiparkinsonian drugs. Constipation is a universal problem and is taken for granted by many patients. Many have a tendency to delay evacuation and to rely on suppositories and enemas to do so.[12] Constipation may be a source of abdominal distention, ileus, or obstruction. Distention of the rectosigmoid may result in urinary retention and lead to urinary tract infection. These problems need to be detected before surgery because they can be compounded by the anesthesia and by the postoperative analgesia.

NEUROLOGIC CONSIDERATIONS

Many neurologic illnesses resemble idiopathic Parkinson's disease. These disorders present special management problems that must be anticipated. Perhaps the two most important disorders to differentiate from Parkinson's disease are multiple systems atrophy and progressive supranuclear palsy.[17,18] Like Parkinson's disease, they are both progressive neurodegenerative disorders of unknown cause in which slowness, rigidity, and gait impairment are prominent. In contrast to Parkinson's disease, tremor is often absent, the course is more rapid, and the response to therapy is poor. Multiple systems atrophy features prominent autonomic failure, which may influence the surgical decision and the strategy of anesthesia. Signs of autonomic failure include impotence, unexplained urinary dysfunction, postural hypotension, abnormal conduction or repolarization on electrocardiography, and impaired sweating.[17]

Progressive supranuclear palsy features loss of supranuclear gaze control (eg, decreased vertical and later horizontal gaze) that is described by patients as "trouble reading" not related to a refraction error. Patients note trouble walking down stairs (failure of downgaze) and, when the disease is advanced, difficulty looking for items on a table. In addition, patients develop axial dystonia out of proportion to the appendicular rigidity, which is the opposite of what is normally encountered in Parkinson's disease. Rigidity of the neck may make endotracheal intubation difficult and does not respond well to the usual perioperative muscle relaxants. Patients with multiple systems atrophy and progressive supranuclear palsy may be more prone to sleep apnea and other respiratory abnormalities than are patients with Parkinson's disease, and so may be more sensitive to sedatives and hypnotics. This diagnostic outline is meant to raise an index of suspicion for multiple systems atrophy and progressive supranuclear palsy when patients with parkinsonism are evaluated before surgery.

Cervical spondylosis is common in Parkinson's disease, in part because of the affected age group and the accelerated osteoarthritic changes that stem from akinesia. Clinically significant cervical spondylosis may be adversely affected by difficult intubation. Although it is not a contraindication to intubation, this may influence the route (nasotracheal versus oral) and preparation. Clinical signs of cervical spondylosis include neck and shoulder pain, pain radiating down the arms, leg and gait spasticity, hyperactive reflexes in the legs, brisk to patchy reflexes in the arms, and extensor plantar responses. Of note is that similar findings caused by cerebral, rather than cervical, pathology are common in progressive supranuclear palsy.

The presence of dementia significantly increases the risk of perioperative confusion and delirium. Dementia is found in about 15% to 20% of patients with Parkinson's disease and remains undetected in its early stages. The Mini-Mental Status examination is a simple and expeditious but relatively insensitive tool for dementia screening.[19] Early on, a history of ill-defined occupational, personal, and financial difficulties; loss of interest in hobbies; vague memory complaints; and personality changes may be more sensitive indicators of dementia than is the Mini-Mental Status examination. Pseudodementia related to depression is probably a more common cause of these complaints than is senile dementia of the Alzheimer's type. Depression affects over 40% of patients at some point in the illness and is usually accompanied by vegetative signs such as poor sleep and appetite, weight loss, and asthenia.

PHARMACOTHERAPEUTIC ISSUES

Drug interactions that may have been tolerated before surgery can become critical afterward and, thus, must be identified in the initial evaluation. Parkinsonian drug therapy is reviewed briefly and the ways in which it may need to be altered in surgical patients is discussed. Table 41-1 lists commonly prescribed drugs that may aggravate parkinsonian signs and should be avoided in patients with Parkinson's disease.

The mainstay of therapy for Parkinson's disease is still levodopa. It is administered in the form of carbidopa/levodopa to reduce the incidence of peripheral side effects such as nausea and hypotension.[20] Carbidopa is a peripheral dopa decarboxylase inhibitor that blocks the conver-

TABLE 41–1. Drugs That May Be Contraindicated in Patients With Parkinson's Disease

Drug Category	Generic Name
Dopamine antagonists	
Antipsychotics	Haloperidol
	Perphenazine
	Chlorpromazine
	Trifluoperazine
	Fluphenazine
	Thiothixene
	Thioridazine
	Loxapine
Antiemetics	Prochlorperazine
	Metoclopramide
	Thiethylperazine
	Droperidol
Antidepressants	Combinations of perphenazine and amitriptyline (Triavil, Etrafon)
	Phenelzine (monoamine oxidase inhibitor)
	Tranylcypromine (monoamine oxidase inhibitor)
Narcotics	Meperidine
	Fentanyl
Antihypertensives and miscellaneous postoperative medications	Reserpine
	Tetrabenazine
	α-Methylparatyrosine
	Rauwolfia serpentina
	Deserpidine
	Rescinnamine
	Rauwiloid
Drugs with lesser potential to aggravate symptoms	α-Methyldopa
	Phenytoin
	Valproic acid
	Lithium carbonate
	Buspirone

sion of levodopa to dopamine. Peripheral conversion of levodopa to dopamine is believed to be responsible for many of levodopa's side effects. To effectively block peripheral dopa decarboxylase, doses of carbidopa should be at least 75 mg/d, that is, three tablets of carbidopa/levodopa (25/100) or two tablets of controlled-release carbidopa/levodopa (50/200; Sinemet CR). Dopamine agonists such as bromocriptine and pergolide are more potent than levodopa but not as effective at alleviating symptoms, particularly when they are used alone.

The hypotensive effect of levodopa probably results from a central mechanism and may be more pronounced in patients with high baseline blood pressures.[20] The hypotensive effect of dopamine agonists is caused by several mechanisms: (1) relaxation of vascular smooth muscle in the splanchnic and renal circulation, (2) inhibition of noradrenergic nerve endings, and (3) central inhibition of sympathetic activity.[21] Dopamine agonists have a higher incidence of severe hypotension and other side effects than does levodopa. Accordingly, and unlike levodopa, the administration of dopamine agonists can be halted the night before surgery and resumed when the patients are stable.

Levodopa and dopamine agonists can also precipitate cardiac arrhythmias and delirium.[16] These complications tend to be minor and manageable, and do not require routine discontinuation of drug therapy. If concern exists regarding perioperative hypovolemia, the dosage of dopamine agonists should be reduced over 2 to 3 weeks before reductions in the levodopa dosage are considered. If the baseline dose of levodopa is high (eg, greater than 800 mg/d), it too may be decreased slowly to about 300 to 400 mg/d. This should be attempted only if the risks of hypovolemia outweigh the postoperative discomfort that patients are likely to experience as a consequence of increased symptoms.

Ancillary antiparkinsonian therapy such as anticholinergics and amantadine may increase the risk of postoperative delirium but should not be stopped abruptly or withheld for extended periods. Abrupt withdrawal of these and other antiparkinsonian medications may result in acute exacerbation and relative unresponsiveness of parkinsonian symptoms. If patients are not demented and exhibit no signs of delirium, the likelihood of this complication is small and the drug regimen need not be changed. If dementia or delirium is suspected, therapy with these drugs should be tapered or stopped over 2 to 4 weeks.

Special consideration should be given to the use of selegiline, an MAO B inhibitor that does not cause the hypertensive reactions to tyramine and other amino acids that are characteristic of nonselective MAO A or AB inhibitors (see Table 41-1). Selegiline is used to enhance the efficacy of levodopa but can also accentuate its side effects. Because of its long biologic half-life, it can be discontinued without tapering. Meperidine and selegiline should not be used con-

comitantly because of potentially serious adverse reactions (delirium). Based on studies in laboratory animals, selegiline also should not be used in patients with active peptic ulcer disease. The use of nonselective MAO inhibitors in combination with the selective serotonin reuptake inhibitor, fluoxetine, can lead to acute "serotonergic" reactions characterized by delirium, rigidity, and fever.[22] A similar interaction with selegiline has not been reported. In Parkinson's disease, however, fluoxetine may aggravate parkinsonian symptoms[23] and, in combination with selegiline, may lead to acute mania.[24]

Therapy with nonselective MAO inhibitors should be discontinued at least 2 weeks before surgery. Selegiline therapy does not need to be stopped routinely before surgery for the reasons mentioned earlier. Nonetheless, as a general precaution, we recommend discontinuing selegiline therapy 1 week before surgery to reduce the risk of perioperative drug interactions. The symptomatic effect of selegiline on Parkinson's disease symptoms is modest compared with that of levodopa and dopamine agonists; discontinuing its use for a few days generally does not result in serious motor deterioration.

For prolonged cerebral stereotactic procedures that are performed with patients awake, consideration should be given to providing small doses of carbidopa/levodopa orally with minuscule amounts of water, or to providing an intraduodenal infusion to maintain patient comfort (as described later).

ANESTHESIA MANAGEMENT

The specific choice of anesthetics is made by the anesthesiologist in consultation with the treating neurologist. The choice of general over regional anesthesia should be determined by the usual considerations discussed in Chapter 1. When appropriate, local or regional anesthesia are preferred over general anesthesia with the proviso that the first two provide less control of parkinsonian or drug-induced hypoventilation than does the last. Neuroleptanesthesia is not recommended because of the use of agents (eg, droperidol) that antagonize dopamine transmission in the brain and elsewhere. Experience has shown that the potential arrhythmogenic and myocardial depressant effects of chronic dopamine-induced depletion of myocardial catecholamines is small. In brief, the anesthetic strategy should maintain a balance between inadequate anesthesia with its accompanying autonomic nervous system stimulation and a needlessly deep anesthesia with its concomitant cardiopulmonary depressant effects.[16]

Good anesthetic control of patients with Parkinson's disease has been reported using thiopental or diazepam for induction followed by enflurane and nitrous oxide for anesthesia/analgesia.[16] More recently, Hyman and colleagues[25] reported a favorable experience using nitrous oxide and sufentanil infusion anesthesia and vecuronium for muscle relaxation in patients undergoing autologous transplantation of adrenal medulla to brain. Fentanyl analgesia should be used with caution because it can increase muscle tone, a problem that is already present in patients with Parkinson's disease. General precautions such as anticipating tachycardia in response to pancuronium or hypotension in response to d-tubocurarine are particularly important in patients with Parkinson's disease. During surgery, a fine body tremor may be misinterpreted as ventricular fibrillation on the cardiac monitor since the typical parkinsonian tremor may be absent from the limbs.[26]

Intraoperative and perioperative nasogastric suction may help reduce the risks and consequences of nausea and vomiting, particularly in patients with Parkinson's disease, in whom most antiemetics are contraindicated. After surgery, the effect of competitive muscle relaxants must be fully reversed to prevent compromise of ventilatory function.

POSTOPERATIVE CARE

GENERAL MEDICAL CONSIDERATIONS

The postoperative care of patients with Parkinson's disease is similar to that of other elderly patients (see Chapter 42). Special emphasis should be placed on airway protection, chest physiotherapy with incentive spirometry and postural drainage, early mobilization, and prevention of aspiration. Patients with Parkinson's disease may require longer to wake up from anesthesia but should be awake by the evening of the day of surgery. Operative and postoperative complications such as pain, infection, and blood loss can lead to a protracted, poor response to antiparkinsonian medication. This poor response is also seen in ambulatory patients with minor medical problems such as urinary tract infections. The mechanisms in both cases are unknown but attempts to fine-tune symptoms at this time are futile and ill-advised. Patients generally recuperate on their own within days to weeks after surgery without a change in medication.

Postoperative psychosis can develop on awakening from anesthesia or as long as 5 to 7 days after surgery; many patients exhibit the first signs after returning home.[27] Immediate postoperative delirium may be caused by the intraoperative use of atropine, by acute metabolic derangement, or by the withdrawal reactions noted earlier. Delayed-onset delirium does not appear to be related to a particular anesthetic or to the choice of antiparkinsonian drug therapy, and clears spontaneously within 3 days.[27]

Parkinsonian motor symptoms, including so-called off spells, can be severely debilitating after surgery. Although the symptoms can mimic other postoperative problems, they should not be assumed to be caused by parkinsonism until medical and surgical postoperative complications have been ruled out. "Off" symptoms include profound feelings of weakness, shortness of breath (air hunger), urinary retention, anxiety, and intense tremor. These adrenergically charged reactions, if they are persistent, can be arrhythmogenic. "On" spells consist of abnormal involuntary movements and muscle contractions known as dyskinesias and dystonias. The latter can be particularly painful.

Constipation should have been dealt with aggressively before operation; it should be managed gingerly after surgery when vital signs may be unstable. Aggressive postoperative treatment of constipation with enemas or disimpaction can elicit vagal reflexes with concomitant bradycardia and hypotension. Several articles elaborate on specific interventions that address these and other important nursing issues.[28,29]

Postoperative dysphagia or unconsciousness may make the administration of oral antiparkinsonian therapy impractical or nearly impossible. With excellent nursing care, patients with mild to moderate Parkinson's disease who were receiving small doses of medication can probably remain unmedicated for a week or longer if necessary. At some point, however, they lose the long duration response to levodopa and may reach levels of disability that can compromise their respiratory function and overall recovery. If the gastrointestinal tract is functional, levodopa can be given directly into the duodenum using a levodopa/carbidopa solution fed through a Silastic tube with a weighted mercury tip. This technique is discussed later. In patients with advanced disease and a functional gastrointestinal tract, enteral administration of liquid carbidopa/levodopa should be started as soon as possible after surgery.

Dopamine Withdrawal Syndrome

Sudden withdrawal of all antiparkinsonian therapy in Parkinson's disease can lead to a dopamine withdrawal syndrome that clinically resembles the better-known neuroleptic malignant syndrome.[30] The onset of this potentially fatal syndrome usually occurs 24 to 72 hours after abrupt withdrawal of a dopaminomimetic drug. It is thought to be mediated by acute cerebral dopamine depletion. In contrast, neuroleptic malignant syndrome has been linked to an aberrant and acute antagonism (blockage) of cerebral dopamine receptors for which there may be individual (genetic?) predisposition. Fully developed, it is characterized by alterations in mental status (delirium or coma), hyperpyrexia, autonomic instability, muscular rigidity, acidosis, rhabdomyolysis, and renal failure.[31] Prompt resumption of antiparkinsonian therapy is the key to treatment. Other therapeutic measures are discussed later. The differential diagnosis includes malignant hyperthermia from exposure to anesthetics; sepsis; exposure to antiemetics and drugs used to alleviate gastric paresis (eg, metoclopramide); tricyclic antidepressants with lithium; stimulants (eg, cocaine, amphetamines); and some anticonvulsants.[31]

PHARMACOTHERAPEUTIC MANAGEMENT

Liquid levodopa has been used in numerous patients with Parkinson's disease to treat motor fluctuations.[32,33] It has been administered either by constant enteral infusion or by intermittent oral bolus. Postoperative patients with Parkinson's disease who are intubated or unconscious may also benefit from these delivery strategies. The solution can be prepared by pulverizing and dissolving 10 tablets of regular carbidopa/levodopa 10/100 in 1000 mL of tap water with 1 g of ascorbic acid to yield a 1-mg/mL solution of levodopa. Depending on how well the tablet is pulverized, the solution may need to be filtered (using a regular coffee filter) to remove particulate matter. The solution is stable for at least 24 hours if it is kept refrigerated and protected from light. Levodopa is relatively insoluble in a basic medium and does not dissolve at concentrations greater than 2 mg/mL. Ascorbic acid serves to acidify the solution and prevent the oxidation of levodopa and dopamine. Although carbidopa is much less soluble than levodopa, enough apparently gets into solution to block nausea and vomiting.[32] Dosing guidelines can be extrapolated from the following example: if a patient uses 100 mg of levodopa every 4 hours, the infusion rate can start at 25 mL/h and be adjusted according to the clinical response.

Few options are available for treating Parkinson's disease symptoms in postoperative patients who have nonfunctional gastrointestinal tracts. Repeated parenteral injections of anticholinergics such as benztropine have been advocated but the use of these agents can slow recovery of gastrointestinal function and, in the elderly, cause delirium. Subcutaneous injections and infusions of soluble dopamine agonists such as apomorphine and lisuride have been used successfully in Europe and Canada for this purpose.[34,35] These drugs are not available in the United States, however, and their use is limited by the need for oral administration of a peripheral dopamine blocker to control the nausea they produce. Domperidone is the antiemetic of choice for this purpose. It is a peripheral dopamine blocker that improves gastric emptying. Its approval for use in this country is under consideration by the Food and Drug Administration but it is unclear whether it will be available in oral as well as parenteral forms.

The treatment of postoperative emesis presents another dilemma in patients with Parkinson's disease. In mild cases, nasogastric suction and small doses of diphenhydramine (Benadryl) or benzodiazepines (weak antiemetics) may work at the expense of sedating patients. Conventional antiemetics may aggravate parkinsonism by virtue of their dopamine antagonism. Other limiting side effects include sedation, dysphoria, and hallucinations. In patients with mild Parkinson's disease who are not psychotic and in whom nasogastric suction fails, the short-term use of these agents in low doses may be tolerated with only modest aggravation of parkinsonian signs. In this case, we favor the cautious use of metoclopramide and thiethylperazine before prochlorperazine maleate (Compazine) or droperidol. Patients with advanced disease and those with marked dystonic clinical features may not tolerate even small doses of these agents.

Nausea and vomiting in levodopa-treated patients are thought to be mediated by the stimulation of dopamine receptors in the area postrema of the brain stem. In contrast, perioperative emesis is multifactorial.[36] Ondansetron, a selective 5-HT$_3$ serotonin receptor blocker, is effective in the treatment of perioperative nausea and vomiting in patients without Parkinson's disease.[37] Although ondansetron does not block dopamine receptors, it may be effective in treating postoperative emesis in patients with Parkinson's disease through alternate mechanisms.[37] Unlike conventional antiemetics, a recent report suggests that ondansetron may be devoid of extrapyramidal side effects in Parkinson's disease.[38] Finally, domperidone may be another promising candidate to alleviate postoperative nausea in patients with Parkinson's disease without aggravating parkinsonism.[36]

POSTOPERATIVE SITUATIONS UNIQUE TO PARKINSON'S DISEASE

TRANSIENT ANTIPARKINSONIAN TREATMENT FAILURE

Patients with Parkinson's disease often experience transient periods of poor response to therapy after surgery. This phenomenon is poorly understood but, similar to emesis, is multifactorial. Suspected causes include a lingering depressant effect of general anesthetics and analgesics, and a slowing of gastric emptying that results in delayed and incomplete levodopa absorption. These partial explanations notwithstanding, there is, at best, a modest correlation between the complexity, duration, and smoothness of operative procedures and patients' postoperative antiparkinsonian responses. It seems that the stress of anesthesia makes the clinical heterogeneity of the illness more apparent. Patients with disorders similar to Parkinson's disease (ie, multiple system atrophy, progressive supranuclear palsy, Parkinson's disease with senile dementia of the Alzheimer's type) tend to do less well than do patients with idiopathic Parkinson's disease. Other than good medical care and reassurance, no specific neurologic measures need to be taken because patients generally return to baseline within 1 or 2 months. A few complain that they never return to their preoperative level of function, an unexplained situation that may be related to the unmasking of disease progression.

POSTOPERATIVE DELIRIUM

Delirium is a major concern in the postoperative care of patients with Parkinson's disease and of the elderly in general.[39] Antiparkinsonian drugs may act synergistically with various anesthetics and analgesics to promote a protracted alteration in mental status. The use of intraoperative atropine is another source of delirium. In most patients, the delirium is quiet and manifested only by confusion and hallucinosis without agitation. In these cases, observation and supportive care by staff and family may be sufficient. Polypharmacy, particularly antiparkinsonian polypharmacy, should be avoided or simplified using the guidelines outlined earlier. Although levodopa therapy should not be withdrawn entirely, ancillary therapy with anticholinergics, amantadine, and selegiline can be withdrawn as the situation warrants. If additional intervention is necessary, the use of dopamine agonists can also be reduced or withdrawn over a few days while remaining vigilant for signs of the dopamine withdrawal syndrome.

If these maneuvers fail, or if patients are in danger of hurting themselves or others, the use of a low-potency neuroleptic such as mesoridazine, molindone, or thioridazine should be considered. These compounds are used for their sedative, anxiolytic, and antipsychotic effects. Mesoridazine offers the advantage of being available in parenteral (25 mg/mL) and liquid (1 mg/mL) forms. It can be given at low doses (1 to 2 mg/d) initially and titrated quickly to control behavior while vital signs and extrapyramidal motor function are monitored. Molindone is available in 5-mg, 10-mg, and larger tablet sizes, and should be used in the lowest possible dosage. Hypotension associated with low-potency neuroleptics is mostly orthostatic and, thus, less of a problem in bedridden patients. Other neuroleptics such as haloperidol and fluphenazine hydrochloride (Prolixin) are more potent and less likely to alter vital signs, but more likely to worsen parkinsonian signs.

Clozapine has been used successfully for the treatment of psychosis in patients with Parkinson's disease.[40] Its use in Parkinson's disease has not been approved by the US Food and Drug Administration, and it carries the risk of agranulocytosis.[41] Its introduction may be associated with several days of increased confusion, hypotension, and significant sedation. Its onset of antipsychotic action can be delayed for

days. Its use, therefore, is more appropriate in the outpatient setting. Psychotic patients with Parkinson's disease respond poorly or adversely to general sedatives such as benzodiazepines and barbiturates. The onset of action of bupropion is too long (more than 5 days) to be useful in an acute situation. Diphenhydramine (Benadryl) and promethazine (Phenergan), both in doses of 12.5 to 25 mg repeated as often as every 6 hours, may be useful as general sedatives. Phenergan can worsen parkinsonian symptoms and, although it is a weak dopamine blocker, has no antipsychotic properties.

Ondansetron was reported to attenuate or eliminate hallucinosis in seven patients with Parkinson's disease.[37] The drug was well tolerated with no worsening of cognition or parkinsonian signs as the oral dose was gradually increased up to 12 to 20 mg/d. Ondansetron is also available for parenteral use. Although the authors conclude that this may be a safe alternative to the unsatisfactory choices outlined earlier, the results must be confirmed in a larger group of patients using a controlled design.

TREATMENT OF THE DOPAMINE WITHDRAWAL SYNDROME

Proper treatment of the dopamine withdrawal syndrome requires early recognition and transfer to a critical care unit for monitoring. Therapy involves aggressive cooling measures, vigorous hydration, and stabilization of the cardiovascular and renal systems. Immediate withdrawal of any dopamine antagonists (see Table 41-1) and resumption of antiparkinsonian therapy are critical. If patients do not respond to levodopa within the first few hours, the use of bromocriptine can be considered because it has been shown to be effective in the treatment of selected patients without Parkinson's disease who have the neuroleptic malignant syndrome.[31] In this setting, dosages as high as 100 mg/d have been recommended. In critically ill patients with Parkinson's disease, the acute introduction of more than 20 to 40 mg of bromocriptine cannot be advocated, however. Even at these dosages, patients face the potential complications of severe nausea, emesis, hypotension, and psychosis. Alternatives to consider include muscle relaxants such as diazepam, 3 to 5 mg by intravenous bolus, and dantrolene, 1 mg/kg by rapid intravenous push repeated every 1 to 3 minutes as needed up to a maximum of 10 mg/kg. For patients with severe peripheral vasoconstriction, a nitroprusside drip has been recommended (0.5 to 1 mg/kg/min by constant infusion).[31] Careful monitoring of renal function, cardiac function, rhabdomyolysis, myoglobinuria, acidosis, and the continuing threat of superimposed infection is also necessary.

SPECIAL PROCEDURES

The perioperative care of patients with Parkinson's disease who are undergoing neurosurgical procedures such as fetal mesencephalic transplantation, stereotactic thalamotomy, and pallidotomy involves the same principles outlined earlier as well as other subspecialty considerations that are beyond the scope of this chapter. Other sources are available that cover the overlapping topic of the perioperative and intensive care unit treatment of general neurology patients.[21,42]

Acknowledgment

This work was supported in part by a Center of Excellence Grant from the American Parkinson's Disease Association.

REFERENCES

1. Nobrega FT, Glattre E, Kurland LT, Okazaki H. Genetics and epidemiology in Parkinson's disease: comments on the epidemiology of parkinsonism including prevalence and incidence statistics for Rochester, Minnesota, 1935–1966. In: Barbeau A, Brunette JR, eds. Progress in neuro-genetics, vol 1. Amsterdam, Excerpta Medica, 1969:474–485.
2. Rajput AH, Offord KP, Beard CM, Kurland LT. Epidemiology of parkinsonism: incidence, classification, and mortality. Ann Neurol 1984;16:278–282.
3. Forno LS. Pathology of Parkinson's disease. In: Marsden CE, Fahn S, eds. Movement disorders. London, Butterworths, 1982: 25–40.
4. Hornykiewicz O, Kish SJ. Biochemical pathophysiology of Parkinson's disease. Adv Neurol 1987;45:19–34.
5. Tanner CM. Epidemiology of Parkinson's disease. Neurol Clin North Am 1992;10:317–327.
6. Cohen G. The pathobiology of Parkinson's disease: biochemical aspects of dopamine neuron senescence. J Neural Transm 1983;19:89–103.
7. Jenner P, Dexter DT, Sian J, et al. Oxidative stress as a cause of nigral cell death in Parkinson's disease and incidental Lewy body disease. Ann Neurol 1992;32(Suppl):82–87.
8. Cummings JL. Intellectual impairment in Parkinson's disease: clinical, pathologic, and biochemical correlates. J Geriatr Psychiatry Neurol 1988;1:24–36.
9. Mayeux R, Stern Y, Rosenstein R, et al. An estimate of the prevalence of dementia in idiopathic Parkinson's disease. Arch Neurol 1988;45:260–262.
10. Mayeux R, Stern Y, Rosen J, et al. Depression, intellectual impairment and Parkinson's disease. Neurology 1981;31:645–650.
11. Juncos JL. Levodopa: pharmacology, pharmacokinetics and pharmacodynamics. Neurol Clin North Am 1992;487–509.
12. Juncos JL. Diet and related variables in the management of Parkinson disease. In: Schneider JS, Gupta M, eds. Current concepts in Parkinson's disease. Toronto, Hogrefe & Huber Publishers, 1993:365–402.
13. Paulson G, Tafrate R. Some "minor" aspects of parkinsonism, especially pulmonary function. Neurology 1970;20:14–17.
14. Vincken WG, Bauthier SG, Dohlfuss R, et al. Involvement of upper airway muscles in extrapyramidal disorders: a cause for airflow limitation. N Engl J Med 1984;311:438–442.
15. Mier M. Mechanisms leading to hypoventilation in extrapyramidal disorders, with special reference to Parkinson's disease. J Am Geriatr Soc 1976;15:230–238.
16. Brindle GF. Anesthesia in the patient with parkinsonism. Prim Care 1977;4:513–528.
17. Barr A. The Shy-Drager syndrome. In: Vinken PJ, Bruyn GW, Klawans HL, eds. Handbook of clinical neurology, vol 38. New York, Elsevier-North Holland, 1979:233–256.
18. Steele JC. Progressive supranuclear palsy. Brain 1972;95:693–704.
19. Folstein MF, Folstein SE, McHugh PR. "Mini-mental state": a practical method for grading the state of patients for the clinician. J Psychiatr Res 1975;12:189–198.
20. Irwin RP, Nutt JG, Woodward WR, et al. Pharmacodynamics of the hypotensive effect of levodopa in parkinsonian patients. Clin Neuropharmacol 1992;15:365–374.
21. Merli GJ, Bell RD. Preoperative management of the surgical patient with neurologic disease. Med Clin North Am 1987;71:511–527.
22. Brod TM. Fluoxetine and extrapyramidal side effects. Am J Psychiatry 1989;146:399–400.
23. Jansen Steur ENH. Increase of Parkinson disability after fluoxetine medication. Neurology 1993;43:211-213.
24. Suchowersky O, deVries J. Possible interactions between deprenyl and fluoxetine. Can J Neurol Sci 1990;17:352–353.
25. Hyman SA, Rogers WD, Smith DW, et al. Perioperative management for transplant of autologous adrenal medulla to the brain for parkinsonism. Anesthesiology 1988;69:618–622.
26. Reed AP, Han DG. Intraoperative exacerbation of Parkinson's disease. Anesth Analg 1992;75:850–853.
27. Golden WE, Lavender RC, Metzer WS. Acute postoperative confusion and hallucinations in Parkinson disease. Ann Intern Med 1989;111:218–222.
28. Berry P, Ward-Smith PA. Adrenal medullary transplant as a treatment for Parkinson's disease: perioperative considerations. J Neurosci Nurs 1988;20:356–361.
29. Delgado JM, Billo JM. Care of the patient with Parkinson's disease: surgical and nursing interventions. J Neurosci Nurs 1988; 20:142–150.
30. Guze BH, Baxter LR. Neuroleptic malignant syndrome. N Engl J Med 1985;313:163–166.
31. Kaufman CA, Wyatt RJ. Neuroleptic malignant syndrome. In: Meltzer H, ed. Psychopharmacology: the third generation of progress. New York, Raven Press, 1987.
32. Kurlan R, Nutt JG, Woodward WR, et al. Duodenal and gastric delivery of levodopa in parkinsonism. Ann Neurol 1988;22: 589–595.
33. Sage JI, Schuh L, Heikkila RE, Duvoisin RC. Continuous duodenal infusions of levodopa: plasma concentrations and motor fluctuations in Parkinson's disease. Clin Neuropharmacol 1988;11:36–44.

34. Frankel JP, Lees AJ, Kempster PA, Stern GM. Subcutaneous apomorphine in the treatment of Parkinson's disease. J Neurol Neurosurg Psychiatry 1990;53:96–101.

35. Broussolle E, Marion MH, Pollack P. Continuous subcutaneous apomorphine as replacement for levodopa in severe parkinsonian patients after surgery. Lancet 1992;340:860.

36. Mitchelson F. Pharmacological agents affecting emesis: a review (part 1). Drugs 1992;43:295–315.

37. Scuderi P, Wetchler B, Sung Y-F, et al. Treatment of postoperative nausea and vomiting after outpatient surgery with the 5-HT$_3$ antagonist ondansetron. Anesthesiology 1993;78: 15–20.

38. Zoldan J, Friedberg G, Goldberg-Stern H, Melamed E. Ondansetron for hallucinosis in advanced Parkinson's disease. Lancet 1993;341:562–563.

39. Lipowski ZJ. Delirium in the elderly patient. N Engl J Med 1989;320:578–582.

40. Pfeiffer RF, Kang J, Graber B, et al. Clozapine for psychosis in Parkinson's disease. Mov Disord 1990;5:239–242.

41. Alvir JMJ, Lieberman JA, Safferman AZ, et al. Clozapine-induced agranulocytosis: incidence and risk factors in the United States. N Engl J Med 1993;329:162–167.

42. Ropper AH, ed. Neurological and neurosurgical intensive care. New York, Raven Press, 1993.

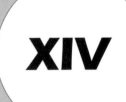

SURGERY IN THE ELDERLY

Medical Management of the Surgical Patient, Third Edition,
edited by Michael F. Lubin, H. Kenneth Walker, and Robert B. Smith III.
J.B. Lippincott Company, Philadelphia, PA © 1995.

ELDERLY PATIENTS

Michael F. Lubin

The aging of the American population has become well recognized in the past two decades as geriatric medicine has become more influential in the medical community. It is clear that there will be many more elderly patients in the future. There has been much discussion in the literature about the implications of this increase: What kind of, and how much, care should be provided to these patients? Which invasive procedures are indicated and when? What is the efficacy of intensive care facilities in the elderly population?

One of the most important of these areas is the surgical care of elderly patients. The literature in this area is extensive and growing rapidly. It indicates that, with careful planning and care, the elderly can undergo surgery safely and with about the same risk as many younger patients. This chapter discusses the following topics as they pertain to the elderly population: (1) physiologic decrements of aging, (2) risks of surgery, (3) preoperative evaluation, (4) anesthesia, (5) common surgical procedures, and (6) postoperative care.

PHYSIOLOGIC DECREMENTS OF AGING

Although physicians see many elderly patients who appear old and sick with many underlying health problems, a large percentage of the elderly population is well. These persons can function entirely normally and are not limited in their activities. Despite this degree of functional normality, however, all older people experience various decrements in physiologic function that are of importance in planning their care, particularly when they are under stresses such as surgery.[1] These decrements make even healthy older patients more fragile and more likely to suffer postoperative complications and death than are their younger counterparts, and physicians must take them into account in their evaluations.

The cardiovascular system has been studied and reviewed extensively.[2-5] Although the ability of aging heart muscle to contract is unaffected, the relaxation phase is prolonged. Other important changes include decreases in maximal heart rate and cardiac output with exercise. The decreases in output are largely the result of increased afterload because of increased stiffness of the arteries and decreased responsiveness to catecholamine stimulation. These changes are important when patients undergo the stresses of surgery.

Although there is evidence in population studies for an increase in blood pressure with age, there is great controversy about its cause. Some think this truly is an age-related change. Others believe it is the result of atherosclerotic changes in the vessels, which is a specific disease process that can be prevented.

Age-related decreases in pulmonary function are marked and have important physiologic consequences in patients undergoing surgery. The elasticity of the lung tissue decreases and compliance increases.[6] These changes result in an increase in residual volume and uneven ventilation. Increases in closing volume also result in ventilation–perfusion abnormalities.

Because of the uneven ventilation, arterial oxygen tension decreases in a predictable way. Sorbini and colleagues[7] found a linear relationship with age: the PO_2 of persons younger than 30 years was 94 mmHg, whereas that of persons older than 60 years was only 74 mmHg. The authors were able to estimate PO_2 by using the following equation:

$$PO_2 \text{ (mmHg)} = 109 - 0.43 \times age$$

Other pulmonary changes are measurable on standard pulmonary function testing. There is a linear decrease in vital capacity of about 25 mL per year beginning in the third decade.[8] Measurements of airflow decrease as well, with decrements in maximum minute ventilation, forced expiratory volume in 1 second, and maximum mid-expiratory flow rate. It is not surprising that pulmonary problems are among the most frequent and important complications in this population.

The effects of aging on the kidneys are important because of the function of these organs in maintaining tonicity and water and salt balance. They also perform a crucial role in the elimination of many drugs.[9,10] Grossly, the kidneys decrease 20% to 30% in weight between the ages of 30 and 80 years. There is a significant decrease in the number of glomeruli and an increase in interstitial fibrosis.

Along with these anatomic changes comes an important decrease in creatinine clearance. Because of a concomitant decrease in the lean mass of the body, however, there is generally no increase in the serum creatinine level, which can be misleading to those unaware of these changes. Two groups have developed estimates of creatinine clearance (C_{cr}) as a function of age. The following equations can be used[11,12]:

$$C_{cr} \text{ (mL/min)} = \frac{(140 - age) \times weight \text{ (kg)}}{72 \times Cr_s}$$

$$C_{cr} \text{ (mL/min)} = 135 - 0.84 \times age$$

These decreases in clearance in the absence of increases in serum creatinine must be taken into account when drugs that are primarily excreted by the kidney are administered.

In addition to decreases in creatinine clearance, tubular function is also affected by age, and there are decreases in concentrating and diluting ability that can lead to overhydration, dehydration, hypernatremia, or hyponatremia if careful attention is not paid to fluid administration. Other important physiologic changes affect water balance. These include a decrease in thirst perception so that elderly patients with volume depletion drink less and more slowly to replete the deficit. Data suggest that certain disorders in antidiuretic hormone physiology predispose at least some ap-

parently normal elderly patients to excessive antidiuretic hormone secretion, resulting in unexpected hyponatremia.

Although the cardiovascular, pulmonary, and renal systems are vital in the survival of surgical patients, other systems undergo important physiologic changes that affect patients' recovery as well. Osteoporosis is common, particularly in white women. Care must be taken in transferring patients to prevent fracture of brittle bones. Skin changes are equally as important and often overlooked. The epidermis and dermis undergo degenerative changes, and the potential for decubitus ulcer development is high if care is not taken to reposition patients frequently. This may even need to be done in the operating room if the procedure is long.

The final important areas of altered physiology are the distribution, metabolism, and elimination of drugs. Drug distribution is affected by the alterations in body composition. Lean body mass, plasma volume, and total body water decrease. Extracellular water decreases 40% and body fat increases about 35%. These changes alter drug action depending on the water and lipid solubility of the agent. For water-soluble drugs, there is a smaller volume of distribution, resulting in a higher concentration at the same dose. For lipid-soluble drugs, there may be relatively larger volume; this often results in prolonged action of the drug.

Metabolism in the liver is altered for some drugs. These changes are variable and not easily predicted. Some important drugs that have a decreased metabolic clearance in the elderly are the benzodiazepines, warfarin, and phenytoin. Renal clearance is invariably decreased in all older patients because of the changes in renal function already discussed. Thus, drugs such as digoxin, antibiotics, and others that are cleared primarily by the kidney must be adjusted for this decrease.

RISKS OF SURGERY

The safety of surgery in the elderly has been discussed for many years. In a 1967 lecture entitled, "Is Risk of Indicated Operation Too Great in the Elderly?," Alton Ochsner said, "In 1927 as a young professor of surgery at Tulane Medical School, I practiced and taught that an elective operation for inguinal hernia in a patient over 50 years old was not justified."[13] Now the literature has titles such as, "Surgical Procedures Involving Cardiopulmonary Bypass in Patients 70 or Older,"[14] and "Resection of Abdominal Aortic Aneurysm in the Over 80 Age Group."[15]

The first reports of the results of surgery in geriatric patients appeared in the late 1930s. These studies reported an overall mortality rate of 20%, whereas the rate for abdominal surgery was over 30%. In more recent years, there have been reports of patients in their 80s and 90s having surgery.[16-19] Investigators describe mortality rates ranging from 30% to 40% for emergency surgery to an average of about 10% for elective surgery, with a few reporting rates under 5%. A recent publication looked at major surgery in a nursing home population and found a mortality rate of only 4%; all the deaths occurred in patients undergoing emergency surgery.[20] There have also been several reports of small series of selected patients older than 100 years who have successfully undergone surgical procedures.[21,22]

The profusion of reports in the literature prompted Linn and Linn[23] in 1982 to review 108 studies of surgery in the elderly from 1930 to 1980. They found flaws and omissions in many of the studies. There were differences in lower age limits, methods used to calculate mortality, lengths of follow-up, mixes of emergency versus elective operations, and types of operations. They came to two main conclusions: (1) emergency surgery is much riskier than elective surgery; and (2) since 1941, the trend has been toward increasing mortality for elective, but not emergency, procedures.

The first conclusion is clearly true; Linn and Linn found an overall mortality rate of 28% for general emergency surgery and a mortality rate of 43% for specialty emergency procedures. Mortality rates for elective surgery averaged about 9%. These basic findings have been replicated in many papers.

Their second conclusion is much more controversial and misleading. The authors divided the studies by decade, which yielded the rates shown below:

Years	Mortality (%)
1931 to 1940	11.0
1941 to 1950	5.0
1951 to 1960	7.3
1961 to 1970	9.2
1971 to 1980	9.5

They proposed two possibilities for this trend toward increasing mortality. The first is that surgical care is deteriorating and the second is that surgeons are treating patients with greater risks. They did not indicate that one was more likely than another. It is clear from Dr. Ochsner's earlier comment, however, and from the subsequent titles listed, that surgeons are performing more extensive operations on sicker patients.

The extent of the increase in risk for older patients related to age alone is uncertain. Many studies have examined this issue, the first of which was published in 1977 by Goldman and colleagues.[24] They evaluated more than 1000 patients, 324 of whom were older than 70 years, and found an independent, statistically significant increase in risk for the older patients. Sikes and Detmer[25] performed a study comparing the mortality for different age groups from birth to the age of 94 years. They found that rates increased slowly from 2.6% in those younger than 64 years to 3.5% in those aged 70 to 74 years. From that point, however, the

rates increased from 4.4% to 10.3% for those aged 90 to 94 years. The authors figured an adjusted mortality rate for procedure; they did not, however, adjust for comorbid conditions.

Other studies have separated some important factors in the surgical mortality of elderly patients. In 1978, Turnbull and associates[26] studied mortality in patients older than 70 years and found a rate of only 4.8% for surgical procedures. One hundred ninety-three deaths occurred in the group: 79 patients died of metastatic disease from the original tumor or from treatment and 48 were believed to have died of the tumor directly. Therefore, 25% died of cancer, even though they were included in the surgical mortality rate. The authors calculated the surgical mortality rate again after excluding those patients who died of far-advanced cancer and "multiple organ decompensation" and found a rate of only 2.8%. Only 6 of 4050 patients died during surgery or in the first 24 hours afterward, 3 of cardiorespiratory failure and 3 of uncontrolled bleeding.

In another study of 75 patients aged 90 years and older, 11 patients died. Three patients had extensive carcinomas, for an adjusted death rate of 10.6%.[27] The other causes of death were two cases of bowel perforation and peritonitis, two cases of pneumonia, one case of myocardial infarction, one case of stroke, and one case of sudden death (presumed myocardial infarction or pulmonary embolism). In 42 elective cases, there was only 1 death, for a mortality rate of 2.3%. There were 5 deaths each in the 32 urgent cases (16% mortality rate) and 11 emergent cases (45% mortality rate).

Comparing crude death rates can be difficult. Seymour and Pringle[28] suggested that in comparing mortality, "nonviable" cases should be separated from potentially viable cases. In their study, mortality decreased from 12% to 5.8%. This must be done for the younger population as well for proper comparison, although the effect on mortality rates in the elderly will be much larger than in younger patients.

Additional studies have concluded that surgery is safe and effective for cardiopulmonary bypass,[14,29,30] resection of abdominal aneurysms,[15,31,32] lung resection,[33,34] abdominal surgery,[35–38] orthopedic procedures,[39] and major gynecologic surgery.[40] Finally, a recent study in Canada evaluated almost 9000 patients older than 65 years who underwent surgical procedures. Using correlation and multiple regression analysis, these researchers found severity of illness to be a much better predictor of outcome than age.[41] A strong case can be made for the safety of surgery, even in the very old, if appropriate precautions are taken.

Another strong argument in favor of surgery was provided by Andersen and Ostberg.[42] They compared the survival rates of 7922 surgical patients older than 70 years with a matched sample of the general population. They found improved survival in the surgical patients over 2 to 16 years of follow-up, indicating that surgery appears to result in long-term improvement in survival. A more recent study demonstrated the same results in an elderly population followed up at the Mayo Clinic.[43] Surgical intervention appears to have no negative effect on overall long-term survival.

Another important question has been raised by several authors. Can, could, or should physicians turn some of the emergency surgical cases into elective procedures? It has been shown that the elderly can undergo emergency surgery and return to their previous living situation.[44] The mortality in emergency procedures, however, is much higher than in elective ones. Seymour and Pringle[45] reviewed this question, using hernias, peptic ulcers, and colorectal carcinomas as pertinent areas of study. They found that 17% of surgical procedures in persons aged 45 to 64 years were emergencies. In patients older than 75 years, however, emergencies accounted for 37% of cases. Femoral hernias were associated with a large increase in emergency procedures, as were inguinal hernias. Peptic ulcers showed the same kind of trends as did the hernias, although not as striking. Finally, similar results were found in colorectal carcinoma, such that the rate of emergency operations for rectal carcinoma was highest in the oldest age group.

From these data, the authors did a prospective study of 74 emergency operations. They believed that the emergency procedure could have been avoided in one third of the patients. Of the 10 patients with strangulated hernias, the condition had been diagnosed in 8 cases before the emergency developed. Nine of 36 patients with acute abdomens had diseases that may have been amenable to surgical therapy, and 7 of 22 patients with cancer had symptoms for 3 months before their emergency operations. Although the conclusions of these authors were based on speculation rather than statistics, it seems fair to say that at least some elderly patients are not undergoing elective surgery for known or diagnosable conditions until they have reached an emergency state, with significantly increased mortality.

Recent studies confirm the increased mortality of emergency surgery in older patients. Keller and colleagues[46] found a 20% mortality rate in emergency surgery versus a 2% mortality rate in elective surgery. Schöön and Arvidsson,[47] studying surgery in patients older than 80 years, found that only 1 of 43 deaths seen within 30 days of surgery occurred after elective procedures.

BARRIERS TO EARLY SURGERY

The reticence to perform elective operations on elderly patients may have several causes. The first is the mistaken belief among physicians that elderly people in general are not good surgical candidates. This can be disproved easily and convincingly. The second problem is that the higher mortality rates in sick elderly patients are related more to comorbid conditions than to their age. This also is true in younger patients. The most common problems in the elderly are dementia, chronic obstructive pulmonary disease, diabetes, coronary artery disease, heart failure, and hypertension. The increased risk from these and other diseases must be evaluated, therapy instituted for those whose conditions can be improved, and surgery avoided in those judged to be at unacceptably high risk.

The last barrier to early surgery is the patient's reluctance. Many elderly patients are frightened of undergoing surgery, feeling that they have little chance of survival. Families often have the same concerns. Physicians can assure them that this definitely is not true. The elderly are frequently concerned that surgery will not improve their quality of life, will make them more dependent on others, or will cause them to have to live in a care facility.[48–50] In addition, they often do not want to undergo the anticipated pain, discomfort, and rigors of surgery and the necessary recovery period to treat a process that may not bother them very much, if at all. This obstacle is often extremely difficult, if not impossible, to overcome.

POSTOPERATIVE MORTALITY

Although the elderly can undergo surgery without undue risk, some patients do die. The disease processes that cause the mortality are not surprising but it is helpful in evaluating patients before surgery and in caring for them afterward to know which complications may be prevented or need to be treated.

In a study of mortality statistics, Palmberg and Hirsjarvi[51] reviewed many surgical cases in elderly patients. They found that 33% died of pulmonary emboli, 20% died of pneumonia, 11% died of "cardiac collapse" (with no pathologic evidence of myocardial infarction), and 9% died of their primary illness. Aspiration, strokes, and gastrointestinal bleeding each contributed 6%, and myocardial infarction contributed only 2%.

Other authors have found similar results, although the rates of myocardial infarction are usually in the range of 20% to 30%. Pneumonia is the cause of death in about 15% to 30% of cases, whereas pulmonary emboli contribute 10% to 20%. Sepsis is also seen regularly.[18,26] The highest death rates occur in patients undergoing abdominal procedures, particularly those with perforation, obstruction, or bowel infarction. The study published by Djokovic and Hedley-Whyte,[17] however, reported no deaths resulting from pulmonary emboli. They attributed this to their "almost universal preoperative initiation of measures such as low dose heparin therapy to prevent intraoperative venous thrombosis."

The statistics for patients with comorbid diseases are interesting.[51] Mortality in those with dementia was a surprising 45%. This is probably the result of patient selection because only surgery that is absolutely necessary because of life-threatening conditions is likely to be done in these patients. In addition, patients with dementia cannot cooperate very well with postoperative care. The mortality rate was 26% in those with diabetes and 17% in those with cardiac disease. Although the rate for cardiac disease seems relatively low compared with other disease states, cardiac disease is common. For this reason, patients who have cardiac disease alone, or in combination with diabetes, gangrene, dementia, or pulmonary disease, accounted for 44 of the 54 deaths.

PREOPERATIVE EVALUATION

In many ways, the preoperative evaluation of the elderly differs little from that of younger patients and involves primarily a good history and physical examination. Older patients do present some unique problems, however.

First, physicians must remember all the expected physiologic decrements. Although elderly patients can often withstand the initial stresses of surgery, once a complication develops, they have less reserve and are much less likely to survive. Wilder and Fishbein[52] found the mortality rate to be 62% among those with complications but only 13% among those who appeared to be having a smooth postoperative course. The most important decrements are in cardiac, pulmonary, and renal function. Any underlying disease in any of these organ systems markedly diminishes the ability to survive a complication.

Evaluating the histories of older patients is fraught with difficulty. Because the elderly are often impatient with long, meticulous history taking, this should be done quickly and efficiently. In addition, elderly patients are often hard of hearing, and their memory of, and attention to, specific symptoms may be less than ideal. These patients often minimize their symptoms out of fear of the consequences of the disease or because they feel that old age is necessarily accompanied by infirmity.

Symptoms may be less apparent and less specific than in younger patients, particularly in regard to infections and pain, which can be especially difficult to document.[53] Often, patients or their families complain of nonspecific problems such as confusion, malaise, incontinence, falls, or refusal to eat.

Even specific complaints may be confusing. The presence of angina may be represented by prominent shortness of breath or epigastric discomfort rather than by classic substernal chest pain. Chest pain may be a manifestation of intraabdominal processes rather than cardiac in origin. Abdominal pain is often poorly localized and may seem to be less severe than would be expected. This can delay diagnosis in such important diseases as appendicitis, mesenteric insufficiency, and perforations of ulcers or diverticula.

Many diseases that cause fever in younger people may not do so in the elderly but present instead as malaise or altered states of consciousness. This is particularly true of pneumonia and urinary tract infection. Although many patients complain of dyspnea for which no cause can be found, it is important to make the diagnosis of heart failure or coronary disease. A heavy smoking history and symptoms of chronic bronchitis or emphysema are also important to elicit. Similarly, many elderly patients have urinary and bowel complaints, and physicians must be aware of the possibilities of obstructive problems in these systems. A careful history of medication use is crucial, and care must be taken to inquire about the nonprescription drugs that are frequently taken by the elderly.

Taking note of visual and hearing impairments is important so that sensory stimuli can be provided for patients who are at high risk for confusion and disorientation, which can present significant problems in postoperative care. Confused and disoriented patients remove nasogastric tubes and intravenous lines, disrupt wounds, fall from beds, and break bones. Studies have shown that these patients have significantly higher in-hospital mortality and poorer survival after hospital discharge.[51-54]

Physical examination also presents difficult problems. Acutely ill elderly patients may cooperate poorly; examinations should be direct and performed as expeditiously as possible. Nutritional assessment, including the state of hydration, is a primary area of concern that is often overlooked or addressed in a cursory fashion. Fluid status can be difficult to assess in these patients. The most important pitfalls are found in evaluating skin turgor and peripheral edema. Turgor is difficult to assess because of senile skin changes; the skin over the forehead appears to be the most reliable area to check. Neck veins can be helpful. Peripheral edema can be misleading because many elderly patients have venous insufficiency and are often sedentary, accumulating dependent fluid. Vigorous diuresis to remove the edema may leave patients with significant intravascular depletion, predisposing to intraoperative hypotension and renal failure. Blood urea nitrogen:creatinine ratios can also be helpful in those who are not malnourished.

Protein-calorie malnutrition has also been shown to increase postoperative complications and decrease survival; hyperalimentation can reverse these trends[55] (see Chap. 2). From the ages of 65 to 94 years, the percentage of underweight men increases from 20% to 50% and the percentage of underweight women increases from 20% to 55%.[56] Elderly patients are often malnourished for a multitude of reasons: underlying disease states such as heart disease, diabetes, or pulmonary disease; drugs that interfere with digestion, absorption, appetite, and taste or smell; inadequate dentition; physical disability resulting in the inability to shop, cook, or feed themselves; and poverty.

The recognition, evaluation, and treatment of protein-calorie malnutrition, therefore, is an important part of the preoperative work-up. Recognition and evaluation can be carried out in the same manner as in younger patients. In addition, Kaminski and colleagues[57] have shown that older patients can tolerate aggressive enteral and parental hyperalimentation as well. Decisions regarding hyperalimentation should be made by assessing patients and their problems, not by looking at age.

Biochemical deficiencies also occur with increased frequency in the elderly. Older patients have often been shown to be deficient in vitamin A, pyridoxine, calcium, and iron. The last two are absorbed less well in the elderly. Vitamin C and zinc appear to have a role in wound healing, and some studies indicate that at least some patients have decreased levels. Some surgeons routinely supplement both in operative patients.

Cardiac status, particularly in reference to signs of heart failure, requires careful evaluation. Although systolic murmurs are common, significant aortic stenosis is also an important risk factor that should be identified. Low systolic blood pressure, narrow pulse pressure, enlarged and sustained PMI pulsation, and left ventricular hypertrophy on the electrocardiogram can be helpful in this regard. Significant controversy still exists regarding the treatment of carotid bruits. Cerebral arterial bruits in the absence of symptoms concern physicians, but there is still inadequate evidence to justify the routine use of diagnostic or therapeutic interventions.[58–60] Evidence of pulmonary disease helps to identify those patients who are at risk for atelectasis and pneumonia. The final significant examination should be for evidence of dementia and confusion because patients so afflicted do poorly after surgery. In Palmberg's[51] study, mortality was 45% in those with dementia; in Wickstrom's[61] study, 7 of 11 patients who died had senile dementia.

Laboratory assessment, as in all other patients, remains controversial. For a detailed discussion of preoperative testing, see Chapter 3. Some authors still recommend using all the standard laboratory tests (ie, complete blood counts, electrolyte determinations, chemistry panels, urinalyses, chest radiographs, and electrocardiograms). Some recommend routinely performing pulmonary function tests, and Del Guercio and colleagues[62] have even recommended the standard use of diagnostic Swan-Ganz catheterization following a staging system that they developed.

In well older patients, most experts believe that preoperative testing can be limited to a hematocrit determination, a test of renal function (usually a creatinine level), an electrocardiogram, and a chest radiograph. Because elderly patients often have underlying diseases and take many medications, including nonprescription drugs such as aspirin, many have indications for other preoperative tests.

Seymour and colleagues[63] studied electrocardiograms in 222 surgical patients older than 65 years. The tests were normal in only 21% of patients and showed major abnormalities in 53%. Twenty-seven patients had postoperative cardiovascular complications, including 22 with heart failure, 3 with definite myocardial infarctions, and 2 with suspected myocardial infarctions. In men, however, there was no correlation between preoperative abnormalities and postoperative complications, whereas in women there did seem to be some minor predictive value; the tests were not clinically helpful, however. Many nonspecific changes appeared in the electrocardiograms after surgery. The authors suggested that preoperative electrocardiograms should be done to provide a baseline for the interpretation of postoperative electrocardiographic changes and for preoperative identification of patients with myocardial infarctions or arrhythmias in whom surgery should be deferred.

A study of chest radiographs was done by Tornebrandt and Fletcher.[64] They evaluated 100 consecutive patients older than 70 years before elective surgery. Of 91 chest radiographs done, 43 were abnormal: 28 showed cardiomegaly, 11 showed pulmonary hypertension, 7 showed chronic pulmonary disease, and 1 showed a pleural effusion. Of the 27 patients who had no indication for the test, 10 had abnormal findings: 5 with cardiomegaly, 2 with atelectasis, and 1 each with emphysema, pulmonary hypertension, and tracheal deviation. Ten percent of the patients developed postoperative complications for which comparison films were helpful. The authors did not attempt to determine whether the abnormal findings were predictive of postoperative complications, so it is difficult to determine whether the routine use of chest radiographs really makes a difference in patient care. Because of the high incidence of cardiopulmonary complications, however, a recent, if not preoperative, chest radiograph is probably useful.

Although some authors recommend routine preoperative pulmonary function testing in the elderly, there are no definitive data to support this practice.[65,66] It seems reasonable to use the same indications applied to younger patients (see Chap. 12). Arterial blood gases may be more important. The Po_2 falls progressively in normal, nonsmoking patients from an average of 94 mmHg in those younger than 30 years to only 74 mmHg in those older than 60 years. There is a wide range of normal findings in elderly patients, however, and it is impossible to know whether a given patient's baseline Po_2 is 74 or 92 mmHg. Those with a smoking history or evidence of chronic obstructive pulmonary disease are even more affected. Because there is such a high incidence of cardiopulmonary complications after surgery, many patients may benefit from having a baseline preoperative Po_2 determination to aid in postoperative diagnosis and therapy.

Although a discussion of the specific treatment of disease states is beyond the scope of this chapter, some unique points must be emphasized in pulmonary care. Patients should stop smoking before the procedure. It has been shown that stopping smoking for 8 weeks before surgery significantly decreases the incidence of postoperative complications. Patients should also be educated about incentive spirometry, coughing, and deep breathing. Finally, meticulous attention to pulmonary toilet both before admission and before surgery helps to reduce postoperative complications.

The indications for invasive monitoring are still debated. Del Guercio and Cohn[62] studied 148 consecutive patients who had been cleared for surgery by routine assessment. They used a staging system that required Swan-Ganz catheterization in all patients and multiple cardiopulmonary function measurements. The authors reported that many patients had unsuspected abnormalities that put them at increased risk, and they were able to identify a group that was at extremely high risk for mortality even though these patients had been cleared to undergo surgery. Surgery was canceled or modified in some cases, and all those who underwent the original procedure died.

This study does not help in determining which patients need this kind of invasive testing, however. The study was not controlled and the authors included several young patients who were diseased, whom they called "physiologically old." About one third of the patients were younger than 60 years and about half were younger than 70 years. The data suggest that some patients can benefit from this type of invasive evaluation but do not indicate which patients these are. In addition, complications from procedures must be considered.

A newer study by Schrader and colleagues[67] has provided important information. They evaluated 46 patients older than 90 years who underwent surgery. None of their patients had invasive monitoring and together they underwent 51 procedures, many of which were major surgery. There were seven major complications, only one of which might have been predicted by the preoperative use of Swan-Ganz catheterization. Most important, there were no perioperative deaths in their entire series. Although there are patients who need intensive preoperative monitoring and evaluation, age alone is not a primary indication for these tests.

ANESTHESIA

Although specifics of anesthetic care are beyond the scope of this chapter, some information is interesting and helpful to nonanesthesiologists. There is a continuing debate over the choice of regional or general anesthesia, although there seems to be no appreciable difference in mortality.[61,68–71]

General anesthesia has several advantages. Patients are unconscious and, therefore, unable to move. They feel no anxiety during the procedure. In addition, the ability to control respiration through endotracheal intubation may be helpful in the elderly because of their decreased respiratory function. Some drawbacks also exist, however. The incidence of pulmonary complications may be increased with general anesthesia. The incidence of mental disturbances also may be higher,[68] although some small studies have shown no differences.[72] The extent of this effect is uncertain but if it is present, it is probably not large and may be outweighed by other considerations.

Regional methods have advantages as well. Some patients prefer to be awake for their procedures. Some anesthesiologists believe that regional anesthesia is associated with less suppression of respiration, less hypoxia, and perhaps fewer respiratory complications, although this is unclear.[68] Disadvantages include difficulties with moving or anxious patients and a somewhat higher incidence of intraoperative and postoperative hypotension.[69] Interestingly, in Hole's[68] study of epidural versus general anesthesia in hip surgery, an equal number of patients in each group (4 of 29 and 4 of 31) did not want the same kind of anesthesia if they were to be operated on for the other hip.

EVALUATION OF RISK

Numerous investigators have attempted to find ways to measure the risks of surgery based on the data gleaned from older patients' histories, physical examinations, and laboratory data. As in all other patients, assessment of preoperative risk can begin with the indices of cardiac risk that were developed by Goldman and Detsky and are discussed in detail in Chapter 4.[24,73] The areas of importance include recent myocardial infarction, severe or unstable angina, congestive heart failure, significant aortic stenosis, arrhythmia, poor general medical status, and emergency operation.

Although the indices developed by Goldman and Detsky are the best ways of approaching the calculation of cardiac risk, both have limited sensitivity and miss many patients with complications who were considered to be at low risk. Gerson[74] found that adding supine bicycle exercise to the preoperative evaluation increases the sensitivity of these indices. He determined that inability to raise the heart rate above 99 beats/min during 2 minutes of exercise is predictive of increased risk in the elderly population. Gerson suggested that patients who have a major risk factor on the Goldman index are at increased risk. Those who do not have a major risk factor should be evaluated with exercise testing. If their heart rates do not rise above 99 beats/min, these patients are considered to be at increased risk as well. A second study by Gerson and colleagues[75] found that this test is also useful for identifying elderly patients who are at risk for pulmonary complications.

COMMON SURGICAL PROBLEMS

CARDIOVASCULAR SURGERY

Cardiovascular surgery is feasible in elderly patients. Many studies have shown that coronary bypass, valve replacement, and vascular surgery can be performed in the elderly with acceptable mortality.[76] This is true even in patients with severe cardiovascular disease because the mortality from the underlying disease is very high. Mortality is much higher (frequently around 80%) when these patients require emergency surgery, however.

Coronary Bypass Surgery

Elderly patients undergoing coronary artery bypass grafting procedures have been evaluated extensively.[77,78] Many of the studies were done on patients between 80 and 90 years of age. The mortality is low, perhaps a few percent, in patients who have no other underlying diseases and are undergoing elective procedures. This is comparable to the mortality in younger patients. Elderly patients with conditions such as unstable angina, recent myocardial infarction, reduced cardiac function, and left main coronary artery disease are at higher risk, perhaps higher than that of younger patients (about 10% to 12%). As expected, however, older patients have more complications because of their decreased reserve.

Several studies have been done on patients with New York Heart Association (NYHA) class IV heart disease. Despite mortality rates in the range of 15% to 20%, these patients should be considered for coronary artery bypass grafting procedures because their prognosis without surgery is extremely poor. Patients with particularly high mortality include those who undergo emergency procedures and those who require intraaortic balloon pulsation.

Other important factors in the decision to perform surgery are the potential for long-term survival and functional improvement. Both of these areas have been studied, and data indicate that a large percentage of elderly patients who survive surgery have increased longevity and are able to function at a higher level. Many patients have gone from NYHA class IV to NYHA classes I and II.

Valvular Surgery

Many elderly patients have significant valve pathology, particularly aortic stenosis and mitral insufficiency. The results of surgical procedures in these patients are mixed.[79–82] Surgery can provide significant benefit if patients are properly selected and cared for well.

Aortic valve replacement can be a life-saving and life-

sustaining procedure. When the disease is detected early, particularly before the onset of significant myocardial dysfunction, elderly patients can have remarkable results from aortic valve replacement. Studies have shown significant increases in long-term survival and impressive increases in functional capacity. Operative mortality in patients without severe myocardial dysfunction can be as low as a few percent.

Overall mortality for patients undergoing aortic valve replacement has been around 10%. Those who survive surgery have had excellent long-term survival. In one study, the 5-year survival rate was 70% (including operative mortality) compared with about 20% for patients who did not undergo surgery. Functional improvement also can be dramatic, with some studies showing almost all patients improving to NYHA classes I and II.

Mitral valve replacement is not as successful. Patients with mitral valve disease often can go for long periods without symptoms. Even after symptoms develop, they can be controlled reasonably well with medication. Thus, by the time most elderly patients are considered for surgery, there is often significant underlying myocardial dysfunction. The mortality rate in mitral valve surgery is commonly around 20% and can be as high as 50% in those with significant heart failure, previous mitral procedures (valvulotomy), and pulmonary hypertension. Most patients appear to die of low output states accompanied by multiple organ failure. There is good evidence, however, that long-term survival in patients who survive surgery is about the same as that of the general population. A clear difference in mortality exists between patients with mitral stenosis, who do better, and patients with mitral regurgitation, who do less well.

Results of combined surgical procedures show an increase in mortality as well. Patients who receive aortic and mitral valves have a modestly increased mortality. Those who undergo coronary bypass procedures and mitral valve replacement appear to have a greatly increased risk of death, and some authors suggest that this combination of procedures be avoided if possible.

Vascular Surgery

Because atherosclerosis is a disease of aging, many elderly patients are candidates for vascular surgery. Several different procedures have been studied, particularly aortic aneurysm repair and carotid endarterectomy.

Many studies have addressed the treatment of aortic aneurysms.[83,84] Emergency aneurysmectomy is a deadly procedure. Mortality ranges from 40% to 80% and usually is at the high end. In contrast, mortality for elective procedures generally is about 5% to 10%. The mortality for symptomatic aneurysm repair usually falls somewhere in between.

Patients who have diagnosed abdominal aneurysms

larger than 6 cm should be seriously considered for elective aortic replacement if they do not have a high risk of mortality because of underlying diseases. There is a high risk of rupture in these patients and high mortality from emergency replacement surgery.

Results of surgery in older patients with carotid artery disease are still not clearcut. As in younger patients, there are few definitive surgical indications for patients with carotid disease. Many elderly patients, particularly those with hemispheric symptoms, can obtain relief with acceptable, although somewhat increased, morbidity (perioperative stroke) and mortality. Most authors indicate that a substantial amount of the morbidity from stroke appears to result from the significant intracranial vascular disease that is more prevalent in this aged population.

Peripheral arterial reconstruction is often helpful in the elderly and can be done with little increase in morbidity and mortality rates compared with younger patients. There is a higher risk of perioperative myocardial infarction, however, because of the high prevalence of coronary disease in patients with peripheral vascular disease. The procedures usually increase the functional state and can prevent the loss of limbs.

ORTHOPEDIC SURGERY

Arthritis, particularly of the hip, is an important factor limiting the mobility and independence of elderly patients. Fractures are also an important cause of morbidity and mortality, and often result in immobility, dependency, and institutionalization.

Hip Fracture

About 250,000 hip fractures occur in the United States each year, most in elderly women. These patients should be treated surgically if possible. Morbidity from the procedure in unselected populations is low (about 5%), considering that many of these patients have chronic diseases and are debilitated. Although mortality is not particularly high for the procedure and perioperative period, these patients often suffer great loss of mobility and become more dependent on others for a variable length of time. It has been shown that the postoperative functional state depends heavily on the functional state before the fracture and not on patients' chronologic age. About 70% of those who were able to walk before the fracture are able to walk in some way after the operation. Although some patients must be admitted to nursing homes after the procedure, most of those who lived independently or with some assistance before the fracture are able to continue to do so.

Many factors affect the postoperative morbidity and mortality of patients with femoral fractures. The surgical procedures themselves are neither elective not emergent. It is important that patients receive adequate preoperative care to ensure appropriate fluid resuscitation and optimal cardiopulmonary physiology.

Many patients have some impairment of mentation after surgery and this complication must be anticipated. Because many patients also have postoperative pulmonary complications, appropriate preparation and prophylactic measures should be taken before and after surgery. Another common, difficult, and preventable complication is pressure sores. These should be prevented if at all possible because they contribute to increased length of hospitalization, perioperative mortality, and admission to nursing homes instead of more independent living arrangements.

Elective Hip Replacement

The case for elective hip replacement is also strong, particularly because this procedure can be performed in a well-selected population.[85] Most patients who undergo this operation have painful and disabling joint disease. In one study of 100 patients in their 80s, 92 returned home. In this population, there were only two deaths, one from myocardial infarction and the other from pulmonary embolus.[86] Deep venous thrombosis and urinary tract infection were the most common postoperative complications, as in most studies of hip repair. Most patients have good to excellent results and are satisfied with the outcome of this surgery.

Other elective joint replacement procedures have been done in older patients. Knee joints are commonly affected by osteoarthritis. Because the elderly are less mobile than are younger patients, they may be better candidates for replacement because loosening with use is a major problem with this procedure. Ankle, shoulder, and elbow replacement have all been done in selected patients with good results.

Rehabilitation units for geriatric patients with orthopedic problems are just beginning to be evaluated. Some evidence suggests that these units can increase patients' self-sufficiency and independence. Units have been developed for the rehabilitation of hip fracture and replacement and of amputations. The most important obstacle to rehabilitation is alteration in mental status; patients with signs of dementia do poorly.

ABDOMINAL SURGERY

Much work has been done to evaluate abdominal surgery in the elderly population because this is a major site for operations. More important, the morbidity and mortality from abdominal surgery can be high. Increasing age, emergent procedures, malignancy, poor physical status, and the site of surgery in the abdomen are significantly associated with a poorer prognosis. One other factor that appears to be important in abdominal surgery in older patients is infection. The risks of infection are much higher in abdominal surgery than in surgery at most other sites. The risk of infection is higher in the elderly than in younger patients and their ability to overcome infection is lower.

Gallbladder Disease

One of the more common problems in elderly patients is determining the best approach to the treatment of asymptomatic gallstones. This decision is made more (or less) difficult by data regarding the results of emergency surgery for acute cholecystitis. The mortality rate ranges from 12% to 20% in patients who undergo emergency surgery for gallbladder disease, compared with 3% to 5% in those who have elective surgery.[87,88] One group has suggested that there is no indication for emergency cholecystectomy in the elderly; they recommend that patients be stabilized if at all possible with fluids and antibiotics before undergoing operation. The efficacy of this approach has not been proven, and others believe that the only therapy for symptomatic gallbladder disease is immediate surgery. There is general agreement, however, that medical therapy alone is not an option in these patients.

Many elderly patients who present with symptomatic gallbladder disease already have gangrene and empyema. Many have been found to have perforations, which can lead to subphrenic abscesses. This is not surprising because these patients often have fewer and less severe symptoms, despite the presence of more severe disease.

The important complications in patients who undergo surgery for gallbladder disease are not surprising. Many have sepsis with common gram-negative organisms, wound infections, and pulmonary complications, as would be expected in patients undergoing upper abdominal surgery.

Appendicitis

Appendicitis is one of the most frequently missed diagnoses in the elderly population. This is important because this otherwise potentially fatal disease can be cured if it is recognized in time.[89,90] The possibility of appendicitis is rarely considered in older patients but should always be a part of the differential diagnosis of abdominal pain. Although symptoms are usually less severe than in younger patients,

the elderly generally have abdominal pain, nausea, and fever. They frequently have abdominal tenderness as well.

Perforation has already occurred in many elderly patients before operation is undertaken. Although nonspecific and muted symptoms often delay the diagnosis, other factors also are involved. The appendix atrophies with age and the walls thin. The blood supply to the organ is also compromised with age. Thus, with infection and increased pressure in the appendix, blood supply is quickly impeded and the thinned wall more easily perforates.

Mortality in this disease depends heavily on patients' underlying health and, most importantly, on the progression of the disease. In patients who undergo operation early, mortality is low. As perforation, abscess, and sepsis appear, however, mortality increases from 5% to as high as 20% to 25%.

Colon Resection

Elective resection of the colon is a reasonably safe procedure in the elderly. Although most resections are for carcinoma (see later discussion), other indications include diverticular disease, polyps, and other benign disorders. Mortality for elective resections is usually under 5%.[91]

GYNECOLOGIC SURGERY

Major gynecologic surgery has been done for many years in elderly women.[92,93] Elective vaginal hysterectomy for such indications as prolapse has been shown to be safe, with mortality rates around 1%. Abdominal hysterectomy has a higher mortality rate (about 5%). Studies have shown that elderly women who undergo surgery for pelvic malignancy have substantial postoperative survival. Therefore, age alone should not be considered a contraindication to surgery for pelvic cancer.

CANCER SURGERY

Because cancer risk increases with age, the elderly have a disproportionate number of cancers, and surgery is still the primary therapeutic approach in most cases. The decision to perform cancer surgery in elderly patients, however, depends on several other factors. The first involves combined consideration of the life expectancy without surgery and the natural history of the underlying cancer. Radical surgery for prostate cancer in an ill 90-year-old man is probably not indicated, whereas resection of a bowel cancer in a vigorous 70-year-old woman is clearly indicated. The second factor is the availability of nonsurgical therapy. The final factor is the risk of the proposed surgery in relation to the chance of cure or prolongation of life.

Lung Cancer

Most lung cancers occur in older patients. Because there is no good effective nonsurgical therapy, resection is the treatment of choice.[94,95] Given equivalent levels of pulmonary function, the elderly generally do well in comparison to younger patients with lung resection. The mortality rate from surgery in elderly patients overall is about 15%. The five-year survival rate in a group of patients older than 70 years in one study was good (32%). However, none of the patients in the study had other severe underlying diseases. Some studies of patients treated without operation have reported 1-year survival rates of 0%.

Colon Cancer

Most of the colon surgery performed in the elderly is for cancer. As with lung cancer, no reasonable nonsurgical therapy is available for these patients. Several studies done in patients older than 75 years show mortality rates of 2% to 9% for colon resection. The lower figures usually predominate, however, because most operations are elective.[96,97] In one study, all nine patients in their 90s survived the surgery. Most patients who are admitted to the hospital from home are able to return home. Most important, postoperative survival compares well with that of younger patients with bowel cancer. Because of the relatively long natural history of bowel cancers in general, the survival of older patients may not differ from that of their normal disease-free cohort because they often die of other causes.

Other Cancers

Esophageal cancer is a deadly disease that cannot be treated without surgery. One study from Japan showed that surgical results are reasonably good in the elderly.[98] This study reported a moderate increase in mortality in older patients that appeared to result from an increase in pulmonary complications. The survival of the elderly group followed up for 5 years was about 25%, essentially identical to that of patients younger than 60 years.

Similar results have been found in several studies of gastric cancer.[99] Mortality is often somewhat greater in the elderly; however, many of their cancers are found at a later stage of disease. Their survival rates compare favorably with those of younger populations and, because nonsurgical therapy offers nothing, surgical intervention is indicated if the perioperative mortality is deemed to be reasonable.

Studies of the treatment of breast cancer have shown 5-year survival rates of around 50%.[100] Because the risks of curative surgery are low in this disease process, operation should be offered to most patients.

POSTOPERATIVE CARE OF ELDERLY PATIENTS

As with preoperative care, the postoperative care of elderly patients is basically the same as that of younger patients. Meticulous attention to detail and awareness of potential problems, however, result in a better chance of survival and a lower potential for postoperative complications in these patients.

Even in the recovery room, attention to the details of care is important. Hypothermia is common because of cool operating rooms, room-temperature intravenous infusions, and cold blood transfusions.[101,102] Some elderly patients are particularly susceptible because of faulty temperature regulation. Hypothermia itself depresses heart function. In addition, on rewarming, the increased metabolic activity and cardiac output needed places an added stress on the heart.

Narcotic-induced ventilatory depression can last longer than usual in the elderly. A significant decrease in PO_2 can occur after surgery, particularly in patients who have had general anesthesia.[103] This appears to be caused by a combination of shunting and an increase in ventilation–perfusion mismatching, and the effect increases with increasing age. Campbell[65] has stated that the continued use of mechanical ventilation into the postoperative period may help prevent some of these complications in patients in whom they are expected. In this way, adequate ventilation and good tracheobronchial toilet can be provided even with the use of narcotic analgesics. No objective evidence exists to support or refute this method of care.

It is important that elderly patients be sitting in chairs and moving as soon as possible after surgery. This helps to increase ventilation, clear secretions, and decrease atelectasis. Another important factor in preventing pulmonary complications is adequate pain relief. Patients who are in pain, particularly from thoracic or abdominal surgery, are less likely to cough, breathe deeply, and cooperate with respiratory therapy.

Postoperative changes in mental state are common in elderly patients, and mortality rates are about twice as high in patients with delirium.[54,104] It has been estimated that 10% to 15% of older patients become delirious after surgery.

Bedford[105] reported that 33% of 4000 patients who exhibited delirium during their hospital admission died within 1 month.[54]

Some authors believe that this postoperative complication results from the effects of the general anesthetic on the cerebral cortex. Blundell[106] studied 86 surgical patients older than 70 years. She found that the main effects were on memory and intellectual abilities that require organization of thought. These effects often lasted for several weeks. There were also some minor effects on psychiatric well-being, which were essentially resolved by discharge from the hospital.

Hole and coworkers[68] think that the effect may be on oxygenation of the brain. They argue that there is a decrease in cardiac output with positive-pressure ventilation and that hyperventilation, which results in hypocapnia, causes a further decrease in blood flow from the resulting cerebral vasoconstriction. Others believe that it may be an effect of the anesthetic agents themselves.

Several factors appear to influence postoperative changes in mentation. Patients who undergo regional anesthesia appear to be affected to a lesser degree, those who have shorter procedures are often less affected, and those who are febrile and are given other drugs are more frequently affected. Blundell believed that moving patients to hospitals was not a significant factor; she used a small control group to evaluate this effect. This conclusion, however, is hard to reconcile with the fact that these types of mental changes are common in hospitalized patients, even those who have not undergone surgery.

Heart failure and myocardial infarction are two important and deadly postoperative complications. Heart failure can be prevented, at least in part, by meticulous attention to intravenous infusions and urine output. At times, invasive monitoring with Swan-Ganz catheterization is essential.

Although myocardial infarction cannot be prevented, it is possible to anticipate its occurrence and to be able to recognize its unusual presentations in the elderly. In a study of 387 patients older than 65 years, Pathy[107] found that the classic presentation was seen in only 19%. The most common presentation was sudden dyspnea or exacerbation of heart failure (20%). Other frequent presentations were acute confusion (13%), strokes, peripheral emboli, and weakness.

Pulmonary embolism is a common complication that is theoretically preventable. The administration of low-dose heparin before and after surgery may be helpful in some procedures, although it has limited effectiveness in hip repair and open prostatectomy.[17] Lee and colleagues[108] have used venous impedance plethysmography to identify elderly patients with deep venous thrombosis and have also used external intermittent pneumatic compression to prevent thrombosis and pulmonary embolism, with excellent results. Methods of preventing deep venous thrombosis and pulmonary embolism are discussed in detail in Chapter 22.

Because of their frailty and decreased physiologic reserve, mortality is greatly increased in older patients who have surgical complications, and prevention and early intervention are crucial to their well-being. As in all care of the elderly, careful attention to detail in all aspects of postoperative care will result in lower morbidity and mortality.

REFERENCES

1. Boss GR, Seegmiller JE. Age-related physiological changes and their clinical significance. West J Med 1981;135:434–440.
2. Gerstenblith G, Lakatta EG, Weisfeldt ML. Age changes in myocardial function and exercise response. Prog Cardiovasc Dis 1976;19:1–21.
3. Weisfeldt ML. Aging of the cardiovascular system. N Engl J Med 1980;303:1172–1173.
4. Port S, Cobb FR, Coleman RE, Jones RH. Effect of age on the response of the left ventricular ejection fraction to exercise. N Engl J Med 1980;303:1133–1137.
5. Strahlman ER, ed. Clinical conferences at the Johns Hopkins Hospital: presbycardia. Johns Hopkins Med J 1981;149:203–208.
6. Kent S. The aging lung, part 1: loss of elasticity. Geriatrics 1978;33:124–130.
7. Sorbini CA, Grassi V, Solinas E, Muiesan G. Arterial oxygen tension in relation to age in healthy subjects. Respiration 1968;25:3–13.
8. Muiesan G, Sorbini CA, Grassi V. Respiratory function in the aged. Bull Physiopathol Respir 1971;7:973–1007.
9. McLachlan MSF. The aging kidney. Lancet 1978;2:143–146.
10. Friedman SA, Raizner AE, Rosen H, et al. Functional defects in the aging kidney. Ann Intern Med 1972;76:41–45.
11. Cockcroft DW, Gault MH. Prediction of creatinine clearance from serum creatinine. Nephron 1976;16:31–41.
12. Hollenberg NK, Adams DF, Solomon HS, et al. Senescence and the renal vasculature in normal man. Circ Res 1974;34:309–316.
13. Ochsner A. Is risk of indicated operation too great in the elderly? Geriatrics 1967;22:121–130.
14. Berman ND, David TE, Lipton IH, Lenkei SC. Surgical procedures involving cardiopulmonary bypass in patients aged 70 or older. J Am Geriatr Soc 1980;28:29–32.
15. Petracek MR, Lawson JD, Rhea WG, et al. Resection of abdominal aortic aneurysms in the over-80 age group. South Med J 1980;73:579–581.
16. Marshall WH, Fahey PJ. Operative complications and mortality in patients over 80 years of age. Arch Surg 1964;88:896–904.
17. Djokovic JL, Hedley-Whyte J. Prediction of outcome of surgery and anesthesia in patients over 80. JAMA 1979;242:2301–2306.
18. Denney JL, Denson JS. Risk of surgery in patients over 90. Geriatrics 1972;27:115–118.
19. Michel SL, Stevens L, Amodeo P, Morgenstern L. Surgical procedures in nonagenarians. West J Med 1984;141:61–63.
20. Keating HJ III. Major surgery in nursing home patients: proce-

dures, morbidity and mortality in the frailest of the frail elderly. J Am Geriatr Soc 1992;40:8–11.

21. Katlic M. Surgery in centenarians. JAMA 1985;253:3139–3141.

22. Cogbill TH, Strutt PJ, Landercasper J. Surgical procedures in centenarians. Wis Med J 1992;91:527–529.

23. Linn BS, Linn MW. Evaluation of results of surgical procedures in the elderly. Ann Surg 1982;195:90–96.

24. Goldman L, Caldera DL, Nussbaum SR, et al. Multifactorial index of cardiac risk in noncardiac surgical procedures. N Engl J Med 1977;297:845–850.

25. Sikes ED, Detmer DE. Aging and surgical risk in older citizens of Wisconsin. Wis Med J 1979;78:27–30.

26. Turnbull AD, Gundy E, Howland WS, Beattie EJ. Surgical mortality among the elderly: an analysis of 4050 operations (1970–1974). Clin Bull 1978;8:139–142.

27. Adkins RB, Scott HW. Surgical procedures in patients aged 90 years and older. South Med J 1984;77:1357–1364.

28. Seymour DG, Pringle R. A new method of auditing surgical mortality rates: application to a group of elderly general surgical patients. BMJ 1982;284:1539–1542.

29. Silvay G, Bodner N, Koffsky B, et al. Open heart surgery in patients in the eighth and ninth decades of life. J Am Geriatr Soc 1988;36:1123–1124.

30. Edmunds LH Jr, Stephenson LW, Edie RN, et al. Open-heart surgery in octogenarians. N Engl J Med 1988;319:131–136.

31. Bernstein EF, Dilley RB, Randolph HF III. The improving long-term outlook for patients over 70 years of age with abdominal aortic aneurysms. Ann Surg 1988;207:318–322.

32. Salo JA, Perhoniemi VJ, Lepantalo MJA, et al. Prognosis of patients over 75 years of age with a ruptured abdominal aortic aneurysm. World J Surg 1989;13:484–487.

33. Berggren H, Ekroth R, Malmberg R, et al. Hospital mortality and long-term survival in relation to preoperative function in elderly patients with bronchogenic carcinoma. Ann Thorac Surg 1984;38:633–636.

34. Didolkar MS, Moore RH, Takita H. Evaluation of the risk in pulmonary resection for bronchogenic carcinoma. Am J Surg 1974;127:700–703.

35. Reiss R, Deutsch AA, Nudelman I. Abdominal surgery in elderly patients: statistical analysis of clinical factors prognostic of mortality in 1,000 cases. Mt Sinai J Med 1987;54:135–140.

36. Sandler RS, Maule WF, Baltus ME, et al. Biliary tract surgery in the elderly. J Gen Intern Med 1987;2:149–154.

37. Pigott JP, Williams GB. Cholecystectomy in the elderly. Am J Surg 1988;155:408–410.

38. Rømrbæk-Madsen M. Herniorrhaphy in patients aged 80 years or more: a prospective analysis of morbidity and mortality. Eur J Surg 1992;158:591–594.

39. Laskin RS, Gruber MA, Zimmerman AJ. Intertrochanteric fractures of the hip in the elderly: a retrospective analysis of 236 cases. Clin Orthop 1979;141:188–195.

40. Kennedy AW, Flagg JS, Webster KD. Gynecologic candor in the very elderly. Gynecol Oncol 1989;32:49–54.

41. Dunlop WE, Rosenblood L, Lawrason L, et al. Effects of age and severity of illness on outcome and length of stay in geriatric surgical patients. Am J Surg 1993;165:577–580.

42. Andersen B, Ostberg J. Long term prognosis in geriatric surgery: 2–17 year follow-up of 7922 patients. J Am Geriatr Soc 1972;20:255–258.

43. Hosking MP, Warner MA, Lobdell CM, et al. Outcomes of surgery in patients 90 years of age and older. JAMA 1989;261:1909–1915.

44. Salem R, Devitt P, Johnson J, Firmin R. Emergency geriatric surgical admissions. BMJ 1978;2:416–417.

45. Seymour DG, Pringle R. Surgical emergencies in the elderly: can they be prevented? Health Bull (Edinb) 1981;41:112–131.

46. Keller SM, Markovitz LJ, Wilder JR, et al. Emergency and elective surgery in patients over the age 70. Am Surg 1987;53:636–640.

47. Schöön IM, Arvidsson S. Surgery in patients aged 80 years and over. Eur J Surg 1991;157:251–255.

48. Pomorski ME. Surgical care for the aged patient: the decision-making process. Nurs Clin North Am 1983;18:365–372.

49. Neugent MC. Social and emotional needs of geriatric surgery patients. Social Work Health Care 1981;6:69–75.

50. Reiss R. Moral and ethical issues in geriatric surgery. J Med Ethics 1980;6:71–77.

51. Palmberg S, Hirsjarvi E. Mortality in geriatric surgery. Gerontology 1979;25:103–112.

52. Wilder RJ, Fishbein RH. The widening surgical frontier. Postgrad Med 1961;29:548–551.

53. Samiy AH. Clinical manifestations of disease in the elderly. Med Clin North Am 1983;67:333–344.

54. Hodkinson HM. Mental impairment in the elderly. J R Coll Physicians Lond 1973;7:305–317.

55. Mullen JL, Buzby GP, Matthews DC, et al. Reduction of operative morbidity and mortality by combined preoperative and postoperative nutritional support. Ann Surg 1980;192:604–613.

56. Master AM, Lasser RP. Tables of average weight and height of Americans aged 65 to 94 years. JAMA 1960;172:658–662.

57. Kaminski MV, Nasr NJ, Freed BA, Sriram K. The efficacy of nutritional support in the elderly. J Am Coll Nutr 1982;1:35–40.

58. Corman LC. The preoperative patient with an asymptomatic cervical bruit. Med Clin North Am 1979;63:1335–1340.

59. Evans WE, Cooperman M. The significance of asymptomatic unilateral carotid bruits in preoperative patients. Surgery 1978;83:521–522.

60. Berens ES, Kouchoukos NT, Murphy SF, et al. Preoperative carotid artery screening in elderly patients undergoing cardiac surgery. J Vasc Surg 1992;15:313–323.

61. Wickstrom I, Holmberg I, Stefansson T. Survival of female geriatric patients after hip fracture surgery: a comparison of 5 anesthetic methods. Acta Anaesthesiol Scand 1982;26:607–614.

62. Del Guercio LRM, Cohn JD. Monitoring operative risk in the elderly. JAMA 1980;243:1350–1355.

63. Seymour DG, Pringle R, MacLennan WJ. The role of the preoperative electrocardiogram in the elderly surgical patient. Age Ageing 1983;12:97–104.

64. Tornebrandt K, Fletcher R. Pre-operative chest x-rays in elderly patients. Anaesthesia 1982;37:901–902.

65. Campbell JC. Detecting and correcting pulmonary risk factors before operation. Geriatrics 1977;32:54–57.

66. Tisi GM. Preoperative evaluation of pulmonary function. Am Rev Respir Dis 1979;119:293–310.

67. Schrader LL, McMillen MA, Watson CB, et al. Is routine pre-

operative hemodynamic evaluation of nonagenarians necessary? J Am Geriatr Soc 1991;39:1–5.

68. Hole A, Terjesen T, Breivik H. Epidural versus general anesthesia for total hip arthroplasty in elderly patients. Acta Anaesthesiol Scand 1980;24:279–287.

69. Guillen J, Aldrete JA. Anesthetic factors influencing morbidity and mortality of elderly patients undergoing inguinal herniorrhaphy. Am J Surg 1970;120:760–763.

70. Miller R, Marlar K, Silvay G. Anesthesia for patients aged over ninety years. NY State J Med 1977;77:1421–1425.

71. Davis FM, Woolner DF, Frampton C, et al. Prospective, multicentre trial of mortality following general or spinal anaesthesia for hip fracture surgery in the elderly. Br J Anaesth 1987;59:1080–1088.

72. Asbjørn J, Jakobsen BW, Pilegaard K, et al. Mental function in elderly men after surgery during epidural analgesia. Acta Anaesthesiol Scand 1989;33:369–373.

73. Detsky A, Abrams H, McLaughlin J, et al. Predicting cardiac complications in patients undergoing non-cardiac surgery. J Gen Intern Med 1986;1:211–219.

74. Gerson MC, Hurst JM, Hertzberg VS, et al. Cardiac prognosis in noncardiac geriatric surgery. Ann Intern Med 1985;103:832–837.

75. Gerson MC, Hurst JM, Hertzberg VS, et al. Prediction of cardiac and pulmonary complications related to elective abdominal and noncardiac thoracic surgery in geriatric patients. Am J Med 1990;88:101–107.

76. Mannion JD, Armenti FR, Edie RN. Cardiac surgery in the elderly patient. Cardiovasc Clin 1992;22:189–207.

77. Ko W, Gold JP, Lazzaro R, et al. Survival analysis of octogenarian patients with coronary artery disease managed by elective coronary artery bypass surgery versus conventional medical treatment. Circulation 1992;86(Suppl II):191–197.

78. Glower DD, Christopher TD, Milano CA, et al. Performance status and outcome after coronary artery bypass grafting in persons aged 80 to 93 years. Am J Cardiol 1992;70:567–571.

79. Olsson M, Granstrom L, Lindblom D, et al. Aortic valve replacement in octogenarians with aortic stenosis: a case-control study. J Am Coll Cardiol 1992;20:1512–1516.

80. Pasic M, Carrel T, Laske A, et al. Valve replacement in octogenarians: increased early mortality but good long-term result. Eur Heart J 1992;13:508–510.

81. Davis EA, Gardner TJ, Gillinov M, et al. Valvular disease in the elderly: influence on surgical results. Ann Thorac Surg 1993;55:333–338.

82. Nair CK, Biddle WP, Kaneshige A, et al. Ten-year experience with mitral valve replacement in the elderly. Am Heart J 1992;124:154–159.

83. Tabayashi K, Ohmi M, Syohji Y, et al. Thoracic aortic operations in patients aged 70 years or older. Ann Thorac Surg 1992;54:279–282.

84. Dean RH, Woody BA, Carn E, et al. Operative treatment of abdominal aortic aneurysms in octogenarians: when is it too much too late? Ann Surg 1993;217:721–728.

85. Ekelund A, Rydell N, Nilsson OS. Total hip arthroplasty in patients 80 years of age and older. Clin Orthop 1992;281:101–106.

86. Phillips TW, Grainger RW, Cameron HS, et al. Risks and benefits of elective hip replacement in the octogenarian. Can Med Assoc J 1987;137:497–500.

87. Harness JK, Strodel WE, Talsma SE. Symptomatic biliary tract disease in the elderly patient. Am Surg 1986;52:442–445.

88. Margiotta SJ, Horwitz JR, Willis IH, et al. Cholecystectomy in the elderly. Am J Surg 1988;156:509–512.

89. Smithy WB, Wexner SD, Dailey TH. The diagnosis and treatment of acute appendicitis in the aged. Dis Colon Rectum 1986;29:170–173.

90. McCallion J, Canning GP, Knight PV, et al. Acute appendicitis in the elderly: a 5-year retrospective study. Age Ageing 1987;16:256–260.

91. Cohen H, Willis I, Wallack M. Surgical experience of colon resection in the extreme elderly. Am Surg 1986;52:214–217.

92. Schneider J, Benito R. Extensive gynecologic surgical procedures upon patients more than 75 years of age. Surg Gynecol Obstet 1988;167:497–500.

93. Lichtinger M, Averette H, Penalver M, et al. Major surgical procedures for gynecologic malignancy in elderly women. South Med J 1986;79:1506–1510.

94. Roxburgh JC, Thompson J, Goldstraw P. Hospital mortality and long-term survival after pulmonary resection in the elderly. Ann Thorac Surg 1991;51:800–803.

95. Thomas P, Sielezneff I, Ragni J, et al. Is lung cancer resection justified in patients aged over 70 years? Eur J Cardiothorac Surg 1993;7:246–251.

96. Whittle J, Steinberg EP, Anderson GF, et al. Results of colectomy in elderly patients with colon cancer, based on Medicare claims data. Am J Surg 1992;163:572–576.

97. Fitzgerald SD, Longo WE, Daniel GL, et al. Advanced colorectal neoplasia in the high-risk elderly patient: is surgical resection justified? Dis Colon Rectum 1993;36:161–166.

98. Sugimachi K, Inokuchi K, Ueo H, et al. Surgical treatment for carcinoma of the esophagus in the elderly patient. Surg Gynecol Obstet 1985;160:317–319.

99. Coluccia C, Ricci EB, Marzola GG, et al. Gastric cancer in the elderly: results of surgical treatment. Int Surg 1987;72:4–10.

100. Amsterdam E, Birkenfeld S, Gilad A, et al. Surgery for carcinoma of the breast in women over 70 years of age. J Surg Oncol 1987;35:180–183.

101. Vaughn MS, Vaughn RW, Cork RC. Postoperative hypothermia in adults: relationship of age, anesthesia, and shivering to rewarming. Anesth Analg 1981;60:746–751.

102. Heymann AD. The effect of incidental hypothermia on elderly surgical patients. J Gerontol 1977;32:46–48.

103. Kitamura H, Sawa T, Ikezono E. Postoperative hypoxemia: the contribution of age to the maldistribution of ventilation. Anesthesiology 1972;36:244–252.

104. Lipowski ZJ. Transient cognitive disorders (delirium, acute confusional states) in the elderly. Am J Psychiatry 1983;140:1426–1436.

105. Bedford PD. General medical aspects of confusional states in elderly people. BMJ 1959;2:185–188.

106. Blundell E. A psychological study of the effects of surgery on eighty-six elderly patients. Br J Soc Clin Psychol 1967;6:297–303.

107. Pathy MS. Clinical presentation of myocardial infarction in the elderly. Br Heart J 1967;29:190–199.

108. Lee BY, Thoden WR, Trainor FS, Kavner D. Noninvasive detection and prevention of deep-vein thrombosis in the geriatric patient. J Am Geriatr Soc 1980;28:171–175.

SECTION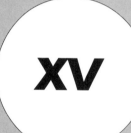

OBESITY

Medical Management of the Surgical Patient, Third Edition,
edited by Michael F. Lubin, H. Kenneth Walker, and Robert B. Smith III.
J.B. Lippincott Company, Philadelphia, PA © 1995.

CHAPTER

OBESITY   43

John G. Kral

For practical purposes, "obesity" and "overweight" can be equated because overweight is mostly composed of excess adipose tissue. The severity of the disease is proportional to the excess weight, and mortality increases exponentially with weight gain. "Ideal" or "desirable" body weight (for height) is defined by mortality statistics from large population studies and does not reflect value judgments in favor of leanness or against obesity. The nadir of the J-shaped weight–mortality relationship reflects biologic "normalcy" (minimum morbidity), so it follows that lower and higher weights are pathologic, whatever the cause. Obesity begins at a weight 20% above the nadir, based on the opinion of a National Institutes of Health consensus conference.

The most practical way to express weight is through the body mass index (BMI), which normalizes weight to height, allowing comparisons between populations with different stature, such as between men and women, and between races. BMI is calculated by dividing weight in kilograms by height in meters squared (kg/m^2). The "normal" range of BMI is about 20 to 25. Because body fat, however it is measured, is tightly correlated to the BMI, this can serve as a surrogate for actual determination of body fat.

The severity of obesity in terms of mortality has been classified into three grades according to BMI. Grade I corresponds to a BMI of 26 to 29.9 and grade III to a BMI of 40 or more (Fig. 43-1). This convenient scheme has been suggested as a guide for choosing among treatment strategies.[1]

The disease of obesity has reached epidemic proportions in industrialized countries and there are many indications that it is increasing in prevalence.[2] According to the latest surveys, nearly one third of women and one fourth of men in the United States are obese[3]; in subsets of the population, the prevalence exceeds 50%.[4] It follows that at least 30% of all surgical patients, without taking diagnosis into account, may be obese. The prevalence of obesity actually is likely to be even greater among surgical patients than in the general patient population. Virtually all organs are affected by obesity, and the diseases topping US mortality statistics are significantly associated with obesity (italic entries):

Ten leading causes of death in the United States in 1989

- *Heart disease*
- *Cancer*
- *Stroke*
- Trauma
- *Chronic lung disease*
- Pneumonia and influenza
- *Diabetes*
- *Suicide*
- Liver disease
- *Arterial disease*

Numerous obesity-related diseases are treated surgically (Table 43-1) and physicians should be familiar with the medical care of obese surgical patients. This chapter dis-

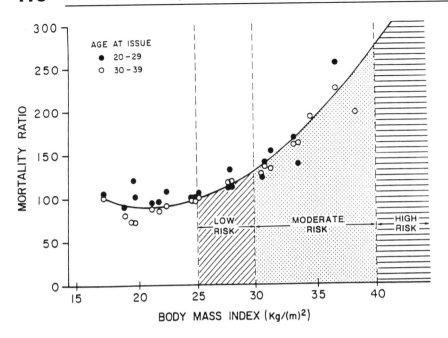

FIG. 43-1. Relationship between body mass index and mortality ratio (percentage) for persons aged 20 to 29 and 30 to 39 derived from life insurance statistics. (Copyright 1976, George A. Bray, with permission)

cusses the pathophysiology of obesity and suggests methods for evaluating and treating comorbid conditions.

ETIOLOGY

The ingestion of calories in excess of expenditure has many causes, although the overall etiology remains obscure. Only a few obese patients have identifiable primary endocrine abnormalities causing their condition. In severely obese patients, an endocrine work-up to exclude such conditions as hypothyroidism, Cushing's syndrome, and prolactinoma is seldom warranted. Genetic syndromes resulting in obesity are exceedingly rare and are often fatal before patients have had time to develop any surgical disease.

TABLE 43–1. Obesity-Related Diseases Treated Surgically

Metabolic	Neoplastic
Cholelithiasis	Cancer
Thromboembolism	Endometrial, breast,
Peripheral vascular	prostate
Urolithiasis	Colorectal
Mechanical	Renal
Osteoarthritis	Fibroadenoma of the breast
Varicose veins	**Gynecologic**
Esophagitis	Uterine fibroma
Hiatus hernia	Ovarian cysts
Abdominal wall hernia	Cesarian section
	Stress urinary incontinence

Body weight and BMI are genetically determined, as are metabolic rate and fat cell number.[5,6] Furthermore, taste preferences and eating behavior already present at birth are predictors of overweight. Ascribing obesity to a character disorder, the sins of gluttony and sloth, is not only a gross simplification but also patently wrong in most cases.

Significant environmental factors contribute to the increasing prevalence of obesity in the United States; increasing consumption of fatty foods and overall reduction in physical activity are also important determinants of overweight.

Nevertheless, the cause of most forms of obesity is unknown, making causal, curative treatment infeasible. Furthermore, once it is established, the obese state is exceedingly resistant to therapy because of poorly understood mechanisms.[7] Some of the pathophysiologic changes that occur during the development of obesity seem to perpetuate the disease, and it is not known whether some of these changes are irreversible. The goal of medical therapy for obese patients who are undergoing surgery is to identify significant comorbid diseases and then to ensure their optimal physical condition.

PATHOPHYSIOLOGY

Obesity is an independent risk factor for numerous serious systemic and organ-specific diseases. It is not known whether obesity may have a primary role in the development of some forms of diabetes, hypertension, congestive heart failure, and even cancer. The distribution of adipose tissue has been hypothesized to be a significant determinant of complications of obesity, although the mechanism is unknown. The metabolic syndrome, or syndrome X, associates non–insulin-dependent diabetes, hypertension, hyperlipoproteinemia, and obesity with a central (visceral, abdominal, upper body) distribution of fat. A series of recent studies has demonstrated the importance of early growth in adult distribution of adipose tissue and the development of comorbid conditions.[8]

Initially, various simple anthropometric measures were shown to differentiate between upper body, central, or android, obesity and femoral-gluteal, or gynoid, obesity. The simplest is the waist/hip ratio, which is obtained by dividing the minimum girth at the waist by the maximum girth below the waist in the standing position. There are no published normal, control, or reference values for the waist/hip ratio that can be applied to evaluate risk in particular patients. As a general rule, however, ratios greater than 0.82 in women and 0.92 in men indicate greater risk of present or future morbidity. Computed tomography has been used in research studies to measure the amount of intraabdominal or "visceral" adipose tissue compared with the amount of subcutaneous adipose tissue, leading to refinements in the predictive power of the relative distribution of fat in identifying the risks for developing comorbid conditions. Preliminary data indicate that the absolute amount of visceral fat rather than the relative distribution of fat, the total amount of body fat, or the body weight is the strongest predictor.[9]

CARDIOVASCULAR COMPLICATIONS OF OBESITY

Cardiomegaly; increased cardiac output, stroke volume, and blood volume; and excess extracellular fluid all increase the surgical risk of obese patients. It has been suggested that the hyperdynamic circulation of these patients reflects an adaptation to increased metabolic needs of the excess tissue. This adaptation leads to increased cardiac index and output, stroke volume, and left and right ventricular work; higher right and left heart filling pressures; and increased pulmonary artery pressure.[10]

Whereas hemodynamic variables are in the high part of the normal range in obese patients before operation, significant decreases occur in the cardiac index and in right and left ventricular stroke work during operation that continue during the postoperative period.[11] Obese patients react to the stress of anesthesia and surgery with left ventricular dysfunction. Intraoperative depression of cardiac output that persists after operation and is not followed by a normal elevation of these parameters predicts poorer outcome in trauma victims not stratified for weight. This response pattern may explain the increased operative risk of obese patients undergoing elective surgery, who often manifest left ventricular dysfunction at rest.[12]

It is not known whether increased intraabdominal fat is associated with greater perioperative morbidity than is peripheral fat. Left, right, and biventricular cardiac dysfunction is prevalent among asymptomatic candidates for obesity surgery, and is significantly more common in patients with visceral than with peripheral fat distribution.[13] The increased cardiac size, from increased filling and wall thickness (resulting from greater stroke work causing hypertrophy) is associated with elevated systemic arterial pressure. This constellation leads to susceptibility to congestive heart failure and to cardiac arrhythmias when obese patients who have limited reserves are stressed during operation, along with interrelated problems of pain, posture, and hypoxia.

PULMONARY COMPROMISE

The cardiac abnormalities described occur in conjunction with pulmonary dysfunction. Isolated cor pulmonale, however, is uncommon in severe obesity and seems to be caused by pulmonary embolization rather than progressive insufficiency.[14]

The sheer mechanical burden of excess adipose tissue on the chest wall and in the abdomen, pushing on the diaphragm, compresses the lungs (Table 43-2). The role of increased fatty infiltration of the diaphragm and intercostal muscles is less clear in the pulmonary pathophysiology of obesity.[15] The combined effects of decreased chest wall compliance and increased adipose tissue lead to the typical reduction of functional residual capacity and total lung volume that is seen in severe obesity.

A related phenomenon is premature airway closure leading to alveolar hypoxia, which in turn leads to pulmonary vasoconstriction and pulmonary hypertension. Obesity-related hypertension ("obitension") is somewhat controversial. Some question its existence, and proponents are unable to agree on its pathogenesis.[16] Given the prevalence

---

TABLE 43–2. Increased Body (Fat) Mass Causes Hypoxemia in Obesity

Increased Oxygen Consumption
↑ Chest load
↑ CO_2
↑ Respiratory rate

Decreased Oxygenation
↓ Lung volume, ↓ functional residual capacity
↓ Inspiratory strength
↓ Brain stem CO_2 response
↑ Small airway closure, ↑ shunts

of hypoxia in obese patients and the sequence described earlier, it is possible that obitension is pulmonary in origin.

Of immediate perioperative concern are the two pulmonary syndromes, sleep apnea and obesity hypoventilation.[17] The restrictive respiratory pattern caused by excess fat that leads to obesity hypoventilation is often found in patients with other pulmonary risk factors, such as smoking, asthma, or fibrosis, and can occur alone or in conjunction with sleep apnea. Sleep apnea is clearly weight-related, sometimes appearing at a threshold level of weight. It can be peripheral (obstructive) or, rarely, central in origin and contributes significantly to the increased prevalence of sudden death in obese patients. The obstruction can be caused by a large tongue or tonsils, or sometimes by a deviated nasal septum or other nasopharyngeal pathology. Loud snoring is the hallmark of this condition. Disordered sleep often leads to severe daytime somnolence, headaches, and even depression.

The increased blood volume in obesity is not associated with a commensurate increase in chest volume, so the relative increase in central circulation causes alveolar compression. There is an increased venous admixture from the ventilation–perfusion mismatch caused by atelectatic lung. Chronic hypoxemia in turn leads to polycythemia, a harbinger of thromboembolism.

THROMBOEMBOLISM

The most prevalent serious complication of surgery in obese patients is thromboembolism. Tables 43-3 and 43-4 outline factors of pathogenetic importance for the increased incidence of pulmonary embolism and thrombotic conditions in obese patients. Many of these factors are interrelated; cause and effect cannot be determined. For example, several chemical abnormalities are associated with type II diabetes,[18,19] yet may be caused by fatty infiltration of the liver, which in turn is more prevalent in type II diabetes. In

TABLE 43–4. Increased Body Fat Mass Predisposes to Thromboembolism in Obesity

↑ Intraabdominal pressure
    Varicose veins
↑ Blood volume/intrathoracic pressure
    Cardiopulmonary failure
    Polycythemia
↑ Serum-free fatty acids
    Glucose intolerance/hyperinsulinemia
    Fatty liver
↓ Locomotion
    Hypostasis

principle, obesity is associated with elevated levels of thrombosis-promoting factors and decreases in fibrinolysis. These changes are significantly related to abdominal fatness.[8] In addition, hemodynamic abnormalities associated with comorbid conditions (hypertension), as well as mechanical (intraabdominal pressure) and possibly behavioral (smoking, sedentary life-style) factors, all contribute to explaining the high incidence of thromboembolism in obese patients.

KIDNEY FAILURE

Both functional and morphologic renal abnormalities have been described in obese patients.[20] Just as with other obesity-related morbidity, it is difficult to separate the contributing factors. Thus, glucose intolerance and frank diabetes as well as hypertension are associated with glomerular hyperfiltration and with renovascular hypertrophy and fibrosis.[21,22] Gout is prevalent in obese patients and is a cause of renal pathology. Several reports describe nephrosis in severely obese patients but there are no data implicating obesity as an independent risk factor for kidney failure.

The prevalence of obesity among kidney transplant recipients does not reflect the overall prevalence of kidney failure among obese patients because many transplant centers exclude these patients from their programs and nephrologists are reluctant to refer them. Recent studies have demonstrated poorer outcome in obese patients after renal transplantation compared with control patients of normal weight.[23,24] Only one study obtained different results, possibly because it used a lower threshold for obesity (120% of ideal body weight versus 140% in the former studies).[25] This study found preoperative weight to be a highly significant predictor of posttransplant weight gain, which was not the case in one of the other studies. Reasons for poorer graft survival and higher mortality in obese patients may include impaired glucose metabolism associated not

TABLE 43–3. Comorbid Conditions Contributing to Thromboembolism in Obesity

Condition	Chemical Abnormality
Dyslipidemia	↑ Serum triglycerides
	↑ Serum low-density lipoprotein cholesterol
	↓ Serum high-density lipoprotein cholesterol
	↑ Blood-viscosity
Diabetes	↑ Serum antithrombin III
	↑ Serum fibrinogen
	↑ Serum fibronectin
	↓ Tissue plasminogen activity
Hypertension	
Renal failure	

only with obesity but also with the administration of steroids and cyclosporin A, which may act synergistically with obesity.

FLUID AND ELECTROLYTE ABNORMALITIES

Extracellular water increases with expanding fat mass through unknown mechanisms.[26] Irreversibility of the elevated ratio of extracellular to intracellular fluid with massive weight loss implies an intrinsic abnormality[27] unrelated to right ventricular failure or edema.[28] The increase in extracellular fluid influences distribution volumes of medications as well as volume status.

Obese patients often have histories of diuretic use, either for surreptitious treatment of "swelling" or as part of legitimate therapy for hypertension. This use of diuretics as well as repeated bouts of fasting, low-calorie diets, or even bulimia may contribute to the depletion of total body potassium levels. Such depletion is not obvious from serum concentrations, in which a reduction from 4 to 3 mEq/L may be associated with a body loss of 1000 mEq of potassium.

Once again, comorbid conditions such as type II diabetes (hyperinsulinemia)[29] and hypertension can contribute to other abnormalities, although one study suggests the presence of an intrinsically low total body potassium level in obese patients.[30] Fatty liver, a corollary of hyperinsulinemia, is associated with decreased protein synthesis[31] and may be accompanied by reductions in serum albumin, which in turn predispose to fluid and electrolyte abnormalities.

METABOLIC DISEASE

Obesity is associated with metabolic disturbances such as diabetes, lipid abnormalities, and gout, all of which can cause multiorgan dysfunction. Considerable controversy surrounds the primacy of obesity in this context and the pathogenetic mechanism linking obesity to these abnormalities. It is likely that advances in genetic research will demonstrate shared and complex heritability of fat accumulation, carbohydrate and lipid metabolism, and energy balance.[6]

Diabetes is more prevalent among obese patients than among those of normal weight. β Cells in Langerhans islets are larger in obese patients. Glucose tolerance is almost universally impaired in obesity, and there is down-regulation of insulin receptors in all tissues studied. Furthermore, glucose transport is defective. These abnormalities are reversible,[32,33] however, demonstrating that they do not have a causal role in obesity, although they likely contribute to perpetuating the obese state and are instrumental in causing comorbid complications.

SUSCEPTIBILITY TO INFECTION

Obese patients are at greater risk for wound infection than are patients of normal weight. Studies on absenteeism have suggested that obese patients are more prone to other infections, too, but it is not known whether there is a primary immune defect in obesity. Intuitively, expecting susceptibility to pneumonia from respiratory compromise and to cellulitis from intertriginous changes under an abdominal panniculus or in the edematous skin of the lower leg would be reasonable without postulating any immune compromise. Evidence exists, however, for impaired immunocompetence in obese patients, although the mechanisms are not known.[34] Once again, obesity-related impairment in glucose metabolism may be implicated: defective leukocyte function has been demonstrated in the prediabetic state.[35,36] Patients with diabetes are notorious for their susceptibility to infections, so it is possible that such susceptibility in obese patients is a reflection of the intrinsically deranged glucose metabolism in obesity, regardless of severity.

EVALUATION OF OBESE PATIENTS

Because of their size, obese patients pose a significant diagnostic challenge for purely physical reasons. In severe obesity, there is considerable occult pathology that may become manifest only during the added challenge of an operation. Limited physiologic reserves elude detection during routine activities of daily living that have gradually been adapted to the constraints imposed by excess weight. Thus, patients' histories may be noncontributory. In addition, risk factors for obesity must be considered:

- Male gender
- Adult onset
- Visceral distribution of fat (increased waist-to-hip ratio)
- Smoking
- BMI greater than 26
- Manifest comorbid conditions (eg, diabetes, hypertension)
- Family history of complicated obesity (eg, myocardial infarction, stroke, diabetes)

BASIC PREOPERATIVE EVALUATION

The goal of the preoperative evaluation is to detect any preexisting pathology and optimize a patient's physical condition. It can also provide a baseline for the interpretation of postoperative findings. Last, it serves as a predictor, allowing the team to focus its monitoring efforts on potentially critical areas.

In the performance of standard electrocardiograms, chest radiographs, blood counts, and electrolyte levels, some specific findings that require particular attention may be overlooked in routine practice. A prolonged QT interval is an electrocardiographic marker of sudden cardiac arrest. A prolonged QT interval was found in retrospect in most severely obese patients who died of malignant arrhythmias in one study.[37] Similar findings have been associated with fatal[38] and nonfatal[39] dieting. Electrocardiographic signs of left ventricular hypertrophy also carry an increased risk of sudden cardiac death,[40] with an increased prevalence of ventricular ectopy in obese patients.[41]

Obtaining a routine chest radiograph in obese patients can be difficult for reasons of sheer size. Attention must be paid to achieving adequate penetration and evaluation of the whole lung. Obtaining well-penetrated images of both bases, in which small amounts of pleural fluid indicating incipient heart failure may be present, sometimes requires an extra set of films.

Standard blood tests are often challenging to obtain in obese patients because venipuncture is difficult. Prolonged stasis during sampling and the stress of pain from multiple needlesticks may influence such parameters as serum potassium, hematocrit, and blood glucose levels. A spurious elevation in the potassium level may raise an otherwise low level into the normal range. Among other routine blood tests, it is noteworthy that a leukocyte count in the high-normal range (greater than 9000/µL) is a strong predictor of risk for acute myocardial infarction independent of tobacco smoking.[42] Obese patients commonly have high-normal white blood cell counts and seem to have exaggerated and unexplained postoperative elevations of the white blood cell count.

Elevations of liver enzyme levels are common among obese patients and do not indicate severe liver disease but rather fatty infiltration of the liver.[43] Nevertheless, a fatty liver is more vulnerable than is a normal one, and this must be considered in anesthetic management.[44]

SPECIAL TESTS

Cardiopulmonary evaluation is particularly important in obese surgical patients who are at least 40% overweight. With or without histories indicative of cardiac or pulmonary disease, routine arterial blood gas determinations should be obtained with patients in the supine position and breathing room air. Peak flow spirometry, or simply having patients blow out a match at arm's length, are practical tests for evaluating pulmonary reserve to determine whether more complex testing is indicated. Routine performance of standard spirometry has been questioned in one cost/benefit analysis.

Indications for abbreviated sleep studies (ie, without polysomnography and electroencephalography) should be liberal in obese patients who have histories of snoring and daytime somnolence and any witnessed episodes of apnea. Evaluation should include otorhinolaryngologic consultation to rule out nasopharyngeal pathology.

The issue of cardiovascular compromise is particularly important in obese patients. Standard diagnostic techniques such as exercise testing and echocardiography are limited in severely obese patients, who simply are unable to achieve prerequisite levels of exercise stress to make such studies meaningful. Excess adipose tissue limits the sensitivity of ultrasound of the chest, although newer intraesophageal probes may prove helpful. In lieu of exercise testing, dipyridamole-thallium can be used to achieve stress levels of myocardial perfusion and detect areas of reduced flow. Other quantitative radionuclide cardiographic techniques are able to detect abnormalities of ventricular function, although it has not been determined whether such abnormalities are predictors of outcome. Calibration standards and dosimetry present problems in the most obese patients. In spite of these difficulties, echocardiography has been valuable in demonstrating cardiac abnormalities in severely obese patients.[12,45]

Thorough lipid evaluations are valuable in obese patients. In addition to elevated levels of serum cholesterol, decreased levels of high-density lipoproteins and increased levels of serum triglycerides are markers of coronary heart disease risk.[46] The controversy over the importance of triglycerides as an independent risk factor for coronary heart disease notwithstanding, their association with impaired glucose metabolism in obesity increases the significance of elevated levels.

TREATMENT AND PREVENTION

It is logical to recommend nutritionally sound weight loss before elective operation, particularly if this would correct comorbid conditions such as diabetes, congestive heart failure, or respiratory insufficiency. As with smoking cessation, however, which is doubly important for obese patients, it is unrealistic to expect full cooperation with this recommendation. Nevertheless, the consistently poor results of obese patients in achieving and maintaining weight loss in daily life should not deter physicians from urging preoperative weight loss. This cannot be a universal requirement because weight loss may be detrimental to some diseases being treated. Care must be taken to avoid imposing a catabolic state and adding to the catabolism of surgery.

Increasing physical activity, preferably through an exercise program, is an excellent preventive measure in sedentary obese patients. Combined with smoking cessation and chest physical therapy, exercise training dramatically reduces the risks of postoperative pulmonary complications. Patients with sleep apnea benefit from nasal continuous positive airway pressure, which is preferable to tracheostomy.[17] Patients with upper airway obstruction experience great improvement with weight loss. Although surgical correction of a deviated nasal septum may be beneficial, there is little role for uvulopalatopharyngoplasty in obese patients who have snoring and intermittent hypercapnia.

Several measures can be taken to help prevent thromboembolism. Before elective operations, the administration of low-dose warfarin can restore levels of antithrombin III and should be considered in obese patients with a prior history of thrombosis.[47] The routine use of minidose heparin (with the dose adjusted for body weight), antiembolic stockings, intermittent venous compression, and early extubation and ambulation has drastically reduced the prevalence of thromboembolism in severely obese patients. The infusion of dextrose solutions in the postoperative period to suppress free fatty acid release has also been recommended, although the antilipolytic effects of insulin may be just as effective. Some surgeons treating severely obese patients administer excess fluid before operation to achieve hemodilution to rheologically optimal hematocrit levels (28% to 32%) as a potential antithrombotic measure. Theoretically, this could lead instead to a hypercoagulable condition resulting from the dilution of thrombolytic factors.[48] This has not been demonstrated, however, in any of the large series of obesity operations in which fluid loading has been a routine practice.

Postoperative infections can be prevented effectively through several approaches, used alone or in combination. Local treatment of skin infections and routine use of antibacterial soap for showering and shampooing the evening before and morning of surgery are simple first steps. The routine use of prophylactic antibiotics (such as 1 to 2 g of cefazolin) is justified to prevent wound infections in obese patients regardless of the type of operation planned. The efficacy of paper drapes, vigorous irrigation, and local antibiotics has not been evaluated in prospective, randomized trials in obese patients but has been demonstrated historically in operations with a high risk of infection. Surgical techniques involving adequate exposure are particularly important in obese patients. Sutures and drains should not be placed in the subcutaneous adipose tissue.

Table 43-5 summarizes the steps that can be taken to reduce surgical risks in obese patients. Specific anesthesiologic measures are not considered in this chapter but have been outlined elsewhere.[49,50]

TABLE 43–5. Perioperative Risk Reduction in Obese Patients

Rule Out Treatable Conditions
Congestive heart failure
Respiratory insufficiency
  Obstructive sleep apnea
  Hypercapnia
Diabetes out of control
Smoking
Congestive heart disease
Chronic skin infection

Treat Complicating Conditions
Diuresis
Weight loss
Glycemic control
Airway obstruction
Antibiotics—local control of skin infections
Malnutrition

Prevent Known Risks
Pulmonary
  Breathing exercises
  Early ambulation/prothrombin time
  Oxygen
  Elevate head and upper body
Thrombosis
  Intermittent compression stockings/TEDs
  Ambulate
  Fluid load
  Heparin
Infection
  Prophylactic
    Showers
    Antibiotics
  Irrigation
  Paper drapes
  Technique
    No subcutaneous sutures
    Exposure
Others
  Aspiration
    Elevate head and upper body
    Nasogastric intubation
    Gastric acid suppression
  Monitor
    Central venous pressure
    Arterial blood gases
    Swan-Ganz

Miscellaneous
Access
Antecubital/internal jugular/subclavian veins
Acid–base
Glycemic control
  Chemstrips
  Humulin (subcutaneous)
Nutritional support
  Total parenteral nutrition/lipids?
  Fluid volume

POSTOPERATIVE CARE

It is particularly important that obese patients be mobilized as soon as possible after operation to prevent thromboembolism, atelectasis, and other pulmonary complications. Similarly, earliest possible extubation, adhering to stringent extubation criteria, helps to activate patients, promoting coughing and deep breathing. Having patients walk and perform knee bends within 4 hours of extubation significantly reduces the risk of postoperative pulmonary complications.

Early ambulation also has great psychologic importance for obese patients because they frequently are sedentary. When they realize that they are able to ambulate without excessive pain, it helps them to overcome their intrinsic fear of moving and the common tacit assumption that they must remain in bed. Postponing ambulation to the first postoperative day may disproportionately prolong the recuperative process and length of hospitalization.

Anecdotally, it seems as if patients who are mobilized early require less pain medication, although it is difficult to separate cause and effect. Nevertheless, pain medications and sedatives may have profound depressive effects on respiration in obese patients, who have marginal respiratory reserves. It is difficult to balance the requirement for increased doses of narcotics adjusted for increased body mass to facilitate beneficial ambulation against the risk of sedating patients and increasing the risk of hypercarbia, hypoxia, and acidosis.

SURGERY FOR OBESITY

Two main types of operations are performed to treat severe obesity (ie, a BMI of at least 40 or a BMI of at least 35 and severe comorbid conditions such as hypertension, diabetes, or pulmonary compromise). Gastric restriction limits the amount of food that is eaten and the rate at which it is consumed. Vertical banded gastroplasty and adjustable gastric banding are gastric restrictive operations. The other main type of surgery is a combination of restriction and bypass of varying lengths of the gastrointestinal tract, as in gastric bypass or "long-limb" gastric bypass.

These operations achieve medically significant weight loss in most patients who are followed up for 5 years or more. Typical results are losses of 40% to 45% of excess weight after gastric restriction and 55% to 65% after gastric bypass operations. Such operations should be undertaken only by surgeons who are committed to extensive patient education in an environment that is conducive to interdisciplinary collaboration. Many of the management principles outlined in this chapter have evolved from the practice of surgeons dedicated to the surgical treatment of medically significant obesity. The National Institutes of Health Consensus Development Conference on Gastrointestinal Surgery for Severe Obesity provides a recent extensive review of the topic.[51]

SUMMARY

Obesity is a prevalent disease in industrialized nations and is associated with numerous conditions that require operation. Obese patients are at greater risk for perioperative complications than are patients of normal weight. With proper perioperative evaluation and care, the risk of complications can be reduced so that obesity does not contraindicate necessary surgery. Identifying risk factors in obese patients, understanding the pathophysiology of obesity, and exhibiting compassion toward obese patients rather than the punitive attitude that is prevalent among health care practitioners will significantly enhance the quality of care these patients receive.

REFERENCES

1. Garrow JS. Treat obesity seriously: a clinical manual. London, Churchill Livingstone, 1981:1–249.
2. Gortmaker SL, Dietz WH, Sobol AM, Wehler A. Increasing pediatric obesity in the United States. Am J Dis Child 1987;141:535–540.
3. Kuczmarski RJ. Prevalence of overweight and weight gain in the United States. Am J Clin Nutr 1992;55(Suppl):495S–502S.
4. VanItallie TB. Health implications of overweight and obesity in the United States. Ann Intern Med 1985;103:983–988.
5. Stunkard A, Harris JR, Pedersen NL, McClearn GE. A separated twin study of the body mass index. N Engl J Med 1990;322:1483–1487.
6. Bouchard C, Tremblay A, Nadeau A, et al. Genetic effect in resting and exercise metabolic rates. Metabolism 1989;38:364–370.
7. NIH Technology Assessment Conference Panel. Methods for voluntary weight loss and control. Ann Intern Med 1992;116:942–949.
8. Law CM, Barker DJP, Osmond C, et al. Early growth and abdominal fatness in adult life. J Epidemiol Community Health 1992;46:184–186.
9. Sjostrom L. A CT based multicompartment body composition technique and anthropometric predictions of lean body mass, total and subcutaneous adipose tissue. Int J Obes 1991;15(Suppl 2):19–30.
10. Alexander JK. Obesity and cardiac performance. Am J Cardiol 1964;14:860–865.
11. Agarwal N, Shibutani K, SanFillipo J, et al. Hemodynamic and respiratory changes in surgery of the morbidly obese. Surgery 1982;92:226–234.

12. Zarich SW, Kowalchuk GJ, McGuire MP, et al. Left ventricular filling abnormalities in asymptomatic morbid obesity. Am J Cardiol 1991;68:377–381.

13. Tang S, Kral JG, Barnard JT, Pierson Jr RN. Android fat distribution predicts ventricular dysfunction in obese women. Eur J Clin Invest 1988;18:A10.

14. Alexander KL, Amad KH, Cole VW. Observations on some clinical features of extreme obesity with particular reference to the cardiorespiratory effects. Am J Med 1962;32:512–524.

15. Fadell EJ, Richman AD, Ward WW, Hendon JR. Fatty infiltration of respiratory muscles in the pickwickian syndrome. N Engl J Med 1962;266:861–863.

16. Dustan HP. Obesity and hypertension. Ann Intern Med 1985; 103:1047–1049.

17. Sugerman H. Pulmonary function in morbid obesity. Gastroenterol Clin North Am 1987;16:225–237.

18. Dejgard A, Andersen T, Gluud C. The influence of insulin on the raised plasma fibronectin concentration in human obesity. Acta Med Scand 1986;220:269–272.

19. Rillaerts E, Van Gaal L, Xiang DZ, et al. Blood viscosity in human obesity: relation to glucose tolerance and insulin status. Int J Obes 1989;13:739–745.

20. Cohen AH. Massive obesity and the kidney. Am J Pathol 1975; 81:117–130.

21. Carr S, Mbanya JC, Thomas T, et al. Increase in glomerular filtration rate in patients with insulin-dependent diabetes and elevated erythrocyte sodium-lithium countertransport. N Engl J Med 1990;322:500–505.

22. Schmeider RE, Messerli FH, Garavaglia G, Nunez B. Glomerular hyperfiltration indicates early target organ damage in essential hypertension. JAMA 1990;264:2775–2780.

23. Holley JL, Shapiro R, Lopatin WB, et al. Obesity as a risk factor following cadaveric renal transplantation. Transplantation 1990;49:387–389.

24. Gill IS, Hodge EE, Steinmuller DR, et al. The impact of obesity on renal transplantation. Transplant Proc 1992;25: 1047.

25. Merion RM, Twork AM, Rosenberg L, et al. Obesity and renal transplantation. Surg Gynecol Obstet 1991;172:367–376.

26. Waki M, Kral JG, Mazariegos M, et al. Relative expansion of extracellular fluid in obese versus non-obese women. Am J Physiol 1991;261:E199–E203.

27. Mazariegos M, Kral JG, Wang J, et al. Body composition and surgical treatment of obesity: effects of weight loss on fluid distribution. Ann Surg 1992;216:69–73.

28. Raison J, Achimastos A, Asmar R, et al. Extracellular and interstitial fluid volume in obesity with and without associated systemic hypertension. Am J Cardiol 1986;57:223–226.

29. De Fronzo RA, Cooke RE, Andres R. The effects of insulin on renal handling of sodium, potassium, calcium, and phosphate in man. J Clin Invest 1975;55:845–855.

30. Colt EWD, Wang J, Stallone F, et al. A possible low intracellular potassium in obesity. Am J Clin Nutr 1981;34:367–372.

31. Kral JG, Lundholm K, Sjostrom L, et al. Hepatic lipid metabolism in severe human obesity. Metabolism 1977;26:1025–1031.

32. Friedman JE, Dohm GL, Leggett-Frazier N, et al. Restoration of insulin responsiveness in skeletal muscle of morbidly obese patients after weight loss: effect on muscle glucose transport and glucose transporter GLUT4. J Clin Invest 1992;89:701–705.

33. Pories WJ, MacDonald Jr KG, Flickinger EG, et al. Is type II diabetes mellitus (NIDDM) a surgical disease? Ann Surg 1992; 215:633–643.

34. Weber DJ, Rutala WA, Samsa GP, et al. Impaired immunogenicity of hepatitis B vaccine in obese persons. (Letter) N Engl J Med 1986;314:1393.

35. Krishnan EC, Trost L, Aarons S, et al. Study of function and maturation of monocytes in morbidly obese individuals. J Surg Res 1982;33:89–97.

36. Kolterman OG, Olefsky JM, Kurakara C, et al. A defect in cell-mediated immune function in insulin-resistant diabetic and obese subjects. J Lab Clin Med 1980;96:535–543.

37. Drenick EJ, Fisler JS. Sudden cardiac arrest in morbidly obese surgical patients unexplained after autopsy. Am J Surg 1988; 155:720–726.

38. Isner JM, Sours HE, Paris AL, et al. Sudden unexpected death in avid dieters using the liquid-protein modified-fast diet: observations in 17 patients and the role of the prolonged Q-T interval. Circulation 1979;60:1401–1412.

39. Drenick EJ, Blumfield DE, Fisler JS, Lowy S. Cardiac function during very low calorie reducing diets with dietary protein of good and poor nutritional quality. In: Blackburn GL, Bray GA, eds. Management of obesity by severe caloric restriction. Littleton, MA, PSG Publishing, 1985:223–234.

40. Messerli H, Ventura HO, Elizardi DJ, et al. Hypertension and sudden death: increased ventricular ectopic activity in left ventricular hypertrophy. Am J Med 1984;77:18–22.

41. Messerli FH, Nunez BD, Ventura HO, Snyder DW. Overweight and sudden death: increased ventricular ectopy in cardiopathy of obesity. Arch Intern Med 1987;147:1725–1728.

42. Ernst E, Hammerschmidt DE, Bagge U, et al. Leukocytes and the risk of ischemic diseases. JAMA 1987;257:2318–2324.

43. Palmer M, Schaffner F. Effect of weight reduction on hepatic abnormalities in overweight patients. Gastroenterology 1990; 99:1408–1413.

44. Vaughan RW. Biochemical and biotransformation alterations in the obese. In: Brown BR Jr, ed. Anesthesia and the obese patient. Philadelphia, FA Davis Co, 1982:55.

45. Terry BE. Morbid obesity: cardiac evaluation and function. Gastroenterol Clin North Am 1987;16:215–223.

46. Criqui MH, Heiss G, Cohn R, et al. Plasma triglyceride level and mortality from coronary heart disease. N Engl J Med 1993;328:1220–1225.

47. Bern MM, Bothe Jr A, Bistrian B, et al. Effects of low-dose warfarin on antithrombin III levels in morbidly obese patients. Surgery 1983;94:78–83.

48. Janvrin SB, Davies G, Greenhalgh RM. Postoperative deep vein thrombosis caused by intravenous fluids during surgery. Br J Surg 1980;67:690–693.

49. Vaughan RW. Anesthesia and morbid obesity. In: Bjorntorp B, Brodoff JB, eds. Obesity. Philadelphia, JB Lippincott Co, 1992: 720–730.

50. Brown Jr BR, ed. Anesthesia and the obese patient. Philadelphia, FA Davis, 1982.

51. NIH Consensus Development Conference. Gastrointestinal surgery for severe obesity. Am J Clin Nutr 1992;55(Suppl 2): 487S–619S.

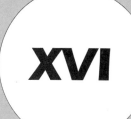

PSYCHIATRIC DISORDERS

Medical Management of the Surgical Patient, Third Edition,
edited by Michael F. Lubin, H. Kenneth Walker, and Robert B. Smith III.
J.B. Lippincott Company, Philadelphia, PA © 1995.

CHAPTER

44

PSYCHOLOGIC AND EMOTIONAL REACTIONS TO ILLNESS AND SURGERY

Alan Stoudemire

Patients who are faced with major physical illness and surgery are beset by numerous basic stresses that may challenge their psychologic equilibrium. Patients not only anticipate and fear the prospect of pain, disability, and perhaps even death but must struggle with other stresses that may threaten their sense of personal control, autonomy, identity, and independence. Patients who are admitted to hospitals suddenly enter highly regimented bureaucratic and technologically oriented systems over which they have little control and do not fully understand. Their personal and physical privacy is suddenly invaded by questions, examinations, and procedures. Patients must temporarily relinquish a great deal of control over their lives to the hospital routine, which they may find bewildering, confusing, anxiety provoking, and at times even humiliating.

In addition, patients are separated from their loved ones and family and may be geographically far away from home. Elderly patients in particular may not have family readily available, and older patients with cognitive impairment may become confused, disoriented, and agitated. Patients may face considerable financial strain if their insurance coverage is limited or if they will be out of work. Finally, uncertainty about the diagnosis and prognosis of their condition may exacerbate the anxiety and fear that patients experience.

Patients who are facing extensive surgical procedures that involve ostomy formation or amputation, or other types of surgery that result in some form of disfigurement are concerned about their appearance and body image, and about the way in which the surgery will affect their sexual functioning and attractiveness. For example, women undergoing mastectomy may fear losing love and sexual desirability. Patients undergoing ostomy placement may react to surgery by fearing that they will appear ugly and repulsive, and will be rejected. Patients undergoing urologic procedures may face the prospect of sexual dysfunction or impotence. Grief reactions manifested by depressive symptoms may be encountered as patients "mourn" the loss of body image, body parts, or physical functioning and mobility.

The reaction to these stresses varies among patients and depends on several factors, including preexisting psychologic strength, amount of family support available, financial resources, type and extent of illness, surgical procedures involved, and overall prognosis. Despite the stressful nature of illness, hospitalization, and surgery, most patients may be expected to do well. Physicians should be alert, however, for signs and symptoms suggesting that a patient's ability to adapt to the stress of illness is being overwhelmed, indicating some degree of psychologic decompensation.

BEHAVIORAL REGRESSION

A helpful concept to consider in assessing psychologic reactions to illness, particularly when they appear to be maladaptive or pathologic, is the concept of behavioral "regres-

427

sion." Regression means that patients, in reaction to the stress of illness and accompanying enforced dependency on others, may resort to more infantile or childlike ways of thinking, feeling, and behaving. In most situations, this period of regression is limited, as patients recover or adapt to their illnesses. Under certain circumstances, however, patients may undergo more severe and prolonged regression, particularly those with preexisting psychiatric disorders, marginal abilities to cope under severe stress, or little or no social support. Regressive behavior is characterized by withdrawal, helplessness, clinging, excessive dependency, and fear. Patients may also whine and complain, and be angry, irritable, and demanding. Serious forms of regression may lead to profound emotional withdrawal, passivity, depression, and, occasionally, overtly psychotic behavior. Even the strongest and most psychologically healthy person may at times be overwhelmed emotionally in the context of severe and overwhelming stress, resulting in regressive forms of behavior.

Understanding the concept of behavioral regression under stress and its behavioral manifestations is helpful in understanding the physician's role in managing such reactions. Because regression involves the display of frightened and childlike behavior, patients' reactions to physicians may resemble those of children to frustrating parents because physicians, in the view of patients, may take on the roles of powerful and authoritative parent figures. Although such dependency may make some patients compliant with treatment and thankful for physicians' help, other reactions may occur that are much more difficult for physicians to manage. Patients may displace their anger, fear, and frustration onto physicians and become resistant, difficult, defiant, ungrateful, and critical; they may even threaten litigation. Although reasonable limits should be set on such behavior, physicians ideally should attempt to help patients understand the feelings that usually underlie such behavior and empathize with those feelings as much as possible rather than respond with anger and defensiveness.

Physicians must give steady and consistent emotional support to patients who are in regressive emotional turmoil by providing information, advice, encouragement, and realistic reassurance. These efforts, termed *ego support*, are directed toward preventing extensive behavioral regression by suppressing anxiety and strengthening patients' psychologic defenses and coping mechanisms. Severe regression should be prevented by encouraging patients to pursue rehabilitation efforts, helping them to become as independent as possible, and allowing them to participate as much as is reasonable in decisions regarding their care. The last approach gives patients some sense of control over their treatment.

One of the more common difficulties for physicians is patients who exhibit profound emotional reactions to an illness such as crying or becoming deeply depressed, helpless, and dependent. Physicians who are uncomfortable with these types of intense emotion may actively discourage patients from talking about their feelings, avoid such patients, or offer unrealistic, patronizing reassurance. Such intense emotions, however, are often best handled by allowing carefully titrated brief periods of catharsis (allowing patients to "ventilate," "blow off steam," or cry) and by empathizing with patients' feelings. Such periods of emotional catharsis are usually transient and provide relief for patients. Patients may also be relieved that physicians are interested and open to their feelings. Severe regressive behaviors that are persistent or accompanied by evidence of severe depression, anxiety, or significant psychopathologic reactions (particularly those that create conflict or tension in the doctor-patient relationship) are indications for psychiatric referral.[1]

IDENTIFICATION OF HIGH-RISK GROUPS

Several characteristics place patients at relatively higher risk for the development of psychiatric complications during illness or surgery. Although no particular patient profile is totally predictive, there are criteria for identifying and monitoring high-risk patients.

Groups of psychologically high-risk patients have been delineated by Baudry and Weiner[2] and subsequently developed by Strain.[3] High-risk groups include the following:

- Patients with histories of psychotic decompensation (including delirium) or psychiatric consultation during previous physical illnesses or surgeries
- Patients who refuse or are resistant to undergo surgery either through threatening to leave the hospital against medical advice or refusing to sign a consent form
- Patients with histories of difficult and hostile relationships with nursing and medical or surgical staff
- Patients with unrealistic or magical expectations of their surgery (excessive denial)
- Patients who present special diagnostic problems, such as histories of multiple surgeries for questionable or vague indications with negative results (malingering, hysterical, factitious, or hypochondriacal patients)
- Patients who show blasé, apathetic reactions or a lack of appropriate concern and anxiety.

To these, I would add:

- Patients with histories of alcohol and substance abuse or those who are taking multiple psychotropic or analgesic agents
- Elderly patients with cognitive impairment (who are at risk for postoperative delirium)

- Patients with histories of medical litigation or questionable disability suits
- Patients with histories of chronic pain complaints of obscure cause

VALUE OF PREOPERATIVE PSYCHOLOGIC ASSESSMENT

Numerous studies have demonstrated the potential value of preoperative preparation of patients to promote increased tolerance to the stresses of the surgical procedure.[3] Educational efforts provide patients with information that helps them anticipate surgery and tend to diminish uncertainty and alleviate anxiety. Patients who receive information and are familiar with the staff and the medical–surgical routine are better able to anticipate and prepare for whatever discomfort the procedure may entail. Such preparation is particularly important for children. In two studies, preoperative preparation by the anesthesiology staff resulted in a reduction in requests for narcotics and earlier discharge from the hospital among the patients involved compared with other patients.[4,5] Other investigators have reported decreased postoperative delirium in groups of patients who received preoperative preparation by a psychiatrist.[6,7] Several additional studies have claimed improved recovery rates in patients who received instruction designed to facilitate coping with the stress of surgery.[8,9] Although surgeons may have a limited amount of time to devote to extensive educational efforts, some programs can be administered by ancillary medical or nursing personnel with the aid of audiovisual guides.

Although significant methodologic problems exist for most studies that claim effectiveness of psychiatric and behavioral interventions in improving postoperative outcomes (primarily pertaining to control of multiple variables that could affect outcome, matching of appropriate control subjects, standardization of interventions, objective rating of results, and pressure from third-party carriers for early discharge), data suggest that appropriate screening and evaluation of high-risk patients and provision of adequate information to decrease anticipatory anxiety and postoperative confusion will yield therapeutic benefits and perhaps decrease the likelihood of major psychiatric complications.

REFERENCES

1. Green SA. Principles of medical psychotherapy. In: Stoudemire A, Fogel BS, eds. Psychiatric care of the medical patient. New York, Oxford University Press, 1993:3–18.
2. Baudry F, Weiner A. The surgical patient. In: Strain J, Grossman S, eds. Psychological care of the medically ill: a primer in liaison psychiatry. New York, Appleton-Century-Crofts, 1975: 123–137.
3. Strain J. The surgical patient. In: Cavenar J, ed. Psychiatry. Philadelphia, JB Lippincott, 1986:1–11.
4. Egbert LD, Battit GE, Welch CD, Bartlett MK. Reduction of postoperative pain by encouragement and instruction of patient. N Engl J Med 1964;270:825–827.
5. Egbert LD, Bartlet GE, Taldorf H, Beecher HK. The value of preoperative visits by the anesthetist. JAMA 1963;185:553–555.
6. Layne OL Jr, Yudofsky SC. Postoperative psychosis in cardiotomy patients: the role of organic and psychiatric factors. N Engl J Med 1971;284:518–520.
7. Lazarus HR, Hagens TH. Prevention of psychosis following open-heart surgery. Am J Psychiatry 1968;124:1190–1195.
8. Andrew JM. Recovery from surgery, with and without preparatory instruction, for three coping styles. J Pers Soc Psychol 1970;15:223–226.
9. Reading AE. The short-term effects of psychological preparation for surgery. Soc Sci Med 1979;13A:641–654.

Medical Management of the Surgical Patient, Third Edition,
edited by Michael F. Lubin, H. Kenneth Walker, and Robert B. Smith III.
J.B. Lippincott Company, Philadelphia, PA © 1995.

CHAPTER

45

DEPRESSION

Alan Stoudemire

Along with delirium, depressive disorders are the most common psychiatric problems seen in medical–surgical patients. The causes of depression in medically ill patients may be multiple but important issues include dealing with loss; helplessness; chronic disability and pain; injuries to self-esteem; and financial, marital, or interpersonal strain after illness. In some instances, depressive symptoms can result from underlying physical illness (eg, hypothyroidism, occult pancreatic carcinoma) or be induced by medications (eg, reserpine).

The issue of loss tends to be a recurrent theme in many depressed patients. Patients may perceive the loss of a body part (amputation, mastectomy); sexual functioning (spinal cord injury, radical prostatectomy); bodily function (ostomy placement); or body image (burns). The progressive loss of autonomy, independence, and control over one's life that physical illness brings can lead to depression. Self-esteem can be damaged if patients perceive themselves as unattractive or unproductive. Patients who feel helpless and overwhelmed by an inability to control, predict, or master the consequences of their illnesses may become passive, withdrawn, and resigned. Alternately, they may react with embittered anger and hostility.

The financial stress induced by illness also brings with it a certain degree of depression, especially if financial strain makes patients feel they are a burden to their families or will never recover from illness-induced indebtedness. The stress of illness brings tension to marital and family relationships, estranging some patients from their loved ones. In searching for the psychologic precipitants of depression, physicians must look beyond the immediate circumstances of patients' illnesses to evaluate the extent of their abilities to cope with the many stresses of illness, the amount of family support available, the degree of financial and occupational strain, and other conflicts, pressures, or losses with which they may be struggling.

Most depressive reactions in medical–surgical patients are relatively short, resolve after surgery, and do not cause major disturbances in social, occupational, interpersonal, physical, or psychologic functioning. In some cases, however, depressive symptoms may not resolve and may deteriorate into what is now termed *major depression*. Major depression is the new term for what was previously referred to as endogenous or melancholic depression. It is characterized by markedly dysphoric mood and the inability to derive pleasure in life, or a loss of interest in life. The mood disturbance usually significantly disrupts patients' occupational, social, and interpersonal functioning.

Physical or "vegetative" symptoms can include sleep disturbances (often fragmented sleep with early morning awakening), appetite disturbance (loss or increase in appetite), weight changes (usually weight loss), crying spells, fatigue, lassitude, irritability, constipation, decreased sexual interest, and impotence. Self-esteem is usually low. Patients are pessimistic about the future and may be cynical, bitter, and angry. Feelings of hopelessness, helplessness, and guilt may abound. Patients may have suicidal thoughts and perhaps overt plans. Cognitive functioning may be affected, especially in the elderly, and can resemble dementia, a condition that is termed *depressive pseudodementia* and that is marked primarily by problems with attention, concentration, and memory.[1,2] Other common symptoms include marked anorexia, weight loss, disinterest, apathy, and guilty ruminations, a form of depression formerly categorized as melancholic. Some patients progress to psychotic proportions with paranoia, hallucinations, delusions of guilt, somatic delusions (often involving the delusion of having venereal diseases including the acquired immunodeficiency syndrome), and obsessive-compulsive behavior. Such depression is termed major depression with psychotic features.

Sometimes depression is masked by patients' denial or limited ability to verbalize their feelings. Patients with limited cultural and educational backgrounds, and particularly the elderly, may have "somatizing" depression and a host of complaints referable to almost every organ system (eg, headaches, nausea, gastrointestinal distress, and muscle aches and pains) in addition to the classic neurovegetative symptoms of depression. This somatic form of depression may be the predominant way in which most patients present with mood disturbance in the primary care setting. Physicians should not tacitly accept patients' denial that they are depressed as excluding the diagnosis. After a reasonable medical evaluation has been done to rule out an organic cause for patients' physical complaints, a therapeutic trial of antidepressant medication may be in order.

ASSESSMENT OF SUICIDE RISK

One of the myths surrounding the assessment of suicide risk in depressed patients is that asking about suicidal ideation will bring the idea to patients' minds, thereby increasing the chance of suicide. Actually, the opposite is true: openly broaching the subject of suicide and allowing patients to express their possible motives, ideas, and specific plans is the best way to defuse a planned or potential suicide attempt. Therefore, open, thorough, and detailed questioning regarding suicidal ideation should be a part of every assessment of a depressed patient.

Several factors may help identify patients who are at higher risk for suicidal intention. Older men and persons who live alone, have suffered a recent major loss, have a chronic debilitating illness (eg, renal disease requiring dialysis), or have a previous history of depression and suicidal attempts are of special concern. Women tend to attempt suicide more often but men more often succeed in their attempts. Table 45-1 lists major risk factors for suicide.[3]

Questioning of the family is crucial because the most se-

TABLE 45–1. Major Risk Factors for Suicide

Older, divorced, or widowed men
Whites
Unemployment
Poor physical health
Past suicide attempts
Family history of suicide, especially parent
Psychosis
Alcoholism or drug abuse
Chronic, painful disease
Sudden life changes
Living alone
Anniversary of significant loss

(Dubin WR. Psychiatric emergencies: recognition and management. In: Stoudemire A, ed. Clinical psychiatry for medical students. Philadelphia, JB Lippincott, 1990:513)

riously suicidal patients are those who may have already made up their minds and are determined that no one intervene. Patients who begin to set their affairs in order, make out a will, and suddenly "get better" inexplicably (because they feel they finally have figured a way out of their situation) should be evaluated carefully. In direct questioning of patients, it is important to be specific in asking about the method of suicide; plans involving guns, hanging, or carbon monoxide leave little chance for rescue or recovery. Patients who have schizophrenia or brain syndromes (eg, delirium, dementia) and those who abuse alcohol or drugs are more likely to commit suicide because of impaired judgment and impulsiveness. Depressed patients, particularly those with excessive guilt, low self-esteem, and feelings of helplessness and hopelessness, are at extremely high risk.

If a significant suicidal risk exists, immediate psychiatric consultation is indicated before patients are discharged from the hospital. Mobilization of family, friends, or significant others is also important so that patients are not left alone until a psychiatric assessment and disposition can be arranged. The broad grounds for psychiatric commitment usually state that patients must have a mental illness and be dangerous to themselves or to others, or be too gravely incapacitated to care for themselves. Commitment codes and procedures vary among states, and psychiatric consultation is advised before pursuing commitment procedures. Table 45-2 lists criteria for hospital admission for suicidal patients.

PAIN AND DEPRESSION

In general, especially in the acute surgical setting, pain medications tend to be underused. Terminally ill patients are sometimes undermedicated as well. The reasons for un-

TABLE 45–2. Criteria for Hospital Admission for Suicidal Patients

Patients show no improvement with medication and interviews.

Patients improve but remain so psychotic that they cannot care for their daily needs (ie, work, housing, grooming).

Patients pose a physical threat to themselves or others.

Patients are having command hallucinations.

Physicians are in doubt about the severity of the condition.

Patients are toxic from drugs, alcohol, or prescribed medications.

Patients are psychotic and have exhausted caregivers or all sources of external support.

(Dubin WR. Psychiatric emergencies: recognition and management. In: Stoudemire A, ed. Clinical psychiatry for medical students. Philadelphia, JB Lippincott, 1990:512)

dermedication include exaggerated fear of addiction, underestimation of effective unit doses, and overestimation of the duration of narcotic action.[4] Actually, there is little likelihood of addiction in patients who are experiencing acute postoperative pain unless there is a history of narcotic abuse or a severe personality disorder. Addiction should not be a concern in terminally ill patients.[5]

A brief note should be made of the possible drug interactions between narcotics and other psychotropic agents. Concurrent use of antipsychotic agents in patients receiving haloperidol and thiothixene for delirium tends to enhance the effects of narcotics and sedative-hypnotics. The respiratory depressant effect of narcotics is increased by the concurrent use of antipsychotics and sedative-hypnotics. In the treatment of pain, however, if respiratory depression is not a particular concern, antipsychotic and narcotic drugs tend to have a synergistic effect on pain suppression.

The relationship between pain, particularly chronic pain, and depression is a question that arises frequently in medical–surgical patients. High rates of pain complaints attributable to almost every organ system have been observed in depressed patients (eg, headaches, abdominal pain, joint pain, back pain, and chest pain).[6] Somatic pain complaints in the presence of an obviously depressed mood have been described as masked depression and the symptoms as depressive equivalents.

Clinicians have also noted the high frequency of depressive complaints among patients with chronic pain (sleep disturbance, appetite changes, irritability, decreased libido, social withdrawal, and somatic preoccupation). Whether this symptom constellation constitutes true clinical depression is a matter of controversy. Arguments in this area soon become circular: chronic pain may be accompanied by a plethora of somatic and vegetative features, and patients with primary depressive disorders are often plagued by many pain complaints. Chronic pain can cause significant reactive depression, and primary depressions can lead to chronic pain behavior.[7]

Patients seen at pain clinics tend to be a highly heterogenous group. They may vary in the degree to which demonstrable organic pathologic states are present. Pain is a subjective phenomenon, and the manner in which patients deal with chronic pain depends on psychologic coping mechanisms, earlier developmental experiences in coping with illness and pain, socioeconomic factors, and underlying biologic factors such as vulnerability to depression. Some patients may have depression with pain complaints as the somatic manifestation of the mood disorder, whereas other patients have secondary depression induced by the chronic stress of pain. The matter is confounded further by the fact that many of these disorders overlap to some degree. Invariably, however, if major depression is the basis for patients' pain complaints or amplifies their symptoms, antidepressant therapy will result in improved mood and diminished pain.[7,8] Whether antidepressant agents elevate mood or have a direct analgesic effect is not fully understood because common biochemical mechanisms have been postulated for coexisting pain and depressive syndromes, probably through simultaneous effects on biogenic amines and enkephalins. The treatment of acute and chronic pain in medical patients is reviewed in more detail elsewhere.[5,9]

SECONDARY MOOD DISORDERS

Medical conditions and medications may induce depression or mimic symptoms of depression. This possibility should be ruled out before a patient's condition is attributed to a purely psychiatric cause. Medications that have been implicated in inducing mood disorders include steroids, reserpine, α-methyldopa, propranolol, carbonic anhydrase inhibitors, and the long-term use and abuse of sedative-hypnotics, benzodiazepines, and narcotics. More recent data, however, have questioned whether β-blockers such as propranolol actually induce depression, although idiosyncratic reactions remain possible.

Medical conditions, particularly those that are insidious, may also present as depression. Illnesses that tend to present in this manner include endocrinopathies (eg, Cushing's syndrome, hypothyroidism, hypocalcemia, hypercalcemia); occult cancers (eg, lymphoma, pancreatic carcinoma, glioma); hepatitis; and mononucleosis. A basic history and physical examination with screening laboratory tests rules out most organic mood syndromes if physicians are sensitive to these diagnostic possibilities. Table 45-3 lists the major causes of secondary depressive disorders in medical patients.[10]

TABLE 45–3. Major Causes of Depressive Disorders in Medical Patients Due to Medications and General Medical Conditions

Medications
Antihypertensives (reserpine, methyldopa, propranolol)
Barbiturates
Corticosteroids
Guanethidine
Indomethacin
Levodopa
Psychostimulants (amphetamine and cocaine in the postwithdrawal phase)

Medical Illnesses
Carcinoid syndrome
Carcinomas (pancreatic)
Cerebrovascular disease (stroke)
Collagen vascular disease (systemic lupus erythematosus)
Endocrinopathies (Cushing's syndrome, Addison's disease, hypoglycemia, hypercalcemia and hypocalcemia, hyperthyroidism and hypothyroidism)
Lymphomas
Parkinson's disease
Pernicious anemia (vitamin B_{12} deficiency)
Viral illnesses (hepatitis, mononucleosis, influenza)

(Stoudemire A. Organic mental disorders. In: Stoudemire A, ed. Clinical psychiatry for medical students. Philadelphia, JB Lippincott, 1990:75)

INDICATIONS FOR PSYCHOPHARMACOLOGIC TREATMENT OF DEPRESSION

Indications for the use of antidepressant drugs are clearest in patients with symptoms of major depression. Prominent somatic or vegetative signs and symptoms in addition to profound mood disturbance are relatively clear indications of an underlying biologic disruption in central nervous system mood regulation. Other clinical indications that depression may have a biologic determinant include a previous history of depression or recurrent depression, a previous response to antidepressant or electroconvulsive therapy (ECT), and a family history of depression or suicide. All patients who respond to antidepressants, however, do not necessarily have prominent somatic features and may be plagued by severe cognitive signs of depression (low self-esteem, guilt, uncertainty, pessimism, and suicidal thoughts) in addition to their dysphoric mood. These patients may benefit from a trial of drug treatment as well.

In the early 1980s, a version of the dexamethasone suppression test was evaluated as a diagnostic probe for the diagnosis of depression.[11] In its most simple form, dexamethasone is given in a dose of 1 mg at 11:00 PM, and serum cortisol levels are drawn that same day at 4:00 PM and the next day at 4:00 PM. Nonsuppression, usually defined as failure to suppress cortisol below 5 µg/mL, correlates with

the diagnosis of melancholia and suggests a strong biologic component to the depressive disorder. The associated neuroendocrine disorder has been theoretically related to a disinhibition of the hypothalamic-pituitary-adrenal axis, possibly because of central neurotransmitter effects. The sensitivity of the test has been reported to be 50% to 60% (indicating a high number of false-negative results) and the specificity to be 90% to 95% (indicating a low number of false-positive results). The test may be confounded by almost any major medical illness (eg, heart failure, renal failure, liver disease, fever) and by barbiturate, phenytoin, carbamazepine, steroid, or benzodiazepine use. As a result, this test has almost no real use in a medically ill population and, even under ideal circumstances, is limited by low sensitivity. In general, the dexamethasone test should not be used for the diagnosis of depression outside of research settings.

The pharmaceutical armamentarium of antidepressant agents includes the cyclic antidepressants; monoamine oxidase (MAO) inhibitors; and, in patients with bipolar affective disorder (manic-depressive illness), lithium carbonate, carbamazepine, and sodium valproate. The cyclic antidepressants are the drugs of choice. MAO inhibitors, lithium, carbamazepine, and valproate are primarily used by psychiatrists to treat mood disorders. The cyclic antidepressants include the traditional tricyclics such as amitriptyline and imipramine; selective serotonin reuptake inhibitors include fluoxetine (Prozac) and sertraline (Zoloft).

The dose ranges and general properties of the cyclic antidepressants are shown in Table 45-4 but the average maintenance dosage for most tricyclic antidepressants is between 75 and 150 mg/d. Prominent exceptions include trazodone (Desyrel), for which the maintenance dosage may range from 300 to 600 mg/d, and protriptyline, for which the average daily dosage is 40 mg/d.

In general, therapy with tricyclics such as nortriptyline (Pamelor) should be started at low bedtime dosages (25 mg) and gradually increased every third night over 10 to 14 days to a maintenance dosage of about 75 to 150 mg/d (with the exceptions noted earlier). Although more rapid dosing is possible, this regimen allows patients more time to adapt to side effects. If adverse drug effects are experienced too suddenly as a result of rapid loading, patients may stop taking the medication. Elderly patients usually require lower maintenance dosages because of their sensitivity to side effects. Fluoxetine therapy is usually begun at a dosage of 10 to 20 mg every morning because of its activating effect, although about 15% of patients experience a sedative effect with this drug and prefer to take it at night. If patients do not respond to fluoxetine after 4 weeks of therapy, the dosage may be increased to 40 mg/d. Because of its long half-life (8 to 12 days for its principal metabolite), fluoxetine takes 3 to 4 weeks to reach steady-state levels.

Sertraline (Zoloft) administration is begun at a dosage of

TABLE 45–4. Properties of Selected Cyclic Antidepressants*

Agent	Effect on Serotonin Reuptake	Effect on Norepinephrine Reuptake	Sedating Effect	Anticholinergic Effect	Orthostatic Effect	Dose Range[¶] (mg)
Amitriptyline[†]	++++	++	++++	++++	++++	75–300
Imipramine[†]	++++	++	+++	+++	++++	75–300
Nortriptyline	+++	+++	++	++	+	40–150
Protriptyline	+++	++++	+	+++	+	10–60
Trazodone	+++	±	+++	±[‡]	++	200–600
Desipramine	+++	++++	+	+	++	75–150
Amoxapine[§]	++	+++	++	++	++	75–600
Maprotiline	+	++	++	+	++	150–200
Doxepin	+++	++	+++	++	++	75–300
Trimipramine[§]	+	+	++	++	++	50–300
Fluoxetine	++++	–	–	–	–	20–60
Sertraline	++++	–	–	–	–	50–200
Bupropion	–	–	–	±	–	150–450

–, none; +, slight; ++, moderate; +++, marked; ++++, pronounced; ±, indeterminant.
*Relative potencies (some ratings are approximated) based partly on affinities of these agents for brain receptors in competitive binding studies (Richelson E. Pharmacology of antidepressants in use in the United States. Clin Psychiatry 1982;43:4–11).
[†]Available in injectable form.
[‡]Most in vivo and clinical studies report the absence of anticholinergic effects (or no difference from placebo). There have been case reports, however, of apparent anticholinergic effects.
[§]Amoxapine and trimipramine have dopamine receptor–blocking activity.
[¶]Dose ranges are for treatment of major depression. Lower doses may be appropriate for other therapeutic uses. Lower and middle dose ranges are those recommended in the general medical setting.
(Stoudemire A, Fogel BS, Gulley LR, Moran MG. Psychopharmacology in the medically ill. In: Stoudemire A, Fogel BS, eds. Psychiatric care of the medical patient. New York, Oxford University Press, 1993:160)

25 to 50 mg each morning but may be increased over 4 to 6 weeks up to 200 mg/d. Most patients respond at dosages between 50 and 100 mg. Because of its short half-life of 24 hours, steady-state levels are reached within a week. Bupropion (Wellbutrin) is a new drug with structural similarities to amphetamines and a short half-life that must be taken three times a day. Bupropion is contraindicated in patients at risk for seizures.

A lag time of 3 to 4 weeks may be seen before a true mood-elevating effect is achieved with these drugs, and patients should be counseled not to expect overnight improvement. Improvements in certain biologic abnormalities, such as sleep disturbance, agitation, and anxiety, may be seen early on and precede the onset of antidepressant activity. Sleep improvement, in particular, is an excellent parameter to monitor for response to treatment and to assess whether the dosage is sufficient.

The ideal duration of therapy with these drugs after an effective antidepressant effect has been achieved is unclear, although the general consensus is that antidepressant medication should be administered for 6 to 12 months and then gradually tapered, observing for signs of relapse. Psychotherapy or some form of counseling to address the conflicts, stresses, or other precipitants that caused the depression also usually is necessary, although this may be relatively brief and confined to the early stages of treatment.

SIDE EFFECTS

The most bothersome side effects of tricyclic antidepressants such as nortriptyline are anticholinergic in nature and similar to, but more pronounced than, the anticholinergic side effects described for the antipsychotic drugs. The relative anticholinergic potential and sedating side effects of the cyclic antidepressants are listed in Table 45-4. Trazodone has been described as being devoid of anticholinergic side effects but may cause priapism and urinary retention in men, although this is uncommon. Fluoxetine, sertraline, and bupropion offer major advantages in the medically ill because they lack anticholinergic, orthostatic, and quinidine-like side effects.

The hypotensive effects of the older tricyclic antidepressants, such as amitriptyline, are often a primary concern and frequently limit or contraindicate their use in elderly patients, who are most prone to the development of orthostatic hypotension. One of the better predictors for the development of orthostatic hypotension is the degree of orthostatic hypertension that is present before treatment. Although orthostatic effects can be partly offset by slow, low dosing, the development of hypotension that may precipitate falls and cerebrovascular and cardiac events may prohibit the achievement of therapeutic drug levels.

Demethylated or secondary tricyclic antidepressants such as nortriptyline are less likely to cause orthostatic hypertension than are amitriptyline (Elavil) and imipramine (Tofranil). It is difficult to predict the degree of orthostatic hypotension that may develop with any of these drugs, however, and patients at high risk (particularly the elderly) should be monitored in the hospital until stable levels are reached, a noticeable therapeutic response is achieved, and blood pressure remains stable. Patients with impaired left ventricular function are particularly prone to the development of orthostatic hypotension with tricyclic antidepressant therapy but not with the newer agents fluoxetine, sertraline, and bupropion.[12] Patients with congestive heart failure or liver failure usually require reduced dosages.

Problems may also arise in patients with cardiovascular disease, particularly those with conduction delays. On the electrocardiogram, the tricyclic antidepressants as a group tend to increase the PR interval, QRS duration, and QT$_c$ time, and to flatten the T wave. In patients with preexisting bundle branch block or in cases of overdose, high degrees of atrioventricular block may develop. Patients with conduction delays, therefore, may progress to higher degrees of bundle branch block. Tricyclics have a quinidine-like effect on the heart and, thus, tend to increase conduction time. If type I antiarrhythmic agents (eg, procainamide, disopyramide) are used concurrently with tricyclic antidepressants, effects on conduction may be additive. As a serendipitous effect, premature ventricular contractions can be expected to decrease with treatment, particularly with imipramine.[13] As noted earlier, fluoxetine, sertraline, and bupropion do not have significant effects on cardiac conduction.

The other area of importance in considering the effects of tricyclic antidepressants on the heart concerns the potential exacerbation of congestive heart failure. Recent studies have demonstrated, however, that even in the presence of chronic heart disease, patients can be treated relatively safely without adverse effects on rhythm or hemodynamic function unless myocardial performance is severely impaired or patients are highly unstable or decompensating.[13]

Other side effects of interest are a tendency of tricyclic antidepressants to block the antihypertensive effects of guanethidine, methyldopa, and clonidine, and to potentiate the hypotensive effect of prazosin. The cyclic antidepressants may inhibit the metabolism of anticoagulants, leading to increased prothrombin times. Therefore, a clear distinction should be made between the older tricyclic class of drugs and the newer drugs such as fluoxetine, paroxetine, sertraline (all selective serotonin reuptake inhibitors), and

bupropion. The latter drugs, which lack anticholinergic, quinidine-like, and orthostatic hypotensive side effects, are generally much safer to use in medically frail patients.

Both antipsychotic and antidepressant agents are metabolized by the cytochrome P-450 system, which is present in diseased as well as healthy hepatic tissue.[14] Dosages of cyclic antidepressants in patients with liver disease are generally the same as in other patients, although downward adjustments may be necessary in advanced disease. Serum levels are helpful in monitoring patients with liver disease and congestive heart failure, in whom drug levels may be increased. Because of their anticholinergic effects, tricyclic antidepressants may induce narrow-angle glaucoma crisis, delay gastric emptying, and exacerbate symptoms in patients with dysphagia. Most antidepressants have the capacity to lower the seizure threshold in patients with seizure disorders, but exacerbation of seizures is usually not a problem if seizures are under good control and therapeutic levels of anticonvulsant agents are maintained. The only exception is bupropion (Wellbutrin), which has a seizure frequency up to three times higher (4:1000) than that of other antidepressants and is contraindicated in patients with epilepsy or other risk factors for seizures (eg, head trauma). Cigarette smoking and the use of oral contraceptives, alcohol, and barbiturates lower antidepressant levels through hepatic enzyme induction.

Although the specific uses and indications for MAO inhibitors and lithium carbonate are not discussed here, several aspects of these drugs that may be pertinent to the medical–surgical evaluation of patients taking these drugs are considered briefly.

The MAO inhibitors may be used in the medical population but should not be given to patients who are taking guanethidine or sympathomimetic agents of any kind (eg, methylphenidate, metaraminol, ephedrine, phenylpropanolamine, epinephrine) or to those who are using narcotics or alcohol. MAO inhibitors may also cause orthostatic hypotension.[15] In addition, patients with congestive heart failure, liver disease, or pheochromocytoma should be excluded from such therapy. These drugs also have anticholinergic and orthostatic hypotensive effects. The possible precipitation of hypertensive crisis through the ingestion of tyramine-containing foods is well known. Hypertensive reactions have been reported with the concurrent use of MAO inhibitors and reserpine and methyldopa.[16]

Lithium carbonate is indicated for patients with bipolar (manic-depressive) mood disorders. Lithium is excreted by the kidney, and rates of excretion are affected by advancing age and other conditions that alter renal blood flow. Renal function should be measured before treatment is initiated, and electrolyte studies, an electrocardiogram, and thyroid function tests should be performed. Lithium excretion decreases with advancing age, and lower dosages are sometimes required in older patients. Because the elderly can exhibit sensitivity to lithium's side effects, lithium toxicity may appear even at levels that are normal for younger patients. Lithium-induced electrocardiographic changes include inversion and flattening of the T wave. Sinus node dysfunction, sinoatrial block, and ventricular irritability have been described even at therapeutic blood levels, although such effects are extremely rare.[17]

Stimulants such as methylphenidate occasionally have been suggested for use in depressed medical patients, particularly those who cannot tolerate cyclic antidepressants and MAO inhibitors or who refuse ECT. The recommended dosage of methylphenidate is 10 mg twice daily.[18] These drugs may cause agitation, restlessness, insomnia, and rebound depression. They are used primarily in patients who refuse or cannot tolerate other modalities or in combination with narcotics to prevent excessive sedation in patients with intractable pain or limited life-spans.

USE OF ELECTROCONVULSIVE THERAPY IN THE MEDICALLY ILL

Electroconvulsive therapy is the treatment of choice for patients who cannot tolerate the side effects of antidepressants; who have psychotic, severely melancholic, delusional, severe obsessional depression; or who are so acutely suicidal that waiting for the lag time of the cyclic antidepressants to take effect would be dangerous. The only contraindications to ECT are the presence of central nervous system mass lesions, recent myocardial infarction, or a history of unstable malignant ventricular arrhythmia. Prolonged apnea may occur with severe liver disease or the use of phenelzine, lithium, and cholinesterase inhibitors. Severe chronic obstructive pulmonary disease may complicate ventilation and respiratory recovery. Patients previously treated with MAO inhibitors should discontinue the use of these drugs 1 week before ECT is performed. ECT usually causes reflex bradycardia immediately after seizure onset, followed by tachycardia (120 to 200 beats/min) and increases in systolic (200 to 250 mmHg) and diastolic (110 to 150 mmHg) blood pressure. These adrenergic-mediated reactions can be safely blunted by the use of β-blockers such as labetalol in patients in whom this transient tachycardia and hypertension would create risk.

The most common arrhythmias associated with ECT are premature ventricular contractions, with most noted after the seizure occurs and before spontaneous breathing resumes.[19] Patients at risk for malignant arrhythmias should have a cardiologist in attendance with the option of temporary pacemaker insertion. Reviews of special considerations in medically compromised patients who receive ECT can be found elsewhere.[20,21]

With modern anesthesia to induce sedation and muscle relaxation to keep the seizure centrally focused, ECT is a relatively benign procedure and is the safest treatment for many elderly medically compromised patients because the risk can be carefully controlled with the use of a trained anesthetist or anesthesiologist, cardiac monitoring, and adequate oxygenation.

REFERENCES

1. Wells CE. Pseudodementia. Am J Psychiatry 1979;136:895–900.
2. McAllister TW. Overview: pseudodementia. Am J Psychiatry 1983;140:528–533.
3. Dubin WR. Psychiatric emergencies: recognition and management. In: Stoudemire A, ed. Clinical psychiatry for medical students. Philadelphia, JB Lippincott, 1990:497–526.
4. Marks RM, Sachar EJ. Undertreatment of medical inpatients with narcotic analgesics. Ann Intern Med 1973;78:173–181.
5. Goldberg RJ. Acute pain management. In: Stoudemire A, Fogel BS, eds. Psychiatric care of the medical patient. New York, Oxford University Press, 1993:323–339.
6. Knorring L. The experience of pain in depressed patients. Neuropsychobiology 1975;1:155–165.
7. Hameroff SR, Cork RC, Scherer K, et al. Doxepin effects on chronic pain, depression and plasma opioids. J Clin Psychiatry 1982;43:22–27.
8. Ward NG, Bloom VL, Friedel RO. The effectiveness of tricyclic antidepressants in the treatment of coexisting pain and depression. Pain 1979;7:331–341.
9. Portenoy RK. Chronic pain management. In: Stoudemire A, Fogel BS, eds. Psychiatric care of the medical patient. New York, Oxford University Press, 1993:341–366.
10. Stoudemire A. Organic mental disorders. In Stoudemire A, ed. Clinical psychiatry for medical students. Philadelphia, JB Lippincott, 1990:72–103.
11. Carroll BJ. Dexamethasone suppression test: a review of contemporary confusion. J Clin Psychiatry 1985;46:13–24.
12. Glassman AH, Johnson LL, Giardina EGV, et al. The use of imipramine in depressed patients with congestive heart failure. JAMA 1983;250:1997–2001.
13. Veith RC, Raskind MA, Caldwell JH, et al. Cardiovascular effects of tricyclic antidepressants in depressed patients with chronic heart disease. N Engl J Med 1982;306:954–959.
14. Siris SG, Rifkin A. The problem of psychopharmacotherapy in the medically ill. Psychiatr Clin North Am 1981;4:379–390.
15. Robinson DS, Nies A, Corcella J, et al. Cardiovascular effects of phenelzine and amitriptyline in depressed outpatients. J Clin Psychiatry 1982;43:8–15.
16. Zisook S. A clinical overview of monoamine oxidase inhibitors. Psychosomatics 1985;26:240–251.
17. Stoudemire A, Fogel BS, Gulley LR, Moran MG. Psychopharmacology in the medically ill. In: Stoudemire A, Fogel BS, eds. Psychiatric care of the medical patient. New York, Oxford University Press, 1993:155–206.

18. Katon W, Raskind M. Treatment of depression in the medically ill elderly with methylphenidate. Am J Psychiatry 1980;137: 963–965.

19. McKenna G, Engle RP, Brooks H, et al. Cardiac arrhythmias during electroshock therapy: significance, prevention and treatment. Am J Psychiatry 1970;127:530–533.

20. Weiner R. ECT in the physically ill. J Psychiatr Treat Eval 1983; 5:457–462.

21. Weiner RD, Coffey CE. Electroconvulsive therapy in the medical and neurologic patient. In: Stoudemire A, Fogel BS, eds. Psychiatric care of the medical patient. New York, Oxford University Press, 1993:207–224.

CHAPTER

46

ANXIETY AND SOMATOFORM DISORDERS

Medical Management of the Surgical Patient, Third Edition,
edited by Michael F. Lubin, H. Kenneth Walker, and Robert B. Smith III.
J.B. Lippincott Company, Philadelphia, PA © 1995.

Alan Stoudemire

ANXIETY

Most patients are justifiably anxious in reaction to the diagnosis of illness and the performance of diagnostic tests and surgical procedures. Most anxiety reactions remit when the illness resolves or the condition stabilizes but anxiety may be chronic if persistent uncertainty exists about the course and prognosis or if treatment is periodically stressful (eg, dialysis, chemotherapy). Most patients with anxiety should be given periodic opportunities to express their questions, fears, and concerns. Physicians should be attentive, open, empathic, and supportive of patients' concerns, and should provide information, advice, encouragement, and reassurance at appropriate times, being careful not to sugarcoat responses, suppressing fears and feelings that patients may need to express.

As with depression, underlying medical conditions and medications should be considered before patients' symptoms of anxiety are attributed to psychiatric factors. Medical conditions that may present with anxiety as the primary complaint include hyperthyroidism, hypercalcemia, hypoglycemia, mitral valve prolapse, cardiac arrhythmias, angina, pulmonary failure, and vitamin B_{12} deficiency (in which peripheral neuropathy may mimic symptoms of anxiety). Patients with mitral valve prolapse in particular may have a variety of symptoms most likely associated with arrhythmia-related dyspnea, fatigue, and palpitations. Such patients have been reported to have a higher prevalence of

panic disorder but this association has recently been questioned.[1]

Certain drugs and medications should also be considered. In particular, psychostimulants such as amphetamines and cocaine may cause anxiety. Caffeine is probably the most common culprit in anxiety and irritability. Other medications that may be contributory are the theophylline derivatives used in the treatment of chronic obstructive pulmonary disease and asthma. Anxiety may also be a prominent symptom associated with withdrawal from alcohol, benzodiazepines, and sedative-hypnotics.

If patients are unduly anxious or agitated, or if their level of anxiety interferes with their social interactions or medical treatment, the adjunctive use of minor tranquilizers such as benzodiazepines may be considered, as long as several key points are kept in mind. First, in most patients, benzodiazepines should be used in relatively low dosages for short periods (2 to 4 weeks). These prescribing limitations should be made clear to patients before treatment is begun. If more than 1 month of treatment with benzodiazepines is contemplated, psychiatric consultation or referral may be warranted before therapy is instituted. Depression should be ruled out first to ensure that patients' symptoms of anxiety are not secondary manifestations of mood disorders for which antidepressants would be the treatment of choice.

The half-life of the benzodiazepines ranges from short (5 to 15 hours: alprazolam, lorazepam, oxazepam) to long (20 to 100 hours: diazepam). Lorazepam and oxazepam are primarily metabolized by glucuronide conjugation and are not as affected by the presence of liver disease, age, or the concurrent use of cimetidine (which may prolong the half-life of benzodiazepines), although the last effect may be of little clinical significance.[2] Longer acting drugs such as diazepam, halazepam, and prazepam are primarily metabolized by hepatic microsomal oxidation. Actually, these are minor pharmacologic differences that are rarely of major importance because the amount and frequency of dosing can be reduced to adjust serum levels, even in patients with liver disease.[3] If intramuscular administration is required, lorazepam and midazolam are the only benzodiazepines that are reliably absorbed through this route.

Benzodiazepines should not be administered to patients with alcoholism or central or peripheral sleep apnea. A withdrawal syndrome with seizures can develop after the abrupt discontinuation of drug therapy in patients who have received high doses or long-term treatment, and dosages should be tapered slowly in such cases.

PANIC ATTACKS

Recent work has also focused on treating panic and phobic disorders with pharmacologic agents.[4] Panic attacks (or anxiety attacks) may present with a constellation of symptoms, including hyperventilation, numbness, tingling, dizziness, palpitations, tachycardia, a feeling of impending doom or death, shortness of breath, and frantic behavior. Phobias, particularly agoraphobia, may develop around the panic attack, and phobic responses may eventually trigger a panic reaction. Panic attacks and agoraphobia have been found to respond to tricyclic antidepressants such as imipramine and to monoamine oxidase inhibitors. The diagnosis may be important if patients are noted to be particularly phobic about surgery, and an occult coexisting panic disorder may be present. Depression frequently accompanies panic disorder. These patients should be referred for treatment by a psychiatrist.

For other physicians, benzodiazepines and tricyclics (eg, imipramine, nortriptyline) are the drugs of choice for the pharmacologic treatment of patients in the primary care setting. If a benzodiazepine is used, many clinicians now prefer the long-acting agent clonazepam (Klonopin) over alprazolam (Xanax). There appear to be fewer problems with withdrawal reactions with clonazepam. If tricyclics are used as primary therapy or in conjunction with benzodiazepines, dosages should be low initially (10 mg/d) and increased by as little as 10 mg/wk, because patients with panic disorder are exquisitely sensitive to transient exacerbations of their symptoms when these drugs are first administered. Once patients are in remission, treatment usually must continue for at least 6 to 12 months before

medication dosages can be tapered. Behavioral therapy may be required if symptoms are associated with panic disorder. Caffeine and other stimulants should be strictly prohibited.

INSOMNIA

Many patients experience anxiety and insomnia during hospitalization and require medication to help them sleep. Benzodiazepines are generally the drugs of choice in this situation because they are effective in inducing and maintaining sleep, with little likelihood of inducing respiratory depression, and have a wide safety margin. Flurazepam (Dalmane), temazepam (Restoril), triazolam (Halcion), estazolam (ProSom), and quazepam (Doral) are benzodiazepines that have been developed primarily as soporifics.[5] These drugs differ primarily in their half-lives but temazepam is the only one that is metabolized by glucuronide conjugation. Flurazepam has a half-life of 50 to 100 hours; thus, daytime sedation may impair psychomotor performance, particularly in the elderly. Temazepam has a half-life of 13 to 16 hours but is relatively slowly absorbed and should be given at least 1 hour before the desired time of sleep. Triazolam, which has become a controversial drug, has a half-life of 2 to 3 hours; therefore, most of this agent is metabolized by the next morning, decreasing the possibility of significant daytime sedation. Because the medication peaks rapidly, however, amnestic episodes have been described if patients awaken in the night, as have rebound insomnia and daytime anxiety. Appropriate dosages are as follows: flurazepam, 15 to 30 mg; temazepam, 15 to 30 mg; triazolam, 0.125 and 0.25 mg; estazolam 1 and 2 mg; and quazepam 7.5 and 15 mg. The minimum dose should be given to elderly patients because half-lives are prolonged in this population.[6,7]

BUSPIRONE AND CHRONIC ANXIETY

Buspirone is a nonbenzodiazepine anxiolytic that is not sedating or habit forming, does not cause respiratory suppression, and is not associated with a withdrawal syndrome. It is indicated for chronic generalized anxiety (anxiety neurosis), which is manifested by multiple nonspecific somatic complaints in the primary care setting. A lag time in onset is typical and the drug may take 2 to 4 weeks to become effective. Average maintenance dosages are 5 to 10 mg three times daily and may be increased to as much as 10 to 20 mg three times daily over several weeks for more severe cases of chronic anxiety. There are no major drug interactions of significance, although buspirone may raise

TABLE 46–1. Somatoform Disorders, Factitious Disorders, and Malingering: A Comparison of Clinical Features

Diagnostic Subtype	Clinical Presentation	Demographic/ Epidemiologic Features	Diagnostic Features	Management Strategies	Prognostic Outlook	Associated Disturbances	Primary Differential Presentation	Psychologic Processes Contributing to Symptoms	Motivation for Symptom Production
Somatoform Disorders									
Somatization disorder	Polysymptomatic Recurrent/chronic "Sickly" by history	Younger age Female predominance 20:1 Familial pattern 5%–10% incidence in primary care populations	Review of systems profusely positive Multiple clinical contacts Polysurgical	Therapeutic alliance Regular appointments Crisis intervention	Poor to fair	Histrionic personality Sociopathy Substance/alcohol use Many life problems Conversion	Physical disease Depression	Unconscious Cultural/developmental	Unconscious psychologic factors
Conversion disorder	Monosymptomatic Mostly acute Simulates disease	Female predominance, younger age Rural/lower social class Less educated/ psychologically unsophisticated	Simulation incompatible with known physiologic mechanisms or anatomy	Suggestion and persuasion Multiple techniques	Excellent except chronic conversion	Drug/alcohol dependence Sociopathy Somatization disorder Histrionic personality	Depression Schizophrenia Neurologic disease	Unconscious Psychological stress or conflict may be present	Unconscious psychologic factors
Pain disorder, psychologic type	Pain syndrome simulated	Female predominance 2:1 Older: 4th or 5th decade Familial pattern Up to 40% of pain populations	Simulation or intensity incompatible with known physiologic mechanisms or anatomy	Therapeutic alliance Redefine goals of treatment Antidepressant medications	Guarded, variable	Depression Substance/ alcohol use Dependent/ histrionic personality	Depression Psycho- physiologic Physical disease Malingering/ disability syndrome	Unconscious Acute stressor/ developmental Physical trauma may predispose	Unconscious psychologic factors
Hypochondriasis	Disease concern or preoccupation	Previous physical disease Middle or older age Male/female ratio equal	Disease conviction amplifies symptoms Obsessional	Document symptoms Psychosocial review Psychotherapeutic	Fair to good Waxes and wanes	Obsessional "neurosis" Depression-anxiety	Depression Physical disease Personality disorder Delusional disorder	Unconscious Stress—bereavement Developmental factors	Unconscious psychologic factors
Body dysmorphic disorder	Subjective feelings of ugliness or concern with bodily defect	Adolescence or young adult ? Female predominance Largely unknown	Pervasive bodily concerns	Therapeutic alliance Stress management Psychotherapies Antidepressant medications	Unknown	Anorexia nervosa Psychosocial distress Avoidant/compulsive personality disorder	Delusional psychosis Depression Somatization disorder	Unconscious Self-esteem factors	Unconscious psychologic factors

TABLE 46–1. (Continued)

Diagnostic Subtype	Clinical Presentation	Demographic/ Epidemiologic Features	Diagnostic Features	Management Strategies	Prognostic Outlook	Associated Disturbances	Primary Differential Presentation	Psychologic Processes Contributing to Symptoms	Motivation for Symptom Production
Factitious Disorders									
Factitious with physical symptoms or signs or disease	Feigned or simulated physical symptoms or signs or disease	Female, younger, socially conforming Employed in medical field Social supports often available	Feigned illness No external goal of simulation is obvious Organ mode of presentation varies but is physical	Confront as appropriate Redefine illness as psychiatric Psychiatric referral	Fair to good except Munchausen subtype	Depression Borderline or other personality disorder	Malingering Conversion disorder Hypochondriasis Depression Schizophrenia	Unconscious Developmental/ family factors Masochism, dependency, and mastery are used	Conscious effort to assume patient status
Factitious with psychologic symptoms	Multiple hospitalizations	Female, younger, socially conforming Employed in medical field Social supports often available	Feigned illness No external goal of simulation is obvious Mode of presentation varies but is psychiatric	Confront as appropriate Redefine illness as psychiatric Psychiatric referral	Fair to good except Munchausen subtype	Schizophrenia Borderline or other personality disorder	Malingering Conversion disorder Hypochondriasis Depression Schizophrenia	Unconscious Developmental/ family factors Masochism, dependency, and mastery are used	Conscious effort to assume patient status
Munchausen syndrome	Multiple hospitalizations	Male, younger, socially nonconforming Social supports unavailable	Feigned illness Pathologic liar Geographic wandering Antisocial features Frequently leaves against medical advice	Recognize Confront Avoid invasive or iatrogenic procedures or treatments Social work referral	Poor	Antisocial, histrionic, or borderline personality	Malingering Conversion disorder Hypochondriasis Depression Schizophrenia	Unconscious Developmental/ family factors Masochism, dependency, and mastery are used	Conscious effort to assume patient status
Malingering									
Malingering	Feigned or simulated with physical or psychologic symptoms	? Male predominance Psychosocial stress or failure present	Feigned illness External incentives for disease present	Confront Consider psychiatric or psychosocial problems	Poor	Antisocial personality Substance abuse/ dependence	Factitious disorder Personality disorder Ganser syndrome Munchausen syndrome Major psychosis Disability syndrome	Conscious but may display other psychopathology	Conscious response to external incentives

(Folks DG, Ford CV, Houck CA. Somatoform disorders, factitious disorders, and malingering. In: Stoudemire A, ed. Clinical psychiatry for medical students, ed 2. Philadelphia, JB Lippincott, 1994:278–279) levels of haloperidol (Haldol) and should not be used with monoamine oxidase inhibitors.

SOMATOFORM DISORDERS, FACTITIOUS DISORDERS, AND MALINGERING

Several other psychiatric disorders may be seen in medical–surgical patients, although the emphasis here is on their recognition because their treatment, when and if possible, is usually difficult and requires psychiatric consultation. The importance of appropriate recognition is underscored by the fact that these patients often are a great burden on the medical system and tend to receive many unnecessary medications, tests, and surgery.

Somatoform disorders include hypochondriasis, somatization disorder, conversion disorder, and body dysmorphic disorder. Hypochondriasis is diagnosed when patients develop fixed obsessions with having particular illnesses or insist that particular symptoms represent feared illnesses despite repeated tests and reassurances to the contrary. Such patients may "doctor shop" and alternately frustrate and exhaust one physician after another. These patients have little interest in being cured. One hypothesis for their behavior is the unconscious need to maintain a dependent (but often with a mixture of hostility and dependency) tie to an authority figure (the physician) through somatic complaints to enable them to receive attention and care that is usually not available in other areas of their life. Other models view hypochondriasis as a form of obsessional neurosis with a somatic fixation. When they are treated, patients with hypochondriasis are best managed through regular periodic office visits that are scheduled irrespective of the presence or severity of symptoms, thereby enabling them to maintain contact with physicians. These patients typically are not agreeable to psychiatric therapy or referral, so most are treated by primary care physicians.[8] Major depression should be ruled out to ensure that patients' somatic preoccupations are not symptoms of depression.

Somatization disorder is similar to hypochondriasis. Although patients may chronically complain of many physical symptoms affecting almost every organ system, they usually are not obsessed with the idea of having life-threatening illnesses. These persons often have lifelong histories of being sickly, passive, and dependent children. The sick role, as with hypochondria, may serve to meet dependency needs. The disorder predominates in women. The goals of treatment are supportive care and containment of medical utilization by prevention of unnecessary tests, procedures, and surgeries.[9]

In diagnosing hypochondriasis and somatization disorder, physicians should be careful not to overlook an underlying depression or anxiety disorder because depression and anxiety often present with prominent somatization, somatic obsessions and preoccupations, and hypochondriacal concerns. Psychiatric consultation may be helpful in sorting such patients with masked depressions because the prognosis for improvement is much better if a mood disturbance is the primary problem.

Conversion disorder refers to the loss or alteration of a physical function usually referable to neurologic dysfunction that cannot be explained on the basis of known anatomic or pathophysiologic mechanisms. It may be more common in patients with histrionic (hysterical) personalities and reflects the repression of unconscious drives, feelings, or conflicts over dependency, aggression, and sexuality.

Finally, the diagnosis of factitious disorders and malingering should be contrasted. Factitious disorders (ie, Munchausen syndrome) are psychiatric conditions in which patients self-induce or manufacture symptoms with the intent of gaining medical attention. Examples are patients who present to numerous hospitals with chest or abdominal pain and submit to repeated tests, procedures, and surgery. Other patients may self-inject feces and surreptitiously warm thermometers to create the appearance of fever. In factitious disorders, there is no clear goal or reward involved other than seeking to be a patient and to maintain the sick role. In contrast, malingerers fabricate symptoms with clearly identified goals in mind (ie, disability or financial compensation), and their behavior is sociopathic.

Finally, body dysmorphic disorder involves distortion in body image in which patients become excessively and obsessively preoccupied with the perception that some aspect of their body is ugly or defective. To neutral observers, the so-called bodily defects are considered trivial or inconsequential but to patients they are a source of extreme distress. Such patients are likely to seek corrective surgery from cosmetic surgeons with unrealistic expectations. Because the disorder is predominantly psychologic in nature and involves obsessional features and an intrapsychic distortion in body image, patients are rarely satisfied with corrective procedures. Therefore, recognition of this condition is essential for specialists such as plastic surgeons and dermatologists, who are most likely to encounter these patients. Table 46-1 contrasts the major clinical characteristics of the somatoform disorders, factitious disorders, and malingering.

REFERENCES

1. Schuckit MA. Anxiety related to medical disease. J Clin Psychiatry 1983;44:31–37.
2. Greenblatt DJ, Shader RI, Abernethy DR. Current status of benzodiazepines. N Engl J Med 1983;309:410–416.

3. Brown JT, Mulrow CD, Stoudemire A. The anxiety disorders. Ann Intern Med 1984;100:558–564.

4. Sheehan DV. Current concepts in psychiatry: panic attacks and phobias. N Engl J Med 1982;307:156–158.

5. Berlin RM. The management of insomnia in hospitalized patients. Ann Intern Med 1984;100:398–404.

6. Stoudemire A, Fogel BS, Gulley LR, Moran MG. Psychopharmacology in the medically ill. In: Stoudemire A, Fogel BS, eds. Psychiatric care of the medical patient. New York, Oxford University Press, 1993:155–206.

7. Goldberg RJ, Posner D. Anxiety in the medically ill. In: Stoudemire A, Fogel BS, eds. Psychiatric care of the medical patient. New York, Oxford University Press, 1993:87–104.

8. Folks DG, Houck CA. Somatoform disorders, factitious disorders and malingering. In: Stoudemire A, Fogel BS, eds. Psychiatric care of the medical patient. New York, Oxford University Press, 1993:267–288.

9. Folks DG, Ford CV, Houck CA. Somatoform disorders, factitious disorders, and malingering. In: Stoudemire A, ed. Clinical psychiatry for medical students. Philadelphia, JB Lippincott 1990:237–268.

Medical Management of the Surgical Patient, Third Edition,
edited by Michael F. Lubin, H. Kenneth Walker, and Robert B. Smith III.
J.B. Lippincott Company, Philadelphia, PA © 1995.

CHAPTER

47

SUBSTANCE ABUSE

Ted Parran, Jr.

Problems of drug and alcohol abuse are ubiquitous in hospitalized patient populations. A prevalence study at Johns Hopkins Hospital in 1986 demonstrated active alcoholism in 23% of surgical patients, with subgroup rates ranging from 14% in patients on the urology service, to 28% in those on the orthopedic service, to 43% in those on the otorhinolaryngology service.[1] Although this study did not evaluate the prevalence of drug abuse, consideration of the abuse of drugs other than alcohol could only increase the overall rate of affected patients on surgical services. Detection rates by physician staff of patients with substance abuse problems are low in general and lowest on surgery and obstetrics-gynecology services. Data indicate that under 25% of affected patients are identified on these specialty services. In addition, less than half the substance-abusing patients who are identified receive any form of intervention, counseling, or even a medical treatment plan that addresses the substance abuse issues. Therefore, only about 10% of surgical patients with substance abuse problems have their abuse addressed in any way by their physicians.

In a few special populations of surgical patients, problems of substance abuse are of even greater magnitude. Trauma service data indicate that between 30% and 75% of all injured patients have positive results on toxicology testing for legal levels of alcohol intoxication or for drugs of abuse at the time of hospital admission.[2–5] Our experience after a year of testing each consecutive level 1 trauma admission indicates an alcohol intoxication rate of 63%, an il-

licit drug use rate of 48%, and a combined rate of 78%. Follow-up interviews with these patients reveal that most have serious drug and alcohol abuse or dependence, with only 8% being substance users who happened to suffer a major trauma.

A significant literature is emerging that examines the potential for increased morbidity, mortality, and hospitalization costs associated with drug and alcohol abuse in surgical patients. Although there are some conflicting reports and a vast diversity of research design, a consensus appears to be emerging that these patients do carry an increased burden of morbidity, mortality, and cost associated with their treatment. Some of them have been shown to have increased intraoperative and postoperative complication rates (ie, neurosurgical patients with alcoholism and subdural hematoma, patients with alcoholism who undergo transurethral prostatectomy, patients with alcoholism and drug dependency who undergo plastic surgery and burn treatment, and patients with alcoholism who undergo bowel resection or hysterectomy).[6–10] They have also been shown to have increased postoperative morbidity and, in many studies, increased mortality. Finally, theoretic and actual anesthesia risks in surgical patients who abuse drugs and alcohol have recently been reviewed.[11]

Clinically important issues involved in the treatment of substance abuse in surgical patients are considered further in the following order: screening and diagnosis strategies, medical therapy considerations by drug class, brief intervention and treatment planning, and postoperative pain management issues.

SCREENING APPROACHES

The need for better and more widespread screening for substance abuse problems in hospitalized patients is obvious.[12–14] Because the prevalence of these patients is between 20% and 40% on surgical services, and because the diagnosis is overlooked in 50% to 80% of cases, the need for active screening of all patients is indisputable. A good screening test should be clinically powerful (with high sensitivity and an acceptable level of specificity), simple to use, and easy to master and remember, and should have a high degree of patient and physician acceptability. Several good approaches have been developed and tested over the past 20 years, and three are perhaps most appropriate to surgical settings: the CAGE questionnaire, the Trauma Survey, and toxicology testing.[12,15,16]

The CAGE questions were first published in the early 1970s and have been widely studied in various patient populations (Table 47-1). The questions are easy to remember and simple to ask, tend not to engender defensiveness and discomfort in patients or physicians, and are far more sensitive and specific in identifying clinically important substance abuse problems than are typical questions regarding amount and frequency of use. The CAGE questionnaire also can be used to ask family members about patients, especially when patients are unable to be meaningfully interviewed. In hospitalized patients, each positive response to a CAGE question indicates a 30% to 40% likelihood of a substance abuse problem. Therefore, two positive responses to four questions indicates an 80% sensitivity and specificity for substance abuse.

It is thought that young men tend to produce false-negative results when they are tested with the CAGE questionnaire. Skinner and colleagues[16] observed that young men with substance abuse problems often suffer repetitive traumatic injury. They developed the Trauma Survey (Table 47-2) for use in this population, and positive responses to

TABLE 47–2. Trauma Scale Questionnaire

Since your 18th birthday,
   Have you had any fractures or dislocations of your bones or joints?
   Have you been injured in a road traffic accident?
   Have you injured your head?
   Have you been injured in a non–sports-related assault or fight?
   Have you been injured after drinking?

two of its five categories indicate the likelihood of a substance abuse problem. The Trauma Survey is more clinically useful than are the results of laboratory tests (ie, liver tests or the mean corpuscular volume) or standard questions regarding the amount and frequency of use, especially in populations of young men.

The prevalence of positive results on toxicology testing at the time of hospital admission is startlingly high in some patient populations, especially trauma patients. A consensus is gradually emerging among trauma services that the use of routine admission toxicology testing is a reasonable trauma protocol standard.[5] Although this is not the case in all surgical patient populations, the single most clinically useful laboratory test after positive results are obtained with a CAGE questionnaire or Trauma Survey is toxicology testing for a blood alcohol level and urine screening for drugs of abuse. Most risk management experts consider this "for cause" toxicology testing ("for cause" because the clinical history indicates the likelihood of a medical illness of chemical dependence) to be justified and defensible, even without special informed written consent by patients.

Substance abuse screening tools are available and are practical, clinically powerful, and easy to use. Their use should be extended into patient care in general and into surgical populations in particular. Once the use of effective screening is more widespread, detoxification management, presentation of the diagnosis, referral for counseling and treatment, and management of special considerations such as postoperative pain become critical for the surgical team and its medical consultants.

TABLE 47–1. CAGE Questionnaire*

Have you ever felt the need to <u>C</u>ut down on your drinking[+]
Have people <u>A</u>nnoyed you by criticizing your drinking[+]
Have you ever felt bad or <u>G</u>uilty about your drinking[+]
Have you ever had a drink[+] first thing in the morning to steady your nerves or to get rid of a hangover (<u>E</u>ye opener)?

*The family CAGE (fCAGE) involves asking if "anyone in your family" has felt the need to. . . .
[+]Many clinicians substitute "drinking or drug use" when using the CAGE questionnaire.

MEDICAL CONSIDERATIONS BY DRUG CLASS

The medical considerations involved in caring for surgical patients with substance abuse problems are vast. The primary areas addressed here are basic pharmacology, management of intoxication and toxicity, management of withdrawal, and other considerations (ie, nutritional, metabolic).[17] The various drugs are discussed by class: alcohol and sedative-hypnotics, cocaine and stimulants, and opiates.

ALCOHOL AND SEDATIVE-HYPNOTICS

Alcohol and sedative-hypnotic agents (eg, benzodiazepines, barbiturates) are involved in most of the substance abuse that is encountered in surgical patients.[18] Intoxication with these agents is associated with dose-related and tolerance-related disinhibition, loss of judgment, delay in psychomotor coordination, decrease in cognitive ability, and impairment of short-term memory formation. At high levels of intoxication, consciousness, respiratory drive, and cardiovascular function are depressed.[17] Signs of acute toxicity are altered mental status, lethargy and stupor, dilated pupils, slowed respiration, and decreased reflexes, including the gag reflex. The mixing of sedatives can markedly potentiate their toxicity, resulting in a dramatically narrowed toxic/therapeutic ratio and death. This should be considered in the management of agitated behavior, the treatment of withdrawal, or the consideration of anesthesia or analgesia. The necessity of obtaining accurate toxicology data for use in these types of management decisions cannot be overemphasized. The treatment of toxicity involves cardiovascular and respiratory monitoring and support, the cessation of gastrointestinal absorption, and attempts to increase drug excretion. Some investigators have used high doses of naloxone (Narcan) in these patients, with conflicting results.

The alcohol and sedative-hypnotic withdrawal syndromes are similar and can be considered in terms of four categories of symptoms and signs (Table 47-3). Category 1 withdrawal involves increases in heart rate, blood pressure, and reflexes accompanied by tremors, diaphoresis, headache, nausea or diarrhea, insomnia, and anxiety. Category 2

withdrawal is benign alcohol hallucinosis, a clinical picture of visual, tactile, or auditory hallucinations coupled with a clear sensorium. Category 3 withdrawal is the so-called rum fits or withdrawal seizures. These grand mal seizures can be single or multiple discrete seizures, can progress to status epilepticus in the case of barbiturate and perhaps benzodiazepine withdrawal, and tend to be of short duration with accordingly short postictal periods. Category 4 withdrawal is a delayed-type withdrawal that is also known as delirium tremens, or DTs. This is characterized by the hyperautonomic signs and symptoms of category 1 coupled with delirium consisting of global confusion hallucinations and agitation.

The first three categories of withdrawal tend to begin within 12 to 24 hours of the last drink or drug ingestion, rapidly escalate to peak symptoms in another 12 to 24 hours, and ease over an additional 48 to 72 hours. Delayed withdrawal begins 3 to 5 days after the last use and then follows a similar time frame. The only significant exceptions to this involve the long-acting benzodiazepine medications such as diazepam, chlordiazepoxide, clorazepate (Tranxene), and clonazepam (Klonopin). Because of their extended half-lives or active metabolites, the onset of withdrawal from these agents can be delayed for 3 to 6 days after cessation of use, and symptoms often persist for an additional 10 days to 3 weeks.

The likelihood that patients will experience one or more categories of withdrawal symptoms is dependent on their previous withdrawal experience. Patients who have not had previous withdrawal symptoms on abrupt discontinuation of drug use are unlikely to go through withdrawal during their hospitalization for surgery. Patients who have had category 3 withdrawal seizures in the past have as much as a 30% risk for recurrent seizures during each subsequent withdrawal episode. The easiest way to predict which patients are at risk for significant withdrawal, and hence which patients require moderate to vigorous withdrawal prophylaxis while they are hospitalized on a surgical service, is to closely interview patients and their families and to review the medical records for data regarding the presence of previous withdrawal symptoms.

The treatment of alcohol withdrawal varies among hospital services. One approach that we recommend for surgical patients is to first evaluate pulmonary function, liver function, and previous withdrawal symptomatology. If patients have reasonable liver function (ie, the prothrombin time is less than 1.3 times control) and pulmonary function (ie, the FEV_1 is greater than 1 to 1.3 L), we use long-acting benzodiazepines to treat withdrawal symptoms (Table 47-4). If either hepatic or pulmonary function is impaired, we administer short-acting benzodiazepines. It also is useful to assess the intensity of withdrawal signs and symptoms. In patients with mild category 1 or 2 symptoms, the low-dose intermittent use of benzodiazepines as needed is reasonable. If the symptoms are intense or severe in any category,

TABLE 47–3. Alcohol and Sedative-Hypnotic Withdrawal*

Class	Signs and Symptoms	Time Course[+]	
		Onset	Duration
Class I	Increased heart rate, blood pressure, and reflexes Diarrhea, nausea, and vomiting Tremor, anxiety, and insomnia	12–24 h	72–96 h
Class II	Visual >auditory >tactile hallucinations	12–24 h	72–96 h
Class III	Grand mal seizures	12–96 h	6–24 h
Class IV	Class I signs with delirium-disorientation, confusion, hallucinations, agitation, anxiety, insomnia	3–6 d	72–96 h

*Applies to alcohol and short-acting sedative-hypnotics. See text for time course differences with long-acting sedative-hypnotics.
[+]Onset relates to initiation of syndrome after last use of the involved drug. Duration relates to duration of syndrome after initiation.

TABLE 47–4. Strategies for Alcohol Withdrawal Management

Withdrawal Symptoms	Pulmonary or Hepatic Function	
	Impaired	Not Impaired
Mild class I symptoms	Low-dose, short-acting benzodiazepine: protocol A	Low-dose, long-acting benzodiazepine: protocol C
Severe Class I, or class II, III, or IV symptoms	Intensive short-acting benzodiazepine: protocol B	Intensive long-acting benzodiazepine: protocol D

a higher-dose intensive benzodiazepine regimen is suggested (Table 47-5).

Periodically, patients are seen who have received large doses of benzodiazepines or barbiturates as outpatients. In this case, therapy with these medications either should be maintained without change or discontinued and replaced with phenobarbital. The mixing of acute doses of benzodiazepines and phenobarbital is strongly discouraged because of the risk of iatrogenic overdose and respiratory depression. One phenobarbital dosing schedule is outlined in Table 47-5, and can be applied to the treatment of alcohol or sedative-hypnotic withdrawal.

Several electrolyte and nutritional issues must be considered when patients with alcoholism are treated on the surgical service. Thiamine deficiency is seen in this population and can have catastrophic and permanent neurologic consequences. Thiamine should be given intramuscularly at a dosage of 100 mg for 3 days if necessary. In addition, pa-

TABLE 47–5. Alcohol Withdrawal Protocols

Protocol A	Lorazepam 0.5 mg PO, IM, or IV each 4–8 hours per specific signs or symptoms of withdrawal. Discontinue after 72–96 hours.
Protocol B	Lorazepam 0.5 to 2 mg PO/IM or IV each 1–4 hours until specific signs or symptoms of withdrawal are suppressed or patient is sleepy. Restart protocol if withdrawal reemerges.
Protocol C	Diazepam 5 mg PO or IV each 4–8 hours per specific signs or symptoms of withdrawal. Discontinue after 72–96 hours.
Protocol D	Diazepam 10 mg PO or IV each 1 hour until specific sign of withdrawal is suppressed or patient is sleepy. Restart protocol if withdrawal reemerges.
Protocol E	Sedative-hypnotic withdrawal protocol. Phenobarbital 90 mg PO or IM each 2–4 hours until therapeutic (antiseizure) blood level is achieved. Then titrate daily phenobarbital dose to maintain a therapeutic blood level.

tients with alcoholism frequently have vitamin C, vitamin B complex, and folic acid deficiencies. These should be supplemented by the oral, intravenous, or intramuscular route. Multiple electrolyte abnormalities occur in this population and careful evaluation of the serum sodium, potassium, phosphorus, glucose, and magnesium levels is essential. Abnormalities in each of these electrolytes can lead to altered mental status, seizures, or cardiac arrhythmias.

A review of all the medical complications of alcohol abuse and dependence is beyond the scope of this chapter but a few problems deserve special mention. Hematologic problems include alcohol-associated anemias, thrombocytopenia, and clotting factor abnormalities. Alcohol-associated liver disease can complicate the selection and dosage of anesthetics. Finally, it is important to screen for congestive heart failure symptoms related to alcoholic cardiomyopathy before surgery is undertaken.[19]

COCAINE AND OTHER STIMULANTS

Cocaine is the most commonly abused stimulant, although the various schedule II amphetamines are still abused by some patient populations and methamphetamine (known as crystal, crystal-meth, or ice) has recently begun to be manufactured and abused in large amounts. Common properties of stimulants involve inhibition of the reuptake of norepinephrine systemically and dopamine centrally.[17] This produces systemic effects of markedly elevated heart rate, blood pressure, reflexes, and level of smooth muscle spasticity.[20] Cardiac arrhythmias; brain, heart, intestinal, uterine, and muscular ischemia; and seizures are common during stimulant binges and are thought to be caused by norepinephrine surges. Of special medical significance in patients who abuse cocaine is the markedly increased risk for trauma, sexually transmitted diseases, tuberculosis (including resistant strains), and the human immunodeficiency virus as a result of intravenous drug use or multiple sexual encounters.[21]

Centrally, the excess levels of dopamine associated with cocaine and other stimulant use produce intense feelings of euphoria, stamina, power, and control associated with sleeplessness, loss of appetite, and physical restlessness.[20] These effects rapidly abate and are replaced by dysphoric and depressive feelings. The evanescent nature of the "high" associated with stimulant use results in frequent repeated administration of the drugs and the typical binge–crash pattern of stimulant abuse and addiction. Urine toxicology testing for cocaine and metabolites remains positive in proportion to the duration and intensity of use. Toxicology often reveals casual use for 18 to 24 hours, whereas serial screenings (ie, every 12 hours) after a binge of several days can remain positive for as long as 4 days. Toxicology testing for amphetamine use often produces false-positive results in patients who are taking nonprescription cold preparations. These results should be confirmed with gas chromatography.

Toward the end of a binge, which can last from 12 to 96 hours, patients typically report more and more intense feelings of agitation, depression, and even paranoia that may last for several hours. It is during this unstable, agitated phase that much of the violence associated with stimulant abuse occurs. Patients then crash and begin a period of several hours to a few days of hypersomnia and hyperphagia (Table 47-6). This has been called phase 1 withdrawal. Phase 2 withdrawal is characterized by restlessness, edginess, mood swings, sleep disturbance, and stimulant cravings, and can affect patients intermittently for several weeks to months.

The symptoms of category 2 withdrawal are thought to be mediated on the basis of dopamine depletion. Therefore, the primary interventions include the administration of dopaminergic agents such as amantadine and bromocriptine or antidepressant drugs such as desipramine. Although each of these medications has been studied for efficacy in cocaine withdrawal, none has been demonstrated to have a significant therapeutic effect. As a consequence, some substance abuse treatment providers do not prescribe any drugs for the symptoms of cocaine or stimulant withdrawal. Symptoms that should be medicated are those seen during the period of agitated paranoia at the end of a binge. At this point, patients tend to respond to intramuscular sedatives, ranging from 100 mg of hydroxyzine for relatively mild cases to 2 mg of lorazepam or 2 mL of droperidol for more agitated patients as a one-time dose.

Finally, the implications of a stimulant binge should be considered in planning anesthesia. Patients with substance abuse problems and major trauma often have not had much to eat or drink for several hours to days. Their urinalyses commonly show maximally concentrated specimens with ketones, traces of protein, and much sediment. Serum creatinine and, especially, blood urea nitrogen determinations frequently do not reflect the true degree of volume depletion secondary to starvation effects. Therefore, accurate assessment of volume status is important. Another concern in undertaking surgery in these patients is the possible existence of a catecholamine-depleted state after a binge. Although no empiric evidence exists on this subject, catecholamine-stimulating pressors may not be as effective in these patients. Ruling out binge-associated cardiac ischemia, arrhythmia, pneumothorax, and rhabdomyolysis is important before surgery.[21]

OPIATES

All opiates are abused by some patients, including propoxyphene, codeine, oxycodone, meperidine, methadone, hydromorphone, morphine, heroin, opium, pentazocine, butorphanol, nalbuphine, and buprenorphine (Table 47-7). All opiates (except for methadone and perhaps buprenorphine) are rapidly metabolized and cleared, so their presence is rarely identified by urine toxicology testing performed more than 24 hours after the last use. Based on their observed actions, opiates are classified into the following categories: mu-agonists, kappa-agonists, and sigma-agonists.[22] The mu-agonists produce supraspinal anesthesia; euphoria; myosis; sedation; dose-related respiration, pulse, and blood pressure depression; tolerance; physiologic dependence; and a withdrawal syndrome associated with drug cravings. The kappa-agonists produce spinal anesthesia and physiologic tolerance. These drugs cause significantly less euphoria, myosis, and sedation. Respiratory depression, bradycardia, and hypotension are also less frequent with kappa-agonists. Withdrawal syndromes from mu-agonists are associated with much more drug craving. The kappa-agonists also act as mu-receptor antagonists, precipitating withdrawal in mu-agonist–dependent patients. At higher therapeutic doses, kappa-agonists tend to produce more and more dysphoric symptoms, which can limit their usefulness in the treatment of extremely severe pain.

Opiate intoxication produces a clinical picture of transient nausea; dry mouth; constipation; sleepiness; euphoria; a feeling of tranquility; constricted pupils; warm, dry skin; and depressed respirations, heart rate, and blood pressure. Opiate toxicity presents as depressed mentation ranging from obtundation or coma to myotic pinpoint pupils, bradycardia, hypotension, apnea, and death.[17] This toxic state can be easily reversed by the administration of naloxone (Narcan). The intravenous administration of 0.4 mg

TABLE 47–6. Stimulant Withdrawal

	Symptoms and Signs	Duration
Binge	Repetitive compulsive self-administration of cocaine; dilated pupils; increased pulse, increased blood pressure, decreased sleep, decreased eating; restlessness, grandiosity, pressured thoughts	Hours to several days
Agitated phase	Intense dysphoria, excitement, agitation, paranoia, rare cardiovascular instability	Up to several hours
Phase I ("crash")	Restlessness, anxiety, mood lability	12 to 72 hours
Phase II ("cravings")	Mood swings, concentration difficulties, strong urges regarding cocaine	Weeks to months

TABLE 47–7. Strategies for Opiate Withdrawal Management

Receptors	Actions	Agonists	Antagonists
mu	Supraspinal analgesia, euphoria, sedation, respiratory depression, physical withdrawal with drug cravings	Morphine Meperidol Methadone Oxycodone Codeine Propoxyphene Hydromorphone Buprenorphine* Heroin	Naloxone Naltrexone Pentazocine Nalbuphine
kappa	Spinal analgesia, miosis, sedation, physical withdrawal without drug cravings	Pentazocine Nalbuphine* Butorphanol	Naloxone Naltrexone
sigma	Mydriasis, dysphoria, respiratory stimulation	Butorphanol Pentazocine* Nalbuphine*	Naloxone Naltrexone

*Partial agonist for indicated receptor.

usually produces a response in vital signs and pupillary dilation, although patients with greater degrees of intoxication sometimes require multiple doses. The duration of intoxication with most opiates is 1 to 3 hours, and the duration of naloxone's antagonistic effect is 20 to 40 minutes, so close patient observation and repeated dosing is important. Methadone has a much longer duration of intoxication and toxicity, and patients who have overdosed on this drug must be monitored for at least 12 to 24 hours. Naltrexone (Trexan) is an oral form of naloxone that has a half-life of 18 to 24 hours. It occasionally is useful in patients with toxicity, especially if methadone is involved. Because naloxone and naltrexone are mu-receptor and kappa-receptor antagonists, their administration in the proper dosage not only reverses opiate toxicity but also precipitates opiate withdrawal in patients who are physically dependent. This withdrawal syndrome lasts for only 20 or 30 minutes in the case of naloxone but can last for as long as 24 hours after the administration of naltrexone.

By stage, the signs and symptoms of opiate withdrawal are as follows:

1. Lacrimation, rhinorrhea, diaphoresis, yawning, restlessness, insomnia
2. Mydriasis, piloerection, muscular fasciculation, myalgia, arthralgia, abdominal pain
3. Tachycardia, hypertension, tachypnea, fever, anorexia, nausea, extreme restlessness
4. Diarrhea, emesis, dehydration, hyperactive bowel sounds, hypotension, fetal position

These vary in intensity depending on the type of opiate used, the dose taken, and the duration of use. The symptoms of craving, restlessness, and insomnia tend to be especially long-lasting.[23] Nonmethadone opiate withdrawal generally begins 6 to 12 hours after the last use, progresses to a peak within 36 hours of initiation, and resolves over an additional 36 hours. Except as noted earlier, opiate withdrawal symptoms resolve within 4 days of the last drug use. Methadone withdrawal begins about 48 hours after the last use, gradually builds for a week or so, and then abates over another 5 to 7 days.

The treatment of opiate withdrawal involves the use of clonidine, methadone, or buprenorphine.[23–25] The following clonidine protocol has been used extensively in patients with heavy physical dependence on opiates who are hospitalized in detoxification units:

1. Administer clonidine, 0.1 mg orally every 4 hours for 36 hours.
2. Administer clonidine, 0.1 mg orally every 6 hours for 24 hours.
3. Administer clonidine, 0.1 mg orally every 8 hours for 24 hours.
4. Administer clonidine, 0.1 mg orally every 12 hours for 24 hours.
5. Discontinue clonidine therapy.
6. Do not administer clonidine if patients are asleep or if the systolic blood pressure is less than 90 mmHg.

Adjunct medications are often helpful, including ibuprofen and acetaminophen for myalgia, dicyclomine for abdominal symptoms, hydroxyzine for anxiety, and amitriptyline with diphenhydramine for sleep. Patients with hemodynamic instability, advanced age, or acute or chronic pain syndromes often do not tolerate this clonidine regimen.

It is in this group of patients that methadone has historically been used.[23] Difficulties with methadone therapy include the need to first stabilize patients on it and then taper them off relatively slowly, legal issues surrounding the outpatient prescription of methadone, and the referral to methadone maintenance programs of patients who have begun such treatment in the hospital. Methadone has 30% more bioavailability when it is given intramuscularly than when it is given orally. Therefore, patients who cannot take oral medications should be given two thirds of their usual daily oral dose in two divided intramuscular doses every 12 hours. Methadone is administered as follows:

1. Administer 5 to 10 mg of methadone orally every 12 hours.
2. Monitor for ablation of withdrawal symptoms.
3. Increase the dose by 5 to 10 mg until symptoms are suppressed (stabilization dose).
4. Taper the methadone over 5 to 20 days be decreasing the dose by 5% to 20% per day.
5. Treat reemergent withdrawal symptoms with clonidine patches.

The advent of short-term, inpatient buprenorphine tapering protocols such as the one that follows has markedly decreased the number of patients in whom methadone therapy must be initiated during their hospitalization[25,26]:

1. Administer buprenorphine, 0.2 to 0.5 mg subcutaneously every 4 hours for 48 hours.
2. Administer buprenorphine, half the above dose every 4 hours for 48 hours.
3. Administer buprenorphine, one half the second dose every 4 hours for 48 hours.
4. Discontinue buprenorphine administration.

It appears that the withdrawal syndrome from buprenorphine, especially when it is given in this short-term, low-dose tapering method, is mild and often clinically trivial. Therapy is begun at a dosage designed to relieve withdrawal symptoms (and pain if appropriate) without making patients sleepy or sedated. Because 0.3 mg of buprenorphine is equivalent to 10 mg of morphine, we usually start with doses between 0.2 and 0.4 mg. Once this initial therapeutic dose is identified, it is relatively easy to discontinue drug treatment gradually over 5 or 6 days.

Common medical complications in patients who are dependent on opiates are related to the degree of opiate tolerance and the delivery system used. The degree of tolerance that patients have for opiate effects can markedly affect decisions relating to anesthesia and analgesia management (see later discussion). A significant proportion of the estimated 1.1 million opiate-dependent persons in our country use, at least intermittently, the intravenous route. Careful observation for track marks, abscesses, and cellulitis is critical. Viral hepatitis is a ubiquitous problem, with seropositivity for hepatitis B and C being the rule rather than the exception. Human immunodeficiency virus seropositivity also is high, ranging from 6% to 60% depending on the metropolitan area being studied. Other infectious problems include endocarditis, osteomyelitis, bacterial pneumonia, and tuberculosis. In some inner cities, patients who abuse intravenous drugs have a 35% positive rate on PPD testing. All intravenous drug users who are hospitalized require hepatitis testing, human immunodeficiency virus testing (with consent), and PPD testing with an anergy panel. Finally, many opiate-dependent patients have ignored or self-treated many symptoms before coming to the hospital. As they come out from under their self-induced opiate anesthetic, serious and at times far-advanced illnesses often emerge. It is important to perform a thorough baseline evaluation and to investigate all emerging symptom complexes.

PRESENTING THE DIAGNOSIS AND FORMING A TREATMENT PLAN

After detoxification has been accomplished, physicians are often reluctant to address important issues in patients with substance abuse problems.[1,27] There are many reasons for this, including discomfort with this disease in general, lack of training in dealing with these types of patients, lack of institutional and departmental support, and a prevailing sense of therapeutic futility. This feeling of hopelessness and of being overwhelmed by the magnitude of skills needed to treat chemically dependent patients is not supported by recent research. Data from brief intervention studies indicate that traditional skills used in presenting other difficult diagnoses to patients (ie, cancer, acquired immunodeficiency syndrome) are also effective in presenting the diagnosis of substance abuse.[28]

Simple and effective strategies for presenting the diagnosis of alcohol or drug dependence are being taught in most medical schools and many residency programs. Two such strategies are the Eight Basic Actions outlined by Barker and Whitfield,[29] and the SOAPE mnemonic by Clark.[30] The primary points of these and other strategies include the need to be clear, concise, and specific about the diagnosis; to appear comfortable during the discussion; to avoid blaming patients and to show support for their present or future willingness to work toward sobriety; to be optimistic about eventual success; and to urge a treatment plan based on abstinence with close follow-up and reinforcement.[31]

Several specific pitfalls should be avoided when presenting the diagnosis and forming a treatment plan. The discussion should be kept extremely brief if patients are intoxicated and followed up at a later date. Patients often try to direct the discussion into various reasons or explanations for their problems. Efforts should be made to keep the discussion focused on the diagnosis itself and to avoid speculations about the cause or origin of substance abuse. Because arguments tend to be fruitless, an attempt should be made to defuse them with empathy, respect, and a thorough explanation of the disease as a chronic, progressive illness. Outpatient prescribing of anxiolytics is strongly discouraged and prescribing of opiate analgesics should be for a specific, self-limited period. Finally, physicians should strive to appear certain, comfortable, and caring.[31]

In many cases, this simple approach is unsuccessful. Consultation is often needed for these more complicated situations. Given the prevalence of substance abuse problems in surgical patients, it is reasonable for departments of surgery to insist that chemical dependency consultation services be provided by their hospital systems. With the prevalence exceeding 50% on some trauma services, substance abuse consultation is essential for adequate patient care.[5]

PAIN MANAGEMENT STRATEGIES

The management of acute and chronic pain is a difficult and complicated area of patient care that cannot be summarized in this chapter. Physicians have varying philosophies about pain management, the prescription of opiate analgesics, and the use of pain management consultants. In contrast, the commonalities of addictions are strong, and patients who develop difficulties with the use of one mood-altering drug commonly develop problems with other mood-altering drugs to which they are exposed. Patients with substance abuse problems who are prescribed mood-altering drugs create significant problems for physicians. Issues concerning the prescribing of controlled drugs are the leading cause for state medical boards to investigate and take action against physicians. Several basic management principles can be outlined.

Before opiate analgesics are prescribed for all patients, and especially for patients with substance abuse problems, a clear diagnosis must be identified. Then a therapeutic plan with specific treatment goals, methods of monitoring symptoms, and expected time course must be outlined and documented in the chart.[32] Several important factors should be considered once a decision to prescribe has been reached. First, the provision of reasonable relief for acute, self-limited pain is a justifiable expectation for all patients, regardless of their chemical dependency status. Second, patients who have misused mood-altering chemicals in the past may

have higher medication tolerance than other patients and, thus, require higher doses of medication. Third, patients with substance abuse problems may misuse their prescription analgesics. Therefore, it is important to prescribe adequate dosages of analgesics while at the same time limiting the amount of drug dispensed, to provide no refills on any controlled prescription, and to refuse to prescribe more medication than originally intended unless the diagnosis changes. Frequent brief visits to renew the prescription, monitor the response to treatment, and maintain patient commitment to discontinuing opiate therapy at the predetermined time is an appropriate pattern of management. The more common practice of providing large prescriptions and rare follow-up appointments often results in frequent attempts to obtain early refills. When opiate analgesics are prescribed for patients with previous opiate dependence, physicians should attempt to use medications from a different class than the one previously abused. For example, a former heroin (mu-agonist) user who requires opiate-type analgesia should be treated with kappa-agonists if at all possible. This provides adequate pain relief with less risk of rekindling the former addiction.

The use of opiate analgesics is highly questionable in the treatment of chronic pain, especially if it is of unclear origin and even more so if it is chronic cryptogenic pain in patients with histories of substance abuse. Opiate therapy should be initiated in this setting with great reluctance and can be considered to be contraindicated. In cases in which long-term opiate therapy has already been initiated in patients with chronic cryptogenic pain and substance abuse, it is reasonable to gradually taper the medication at a rate of 5% to 10% per week. Many practitioners ask their patients to sign a treatment plan or contract in which they agree to be admitted to the hospital for detoxification if this type of medication tapering regimen is not completed successfully. Patients who refuse such interventions present difficult choices; some authorities suggest that they be referred to methadone maintenance programs. These management decisions are extremely difficult and influenced by many factors, including the personalities and philosophies of patients and physicians. Although treatment approaches are never clearcut, the considerations outlined can help guide the decision-making process.

REFERENCES

1. Moore RD, Levine DM. Prevalence, detection, and treatment of alcoholism in hospitalized patients. JAMA 1989;261:403–407.
2. Clark DE, McCarthy E, Robinson E. Trauma as a symptom of alcoholism. Ann Emerg Med 1985;14:274–277.
3. Antti-Poika I. Heavy drinking and accidents. Br J Accident Surg 1988;19:198–200.

4. Anda RH. Alcohol and fatal injuries among U.S. adults. JAMA 1988;260:2529–2532.

5. Soderstrom CS. A National Alcohol and Trauma Center survey. Arch Surg 1987;122:1067–1071.

6. Sonne NM, Tonnesen H. The influence of alcoholism on outcome after evaluation of subdural hematoma. Br J Neurosurg 1992;6:125–130.

7. Tonnesen H. Influence of alcoholism on morbidity after transurethral prostatectomy. Scand J Urol Nephrol 1988;22:175–177.

8. Brezel BS, Stein JM. Burns in substance abusers. J Burn Care Rehabil 1988;9:169–171.

9. Felding CF, Jensen LM, Ronnesen H. Influence of alcohol intake on postoperative morbidity after hysterectomy. Am J Obstet Gynecol 1992;166:667–670.

10. Tonnesen H, Petersen KR. Postoperative morbidity among symptom-free alcohol misusers. Lancet 1992;340:334–337.

11. Wood PR, Soni N. Anaesthesia and substance abuse. Anaesthesia 1989;44:672–680.

12. Hays JT, Spickard WA. Alcoholism: early diagnosis and treatment. J Gen Intern Med 1987;2:420–427.

13. Rydon P, Reid A. Detection of alcohol related problems in general practice. J Stud Alcohol 1992;53:197–202.

14. Lewis CM. Perioperative screening for alcoholism. Ann Plast Surg 1992;28:207–209.

15. Ewing JA. Detecting alcoholism. JAMA 1984;252:1905–1907.

16. Skinner HA. Identification of alcohol abuse using a history of trauma. Ann Intern Med 1984;101:847–851.

17. Kantzian EJ, McKenna GJ. Acute toxic and withdrawal reactions associated with drug abuse. Ann Intern Med 1979;40:361–372.

18. Turner RC, Lichstein PR. Alcohol withdrawal syndromes. J Gen Intern Med 1989;4:432–444.

19. Eckardt MJ, Hartford TC, Kaelber CT. Health hazards associated with alcohol consumption. JAMA 1981;246:648–666.

20. Gavin FH, Ellinwood EH. Cocaine and other stimulants. N Engl J Med 1988;318:1173–1182.

21. Cregler LL, Marck H. Medical complications of cocaine abuse. N Engl J Med 1988;315:1495–1500.

22. Jaffe JH, Martin WR. Opioid analgesics and antagonists. In: Gilman AG, Goodman LS, Rall TW, Murad F, eds. Pharmacological basis of therapeutics. New York, MacMillan, 1985:491–531.

23. Fultz JM, Senay EC. Guidelines for the management of hospitalized narcotic addicts. Ann Intern Med 1975;82:815–818.

24. Gold MS, Pottash CA, Kleber HD. Opiate withdrawal using clonidine. JAMA 1980;243:343–346.

25. Parran TV, Jasinski DR. Buprenorphine detoxification of medically unstable narcotic dependent patients. Substance Abuse 1990;11:197–202.

26. Bickel WK, Johnson RE. Clinical trial of buprenorphine. Clin Pharmacol Ther 1989;43:72–78.

27. Clark WD. Alcoholism: blocks to diagnosis and treatment. Am J Med 1981;71:275–286.

28. Babor TF, Good SP. Screening and early intervention. Australian Drug and Alcohol Review 1987;6:325–339.

29. Barker LR, Whitfield CL. Alcoholism. In: Barker LR, Burton JR, Ziere PD, eds. Principles of ambulatory medicine. Baltimore, Williams & Wilkins, 1986:258–259.

30. Clark WD. The medical interview: focus on alcohol problems. Hosp Pract 1985;20:59–68.

31. Parran TV. Developing a treatment plan for the chemically dependent primary care patient. In: Bigby JA, ed. Substance abuse education in general internal medicine: a manual for faculty. Society of General Internal Medicine and the Ambulatory Pediatric Association, Bureau of Health Professions HRSA, 1993:1–11.

32. Parran TV, Bigby JA. Prescription drug abuse. In: Substance abuse education in general internal medicine: a manual for faculty. Society of General Internal Medicine and the Ambulatory Pediatric Association, Bureau of Health Professions HRSA, 1993:1–35.

Medical Management of the Surgical Patient, Third Edition,
edited by Michael F. Lubin, H. Kenneth Walker, and Robert B. Smith III.
J.B. Lippincott Company, Philadelphia, PA © 1995.

CHAPTER

48

COMPETENCY AND INFORMED CONSENT

Alan Stoudemire

Issues of competency to give informed consent may occasionally arise in medical–surgical patients who have psychiatric illnesses, in older debilitated patients, in minors, and in medical–surgical emergencies. Physicians need a basic working knowledge regarding the medicolegal issues involved in competency and informed consent even though legal and administrative consultation should always be sought in ambiguous situations. Hospital policies and state laws vary as well.

Competency to consent to treatment is most commonly defined as the capacity to comprehend relevant information regarding treatment, the ability to weigh the benefits of the proposed treatment, and the capacity to reach a reasonable decision.[1] Competency must always precede consent because consent cannot be legally given unless competency first exists. In medical situations, competency must be determined in the context of the clinical circumstances at hand. Competency standards are defined legally in specific regard to the matter to be considered (ie, to make a will, to stand criminal trial, to make a contract, to have a guardian appointed). For example, patients may be found to be competent in one area and incompetent in another. In the medical–surgical setting, the usual issue is whether patients are competent to consent to diagnostic or surgical procedures.[2]

Competency in the medical–surgical setting depends on the ability of patients to understand the nature of their illnesses, the benefits of proposed treatments, the risks of treatment, and the consequences of refusing treatment, and

to rationally consider alternate treatments that may be available. Patients must also be able to understand the consequences of refusing treatment (informed refusal).

Physicians frequently confuse the issue of competency with situations involving psychosis, civil commitment, and insanity defenses in criminal acts.[1] Patients may have schizophrenia, dementia, or a variety of other psychiatric illnesses and still be competent in the legal sense to make informed decisions regarding their medical care if they are able to comprehend the necessary information regarding the proposed treatment being proposed.

Another misconception is the belief that psychiatrists determine whether patients are competent. The courts, not psychiatrists, determine competency. Psychiatrists may render professional opinions regarding competency for the courts to consider, but the courts make the final decision regarding whether patients are competent.

Clinical situations involving competency may be broadly divided into emergencies (life-threatening conditions) and nonemergencies. In emergencies, physicians may act to save patients' lives before consent has been given if patients are unable to provide consent because of their illness (eg, unconsciousness because of an epidural hematoma), although a reasonable effort to contact the next of kin or legal guardian to obtain consent must be made. If the life-threatening nature of the situation is clearly defined and documented, there is little likelihood of legal consequence for proceeding if a reasonable effort has been made to ob-

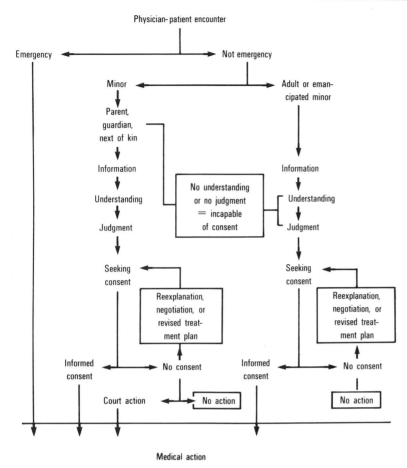

FIG. 48-1. Seeking and obtaining informed consent. (Groves JE, Vaccarino JM. Legal aspects of consultation. In: Hackett TP, Cassem NH, eds. Massachusetts General Hospital Handbook of General Hospital Psychiatry, ed 2. Littleton MA, PSG Publishing, 1987:601)

tain consent from the next of kin. If any confusion or ambiguity exists, a legal opinion should always be obtained before proceeding if possible.

Nonemergencies are an entirely different matter. If patients are incompetent to give consent, consent should be sought from the next of kin. Physicians should be aware that the legally identified persons considered to be next of kin vary from state to state. If no one takes responsibility for patients, psychiatric consultations and petitions to the court must be made to have patients declared incompetent to make medicolegal decisions. Emergency guardians usually are appointed by the courts or the courts otherwise allow physicians to proceed.

In the past, physicians were reasonably assured of not encountering subsequent legal difficulties if they acted in good faith with sound clinical judgment and in patients' best interests. The current atmosphere of medical litigation, however, warrants extreme caution and legal advice if questions of competency and consent arise.[3] Figure 48-1 presents one basic approach to informed consent in the medical setting.[1,4]

REFERENCES

1. Groves JE, Vaccarino JM. Legal aspects of consultation. In: Hackett TP, Cassem NH, eds. Massachusetts General Hospital Handbook of general hospital psychiatry, ed 2. Littleton, MA, PSG Publishing, 1987:591–604.
2. Deaton RJS, Colenda CC, Bursztajn HJ. Medical-legal issues. In: Stoudemire A, Fogel BS, eds. Psychiatric care of the medical patient. New York, Oxford University Press, 1993:929–938.
3. Overman WH. Medical legal issues in dementia. In: Stoudemire A, Fogel BS, eds. Psychiatric care of the medical patient. New York, Oxford University Press, 1993:939–952.
4. Dubin WR. Psychiatric emergencies: recognition and management. In: Stoudemire A, ed. Clinical psychiatry for medical students. Philadelphia, JB Lippincott, 1990:497–526.

PART

2

SURGICAL
PROCEDURES AND
THEIR COMPLICATIONS

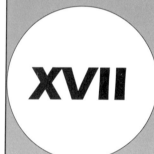

GENERAL SURGERY

Medical Management of the Surgical Patient, Third Edition,
edited by Michael F. Lubin, H. Kenneth Walker, and Robert B. Smith III.
J.B. Lippincott Company, Philadelphia, PA © 1995.

LYSIS OF ADHESIONS

David V. Feliciano

Adhesions from previous abdominal operations are the most common cause of mechanical small bowel obstruction in adults. Attempts to limit the number and magnitude of postoperative adhesions through instillation of agents such as heparin and hydroxyethyl starch into the peritoneal cavity have proved unsuccessful. Patients with adhesive small bowel obstruction present with either partial or complete obstruction. In patients who are still passing flatus and who have only moderate cramping, minimal abdominal distention, and no signs of peritonitis, a trial period of nasogastric tube suction, hydration, and observation is worthwhile. Laparotomy has been avoided in 40% of such patients in some series. Patients with histories of complete bowel obstruction or with closed loop obstruction (steady pain), elevated temperature, signs of peritonitis on examination, progressive leukocytosis, or a "stepladder" appearance of dilated intestinal loops on flat plate radiographs of the abdomen should undergo urgent operation. Ischemia and even gangrene of the obstructed bowel can occur in the absence of the classified symptoms and signs.

Dehydration and electrolyte abnormalities (hyponatremic hypokalemic metabolic alkalosis) are common in patients with repeated episodes of vomiting related to proximal obstruction of the small bowel. Preoperative correction of these problems is appropriate in all patients and assists in maintaining hemodynamic stability through the perioperative period.

Rapid-induction general endotracheal anesthesia is used, and adhesions are divided by the finger fracture technique, scissors, or electrocautery. An iatrogenic enterotomy increases postoperative morbidity because of the overgrowth of colonic-type bacteria in the obstructed loop. Vigorous antibiotic irrigation and open packing of the skin and subcutaneous tissue of the laparotomy incision are appropriate if this complication occurs. The procedure may last only 1 hour if a single adhesive band has caused the obstruction. In patients with multiple previous laparotomies and dense adhesions, lysis may take 4 to 6 hours to complete. The stress of the procedure depends on the duration of the obstruction, the magnitude of dehydration and electrolyte abnormalities, the type of adhesions, and the absence or presence of ischemia. In elderly patients with prolonged bowel obstruction and gangrene, stress is considerable because of sepsis. Administration of one or two units of blood may be needed during difficult and prolonged lysis procedures.

USUAL POSTOPERATIVE COURSE

Expected postoperative hospital stay: 7 to 10 days

Operative mortality: Up to 5% overall; up to 15% for strangulation obstruction

Special monitoring required: Hyponatremic hypokalemic

metabolic alkalosis and dehydration may be present post-operatively if an emergency operation was necessary. In hypokalemic patients who are voiding, 15- to 20-mEq aliquots of potassium chloride are administered every hour through a central venous line, if necessary. Fluid replacement with 0.45% sodium chloride (approximates gastric juice) is based on central venous pressure and urine output. Rehydration is suggested by a urine output of 0.5 to 1 mL/kg/h in adults.

Patient activity and positioning: Patients may be out of bed on the day after the operation. If significant abdominal distention is present, upright positioning aids in ventilation.

Alimentation: Nasogastric tube decompression may be prolonged in patients with marked preoperative dilation of multiple loops of bowel or severe perioperative electrolyte abnormalities, as well as in those who undergo difficult and lengthy operations. In patients with obvious nutritional deficiencies at the time of operation, postoperative intravenous hyperalimentation is started once electrolyte abnormalities are corrected.

Antibiotic coverage: All patients receive cephalosporin or advanced penicillin preoperatively and 24 hours postoperatively. If at surgery the obstructed small bowel is seen to be gangrenous or perforated, antibiotic administration is continued for 5 to 7 days postoperatively.

ing the lysis of adhesions are at significantly increased risk for the development of a postoperative wound infection. Open packing of the subcutaneous tissue and skin at the time of the lysis is appropriate. Delayed primary closure of the wound can be performed on the sixth postoperative day, with a 10% to 20% risk of infection.

Breakdown of enterotomy repair or small bowel anastomosis: A variety of factors may lead to a leak from a repaired enterotomy site or small bowel anastomosis. An enterocutaneous fistula through the abdominal wound or drainage tract is treated with oral intake prohibition, sump drainage, intravenous hyperalimentation, antibiotics, and somatostatin analogue (Sandostatin). A low-output fistula (less than 500 mL/24 h) in the distal ileum has an excellent likelihood of closing with this management. If an intraabdominal abscess occurs, either percutaneous drainage or another laparotomy with resection and reanastomosis is indicated.

AFTER DISCHARGE

Recurrent obstruction: Repeated episodes of adhesive obstruction occur in 30% of patients within 10 years and should be managed as described.

POSTOPERATIVE COMPLICATIONS

IN THE HOSPITAL

Prolonged ileus: As noted, peristalsis may return slowly in some patients. Because recurrent obstruction of the small bowel is always a concern, the administration of *low volumes* of a bowel-cleaning agent (eg, GoLYTELY) in patients with bowel sounds after the first week may be useful. Passage of this agent rectally without severe cramping suggests that merely an adynamic ileus is present. Barium may also be administered to rule out a recurrent mechanical bowel obstruction, but it may be difficult to remove if the ileus persists after the study.

Wound infection: Patients who require prolonged preoperative in-hospital observation or who underwent previous laparotomy during the same admission or enterotomy dur-

BIBLIOGRAPHY

Bizer LS, Liebling RW, Delany HM, Gliedman ML. Small bowel obstruction: the role of nonoperative treatment in simple intestinal obstruction and predictive criteria for strangulation obstruction. Surgery 1981;89:407–413.

Butler JA, Cameron BL, Morrow M, et al. Small bowel obstruction in patients with a prior history of cancer. Am J Surg 1991;162:624–628.

Landercasper J, Cogbill TH, Merry WH, et al. Long-term outcome after hospitalization for small-bowel obstruction. Arch Surg 1993;128:765–771.

Nubiola P, Badia JM, Martinez-Rodenas F, et al. Treatment of 27 postoperative enterocutaneous fistulas with the long half-life somatostatin analogue SMS 201-995. Ann Surg 1989;210:56–58.

Stewart RM, Page CP, Brender J, et al. The incidence and risk of early postoperative small bowel obstruction: a cohort study. Am J Surg 1987;154:643–647.

Medical Management of the Surgical Patient, Third Edition,
edited by Michael F. Lubin, H. Kenneth Walker, and Robert B. Smith III.
J.B. Lippincott Company, Philadelphia, PA © 1995.

CHAPTER

ABDOMINAL TRAUMA

50

David V. Feliciano

In patients with blunt abdominal trauma, emergent or urgent laparotomy is performed for hypotension and abdominal hemorrhage (frequently confirmed by diagnostic peritoneal lavage or ultrasound), overt peritonitis, or obvious signs of abdominal visceral injury without the need for further advanced diagnostic studies. Included are patients with significant proctorrhagia after pelvic fracture; those with evidence of a ruptured hemidiaphragm or air in the peritoneal cavity or retroperitoneum on plain radiographs; and those with evidence of a ruptured duodenum, intraperitoneal rupture of the bladder, or significant injury to the renal artery or kidney on contrast-enhanced radiographs. All other stable patients whose abdominal examinations are compromised by an abnormal sensorium (related to alcohol, drugs, head injury), abnormal sensation (due to spinal cord injury), or adjacent injuries are best evaluated by abdominal computed tomography.

In patients with stab wounds to the abdomen, emergent or urgent laparotomy is performed for abdominal distention and hypotension, overt peritonitis, significant evisceration, or obvious signs of abdominal visceral injury without the need for further advanced diagnostic studies. Included in the last group are patients with hematemesis, proctorrhagia, or hematuria; those with evidence of diaphragmatic defect on finger palpation before insertion of a thoracostomy tube; and those with evidence of an injury to the kidney, ureter, or bladder on contrast-enhanced radiograph. All other stable patients undergo local exploration of

the stab wound to verify peritoneal penetration. In asymptomatic patients with peritoneal penetration, a 24-hour period of observation is appropriate. An alternate approach is to use diagnostic peritoneal lavage after local wound exploration verifies peritoneal penetration. The diagnosis of intraabdominal injury is delayed 10 to 12 hours in patients with false-negative results on initial physical examination or diagnostic peritoneal lavage.

Gunshot wounds shown to traverse the abdominal cavity on either physical examination or plain radiographs of the trunk cause visceral or vascular injuries in 96% to 98% of patients. This incidence of injury with penetration of the peritoneal cavity or the visceral or vascular compartment of the retroperitoneum is significantly greater than that seen with penetrating stab wounds. Therefore, a policy of emergency laparotomy is followed in most trauma centers whenever a missile appears to have traversed the abdominal cavity.

General anesthesia is used for trauma laparotomy. After evacuation of blood and clot from the peritoneal cavity, areas of hemorrhage are controlled by manual compression, packing with laparotomy pads, or vascular clamps. Perforations in the gastrointestinal tract are then sealed with noncrushing clamps. The sequence of operative repairs or resections depends on the combination of injuries. Laparotomies for trauma are usually completed in 3 hours or less because longer procedures in previously hypotensive patients can lead to hypothermia, persistent metabolic

461

acidosis, and coagulopathies. The need for transfusion is extremely variable, ranging from less than 25% of patients with stab wounds to 50% of patients with gunshot wounds. The stress of the operative procedure depends on the number of organs injured and the magnitude of blood loss in the perioperative period.

USUAL POSTOPERATIVE COURSE

Expected postoperative hospital stay: 5 to 7 days after laparotomy for a stab wound and 7 to 9 days after laparotomy for a gunshot wound or blunt trauma, depending on associated injuries

Operative mortality: In patients undergoing laparotomy for stab wounds of the abdomen, the mortality rate is 1% to 2%. The mortality increases to 3% in patients with routine gunshot wounds (no vascular injury) and to 12% in patients with abdominal vascular injuries. The mortality after laparotomy for blunt abdominal trauma is related to the presence of associated injuries to the head and chest, and to the magnitude of intraabdominal visceral injuries. For example, the mortality after laparotomy for major blunt hepatic injuries in referral trauma centers ranges from 14% to 31%.

Special monitoring required: Patients with known cardiac or pulmonary compromise and those who undergo difficult procedures associated with excessive blood loss require postoperative hemodynamic monitoring with pulmonary artery catheters.

Patient activity and positioning: Patients may be out of bed on the day after the operation, depending on hemodynamic stability.

Alimentation: Early enteral feeding through a nasojejunal tube or needle-catheter jejunostomy placed at laparotomy is the standard of care in many centers for patients with major abdominal injury (Penetrating Abdominal Trauma Index 15 to 40 or Injury Severity Score greater than 25 for blunt trauma). Full caloric requirements can be met at 2½ to 3 days in properly selected patients. Early enteral feeding has reduced septic morbidity after laparotomy for abdominal trauma in several studies.

In patients with extensive resection of the midgut, marked abdominal distention, or exposure of the midgut under a plastic silo (abdominal wall not closed), early intravenous hyperalimentation may be used in place of enteral feeding. Full caloric requirements can be met at 2 to 2½ days in properly selected patients. Disadvantages of intravenous feeding include the fixed rate of long-term catheter infection (3% to 10%), a higher overall rate of postoperative infection exclusive of catheter infection (possible gut-origin sepsis), and the development of hepatic cholestasis and fatty infiltration.

Antibiotic coverage: Postoperative antibiotics are not routinely administered to patients with blunt abdominal trauma unless rupture of the gastrointestinal tract is found at laparotomy or a chest tube is in place. Cephalosporin or advanced penicillin with aerobic and anaerobic coverage is continued for 24 hours in patients who have undergone laparotomy for a penetrating abdominal wound within 8 to 12 hours of injury. Patients with a long delay between injury and laparotomy and those with extensive fecal contamination are treated for 5 to 7 days for established peritonitis.

Drains: Suction drains are placed by most surgeons in patients who have undergone repair or resection of a major hepatic injury, repair of a major duodenal or renal injury, or distal pancreatectomy. The duration of drain placement depends on the injury but ranges from 5 to 7 days in most centers.

POSTOPERATIVE COMPLICATIONS

IN THE HOSPITAL

Wound infection: Infection occurs in 2% to 3% of patients without colon injuries and is treated as described in the section on lysis of adhesions. If the colon is perforated and moderate to extensive contamination is present, the subcutaneous tissue and skin are packed open in 50% to 75% of patients. This decreases the wound infection rate in these high-risk patients to 5% to 6%.

Intraabdominal abscess: Abscesses occur in 2.5% to 3% of patients undergoing laparotomy for abdominal trauma, usually in those with perforation of the gastrointestinal tract (3.9% to 4% versus 1% to 1.5%). Percutaneous drainage by an interventional radiologist is an appropriate first step, followed by reopening of an old drain tract or extraperitoneal surgical drainage if the percutaneous approach fails. Reopening of the midline incision is rarely necessary and carries the highest mortality.

Postoperative hemorrhage: Hemorrhage requiring reoperation occurs in 2% to 2.5% of patients, almost all of whom had severe hepatic injury or intraoperative coagulopathy at the first procedure.

AFTER DISCHARGE

Adhesive small bowel obstruction: Much as in patients who have undergone elective abdominal procedures, late adhesive obstruction occurs in 10% to 25% of patients.

BIBLIOGRAPHY

Feliciano DV. Abdominal trauma. In: Schwartz SI, Ellis H, eds. Maingot's abdominal operations. Norwalk, CT, Appleton & Lange, 1989;457.

Feliciano DV. Diagnostic modalities in abdominal trauma. Peritoneal lavage, ultrasonography, computed tomography scanning, and arteriography. Surg Clin North Am 1991;71:241–256.

Feliciano DV, Burch JM, Spjut-Patrinely V, et al. Abdominal gunshot wounds. An urban trauma center's experience with 300 consecutive patients. Ann Surg 1988;208:362–370.

Feliciano DV, Gentry LO, Bitondo CG, et al. Single agent cephalosporin prophylaxis for penetrating abdominal trauma: results and comment on the emergence of the enterococcus. Am J Surg 1986;152:674–681.

Feliciano DV, Spjut-Patrinely V, Burch JM. Enteral vs. parenteral nutrition in patients with severe penetrating abdominal trauma. Contemp Surg 1991;39:30–36.

CHAPTER

51

SMALL BOWEL RESECTION

Medical Management of the Surgical Patient, Third Edition,
edited by Michael F. Lubin, H. Kenneth Walker, and Robert B. Smith III.
J.B. Lippincott Company, Philadelphia, PA © 1995.

David V. Feliciano

Small bowel resection is performed in a variety of settings, the most common of which are traumatic perforation, thrombotic or embolic infarction, regional enteritis, and concomitant colectomy. Less common indications for resection include benign or malignant neoplasms (leiomyoma, hemangioma, carcinoid, lymphoma, adenocarcinoma, sarcoma); fistula resulting from a previous repair or resection; symptomatic Meckel's diverticulum; neutropenic enterocolitis; and spontaneous perforation in patients with cancer who are receiving chemotherapy and corticosteroids.

Segmental resection and end-to-end anastomosis with suture or staples usually can be performed in 20 minutes. With diffuse ischemia or peritonitis, resection and the creation of adjacent stomas allows for the instillation of succus entericus into the distal limb if necessary.

With the exception of those performed for a neoplasm in the adjacent right colon, most resections of the small bowel for trauma, infarction, or inflammatory bowel disease cause moderate to severe stress. General anesthesia is used, the length of the procedure depends on the indication, and blood transfusions are necessary only in patients with trauma, extensive inflammation, or infiltrating neoplasms.

Special monitoring required: Many patients with major abdominal trauma or midgut infarction require postoperative hemodynamic monitoring with a pulmonary artery catheter. Serial measurements of arterial pH are also worthwhile if bowel with borderline viability is left in the abdomen at the first operation.

Patient activity and positioning: Patients may be out of bed on the day after operation, depending on hemodynamic stability.

Alimentation: For routine procedures, clear liquids are begun with the return of bowel function and advanced as tolerated. In cases involving multiple intraabdominal injuries or major resection of the midgut secondary to infarction, intravenous hyperalimentation is begun as soon as patients are hemodynamically stable.

Antibiotic coverage: All patients receive cephalosporin or advanced penicillin preoperatively and for 24 hours postoperatively. In the presence of established peritonitis from infarction or perforation of regional enteritis, a Meckel's diverticulum, neutropenic enterocolitis, or chemotherapy, the antibiotic is continued for 5 to 7 days postoperatively.

USUAL POSTOPERATIVE COURSE

Expected postoperative hospital stay: 5 to 7 days

Operative mortality: 2% to 3% for elective resection, 12% for penetrating trauma with two other organ injuries, 25% for superior mesenteric artery embolism, and 60% for superior mesenteric artery thrombosis

POSTOPERATIVE COMPLICATIONS

IN THE HOSPITAL

Wound infection: See Chapter 49.

Breakdown of enterotomy repair or small bowel anastomosis: See Chapter 49.

Recurrent infarction: If bowel with questionable viability is left in the abdomen or a borderline stoma is brought to the skin at the first operation, further ischemic changes may occur and necessitate reoperation. Many surgeons choose to close only the skin of the abdominal incision at the first operation and perform a second operation (second-look procedure) 12 hours later to reassess the questionably viable bowel. Others monitor the color of a stoma or serial arterial pH levels to assist in determining whether reoperation is necessary.

Prolonged ileus: Peristalsis may return slowly in patients with multiple intraabdominal injuries, a superior mesenteric artery embolus or thrombus, chronic obstruction from enteritis or a neoplasm, or diffuse peritonitis from a perforation. Continuous nasogastric suction, intravenous hyperalimentation, and patience are indicated. If there is serious concern about a possible early mechanical small bowel obstruction instead of an ileus, the use of an oral colon-cleaning agent or barium is indicated as described in Chapter 49.

AFTER DISCHARGE

Obstruction: Early in-hospital adhesive small bowel obstruction occurs in 2% to 3% of patients who undergo small bowel resection. Late episodes of adhesive obstruction occur in 10% to 25% of patients.

Nutritional deficiency: Massive resection of the midgut may lead to chronic diarrhea and nutritional deficiencies, particularly if the ileocecal valve has been sacrificed. In-hospital and subsequent home hyperalimentation is indicated in such patients. Progressive hyperplasia of the lining of the remaining midgut may allow for resumption of enteral feedings over time.

BIBLIOGRAPHY

Broe PJ, Bayless TM, Cameron JL. Crohn's disease: are enteroenteral fistulas an indication for surgery? Surgery 1982;91:249–253.

Crohn BB, Ginzburg L, Oppenheimer GD. Regional ileitis: a pathologic and clinical entity. JAMA 1932;251:73–81.

Farnell MB. Neutropenic enterocolitis: a surgical disease? Infections in Surgery 1987;6:120–131.

Levy PJ, Krausz MM, Manny J. Acute mesenteric ischemia: improved results: a retrospective analysis of ninety-two patients. Surgery 1990;107:372–380.

Torosian MH, Turnbull ADM. Emergency laparotomy for spontaneous intestinal and colonic perforations in cancer patients receiving corticosteroids and chemotherapy. J Clin Oncol 1988;6:291–296.

Medical Management of the Surgical Patient, Third Edition,
edited by Michael F. Lubin, H. Kenneth Walker, and Robert B. Smith III.
J.B. Lippincott Company, Philadelphia, PA © 1995.

CHAPTER

52 APPENDECTOMY

David V. Feliciano

Appendectomy is performed for acute appendicitis (simple, suppurative, gangrenous, gangrenous with perforation); as an interval procedure after recovery from an appendiceal abscess; for small (less than 2.5 cm) carcinoid tumors or benign mucoceles; and prophylactically during laparotomy for other conditions. The accuracy of diagnosis in acute appendicitis has increased from 80% to over 90% in several recent series using diagnostic adjuncts such as graded-compression ultrasound, barium enema, and laparoscopy. In addition, percutaneous drainage of periappendiceal abscesses may allow for a subsequent single operation to remove the perforated appendix (interval appendectomy).

With the patient under general anesthesia, appendectomy may be performed through a right lower quadrant muscle-splitting incision or by a laparoscopic approach using four ports. With simple, suppurative, or gangrenous appendicitis, the stress of operation is minimal. For patients with perforated gangrenous appendicitis and diffuse peritonitis, or with large intraabdominal abscesses, stress may be moderate or even major. The duration of a simple appendectomy is 45 minutes, but this increases to 60 to 75 minutes in obese patients with retrocecal appendicitis and rupture. In some of these patients, the usual 6- to 7-cm incision must be extended to gain exposure of the posterior cecum and ascending colon. Blood transfusion is never required.

USUAL POSTOPERATIVE COURSE

Expected postoperative hospital stay: 1 to 2 days for simple, suppurative, or gangrenous (without rupture) appendicitis; 7 to 10 days for perforated appendicitis with diffuse peritonitis or an intraabdominal abscess

Operative mortality: 0.1% for simple or suppurative appendicitis, 0.6% for gangrenous appendicitis, and 5% for perforated appendicitis

Special monitoring required: Patients with sepsis syndrome or shock secondary to perforated appendicitis require postoperative hemodynamic monitoring with a pulmonary artery catheter.

Patient activity and positioning: Patients with non-perforated appendicitis may be out of bed the day of operation and resume activity gradually during the first 2 weeks after hospital discharge. Those with perforated appendicitis historically remain in bed in the semi-Fowler position to encourage pelvic localization of pus.

Alimentation: Clear liquids are given on the day of operation, and food intake is advanced as tolerated in patients with nonperforated appendicitis. In those with perforated appendicitis, clear liquids are permitted with the return of bowel function and intake is advanced as tolerated.

Antibiotic coverage: All patients with suspected appendicitis receive cephalosporin or advanced penicillin preoperatively. Those with simple or suppurative appendicitis require no further antibiotic coverage. All patients with gangrenous appendicitis receive antibiotics for 24 hours postoperatively, and those with perforated appendicitis and secondary peritonitis or intraabdominal abscess continue to receive antibiotics for 5 to 7 days postoperatively.

Drains: Closed suction drains are placed in well-defined abscess cavities in the pericecal or pelvic area for 5 to 7 days postoperatively. A decision for removal is based on a postoperative computed tomographic scan or a sinogram performed through the drains.

Wound closure: Open packing of the subcutaneous tissue and skin is indicated in adult patients with extensive gangrenous or perforated appendicitis. Delayed primary closure of the wound can be performed on the sixth postoperative day and has a 10% to 20% risk of infection.

POSTOPERATIVE COMPLICATIONS

IN THE HOSPITAL

Diffuse peritonitis: Diffuse peritonitis that is present at the time of appendectomy may lead to sepsis syndrome or septic shock in the early postoperative period or to intraabdominal abscess in the late postoperative period.

Wound infection: Wound infection occurs primarily when attempts are made to close the subcutaneous tissue and skin in patients with gangrenous or perforated appendicitis. Treatment includes the administration of antibiotics based on Gram stain results, the application of local heat, and opening of a portion of the incision.

Intraabdominal abscess: Intraabdominal abscess may develop in up to 20% of patients with gangrenous or perfora-

ted appendicitis. Diagnosis and treatment are by clinical examination and transrectal drainage for pelvic abscess, or computed tomography and percutaneous drainage or reoperation for paracecal or subphrenic abscess).

Fecal fistula: Less than 1% of patients experience blow out of the appendiceal stump leading to a fecal fistula through the incision or a drain. Spontaneous closure usually occurs within 2 to 3 weeks.

AFTER DISCHARGE

Late diagnosis of a carcinoid tumor or appendiceal carcinoma: A late pathology report may describe the presence of a carcinoid tumor larger than 2.5 cm or an appendiceal carcinoma in the resected specimen. Reoperation for a formal right hemicolectomy is indicated.

BIBLIOGRAPHY

Berry J Jr, Malt RA. Appendicitis near its centenary. Ann Surg 1984;200:567–575.

Fitz RH. Perforating inflammation of the vermiform appendix, with special reference to its early diagnosis and treatment. Trans Assoc Am Physicians 1886;1:107–144.

Kniskern JH, Eskin EM, Fletcher HS. Increasing accuracy in the diagnosis of acute appendicitis with modern diagnostic techniques. Am Surg 1986;52:222–225.

Nitecki S, Karmeli R, Sarr MG. Appendiceal calculi and fecaliths as indications for appendectomy. Surg Gynecol Obstet 1990;171:185–188.

Schirmer BD, Schmieg RE, Dix J, et al. Laparoscopic versus traditional appendectomy for suspected appendicitis. Am J Surg 1993;165:670–675.

Medical Management of the Surgical Patient, Third Edition,
edited by Michael F. Lubin, H. Kenneth Walker, and Robert B. Smith III.
J.B. Lippincott Company, Philadelphia, PA © 1995.

CHAPTER

53

COLON RESECTION

David V. Feliciano

Open or laparoscopic colon resection is performed for a variety of conditions, the most common of which are benign or malignant neoplasms (tubular or villoglandular adenomas, adenocarcinoma, carcinoid, lymphoma); complications of diverticular disease (perforation with peritonitis or abscess, stricture, bleeding); extensive traumatic perforations; angiodysplasia or arteriovenous malformation with lower gastrointestinal bleeding; and inflammatory bowel disease (ulcerative colitis, segmental colonic Crohn's disease, toxic megacolon). Less common indications for resection include volvulus of the sigmoid colon or cecum; thrombotic, embolic, or low-flow infarction; and premalignant conditions (familial polyposis, Gardner's syndrome).

Hemicolectomy or segmental resection for malignant neoplasms involves excision of the area of the tumor, at least 10 cm of normal proximal colon or small bowel, and 5 cm of normal distal colon, as well as the regional lymphatics that accompany the major veins. In contrast, segmental resection for complications of diverticular disease, Crohn's disease, colonic volvulus, or infarction involves only grossly diseased bowel without excision of regional lymphatics. Subtotal abdominal colectomy with ileorectostomy is performed for patients with nonfamilial synchronous scattered benign or malignant neoplasms. It is also used in some patients with megacolon secondary to obstructing neoplasms of the sigmoid or rectosigmoid colon or of the upper rectum. A near-total abdominal colectomy with preservation of a seromuscular short rectal cuff to preserve anal continence through the creation of an ileal pouch–anal anastomosis is indicated in patients with severe chronic ulcerative colitis, familial polyposis, or Gardner's syndrome.

In patients who have undergone preoperative colon preparation with cleaning agents and nonabsorbable antibiotics, a sutured or stapled anastomosis is performed after resection. Because of the tedious nature of intracorporeal suture techniques in laparoscopic colon surgery, a limited incision is made in the body wall after resection to perform an extracorporeal anastomosis. Emergency resections involving the right half of the colon—such as might be performed for perforated cecal diverticulitis, angiodysplasia with bleeding, traumatic perforation, cecal volvulus, or low-flow infarction—are often reconstructed with an ileocolostomy, even without preoperative or intraoperative bowel preparation, because surgeons consider such an operation to be a small bowel–type anastomosis. Emergency resections involving the entire colon (for an unknown site of bleeding or megacolon secondary to an obstructing neoplasm of the sigmoid or rectosigmoid colon) are also reconstructed with an ileorectostomy by some surgeons for the same reason. Emergency resections involving the transverse colon or left half of the colon are usually followed by creation of a proximal end colostomy and a mucous fistula (distal stoma in body wall) or Hartmann pouch (distal end of bowel closed and left in abdomen).

Elective colon resection, even near-total colectomy, is a controlled operation with little blood loss and only moderate stress to the patient. Emergency colon resection for perforated sigmoid diverticulitis, bleeding angiodysplasia, extensive traumatic perforation, toxic megacolon, or infarction from volvulus or low flow may be associated with moderate blood loss and is a significant stress, particularly in elderly patients.

USUAL POSTOPERATIVE COURSE

Expected postoperative hospital stay: 7 to 10 days

Operative mortality: 2% to 6% for elective resection in elderly patients; 4% to 9% for emergency right colon or subtotal resection with primary anastomosis; 20% to 30% for subtotal resection in the presence of a perforated toxic megacolon or unknown site of lower gastrointestinal hemorrhage

Special monitoring required: Postoperative hemodynamic monitoring with a pulmonary artery catheter is necessary in many elderly patients with emergency resection of the colon and in younger patients with major abdominal trauma, including injury to the colon.

Patient activity and positioning: Depending on hemodynamic stability and the presence of other injuries, patients may be out of bed on the day after operation.

Alimentation: For routine procedures, patients are permitted clear liquids with the return of bowel function and intake of food is advanced as tolerated. Patients with emergency subtotal resection for obstruction, bleeding, toxic megacolon, or multiple intraabdominal injuries receive intravenous hyperalimentation as soon as they are hemodynamically stable.

Antibiotic coverage: Gavage cleaning of the colon in combination with nonabsorbable antibiotics (neomycin and erythromycin base at 1 PM, 2 PM, and 11 PM the day before surgery) is the standard colon preparation. All patients also receive intravenous cephalosporin, advanced penicillin, metronidazole, or a combination of antibiotics before and at least 24 hours after surgery. Antibiotics are continued for 5 to 7 days postoperatively in patients with established peritonitis from perforated sigmoid or cecal diverticulitis, perforated toxic megacolon, gangrenous colon from volvulus or vascular catastrophe, or delayed operation for traumatic perforation.

Delayed wound closure: Open packing of the skin and subcutaneous tissue of the incision is indicated with gangrenous or perforated colon. Delayed primary closure is appropriate at 5 to 6 days in patients with clean, deep wounds that would otherwise require 6 to 12 weeks of dressing changes at home.

Drains: Colectomies above the peritoneal reflection are not drained unless a well-defined abscess cavity from a perforation is present. Many surgeons drain the deep pelvis after low anterior resection of the rectosigmoid colon or upper rectum.

POSTOPERATIVE COMPLICATIONS

IN THE HOSPITAL

Wound infection: See Chapter 49.

Breakdown of anastomosis: Disruption of an ileocolostomy or colocolostomy in the early postoperative period is a rare but potentially lethal complication. Patients with obvious fecal peritonitis require early reoperation. After 5 to 7 days, a partial leak leads to a contained perianastomotic or pelvic abscess or a colocutaneous fistula through a drainage site or the abdominal incision. Percutaneous drainage of an intraperitoneal abscess may be a worthwhile first step, although a fecal fistula is an obvious risk. Operative transrectal drainage is appropriate for a pelvic abscess that is palpable on rectal examination. Ileocolocutaneous or colocutaneous fistulas are treated with prohibition of oral intake, intravenous hyperalimentation, administration of a somatostatin analogue, and protection of the surrounding skin. In the absence of a foreign body, intraabdominal infection, a short tract (epithelialization), residual neoplasm, or distal obstruction ("FIEND"), the fistula is expected to close without reoperation.

Pseudomembranous enterocolitis: The sudden onset of tenderness over the remaining colon in association with diarrhea and systemic toxicity is strongly suggestive of pseudomembranous enterocolitis. A specimen of stool is sent for *Clostridium difficile* enterotoxin, and empiric vancomycin is administered intravenously.

AFTER DISCHARGE

Change in bowel movements: Patients who have undergone resection of the ileocecal valve or an extensive portion of the left colon (left hemicolectomy, subtotal or total colectomy with anastomosis) have an increased number of bowel movements. These usually decrease over time; the average number of bowel movements in one series of patients with subtotal colectomy and ileorectostomy was two per day after 6 months.

Patients with total colectomy, creation of an ileal pouch, and an ileal pouch–anal anastomosis average five or six bowel movements in 24 hours. Complete daytime continence is present in 75%. Nighttime continence is present in only 45% during the first several years, but improves to 75% after 4 years.

Recurrent tumor: After resection for colorectal carcinoma, the patient is monitored by colonoscopy every 6 months and carcinoembryonic antigen levels every 2 months for 2 years, after which time follow-up intervals may be lengthened. Reoperation is indicated if colonoscopy reveals recurrent tumor or the carcinoembryonic antigen level is increased but less than 10 ng/mL, and if no distant metastases are seen with computed tomography. The role of radiolabeled monoclonal antibody directed against tumor-associated antigens as a surveillance tool is being studied extensively.

BIBLIOGRAPHY

Halevy A, Levi J, Orda R. Emergency subtotal colectomy: a new trend for treatment of obstructing carcinoma of the left colon. Ann Surg 1989;210:220–223.

Kelly KA. Anal sphincter-saving operations for chronic ulcerative colitis. Am J Surg 1992;163:5–11.

Peoples JB, Vilk DR, Maguire JP, et al. Reassessment of primary resection of the perforated segment for severe colonic diverticulitis. Am J Surg 1990;159:291–294.

Riseman JA, Wichterman K. Evaluation of right hemicolectomy for unexpected cecal mass. Arch Surg 1989;124:1043–1044.

Walsh RM, Aranha GV, Freeark RJ. Mortality and quality of life after total abdominal colectomy. Arch Surg 1990;125:1564–1566.

Medical Management of the Surgical Patient, Third Edition,
edited by Michael F. Lubin, H. Kenneth Walker, and Robert B. Smith III.
J.B. Lippincott Company, Philadelphia, PA © 1995.

ABDOMINOPERINEAL RESECTION

David V. Feliciano

Abdominoperineal resection (Miles' operation) with a permanent end colostomy is performed to remove malignant neoplasms (adenocarcinoma, carcinoid, lymphoma, squamous cell carcinoma remaining after chemotherapy or radiotherapy, cloacogenic carcinoma, basal cell carcinoma, and malignant melanoma) or extensive Crohn's disease with fistulas of the mid-rectum, low rectum, or perianal area. The operation is conducted through both a low midline laparotomy incision and a circumferential perianal incision, and is essentially a posterior exenteration of the pelvis. Included in the excision are the rectosigmoid colon, the rectum, the pelvic mesocolon, the lymph nodes associated with the three sets of hemorrhoidal vessels, the levator muscles out to the ischial tuberosities, the anus, and the perianal skin. Many surgeons use low anterior resection with an anastomosis in patients with adenocarcinoma of the upper or mid-rectum because it produces essentially equivalent survival and precludes the need for colostomy. The surgeon must be able to excise a 2-cm margin of normal bowel beyond the rectal tumor and to have enough rectum left at or above the levator muscles to allow the performance of a stapled or hand-sewn anastomosis.

The rectum alone is excised (without the mesocolon or lymph nodes), and a seromuscular short rectal cuff is preserved to maintain anal continence through the creation of an ileal pouch–anal anastomosis in patients with severe chronic ulcerative colitis, familial polyposis, or Gardner's syndrome, but not in those with Crohn's disease. This oper-

ation is most commonly performed as part of a near-total abdominal colectomy and differs significantly from the exenterative procedure described in this chapter.

If preoperative external-beam radiotherapy has been used to shrink a large rectal tumor and sterilize areas of adherence to the sacrum posteriorly or to the vagina or prostate gland anteriorly, abdominoperineal resection is delayed for 4 to 6 weeks. The operation is performed after preoperative colon preparation with cleaning agents and nonabsorbable antibiotics. The ideal site for the permanent end colostomy in the left lower quadrant is marked by the surgeon or enterostomal therapy nurse the night before operation. The procedure is often performed by two surgical teams simultaneously. The team performing the laparotomy mobilizes the rectosigmoid colon, rectum, and mesocolon with vessels and lymph nodes off the sacrum, divides the colon with a stapler, and creates a proximal end sigmoid colostomy. The second team excises the perianal skin, anus, and levator muscles, and removes the entire specimen through the perineum.

Extensive resection of a mid-rectal tumor may remove the pelvic peritoneum. Some surgeons leave the pelvis open and allow the small bowel to fall into the hollow of the sacrum. Others suture a sheet of absorbable mesh to replace the pelvic peritoneum and support the small bowel above the deep pelvic space. This is particularly useful if further postoperative radiotherapy is necessary because of tumor invasion of the pelvic side wall. Before the remnants of the levators, the subcutaneous tissue, and the skin of the perineal incision are closed, closed suction drains are inserted through the distal medial buttocks into the deep pelvic space for postoperative irrigation. In rare patients, the perineal wound must be left open because of sacral bleeding, which requires the insertion of pelvic packing, or because of extensive contamination associated with Crohn's disease of the anorectum.

Moderate blood loss is common, particularly in patients in whom the neoplasm is affixed to the sacrum or prostate gland. Because the procedure involves two incisions and creates a large dead space in the posterior pelvis that takes time to heal, the stress is moderate to severe in all patients.

USUAL POSTOPERATIVE COURSE

Expected postoperative hospital stay: 7 to 10 days

Operative mortality: 2%

Special monitoring required: Postoperative hemodynamic monitoring with a pulmonary artery catheter occasionally is necessary in elderly patients with excessive blood loss during a difficult procedure.

Patient activity and positioning: Patients may be out of bed the day after surgery, depending on hemodynamic stability.

Alimentation: For routine procedures, patients are permitted clear liquids with the return of bowel function, and food intake is advanced as tolerated.

Antibiotic coverage: Gavage cleaning of the colon in combination with nonabsorbable antibiotics (neomycin and erythromycin base at 1 PM, 2 PM, and 11 PM the day before surgery) is the standard colon preparation. All patients also receive intravenous cephalosporin, advanced penicillin, metronidazole, or a combination of antibiotics, preoperatively and for at least 24 hours postoperatively.

Delayed closure if the perineal wound has been left open: Once the pelvic packing has been removed or perineal cellulitis from previously resected Crohn's disease has resolved, delayed primary closure of the skin or transposition of gracilis muscle flaps into the pelvic space and closure of the skin is performed.

Drains: Irrigation with normal saline at a rate of 1000 mL/12 h is performed through one perineal drain while continuous suction is applied to the other. When the effluent is clear, irrigation is discontinued, suction is applied to both drains for 12 to 24 hours, and the drains are removed.

Bladder catheter: Attempts to remove the bladder catheter are begun 4 or 5 days after operation. Urinary retention is managed with reinsertion of the catheter for another 2 or 3 days.

Colostomy care: The patient is instructed in the care of the permanent end colostomy by an enterostomal therapist.

POSTOPERATIVE COMPLICATIONS

IN THE HOSPITAL

Wound infection: See Chapter 49.

Urinary tract complications: Operative injury to or deliberate excision of a portion of the ureter occasionally occurs in secondary pelvic surgery or during the excision of a large, bulky, or inflamed rectal neoplasm. Repair of the ureter or reimplantation into the dome of the bladder is best performed by a urologist. An unrecognized injury may present as a postoperative ureterocutaneous or cystocutaneous fistula with fluid containing high levels of creatinine leaking through the perineal wound or through drains. A retrograde cystoureterogram is necessary to localize the injury and the need for reoperation is determined by the urologist.

Urinary retention after removal of the bladder occurs more commonly in men than in women. Conservative treatment with reinsertion of the catheter succeeds in 70% of patients and transurethral resection of the prostate is necessary in the remainder after 2 to 3 weeks of outpatient observation with a catheter in place.

Intestinal obstruction: Even with insertion of an absorbable mesh to replace the pelvic peritoneum, adhesive obstruction of the small bowel in the pelvis may occur in the early postoperative period. On occasion, small bowel obstruction may also occur around the colon segment exiting the abdominal wall as a colostomy. Treatment is as described in Chapter 49.

Colostomy complications: Necrosis, retraction, prolapse, and parastomal abscess occur in 5% to 10% of patients and may mandate reoperation.

Pelvic abscess: Pelvic abscess is a rare complication diagnosed by pelvic computed tomography and treated by reopening the perineal incision.

AFTER DISCHARGE

Impotence: Impotence develops in 15% to 100% of men, depending on the level of the tumor and the extent of the resection.

Colostomy complications: Retraction, stricture, or fistula formation occurs in 7% to 8% of patients, and late parastomal hernia occurs in 10% to 12%.

Tumor recurrence in the pelvis: Carcinoma recurs in as many as 32% of patients, with 70% of these cases developing within 2 years of operation. High histologic grade of the original tumor, local spread of the tumor, and metastasis to pelvic nodes are ominous prognostic signs. Computed tomography is used to determine the extent of the recurrence, and repeated transperineal excision, abdominosacral resection, pelvic exenteration, and further radiotherapy all have been used with modest success to relieve pelvic pain and lengthen survival.

BIBLIOGRAPHY

Beahrs JR, Beahrs OH, Beahrs MM, et al. Urinary tract complications with rectal surgery. Ann Surg 1978;187:542–548.

Glaser F, Kuntz C, Schlag P, et al. Endorectal ultrasound for control of preoperative radiotherapy of rectal cancer. Ann Surg 1993;217:64–71.

Hermanek P, Gall FP, Guggenmoos-Holzman G, et al. Pathogenesis of local recurrence after surgical treatment of rectal carcinoma. Dig Surg 1985;2:7–11.

Miles WE. A method of performing abdominoperineal excision for carcinoma of the rectum and of the terminal portion of the pelvic colon. Lancet 1908;2:1812–1813.

Pahlmann L, Glimelius B. Pre- or postoperative radiotherapy in rectal and rectosigmoid cancer. Ann Surg 1990;211:187–195.

Medical Management of the Surgical Patient, Third Edition,
edited by Michael F. Lubin, H. Kenneth Walker, and Robert B. Smith III.
J.B. Lippincott Company, Philadelphia, PA © 1995.

CHAPTER

55

GASTRIC PROCEDURES

David V. Feliciano

Gastric procedures performed with the patient under general anesthesia include those done for complications of peptic ulcer disease (parietal cell vagotomy [PCV], vagotomy and pyloroplasty [VP], vagotomy and antrectomy [VA], hemigastrectomy alone); for benign neoplasms (proximal or distal gastrectomy); and for malignant neoplasms (extended subtotal or total gastrectomy).

PCV, also known as highly selective or proximal gastric vagotomy, denervates the fundus and body of the stomach (parietal cell area). It is used widely for both uncomplicated and complicated (perforation, bleeding) duodenal ulcers, and has an ulcer recurrence rate of 6% to 12% on long-term follow-up. Preoperative preparation is nil, the stress to patients is modest, the open procedure is performed in 1½ hours, and blood transfusion is unnecessary. Laparoscopic division of the posterior vagus nerve combined with an anterior gastric seromyotomy is being evaluated as an alternative to PCV.

VP and VA involve cutting the vagal nerve trunks at the esophageal hiatus and rearranging or resecting the pylorus. With antrectomy, all the gastrin-secreting cells are removed as well and reanastomosis to the duodenum (Billroth I) or jejunum (Billroth II) is necessary. These procedures are used in patients with life-threatening complications of duodenal ulcer disease (bleeding, perforation, obstruction) and are associated with ulcer recurrence rates of 1% to 2% (VA) and 10% to 12% (VP). Preoperative decompression of the stomach for 5 to 7 days and antibiotic irrigation the night before operation is indicated in patients with gastric dilation from pyloric obstruction. Subtotal gastrectomy (removal of the ulcer and the distal stomach) is 96% curative for patients with uncomplicated and complicated gastric ulcers and 100% curative for those with benign tumors (leiomyomas). The stress of these procedures is moderate, they take 1½ to 2 hours to perform, and blood transfusion is required only in patients with anemia or active bleeding.

Extended subtotal gastrectomy (additional removal of the greater and lesser omentum, the celiac nodes, and, sometimes, the spleen) or total gastrectomy is reserved for patients with mid-stomach or proximal adenocarcinomas. With a leiomyosarcoma, only the gastrectomy is performed. Reconstruction is by a Roux (borrowed) limb of proximal jejunum. The stress of surgery is moderate, the procedure is performed in 3 hours, and blood transfusion may be necessary if neoplasms are adherent to the pancreas, liver, or retroperitoneum.

USUAL POSTOPERATIVE COURSE

Expected postoperative hospital stay: 5 days for PCV; 7 to 10 days for VP, VA, or subtotal gastrectomy; and 12 to 14 days for total gastrectomy

Operative mortality: 0% for PCV; 1% to 2% for elective VP, VA, and gastrectomy; 5% to 15% for emergency VP, VA, and gastrectomy; and 3% to 8% for elective total gastrectomy

Special monitoring required: Nasogastric or nasojejunal tube drainage is monitored and replaced intravenously if it is excessive. Serum electrolytes also are measured and replaced as needed. A gastric pH level is checked before patient discharge to verify a properly performed PCV.

Patient activity and positioning: Patients may be out of bed the day after surgery.

Alimentation: Patients are permitted clear liquids with the return of bowel function, and food intake is advanced as tolerated. Patients with VAs or gastrectomies of any type are advised to eat slowly, drink less with meals, and avoid milk products in the early postoperative period as they adjust to the new size of their stomachs and loss of the pylorus. They are also advised to avoid large amounts of foods that are difficult to digest, including oranges, broccoli, and asparagus. Patients who have had total gastrectomies remain on hyperalimentation until anastomoses are healed (see later).

Antibiotic coverage: A cephalosporin or an advanced penicillin is administered preoperatively and for 24 hours postoperatively. If perforation of a duodenal or gastric ulcer is noted at surgery, the antibiotic is continued for 5 to 7 days postoperatively.

Drains: After gastrectomy and reconstruction with a gastrojejunostomy, the duodenal stump is drained with a closed suction drain for 5 to 7 days. After total gastrectomy, the esophagojejunal anastomosis is drained by many surgeons until a healed anastomosis is demonstrated.

Upper gastrointestinal radiography: Upper gastrointestinal radiography is performed with water-soluble dye 7 to 10 days after total gastrectomy to check healing of the esophagojejunal anastomosis. If a small leak is present, patients remain on hyperalimentation until repeated studies are performed in 5 to 7 days.

POSTOPERATIVE COMPLICATIONS

IN THE HOSPITAL

Wound infection: In patients with bleeding or perforated ulcers, gastric acid is neutralized by blood or food. This allows for overgrowth of bacteria, and open packing or delayed primary closure of the subcutaneous tissue and skin is appropriate after many emergency gastric procedures. If a wound infection occurs, treatment is as described earlier.

Duodenal stump leak: Duodenal stump leak occurs in 1% to 2% of patients after gastric resection with gastrojejunostomy. Right upper quadrant pain, fever, tachycardia, and bilious drainage out of the suction drain placed beneath the stump are diagnostic. The leak is treated with prohibition of oral intake, insertion of a sump drain under fluoroscopy, use of intravenous hyperalimentation, and administration of antibiotics and a somatostatin analogue (Sandostatin). Reexploration is indicated only if sepsis does not resolve with insertion of the sump drain.

Stomal dysfunction: Slow gastric emptying occurs in less than 5% of patients after gastrectomy, particularly if gastrojejunostomy has been performed. If output through the nasogastric tube is excessive at 7 days after surgery, upper gastrointestinal radiography with water-soluble contrast is performed. If the agent does not pass through the anastomosis, a second study with barium is performed the next day. Passage of the barium is reassuring, and nasogastric tube decompression and hyperalimentation are continued for 2 to 3 more weeks as needed. Failure of the barium to pass mandates endoscopy to rule out a mechanical obstruction.

AFTER DISCHARGE

Nutritional disturbances: Megaloblastic anemia from loss of intrinsic factor and iron-deficiency anemia from unknown causes occur over time in many patients with previous gastrectomies. Lifelong yearly monitoring of hemoglobin levels is appropriate, with replacement therapy administered as needed. Calcium deficiency and steatorrhea also have occurred.

Dumping syndrome: The passage of a hypertonic food bolus directly into the duodenum or jejunum after an antrectomy may precipitate sweating, weakness, palpitations, nausea, vomiting, and diarrhea due to hormonal changes, as well as an outpouring of extracellular fluid into the upper gastrointestinal tract. Symptomatic dumping occurs in less than 15% of patients. Only 1% of patients may require remedial operations after failing to respond to a change in dietary habits (restriction of fluids, carbohydrates, and extra salt with meals).

Diarrhea: About 10% to 25% of patients have altered bowel movements after truncal vagotomy. Only 1% to 2% require remedial operations after failure to respond to a change in dietary habits (see earlier) or to the use of common medications such as codeine, diphenoxylate, or cholestyramine.

Gastric atony: Delayed gastric emptying is a persistent problem in 1% to 2% of patients and may respond to the administration of metoclopramide, coherin peptide, or erythromycin lactobionate. Remedial operation consists of near-total gastrectomy with Roux-en-Y gastrojejunostomy.

Marginal or recurrent ulcer: A marginal or stomal ulcer develops in about 1% of patients undergoing VA for duodenal ulcer and 4% to 6% of those undergoing gastrectomy for gastric ulcer. Recurrent ulcers develop in 6% to 12% of patients after PCV and in 10% to 12% after VP for duodenal ulcer. Gastric analysis is appropriate to document the persistence of gastric acid after VA, which suggests that an incomplete vagotomy has been performed. A significantly elevated gastrin level is indicative of a Zollinger-Ellison syndrome or retained antrum syndrome after antral resection. H_2 blockers and, if necessary, omeprazole (which is not approved by the US Food and Drug Administration for this indication) are administered to control symptoms. Persistent symptoms despite medical therapy, or life-threatening bleeding or perforation mandate reoperation. Patients with previous PCVs are converted to VAs; those with previous VAs require repeated vagotomy and resection.

Other postgastrectomy complications: The afferent loop syndrome, efferent loop syndrome, and alkaline reflux gastritis occur infrequently, but remedial operations are available for correction.

Gastric stump carcinoma: Carcinoma of the gastric pouch develops in as many as 5% of patients who survive 10 to 15 years after gastrectomy. Late-developing symptoms of pain and anemia in patients who have previously done well after gastrectomy demand endoscopy with biopsy.

BIBLIOGRAPHY

Herrington JL Jr. Remedial operations for postgastrectomy syndromes. Curr Probl Surg 1970;7:1–63.

Ingvar C, Adami HO, Enander LK, et al. Clinical results of reoperation after failed highly selective vagotomy. Am J Surg 1986;152:308–313.

Jordan PH Jr. Surgery for peptic ulcer disease. Curr Probl Surg 1991;28:267–330.

Koo J, Lam SK, Chan P, et al. Proximal gastric vagotomy, truncal vagotomy with drainage, and truncal vagotomy with antrectomy for chronic duodenal ulcer: a prospective, randomized controlled trial. Ann Surg 1983;197:265–271.

Vogel SB, Vair DB, Woodward ER. Alterations in gastrointestinal emptying of 99m-technetium–labeled solids following sequential antrectomy, truncal vagotomy and Roux-Y gastroenterostomy. Ann Surg 1983;198:506–514.

Medical Management of the Surgical Patient, Third Edition,
edited by Michael F. Lubin, H. Kenneth Walker, and Robert B. Smith III.
J.B. Lippincott Company, Philadelphia, PA © 1995.

CHAPTER

CHOLECYSTECTOMY 56

David V. Feliciano

Cholecystectomy is indicated for calculous cholecystitis (acute or chronic); acalculous acute cholecystitis; a gallbladder that continues to produce stones in the common bile duct (obstructive jaundice, gallstone pancreatitis, cholangitis); carcinoma of the gallbladder; and traumatic perforation of the gallbladder. It is also performed after right hepatic artery ligation for hepatic trauma and in preparation for infusion of the hepatic artery with chemotherapeutic agents for metastases. It is included as part of a pancreatoduodenectomy by some surgeons and may be necessary for exposure of the porta hepatis in occasional patients undergoing portacaval shunt procedures.

Cholecystectomy is routinely performed within 24 hours of admission for patients with acute cholecystitis documented on ultrasonography or radionuclide scanning (ie, HIDA scan) unless general anesthesia is contraindicated. If patients with acute cholecystitis are observed for a longer period, the extent of inflammation may make a laparoscopic approach difficult. Patients with obstructive jaundice, gallstone pancreatitis, or cholangitis undergo cholecystectomy after observation to determine whether the bilirubin level will fall, when the amylase level returns to normal, and when hemodynamic stability has been restored, respectively.

General anesthesia is used for both open and laparoscopic cholecystectomy. Open procedures are completed in 1 to 1½ hours, blood transfusions are essentially never necessary, and the stress of the routine procedure is moderate. If gangrenous cholecystitis with perforation is present, the underlying disease causes severe stress during the peri-

operative period. Most patients are discharged from the hospital 2 to 4 days after operation and return to work in 4 to 6 weeks.

A laparoscopic approach is used in 90% to 95% of the more than 700,000 patients who undergo cholecystectomy in the United States each year. Rates of conversion to an open procedure are 5% to 10% for experienced laparoscopic general surgeons, with most conversions necessitated by adhesions, severe inflammation, confusing anatomy, or, rarely, bleeding. Laparoscopic procedures are completed in 1 to 1½ hours, blood transfusions are essentially never necessary, and the stress of the routine procedure is modest. Most patients are discharged from the hospital the day after operation and return to work in 1 to 2 weeks. The major concern about the rapid acceptance of this procedure has been the greater than 2% incidence of injuries to the common bile duct during the surgeon's "learning curve" (the first 13 laparoscopic cholecystectomies in one series). This complication occurs in 0.2% to 0.5% of a surgeon's subsequent procedures, a figure slightly greater than that historically reported for open cholecystectomy.

USUAL POSTOPERATIVE COURSE

Expected postoperative hospital stay: 2 to 4 days for open cholecystectomy; 1 day for laparoscopic cholecystectomy

Operative mortality: Under 0.1% for routine open or laparoscopic cholecystectomy; 10% to 15% for cholecystectomy performed for empyema or gangrene of the gallbladder, emphysematous cholecystitis, or acalculous cholecystitis; 20% to 25% for cholecystectomy performed for toxic cholangitis due to gallstones; 25% to 50% for cholecystectomy performed for hemorrhagic or necrotizing pancreatitis due to gallstones

Special monitoring required: Postoperative hemodynamic monitoring with a pulmonary artery catheter is necessary only in patients with sepsis from empyema or gangrene of the gallbladder, emphysematous cholecystitis, acalculous cholecystitis, toxic cholangitis, or associated hemorrhagic or necrotizing pancreatitis.

Patient activity and positioning: Patients may be out of bed the day after surgery, depending on hemodynamic stability.

Alimentation: For patients undergoing routine open or laparoscopic cholecystectomy, clear liquids are allowed the evening after operation or the first postoperative morning. Patients with more complicated indications for cholecystectomy are permitted clear liquids with the return of bowel function, and food intake is advanced as tolerated. Patients with associated hemorrhagic or necrotizing pancreatitis receive intravenous hyperalimentation as soon as they are hemodynamically stable.

Antibiotic coverage: Antibiotics are not administered to patients younger than 60 to 70 years who are undergoing cholecystectomy for cholelithiasis with chronic cholecystitis. Older patients or those with acute cholecystitis, resolving acute cholecystitis, obstructive jaundice, known choledocholithiasis, or secondary toxic cholangitis receive perioperative cephalosporin, advanced penicillin, or an aminoglycoside–anaerobic agent combination. The duration of postoperative antibiotic administration depends on the underlying condition.

POSTOPERATIVE COMPLICATIONS

IN THE HOSPITAL

Wound infection: Subcutaneous wound infections occur in 1% to 5% of all patients undergoing open cholecystectomy, but in only 1% of those undergoing laparoscopic cholecystectomy.

Subhepatic biloma or abscess: A biloma may rarely occur from necrosis of the cystic duct stump or unrecognized division of a duct of Luschka (gallbladder–liver connection); it is treated with percutaneous drainage. Subhepatic abscesses are extraordinarily rare and almost always occur when cholecystectomy is performed in conjunction with another intraabdominal procedure.

Bile duct injury: An injury recognized during open or laparoscopic cholecystectomy is repaired with absorbable sutures, and a T-tube is inserted if an end-to-end anastomosis is required. An unrecognized injury during laparoscopic cholecystectomy leads to postoperative ileus and abnormal liver function test results. With early recognition in the postoperative period, immediate laparotomy is performed with biliary reconstruction as indicated. With delayed recognition, an endoscopic retrograde cholangiopancreatogram (ERCP) and percutaneous biliary stent placement and subhepatic drainage are performed before biliary reconstruction.

Bowel injury: Injury to either the duodenum or the jejunum occurred in 0.3% of patients undergoing laparoscopic cholecystectomy in one series. Sepsis and ileus are usually present within 24 hours, and a laparotomy is performed with closure as indicated.

Bleeding: Bleeding from the bed of the gallbladder or a branch of the cystic artery occurred in 0.3% of patients undergoing laparoscopic cholecystectomy in one series. Either an open or a laparoscopic approach can be used to control the source of hemorrhage.

Retained or residual common bile duct stone: Failure to perform operative cholangiography may lead to a retained common bile duct stone after either open or laparoscopic cholecystectomy. Even with intraoperative diagnosis of a common bile duct stone, an open or laparoscopic attempt at stone removal (choledocholithotomy) may fail, and a known residual stone will be left in place. A postoperative ERCP with sphincterotomy is indicated to allow for passage of the retained or residual stone if no T-tube has been left in the common bile duct at the first operation. If a T-tube is in place, early irrigation with heparinized saline or monoctanoin aids in the dissolution of cholesterol stones. Stones that do not respond to irrigation or attempted dissolution are approached through the T-tube tract by an interventional radiologist after 6 weeks.

AFTER DISCHARGE

Retained or residual common bile duct stone: See earlier discussion.

BIBLIOGRAPHY

Burch JM, Feliciano DV, Mattox KL, et al. Gallstone pancreatitis: the question of time. Arch Surg 1990;125:853–860.

Graham SM, Flowers JL, Scott TR, et al. Laparoscopic cholecystectomy and common bile duct stones: the utility of planned perioperative endoscopic retrograde cholangiography and sphinctero-tomy—experience with 63 patients. Ann Surg 1993;218:61–67.

Paulino-Netto A. A review of 391 selected open cholecystecto-mies for comparison with laparoscopic cholecystectomy. Am J Surg 1993;166:71–73.

Roslyn JJ, Binns GS, Hughes EFX, et al. Open cholecystectomy: a contemporary analysis of 42,474 patients. Ann Surg 1993;218:129–137.

Southern Surgeons Club. A prospective analysis of 1518 laparo-scopic cholecystectomies. N Engl J Med 1991;324:1073–1078.

Medical Management of the Surgical Patient, Third Edition,
edited by Michael F. Lubin, H. Kenneth Walker, and Robert B. Smith III.
J.B. Lippincott Company, Philadelphia, PA © 1995.

CHAPTER

57

COMMON BILE DUCT EXPLORATION

David V. Feliciano

Common bile duct exploration is indicated for palpable or radiologically confirmed gallstones in the duct (choledocholithiasis) that are asymptomatic or causing obstructive jaundice, gallstone pancreatitis, or toxic cholangitis; to diagnose and treat obstructive jaundice from a benign or malignant stricture; to diagnose and treat sphincter stenosis; or to repair an injury caused by operation or trauma.

Common bile duct exploration is essentially performed at first operations only for these conditions, especially choledocholithiasis. Mandatory indications to explore the common bile duct at the time of either open or laparoscopic cholecystectomy include a palpable or radiologically confirmed stone or marked dilation (more than 2 to 2.5 cm) of the duct. All other indications are relative, and a cystic duct cholangiogram is usually performed first to verify the presence of a stone or other obstruction.

General anesthesia is used for both open and laparoscopic common bile duct exploration. The procedure adds 60 minutes to a routine open cholecystectomy because of the need to expose and open the duct (choledochotomy), extract the stones and perform choledochoscopy, insert a T-tube, close the duct around the T-tube, and perform a completion T-tube cholangiogram. Laparoscopic common bile duct exploration also adds 30 to 60 minutes to a routine cholecystectomy. The ideal approach involves balloon dilation of the cystic duct, passage of a flexible fiberoptic endoscope through the cystic duct, and basket extraction of common duct stones under direct vision. Laparoscopic choledochot-

omy is technically demanding and not widely used. Blood transfusion is essentially never necessary with routine open or laparoscopic cholecystectomy. In contrast, common bile duct exploration to diagnose and treat obstructive jaundice from a benign (ie, previous operative injury) or malignant stricture often is associated with moderate blood loss that requires transfusion. Routine exploration creates modest stress for patients who also are undergoing cholecystectomy, whereas exploration for a benign or malignant stricture may cause severe stress from blood loss and extended duration of the procedure.

USUAL POSTOPERATIVE COURSE

Expected postoperative hospital stay: 5 to 10 days

Operative mortality: 2% to 3% for elective operations; 15% and 40% for urgent and emergency operations, respectively, to relieve ascending cholangitis; 20% in patients undergoing exploration and biliary bypass to relieve obstructive jaundice from a malignant stricture

Special monitoring required: Postoperative hemodynamic monitoring with a pulmonary artery catheter is necessary only in patients with toxic cholangitis, patients undergoing a complicated reoperation to correct a benign biliary stricture, and patients undergoing a biliary bypass procedure who are debilitated from an unresectable malignant stricture.

Patient activity and positioning: Patients may be out of bed on the day after operation, depending on hemodynamic stability.

Alimentation: For patients undergoing laparoscopic cholecystectomy, clear liquids are permitted on the evening after operation or on the first postoperative morning. For those with open procedures, clear liquids are given with the return of bowel function and food intake is advanced as tolerated.

Antibiotic coverage: All patients undergoing common bile duct exploration receive perioperative cephalosporin, advanced penicillin, or an aminoglycoside-anaerobic agent combination. Patients with toxic cholangitis are maintained on the appropriate antibiotic (determined by bile culture) until sepsis resolves and fever has been absent for 48 hours.

T-tube: The T-tube left in the common bile duct after an open choledochotomy is connected to gravity drainage. A T-tube cholangiogram is performed on postoperative day 6 or 7 to document the absence of retained stones and the free flow of contrast into the duodenum. About 12 hours after a normal cholangiogram, the portion of the T-tube outside the body is clamped or tied off, leaving 2 to 3 inches of tubing covered with a piece of tape. The clamp or tie is released only if patients develop cholangitis, right upper quadrant pain, or a bile leak around the T-tube. A T-tube inserted at the time of a routine choledochotomy is removed in an outpatient setting 2 weeks after the exploration. Patients are warned to expect a small amount of bile leakage from the T-tube site for 2 or 3 days.

POSTOPERATIVE COMPLICATIONS

IN THE HOSPITAL

Wound infection: See Chapter 56.

Subhepatic abscess: See Chapter 56.

T-tube displacement: Early displacement of the T-tube may precipitate bile peritonitis that is not responsive to percutaneous drainage and reoperation may be necessary. Late displacement when adhesions are present may be treated with insertion of a percutaneous drain near the choledochotomy site.

Retained or residual common bile duct stone: See Chapter 56.

Pancreatitis: Operative manipulation of the distal common bile duct may precipitate transient, mild postoperative pancreatitis. This is usually self-limited if the common bile duct has been cleared of stones.

AFTER DISCHARGE

Stricture: Attacks of cholangitis manifested by pain, fever, jaundice, and elevation of the alkaline phosphatase level are strongly suggestive of biliary stricture. The diagnosis is confirmed by ultrasound or computed tomography to rule out a neoplasm and by a transhepatic cholangiogram or endoscopic retrograde cholangiopancreatogram to localize the area of obstruction. Transhepatic balloon dilation of the area of stricture may obviate the need for reoperation with biliary reconstruction.

Common bile duct stone: In patients who are not of Asian descent, late cholangitis caused by a common bile duct stone is almost always the result of failure to clear stones from the common bile duct at the first operation. Either endoscopic sphincterotomy or transhepatic extraction is indicated. Patients of Asian descent have a much higher incidence of spontaneously formed intrahepatic ductal stones that may migrate into the common bile duct long after operation. In addition to endoscopic sphincterotomy, a variety of radiologic procedures for irrigation and extraction of impacted stones are usually attempted, although reoperation with a biliary-enteric bypass may be necessary.

BIBLIOGRAPHY

Boey JH, Way LW. Acute cholangitis. Ann Surg 1980;191:264–270.

Hauer-Jensen M, Karesen R, Nygaard K, et al. Predictive ability of choledocholithiasis indicators: a prospective evaluation. Ann Surg 1985;202:64–68.

Hunter JG. Laparoscopic transcystic bile duct exploration. Am J Surg 1992;163:53–58.

Neoptolemos JP, Carr-Locke DL, Fossard DP. Prospective randomized study of preoperative endoscopic sphincterotomy versus surgery alone for common bile duct stones. BMJ 1987;294:470–474.

Stoker ME, Leveilee RJ, McCann JC, et al. Laparoscopic common bile duct exploration. J Laparoendosc Surg 1992;2:15–21.

Medical Management of the Surgical Patient, Third Edition,
edited by Michael F. Lubin, H. Kenneth Walker, and Robert B. Smith III.
J.B. Lippincott Company, Philadelphia, PA © 1995.

CHAPTER

58

PANCREATODUODENAL RESECTION

David V. Feliciano

Pancreatoduodenal resection is performed for attempted cure of periampullary carcinomas (head of pancreas, ampulla of Vater, duodenal wall, or distal common bile duct); malignant islet cell neoplasms; mucinous cystic neoplasms or mucinous cystadenocarcinoma of the head of the pancreas; benign masses from chronic pancreatitis in the head of the pancreas with secondary pancreatic duct, common bile duct, or duodenal obstruction; and, rarely, major trauma to the pancreatoduodenal complex.

Patients with obstructive jaundice (dilated hepatic ductal system) and no evidence of gallstones on ultrasound or computed tomography (CT) should undergo abdominal CT to determine whether there is a mass in the periampullary area and whether hepatic metastasis or regional invasion has occurred. Further work-up to localize the area of obstruction in patients without a periampullary mass should include an endoscopic retrograde cholangiopancreatogram or transhepatic cholangiogram. Preoperative fine-needle aspiration if a mass is present and a celiac-superior mesenteric arteriogram to rule out local vascular invasion are also performed in some centers.

Percutaneous transhepatic drainage of the obstructed biliary ductal system in the preoperative period is no longer performed because prospective trials have not demonstrated improvement in postoperative survival. The preoperative administration of parenteral vitamin K and the insti-

tution of intravenous or supplemental enteral alimentation are appropriate in patients with 10% loss of body weight, albumin levels less than 2.5 mg/dL, or anergy on delayed hypersensitivity skin testing.

After the induction of general endotracheal anesthesia, many younger surgeons first perform transduodenal needle biopsies of the mass to verify the presence of a malignant tumor. More experienced surgeons are usually comfortable performing pancreatoduodenal resection for local masses in the head of the pancreas with secondary biliary and duodenal obstruction in appropriately staged patients. The mass is staged before resection to verify the absence of hepatic, celiac nodal, and pelvic metastases or regional invasion into the portal vein, superior mesenteric vessels, inferior vena cava, or aorta. Resection for cure includes the head, neck, and, sometimes, a portion of the body of the pancreas; the entire duodenum; the distal common bile duct; and the antrum of the stomach. Some surgeons also perform cholecystectomy and a truncal vagotomy as part of the procedure. Reconstruction is accomplished by anastomosis of the jejunum to the ends of the remaining pancreas, common bile duct, and stomach. An alternate and increasingly popular approach is the pylorus-preserving pancreatoduodenectomy, in which the stomach and a 2-cm cuff of duodenum are preserved to improve patients' long-term nutritional status. Short- and long-term survival rates after this operation are similar to those with standard pancreatoduodenectomy, but a clearcut long-term nutritional advantage remains to be proved.

Experienced surgical teams perform pancreatoduodenectomy in 4½ to 7 hours, with a blood replacement of one to four units. The procedure is extremely stressful because of the underlying disease, the duration of the operation, the complications that are encountered in 50% to 70% of patients, and the nutritional problems that are associated with reconstruction of the upper digestive tract.

USUAL POSTOPERATIVE COURSE

Expected postoperative hospital stay: 10 to 20 days, with a median of 17 days in one large series

Operative mortality: In series reviewing operations performed between 1970 and 1980, the operative mortality rate was about 8% to 9%. Series since the early 1980s have reported an in-hospital mortality rate of 0% to 2.8%. A recent report described 145 consecutive pancreatoduodenectomies over a 33-month period with no operative mortality.

Special monitoring required: Patients with known cardiac or pulmonary compromise and those who have undergone difficult procedures associated with excessive blood loss require postoperative hemodynamic monitoring with a pulmonary artery catheter.

Patient activity and positioning: Patients may be out of bed the day after operation, depending on hemodynamic stability.

Alimentation: Because of the magnitude of the procedure and the compromised nutritional state of many patients, intravenous hyperalimentation is administered routinely. Clear liquids are permitted with the return of bowel function, and food intake is advanced as tolerated. Delayed gastric emptying is common after pancreatoduodenectomy and has been noted in 30% to 40% of patients who undergo the pylorus-preserving procedure. A recent prospective trial in which 200 mg of intravenous erythromycin lactobionate, a motilin agonist, was given every 6 hours from the third to the tenth postoperative day documented a 37% reduction in the incidence of delayed gastric emptying.

Antibiotic coverage: All patients receive an intravenous cephalosporin or advanced penicillin preoperatively and for at least 24 hours postoperatively.

Drains: Closed suction drains are usually placed posterior to the pancreatojejunostomy and choledochojejunostomy, and are removed within 5 to 7 days if no fistula occurs. Some surgeons leave a plastic stent through the pancreatojejunostomy or a T-tube through the choledochojejunostomy, with the timing of removal based on personal preference.

POSTOPERATIVE COMPLICATIONS

IN THE HOSPITAL

Delayed gastric emptying: Delayed gastric emptying occurs in about 30% to 40% of patients after either standard or pylorus-preserving pancreatoduodenectomy. The use of intravenous erythromycin lactobionate appears promising in diminishing the incidence of this complication, and nasogastric suction and intravenous hyperalimentation are indicated when it occurs.

Pancreatic fistula: A leak from the pancreatojejunostomy occurs in 15% to 20% of patients and is treated by prohibiting oral intake, continuing suction drainage, and, on some surgical services, administering 100 to 150 μg of somatostatin analogue (octreotide) every 8 hours.

Intraabdominal abscess: An abscess occurs in 10% of cases and is caused by a leak from the pancreatojejunostomy or the choledochojejunostomy. The diagnosis is suggested by spiking temperatures, ileus, and leukocytosis; CT-guided percutaneous drainage is the appropriate treatment.

Wound infection: See Chapter 49.

Hyperglycemia: Elevated glucose levels are frequently noted, particularly in elderly patients receiving hyperalimentation. Intravenous insulin is administered as necessary until an enteral diet is resumed. Long-term insulin rarely is required.

AFTER DISCHARGE

Recurrent carcinoma: The median survival for patients with positive lymph nodes in the resected specimen is about 12 months. Patients with recurrent carcinoma usually have back pain, weight loss, an abdominal mass, and hepatic metastases, and pain control is often the most important palliation that can be offered.

Marginal ulcer: Although the incidence of an ulcer in the gastrojejunostomy generally ranges from 5% to 10% in long-term survivors, it approached 50% in at least one series. Patients surviving long enough for a marginal ulcer to develop are best treated with H_2 blockers or omeprazole, with thoracoscopic vagotomy reserved for those who do not respond to medication.

Pancreatic insufficiency: Even with a successful pancreatojejunostomy, pancreatic insufficiency may occur and is treated with exocrine replacement.

BIBLIOGRAPHY

Cameron JL, Crist DW, Sitzmann JV, et al. Factors influencing survival after pancreaticoduodenectomy for pancreatic cancer. Am J Surg 1991;161:120–125.

Cameron JL, Pitt HA, Yeo CJ, et al. One hundred and forty-five consecutive pancreaticoduodenectomies without mortality. Ann Surg 1993;217:430–438.

Whipple AO, Parsons WB, Mullins CR. Treatment of cancer of the ampulla of Vater. Ann Surg 1935;102:765–779.

Willett CG, Lewandrowski K, Warshaw AL, et al. Resection margins in carcinoma of the head of the pancreas. Ann Surg 1993;217:144–148.

Yeo CJ, Barry MK, Sauter PK, et al. Erythromycin accelerates gastric emptying after pancreaticoduodenectomy. Ann Surg 1993;218:229–238.

Medical Management of the Surgical Patient, Third Edition,
edited by Michael F. Lubin, H. Kenneth Walker, and Robert B. Smith III.
J.B. Lippincott Company, Philadelphia, PA © 1995.

CHAPTER

MAJOR HEPATIC RESECTION

59

David V. Feliciano

Major hepatic resection is performed to remove malignant neoplasms (hepatoma, cholangiocarcinoma, metastases); benign neoplasms (liver cell adenoma, focal nodular hyperplasia, cavernous hemangioma); and cysts (congenital, multicystic disease, echinococcal). It is also used to treat major injuries. If the remaining hepatic tissue is normal, as much as 80% to 90% of the liver can be removed in children and adults.

Although no precise correlation has been found between preoperative liver function test results and long-term survival after resection for primary malignant neoplasms, high serum transaminase level, alkaline phosphatase level, and prothrombin time are statistically correlated with decreased survival. Less than 25% of patients with operable primary hepatic malignant tumors in North America have cirrhosis, a much lower figure than that reported from Asia.

Preoperative screening before major resection also should include an abdominal computed tomographic (CT) scan and separate celiac and superior mesenteric arteriography or combined CT and arterial portography. These studies determine the extent of the hepatic lesion, its resectability if it is known to be malignant or metastatic, and the blood supply to both lobes.

Major hepatic resection is performed under general anesthesia through an upper abdominal incision using either vascular inflow occlusion (Pringle maneuver or clamping of the porta hepatis) or total vascular isolation (clamping of the porta hepatis, supraceliac aorta, and inferior vena cava

above and below the liver). Division of the hepatic parenchyma is accomplished using finger fracture techniques, blunt knife handle dissection, or the ultrasonic vibrating-aspirating device. Blood loss depends on the extent of the resection and involvement of the retrohepatic vena cava; it ranged from zero to six units and averages two units in current series. The stress of a major hepatic resection is moderate to severe.

USUAL POSTOPERATIVE COURSE

Expected postoperative hospital stay: 7 to 15 days

Operative mortality: 3% to 10% for elective resection; 25% to 30% for emergency resection; 25% to 50% for emergency resection for trauma

Special monitoring required: Patients with known cardiac or pulmonary compromise and those who have undergone difficult resections associated with extensive blood loss require postoperative hemodynamic monitoring with a pulmonary artery catheter.

Patient activity and positioning: Patients may be out of bed on the day after operation, depending on hemodynamic stability.

Alimentation: Hypoglycemia can usually be prevented by the infusion of a 10% glucose solution after extensive resection. If hypoalbuminemia occurs and colloid osmotic pressure decreases, periodic infusions of salt-poor albumin may be indicated. Early nutritional support through the gastrointestinal tract is mandatory. Besides the theoretic benefit of lowering the incidence of gut-origin sepsis, use of the gastrointestinal tract appears to generate a hepatotrophic substance that maintains the integrity of the liver. This is in contrast to the cholestasis and fatty infiltration that occur in patients who are maintained on intravenous hyperalimentation for prolonged periods.

Antibiotic coverage: Perioperative coverage for 24 hours with cephalosporin or advanced penicillin is routine, although the precise benefit is unclear in patients without preoperative cholangitis.

Drains: Suction drains are left in the subphrenic and subhepatic spaces for 5 to 7 days or until drainage decreases to 30 to 50 mL/d.

POSTOPERATIVE COMPLICATIONS

IN THE HOSPITAL

Perihepatic abscess: Abscesses in the subphrenic or subhepatic area occur in 2% to 10% of patients and are treated with CT-guided percutaneous drainage.

Pleural effusion: Sympathetic pleural effusions occur in 2% to 10% of patients and are treated conservatively unless pulmonary compromise is present.

Prolonged postoperative fever: Prolonged postoperative fever is a common problem in patients undergoing emergency resection in which mass ligation techniques are used. A CT scan with contrast should be used to monitor the viability of the remaining liver and rule out the presence of a perihepatic abscess.

Postoperative bleeding: A second laparotomy for bleeding from the raw edge of the remaining liver is necessary in only 2% to 3% of patients after elective operation and 5% to 7% of patients after emergency resection for severe hepatic injuries.

Hepatic failure: Metabolic failure characterized by progressive elevation of the transaminase, bilirubin, and alkaline phosphatase levels and of the prothrombin time occurs in 5% of patients after extensive resection and is usually reversible with enteral nutrition and support in the intensive care unit.

AFTER DISCHARGE

Recurrent carcinoma: The median survival for patients without cirrhosis who undergo curative resection for hepatocellular carcinoma is about 24 months; this decreases by 11 to 12 months for patients with cirrhosis. The overall 5-year survival of patients undergoing hepatic resection for colorectal metastases is 20% to 30%. Patients with recurrent carcinoma usually have weight loss, abdominal distention, an abdominal mass, and progressive jaundice.

BIBLIOGRAPHY

Emre S, Schwartz ME, Katz E, et al. Liver resection under total vascular isolation: variations on a theme. Ann Surg 1993;217:15–19.

Karl RC, Morse SS, Halpert RD, et al. Preoperative evaluation of patients for liver resection: appropriate CT imaging. Ann Surg 1993;217:226–232.

Nagorney DM, van Heerden JA, Ilstrup DM, et al. Primary hepatic malignancy: surgical management and determinants of survival. Surgery 1989;106:740–749.

Savage AP, Malt RA. Elective and emergency hepatic resection: determinants of operative mortality and morbidity. Ann Surg 1991;214:689–695.

Sparkman RS. The world's first successful elective liver resection. Surg Rounds 1984;7:54–58.

Medical Management of the Surgical Patient, Third Edition,
edited by Michael F. Lubin, H. Kenneth Walker, and Robert B. Smith III.
J.B. Lippincott Company, Philadelphia, PA © 1995.

CHAPTER

60

ANAL OPERATIONS

David V. Feliciano

Anal operations, including hemorrhoidectomy, excision of anal fissure and lateral subcutaneous internal sphincterotomy, drainage of a perianal or ischiorectal abscess, and anal fistulotomy, are among the most common operations performed by general surgeons.

Hemorrhoids are abnormally dilated veins of the hemorrhoidal venous plexus that are classified according to their location above (internal) or below (external) the dentate line. Most hemorrhoids cause minimal symptoms and are managed by sitz baths, topical anesthetics, stool softeners, and a high-fiber diet. In the absence of contraindications such as inflammatory bowel disease, portal hypertension, blood dyscrasias, local cellulitis, and uncontrollable diarrhea, hemorrhoidectomy is indicated for patients with persistent bleeding or pain or for prolapse. Patients with contraindications to operation are treated with injection of sclerosing agents or rubber band ligation (internal hemorrhoids only).

Fissures are openings in the anal mucosa that cause painful defecation. Acute fissures may heal with conservative treatment, but chronic fissures are essentially nonhealing ulcers that often require surgical therapy. A chronic fissure is best excised, with a lateral subcutaneous internal sphincterotomy added to relieve chronic sphincter spasm.

Perianal and ischiorectal abscesses are purulent collections thought to arise from extension of infection in an anal crypt. Perianal abscesses are painful when the patient sits or walks, but not always during defecation. Superficial abscesses present with erythema, swelling, induration, warmth, and tenderness to palpation, whereas deeper abscesses may cause rectal pressure and signs of sepsis. Prompt incision and drainage is the treatment of choice for these lesions, although a fistula may result.

Anal fistulas are openings in the perianal skin that drain purulent material. They arise from spontaneous or surgical drainage of abscesses originating in the anal crypts and may heal spontaneously in some patients. Chronic or long fistulas are treated by fistulotomy, in which the fistula tract is unroofed by cutting through skin and portions of the sphincter muscles and the opened tract is allowed to heal by scarring.

Anal operations are performed under local, caudal, spinal, or general anesthesia, with the patient in the lithotomy, prone, or jackknife position. If local anesthesia is used, many surgeons add epinephrine to decrease blood loss. Most anal operations are performed in 30 to 60 minutes, blood loss is modest, and there is minimal stress to the patient.

USUAL POSTOPERATIVE COURSE

Expected postoperative hospital stay: Ambulatory procedures are routinely performed on patients with anal fissures, perianal abscesses, and fistulas in ano, as long as they are able to return to the surgeon's office on a regular basis in the early postoperative period. After an extensive hemorrhoidectomy, the hospital stay is 3 or 4 days.

Operative mortality: Under 0.1% in patients without portal hypertension

Special monitoring required: The dressing is checked for bleeding every 4 hours during the immediate postoperative period.

Patient activity and positioning: Patients may be out of bed the day of surgery. After removal of the pressure dressing on the first postoperative day, sitz baths of lukewarm water are permitted.

Alimentation: Clear liquids are permitted on the day of operation, and food intake is advanced as tolerated. Psyllium hydrophilic mucilloid (Metamucil) is administered to restore normal bowel function.

Antibiotic coverage: Cephalosporin or advanced penicillin is given to patients undergoing operation for perianal or ischiorectal abscesses or fistulas in ano. Antibiotics are administered until the woody cellulitis surrounding the abscess or fistula tract resolves. All patients with valvular heart disease, prosthetic valves, or vascular grafts receive perioperative antibiotics because of the risk of infection from bacteremia.

Analgesia: Injections of a local anesthetic are frequently performed at the conclusion of anal procedures to relieve pain in the first 6 to 18 hours. Intramuscular narcotics are often administered until the patient has had the first bowel movement after hemorrhoidectomy.

POSTOPERATIVE COMPLICATIONS

IN THE HOSPITAL

Bleeding: Incomplete surgical hemostasis, particularly at the base of a resected hemorrhoid, may lead to postoperative bleeding. Ligation of the bleeding vessel may be possible only by reoperation because exposure at the bedside is too painful. On rare occasions, postoperative bleeding in a patient with cirrhosis may necessitate the use of balloon catheter tamponade followed by the injection of a sclerosing agent.

Urinary retention: Failure to void in the first 4 to 6 hours after operation delays discharge from the ambulatory surgical suite. In-and-out catheter insertion is usually all that is needed in the early postoperative period.

AFTER DISCHARGE

Anal stricture: Excessive excision of anal skin during a hemorrhoidectomy or fissurectomy, or suture closure of the remaining skin may cause an anal stricture as healing occurs. Progressive anal dilation usually solves the problem, although operative release of the stricture occasionally is necessary.

Anal incontinence: A fistula in ano extending into the high intermuscular or supralevator area should not be opened completely at the first operation because damage to the sphincters causes anal incontinence. If this has occurred, a late reoperation with reconstruction of the sphincter mechanism may be necessary.

BIBLIOGRAPHY

Cocchiara JL. Hemorrhoids: a practical approach to an aggravating problem. Postgrad Med 1991;89:149–152.

Dennison AR, Wherry DC, Morris DL. Hemorrhoids: nonoperative management. Surg Clin North Am 1988;68:1401–1409.

Lewis TH, Corman ML, Prager ED, et al. Long-term results of open and closed sphincterotomy for anal fissure. Dis Colon Rectum 1988;31:368–371.

Schouten WR, van Vroonhoven TJ. Treatment of anorectal abscess with or without primary fistulotomy: results of a prospective randomized trial. Dis Colon Rectum 1991;34:60–63.

Williams JG, Rothenberger DA, Nemer FD, et al. Fistula-in-ano in Crohn's disease: results of aggressive surgical treatment. Dis Colon Rectum 1991;34:378–384.

Medical Management of the Surgical Patient, Third Edition,
edited by Michael F. Lubin, H. Kenneth Walker, and Robert B. Smith III.
J.B. Lippincott Company, Philadelphia, PA © 1995.

CHAPTER

61

LAPAROTOMY IN PATIENTS WITH HUMAN IMMUNODEFICIENCY VIRUS INFECTION

David V. Feliciano

Indications for laparotomy in asymptomatic patients with human immunodeficiency virus (HIV) infection, those with acquired immunodeficiency-related complex, or those with full-blown acquired immunodeficiency syndrome are the same as those in patients without these disorders. These include emergency abdominal conditions (perforation of the gastrointestinal tract, intestinal infarction, intraabdominal hemorrhage); urgent abdominal conditions (acute inflammation, obstruction of the small or large intestine, acute gynecologic lesion); and diagnosis and treatment of a malignancy, fever of unknown origin, or abdominal pain of unknown cause.

The diagnostic problem in immunocompromised patients with HIV infection and abdominal pain is the increased incidence of conditions related to the presence of unusual infectious agents (*Candida, Histoplasma, Mycobacterium avium, Cryptococcus,* cytomegalovirus) or malignancies (non-Hodgkin's lymphoma, Kaposi's sarcoma). Because of the hepatosplenomegaly, intraabdominal inflammatory masses, retroperitoneal lymphadenopathy, and enterocolitis related to the processes listed above, diagnostic dilemmas are common in these patients. They require surprisingly few major abdominal operations for acute conditions, however (less than 17% in one study).

Modestly invasive diagnostic procedures such as lapa-

roscopy should be considered in patients with HIV infection and abdominal pain that is not typical of the usual emergent or urgent conditions requiring laparotomy.

Approach to the Patient With HIV Infection and Abdominal Pain (summarized from Barone and colleagues)

1. If diarrhea is present, search for an infectious cause of the pain and observe the abdomen.
2. In patients with organomegaly or ileus, abdominal pain may be related to these problems.
3. Common acute abdominal conditions (appendicitis, cholecystitis) occur in patients with HIV infection and should be treated appropriately.
4. If laparotomy is performed and enteritis is the only finding, mesenteric nodes should be excised for biopsy and culture.

USUAL POSTOPERATIVE COURSE

The significant mortality recorded after laparotomy in patients with HIV infection is believed to be related to their immunocompromised state and the relentless progression of the opportunistic infections and neoplasms that are so prevalent in the last 8 to 12 months of their lives.

489

BIBLIOGRAPHY

Barone JE, Gingold BS, Arvanitis ML, et al. Abdominal pain in patients with acquired immune deficiency syndrome. Ann Surg 1986;203:619–623.

Bartlett JG. HIV infection and surgeons. Curr Probl Surg 1992;29:197–280.

LaRaja RD, Rothenberg RE, Odom JW, et al. The incidence of intra-abdominal surgery in acquired immunodeficiency syndrome: a statistical review of 904 patients. Surgery 1989;105:175–179.

Nugent P, O'Connell TX. The surgeon's role in treating acquired immunodeficiency syndrome. Arch Surg 1986;121:1117–1120.

Potter DA, Danforth DH Jr, Macher AM, et al. Evaluation of abdominal pain in the AIDS patient. Ann Surg 1984;199:332–339.

Medical Management of the Surgical Patient, Third Edition,
edited by Michael F. Lubin, H. Kenneth Walker, and Robert B. Smith III.
J.B. Lippincott Company, Philadelphia, PA © 1995.

CHAPTER

SPLENECTOMY

62

David V. Feliciano

Splenectomy is indicated for acquired thrombocytopenias (immune thrombocytopenic purpura [ITP] with or without a human immunodeficiency virus [HIV] infection, thrombotic thrombocytopenic purpura); congenital or acquired anemias (hereditary spherocytosis, hereditary elliptocytosis, autoimmune hemolytic anemia); staging of Hodgkin's disease; chronic severe secondary hypersplenism with or without splenomegaly (non-Hodgkin's lymphoma, myelofibrosis, Felty's syndrome, hairy cell leukemia, chronic myelogenous or lymphocytic leukemia); splenic vein thrombosis with left-sided (sinistral) portal hypertension; most grade III and IV and all grade V traumatic ruptures; splenic artery aneurysms; and some splenic cysts. The primary indications for splenectomy on university surgical services are thrombocytopenia, anemia, and severe hypersplenism because staging for Hodgkin's disease and operative therapy of traumatic rupture have significantly decreased in frequency in the past 10 years.

General anesthesia is used for both open and laparoscopic splenectomy, although few laparoscopic procedures are reported. Open procedures for routine thrombocytopenia, anemia, or isolated severe blunt rupture are completed in 1 to 1½ hours. A careful search for accessory spleens is mandatory in the first two groups of patients. Blood transfusions are essentially never necessary for routine elective procedures, and platelets usually are not infused in patients with severe thrombocytopenia until the splenic artery has been ligated. The stress of the surgical

procedure is modest even in patients with underlying HIV infection.

Splenectomy is more difficult in patients with chronic severe secondary hypersplenism because of the underlying disease process, frequently associated splenomegaly (500 to 6000 g), and extensive vascular collaterals between the enlarged spleen and the diaphragm and retroperitoneum. Open procedures may take more than 3 hours to complete, blood transfusions of two to four units are common, and the morbidity rate is 20% to 56%, depending on the patient's subgroup classification. Surgical stress is moderate to severe in compromised patients with non-Hodgkin's lymphoma, myelofibrosis, or chronic leukemia.

All patients receive antipneumococcal vaccine before hospital discharge, but usually only children younger than 2 years and selected older adults are given anti-*Haemophilus* vaccine.

USUAL POSTOPERATIVE COURSE

Expected postoperative hospital stay: 5 to 7 days for routine splenectomy; 10 to 21 days for complex splenectomy

Operative mortality: 0% to 2% for elective routine splenectomy; 4% to 33% for elective complex splenectomy; 0% to 40% for trauma splenectomy, depending on associated injuries

Special monitoring required: Platelet counts are monitored after splenectomy for thrombocytopenia and a complete blood count is obtained as necessary in patients with preoperative anemia or pancytopenia. Patients with excessive blood loss during elective complex or trauma splenectomies occasionally require postoperative hemodynamic monitoring with a pulmonary artery catheter.

Patient activity and positioning: Patients may be out of bed the day after operation, depending on hemodynamic stability.

Alimentation: For routine or complex procedures, clear liquids are permitted with the return of bowel function and food intake is advanced as tolerated. For trauma patients with multiple associated injuries (usually Injury Severity Score is over 15), early institution of enteral or intravenous hyperalimentation is appropriate.

Antibiotic coverage: Antibiotics are not administered for routine elective splenectomy unless severe associated granulocytopenia is present. For trauma splenectomy, antibiotics are given for at least 24 hours after surgery in patients with associated perforations of the gastrointestinal tract.

Drains: Drains are not placed after elective routine or trauma splenectomy. The use of closed suction drains after elective complex splenectomy for patients with significant splenomegaly is controversial. The frequent occurrence of left subphrenic seromas after such procedures suggests that drainage would be helpful, but some surgeons believe that any type of drain increases the risk of conversion to a left subphrenic abscess. If a trauma splenectomy is performed as part of a distal pancreatectomy, a closed suction drain is usually left in place for 7 to 10 days.

POSTOPERATIVE COMPLICATIONS

IN THE HOSPITAL

Left lower lobe atelectasis: Left lower lobe atelectasis occurs in 15% to 20% of patients and usually responds to nasotracheal suctioning and chest physiotherapy.

Left subphrenic abscess: Abscesses occur in only 2% to 3% of patients who have elective routine or complex splenectomy but in 5% to 7% of those who have trauma splenectomy. Only 2% to 3% of patients who undergo splenorrhaphy (splenic repair) after trauma or iatrogenic injury develop this complication.

Postoperative hemorrhage: Hemorrhage from the splenic bed occurs in 5% of patients who undergo elective complex splenectomy and is often related to severe persistent thrombocytopenia (nonresponders).

Rebound thrombocytosis: Heparin therapy is suggested if the platelet count exceeds 1 million, but this complication is extremely rare.

Persistent thrombocytopenia: Thrombocytopenia persists in 13% to 30% of patients who undergo splenectomy for ITP. If a radionuclide scan with [111]I-labeled autogenous platelets was not performed before surgery, this study is indicated in the postoperative period to rule out residual accessory spleens not detected at the time of splenectomy. Positive results mandate reoperation if thrombocytopenia persists; patients with normal results should remain on immunosuppressive therapy.

Persistent thrombocytopenia occurs in half the patients with severe preoperative thrombocytopenia from chronic lymphocytic leukemia.

AFTER DISCHARGE

Persistent thrombocytopenia: See earlier discussion.

Overwhelming postsplenectomy infection (OPSI): Splenectomy usually is not performed in children younger than 2 years and is performed infrequently in children younger than 10 years because of the risk of OPSI with encapsulated pneumococci, meningococci, or *Haemophilus* organisms. Most episodes of OPSI occur in the first several years after splenectomy. The relative risk of developing OPSI is lowest when splenectomy is performed for trauma and increases progressively as splenectomy is performed for primary splenic disease, hematologic disease, incidental injury at other operation, and incidental injury at operation for malignancy. The long-term risk in adults is thought to be about 0.5% to 1.45%, and the mortality has decreased to 30% with earlier recognition of the overwhelming bacteremias in patients with previous splenectomy. Neither the administration of antipneumococcal vaccine nor the development of antipneumococcal antibodies is uniformly protective against the development of OPSI.

BIBLIOGRAPHY

Akwari O, Itani KMF, Coleman RE, et al. Splenectomy for primary and recurrent immune thrombocytopenic purpura (ITP): current criteria for patient selection and results. Ann Surg 1987;206:529–541.

Coon WW. The limited role of splenectomy in patients with leukemia. Surg Gynecol Obstet 1985;160:291–294.

Morris DH, Bullock FD. The importance of the spleen in resistance to infection. Ann Surg 1919;70:513–521.

Musser G, Lazar G, Hocking W, et al. Splenectomy for hematologic disease: the UCLA experience with 306 patients. Ann Surg 1984;200:40–45.

Schwartz JS. Pneumococcal vaccine: clinical efficacy and effectiveness. Ann Intern Med 1982;96:208–220.

Medical Management of the Surgical Patient, Third Edition,
edited by Michael F. Lubin, H. Kenneth Walker, and Robert B. Smith III.
J.B. Lippincott Company, Philadelphia, PA © 1995.

CHAPTER

INGUINAL HERNIA REPAIR

63

David V. Feliciano

Inguinal herniorrhaphy is performed for indirect (lateral to the inferior epigastric vessels) or direct (medial to the inferior epigastric vessels in Hesselbach's triangle) groin hernias. Elective procedures for asymptomatic reducible hernias are preferred, but urgent and emergency operations are still required for irreducible hernias and strangulated (ischemic bowel) hernias, respectively.

If routine inguinal herniorrhaphy through a transverse inguinal incision is performed under regional or local anesthesia in an outpatient setting, patients are discharged home when they can void. General anesthesia is appropriate for patients with large hernias that are difficult to reduce, those with multiply recurrent hernias in whom orchiectomy is a consideration, and those who prefer to be asleep. The stress of a routine inguinal herniorrhaphy is minimal and blood transfusions are essentially never required. In contrast, an emergent repair of a strangulated inguinal hernia in which resection of the small bowel is necessary may be life-threatening to elderly patients because of the risk of perioperative sepsis.

The continuing development of laparoscopic inguinal herniorrhaphy is responsible for the variety of operative approaches being performed under general anesthesia. Transperitoneal approaches have included tightening of the internal ring, insertion of a prosthetic plug and patch, and insertion of a patch alone. These are completed in 1 hour in most cases. Preperitoneal repairs are also being evaluated and take more than 2 hours to complete in a surgeon's early experience. The high recurrence rates (6% to 15% at 2 years)

in preliminary studies suggest that further technical improvements are necessary before most patients are offered laparoscopic approaches.

USUAL POSTOPERATIVE COURSE

Expected postoperative hospital stay: Patients who undergo routine inguinal herniorrhaphy under local or regional anesthesia are discharged on the day of surgery. Those who have prolonged inguinal herniorrhaphy under general anesthesia are often discharged the day after operation. If gangrenous bowel was resected during the procedure, a 7-day hospitalization is likely.

Operative mortality: Under 0.1% for elective procedures; increases to 5% to 10% for emergency procedures

Special monitoring required: None

Patient activity and positioning: Patients are ambulatory on the day of surgery. Most surgeons discourage the lifting of heavy objects for 4 to 8 weeks after nonprosthetic repair. When a prosthetic patch is used (Lichtenstein repair), there is no restriction after 3 days.

Alimentation: Patients receive a regular diet on the day of operation. If incarceration or strangulation occurs preoperatively or bowel resection was necessary during the operation, treatment is as for routine laparotomy.

Antibiotic coverage: Recent studies suggest that antibiotic coverage is necessary for routine inguinal herniorrhaphy. If the presence of strangulated bowel or need for bowel resection is suspected preoperatively, cephalosporin or advanced penicillin is administered. This is continued for 24 hours postoperatively if a controlled resection is performed or for 5 to 7 days if peritonitis is present.

Special care: A pressure dressing on the wound minimizes pain, and a scrotal support and ice bag to the scrotum may decrease edema.

POSTOPERATIVE COMPLICATIONS

IN THE HOSPITAL

Inability to void: Some men, including those undergoing operation with local or regional anesthesia, may be unable to void for the first 4 to 6 hours after operation. In-and-out bladder catheterization is indicated before discharge. Elderly patients with prostatism may occasionally require correction of this condition before discharge.

Scrotal hematoma: Extensive dissection of a large or recurrent hernia may lead to the slow development of a scrotal hematoma. Local treatment with ice and elevation is indicated, and the need for surgical decompression is rare.

Wound infection: The incidence of wound infection is under 2% in patients undergoing elective procedures but much higher in those undergoing concomitant resection of gangrenous small bowel. If a prosthetic patch of polypropylene has been used to complete the repair, a wound infection may result in removal of the patch and failure of the repair.

Delayed intestinal perforation: If strangulated bowel appears to recover after removal from the internal inguinal ring, it is returned to the abdominal cavity. On rare occasions, part of the wall of the returned bowel undergoes necrosis, leading to peritonitis. Immediate laparotomy with segmental resection of the involved loop is indicated.

Urinary leak: Unrecognized injury to the bladder has occurred occasionally after repair of a direct inguinal hernia. Leakage of clear fluid from the incision is pathognomonic and demands immediate operative repair.

AFTER DISCHARGE

Hernia recurrence: Historically, primary inguinal herniorrhaphy has been associated with a 5% to 10% recurrence rate. About 25% of recurrences occur in the first year and 50% after 5 years. They are evenly divided between indirect and direct inguinal types. In modern centers using newer techniques, recurrence rates are under 1% at 5 years.

Testicular atrophy: Inadvertent ligation of the spermatic vessels or a significant scrotal hematoma may cause testicular atrophy. No treatment is possible.

BIBLIOGRAPHY

Glassow F. Inguinal hernia repair: a comparison of the Shouldice and Cooper ligament repairs of the posterior inguinal wall. Am J Surg 1976;131:306–311.

Halsted WS. The radical cure of inguinal hernia in the male. Bull Johns Hopkins Hosp 1893;4:17–24.

Lichtenstein IJ, Shore JM. Exploding the myths of hernia repair. Am J Surg 1976;132:307–315.

Lichtenstein IJ, Shulman AG, Amid PK, Montllor MM. The tension-free hernioplasty. Am J Surg 1989;157:188–193.

Ryan JA Jr, Adye BA, Jolly PC, Mulroy MF II. Outpatient inguinal herniorrhaphy with both regional and local anesthesia. Am J Surg 1984;148:313–316.

Medical Management of the Surgical Patient, Third Edition,
edited by Michael F. Lubin, H. Kenneth Walker, and Robert B. Smith III.
J.B. Lippincott Company, Philadelphia, PA © 1995.

VENTRAL HERNIA REPAIR

CHAPTER

64

David V. Feliciano

Ventral hernias encompass a wide variety of abdominal wall defects, including incisional, epigastric, umbilical, and spigelian types. For the purposes of this discussion, the term *ventral hernia* is restricted to the incisional type. A ventral hernia with a small ring predisposes patients to incarceration and possible strangulation of a segment of small or large intestine. Patients with significant ascites are at risk for rupture of a ventral hernia if there is only skin covering the defect. Patients with large ventral hernias have difficulty wearing regular clothes and are often embarrassed by their appearance. For all these reasons, elective repair of ventral hernias is indicated in patients who are healthy enough to undergo mechanical bowel cleaning and general anesthesia.

At the time of operation, the thinned-out skin covering the hernia, the hernia sac itself, and all scar tissue back to normal-appearing rectus or other muscles of the abdominal wall are excised. Once the true size of the hernia defect is seen, a decision is made regarding primary repair versus insertion of a prosthetic patch. Because of the size of many ventral hernias after débridement, patches made of polypropylene (porous) or polytetrafluoroethylene (nonporous) are frequently inserted to fill the musculofascial defect.

Surgical stress is moderate because extensive lysis of adhesions and débridement of the sac is necessary when much of the linea alba has been chronically separated. General anesthesia is used in patients with defects exceeding 4 to 5 cm

in diameter, the procedure may last as long as 2 to 3 hours, and blood transfusion is unnecessary.

USUAL POSTOPERATIVE COURSE

Expected postoperative hospital stay: 5 to 7 days

Operative mortality: Under 1%

Special monitoring required: Nasogastric tube drainage is monitored and replaced intravenously if it is excessive. Serial electrolytes are measured and replaced as needed. The volume of postoperative serum drainage through suction drains placed under the flaps is monitored daily to aid in determining when the drains should be removed.

Patient activity and positioning: Patients may be out of bed on the day after operation. Because of the risk of recurrence, straining and heavy lifting is discouraged for 6 to 8 weeks.

Alimentation: Clear liquids are permitted with the return of bowel function, and food intake is advanced as tolerated.

Antibiotic coverage: All patients receive antistaphylococcic antibiotics preoperatively to prepare for the insertion of a prosthetic mesh. If a mesh is inserted, the antibiotics are continued for 3 days after surgery.

Drains: Two large-bore closed suction drains are placed under the skin flaps to prevent fluid accumulation and encourage adherence of the flaps to the primary or mesh repair. Drainage is monitored as described earlier.

POSTOPERATIVE COMPLICATIONS

IN THE HOSPITAL

Wound infection: The incidence of wound infection is under 2% in patients undergoing elective procedures but much higher in those undergoing concomitant resection of gangrenous small bowel or colon. If a prosthetic patch of polypropylene or polytetrafluoroethylene has been used, a wound infection may necessitate patch removal and result in failure of the repair. Treatment includes the administration of antibiotics based on Gram stain, the application of local heat, and the opening of a portion of the incision.

Wound seroma: If the subcutaneous tissue has been dissected extensively, and especially if a porous prosthetic patch has been inserted, suction drains are necessary to prevent fluid accumulation over the repair. Premature removal of the drains may lead to the formation of a seroma in the wound and significantly increase the risk of a wound infection. Treatment is aspiration under strict sterile technique.

AFTER DISCHARGE

Hernia recurrence: Historically, primary ventral herniorrhaphy has been associated with a 10% to 15% recurrence rate. In modern centers using newer techniques, recurrence rates are under 2% at 5 years.

BIBLIOGRAPHY

Abrahamson J, Eldar S. "Shoelace" repair of large postoperative ventral abdominal hernias: a simple extraperitoneal technique. Contemp Surg 1988;32:24–34.

Bauer JJ, Salky BA, Gelernt IM, Kreel I. Repair of large abdominal wall defects with expanded polytetrafluoroethylene (PTFE). Ann Surg 1987;206:765–769.

Langer S, Christiansen J. Long-term results after incisional hernia repair. Acta Chir Scand 1985;151:217–219.

Poole GV. Mechanical factors in abdominal wound closure: the prevention of fascial dehiscence. Surgery 1985;97:631–640.

Usher FC. New technique for repairing incisional hernias with Marlex mesh. Am J Surg 1979;138:740–741.

Medical Management of the Surgical Patient, Third Edition,
edited by Michael F. Lubin, H. Kenneth Walker, and Robert B. Smith III.
J.B. Lippincott Company, Philadelphia, PA © 1995.

CHAPTER

LUMPECTOMY AND MASTECTOMY

65

David V. Feliciano

Carcinoma of the breast accounts for over 32% of new cancers in women and occurs with a 2½ times greater incidence than either colorectal or lung cancer. The risk of a woman in this country developing breast cancer during her lifetime is about 10%. The surgical treatment of breast cancer has changed considerably since 1980, with a much greater emphasis on selective therapy. Patients with stage I (less than 2 cm) or smaller stage II (more than 4 cm) carcinomas are treated most frequently with lumpectomy or quadrantectomy, sampling of the low axillary nodes, and postoperative radiotherapy with 50 Gy (5000 rad). Data from numerous studies have documented that disease-free survival and actuarial survival rates of these patients at 8 to 10 years are equivalent to those of patients who undergo traditional mastectomy. Women with stage III breast cancer receive preoperative chemotherapy followed by modified radical mastectomy (pectoralis major and, sometimes, pectoralis minor muscles are preserved) and radiotherapy. All surgical specimens are sent for the appropriate hormone receptor assays after lumpectomy or mastectomy. Immediate reconstruction of the amputated breast using myocutaneous transposition flaps is also offered to most women who are likely to need a mastectomy. The surgical stress of a lumpectomy or mastectomy is modest. General anesthesia is used for both lumpectomy combined with axillary dissection and modified radical mastectomy, and each operation lasts about 1½ hours. The addition of breast reconstruction after mastectomy adds another 3 to 5 hours to the operative time. Blood replacement is unusual.

USUAL POSTOPERATIVE COURSE

Expected postoperative hospital stay: 3 or 4 days for lumpectomy and axillary dissection; 5 or 6 days for modified radical mastectomy

Operative mortality: Under 1%

Special monitoring required: The volume of postoperative bleeding through suction drains placed under the flaps of a mastectomy is monitored daily to aid in determining when the drains should be removed.

Patient activity and positioning: Patients may be out of bed the day after operation. Supervised exercises to maintain mobility of the shoulder on the side of the mastectomy also are begun on this day.

Alimentation: Liquids are ingested on the day of surgery, with progression to a regular diet the next day.

Antibiotic coverage: Antibiotics are administered only if there is inflammation in a recent biopsy site in the ipsilateral breast.

Drains: Two or three closed suction drains are placed in the axilla and under the skin flaps to prevent fluid or blood accumulation and encourage adherence of the flap to the chest wall. Drainage is monitored as described earlier.

Psychologic support: Visits from the group Reach to Recovery are of considerable value to patients who have undergone a mastectomy.

POSTOPERATIVE COMPLICATIONS

IN THE HOSPITAL

Wound infection: In obese patients, cellulitis of the mastectomy flaps or actual purulent drainage through suction drains occurs in 4% to 7% of cases. Antibiotics should be administered based on Gram stain, local heat applied, and, occasionally, a portion of the incision opened.

Necrosis of the edge of the skin flap: If the edges of the skin flaps are dissected too thin during a mastectomy, necrosis may result. Débridement and repeated closure is occasionally necessary.

AFTER DISCHARGE

Wound seroma: Serum may accumulate under the skin flaps of a mastectomy if drains are removed prematurely. Needle aspiration and application of a pressure dressing are traditional outpatient treatments, but the use of a small incision and insertion of a soft rubber, open drain often prevents reaccumulation.

Edema of the upper extremity: Edema of the upper extremity occurs in less than 10% of women undergoing standard modified radical mastectomy even when postoperative radiotherapy is used. The primary exception is patients who have extensive nodal involvement around the axillary vein, causing it to become thrombosed in the postoperative period. Edema is treated with elevation and, if necessary, a fitted compression sleeve during the day and an external intermittent compression device at night.

Recurrent cancer: Postoperative radiotherapy administered to various axillary and chest wall ports reduces the incidence of local recurrence by about 15%. Nodules that recur in the old incision are locally excised, but are felt by many to be a marker of distant metastatic disease. Postoperative prophylactic combination chemotherapy is given to premenopausal women with positive lymph nodes. For postmenopausal women with positive lymph nodes *and* positive hormone receptors, tamoxifen is commonly prescribed. If metastases occur, other chemotherapeutic combinations, tamoxifen, or autologous bone marrow transplantation is indicated, depending on the site of the metastases and the age and hormonal status of the patient.

BIBLIOGRAPHY

Fisher B, Redmond C, Poisson R, et al. Eight-year results of a randomized clinical trial comparing total mastectomy and lumpectomy with or without irradiation in the treatment of breast cancer. N Engl J Med 1989;320:822–828.

Haagensen CD, Bodian C. A personal experience with Halsted's radical mastectomy. Ann Surg 1984;199:143–150.

Handley RS. The conservative radical mastectomy of Patey: 10-year results in 425 patients. Breast 1976;2:16–19.

NIH Consensus Conference, June 18-21, 1990. Treatment of early-stage breast cancer. JAMA 1991;265:391–395.

van Heerden JA, Jackson IT, Martin JK Jr, Fisher J. Surgical technique and pitfalls of breast reconstruction immediately after mastectomy for carcinoma: initial experience. Mayo Clin Proc 1987; 62:185–191.

Medical Management of the Surgical Patient, Third Edition,
edited by Michael F. Lubin, H. Kenneth Walker, and Robert B. Smith III.
J.B. Lippincott Company, Philadelphia, PA © 1995.

CHAPTER

66

THYROIDECTOMY

David V. Feliciano

Thyroidectomy is performed for nodules with suspicious cytology on fine-needle aspiration (follicular adenoma), biopsy-proven adenocarcinoma, large goiters with airway compromise or cosmetic concerns, or thyrotoxicosis. Given the 6% to 7% incidence of false-negative results on fine-needle aspiration for adenocarcinoma, nodules enlarging on medical therapy should also be treated with operation. Subtotal thyroidectomy continues to offer an immediate cure and the best chance of restoring a euthyroid state in certain subgroups of patients with thyrotoxicosis. Included among these are children and women of childbearing age with Graves' disease, those who have failed medical or radioiodine therapy for Graves' disease, and those with toxic multinodular goiter (Plummer's disease).

Preoperative preparation with antithyroid drugs, propranolol, and potassium iodide (SSKI) or propranolol alone is indicated in patients with thyrotoxicosis to prevent thyroid storm in the postoperative period. Vocal cord function is checked before the administration of paralytic agents by the anesthesiologist. Thyroidectomy is usually performed under general anesthesia through a low collar incision, which yields excellent cosmetic results. The bilateral parathyroid glands, recurrent laryngeal nerves, and external branches of the superior laryngeal nerves are identified and preserved. Total thyroidectomy is reserved for patients with bilateral intrathyroidal (less than 1.5 cm) or extrathyroidal papillary cancer, follicular cancer with known pulmonary or osseous metastases, or medullary cancer.

Thyroidectomy imposes only a modest stress on patients, most procedures are completed in 2 to 2½ hours, and transfusion is essentially never necessary.

USUAL POSTOPERATIVE COURSE

Expected postoperative hospital stay: Outpatient procedures are appropriate for solitary benign nodules and have been performed for thyrotoxicosis and thyroid cancer in some centers; otherwise, the hospital stay is 1 or 2 days.

Operative mortality: Under 0.1%

Special monitoring required: Respiratory status should be carefully monitored if early postoperative stridor or difficulty in clearing secretions occurs. Patients with thyrotoxicosis who receive appropriate preoperative preparation should undergo routine monitoring.

Patient activity and positioning: The head should be elevated 30 to 45 degrees to minimize edema and venous oozing. Full activity is resumed the morning after operation.

Alimentation: Full liquids are permitted on the day of operation and a regular diet is resumed the next morning.

Antibiotic coverage: None indicated

Drains: Closed suction drains are removed on the first postoperative day.

499

POSTOPERATIVE COMPLICATIONS

IN THE HOSPITAL

Hemorrhage: Although it is extremely rare (less than 0.5%), a hematoma in the area of resection may cause airway obstruction early in the postoperative period. Removal of the skin and strap muscle sutures and evacuation of the hematoma in the recovery room is preferable to tracheostomy. Patients are then returned to the operating room for irrigation of the operative site, control of hemorrhage, and repeated closure of the wound.

Hypoparathyroidism: Transient hypoparathyroidism is seen in 2% to 4% of all patients after thyroidectomy and in 20% to 22% of those who undergo total or repeated thyroidectomy. Permanent hypoparathyroidism occurs in under 0.6% of patients. Symptomatic hypocalcemia (less than 7.5 mg/dL) is characterized by anxiety, perioral or finger tingling, and a positive Chvostek's sign, and usually develops 16 to 24 hours after surgery. Intravenous calcium is given to relieve acute symptoms in the hospital and oral calcium therapy is prescribed at the time of discharge.

Recurrent laryngeal nerve injury: Paralysis of one vocal cord causes hoarseness and difficulty in clearing secretions. This almost always is related to traction on the recurrent nerve and may resolve over a period of days to months. Permanent recurrent nerve palsy occurs in as many as 4.5% of all thyroidectomies, usually resulting from intended sacrifice of a nerve involved with carcinoma.

Thyroid storm: Thyroid storm should not occur after surgery for thyrotoxicosis in adequately prepared patients, but it may be seen in patients with untreated thyrotoxicosis who are undergoing other operations. Symptoms of tremor, agitation, tachycardia, and hyperthermia are treated with intravenous fluids, propranolol, potassium iodide, and steroids.

AFTER DISCHARGE

Recurrent benign nodule or goiter: Recurrence of a benign nodule or goiter can be prevented by the lifelong administration of thyroid hormone.

Recurrent thyroid cancer: To decrease the incidence of recurrent cancer in the neck, lungs, or bone, thyroid hormone replacement is delayed until radioactive iodine is administered.

Late or recurrent hyperthyroidism: Annual thyroid function tests are indicated in patients who are receiving thyroid hormone after operation for goiter or cancer and in those who are originally euthyroid after operation for Graves' disease.

"Permanent" hypoparathyroidism: Vitamin D is added to calcium replacement to enhance absorption. If serial parathyroid hormone levels begin to rise, first the vitamin D and then the calcium supplement should be tapered.

BIBLIOGRAPHY

Feliciano DV. Everything you wanted to know about Graves' disease. Am J Surg 1992;164:404–411.

Foster RS Jr. Morbidity and mortality after thyroidectomy. Surg Gynecol Obstet 1978;146:423–429.

Halsted WS. The operative story of goiter. Johns Hopkins Hosp Rep 1920;19:171–257.

Pederson WC, Johnson CH, Gaskill HV III, et al. Operative management of thyroid disease: technical considerations in a residency training program. Am J Surg 1984;148:350–352.

Medical Management of the Surgical Patient, Third Edition,
edited by Michael F. Lubin, H. Kenneth Walker, and Robert B. Smith III.
J.B. Lippincott Company, Philadelphia, PA © 1995.

PARATHYROIDECTOMY

David V. Feliciano

Parathyroidectomy is performed most commonly in patients with primary hyperparathyroidism and those who are dialysis dependent and have symptomatic secondary hyperparathyroidism. In rare patients who have hypercalcemia on dialysis or after renal transplantation (tertiary hyperparathyroidism), operation is also indicated. A physical examination, chest radiograph, intravenous pyelogram (on rare occasions), and modern parathormone assay distinguish between primary hyperparathyroidism and the hypercalcemia of sarcoidosis, metastases, or a paraneoplastic syndrome. A 24-hour urinary calcium test is occasionally indicated to rule out familial hypocalciuric hypercalcemia. The role of ultrasound for localization of normal and enlarged glands before a first parathyroid exploration by an experienced surgeon is controversial.

Preoperative therapy to lower extraordinarily elevated serum calcium levels in patients with parathyroid comas or suspected carcinomas should include saline infusions, furosemide, and, on occasion, calcitonin. Parathyroidectomy is usually performed under general anesthesia through a low collar incision, although local anesthesia is appropriate for elderly and high-risk patients. All glands are identified by meticulous dissection in a bloodless field. A solitary parathyroid adenoma is present in 80% to 85% of patients and should be excised along with biopsy of one normal gland. Double adenomas are present in 2% to 4% of patients, and excision is appropriate along with biopsy of a normal gland. Sporadic hyperplasia is best treated with subtotal parathyroidectomy (excision of 3½ glands). Patients with secondary or tertiary hyperparathyroidism who are unlikely to be candidates for renal transplantation or to have familial hyperparathyroidism or a multiple endocrine neoplasia (MEN) syndrome should undergo total parathyroidectomy with implantation of a diced half gland into the muscles of their nondominant forearm. The surgical stress of parathyroidectomy is low, and blood transfusions are never given.

USUAL POSTOPERATIVE COURSE

Expected postoperative hospital stay: Outpatient procedures are appropriate for the excision of solitary and double adenomas and have been used for all less than total parathyroidectomies in some centers; otherwise, the hospital stay is 1 or 2 days.

Operative mortality: Essentially 0%

Special monitoring required: The serum calcium level should be measured daily.

Patient activity and positioning: The head should be elevated 30 to 45 degrees to minimize edema and venous oozing. Patients are out of bed the day of operation.

Alimentation: Full liquids are permitted on the day of operation and a regular diet is resumed the next morning.

Antibiotic coverage: None indicated

Drains: Many surgeons no longer place drains. If a closed suction drain is inserted, it is removed on the first postoperative day.

POSTOPERATIVE COMPLICATIONS

IN THE HOSPITAL

Hypoparathyroidism: Early postoperative hypocalcemia may occur in patients who have significant bone resorption before operation or in those who undergo excision of large adenomas or subtotal or total parathyroidectomy. Symptomatic hypocalcemia (less than 7.5 mg/dL) is characterized by anxiety, perioral or finger tingling, and a Chvostek's sign; it usually develops 16 to 24 hours after surgery. Intravenous calcium is given to relieve symptoms in the hospital, and oral calcium therapy may be necessary at the time of discharge in patients with dysfunction of a parathyroid remnant, severe "bone hunger," or total parathyroidectomy with autotransplantation.

Hemorrhage, recurrent laryngeal nerve injury: Hemorrhage and recurrent laryngeal nerve injury occur in less than 0.3% of initial operations performed by experienced parathyroid surgeons. See Chapter 66.

AFTER DISCHARGE

"Permanent" hypoparathyroidism: "Permanent" hypoparathyroidism occurs in only 0.6% to 2% of patients after subtotal or total parathyroidectomy or a second cervical exploration for persistent or recurrent hyperparathyroidism. Vitamin D is added to the calcium replacement to enhance absorption. If serial parathyroid hormone levels begin to rise, first the vitamin D and then the calcium supplement should be tapered.

Persistent or recurrent hyperparathyroidism: Persistent disease (failure of operation) or retrospective misdiagnosis occurs in only 2.5% to 5% of patients. The rate of recurrence after excision of an adenoma is under 1% but increases to 5% to 15% in patients with sporadic hyperplasia who undergo subtotal parathyroidectomy. In patients with renal, familial, or MEN-associated disease who are treated with less than total parathyroidectomy, the recurrence rate for hyperparathyroidism is 15% to 30% in some series. Symptomatic persistent or recurrent hyperparathyroidism should be evaluated first by a careful review of the original operative note and pathology report. Preoperative localization studies include ultrasound of the neck, computed tomography or magnetic resonance imaging of the mediastinum, and thallium-technetium or Sestamibi ^{123}I subtraction scintigraphy. Reoperation by an experienced parathyroid surgeon, particularly after positive localization studies, results in an 85% to 90% cure rate.

BIBLIOGRAPHY

Bauer W, Federman DD. Hyperparathyroidism epitomized: the case of Captain Charles E. Martell. Metabolism 1962;11:21–29.

Edis AJ, Beahrs OH, van Heerden JA, Akwari OE. "Conservative" versus "liberal" approach to parathyroid neck exploration. Surgery 1977;82:466–473.

Feliciano DV. Parathyroid pathology in an intrathyroidal position. Am J Surg 1992;164:496–500.

Kaplan EL, Yashiro T, Salti G. Primary hyperparathyroidism in the 1990's: choice of surgical procedures for this disease. Ann Surg 1992;215:300–317.

Tarazi R, Esselstyn CB Jr, Coccia MR. Parathyroidectomy for primary hyperparathyroidism: early discharge. Surgery 1984;96:1158–1161.

Medical Management of the Surgical Patient, Third Edition,
edited by Michael F. Lubin, H. Kenneth Walker, and Robert B. Smith III.
J.B. Lippincott Company, Philadelphia, PA © 1995.

CHAPTER

TRACHEOSTOMY

68

David V. Feliciano

Tracheostomy historically has been performed for relief of obstruction of the upper airway (trauma, epiglottitis); when prolonged ventilatory support for respiratory failure is likely; for control of secretions in patients with bulbar lesions or closed head injuries; or for sleep apnea. Open surgical tracheostomy now is being replaced with bedside percutaneous dilational tracheostomy in many centers. In patients with acute airway obstruction, cricothyroidotomy ("high tracheostomy") is a better choice than tracheostomy. This is especially true if the individual performing the procedure has little or no surgical training, if the procedure is being performed under less than ideal conditions in the emergency center or intensive care unit, or if there is impending asphyxiation. The delay until tracheostomy is performed in patients with prolonged endotracheal intubation varies from center to center, but prospective data demonstrate the advantage of performing tracheostomy after 7 to 10 days. Recent anecdotal evidence also indicates that patients who cannot be weaned with endotracheal tubes in place often can be weaned rapidly after a tracheostomy is performed. Finally, newer devices are available that enable patients with sleep apnea to be managed without tracheostomies.

After instituting the delivery of 100% oxygen by mask, endotracheal tube, or ventilating bronchoscope, tracheostomy is best performed in the operating room under local anesthesia supplemented by intravenous sedation. The patient's neck is hyperextended and a transverse incision is made over the second tracheal cartilage. The strap muscles are separated in the midline and the anterior trachea from the cricoid cartilage to the fourth tracheal cartilage is cleared. This often necessitates division of the thyroid isthmus between sutures. Either a vertical incision through the second and third cartilages or a three-sided superiorly based flap between the second and third cartilages is made. The tracheostomy tube is then inserted as the anesthesiologist removes the endotracheal tube. The stress of tracheostomy can be considerable if it is performed as an emergent procedure or there is poor coordination between the operating surgeon and the anesthesiologist. Tracheostomy can be performed in 3 to 5 minutes by an experienced surgeon in a sedated patient, but elective tracheostomy performed meticulously in the operating room often requires 25 to 30 minutes. Blood transfusions are never given.

USUAL POSTOPERATIVE COURSE

Expected postoperative hospital stay: The length of the postoperative hospital stay depends on the reason for the tracheostomy. In patients who are converted to tracheostomies to enhance weaning, ventilatory support often is no longer necessary within 1 to 2 weeks.

Operative mortality: The hospital mortality rate for patients undergoing tracheostomy is 50% in some series. The mortality rate related directly to the procedure is under 1% and is always associated with hypoxia or hypoxia-induced cardiac arrhythmias.

Special monitoring required: Both oxygen saturation and end-tidal carbon dioxide monitoring are indicated when intubated and ventilated patients undergo tracheostomy.

Patient activity and positioning: The ventilator tubing should be positioned to prevent undue traction or angling of the tracheostomy tube.

Alimentation: Some patients have difficulty swallowing with a tracheostomy tube in place, presumably because of esophageal compression at the site of the balloon. Passage of a feeding tube with the balloon of the tracheostomy tube partially deflated is appropriate in such a situation.

Antibiotic coverage: Antibiotics are indicated only if the tracheostomy is performed for respiratory failure caused by pneumonia.

Drains: None indicated

POSTOPERATIVE COMPLICATIONS

IN THE HOSPITAL

Hemorrhage: Early bleeding from the soft tissues and thyroid gland near the tracheostomy site results from inadequate surgical hemostasis and can usually be controlled with packing around the stoma. Late transient arterial bleeding in the presence of a pulsating tracheal cannula is suggestive of a tracheal–innominate artery fistula. Hyperinflation of the cuff of the tube occludes the fistula and compresses the artery in most patients. The aspirated blood should be suctioned vigorously as the surgical team is notified. Operative therapy is mandatory and involves resection of the innominate artery and repair of the trachea.

Accidental extubation: An improperly secured tube may become displaced during transport back to the intensive care unit or during a coughing episode. Because the track from the skin to the tracheal stoma is not well formed for 3 to 5 days after a tracheostomy, many surgeons place a silk traction suture through the trachea at the time of operation. This suture is taped to the patient's skin and allows for elevation of the trachea into the wound and easier reintubation if early extubation occurs.

Obstruction: Progressive hypoxia despite passage of a suc-tion catheter through the tube suggests that the remainder of the lumen is occluded or there are thick secretions acting as a ball valve at the tip. If equal breath sounds are present and a tension pneumothorax is unlikely, the tracheostomy tube should be changed over a suction catheter.

Infection: Tracheitis, pneumonia, mediastinitis, and pneumonia have all been reported. Frequent suctioning of the stoma using meticulous sterile technique should decrease the incidence of infection in the airway. Loose closure of the skin wound and frequent suctioning around the tracheostomy tube should reduce the incidence of soft tissue infection.

Tracheoesophageal fistula: Increased secretions and tube feedings in the airway associated with severe coughing related to swallowing suggests the presence of a fistula. Once bronchoscopy and esophagoscopy have confirmed the diagnosis, operative repair involves closure of the holes in both organs and the interposition of a bulky vascularized muscle flap.

AFTER DISCHARGE

Tracheal stenosis: The late development of stridor, wheezing, dyspnea on effort, or airway obstruction from secretions in patients with histories of prolonged tracheostomy placement mandates bronchoscopy. Strictures may occur at the level of the previous stoma, at the balloon site, or at the tip of the tracheostomy tube. Resection of the stricture and end-to-end anastomosis of the trachea are indicated.

BIBLIOGRAPHY

Andrews MJ, Pearson FG. The incidence and pathogenesis of tracheal injury following cuffed tube tracheostomy with assisted ventilation: an analysis of a two-year prospective study. Ann Surg 1971;173:249–263.

Ciaglia P, Firsching R, Syneic C. Elective percutaneous dilational tracheostomy: a new simple bedside procedure. Chest 1985;87:715–719.

Shackford SR. Tracheostomy and cricothyroidotomy. In: Benumof JL, ed. Clinical procedures in anesthesia and intensive care. Philadelphia, JB Lippincott, 1992:211.

Stauffer JL, Olson DE, Petty TL. Complications of endotracheal intubation and tracheostomy: a prospective study of 150 critically ill adult patients. Am J Med 1981;70:65–76.

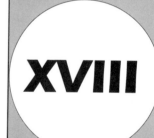

VASCULAR SURGERY

Medical Management of the Surgical Patient, Third Edition,
edited by Michael F. Lubin, H. Kenneth Walker, and Robert B. Smith III.
J.B. Lippincott Company, Philadelphia, PA © 1995.

CHAPTER

69

THORACIC OUTLET DECOMPRESSION

Alan B. Lumsden

Thoracic outlet compression is a condition in which the vascular or neurologic structures are compressed as they exit the thorax and course to the upper extremities. It is manifest by a constellation of vascular and neurologic symptoms. Etiologic factors include compression by the anterior scalene muscle, cervical ribs, subclavius muscle, constricting bands, and other bony anomalies. Neurologic symptoms most frequently occur in the ulnar nerve distribution and include numbness, weakness, and paresthesias. Subclavian vein thrombosis presents as a cyanotic, painful, swollen arm. Arterial manifestations include infarction from emboli, neural compression from a subclavian aneurysm, and Raynaud's syndrome.

The diagnosis is established from the history and physical examination. Standard cervical spine and chest radiographs may show bony anomalies. Nerve conduction studies may confirm neural involvement and help to distinguish peripheral entrapment syndromes. Arteriography and venography delineate vascular compression or show secondary anatomic abnormalities.

The first rib lies inferior to the neurovascular bundle; consequently, anterior scalenectomy and first rib resection is the most commonly performed decompressive procedure. This may be accomplished through either a transaxillary or a supraclavicular approach, dictated by the surgeon's preference and by preoperatively defined anatomic anomalies. The operation is performed under general endotracheal anesthesia and takes 1 or 2 hours. Blood loss is minimal and there is little surgical stress to patients. Possible adjunctive procedures include cervical rib resection, division of the subclavius, and arterial reconstruction.

USUAL POSTOPERATIVE COURSE

Expected postoperative hospital stay: 3 or 4 days

Operative mortality: Under 1%

Special monitoring required: A chest radiograph should be obtained immediately after surgery to rule out pneumothorax from pleural injury. A significant pneumothorax necessitates chest tube placement. Upper limb pulses should be recorded every 4 hours, particularly if vascular repair has been performed. The arm should be examined for evidence of neurologic injury.

Patient activity and positioning: Patients may ambulate on the day of operation. Range-of-motion exercises at the shoulder should be commenced on the first postoperative day.

Alimentation: A regular diet is resumed the night of surgery.

Antibiotic coverage: No antibiotics are required.

Postoperative pain: Retractors placed against the shoulder girdle or brachial plexus may cause local discomfort radiating into the upper arm for several days. Patients should be

507

forewarned of this possibility and adequate analgesia provided.

POSTOPERATIVE COMPLICATIONS

IN THE HOSPITAL

Bleeding: Wound hematomas occur in a small percentage of patients. It is particularly likely if vascular repair has been performed and anticoagulants have been administered.

Pneumothorax: Pneumothorax should be identified during the operation, if possible, by recognizing a hole in the pleura. In this case, the air may be evacuated through a catheter and the wound closed, without the need for an indwelling chest tube. If pneumothorax is recognized on a postoperative chest radiograph, tube thoracostomy is usually required for 1 or 2 days.

Brachial plexus injury: Trauma to the brachial plexus may result from direct operative injury or traction from retractors. It may manifest as motor dysfunction, anesthesia, or hypesthesia. Such injuries are more common in patients undergoing reoperation.

Vascular injuries: Vascular injuries are rare and should be recognized and repaired during the operation.

Phrenic nerve injury: Phrenic nerve palsy may be temporary or permanent and results in dysfunction of the hemidiaphragm. There is no specific therapy.

Lymphatic leak: A chyle fistula may present 2 or 3 days after surgery. It is most common on the left side because of injury to the thoracic duct. Reexploration and ligation of the injured duct is usually necessary.

AFTER DISCHARGE

Continued symptoms: Persistence of symptoms may result from misdiagnosis (eg, symptoms caused by carpal tunnel syndrome); inadequate surgical decompression (unrecognized bony abnormalities, compressive fibrous bands); or intrinsic vascular lesions.

Recurrent symptoms: Recurrent symptoms may be caused by regeneration of the resected rib, the postoperative formation of scar tissue, or the development of fibrous bands. Complete neurologic and vascular reevaluation should be performed before further surgical intervention is undertaken.

BIBLIOGRAPHY

Clagett OT. Research and prosearch. J Thorac Cardiovasc Surg 1962;44:153–166.

Dale WA, Lewis MR. Management of thoracic outlet syndrome. Ann Surg 1975;181:575–585.

Roos DB. The place for scalenectomy and first rib resection in thoracic outlet syndrome. Surgery 1982;92:1077–1085.

Urschel HC Jr, Razzuk MA. Management of the thoracic outlet syndrome. N Engl J Med 1972;286:1140–1143.

Urschel HC Jr, Razzuk MA. Improved management of the Paget-Schrötter syndrome secondary to thoracic outlet compression. Ann Thorac Surg 1991;52:1217–1221.

Medical Management of the Surgical Patient, Third Edition,
edited by Michael F. Lubin, H. Kenneth Walker, and Robert B. Smith III.
J.B. Lippincott Company, Philadelphia, PA © 1995.

CHAPTER

70

PORTAL SHUNTING PROCEDURES

Tarek A. Salam
Atef A. Salam

Decompressive portosystemic shunts play an important role in the treatment of patients with portal hypertension and gastroesophageal varices. The main indication for portal shunting procedures is the prevention of recurrent variceal bleeding in patients with cirrhosis and portal hypertension after failure of endoscopic sclerotherapy. Less often, an emergency shunt procedure is required for acute variceal bleeding that is not controlled by sclerotherapy, vasopressin infusion, or esophageal balloon tamponade. Portal shunting procedures are not indicated for prophylaxis against variceal bleeding in patients who have not yet bled. Ideal candidates for shunt procedures are patients at Child's class A or B risk levels who have favorable venous anatomy. Patients with variceal bleeding and advanced or progressive liver disease should be evaluated for hepatic transplantation. Portal shunting procedures can be divided into two main categories:

Total shunts: With total shunts, the entire portal venous blood flow is shunted into the systemic venous circulation. This includes end-to-side and side-to-side portacaval shunts, central splenorenal shunts, Marion-Clatworthy mesocaval shunts, and interposition mesocaval shunts. The recently introduced transjugular intrahepatic portosystemic shunt also falls into this category. The small graft portacaval interposition shunt is a modification designed to achieve partial rather than total diversion of portal venous flow.

Selective distal splenorenal (Warren) shunt: With the selective distal splenorenal shunt, the gastroesophageal varices are selectively decompressed by way of the upper stomach through the short gastric veins and the disconnected splenic vein into the left renal vein, while enough pressure is maintained in the portal and superior mesenteric veins to drive blood through the diseased liver. The spleen is not removed in this procedure.

Because it is associated with a lower incidence of encephalopathy and hepatic insufficiency, the distal splenorenal shunt is used in most patients. Although collateral veins develop over time after this shunting procedure, with progressive diversion of portal blood flow, there often is no parallel progress of encephalopathy, which remains significantly less than that seen after rapid diversion of portal flow by a total shunt. Unlike portacaval shunts, distal splenorenal shunts do not complicate future liver transplantation. In some patients, however, adequate splenic or renal veins are not available to make this shunt feasible. The selective shunt is not recommended for patients with refractory ascites. A total shunt should be considered under these circumstances. If patients who require total shunts are potential candidates for liver transplantation, mesocaval rather than portacaval shunts should be chosen to preclude dissection in the liver hilus, which would complicate subsequent liver transplantation. All portal shunts cause severe surgical stress and may necessitate multiple perioperative transfusions.

POSTOPERATIVE CARE

Expected postoperative hospital stay: The hospital stay is 7 to 10 days for most patients but is longer if complications occur.

Operative mortality: The operative mortality rate varies from 5% to 30%, depending on the Child's classification and the urgency of the procedure.

Special monitoring required: Intensive care unit monitoring is necessary for the first 2 or 3 days after surgery. Serial monitoring of vital signs, intake and output, central venous pressure, body weight, renal function, hematocrit, and liver function is essential.

Patient activity and positioning: Intensive pulmonary care and early ambulation starting on the first postoperative day are important to minimize atelectasis and subsequent pulmonary complications.

Alimentation: Oral intake is allowed when intestinal peristalsis returns, usually the third to fourth postoperative day. Free sodium intake should be minimized. Dietary protein is not restricted unless patients have signs of encephalopathy.

Antibiotic coverage: A first- or second-generation cephalosporin is usually administered for 24 to 48 hours after surgery, especially if a prosthetic interposition graft has been implanted.

Reaccumulation of ascites: Ascites commonly reaccumulates for several days after operation and should be monitored by daily weighing and abdominal girth measurements. Intravenous colloid solutions coupled with potassium-sparing diuretics (spironolactone, 25 mg three times daily) should be given to maintain a stable urinary output (30 to 50 mL/h).

Postoperative ultrasonography: Shunt patency should be evaluated with ultrasonography.

POSTOPERATIVE COMPLICATIONS

IN THE HOSPITAL

Gastrointestinal bleeding: Recurrence of bleeding after portal shunting can result from postoperative gastritis or peptic ulcer disease. Variceal bleeding as a result of shunt occlusion always must be considered, however, and angiographic evaluation of the shunt may be required.

Ascites: A mild degree of ascites is common in the early postoperative period. Persistent or massive ascites refractory to medical therapy may eventually require a peritoneovenous shunt. Chylous ascites may occur after distal splenorenal shunt placement because of disruption of intestinal lymphatics in the vicinity of the superior mesenteric vessels. A peritoneal tap is diagnostic in such cases, and treatment consists of cessation of oral intake and institution of parenteral hyperalimentation.

Hepatic encephalopathy: The incidence of hepatic encephalopathy after total shunt procedures ranges from 20% to 60%. The rate is significantly lower after distal splenorenal shunt placement because portal perfusion is maintained, particularly in patients without cirrhosis. Therapy consists of dietary protein restriction and the administration of drugs that alter colonic bacterial flora (lactulose, neomycin).

Hepatorenal failure: Serum bilirubin and liver enzyme levels often are elevated mildly during the first postoperative week but usually decline promptly to preoperative baseline levels if the hepatic reserve is adequate. Progressive deterioration of liver function coupled with hypovolemia secondary to dehydration, postoperative bleeding, or massive ascites can result in hepatorenal syndrome, which is associated with a high mortality once it is established.

Ascitic fluid leakage from the abdominal incision: If ascitic fluid leaks from the abdominal incision, the wound may need to be sutured again to prevent massive fluid losses and to reduce the risk of peritonitis.

Chylous ascites: Chylous ascites is an uncommon problem that is seen most often after selective distal splenorenal shunt placement. Patients with unusually resistant chylous ascites may eventually require a peritoneovenous shunt for control.

AFTER DISCHARGE

Shunt occlusion with recurrent variceal bleeding: Sclerotherapy or reoperation should be considered if shunt failure is confirmed by angiography.

Progressive hepatic failure: Progressive hepatic failure is the most common cause of late death in patients with cirrhosis who undergo shunt placement.

Ascites reaccumulation: Salt restriction and diuretic administration usually control ascites, but the possibility of shunt failure must be entertained.

Chronic alcoholism: Continued alcoholism is generally associated with a poor prognosis for long-term survival.

BIBLIOGRAPHY

Henderson JM, Kunter MH, Millikan WJ, et al. Endoscopic variceal sclerosis compared with distal splenorenal shunt to prevent recurrent variceal bleeding in cirrhosis: a prospective randomized trial. Ann Intern Med 1990;112:262–269.

Jim G, Rikkers LF. Cause and management of upper gastrointestinal bleeding after distal splenorenal shunt. Surgery 1992;112:719–727.

Portal hypertension. Am J Surg 1990;160:1–138.

Richter GM, Noeldge G, Palmaz JC, et al. Transjugular intrahepatic portacaval shunt: preliminary clinical results. Radiology 1990;174:1027–1030.

Medical Management of the Surgical Patient, Third Edition,
edited by Michael F. Lubin, H. Kenneth Walker, and Robert B. Smith III.
J.B. Lippincott Company, Philadelphia, PA © 1995.

CHAPTER

71

FEMOROPOPLITEAL BYPASS GRAFTING

Alan B. Lumsden

Femoropopliteal bypass is a procedure in which either a saphenous vein or a prosthetic graft is used to conduct blood from the common femoral artery to the popliteal artery. It is indicated primarily for bypass of atherosclerotic occlusive disease of the superficial femoral or proximal popliteal artery. Such occlusion may be asymptomatic or result in intermittent claudication, rest pain, gangrene, or ischemic ulceration. Intermittent claudication alone is rarely an indication for bypass procedures unless it severely limits life-style or prevents employment; asymptomatic lesions should never be treated.

The preoperative evaluation should include measurement of the ankle-brachial index and performance of arteriography. During the arteriogram, the abdominal aorta, iliac system, and entire lower limb vasculature are carefully documented to define the site and degree of occlusion. The surgeon attempts to determine whether there is adequate inflow to the groin and outflow down the leg to support successful bypass. This decision is based on the cumulative findings of clinical examination, segmental limb pressures, and absence of significant stenoses on arteriography.

Autogenous saphenous vein (either reversed or in situ) is the best conduit, but alternative grafts of Dacron, polytetrafluoroethylene, and umbilical vein are available. Most procedures are performed under spinal anesthesia, but general and epidural anesthesia are suitable. Blood transfusion is usually not required, but a crossmatched sample should be available. The procedure causes little physiologic stress.

USUAL POSTOPERATIVE COURSE

Expected postoperative hospital stay: 4 to 6 days

Operative mortality: 2% to 4%

Special monitoring required: Pedal pulses should be evaluated every 4 hours by palpation or by Doppler ultrasound if they are not palpable.

Patient activity and positioning: Patients ambulate with help on the first postoperative day. To minimize postoperative edema, the legs should remain elevated when patients are not ambulatory. Prolonged bending of the knee should be avoided, because this can cause graft kinking and occlusion.

Alimentation: Clear liquids are allowed on the night of operation and a regular diet is resumed on the first postoperative day.

Antibiotic coverage: First-generation cephalosporin is administered for 24 hours, beginning immediately before operation. A longer course is necessary for patients with open or infected foot lesions.

POSTOPERATIVE COMPLICATIONS

IN THE HOSPITAL

Bleeding: Bleeding is the most common complication and occurs from the anastomosis, surgical incision, or graft tunnel. Intraoperative anticoagulation is contributory. Tense hematomas should be surgically evacuated in the operating room. Smaller hematomas may be observed and will resorb.

Graft thrombosis: Immediate postoperative occlusion (less than 48 hours) usually indicates a technical problem with the anastomosis. Operative revision and graft thrombectomy are indicated.

Leg edema: Leg edema results from operative injury and obstruction of the lymphatic outflow. It occurs to some degree in all patients and can be alleviated by elevating the legs while at rest. Spontaneous improvement occurs over 1 to 2 months.

Wound infection: Wound infection is an uncommon (less than 4%) but limb-threatening complication, particularly when prosthetic grafts have been used. Superficial infections may be treated by wound opening, dressing changes, and culture-directed antibiotic coverage. Deep infections that involve the graft necessitate graft removal, revascularization with autologous tissues (usually vein), and prolonged antibiotic coverage. Amputation is necessary in 70% of patients with infected lower extremity bypass grafts. Spontaneous bleeding from an infected anastomosis may be massive.

AFTER DISCHARGE

Vein graft thrombosis: Vein graft thrombosis occurs in 10% to 15% of patients within 2 years as a result of segmental fibrotic narrowing. It may cause recurrence of symptoms or a reduction in segmental Doppler pressures. Duplex scanning and angiography are indicated for diagnosis. Correction may be performed by either percutaneous balloon angioplasty or surgical revision. Grafts should be monitored with Duplex scanning for 2 years to ensure early detection of stenoses.

Graft occlusion: Graft occlusion may occur suddenly without antecedent symptoms and result in an acutely ischemic limb. This can often be treated successfully by operative thrombectomy and correction of contributing lesions. Lytic therapy with a plasminogen activator is an alternative to opening thrombosed grafts.

More commonly, gradual occlusion results from progressive atherosclerosis in the vessels of the lower limb. Treatment depends on the severity of symptoms and the pattern of occlusive disease.

BIBLIOGRAPHY

Imparato AM, Bracco A, Kim GEB. Comparisons of three techniques for femoral-popliteal arterial reconstruction: 1) vein bypass, 2) open endarterectomy, 3) semi-closed endarterectomy. Ann Surg 1973;177:375–380.

Reichle FA, Rankin KP, Tyson RR, et al. Long-term results of 474 arterial reconstructions for severely ischemic limbs: a 41-year follow-up. Surgery 1979;85:93–100.

Sullivan K, Gardiner GA, Kandarpa K. Efficacy of thrombolysis in infrainguinal bypass grafts. Circulation 1991;83(Suppl I):99–105.

Veith FJ, Gupta SK, Acer E, et al. Six-year prospective randomized comparison of autologous saphenous vein and expanded polytetrafluoroethylene grafts in infrainguinal reconstruction. J Vasc Surg 1986;3:104–114.

Medical Management of the Surgical Patient, Third Edition,
edited by Michael F. Lubin, H. Kenneth Walker, and Robert B. Smith III.
J.B. Lippincott Company, Philadelphia, PA © 1995.

CHAPTER

72

AORTOBIFEMORAL BYPASS GRAFTING

Alan B. Lumsden

Aortobifemoral grafting is used for bypass in patients with atherosclerotic occlusive disease involving the infrarenal aorta and iliac arteries. Typically, this gives rise to thigh and buttock claudication, with impotence in men. Affected patients tend to be in their 40s or 50s, about 10 years younger than patients with femoropopliteal occlusive disease. The operation involves the insertion of a Dacron or expanded polytetrafluoroethylene bifurcated graft. Proximally, the graft is anastomosed to the aorta close to the renal arteries; distally, it extends to the common femoral arteries. Consequently, blood is conducted directly to the infrainguinal vasculature.

This is a physiologically demanding operation that requires general anesthesia. Careful preoperative evaluation of coincidental risk factors is mandatory, particularly in regard to the cardiac system, and should include a careful history of cardiac symptoms, an electrocardiogram (ECG), and dipyridamole (Persantine)-thallium scanning. The procedure takes 3 to 5 hours, and blood transfusion is frequently necessary. During the operation, the use of a cell saver minimizes the need for transfusion.

The operation is performed using a vertical midline abdominal incision, through which the retroperitoneum is divided, exposing the aorta. After systemic heparinization is established by intravenous bolus, the aorta is crossclamped. An appropriately sized graft is sewn to the aorta as close to the renal arteries as is feasible. Each limb of the graft is then passed through a retroperitoneal tunnel to the groins. The

common femoral arteries are exposed through vertical groin incisions and an end-to-side anastomosis is fashioned over the bifurcation of the femoral vessels.

USUAL POSTOPERATIVE COURSE

Expected postoperative hospital stay: 7 to 10 days

Operative mortality: The operative mortality rate ranges from 1% to 3%. The most common cause of death is myocardial infarction, but pulmonary complications such as atelectasis and pneumonia are common. Renal failure occurs occasionally and is associated with significant morbidity.

Special monitoring required: Patients should be placed in the intensive care unit for 1 or 2 days, and vital signs, blood gases, ECG, fluid balance, and hemoglobin, hematocrit, and electrolyte levels should be monitored carefully. Invasive hemodynamic monitoring with a central venous line is routine, and a Swan-Ganz catheter may be necessary in patients with severe cardiac disease.

Patient activity and positioning: Patients are placed at 20 degrees of the reverse Trendelenburg position to maximize pulmonary function. Deep breathing and incentive spirometry are encouraged. Patients may be out of bed the first postoperative day and begin to ambulate the next day.

Alimentation: After laparotomy, an ileus is present for 1 to

3 days. A nasogastric tube is used to decompress the bowel for 24 to 48 hours or until the amount of aspirate is less than 150 mL per shift. Once peristalsis returns (as evidenced by the reappearance of bowel sounds), patients may be given clear liquids and food intake advanced gradually over 2 or 3 days to a regular diet.

Antibiotic coverage: All patients should be treated with perioperative antibiotics. Because the most common organism infecting vascular grafts is a coagulase-negative *Staphylococcus*, a first-generation cephalosporin is a good choice. Antibiotics should be given intravenously immediately before the procedure is begun and continued afterward until all invasive lines and catheters have been removed.

Prevention of pulmonary complications: The most common complications after any laparotomy are atelectasis and pneumonia. Because of their high frequency of tobacco use, patients requiring vascular bypass are at particular risk. Vigorous pulmonary toilet (incentive spirometry, bronchodilators, chest physiotherapy, early ambulation) is an important preventive measure. Epidural anesthesia helps to minimize incisional pain and facilitate deep breathing. Oxygen therapy is routine.

Prevention of cardiac complications: Patients are routinely treated with low-dose intravenous nitroglycerin. Extremes of blood pressure and heart rate are avoided. Creatine phosphokinase isoenzyme levels are monitored, and ECGs are obtained daily. Elective coronary revascularization before aortic surgery may be necessary in patients with severe myocardial ischemia.

POSTOPERATIVE COMPLICATIONS

IN THE HOSPITAL

Cardiac complications: Myocardial infarction is the most common cause of death after aortic surgery. Arrhythmias, pulmonary edema from left ventricular dysfunction, and silent ischemia all may occur.

Pulmonary complications: Pulmonary atelectasis and pneumonia are among the most frequent complications. Mucous plugging of airways may lead to pulmonary collapse. Pulmonary emboli occur occasionally.

Renal complications: Renal failure may occur from a variety of causes, including intraoperative embolization, hypovolemia, suprarenal aortic clamping, hypotension, and blood transfusions. All these factors are particularly deleterious in patients with preoperative renal dysfunction.

Postoperative bleeding: Postoperative bleeding may occur in the retroperitoneum, from the aortic anastomosis, or in the tunnels for each graft limb. Bleeding in the groin may occur from the distal anastomoses. Reoperation may be necessary to evacuate large hematomas and to obtain hemostasis.

Peripheral embolization: Embolization of the lower extremities occurs occasionally. This usually is an intraoperative event and is detected by the loss of peripheral pulses at the conclusion of the procedure.

Acute graft occlusion: Acute graft occlusion is rare and usually reflects a technical problem with insertion of the graft. Reexploration with correction of the underlying problem should be performed.

Infection: Wound infection is rare (less than 1%) but may predispose to late graft infection.

AFTER DISCHARGE

Delayed wound infection: Delayed wound infection is rare and presents with redness, tenderness, and discharge from the groin wound.

Impotence: Retrograde ejaculation and, more rarely, erectile failure are seen in 20% of men.

Graft occlusion: Late graft occlusion (years after surgery) may present with recurrence of symptoms, which may be unilateral or bilateral. Occasionally, acute lower extremity ischemia may result. Operative intervention or fibrinolytic therapy may be necessary.

Anastomotic pseudoaneurysm: Swelling in the groin years after graft implantation most commonly is caused by chronic dehiscence of the suture line resulting in a pseudoaneurysm. Operative repair is necessary.

Aortoenteric fistula: Aortoenteric fistula is a rare complication in which a fistula develops, most frequently between the proximal aortic suture line and the duodenum. Dramatic gastrointestinal bleeding may result, requiring operative intervention for graft removal and repair of the intestinal defect. The interposition of a tissue barrier, such as omentum, between the prosthesis and the duodenum at the initial operation helps to minimize the frequency of this life-threatening complication.

BIBLIOGRAPHY

Brewster DC, Darling RC. Optimal methods of aortoiliac reconstruction. Surgery 1978;84:739–740.

Diehl JT, Cali RF, Hertzer NR, Beven EG. Complications of abdominal aortic reconstruction. Ann Surg 1983;197:49–56.

Malone JM, Moore WS, Goldstone J. The natural history of bilateral aortofemoral bypass grafts for ischemia of the lower extremities. Arch Surg 1975;110:1300–1306.

Szilagyi DE, Elliot JP, Smith RF, et al. A thirty-year survey of the reconstructive surgical treatment of aortoiliac occlusive disease. J Vasc Surg 1986;3:421–436.

Medical Management of the Surgical Patient, Third Edition,
edited by Michael F. Lubin, H. Kenneth Walker, and Robert B. Smith III.
J.B. Lippincott Company, Philadelphia, PA © 1995.

CHAPTER

73

CHRONIC MESENTERIC ISCHEMIA

Alan B. Lumsden

Chronic mesenteric ischemia occurs when there is occlusive disease of the mesenteric arterial circulation. The bowel is supplied by three vessels: the foregut by the celiac artery, the midgut by the superior mesenteric artery, and the hindgut by the inferior mesenteric artery. Typically, symptoms occur when occlusion or significant stenosis involves at least two of the three arteries. Occlusion of the inferior mesenteric artery is common and often asymptomatic; lesions of the celiac artery and the superior mesenteric artery more frequently precipitate symptoms.

Symptoms include weight loss, postprandial mid-abdominal or epigastric pain, and alternate diarrhea and constipation. Patients frequently have histories of cardiovascular disease, including claudication, myocardial infarction, and cerebrovascular disease. The diagnosis is made by arteriography, with a lateral aortogram to demonstrate the origins of the celiac artery and the superior mesenteric artery. Many patients undergo extensive gastrointestinal work-ups before chronic mesenteric ischemia is considered, and some become addicted to analgesic drugs.

Patients with symptoms suggestive of chronic intestinal ischemia and aortograms demonstrating significant stenosis or occlusion of two of the three visceral vessels are candidates for revascularization. Specific preoperative preparation includes cardiac risk stratification because of the high incidence of atherosclerotic heart disease, nutritional evaluation, and hyperalimentation for severely emaciated patients. Revascularization is performed most frequently using a prosthetic graft or saphenous vein originating from the supraceliac aorta and anastomosed to the common hepatic artery and the superior mesenteric artery. Other options include endarterectomy (direct plaque removal) or bypass from the lower abdominal aorta.

The procedure takes 2 to 4 hours. Surgical stress is severe because of the necessity of aortic crossclamping. Blood loss is moderate and transfusion may be necessary. Coordination with the anesthesiologist is essential during the placement and release of aortic clamps to prevent hemodynamic fluctuation.

USUAL POSTOPERATIVE COURSE

Expected postoperative hospital stay: 8 to 10 days

Operative mortality: The operative mortality rate is 3% to 4%. The most common cause of death is myocardial infarction, reflecting the high incidence of intercurrent cardiac disease. Pulmonary complications are next in importance because most of these patients are heavy cigarette smokers.

Special monitoring required: Intensive care is necessary for 2 or 3 days after the operation. Careful hemodynamic monitoring (arterial blood pressure, pulse, electrocardiogram, and Swan-Ganz catheter for those with compromised cardiac function) and strict monitoring of fluid intake and output (urine output, gastrointestinal losses, intravenous fluids) are necessary. A nasogastric tube is required because prolonged postoperative ileus is common.

Patient activity and positioning: Patients should be out of bed and into a chair on the first postoperative day and ambulating twice daily by the next day. The head of the bed is elevated 30 degrees to increase the vital capacity and promote deep breathing. Vigorous coughing, deep breathing, and incentive spirometry (with bronchodilators if necessary) are used to prevent pulmonary complications.

Alimentation: After revascularization, patients often have prolonged ileus. Nasogastric decompression is necessary and intravenous alimentation mandatory. Slow feeding, beginning with clear liquids, is commenced when bowel sounds resume and the nasogastric tube has been removed.

Antibiotic coverage: Patients should receive 24-hour coverage with a cephalosporin, beginning immediately before surgery.

POSTOPERATIVE COMPLICATIONS

IN THE HOSPITAL

Postoperative bleeding: Postoperative bleeding may occur from the arterial anastomoses or dissection site and manifest as low blood pressure or a falling hematocrit level. Intraoperative anticoagulation at the time of aortic clamping is a contributing factor. Reexploration, evacuation of the hematoma, and ligation of the bleeding source may be necessary.

Intestinal edema: Severe intestinal edema has been reported after revascularization. It may result from sudden reperfusion of maximally dilated capillaries distal to the occlusion and contributes to the prolonged ileus that is occasionally encountered. No specific therapy is available. Bowel rest, decompression, and hyperalimentation are necessary until bowel function returns.

Abdominal pain: Mesenteric vasospasm producing recurrent abdominal pain has recently been reported, particularly after bypass with large-caliber prosthetic grafts. This resolves spontaneously after 1 or 2 weeks but may be ameliorated by the postoperative administration of nifedipine.

Myocardial infarction: Myocardial infarction is the most common cause of death after mesenteric revascularization. Prophylactic nitroglycerin should be administered perioperatively.

Acute graft thrombosis: Acute graft thrombosis usually indicates a technical problem with the anastomosis. It presents as acute abdominal pain and may lead to frank intestinal infarction. Operative revision is necessary. Routine postoperative evaluation of the graft is performed using magnetic resonance angiography or duplex ultrasonography.

AFTER DISCHARGE

Graft stenosis: Graft stenosis may occur, most commonly at the anastomoses. This leads to recurrence of symptoms and should be evaluated by repeated angiography.

Graft occlusion: Graft occlusion also may produce recurrent symptoms, although a few grafts undergo asymptomatic occlusion. Patients with symptoms require reoperation and further bypass grafting.

BIBLIOGRAPHY

Beebe HG, Macfarlane S, Raker EJ. Supraceliac aortomesenteric bypass for intestinal ischemia. J Vasc Surg 1987;5:749–753.

Chiene J. Complete obliteration of the celiac and mesenteric arteries: viscera receiving their blood supply through extraperitoneal system vessels. J Anat Physiol 1869;3:65.

Rheudasil JM, Stewart MT, Schellack J, et al. Surgical treatment of chronic mesenteric arterial insufficiency. J Vasc Surg 1988;8:494–500.

Stoney RJ, Ehrenfeld WK, Wylie EJ. Revascularization methods in chronic visceral ischemia caused by atherosclerosis. Ann Surg 1977;186:468–475.

Stoney RJ, Wylie EJ. Recognition and surgical management of visceral ischemia syndromes. Ann Surg 1966;164:714–722.

Medical Management of the Surgical Patient, Third Edition,
edited by Michael F. Lubin, H. Kenneth Walker, and Robert B. Smith III.
J.B. Lippincott Company, Philadelphia, PA © 1995.

CHAPTER

74

CAROTID ENDARTERECTOMY

Thomas F. Dodson

Although carotid endarterectomy is still the most common vascular procedure, its apex of use was reached in 1985, when some 107,000 endarterectomies were performed in the United States. Stroke continues to be the third leading cause of death in this country, and cerebrovascular accident is among the most feared of medical calamities. Therefore, surgical treatment to avert the crisis has inspired passionate debate. Three multicenter trials, reports of which were published in 1991, demonstrated conclusively that carotid endarterectomy is efficacious in the treatment of symptomatic patients with high-grade stenoses. Recent practice guidelines issued by a vascular surgery governing body also suggested that symptomatic patients with low-profile plaques and ulceration or plaques of mixed consistency should be considered for operative intervention. The recommendation for patients who are asymptomatic and have carotid stenoses of varying severity is unclear and is being evaluated in several ongoing trials. Many believe that good-risk asymptomatic patients who have stenoses of 75% to 80% in the internal carotid artery should undergo surgery if the surgeon can offer a combined operative morbidity and mortality rate of less than 3%. Patients with "stroke in evolution" or with completed small strokes and significant carotid lesions fall into other categories for which data are minimal and decision making is difficult.

A carotid endarterectomy can be performed using local, regional, or general anesthesia. Patients with underlying severe heart disease are generally treated best under local an-

esthesia with sedation to minimize the cardiac depression of anesthetic agents. This technique is not recommended, however, in patients who are poorly compliant or unduly anxious. The operation consists of carefully exposing and mobilizing the common carotid artery and its two major branches in the neck. Patients are given heparin, the vessels are clamped, and the carotid artery is opened, extending the incision in the internal carotid artery to just above the atheromatous plaque. Although many surgeons place a shunt at this point to provide blood flow to the brain during the procedure, others do so selectively, depending on several clinical conditions. The atheromatous plaque is then dissected away from the common carotid, the external carotid, and finally the internal carotid, leaving a smooth-appearing lining of media and adventitia. The length of the carotid incision is closed with a continuous suture, using a patch angioplasty in selected patients. The surgical stress of this procedure is low and the operation can usually be completed in 1 or 2 hours. Blood transfusions are rarely required.

USUAL POSTOPERATIVE COURSE

Expected postoperative hospital stay: A 2- or 3-day hospitalization is required. Most complications occur within the first 24 hours.

518

Operative mortality rate: The operative mortality rate is under 1% in patients with no symptoms, about 1% in patients having transient ischemic attacks, and 2% to 5% in patients with strokes in evolution or other critical events.

Special monitoring required: Overnight monitoring is carried out in the intensive care unit, usually with an arterial line to assess fluctuations in blood pressure.

Patient activity and positioning: Patients are usually kept at bed rest on the day of operation and allowed to ambulate the next day.

Alimentation: Liquids or a regular diet is given on the evening after surgery. Except for a sore throat after intubation, the resumption of a normal diet is undisturbed.

Antibiotic coverage: One dose of a cephalosporin is given before the operation and continued for a maximum of 24 hours.

Patient discomfort: Discomfort from the neck incision is minimal and patients may discontinue potent pain medication after the first day.

POSTOPERATIVE COMPLICATIONS

IN THE HOSPITAL

Cardiac complications: Patients with asymptomatic cervical bruits have a higher risk of cardiac ischemic events than of stroke. This fact illustrates that vascular disease involves the entire vascular tree, although to a varying degree. Therefore, although the stress of carotid endarterectomy is characterized as low, patients are at risk for myocardial infarction, cardiac arrhythmias, and other heart-related problems.

Central neurologic complications: For both surgeons and patients, central neurologic complications are ominous. If patients awaken with neurologic deficits or experience the onset of neurologic deficits within a few hours after surgery, immediate reoperation is required. The most common causes of these events are emboli from deposits on the endarterectomized vessel and thrombosis at the operative site. Delayed neurologic events are not as amenable to surgical intervention and may be better managed by confirmation of the diagnosis and provision of supportive treatment. The incidence of surgically related neurologic events is generally no more than 2% in patients operated on for transient ischemic attacks.

Local neurologic complications: The carotid artery is intimately associated with several cranial nerves, all of which are at risk for injury during the procedure. Transient deviation of the tongue toward the side of injury may result from injury or traction on the hypoglossal nerve. Similarly, damage to the vagus nerve, the most commonly injured cranial nerve, may result in either temporary or permanent hoarseness. Injury to the marginal mandibular branch of the facial nerve results in drooping at the corner of the mouth, and damage to the superior laryngeal nerve may cause early fatigability of the voice and impairment in phonation. Trauma to the spinal accessory nerve is an uncommon complication of carotid endarterectomy, but its sequela of shoulder dysfunction is troublesome. Fortunately, most cranial nerve injuries are transient and mild, and recovery can be expected in 6 to 12 months.

Systemic arterial hypertension and hypotension: Blood pressure instability is common in the postoperative period, and an attempt should be made to keep blood pressure in the normal range. Fluid boluses or vasopressors may be necessary to raise the blood pressure, whereas vasodilators may be necessary to lower significant hypertension.

Bradycardia: Slowing of the cardiac rate is common and frequently ascribed to manipulation of the carotid sinus. If the bradycardia is persistent or is associated with hypotension, atropine may be administered.

Postoperative wound hematoma: Postoperative wound hematomas occur in about 5% to 10% of patients. They rarely require surgical intervention, but if a return to the operating room is necessary, the source of bleeding is usually found to be in the subcutaneous tissues rather than the artery itself.

AFTER DISCHARGE

Local complaints: Patients may complain of anesthesia of the ear lobe if the greater auricular nerve has been damaged, and they frequently experience diminished sensation in the region of the neck incision because of the interruption of cervical nerves.

Restenosis of the carotid: About 5% to 10% of patients have significant restenosis of the carotid artery after endarterectomy, although as many as 25% of patients develop greater than 50% stenosis over time. Fortunately, most restenoses are asymptomatic and do not seem to carry the same neurologic threat as do primary atherosclerotic lesions. Reoperation is usually unnecessary in asymptomatic patients except for those with severely tight lesions.

BIBLIOGRAPHY

Eastcott HHG, Pickering GW, Rob CG. Reconstruction of the internal carotid artery in a patient with intermittent attacks of hemiplegia. Lancet 1954;2:994–996.

European Carotid Surgery Trialists' Collaborative Group. MRC European Carotid Surgery Trial: interim results for symptomatic patients with severe (70–99%) or with mild (0–29%) carotid stenosis. Lancet 1991;337:1235–1244.

Mayberg MR, Wilson SE, Yatsu F, et al. Carotid endarterectomy and prevention of cerebral ischemia in symptomatic carotid stenosis. JAMA 1991;266:3289–3294.

Moore WS, Mohr JP, Najafi H, et al. Carotid endarterectomy: practice guidelines. J Vasc Surg 1992;15:469–479.

North American Symptomatic Carotid Endarterectomy Trial Contributors. Beneficial effect of carotid endarterectomy in symptomatic patients with high-grade carotid stenosis. N Engl J Med 1991;325:445–453.

Thompson JE. Complications of carotid endarterectomy and their prevention. World J Surg 1979;3:155–165.

Medical Management of the Surgical Patient, Third Edition,
edited by Michael F. Lubin, H. Kenneth Walker, and Robert B. Smith III.
J.B. Lippincott Company, Philadelphia, PA © 1995.

CHAPTER

75

ABDOMINAL AORTIC ANEURYSM RESECTION

Thomas F. Dodson

In the United States, aortic aneurysm is the tenth leading cause of death in men older than 55 years, and recent evidence suggests that the number of deaths from abdominal aortic aneurysms has increased in the past several decades. There are several potential explanations for the apparent rise in the incidence of these aneurysms, including an aging population, improved detection with ultrasonography and computed tomography, and closer observation of families and first-degree relatives of patients with abdominal aortic aneurysms. The key concept is that this disorder is relatively easily and safely treated in an elective or nonemergent situation. Patients with ruptured aneurysms are difficult to treat, however, and the mortality in these cases ranges from 30% to 50%. Unfortunately, most patients with ruptured aneurysms are unaware that they even had aneurysms.

After an aneurysm of the abdominal aorta is detected, whether by physical examination, plain radiography of the abdomen, computed tomography, magnetic resonance imaging, or B-mode ultrasonography, the urgency and feasibility of elective repair must be determined. Aneurysms less than 5 cm in diameter carry a low risk of rupture, whereas larger lesions have a substantial risk of rupture. Aneurysms 6 to 7 cm or greater in diameter have an even higher propensity to rupture. Because aneurysms usually enlarge annually by 0.3 to 0.5 cm, it is reasonable to monitor small aneurysms (less than 5 cm in diameter) with ultrasound examinations every 6 months. If the aneurysm reaches 5 cm in diameter, operative intervention should be considered. The feasibility of surgery is determined primarily by the functional status of the heart. As many as half of patients with abdominal aortic aneurysms have some evidence of heart disease. Therefore, a cardiac evaluation is the most important step in the preoperative work-up. Other associated problems include chronic lung disease, renal insufficiency, and peripheral vascular disease.

The operation itself is usually performed through a midline incision, although a flank or retroperitoneal exposure is preferred occasionally. After exposure of the aneurysm, patients are heparinized and the aorta is clamped above and below the aneurysm. The dilated segment is opened longitudinally, and the prosthetic graft is placed within the aneurysm sac and sutured both proximally and distally. After the anastomotic suture lines have been checked for bleeding and blood flow has been restored to the lower extremities, the heparin is reversed with protamine. A final "drying up" follows, and the abdominal incision is closed.

The major concern of the vascular surgeon in this setting is blood loss. Fortunately, we have the ability to recapture and reinfuse lost red blood cells by means of an autotransfusion device, a common adjunct to aortic operations. Nevertheless, a net blood loss of 500 to 1000 mL is common, and transfusion may be necessary in the postoperative period. Most abdominal aortic aneurysm procedures are completed in 3 or 4 hours; the operation is viewed as a severe surgical stress.

USUAL POSTOPERATIVE COURSE

Expected postoperative hospital stay: The usual hospital stay is 7 to 10 days, but may be extended if complications occur.

Operative mortality: The mortality rate is 1% to 2% in good-risk patients, 3% to 5% in fair-risk patients, and over 5% in poor-risk patients. *Elective* or *nonemergent* aneurysm repair carries a mortality rate 10 to 25 times *lower* than that in patients with ruptured aneurysms; hence, the emphasis should be on detection, assessment, and planned repair.

Special monitoring required: Intensive care is usually required for 1 or 2 days after surgery, monitoring the blood pressure with an arterial line, the central venous pressure with a central venous pressure line or a Swan-Ganz catheter, and the urine output with a catheter. Hematocrit and electrolyte levels are also observed closely, and blood gas levels are measured periodically to assess oxygenation and ventilation.

Patient activity and positioning: Patients may sit on the side of the bed the morning after operation and ambulate that evening or the next day.

Alimentation: Because disordered bowel function (ileus) is common after aortic procedures, enteral alimentation is withheld for 3 or 4 days. Nasogastric tubes are frequently used in patients undergoing aortic procedures and are removed 1 or 2 days after surgery. In patients with poor nutritional status or underlying severe disease, consideration should be given to peripheral (protein-sparing) or central (hyperalimentation) venous feeding in the early postoperative period.

Antibiotic coverage: An antibiotic effective against skin contamination, generally a cephalosporin, should be administered before surgery and for 24 hours afterward. If invasive monitoring devices are required after this period, it is prudent to continue antibiotic coverage for another 24 hours and then reassess the patient's condition.

Fluid and blood requirements: Numerous factors reduce both urinary output and filling of the heart chambers in the early postoperative period. Appropriate monitoring devices facilitate the correct response to a low central venous pressure or low urine output. The possibility of ongoing blood loss is always a concern in patients who have undergone vascular procedures. Therefore, hematocrit and hemoglobin levels should be measured periodically during the first 24 hours. Generally, major adjustments in fluid and blood products occur in the first 12 to 24 hours, and management after this period is usually somewhat easier.

Pulmonary toilet: Pulmonary toilet, or clearing of airway secretions, is a common concern in patients with vascular disease and large, painful abdominal incisions. This is often exacerbated in long-term smokers with underlying lung disease, and particular attention to frequent coughing, deep breathing, and lung expansion is necessary for an uncomplicated recovery. Judicious but periodic use of pain medication, including patient-controlled devices, is a significant adjunct to postoperative care.

Cardiac analysis: The cardiac subsystem is closely followed by heart chamber pressure analysis, postoperative and daily electrocardiograms, and cardiac enzyme measurements. Because abdominal aortic procedures pose a severe surgical stress, any unexpected clinical deterioration should prompt a reexamination of the myocardial status.

POSTOPERATIVE COMPLICATIONS

IN THE HOSPITAL

Cardiac complications: With careful preoperative evaluation, major postoperative cardiac complications are unusual except in poor-risk patients. Careful attention to filling pressures, cardiac output, and control of hypotension or hypertension facilitates a successful outcome. The treatment of cardiac arrhythmias, particularly those that reduce myocardial perfusion, is an essential element of postoperative care.

Pulmonary complications: Poor pulmonary toilet may lead to retained secretions, atelectasis, and, ultimately, bronchopneumonia. In elderly patients with sleep deprivation, confusion, or airway compromise, aspiration may be a sequela.

Renal complications: Poor renal perfusion in the postoperative period may result from atheromatous embolization to the kidneys during clamping of the aorta; inadequate fluid balance, with a low central venous pressure or low left-sided pressures; or ongoing bleeding, with resultant hypotension. Intraoperative difficulties, including massive bleeding or periods of hypotension, may be manifested postoperatively by diminished renal function. Most renal dysfunction is transient, but some varieties (ie, acute tubular necrosis) may require weeks to resolve.

Colonic ischemia: With careful intraoperative attention to the circulation of the sigmoid colon, colonic ischemia should be an infrequent complication of aortic aneurysm repair. Lower gastrointestinal bleeding, a rising white blood cell count, fever, or unexplained acidosis may presage colonic infarction, however, and vigilance regarding these signs and symptoms should be maintained.

Infection of the operative site: With the use of preoperative antibiotics, the incidence of wound or graft infection is only about 1%.

AFTER DISCHARGE

Anemia: Given the present reluctance to give transfusions and the tendency to accept a lower postoperative hematocrit (except in patients with moderate or severe cardiac disease), anemia is a common occurrence but rarely a long-term problem.

Lassitude: For several reasons, patients are encouraged to leave the hospital as soon as they are able, consistent with good care. In the elderly, a feeling of listlessness or fatigue often persists for several weeks and occasionally for several months. Unless there are mitigating circumstances, however, the symptoms should gradually wane.

Sexual dysfunction: Sexual dysfunction is a known complication of aortic operations and should be discussed frankly before surgery. Pelvic perfusion is at risk during aneurysm surgery, as are the nerves that control ejaculation, which course along the lateral walls of the aorta and cross the proximal common iliac arteries. Thus, iatrogenic impotence and retrograde ejaculation may be reported by sexually active patients after operation. Urologic consultation should be sought if recovery does not ensue after several months.

Aortoenteric fistula: Patients who have undergone retroperitoneal placement of prosthetic grafts are candidates for the development of aortoenteric fistulas, which may occur years after the initial procedure. This should be suspected in patients with either upper or lower gastrointestinal bleeding and previous placement of aortic grafts. Aggressive diagnostic steps and definitive operation may be life-saving.

BIBLIOGRAPHY

Bengtsson H, Bergqvist D, Sternby D-H. Increasing prevalence of abdominal aortic aneurysms: a necropsy study. Eur J Surg 1992;158:19–23.

Hallett JW Jr. Abdominal aortic aneurysm: natural history and treatment. Heart Dis Stroke 1992;1:303–308.

Hollier LH, Taylor LM, Ochsner J. Recommended indications for operative treatment of abdominal aortic aneurysms: report of the Joint Council of the Society for Vascular Surgery and the North American Chapter of the International Society for Cardiovascular Surgery. J Vasc Surg 1992;15:1046–1056.

Katz DA, Littenberg B, Cronenwett JC. Management of small abdominal aortic aneurysms: early surgery vs. watchful waiting. JAMA 1992;268:2678–2686.

Nevitt MP, Ballard DJ, Hallett JW Jr. Prognosis of abdominal aortic aneurysms: a population-based study. N Engl J Med 1989;321:1009–1014.

Szilagyi DE, Smith RF, DeRusso FJ, et al. Contribution of abdominal aortic aneurysmectomy to prolongation of life. Ann Surg 1960;164:678–699.

Medical Management of the Surgical Patient, Third Edition,
edited by Michael F. Lubin, H. Kenneth Walker, and Robert B. Smith III.
J.B. Lippincott Company, Philadelphia, PA © 1995.

CHAPTER

76

LOWER EXTREMITY EMBOLECTOMY

Thomas F. Dodson

Embolic disease of the peripheral arteries is a major problem for internists and vascular surgeons. Most embolic events (80% to 90%) originate in the heart, although a small percentage (5% to 10%) result from proximal arterial lesions. In the remaining few patients, the cause is not identified.

Seventy to 80% of emboli lodge in the limb vessels, with the lower extremities involved in most cases. The femoral artery is the most common artery involved and the most amenable to operative intervention because it can usually be approached under local anesthesia. Evidence of embolization to the popliteal and tibial vessels may require spinal or general anesthesia. The introduction of the Fogarty embolectomy catheter in 1963 marked the beginning of the modern era in treating embolic disorders, but the underlying disease state is still the major impediment to reducing the mortality rate. Although surgeons are able to salvage 90% of affected limbs, hospital mortality in these patients continues to be 20% to 30%.

The key to improved limb salvage is early identification of the problem and prompt definitive treatment. Although the critical duration of limb ischemia continues to be debated, it is clear that patients who have early resolution of their ischemia have more benign courses and increased limb salvage compared to patients who experience lengthy delays. In the past decade, two innovations have been added to the treatment of emboli of the limbs—thrombolytic therapy and angioscopic evaluation or removal of dis-

tal emboli. The role of these new techniques in the treatment of patients with embolic disease is still under evaluation, although thrombolytic therapy holds particular promise in selected circumstances. If embolectomy of the lower extremities can be carried out at the level of the groin under local anesthesia, it should cause only a low degree of surgical stress. More extensive attempts at embolectomy under spinal or general anesthesia may pose a moderate or severe stress, depending on the condition of the myocardium. Blood transfusions are seldom necessary, but blood should be typed before surgery in the event that a more extensive procedure becomes necessary.

USUAL POSTOPERATIVE COURSE

Expected postoperative hospital stay: Five to 7 days of hospitalization are required, depending on the complexity of the operative procedure and the source of the embolic event.

Operative mortality: The mortality rate of the procedure itself is usually low, but the underlying disease state contributes to a 20% to 30% hospital mortality rate.

Special monitoring required: Because of concern about the cardiac subsystem and the need to observe the previously ischemic limb, patients are often monitored in an intensive care unit for a few days. Pulses are palpated or Doppler flow to the operated limb is assessed periodically. It may also be necessary to evaluate motor and sensory function in situations of severe ischemia, and a heightened awareness of the potential for compartment syndrome is essential in such cases. Severe ischemia may also result in muscle breakdown, and this may produce renal damage as well. It is vital that these patients undergo careful monitoring of urinary output, with analysis of the urine for myoglobin, and that mannitol and bicarbonate be prescribed in instances of severe ischemia.

Patient activity and positioning: If the procedure has been limited to a groin incision, patients can often be ambulatory by the next day. More distal incisions usually delay return to full activity, primarily because of patient discomfort and edema of the dependent limb.

Alimentation: Oral feedings begin on the day of operation.

Antibiotic coverage: Usually, one dose of a cephalosporin is given before surgery and the drug is continued for 24 hours afterward.

Postoperative anticoagulation: Heparin is continued after the operation, and warfarin (Coumadin) is added 1 day later. Once patients have had embolic events to the limbs, particularly if the heart is identified as the source, lifelong anticoagulative therapy may be required. It is extremely important that patients be informed about the risks of warfarin therapy, the need for lifelong monitoring of the drug, and the advisability of purchasing Medic-Alert bracelets to notify medical professionals of this therapy in the event of an emergency.

POSTOPERATIVE COMPLICATIONS

IN THE HOSPITAL

Recurrent embolization: Although recurrent embolization is relatively uncommon when anticoagulation is continued after the procedure, it does occur and should be considered in patients who have sudden worsening of the ischemia of the operated limb or who develop ischemia in another limb, the abdominal viscera, or the cerebral circulation.

Compartment syndrome: With severe edema of the revascularized muscles, tissue pressure may exceed the perfusion pressure within compartments of the leg. This can result in muscle necrosis, nerve damage, or thrombosis of the arteries and veins in the related compartment. Early detection is the key to limiting the process, and this can be accomplished by frequent assessment of the motor and sensory function of the limb or by determination of compartment pressures. With diminished motor or sensory function or with significant elevation of compartment pressures, decompressive fasciotomy must be performed.

Myoglobinuria: The appearance of myoglobin in the urine indicates severe ischemia of the affected limb and has potentially serious consequences for renal function. Patients with severe ischemia should be monitored closely for myoglobinuria and treated with attention to adequate hydration and satisfactory urinary output. Alkalinization is necessary in patients with myoglobin release to diminish or prevent precipitation of myoglobin in the renal tubules; mannitol assists with both diuresis and prevention of reperfusion injury.

Metabolic acidosis: Metabolic acidosis is another sign of severe ischemia and may indicate that the attempted embolectomy and revascularization has not been effective. Occasionally, an emergency amputation is the only solution to continued metabolic acidosis and poor tissue perfusion. Hyperkalemia is another concern in cases of severe ischemia, with cell breakdown and release of potassium into the circulation. Again, maintenance of a brisk urinary output in the postoperative period is a helpful adjunct in preventing hyperkalemia.

Leg edema: The extent of edema in the postoperative period often corresponds to the degree of preoperative ischemia as well as the complexity of the procedure necessary to relieve the blockage or reestablish blood flow. Therefore, patients who have had severe ischemia or undergone difficult revascularization procedures frequently have more significant or persistent edema. Elevation of the affected limb continues to be the mainstay of therapy, and patients should be reassured that most of the edema subsides with time.

Wound hematoma: With resumption of heparin therapy after operation, there is an increased risk of hematoma formation in the wound. This is usually not a major problem and rarely requires a return to the operating room for evacuation.

Peripheral nerve deficit: In patients with severe ischemia, peripheral nerve deficits are often the most disabling aspect of their postoperative care. These problems can be manifested by numbness in the sensory distribution of the affected nerve, loss of motor function, or severe neuropathy. Time and analgesics are usually the only allies in this unfortunate complication, although drugs for control of neuropathic pain may be useful.

AFTER DISCHARGE

False aneurysm: False aneurysm is an uncommon complication after embolectomy but must be repaired when it is discovered.

Claudication or rest pain: Symptoms of claudication or rest pain may result if removal of the blockage is incomplete or collateral vessels undergo thrombosis before definitive therapy is achieved. Claudication is usually treated conservatively, whereas rest pain necessitates reevaluation of limb perfusion and an attempt to improve blood flow to the limb.

BIBLIOGRAPHY

Abbott WM, Maloney RD, McCabe CC, et al. Arterial embolism: a 44-year perspective. Am J Surg 1981;143:460–464.

Fogarty TJ, Cranley JJ, Krause RJ, et al. A method for extracting arterial emboli and thrombi. Surg Gynecol Obstet 1963;2:241–244.

Haimovici H. Muscular, renal, and metabolic complications of acute arterial occlusions: myonephropathic–metabolic syndrome. Surgery 1979;85:461–468.

McPhail NV, Fratesi SJ, Barber GG, Scobie TK. Management of acute thromboembolic limb ischemia. Surgery 1983;93:381–385.

Wyffels PL, DeBord JR, Marshal JS, et al. Increased limb salvage with intraoperative and postoperative ankle level urokinase infusion in acute lower extremity ischemia. J Vasc Surg 1992;15:771–779.

Medical Management of the Surgical Patient, Third Edition,
edited by Michael F. Lubin, H. Kenneth Walker, and Robert B. Smith III.
J.B. Lippincott Company, Philadelphia, PA © 1995.

INFERIOR VENA CAVAL INTERRUPTION

77

Thomas F. Dodson

During the past three decades, there has been a startling evolution in the mechanical treatment of patients at risk for pulmonary emboli, beginning with the Mobin-Uddin umbrella filter. Its main drawbacks were a high late vena caval thrombosis rate and occasional detachment from its site of placement. The Greenfield filter was introduced in 1973 to ameliorate the shortcomings of the Mobin-Uddin device and has been largely successful in doing so. It, too, has undergone a transition, and most Greenfield filters now are placed percutaneously in the radiology suite rather than in the operating room. Other devices, purported to embody one advantage or another, are also on the market and are undergoing investigation and clinical use.

With the increased ease with which filter devices can be placed, indications for inferior vena caval interruption have become less strict. Patients with standard indications include those with recurrent embolization despite adequate anticoagulation, those with pulmonary emboli who cannot safely take anticoagulants, those who have had one major embolic event and cannot tolerate another embolus because of their precarious condition, and those who have had serious complications associated with ongoing anticoagulation. Patients with other and more recent indications include those with previous deep venous thrombosis who require major back, abdominal, or extremity operations involving lengthy bed rest; those who are confined to bed for extensive periods and are considered to be at high risk (eg, elderly or obese patients); and those with recent-onset para-plegia or quadriplegia who may be immobile for an extended interval.

Regardless of whether the surgeon places the caval filter in the operating room or the radiologist does so in the radiology suite, the magnitude of stress is minimal. These devices are inserted under local anesthesia by either a cutdown or a percutaneous technique. Blood loss is minimal and blood transfusions are rarely required.

USUAL POSTOPERATIVE COURSE

Expected postoperative hospital stay: Unless anticoagulation is administered or further procedures are planned, patients can go home the evening after the procedure or the next morning.

Operative mortality: The operative mortality rate from the procedure should approach 0%, but the underlying mortality rate from associated conditions is about 10%.

Special monitoring required: No special monitoring is needed in uncomplicated cases. Patients with severe underlying disease may require care in an intensive care unit for treatment of the primary diagnosis.

Patient activity and positioning: Ambulation is allowed on the day of the procedure.

Alimentation: The diet is unrestricted.

Antibiotic coverage: Two doses of a cephalosporin are given, one before surgery and one afterward.

Postoperative anticoagulation: Anticoagulation should be initiated or continued unless contraindicated. The long-term patency rate of the standard stainless steel Greenfield filter is about 96% to 98%, limiting concerns about possible caval thrombosis.

POSTOPERATIVE COMPLICATIONS

IN THE HOSPITAL

Hematoma at the site of cutdown or insertion: Because the filters are placed in a low-pressure system, hematomas are infrequent and rarely a significant problem.

Occlusion of the vein of entry: Jugular vein thrombosis is usually well tolerated except in patients in whom the opposite jugular vein is also occluded. If patients have had a central line in one jugular vein, it is prudent to check the patency of that vein using ultrasound before placing the device into the contralateral jugular vein. Femoral vein thrombosis after either surgical or percutaneous filter placement occurs in 5% to 10% of cases. Limb elevation and anticoagulation (if not contraindicated) are the mainstays of therapy.

Misplacement of the device: The device is misplaced in 4% to 7% of attempts, but use of the guide wire with the Greenfield filter has diminished the frequency of this complication.

Migration of the device: Significant migration of the Greenfield filter is uncommon unless there is incomplete filter expansion resulting from thrombus formation within the carrier at the time of insertion.

Wound infection: Wound infection rarely occurs and probably has an incidence of 1% to 2%.

Caval thrombosis: Unless there is a preexisting clot within the vena cava, caval thrombosis is unlikely.

AFTER DISCHARGE

Recurrent pulmonary embolization: The incidence of recurrent pulmonary embolization with the Greenfield filter is 4%. Given the fact that there are other pathways or even anomalous venous drainage systems, this low but steady incidence is not surprising.

Late venous thrombosis: Late venous thrombosis of the lower extremities may occur either acutely or slowly over time. This probably has more to do with the underlying disorder than with the technique of placement or the nature of the device. It should be treated in the usual manner, including repeated anticoagulation if this is not contraindicated.

BIBLIOGRAPHY

Dalen JE, Alpert JS. Natural history of pulmonary embolism. Prog Cardiovasc Dis 1975;27:259–270.

Goldhaber SZ, Morpurgo M. Diagnosis, treatment, and prevention of pulmonary embolism: report of the WHO/International Society and Federation of Cardiology Task Force. JAMA 1992;268:1727–1733.

Grassi CJ. Inferior vena caval filters: analysis of five currently available devices. AJR 1991;156:813–821.

Greenfield LJ. Evolution of venous interruption for pulmonary thromboembolism. Arch Surg 1992;127:622–626.

Greenfield LJ, McCurdy JR, Brown PP, Elkins RC. A new intracaval filter permitting continued flow and resolution of emboli. Surgery 1973;73:599–606.

Greenfield LJ, Michna BA. Twelve-year clinical experience with the Greenfield vena caval filter. Surgery 1988;104:706–712.

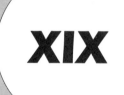

CARDIOTHORACIC SURGERY

Medical Management of the Surgical Patient, Third Edition,
edited by Michael F. Lubin, H. Kenneth Walker, and Robert B. Smith III.
J.B. Lippincott Company, Philadelphia, PA © 1995.

CHAPTER

78

CORONARY ARTERY BYPASS PROCEDURES

Mark W. Connolly

More than 350,000 coronary artery bypass (CAB) procedures are performed annually in the United States. Present indications for surgical revascularization in patients with angiographically significant coronary artery disease are unstable angina refractory to pharmacologic therapy or percutaneous transluminal coronary angioplasty; preservation of "threatened" viable myocardium, particularly in patients with left ventricular dysfunction or acute myocardial infarction; positive results on exercise or thallium stress testing; and significant (greater than 40%) left main disease. Improved survival has been documented in patients with left main disease, triple vessel disease and left ventricular dysfunction (ejection fraction less than 50%), and double vessel disease with positive results on stress testing. In reports from large centers, 10% to 20% of CAB cases are repeated procedures. Contraindications to CAB include low ejection fraction and congestive heart failure or other end-organ systemic disease.

Smooth induction of general endotracheal anesthesia with high-dose opiates and inhalation therapy to prevent hypertension and tachycardia is necessary for acceptable surgical results. After povidone-iodine (Betadine) sterile preparation and draping, a median sternotomy is performed while greater saphenous vein is harvested from the leg. An oscillating saw is used for repeated sternotomies. The left or both internal mammary arteries are dissected from the chest wall. After heparinization, ascending aortic and right atrial cannulas are placed, and cardiopulmonary bypass and systemic cooling to a core temperature of 25° to 32°C is performed. Myocardial arrest is induced by the instillation of antegrade aortic or retrograde coronary sinus

cold blood potassium cardioplegia with topical myocardial cooling. Reversed autologous saphenous vein grafts and, in most patients (over 90%), internal mammary artery grafts are performed. Ten-year patency rates exceeding 90% have been documented with internal mammary artery grafts. The operation generally takes 2 to 4 hours. Blood conservation techniques involving autotransfusion devices are used to minimize homologous blood transfusions. Female gender, small body size, preoperative anemia, advanced age, and the presence of pulmonary or renal disease predispose patients to an increased incidence of blood transfusions.

After revascularization is complete and normothermic systemic temperature is reached, patients are weaned from cardiopulmonary bypass. Inotropic agents and, in patients with low ejection fractions or acute myocardial injuries, intraaortic balloon pumps may be necessary. Protamine is given to reverse the effects of heparin. After hemostasis is obtained and standard closure performed, patients are transferred to the intensive care unit and intubated with mediastinal and pleural drainage tubes and atrioventricular backup pacing.

USUAL POSTOPERATIVE COURSE

Expected postoperative hospital stay: 4 to 7 days

Operative mortality: The operative mortality rate ranges from 1% to 2%, with a higher rate expected in patients with low ejection fractions, acute myocardial infarctions, left

531

main artery disease, repeated sternotomies, or other systemic diseases.

Special monitoring required: Patients stay in the intensive care unit for 12 to 36 hours. Arterial pressure, electrocardiographic signs, Swan-Ganz catheter pressure and cardiac index, urinary output, and chest tube drainage are monitored. Arterial blood gas, serum potassium, and hematocrit levels are obtained every 6 to 8 hours.

Patient activity and positioning: Patients are intubated with their heads elevated 30 degrees for the first 6 to 12 hours. Frequent side-to-side turning is necessary to minimize atelectasis. After extubation, patients are transferred from their beds to chairs. Ambulation is begun and chest tubes are removed on the first or second postoperative day. Frequent ambulation and incentive spirometry are used until patients are discharged from the hospital.

Alimentation: Clear liquids are permitted after extubation, and food intake is advanced to a low-salt, low-fat, low-cholesterol diet as tolerated. Mild gastrointestinal ileus and nausea are common.

Antibiotic coverage: Preoperative prophylaxis with a cephalosporin (or vancomycin in penicillin-allergic patients) is continued for 24 hours after surgery.

Pulmonary toilet: Intensive pulmonary toilet with early ambulation, chest physical therapy, incentive spirometry, and, if necessary, inhalation respiratory treatment is routinely used to prevent atelectasis and pneumonia.

Epicardial pacing wires: Temporary epicardial pacing wires are removed on the third postoperative day.

β-Blockers: A low-dose β-blocking agent is used to decrease atrial tachyarrhythmias.

POSTOPERATIVE COMPLICATIONS

IN THE HOSPITAL

Low cardiac output: Low cardiac output is defined as a cardiac index of less than 2 L/min/m^2. Cardiac output is determined by preload (intravascular volume), heart rate, myocardial contractility, and afterload (systemic vascular resistance). A Swan-Ganz pulmonary artery wedge pressure of 12 to 16 mmHg is achieved with colloid or crystalloid volume infusion. A heart rate of 90 to 100 beats/min is obtained using epicardial pacing, if necessary. Myocardial contractility can be increased with inotropic agents such as epinephrine, dobutamine, or amrinone lactate (a new phosphodiesterase inhibitor). Systemic vascular resistance is increased with norepinephrine (Levophed) or phenylephrine (Neo-Synephrine), or is decreased in the event of hypertension with nitroglycerin and sodium nitroprusside. An in-

traaortic balloon pump inserted percutaneously through the femoral artery may be necessary to decrease afterload and increase diastolic coronary perfusion and cardiac output. Tachycardia is controlled with intravenous β-blockers such as metoprolol (Lopressor) or esmolol.

Bleeding: About 1% to 3% of patients develop postoperative coagulopathy because of defibrinolysis and platelet abnormalities. Chest tube drainage exceeding 200 mL/h for more than 3 hours is treated with rapid rewarming to 37°C and homologous platelet and plasma infusion. Reexploration may be necessary for continued bleeding or cardiac tamponade.

Arrhythmias: Ventricular arrhythmias are treated with correction of serum potassium and magnesium levels and, if necessary, lidocaine infusion. Continued ventricular ectopy is usually a sign of myocardial ischemia. Atrial tachyarrhythmias, which occur in about 30% of patients, are treated with digitalis, β-blockers, or calcium channel blockers. Occasionally, electrical cardioversion may be necessary before patients are discharged from the hospital.

Pericarditis: Symptoms of pericarditis include retrosternal pain, nausea, low-grade fever, and atrial arrhythmias associated with a pericardial rub on auscultation. Patients are treated with intravenous steroids for severe cases and with oral antiinflammatory agents such as indomethacin, ibuprofen, or ketorolac (Toradol) for mild symptoms.

Cerebrovascular accidents: The incidence of cerebrovascular accidents has increased from 1% to 2% to 2% to 4% as older patients have begun to undergo operation. They are caused by air emboli, atheromatous aortic debris, or endomyocardial thrombi. Extracranial and intracranial cerebrovascular disease is also a contributing factor. If this complication is suspected, hyperventilation is used and mannitol and dexamethasone are given to decrease cerebral edema.

Infection: Mediastinitis occurs in 0.5% to 1% of cases and is characterized by fever, lethargy, sternal pain radiating to the back and shoulders, incisional drainage, and sternal instability. The white blood cell count usually is elevated and blood cultures reveal the presence of gram-positive organisms. Operative treatment with sternal débridement and irrigation and muscle flap closure with major pectoralis or rectus abdominis is extremely effective. Organism-specific antibiotic coverage is continued for 4 weeks. Mortality from mediastinitis is extremely rare.

Fluid retention: Cardiopulmonary bypass may result in the accumulation of 4 to 8 pounds of interstitial fluid. The administration of low-dose diuretics for 2 or 3 days reestablishes preoperative weight.

Pulmonary embolus: Pulmonary emboli are extremely rare, but patients known to be sedentary before operation are more susceptible.

Pleural effusion: Pleural effusion usually occurs on the left when the internal mammary artery is used and results from the accumulation of serosanguineous operative fluid after chest tube removal or pleuropericarditis. Symptomatic patients should undergo left thoracentesis before they are discharged from the hospital.

Gastrointestinal symptoms: Nausea, vomiting, intestinal bloating, and ileus occur in 10% to 30% of patients. A clear liquid diet, H_2 blockers, antiemetics, and time should reverse the symptoms in 1 to 3 days.

AFTER DISCHARGE

Incisional pain: Incisional pain usually can be controlled with oral analgesia. Left parasternal numbness may persist for 6 to 12 months if the left internal mammary artery was used.

Sternal clicking: Sternal clicking is increased with exertion and coughing. This generally resolves in 6 to 12 weeks as the sternum heals. Infrequently, the sternum may need to be rewired.

Lower leg edema: Some degree of lower leg edema almost always occurs in the leg from which the saphenous vein was harvested. It is controlled with leg elevation and support hose, and resolves completely in 3 to 6 months.

Ulnar nerve palsy: Ulnar nerve palsy is more prominent in the left forearm and hand because of arm positioning and stretching of the brachial plexus during harvest of the internal mammary artery. This complication resolves completely in 3 to 6 months.

Recurrent angina: Recurrent angina results from incomplete revascularization, graft closure, or progression of native coronary disease. Repeated angiography may be necessary. All patients are administered daily aspirin to prolong graft patency. Repeated angioplasty or bypass surgery is rarely required before 6 to 8 years after the initial procedure.

BIBLIOGRAPHY

Accola KD, Craver JM, Weintraub WS, et al. Multiple reoperative coronary artery bypass surgery. Ann Thorac Surg 1991;52:738–744.

Connolly MW, Guyton RA. Surgical intervention in coronary artery disease. In: Wegner NK, Hellerstein HK, eds. Rehabilitation of the coronary patient, ed 3. New York, Churchill Livingstone, 1992: 323.

Kirklin JW, Barratt-Boyes BG, eds. Cardiac surgery, ed 2, vol 1. New York, Churchill Livingstone, 1993:285.

Medical Management of the Surgical Patient, Third Edition,
edited by Michael F. Lubin, H. Kenneth Walker, and Robert B. Smith III.
J.B. Lippincott Company, Philadelphia, PA © 1995.

CHAPTER

79

MITRAL VALVE REPLACEMENT OR REPAIR

John Parker Gott

The major pathologic conditions necessitating surgical treatment of acquired mitral valve disease vary in incidence among populations. In North America, rheumatic valvular disease is the most commonly encountered condition and may present with stenosis, regurgitation, or both. Stenotic valves are occasionally amenable to open commissurotomy, obviating valve replacement. Degenerative or myxomatous mitral valve disease is the second most frequent condition and is generally associated with pure mitral regurgitation. Operation for rheumatic or degenerative disease is indicated for progressive symptoms of congestive heart failure or objective evidence of deteriorating left ventricular function. Operation is ideally accomplished before or soon after the onset of atrial fibrillation to prevent the long-term morbidity and mortality of chronic atrial fibrillation. Reparative operation as compared with valve replacement for mitral regurgitation appears to have a lower operative mortality, to result in superior postoperative left ventricular function, and to preclude the intrinsic problems associated with available biologic and mechanical prostheses. The benefits of valve repair may justify operation earlier in the course of the disease, lessening the chance for irretrievable loss of left ventricular function.

Ischemic mitral regurgitation often improves with surgical revascularization. Valve operation is usually reserved for patients with moderate to severe regurgitation. Acute infarction generally is not associated with papillary muscle rupture but with acute severe regurgitation and constitutes a surgical emergency. Prompt operation results in patient salvage in a high percentage of cases.

Most mitral valve endocarditides can be cured medically with prolonged antimicrobial treatment. The indications for surgical treatment include progressive heart failure, failure to eradicate the infection, and repeated systemic embolization.

The choice of prosthetic valve replacement requires close communication between patients, cardiologists, and surgeons. Mechanical valves are durable and have low thromboembolic rates, particularly the tilting leaflet designs, but require indefinite anticoagulant therapy. Bioprosthetic valves do not require long-term anticoagulation but are less durable because of degenerative processes (primarily calcification) and are associated with a higher incidence of reoperation for valve failure. The degenerative potential for tissue valves is lower in elderly patients, for whom these bioprostheses are more appropriate choices.

Open mitral valve operations are a major multisystem stress. General endotracheal anesthesia techniques involve combinations of high-dose narcotic agents, benzodiazepines, propofol, and neuromuscular blocking agents. Inhalation agents are used sparingly. Intraoperative epicardial or, preferably, transesophageal echocardiography offers important real-time feedback on valve pathophysiology and subsequent efficacy of mitral valve repair. The median sternotomy incision affords excellent exposure and causes the least postoperative pain and pulmonary embarrassment of any major thoracic incision. The use of meticulous surgical technique to protect the myocardium is critical to prevent postoperative development of the low cardiac output syndrome.

The operative strategy is directed at evaluation of the valve for commissurotomy or repair. If valve conservation is not feasible, replacement is carried out using a technique that spares the posterior leaflet and its chordal mechanism. Adequate excision of the anterior leaflet, chords, and annular and subvalvar fibrocalcific reaction minimizes the chance for interference with mechanical valve motion. Attention to anatomic detail allows proper avoidance of the conduction system, circumflex coronary artery, and aortic valve cusps during valve suture placement.

The duration of the procedure ranges from 2½ to 5 hours; replacement is generally accomplished in less time than repair.

Perioperative blood transfusion has decreased partially as a result of improved technology for blood salvage and reinfusion. Comfort regarding the safety of lower blood counts at the time of hospital discharge is also increasing.

USUAL POSTOPERATIVE COURSE

Expected postoperative hospital stay: The usual length of hospitalization is 5 days, although proper regulation of oral anticoagulants may necessitate a lengthier stay.

Operative mortality: The operative mortality rate ranges from 2% to 6%. The risk increases with the degree of heart failure, which is measured by preoperative functional class or cardiac chamber size, patient age, regurgitation as opposed to stenosis, and duration of crossclamp time. The risk is 10% to 20% or higher for emergent operations, ischemic mitral regurgitation, and cardiogenic shock.

Special monitoring required: The use of thermistor tip pulmonary artery catheters is standard. Left atrial catheters allow more accurate assessment of left-sided filling pressures in the presence of the pulmonary hypertension that is often encountered in mitral valve disease. A second left atrial catheter is occasionally indicated for delivery of pressor agents, particularly norepinephrine. This allows the desired systemic vasoconstrictor effect and minimizes the pulmonary vasoconstrictor effect because most of the drug is metabolized at the first capillary bed it encounters. Intensive care monitoring is continued until satisfactory separation from the ventilator has been achieved and the use of parenteral antiarrhythmics and cardiotonic agents has been discontinued. Telemetry is discontinued after 36 to 48 hours of stable rhythm. Daily prothrombin time determinations are used to regulate warfarin activity.

Patient activity and positioning: Patients are up at their bedsides the day of extubation. Frequent ambulation is strongly encouraged but should be interrupted if bradyarrhythmias or tachyarrhythmias occur or when temporary cardiac pacing wires are removed; in these situations, a few hours of bed rest and frequent vital sign monitoring are prudent. Incentive spirometry is continued until patients are discharged from the hospital.

Alimentation: Clear liquids are permitted after extubation, and food intake is advanced as tolerated. Salt and fluid restriction is advisable because of the physiologic response of the atrial volume receptors and antidiuretic hormone to the postoperative decrease in atrial pressures.

Antibiotic coverage: A cephalosporin with good antistaphylococcic activity based on hospital sensitivities is given 15 to 30 minutes before incision and discontinued within 24 hours after the operation. Depending on the pharmacokinetics of the drug used, a second dose may be administered intraoperatively for patients undergoing longer procedures. Vancomycin is given to penicillin-sensitive patients.

Anticoagulation: Almost all patients who undergo mitral operation are candidates for a period of anticoagulant therapy as prophylaxis against cardioarterial embolism. There are varying degrees of indication. Patients with mechanical prostheses have an absolute indication for anticoagulation as long as the mechanical valves are in place. Patients with documented thromboembolic events, chronic atrial fibrillation, left atrial thrombi seen at operation, or large left atria have a relative indication. Patients who undergo mitral repair with an annuloplasty ring or valve replacement with a bioprosthesis should be considered for 6 to 12 weeks of warfarin therapy to allow time for endothelial incorporation of the foreign material.

POSTOPERATIVE COMPLICATIONS

IN THE HOSPITAL

Arrhythmias: Atrial tachyarrhythmias are more common after mitral (70%) operations than after aortic (40%) or coronary (15% to 20%) operations. The ultimate goal is conversion to sinus rhythm, but control of ventricular response is an immediate goal. Treatment may be with digoxin, calcium channel blockers, β-blockers, procainamide, sotalol, or quinidine in various combinations. Bradyarrhythmias or atrioventricular block is common, usually transient, and treated with atrioventricular sequential pacing using the temporary wires. Oral theophylline may be helpful for increasing the rate of some bradycardias. Permanent pacing is seldom required. Premature ventricular contractions are fairly common and may be suppressed by atrial or atrioventricular sequential pacing to a rate of 90 to 100 beats/min. Repletion of potassium and magnesium is often corrective.

Stroke: Intraoperative cardioarterial embolism of thrombus, calcium particles, or air may lead to stroke. If air is known or strongly suspected to be the cause of a neurologic deficit, hyperbaric oxygen treatment is indicated. Such therapy can completely reverse the neurologic deficit even if it is delayed as long as 24 hours and even if transportation to another facility is required for treatment.

Bleeding: Reoperation for bleeding is necessary in 2% to 3% of cases and is indicated if bleeding greater than 200 mL/h persists after coagulopathy is corrected or if tamponade or massive bleeding supervenes.

Left ventricular rupture: Left ventricular rupture is an increasingly uncommon phenomenon that is usually fatal if it occurs after patients have left the operating room. Multiple technical factors are known to be associated and generally can be avoided during surgery.

Inadequate cardiac output: The syndrome of inadequate cardiac output is recognized when the cardiac index is below 2 L/min/m^2, mixed venous saturation is low, or other signs of low cardiac output are present. Adequate intravascular volume should be ensured and afterload optimized. Atrial or atrioventricular sequential pacing is used if the heart rate is less than 90 beats/min. Pharmacologic or electrical control is used to treat tachyarrhythmias and inotropic support is provided for inadequate myocardial contractility. Intraaortic balloon pump support should be necessary in no more than 1% to 2% of cases. Transesophageal echocardiography is useful to exclude tamponade and to evaluate valvular and ventricular function and aid in diagnosis of tamponade.

Sternal wound infection or mediastinitis: Deep sternal wound infection or mediastinitis should occur in less than 1% of cases. This complication is particularly hazardous in the presence of prosthetic valve material. The mortality rate accompanying the development of prosthetic valve endocarditis (PVE) is high despite the use of antimicrobial agents, débridement, and muscle flaps.

AFTER DISCHARGE

Thromboembolism: The linearized rate for thromboembolism is about 2% per patient-year for bioprostheses and 3% for mechanical valves. Optimizing warfarin therapy (1.5 times control) appears to be the best defense. It is not clear that adding antiplatelet agents lowers the thromboembolism rate significantly.

Bleeding: The linearized rate for significant bleeding associated with anticoagulation is about 3% per patient-year. Again, rigorous patient education and warfarin regulation are the best safeguards.

Prosthetic valve endocarditis: Early onset PVE is evident less than 6 months after operation, is related to intraoperative contamination, has a mortality rate as high as 50%, and is initially treated with antimicrobial agents but usually requires a second valve replacement. Late-onset PVE develops more than 6 months after surgery and emphasizes the need for antimicrobial prophylaxis for dental procedures, operations, and other events associated with bacteremia. Late-onset PVE may occasionally be cured with antimicrobial therapy. Because of the potential for sudden hemodynamic deterioration from valve dysfunction, these patients should be cared for at a center equipped with cardiac surgical services.

Hemolysis: Properly sized and functioning prostheses have low rates of hemolysis. Significant hemolysis should prompt an echocardiographic search for a perivalvular leak. Severe anemia may represent an indication for repeated valve replacement in this setting.

Arrhythmia: Sinus rhythm usually can be restored if atrial fibrillation has been present for less than 1 year before mitral valve operation. If pharmacologic efforts at converting patients to sinus rhythm are not successful, attempts at electrical cardioversion are indicated. Patients should receive anticoagulant therapy for 3 to 4 weeks before electrical cardioversion is attempted. Multivariate analysis has suggested that if the left atrium measures more than 5.2 cm or if symptoms preceded operation by more than 3 years, the chance for successful cardioversion is so low that an attempt is not recommended.

Prosthetic valve dysfunction: Valve thrombosis occurs more often in mechanical valves than in bioprostheses, is diagnosed echocardiographically, and represents a surgical emergency. A second replacement is usually necessary, although operative thrombectomy may suffice in selected cases. With bioprosthetic deterioration, calcific degeneration of the tissue valve is the major finding. Tissue failure and attendant reoperation reaches 20% to 25% at 10 years, and is higher for patients younger than 35 years. The onset of symptoms usually is gradual but sudden, catastrophic failure can occur. Pannus ingrowth may interfere with mechanical valve function and accounts for 20% of causes of valve failure in autopsy series.

Left ventricular outflow tract murmur: After mitral valve repair with the rigid Carpentier ring, there occasionally is a new left ventricular outflow tract murmur and a gradient may be measured. The murmur and gradient usually resolve within a year and most often are not clinically significant.

Congestive heart failure: Congestive heart failure may recur or fail to resolve after operation. A diligent search for failure of mitral valve repair or prosthetic dysfunction is indicated. The usual cause, however, is preexisting left ventricular dysfunction. This is treated medically.

BIBLIOGRAPHY

Arom KV, Nicoloff DM, Kersten TE, et al. St. Jude Medical prosthesis: valve-related deaths and complications. Ann Thorac Surg 1987;43:591–598.

Carpentier A. Cardiac valve surgery: the "French correction." J Thorac Cardiovasc Surg 1983;86:323–337.

Cutler EC, Levine SA. Cardiotomy and valvulotomy for mitral stenosis: experimental observations and clinical notes concerning an operated case with recovery. Boston Med Surg J 1923;188:1023–1027.

Galloway AC, Colvin SB, Baumann FG, et al. A comparison of mitral valve reconstruction with mitral valve replacement: intermediate term results. Ann Thorac Surg 1989;47:655–662.

Medical Management of the Surgical Patient, Third Edition,
edited by Michael F. Lubin, H. Kenneth Walker, and Robert B. Smith III.
J.B. Lippincott Company, Philadelphia, PA © 1995.

CHAPTER

80

AORTIC VALVE REPLACEMENT

John Parker Gott

The onset of symptoms in the presence of significant aortic stenosis is an indication for aortic valve operation. The most frequently encountered symptoms and associated average life expectancy without surgical treatment are as follows: angina pectoris, 5 years; syncope, 3 to 4 years; and congestive heart failure, 1½ to 2 years. The development of symptoms in the setting of aortic stenosis portends entry into a high-risk phase: sudden death occurs in 15% to 20% of these patients. Operation offers improved quality and duration of life and should also be considered for selected asymptomatic patients who have transvalvular gradients exceeding 50 mmHg or valve orifice areas less than 0.8 cm^2.

Aortic insufficiency of gradual onset is usually well tolerated and may remain asymptomatic for years even with deterioration of left ventricular function. A primary goal of treatment is to prevent irreversible loss of this function. Operation is indicated if symptoms develop, because a rapid decline in cardiac function often ensues. Valve replacement is required even in the absence of symptoms if serial quantitative examinations (echocardiography, radionuclide study, or ventriculography) document deteriorating function. Patients with initially moderate to severe impairment of function may still benefit from operation, but the risk for perioperative mortality or long-term failure is elevated. Inability to eradicate aortic valve endocarditis with antimicrobial treatment or the development of supervening congestive heart failure or recurrent embolization mandate surgical treatment. Repair of dissection involving the as-

cending aorta may require aortic valve replacement or suspension.

Options for direct repair of the aortic valve are limited to highly selected patients; the mainstay of surgical treatment is valve replacement. The choice of a replacement device requires an individualized consideration of relative risks. Available bioprostheses offer freedom from long-term anticoagulation but at the expense of a significant potential for valve degeneration necessitating reoperation (about 15% at 10 years and 35% at 15 years in the aortic position). Mechanical prostheses are extremely durable and have a lower risk of valve failure and reoperation but a higher risk of thromboembolic complications and anticoagulant-related bleeding. Fresh or cryopreserved aortic valve homografts offer freedom from long-term anticoagulation and improved durability compared with bioprostheses. A scarce supply and the learning curve associated with the increased technical demands of homograft implantation have limited this approach.

Preoperative coronary arteriography is advisable for patients older than 40 years to allow concomitant revascularization, which has lowered short- and long-term risk in this population. Careful screening for periodontal disease and preoperative tooth extraction (as required for control of oral infection) decrease the risk of prosthetic valve endocarditis.

General endotracheal anesthesia with high-dose narcotics and perioperative monitoring with systemic and pulmonary artery catheters are routine. A median sternotomy incision is used and cardiopulmonary bypass is instituted. Meticulous attention to myocardial protection using one of several cardioplegic techniques has minimized the incidence of postoperative low cardiac output syndrome. The aorta is crossclamped, the valve inspected through an aortotomy and excised, and the annulus débrided of calcium. Valve sutures are placed through the annulus, then through the sewing ring of the prosthesis; the prosthesis is seated and the sutures are tied and cut. The aortotomy is closed and deairing of the cardiac chambers is carried out. Patients are then tapered from cardiopulmonary bypass. Most patients receive blood transfusion (typically, 2 to 4 units). The need is based on the preoperative red blood cell mass and body size of the patient, the blood conservation techniques used, and the degree of postoperative bleeding from coagulopathy and surgical sites. Operative time is 3 or 4 hours.

Aortic valve replacement causes major physiologic stress because of the duration of extracorporeal circulation. Longer operative times are necessary for the few patients who undergo left ventricular outflow enlargement (aortic root enlargement) to enable them to accommodate larger valves for hemodynamic reasons. This is accomplished by dividing the annulus and inserting a gusset of pericardium or a prosthetic patch.

USUAL POSTOPERATIVE COURSE

Expected postoperative hospital stay: The usual hospitalization is 5 days; some patients require a longer stay for regulation of anticoagulant therapy.

Operative mortality: 1% to 2% for a primary operation; 6% to 10% for reoperation

Special monitoring required: Intensive care is necessary until patients are fully awake, extubated, and no longer receiving intravenous inotropic or antiarrhythmic agents (usually within 24 hours). After that point, care is provided in a regular hospital room with 24 to 48 hours of telemetry to monitor the cardiac rhythm.

Patient activity and positioning: Patients are up at their bedsides on the first postoperative day and ambulate at least three times daily thereafter.

Alimentation: Small amounts of clear liquids are allowed 4 hours after extubation. and food intake is advanced to a regular diet as tolerated the next day.

Antibiotic coverage: A prophylactic intravenous cephalosporin antimicrobial is given within the hour preceding skin incision and is discontinued within 24 to 48 hours. Vancomycin is administered to patients with penicillin or cephalosporin allergy.

POSTOPERATIVE COMPLICATIONS

IN THE HOSPITAL

Arrhythmia: Up to 40% of patients develop atrial arrhythmias, usually atrial fibrillation, after aortic valve replacement. To decrease the incidence of atrial arrhythmias early after operation, a low-dose β-blocker (5 to 10 mg of propranolol given orally four times a day) is administered after operation, then tapered over 3 weeks and discontinued. Premature ventricular complexes are common and often respond to correction of potassium and magnesium levels or to atrial pacing at a higher rate. Heart block requiring permanent pacing occurs in less than 5% of cases. Temporary pacing is frequently used for transient conduction abnormalities and for atrial pacing to optimize the heart rate (around 90 beats/min) and, thus, cardiac output in the first 24 to 48 hours after operation.

Bleeding: Reexploration for postoperative bleeding is necessary in 2% to 3% of patients. Most bleeding occurs in response to the coagulopathic state that is associated with the duration of extracorporeal circulation. Assay-guided protamine reversal of heparin, the administration of desmopressin to stimulate platelet function, increase in the ventilatory positive end expiratory pressure, judicious use of platelet transfusion and coagulation factors, and the passage of time usually control this bleeding. Persistent bleeding after correction of coagulopathy (200 mL/h), and bleeding associated with hemodynamic compromise (particularly with signs of tamponade) require operative exploration. The sudden onset of brisk bleeding after a surge in blood pressure may signify disruption of the aortotomy suture line. Prompt reentry for control, in the intensive care unit if necessary, may be life-saving.

Stroke: Atherosclerotic debris from the ascending aorta, calcific deposits that escape from the annulus at the time of valve excision, or air may lodge in the cerebral circulation, resulting in stroke in 1% to 2% of patients. Uncommonly, thrombus from the valve prosthesis becomes an embolus during the in-hospital recovery phase. Treatment is supportive. Physical and occupational therapy are begun.

Low cardiac output syndrome: Pump failure is the most common cause of in-hospital death after aortic valve replacement. While mechanical problems are being excluded (transesophageal echocardiographic examination for prosthetic malfunction or tamponade), treatment is begun to optimize the heart rate and rhythm (about 90 beats/min with atrioventricular synchrony), using the temporary pacing system if necessary. The filling pressures that are required for an adequate preload are often higher than usual (the goal is a capillary wedge pressure of 16 to 18 mmHg) because of the typical hypertrophied, noncompliant left ventricle that is associated with aortic stenosis. Inotropic pharmacologic support is provided and afterload-reducing agents are used if elevated peripheral resistance is contributing to the problem. Mechanical support with the intraaortic balloon pump may be the decisive factor allowing recovery, but it is needed in less than 2% of cases.

Infection: Significant sternal wound infection or mediastinitis occurs in less than 1% of patients. Various combinations of malaise, spiking temperature, tachycardia, increasing wound discomfort, sternal instability, rising white blood cell count, and vasodilation may herald this complication. Early operative drainage, débridement of necrotic tissue, antimicrobial therapy, and wound closure with well-vascularized tissue (muscle or omental flap) are mainstays of care and have improved the survival (94%) associated with this major complication.

AFTER DISCHARGE

Prosthetic valve endocarditis: Postoperative infection of the prosthesis may become evident at any point, but the highest risk occurs within 3 months of operation. This early presentation is assumed to be the result of intraoperative contamination. Infections that are encountered later are caused by bacteremia, emphasizing the importance of lifelong endocarditis prophylaxis in patients with replaced aortic valves. The mortality rate of this devastating complication is 50% to 70%. Successful treatment almost always involves a second replacement of the infected valve. The homograft aortic valve may become the replacement valve of choice in this situation because of its relative resistance to infection and the ability to tailor the tissue to conform to abscess cavities and to replace necrotic areas of the left ventricular outflow tract.

Prosthetic valve dysfunction: Mechanical valves are extremely durable, with a low incidence of intrinsic mechanical failure. Nevertheless, pannus ingrowth, thrombus formation, or suture impingement of leaflet motion can lead to chronic dysfunction or acute catastrophic failure. Suspicion of any of these problems constitutes an emergency and necessitates evaluation at a center with cardiac surgical expertise readily available. Bioprostheses are prone to structural deterioration, most commonly caused by tissue calcifica-

tion. This process tends to be accelerated in young patients (less than 35 years old) and decelerated in elderly patients (more than 65 years old). There is a perception that tissue valves have a "benign" failure mode, with ample clinical warning to allow elective replacement. This view has come into question lately with realization of the significant morbidity and higher mortality that is associated with emergency reoperation for failed tissue valves. This concern should prompt more intense surveillance (symptoms, signs, echocardiography) of such valves when the expected high-risk phase approaches at 10 to 15 years after implantation. Perivalvular leak should raise the question of prosthetic valve endocarditis. A hemodynamically important leak or associated significant hemolysis should prompt reoperation, which may consist of simple closure of the leak. Some cases require a second replacement.

Thromboembolism: Tissue valves are at lower risk for thromboembolism than are mechanical valves, especially after the fourth to sixth postoperative weeks. Mechanical valves have a risk of two thromboembolic events per 100 patient-years. The best defense remains careful patient education and attention to anticoagulation, with an International Normalized Ratio goal of 2.5 to 3.5. This also entails a significant risk of anticoagulant-related bleeding of one to two per 100 patient-years.

BIBLIOGRAPHY

Burdon TA, Miller DC, Oyer PE, et al. Durability of porcine valves at fifteen years in a representative North American patient population. J Thorac Cardiovasc Surg 1992;103:238–252.

Cheung EH, Craver JM, Jones EL, et al. Mediastinitis after cardiac valve operation: impact upon survival. J Thorac Cardiovasc Surg 1985;90:517–522.

Hufnagel CA, Harvey WP. The surgical correction of aortic regurgitation: preliminary report. Bull Georgetown Univ Med Center 1953;6:60–61.

Ivert TSA, Dismukes WE, Cobbs GC, et al. Prosthetic valve endocarditis. Circulation 1984;69:223–232.

Jones EL. Freehand homograft aortic valve replacement: the learning curve: a technical analysis of the first 31 patients. Ann Thorac Surg 1989;48:26–32.

Medical Management of the Surgical Patient, Third Edition,
edited by Michael F. Lubin, H. Kenneth Walker, and Robert B. Smith III.
J.B. Lippincott Company, Philadelphia, PA © 1995.

CHAPTER

REPAIR OF ATRIAL SEPTAL DEFECT

81

John Parker Gott

Operation for correction of atrial septal defect (ASD) is undertaken to prevent or interrupt the progression of pulmonary hypertension, congestive heart failure, and arrhythmia, all of which pose a potential threat to longevity and quality of life. The risk of development of these complications is significant when the pulmonary-to-systemic blood flow (left-to-right shunt) exceeds 1.5 to 1, in which case operation is recommended. ASDs have a diverse morphology. The more straightforward and most common are secundum or foramen ovale (fossa ovalis) defects. The risk for operative mortality is negligible for patients with these defects because the extracorporeal circulation time required for intracardiac repair is brief (less than 30 minutes), the magnitude of surgical stress is low, and the hospital stay is only a few days. Repair of more complicated defects carries a higher operative risk. An example is the ostium primum defect, which accounts for only 5% of ASDs and actually is an atrioventricular canal defect. It requires more extensive operation, often including correction of associated mitral valve insufficiency.

General anesthesia, median sternotomy, cardiopulmonary bypass, and cardioplegic arrest offer the greatest margin of safety for cardiac exposure, precise repair, identification of undiagnosed associated anomalies, myocardial protection, and prevention of air embolism, although other approaches and techniques are used for cosmetic or other considerations. Some defects may be closed primarily; however, if any question exists regarding tension on the suture line or tensile strength of the surrounding atrial tissue, or if the defect is large, a patch of autologous pericardium (preferably) or synthetic material is used for the repair. Patching may decrease the incidence of postoperative atrial arrhythmias by minimizing anatomic distortion of the atrium. The location of all pulmonary veins should be determined during the operation because anomalous drainage occurs in association with ASDs and can be redirected if recognized. In adult patients with normal preoperative hematocrit levels, perioperative transfusion may be expected in less than one third of cases. The operation lasts 2 to 4 hours.

Ideally, repair should be accomplished before symptoms develop, but even patients with advanced symptoms usually have improvement after surgery. About one fifth of adult patients with ASDs develop pulmonary hypertension in response to the left-to-right shunts. Special precaution and detailed invasive monitoring are advised for patients with suspected or known pulmonary hypertension because their risk for repair is significantly increased. If the pulmonary vascular resistance reaches half the systemic resistance, operative mortality approaches 40% and operative survivors often are not rewarded by improvement in symptoms or longevity. Because the onset of pulmonary vascular resistance abnormalities is insidious, unpredictable, and ultimately life-threatening, and because early operation is safe, a low threshold for early repair of ASDs is prudent.

USUAL POSTOPERATIVE COURSE

Expected postoperative hospital stay: 3 to 5 days for an isolated ASD

Operative mortality: The operative mortality rate is under 1% for an isolated ASD and ranges from 3% to 4% for the partial atrioventricular canal type. Associated congestive heart failure, pulmonary hypertension, and other congenital defects increase the risk significantly.

Special monitoring required: Intensive care is required until patients are fully awake and responsive and extubated (usually less than 24 hours). Telemetry should be used for 48 hours because of the significant incidence of atrial arrhythmias. For older patients, left atrial lines or pulmonary artery catheters allow early recognition and prompt treatment of hemodynamic instability, which is infrequent in younger patients.

Patient activity and positioning: Incentive spirometry and early ambulation facilitated by adequate analgesia hasten recovery and minimize inpatient care.

Alimentation: Liquids are allowed a few hours after extubation, and food intake is advanced as tolerated.

Antibiotic coverage: A prophylactic parenteral cephalosporin is given and discontinued within 24 to 48 hours of operation; vancomycin is administered to patients with a history of penicillin or cephalosporin allergy.

Arrhythmias: The incidence of postoperative atrial arrhythmias may be decreased by the administration of a prophylactic regimen of low-dose oral β-blocker after surgery (5 mg of propranolol given orally four times daily and tapered over 3 weeks has been effective).

POSTOPERATIVE COMPLICATIONS

IN THE HOSPITAL

Arrhythmias: Postoperative supraventricular arrhythmias are common, particularly if they were present before surgery, and respond to traditional pharmacologic treatment. Permanent heart block is extremely unusual, even with the partial atrioventricular canal type of repair, in which sutures are placed near the atrioventricular nodal tissue. Transient heart block is treated by the temporary pacing system that should be routinely placed with every cardiac operation; this complication resolves within days.

AFTER DISCHARGE

Thromboembolism: After ASD repair, pulmonary and systemic embolization occur to such a degree in middle-aged and elderly patients that the risk-benefit ratio favors the use of postoperative anticoagulant therapy for 2 to 3 months. This should be continued indefinitely if atrial fibrillation persists.

BIBLIOGRAPHY

Cheng TO. Early thromboembolism after atrial septal defect repair. (Letter) J Thorac Cardiovasc Surg 1990;99:758.

Gibbon JH Jr. Application of a mechanical heart-lung apparatus to cardiac surgery. Minn Med 1954;37:171–180.

Hawe A, Tastelli GC, Brandenburg RO, McGoon DC. Embolic complications following repair of atrial septal defects. Circulation 1969;39:185–189.

Murphy JG, Gersh BJ, McGoon MD, et al. Long-term outcome after surgical repair of isolated atrial septal defect. Follow-up at 27-32 years. N Engl J Med 1990;323:1645–1650.

Medical Management of the Surgical Patient, Third Edition,
edited by Michael F. Lubin, H. Kenneth Walker, and Robert B. Smith III.
J.B. Lippincott Company, Philadelphia, PA © 1995.

CHAPTER

82

PERMANENT PACEMAKER IMPLANTATION

Kamal A. Mansour
Mark W. Connolly

Indications for permanent pacemaker implantation in symptomatic patients are complete heart block, sinus bradycardia, sick sinus syndrome, bundle branch block with a prolonged His bundle–ventricle (H-V) interval, and carotid sinus hypersensitivity. Asymptomatic patients with Mobitz II block below the His system, alternating bundle branch block, and bifascicular block with an H-V interval greater than 100 milliseconds are also candidates for pacemaker implantation.

Epicardial pacing is used during cardiac surgery, in small infants, and when transvenous pacing fails because of high electrical thresholds or electrode displacement. General anesthesia is required and the epicardial leads are manually screwed into the epicardium through subcostal, subxiphoid, or left anterior thoracotomy approaches. The procedure usually takes less than 1 hour and blood transfusions are rarely used. Transvenous pacemaker systems are used in most patients and only local anesthesia is required. Using the Seldinger technique through the subclavian vein, transvenous pacing leads are inserted under fluoroscopic radiographic guidance into the anteroapical right ventricular endocardium. In dual-chamber atrioventricular pacing systems, a lead is also placed into the right apical appendage. Sensing and pacing thresholds are tested with an external analyzer. The generator is placed in a subcutaneous pocket created in the subclavicular area.

USUAL POSTOPERATIVE COURSE

Expected postoperative hospital stay: 3 to 5 days for epicardial pacemakers and 1 day for transvenous pacemakers

Operative mortality: Under 0.5% and related to underlying cardiac disease

Special monitoring required: Electrocardiographic monitoring is required during the procedure and until discharge from the hospital.

Patient activity and positioning: Patients should be out of bed and ambulating as soon as possible. Their underlying cardiac conditions may limit their activity.

Alimentation: Food intake is advanced as tolerated.

Antibiotic coverage: A cephalosporin with sensitivity for gram-positive organisms is given intravenously for 24 hours then orally for 5 more days. Vancomycin is substituted in penicillin-allergic patients.

543

Radiography: A chest radiograph is necessary to check lead placement, and a 12-lead electrocardiogram should be performed with and without pacemaker magnet to verify proper pacemaker function.

POSTOPERATIVE COMPLICATIONS

IN THE HOSPITAL

Cardiac tamponade: Cardiac tamponade may be caused by right ventricular or atrial rupture, or by mediastinal bleeding. Surgical decompression is usually required.

Pericarditis: Pericarditis occurs after epicardial placement and responds to the administration of oral antiinflammatory agents or intravenous steroids.

Wound infection: Wound infection is seen in under 1% of patients. It may require removal of the device and replacement at another site.

Arrhythmia: If arrhythmias occur, pharmacologic therapy should be administered according to the rhythm disturbance.

Lead displacement: Lead displacement is confirmed by chest radiography and requires repositioning of the lead under fluoroscopy.

AFTER DISCHARGE

Exit lead block: Exit lead block occurs when the stimulation threshold exceeds the energy output of the pacemaker. Implantation of a new lead is necessary.

Lead fracture: Lead fracture requires placement of a new lead.

Pulse generator failure: Frequent follow-up by telemetry is necessary to detect battery depletion. Replacement of the old generator through the same incision is required.

Diaphragmatic stimulation: Diaphragmatic stimulation may result from close proximity of the lead tip to the phrenic nerve. It is corrected by lowering the stimulation threshold or by repositioning the lead tip.

Muscle stimulation: Local pectoralis muscle twitch is more common with unipolar systems. This is corrected by decreasing the stimulation threshold, by placing an insulating sleeve around the generator, or by repositioning the generator underneath the pectoralis muscle.

Thrombophlebitis of the left subclavian vein: Thrombophlebitis of the left subclavian vein is more common with dual-lead systems and usually responds to intravenous heparin and warfarin (Coumadin) therapy.

BIBLIOGRAPHY

Furman S. Cardiac pacing and pacemakers. In: Baue AE, ed. Glenn's thoracic and cardiovascular surgery. Norwalk, CT, Appleton & Lange, 1993:1887.

Laqerqren H, Levander-Lindgren M. Ten-year follow-up on 1000 patients with transvenous electrodes. PACE 1980;3:424–435.

Mansour KA, Miller JI, Symbas PN, Hatcher CR Jr. Further evaluation of the sutureless, screw-in electrode for cardiac surgery. J Thorac Cardiovasc Surg 1979;77:858–862.

Medical Management of the Surgical Patient, Third Edition,
edited by Michael F. Lubin, H. Kenneth Walker, and Robert B. Smith III.
J.B. Lippincott Company, Philadelphia, PA © 1995.

CHAPTER

83

IMPLANTABLE CARDIOVERTER DEFIBRILLATOR

The implantable cardioverter defibrillator (ICD) has emerged as an important treatment option for patients with ventricular tachycardia or ventricular fibrillation that is refractory to pharmacologic therapy. Patients with indications for ICD implantation include those with classic sudden death associated with ventricular arrhythmias, mostly ischemic in nature. Although they are unable to prevent ventricular arrhythmias, all devices have the capability of delivering a defibrillation shock. Newer third-generation devices offer "tiered therapy," which integrates antitachycardia pacing and defibrillation shocks to optimize arrhythmia therapy and generator battery life. Five-year survival rates in the range of 90% have been achieved in patients with otherwise poor long-term prognoses.

General anesthesia is required and patients are placed in the supine position. Implantation involves the placement of three components: (1) a rate-sensing ventricular endocardial lead, (2) shock delivery endocardial leads or epicardial or epipericardial patches, and (3) an integrator–pulse delivery generator. Standard "open" techniques use median sternotomy, left anterior thoracotomy, and subxiphoid and subcostal approaches for direct placement of defibrillator patches on the epicardium or pericardium. In nonthoracotomy "closed" lead systems, all sensing and defibrillator leads are placed using the Seldinger technique through the subclavian vein under fluoroscopic guidance into the right ventricular endocardium and superior vena cava. The generator is placed under the rectus abdominis muscle or fascial sheath while a counterincision is made over the deltopectoral groove for lead insertion into the subclavian vein and subcutaneous tunneling. Lead sensing and pacing thresholds and induced ventricular arrhythmia defibrillation thresholds are determined during the operation. Patch and lead repositioning may be required to optimize thresholds. Surgical stress is minimal and the prognosis is primarily related to preoperative left ventricular function. Blood samples for typing and screening are drawn before operation, but patients are rarely transfused. The procedure lasts from 1 to 4 hours.

USUAL POSTOPERATIVE COURSE

Expected postoperative stay: Patients usually remain in the hospital for 2 to 5 days, depending on their overall medical condition, especially preoperative left ventricular function and arrhythmias.

Operative mortality: The operative mortality rate ranges from 1.5% to 5% and is related directly to the associated cardiac condition.

Special monitoring required: Continuous monitoring is necessary with electrocardiography, arterial pressure measurement, pulse oximetry, and central venous access. A Swan-Ganz catheter may be required in selected patients with poor ventricular function. Analytic electrophysiologic equipment specific to the implanted device is used. Previously applied external defibrillation patches may be needed for "rescue" shock if the internally placed system fails to defibrillate an induced arrhythmia. Cardiac telemetry is required until discharge from the hospital.

Patient activity and positioning: Patients usually are out of bed and walking on the first day after operation and any chest tubes that were inserted are removed.

Alimentation: Food intake is advanced to a regular diet as tolerated.

Antibiotics: Cefazolin (Ancef), 1 g intravenously, is administered before surgery and prophylactic coverage is continued for 5 to 7 days afterward with oral cephalexin (Keflex) or ciprofloxacin. Vancomycin is used in patients with penicillin allergy.

Repeated electrophysiologic study: Before patients are discharged from the hospital, follow-up electrophysiologic studies generally are carried out, with documentation of ICD function.

POSTOPERATIVE COMPLICATIONS

IN THE HOSPITAL

Postoperative atrial and ventricular arrhythmias: Postoperative atrial and ventricular arrhythmias occur in 30% of patients.

Other complications: Pericardial effusion, pleural effusion, bleeding, pneumonia, atelectasis, pneumothorax, pulmo-

nary emboli, and subclavian vein thrombosis all may occur occasionally.

Wound infection: Wound infection requires prolonged antibiotic therapy. Device removal and replacement into another subcutaneous site may be necessary after the infection has resolved.

AFTER DISCHARGE

Generator end-of-life: Generator life averages 36 to 50 months, depending on usage. The device must be replaced when it is depleted.

Arrhythmias: Although sudden cardiac death is virtually eliminated by the ICD, many patients continue to require pharmacologic treatment of their arrhythmias.

Elevated defibrillation thresholds: If defibrillation thresholds are elevated, patches or endocardial leads must be repositioned.

BIBLIOGRAPHY

Furman S, Kim SG. The present status of implantable cardioverter defibrillator therapy. J Cardiovasc Electrophysiol 1992;3:602–622.

Lehmann MH, Saksena S. NASPE policy statement: implantable cardioverter defibrillators in cardiovascular practice: report of the Policy Conference of the North American Society of Pacing and Electrophysiology. PACE 1991;14:969–979.

Mirowski M, Reid PR, Mower MM. Termination of malignant ventricular arrhythmias with an implantable automatic defibrillator in human beings. N Engl J Med 1980;303:322–324.

Shepard RB, Goldin MD, Lawrie GM, et al. Automatic implantable cardioverter defibrillator: surgical approaches for implantation. J Cardiovasc Surg 1992;3:208–224.

Medical Management of the Surgical Patient, Third Edition,
edited by Michael F. Lubin, H. Kenneth Walker, and Robert B. Smith III.
J.B. Lippincott Company, Philadelphia, PA © 1995.

CHAPTER

PERICARDIECTOMY

84

Joseph I. Miller, Jr.

The surgical indications for pericardiectomy are pericarditis with significant pericardial effusion and tamponade associated with several conditions. The most common types of pericarditis are idiopathic, uremic, infectious, posttraumatic, neoplastic, and chronic constrictive. Patients usually have marked cardiovascular compromise. The main objective of the operation is to remove as much pericardium as is feasible to alleviate the altered vascular dynamics.

The operation represents a significant surgical stress to patients with already compromised cardiovascular systems. General endotracheal anesthesia is used. The procedure is usually carried out as a closed cardiac procedure, except in patients with chronic constrictive pericarditis who have calcium impregnation into the pericardium. In these patients, the procedure should be carried out as a "pump standby" procedure, with cardiopulmonary bypass available because of possible cardiac perforation. A subxiphoid, left anterior thoracotomy, or median sternotomy surgical approach can be used. A left anterior thoracotomy is the approach of choice in all patients except those with chronic constrictive pericarditis. The usual duration of pericardiectomy is 1½ hours; a more extended period is required in patients with chronic constrictive calcific pericarditis. Transfusion generally is not necessary, although blood should always be available and three or four units may be given if cardiopulmonary bypass is performed.

USUAL POSTOPERATIVE COURSE

Expected postoperative hospital stay: The postoperative hospital stay ranges from 7 to 14 days, depending on the extent of altered cardiovascular dynamics.

Operative mortality: 1% to 5%

Special monitoring required: Patients receive intensive care for 2 or 3 days, with monitoring of cardiovascular signs, respiratory status, and urinary output. Close cardiac monitoring is required to detect arrhythmias, particularly atrial arrhythmias, which are common after pericardiectomy. Most patients are given digitalis if they are not already taking it.

Patient activity and positioning: Patients remain flat in bed for the first 24 hours then are mobilized to a sitting position and assisted out of bed 24 hours later.

Alimentation: Liquids are allowed the morning after operation, and food intake is advanced to a regular diet as rapidly as possible.

Antibiotic coverage: Broad-spectrum antibiotics are begun before operation and continued for 1 week afterward. Cephalosporin is the antibiotic of choice.

Pulmonary care: Patients are given mask oxygen for the first 48 hours after operation to assist oxygenation. Serial monitoring of arterial blood gases and close observation of the pulmonary status are vital. Daily chest radiographs are required until all chest tubes have been removed and again on the day before discharge from the hospital.

Thoracotomy tubes: Two chest tubes are left in place until significant drainage has ceased. This generally requires 4 days. The chest tubes are connected by water seal to 20 cm H_2O suction.

POSTOPERATIVE COMPLICATIONS

IN THE HOSPITAL

Congestive heart failure: Congestive heart failure occurs in about 30% to 35% of patients who have chronic constrictive pericarditis. After release of the pericardium, the heart is unable to pump adequately all the blood returning to it, and patients may develop significant heart failure. This generally requires 6 weeks to 2 months to abate and must be carefully treated with digitalis preparations, diuretics, and a salt-restricted diet.

Arrhythmias: Arrhythmias occur in 15% to 20% of patients and generally consist of atrial tachycardia, atrial flutter, or atrial fibrillation. Management is by digitalization.

Infection: Significant infection develops in 1% to 3% of patients. It occurs most often in patients who are unusually susceptible to superinfection because of immunosuppression, malignancy, or azotemia.

Postpericardiotomy syndrome: Postpericardiotomy syndrome is reported in 15% to 20% of patients. It is recognized by a pericardial friction rub, fever, and precordial chest pain radiating into the neck and back. Initial treatment is with salicylates or indomethacin; steroids may be required. The syndrome is usually short-lived, but symptoms may be prolonged in rare patients.

Bleeding: Bleeding after pericardiectomy is uncommon except in uremic patients who may have altered clotting mechanisms. In these cases, appropriate blood products should be available for postoperative administration.

AFTER DISCHARGE

Arrhythmia: Patients with chronic arrhythmia problems should be followed up at frequent intervals with electrocardiograms.

Persistent pericarditis: Patients with persistent pericarditis after pericardiectomy should be observed closely and treated with salicylates and steroids, if indicated. Occasionally, steroid therapy must be maintained for an extended course and tapered gradually.

BIBLIOGRAPHY

Churchill ED. Pericardial resection in chronic constrictive pericarditis. Ann Surg 1936;104:516–529.

Engle MA, McCabe JC, Ebert PA, Zabriskie J. The post-pericardiotomy syndrome and antiheart antibodies. Circulation 1974;49:401–406.

Franco KL, Breckenridge I, Hammond GL. The pericardium. In: Baue AE, Geha AS, Hammond GL, et al, eds. Glenn's thoracic and cardiovascular surgery, ed 5, vol 2. Norwalk, CT, Appleton & Lange, 1991:1985.

Kloster FE, Crislip RL, Bristow JD, et al. Hemodynamic studies following pericardiectomy for constrictive pericarditis. Circulation 1965;32:415–424.

Miller JI, Mansour KA, Hatcher CR Jr. Pericardiectomy: current indications, concepts, and results in a university center. Ann Thorac Surg 1982;34:40–45.

Medical Management of the Surgical Patient, Third Edition,
edited by Michael F. Lubin, H. Kenneth Walker, and Robert B. Smith III.
J.B. Lippincott Company, Philadelphia, PA © 1995.

PULMONARY LOBECTOMY

Joseph I. Miller, Jr.

Pulmonary lobectomy is most often performed for benign and malignant neoplasms of the lung. It may also be required for pulmonary tuberculosis, refractory lung abscess, residual bronchiectasis, pulmonary sequestration, and other infectious processes.

General anesthesia is administered through an indwelling double-lumen endotracheal tube, such as a Carlens or Robertshaw tube. In general, the operation does not require blood transfusion, although blood should always be available in case technical problems arise. Patients are usually placed in the lateral decubitus position with the operated side superior. The main operative steps after thoracotomy incision consist of control of the arterial supply and venous drainage of the respective lobe, followed by dissection of the fissures and division of the bronchus. The operation takes 1½ to 2 hours for a lower lobectomy and 2 to 2½ hours for an upper lobectomy. The procedure is generally well tolerated and is not a major surgical stress if patients have few associated medical problems and adequate pulmonary function.

USUAL POSTOPERATIVE COURSE

Expected postoperative hospital stay: Patients remain in the hospital for 8 to 10 days, depending on their general condition and the degree of postoperative air leak.

Operative mortality: The operative mortality rate is 1% to 3% for elective surgery and 15% to 25% for emergency intervention.

Special monitoring required: Intensive care unit observation is required for 1 or 2 days to allow careful monitoring of vital signs, chest tube drainage, arterial blood pressure, urinary output, renal function, and ventilatory status.

Patient activity and positioning: Patients generally remain in the semi-Fowler position for the first 24 hours and may sit on the side of the bed the morning after operation. They are allowed to move to a chair at 24 hours and to begin ambulation at 48 hours.

Alimentation: Clear liquids are given the morning after operation, and food intake is advanced to a regular diet as rapidly as tolerated.

Antibiotic coverage: Routine prophylactic antibiotics of the cephalosporin group are given before operation and continued for a minimum of 1 week afterward or until all chest tubes have been removed.

Thoracotomy tubes: Chest tubes are connected to wall suction at 20 cm H_2O until all air leaks have ceased, generally within 4 to 7 days. In patients with infectious processes and those whose procedures involved technical difficulty, air leaks may persist for a longer period. Once they have all sealed, the chest tubes are placed on underwater seal drainage and disconnected from suction. When there has been no leak for 24 hours, the chest tubes are removed on successive days, with the lower tube pulled first and the upper tube pulled second.

Pulmonary care: Chest physical therapy, ultrasonic nebulization, and incentive spirometry are begun on the day of operation and continued four times a day until patients have recovered satisfactorily.

Postoperative radiographs: Daily portable upright chest radiographs are obtained to observe lung reexpansion.

POSTOPERATIVE COMPLICATIONS

IN THE HOSPITAL

Arrhythmia: The arrhythmias most frequently encountered are atrial tachycardia, atrial flutter, and atrial fibrillation. They occur in 5% to 15% of patients and usually are recognized by a decrease in blood pressure or are noted on electrocardiographic monitoring in the intensive care unit.

Intrapleural space: A persistent intrapleural space may exist after lobectomy in 5% to 15% of patients. The space results from technical problems or from disease in the residual lung that prevents it from filling the adjacent pleural cavity. In general, these cavities rarely become infected or cause major difficulties.

Prolonged air leak: Prolonged air leak occurs in 3% to 7% of patients and is defined as any air leak that persists longer than 2 weeks. It is detected by the bubbling of air through the underwater sealed chamber and is managed by continued chest tube suction.

Empyema: Pleural empyema develops in 1% to 3% of patients who undergo lobectomy. It is generally managed by closed chest tube thoracostomy or open rib resection. Appropriate antibiotic therapy is administered based on culture and sensitivity reports.

Bronchopleural fistula: About 3% of patients have a bronchopleural fistula. It generally becomes evident 7 to 14 days after resection and is manifested by fever, cough, and an increasing air leak. Therapy consists of closed chest tube thoracostomy or open rib resection, followed later by a definitive procedure.

Pulmonary embolism: Only 1% of patients have a postoperative pulmonary embolus. Preventive measures include antiembolism stockings perioperatively and early mobilization postoperatively. All patients undergoing open thoracotomy are treated with minidose heparin unless this is contraindicated.

Bleeding: Under 1% of patients experience major postoperative bleeding. It is usually evident from excessive drainage through the chest tubes and the source generally can be traced to injury of an intercostal artery or other blood vessel that bleeds again after surgery. Proper therapy includes transfusion and reoperation to achieve hemostasis, if necessary. Reoperation is generally indicated if the blood loss amounts to 300 mL/h for 2 successive hours.

AFTER DISCHARGE

Arrhythmias: Arrhythmias generally are treated for a minimum of 3 months with the appropriate cardiac medications.

Intrapleural space: An intrapleural space should be observed by serial chest radiographs at monthly intervals for the first 6 months.

Bronchopleural fistula: After patients are stable, bronchopleural fistulas can be tracked on an outpatient basis with serial chest radiographs, volume determination of the size of the cavity, appropriate sinograms, and subsequent definitive operation.

BIBLIOGRAPHY

Dart CH Jr, Scott SM, Takaro T. Six-year clinical experience using automatic stapling devices for lung resections. Ann Thorac Surg 1970;9:535–550.

Kirsh MM, Rotman H, Behrendt DM, et al. Complications of pulmonary resection. Ann Thorac Surg 1975;20:215–236.

Meade RH. A history of thoracic surgery. Springfield, IL, Charles C Thomas, 1961.

Scannell JG. Pulmonary resection: anatomy and techniques. In: Baue AE, Geha AS, Hammond GL, et al, eds. Glenn's thoracic and cardiovascular surgery, ed 5, vol 1. Norwalk, CT, Appleton & Lange, 1991:109.

Medical Management of the Surgical Patient, Third Edition,
edited by Michael F. Lubin, H. Kenneth Walker, and Robert B. Smith III.
J.B. Lippincott Company, Philadelphia, PA © 1995.

PNEUMONECTOMY

Joseph I. Miller, Jr.

The chief indication for pneumonectomy is the presence of a pulmonary neoplasm that involves structures rendering pulmonary lobectomy unfeasible. On rare occasions, pneumonectomy may be indicated for benign conditions, such as residual problems with pulmonary tuberculosis, lung trauma, or complications of a pulmonary lobectomy.

General endotracheal anesthesia is administered with the aid of an indwelling double-lumen tube, such as a Carlens or Robertshaw tube, to ensure proper inflation of the dependent lung and to protect it from blood or secretions draining down from the operated bronchus. Patients are placed in the lateral decubitus position. The procedure takes 1½ to 2 hours. Blood transfusion is rarely required in elective pneumonectomy, but blood should always be available. The main operative steps consist of control of the pulmonary artery and superior and inferior pulmonary veins, and secure closure of the bronchial stump. Pneumonectomy carries a high level of surgical stress and should only be performed in patients who have been demonstrated to have sufficient pulmonary reserve to tolerate the procedure. Results of preoperative pulmonary function tests, therefore, comprise the main patient selection criteria for elective resection. In addition, the cardiac status should be evaluated before operation using an exercise treadmill or thallium scan.

USUAL POSTOPERATIVE COURSE

Expected postoperative hospital stay: 10 to 14 days

Operative mortality: 5% to 15%

Special monitoring required: Patients remain in the intensive care unit for 2 or 3 days to allow close monitoring for arrhythmias, pulmonary reserve, urinary output, and other vital functions. Blood gases are assessed daily or more often, if necessary, to monitor the respiratory status.

Patient activity and positioning: The semi-Fowler position is maintained for the first 24 hours and patients are not allowed to turn onto their operated sides. They are permitted to sit on the side of the bed the morning after operation and are moved to a chair 1 day later. Ambulation is begun the next day.

Alimentation: Oral intake is prohibited for 3 days because division of the vagal trunks frequently produces gastric retention. Patients are allowed to consume liquids after 72 hours, and food intake is rapidly advanced to a regular diet.

Antibiotic coverage: Broad-spectrum antibiotics of the cephalosporin group are given 12 hours before resection and continued for 7 to 10 days afterward.

Gastric decompression: An indwelling nasogastric tube is kept in place for 3 days to allow the postoperative gastric atony to resolve.

Postoperative radiographs: Portable upright chest radiographs are obtained regularly to monitor the filling of the pulmonary cavity, a process that generally requires 6 weeks. The hemogram is checked every other day for about 10 days to assess the hematologic response.

Thoracotomy tube: If a chest tube has been left in place connected to a clamped underwater seal bottle, it is removed within 48 hours after the procedure. Some surgeons prefer to remove the tube in the operating room after stabilization of the mediastinum.

POSTOPERATIVE COMPLICATIONS

IN THE HOSPITAL

Arrhythmias: Atrial tachycardia, atrial flutter, or atrial fibrillation develops in 25% to 40% of patients as a result of increased vagal tone or hypoxia. All patients undergo routine prophylactic digitalization in the operating room when the decision is made to perform a pneumonectomy. Digitalis therapy is continued for a minimum of 6 months after surgery.

Empyema: Empyema generally occurs in 2% to 10% of patients in the early postoperative period, but it can develop several years after surgery. It is recognized by systemic signs of infection plus a change in the air–fluid level in the hemithorax or by the expectoration of brown, purulent material. Treatment of an empyema in the pneumonectomy space requires immediate tube thoracostomy drainage, followed by a subsequent Clagett procedure or thoracoplasty.

Bronchopleural fistula: A bronchopleural fistula develops in 3% of patients, generally between the 7th and 14th postoperative days, the weakest period of bronchial stump healing. It is manifested by fever, cough, drainage, or an air leak. Treatment consists of immediate tube thoracostomy, followed by subsequent irrigation of the space with antibiotics and the performance of a delayed closure with muscle flaps.

Cardiac herniation: Cardiac herniation is a rare complication but one that carries greater than 50% mortality. It can be prevented by adequate closure of the pericardium after intrapericardial pneumonectomy.

Bleeding: Under 1% of patients who undergo pneumonectomy experience postoperative bleeding sufficient to require either immediate reexploration for control or subsequent evacuation of the pleural space. After operation, hemorrhage is recognized by immediate filling of the operated hemithorax and rapid deterioration of the vital signs.

Tension pneumothorax: Tension pneumothorax occurs in under 1% of patients and results from a bronchial leak. It is recognized by a shift of the mediastinum accompanied by acute worsening of the respiratory status. Treatment consists of immediate tube thoracostomy of the involved thorax.

AFTER DISCHARGE

Empyema or bronchopleural fistula: Although empyema and bronchopleural fistulas usually develop in the hospital, they can arise months to years after surgery. They are manifested by systemic signs of toxemia, fever, and cough, and are diagnosed by a chest radiograph that shows a decrease in the level of fluid in the chest or the presence of an air–fluid level. Treatment consists of immediate tube thoracostomy with subsequent definitive repair.

Arrhythmias: Arrhythmias may persist after hospital discharge but generally respond to appropriate digitalis glycoside therapy.

Respiratory insufficiency: Respiratory insufficiency may be observed in patients with borderline pulmonary reserve after resection. These patients may remain severely dyspneic and be unable to function at previous levels of exercise tolerance if borderline function was present before operation.

BIBLIOGRAPHY

Dart CH Jr, Scott SM, Takaro T. Six-year clinical experience using automatic stapling devices for lung resections. Ann Thorac Surg 1970;9:535–550.

Kirsh MM, Rotman H, Behrendt DM, et al. Complications of pulmonary resection. Ann Thorac Surg 1975;20:215–236.

Meade RH. A history of thoracic surgery. Springfield, IL, Charles C Thomas, 1961.

Scannell JG. Pulmonary resection: anatomy and techniques. In: Baue AE, Geha AS, Hammond GL, et al, eds. Glenn's thoracic and cardiovascular surgery, ed 5, vol 1. Norwalk, CT, Appleton & Lange, 1991:111.

Medical Management of the Surgical Patient, Third Edition,
edited by Michael F. Lubin, H. Kenneth Walker, and Robert B. Smith III.
J.B. Lippincott Company, Philadelphia, PA © 1995.

CHAPTER

HIATAL HERNIA REPAIR

87

Kamal A. Mansour

Indications for surgical repair of hiatal hernia include (1) failure of strict medical management (intractability); (2) reflux esophagitis with ulcerations, stricture, or bleeding; (3) recurrent aspiration pneumonia; (4) large sliding hernias; and (5) all paraesophageal hernias. The purpose of surgery is not just to reposition the stomach below the diaphragm but to reestablish gastroesophageal competence. Two approaches (transabdominal and transthoracic) and three primary techniques (Belsey, Hill, and Nissen) are used, depending on the preference of the surgeon. If the procedure is performed well, the magnitude of surgical stress is low. General endotracheal anesthesia is used most often and the operative time is 2 or 3 hours. Intraoperative blood transfusions are rarely required.

USUAL POSTOPERATIVE COURSE

Expected postoperative hospital stay: The postoperative hospital stay ranges from 7 to 10 days, depending on the age and associated medical problems of patients.

Operative mortality: Under 1%

Special monitoring required: Intraoperative assessment of the lower esophageal sphincteric zone is performed by pressure manometric studies.

Patient activity and positioning: If a transthoracic ap-

proach is used, a chest tube is inserted and should be removed in 24 hours, after which ambulation is allowed.

Alimentation: A nasogastric tube usually is left in place for the first 24 hours. Patients are then given clear liquids, and food intake is advanced to a soft diet, which is maintained until hospital discharge.

Antibiotic coverage: A broad-spectrum antibiotic, such as a cephalosporin, is given for 5 to 7 days after transthoracic repair or any procedure in which the gastrointestinal tract is entered.

Chest physiotherapy: Chest physiotherapy is stressed, especially when the transthoracic approach is used, to prevent pulmonary complications.

Barium swallow: A barium swallow is done on the seventh postoperative day to assess the status of the surgical repair and to provide a baseline study for follow-up.

POSTOPERATIVE COMPLICATIONS

IN THE HOSPITAL

Pulmonary complications: Pulmonary complications are caused by retained secretions.

Temporary dysphagia: Edema at the cardia may result in temporary dysphagia, which should improve with observation.

553

Rupture of the stomach: Rupture of the stomach has been reported in cases in which a Nissen fundoplication was left in the chest.

Ulceration: Some cases of bleeding peptic ulcer have occurred along the lesser curvature in association with a Nissen repair; their cause is not definitely known.

Splenic injury: Intraoperative splenic injury requiring splenorrhaphy or splenectomy is common in association with Nissen fundoplication.

AFTER DISCHARGE

Recurrence: Hernia recurrence is reported in 8% (Nissen) to 18% (Belsey) of patients after primary repair. In the presence of symptomatic, radiologic, and endoscopic evidence of recurrent gastroesophageal reflux, another surgical repair is indicated.

Gas-bloat syndrome: Gas-bloat syndrome occurs in 15% of patients after Nissen fundoplication and results from over-distention of the stomach that cannot be relieved by belching or vomiting. It may require repeated esophageal dilation or reoperation.

BIBLIOGRAPHY

Baue AE, Naunheim KS. Hiatal hernia and gastroesophageal reflux. In: Baue AE, Geha AS, Hammond GL, et al, eds. Glenn's thoracic and cardiovascular surgery, ed 5, vol 1. Norwalk, CT, Appleton & Lange, 1991:683.

DeMeester TR, Johnson LF, Kent AH. Evaluation of current operations for the prevention of gastroesophageal reflux. Am Surg 1974;180:511–525.

Mansour KA, Burton HG, Miller JI Jr, Hatcher CR Jr. Complications of intrathoracic Nissen fundoplication. Ann Thorac Surg 1981;32:173–178.

Skinner DB, Belsey RH. Surgical management of esophageal reflux and hiatus hernia: long-term results with 1030 patients. J Thorac Cardiovasc Surg 1967;53:33–54.

Medical Management of the Surgical Patient, Third Edition,
edited by Michael F. Lubin, H. Kenneth Walker, and Robert B. Smith III.
J.B. Lippincott Company, Philadelphia, PA © 1995.

CHAPTER

ESOPHAGOGASTRECTOMY

88

Kamal A. Mansour

Esophagogastrectomy is usually performed for carcinoma of the esophagus, particularly of the middle and lower thirds. Less common indications for this procedure are nondilatable stricture of the distal esophagus that must be managed by resection and rupture of the esophagus that cannot be repaired.

Two separate incisions are usually used: abdominal and right thoracic. A left thoracotomy or left thoracoabdominal incision may be used for carcinoma of the distal esophagus and the gastroesophageal junction. To mobilize the stomach, the left gastroepiploic and left gastric arteries are sacrificed, and the blood supply through the right gastroepiploic and right gastric arteries is preserved. The distal line of resection in the proximal stomach is securely closed and an esophagogastric anastomosis is performed on the anterior surface of the stomach below the line of resection. Surgical stress is great and the procedure carries relatively high morbidity and mortality. Anesthesia is usually endotracheal, using a double-lumen tube to allow the lung on the side of the operation to remain collapsed. The procedure takes 4 to 6 hours and requires 2 to 4 units of blood.

USUAL POSTOPERATIVE COURSE

Expected postoperative hospital stay: 2 weeks

Operative mortality rate: The operative mortality rate varies from 10% to 25%, depending on the experience of the surgeon and the condition of the patient.

Special monitoring required: Patients are observed in the intensive care unit with central venous pressure recordings, cardiac monitoring, and arterial lines.

Patient activity and positioning: Patients may ambulate 24 to 48 hours after operation. While they are in bed, patients should be placed in the head-up position to prevent gastric or bile reflux.

Alimentation: Patients are fed intravenously for the first week and a nasogastric tube is connected to gravity drainage. On about the eighth postoperative day, a barium swallow is obtained. If the anastomosis is satisfactory, oral feedings may be permitted.

Antibiotic coverage: Broad-spectrum antibiotics are administered for 1 week.

Chest tube management: The chest tube is removed as soon as drainage is minimal and the chest radiograph is satisfactory. It should not be left longer in case a leak occurs at the anastomosis.

POSTOPERATIVE COMPLICATIONS

IN THE HOSPITAL

Anastomotic leak: An anastomotic leak should be suspected if patients have undue pain or fever, or if a pleural erosion develops. This must be confirmed immediately by radiopaque contrast medium or barium swallow. If the leak is contained and drains back into the gastrointestinal tract, it may be observed; otherwise, immediate external drainage is indicated.

Gastric slough resulting from a vascular accident: Gastric slough may be fatal if the diagnosis is missed. Persistent tachycardia and a progressively rising white blood cell count are suggestive. In addition, the persistence of a foul or old blood-stained aspirate in the nasogastric tube after 48 hours may be an early sign of gastric necrosis. Prompt reoperation is mandatory.

AFTER DISCHARGE

Dysphagia: Dysphagia is caused by stricture at the anastomotic site and may require repeated transesophageal dilation.

BIBLIOGRAPHY

Adams WE, Phemister DB. Carcinoma of the lower thoracic esophagus: report of a successful resection and esophagogastrostomy. J Thorac Surg 1938;7:621–632.

Mansour KA, Downey RS. Esophageal carcinoma: surgery without preoperative adjuvant chemotherapy. Ann Thorac Surg 1989; 48:201–205.

Sweet RH. Transthoracic resection of the esophagus and stomach for carcinoma: analysis of the postoperative complications, causes of death and late results of operation. Ann Surg 1945;121: 272–284.

Medical Management of the Surgical Patient, Third Edition,
edited by Michael F. Lubin, H. Kenneth Walker, and Robert B. Smith III.
J.B. Lippincott Company, Philadelphia, PA © 1995.

COLON INTERPOSITION FOR ESOPHAGEAL BYPASS

Kamal A. Mansour

Indications for colon replacement of the esophagus include (1) gastroesophageal malignancy, (2) benign nondilatable distal esophageal strictures caused by reflux esophagitis, (3) extensive chemical strictures, (4) benign tumors of the esophagus that are extensive or multiple and are not amenable to simpler measures, (5) congenital atresia of the esophagus for which a primary anastomosis is impossible or impractical, (6) rare cases of achalasia in which Heller myotomy fails or is complicated by malignancy, (7) bleeding varices for which shunting fails or stricture formation follows disconnection operation, and (8) rupture of the esophagus for which conservative repair fails or is impossible.

The right or left colon may be used, based on the right or left branch of the middle colic artery. The prepared colonic segment is passed through a retrosternal tunnel or brought into the posterior mediastinum through the right or left pleural cavity, depending on the surgeon's preference. Regardless of the approach used, the procedure is of great magnitude and is associated with relatively high mortality. A general endotracheal anesthetic is administered and the procedure usually takes 4 to 6 hours. Two to four units of blood are frequently required. Intensive preoperative preparation, including correction of fluid, caloric, and protein deficiencies, substantially improves outcome, particularly for elderly or debilitated patients. Careful mechanical and chemical bowel preparation is also required.

USUAL POSTOPERATIVE COURSE

Expected postoperative hospital stay: About 2 weeks

Operative mortality: The operative mortality rate is about 12%, depending on the age and condition of the patient and the vascularity of the interposed colonic segment.

Special monitoring required: Standard thoracotomy intensive care is provided for the first 2 or 3 days, including daily chest radiographs, electrolyte and arterial blood gas determinations, urinary output monitoring, and central venous pressure measurement.

Patient activity and positioning: Patients are ambulatory 24 to 48 hours after operation.

Alimentation: A nasogastric tube is left in the interposed colon and a feeding jejunostomy or gastrostomy is performed at operation. Patients are supported by intravenous fluids for the first 2 to 4 days until bowel sounds are audible, at which time tube feedings are provided. On the 9th or 10th day, a barium swallow is performed to assess the colonic implant for any evidence of leakage. If the reconstruction is intact, patients are allowed oral liquid feedings, and food intake is progressively advanced to a regular diet over several days.

Antibiotic coverage: A cephalosporin is given for 7 to 10 days and modified as indicated.

557

Physiotherapy: Chest physical therapy and vigorous pulmonary toilet are indicated.

POSTOPERATIVE COMPLICATIONS

IN THE HOSPITAL

Pulmonary complications: Pulmonary complications are frequently relatively minor but may become life-threatening in elderly patients or those with poor respiratory reserve.

Colonic necrosis: Massive necrosis of the colon must be diagnosed early and the involved bowel removed before patients become moribund. The nasocolonic tube aspirate is carefully observed for its color and odor; foul or old blood-stained fluid continuing after 48 hours may be the earliest sign of bowel necrosis.

Minor leaks at the cervical anastomosis: Minor leaks at the cervical anastomosis occur with some regularity but usually resolve with simple drainage. A prolonged delay in oral feeding may be necessary. Patients may require a feeding gastrostomy or, ideally, a feeding jejunostomy.

AFTER DISCHARGE

Fibrous stricture of the cologastric anastomosis: Fibrous stricture of the cologastric anastomosis may require dilation or surgical revision.

Gastric ulceration: Gastric ulceration usually occurs just proximal to the cologastric anastomosis on the lesser curvature. Medical therapy generally suffices but vagotomy and drainage may become necessary.

Redundancy of the colon above the diaphragm: Colonic stasis and a prolonged transit time may result from redundancy of the colon above the diaphragm. If the condition is severe, surgical revision may be required.

BIBLIOGRAPHY

Little AG. Esophageal chemical burns, foreign bodies, and bleeding. In: Baue AE, Geha AS, Hammond GL, et al, eds. Glenn's thoracic and cardiovascular surgery, ed 5, vol 1. Norwalk, CT, Appleton & Lange, 1991:679.

Mansour KA, Hansen HA II, Hersh T, et al. Colon interposition for advanced nonmalignant esophageal stricture. Ann Thorac Surg 1981;32:584–591.

Postlethwait RW, Sealy WC, Dillon ML, Young WG. Colon interposition for esophageal substitution. Ann Thorac Surg 1971;12:89–108.

Robertson CS, Howe CS, Smithwick RH. Use of colon to replace lower esophagus in man: report of case three and one-half years after operation. Proceedings of forum sessions, 38th Clinical Congress of American College of Surgeons. Philadelphia, WB Saunders, 1952:66.

SECTION

XX

PLASTIC AND RECONSTRUCTIVE SURGERY

Medical Management of the Surgical Patient, Third Edition,
edited by Michael F. Lubin, H. Kenneth Walker, and Robert B. Smith III.
J.B. Lippincott Company, Philadelphia, PA © 1995.

FACELIFT

CHAPTER

90

Travis C. Holcombe
M.J. Jurkiewicz

The facelift procedure is generally performed on an outpatient basis, but patients may be hospitalized overnight. It is done most commonly for the aging face but can be performed as part of facial reconstruction after tumor excision, burn scarring, or facial paralysis. The procedure involves periauricular or scalp incision, elevation of the soft tissues of the face and neck, pulling of these structures taut, and excision of the excess tissue. It is usually done under local anesthesia with sedation, although general anesthesia may be preferred for selected patients. The procedure commonly lasts 2 or 3 hours and does not require blood transfusion.

USUAL POSTOPERATIVE COURSE

Expected postoperative hospital stay: Most patients go home the same evening or the next day.

Operative mortality: Under 1%

Special monitoring required: None

Patient activity and positioning: Elevation of the head of the bed is important. Most patients are given pressure garments to wear, at least at night, for a month. Patients are discouraged from vigorous activity for 2 to 3 weeks. All these measures are prescribed to reduce swelling and hematoma formation.

Alimentation: A full liquid diet is provided the first night, and food intake is advanced to a regular diet by the next day.

Antibiotic coverage: No routine antibiotic coverage is required.

POSTOPERATIVE COMPLICATIONS

IN THE HOSPITAL

Hematoma: Hematoma occurs in 1% to 8% of patients. Closed suction drains may be placed at the time of operation to reduce this possibility and are removed the next day. If significant hematoma occurs, part of the incision can be opened and the hematoma evacuated without long-term effect.

AFTER DISCHARGE

Swelling and bruising: Facial swelling and bruising can persist for 2 to 3 weeks. This is bothersome to patients but is usually not a functional problem.

Nerve paralysis: Permanent facial nerve paralysis may result from accidental nerve injury but is extremely rare (under 1%).

Skin slough: Skin slough occurs in roughly 4% of patients, generally along the incision lines, and usually heals uneventfully.

BIBLIOGRAPHY

Barton FE. The aging face: rhytidectomy and adjunctive procedures (overview). Select Read Plastic Surg 1991;6:21.

Georgiade GS, Georgiade NG, Riefkohl R, et al, eds. Textbook of plastic, maxillofacial and reconstructive surgery. Baltimore, Williams & Wilkins, 1992:627–630.

Lemmon ML, Hamra ST. Skoog rhytidectomy: a five year experience with 577 patients. Plast Reconstr Surg 1980;65:283–297.

Medical Management of the Surgical Patient, Third Edition,
edited by Michael F. Lubin, H. Kenneth Walker, and Robert B. Smith III.
J.B. Lippincott Company, Philadelphia, PA © 1995.

CHAPTER

91

AUTOLOGOUS BREAST RECONSTRUCTION FOLLOWING MASTECTOMY

Travis C. Holcombe
M.J. Jurkiewicz

Using abdominal tissue to perform immediate breast reconstruction after mastectomy has become a widely accepted technique. This procedure is indicated for patients with adequate abdominal tissue and few abdominal scars who are in relatively good health. After the mastectomy, a football-shaped incision is made in the lower abdomen to include skin fat and one or both rectus abdominis muscles in the flap (TRAM flap). The recti muscles, supplied by either the superior or inferior epigastric blood supply, maintain viability of the fat and skin. The flap can be brought up still attached to the trunk ("pedicled"), or it can be detached from the trunk and a microvascular anastomosis performed to the axillary vessels ("free"). This is an extensive operation, lasting 5 to 7 hours, including the mastectomy, and 2 or 3 hours longer if the free flap technique is used. General anesthesia is used and blood transfusion is usually required. Numerous closed suction drains are placed to drain excess fluid for about 1 week.

USUAL POSTOPERATIVE COURSE

Expected postoperative hospital stay: 5 to 10 days
Operative mortality: Under 1%
Special monitoring: Great attention must be paid to flap viability after the procedure, especially if the free flap technique is used. In this situation, the flap is checked hourly for 72 hours for warmth, color, and capillary refill.

Patient activity and positioning: The length of the abdominal wall soft tissue is decreased by 50% in this operation, similar to the "tummy tuck" procedure. To allow closure of the abdomen, patients are placed in a back-up, knee-up position; the bed is kept in this position throughout the hospital stay. Patients are out of bed by the first postoperative day and ambulating by the second.

Alimentation: Most patients have some degree of ileus but tolerate a liquid diet by the second day, and food intake is advanced to a regular diet by the fourth day.

Antibiotic coverage: A first-generation cephalosporin is administered perioperatively for 24 to 48 hours.

POSTOPERATIVE COMPLICATIONS

IN THE HOSPITAL

Volume depletion: Because of the extensive dissection performed during this procedure, postoperative fluid needs can be great and monitoring must be compulsive. This is assisted by Foley catheterization for 24 to 48 hours.

Total flap failure: Total flap failure occurs rarely (under 2%) but requires monitoring as described earlier.

Pulmonary embolus: Pulmonary embolus also is rare, but patients are routinely placed in intermittent pneumatic compression garments before operation and this therapy is continued until they are ambulating freely.

AFTER DISCHARGE

Abdominal hernia: Abdominal hernia occurs in 2% to 10% of patients because of the tissue harvest from the abdomen. This generally does not cause an acute problem but may require subsequent repair.

Reconstruction: Nipple and areolar reconstruction is generally performed 6 months after the initial surgery.

BIBLIOGRAPHY

Bostwick J. Plastic and reconstructive breast surgery. St Louis, Quality Medical, 1990:800–882.

Hartrampf CR. The transverse abdominal island flap for breast reconstruction. Clin Plast Surg 1988;15:703–714.

Hartrampf CR, Anton MA, Trimble Bried J. Breast reconstruction with the transverse abdominal island (TRAM) flap. In: Georgiade GS, Georgiade NG, Riefkohl R, et al, eds. Textbook of plastic, maxillofacial and reconstructive surgery. Baltimore, Williams & Wilkins, 1992:851–864.

Medical Management of the Surgical Patient, Third Edition,
edited by Michael F. Lubin, H. Kenneth Walker, and Robert B. Smith III.
J.B. Lippincott Company, Philadelphia, PA © 1995.

REPAIR OF FACIAL FRACTURES

Travis C. Holcombe
M.J. Jurkiewicz

Facial fractures are a common problem in this age of frequent motor vehicle accidents. They often occur in patients with multiple injuries and demand a team approach. Repair of facial fractures is indicated to restore appearance or function, usually related to mastication or vision. The operation entails exposing the fractures (usually through multiple intraoral and extraoral incisions), reducing the fractures, and establishing firm fixation. Plates are the most commonly used fixation devices. Intermaxillary fixation is often used and requires that the jaws remain wired closed. The procedure is performed under general anesthesia. Its duration varies from 1 to 8 hours based on the number and location of the fractures. Blood transfusion is usually not needed.

USUAL POSTOPERATIVE COURSE

Expected postoperative hospital stay: The expected postoperative hospital stay is 2 to 5 days if facial fractures are the only injuries.

Operative mortality: 1% to 2%

Special monitoring required: If the facial fractures are severe (particularly if there are posterior intraoral injuries), intubation may be necessary for 48 to 72 hours until swelling is reduced and the airway is safe.

Patient activity and positioning: Elevating the head of the bed is important to reduce facial swelling for the first week. Patients are encouraged to get out of bed on the first postoperative day. Frequently, periorbital swelling can be so great that vision is temporarily limited, and patients require close nursing care.

Alimentation: Patients with mandibular fractures need pureed diets. Most other patients with facial fractures are most comfortable with soft diets for the first few days.

Antibiotic coverage: Both gram-positive and anaerobic antibiotic coverage should be provided in the form of a first-generation cephalosporin and metronidazole for 24 to 72 hours.

POSTOPERATIVE COMPLICATIONS

IN THE HOSPITAL

Aspiration after vomiting: Aspiration can occur if patients vomit while their jaws are wired together. It is imperative that suction be readily available to patients throughout the hospital stay. Wire cutters also must be kept at the bedside to permit rapid release of the wires and opening of the mouth in the event emergency access to the airway is needed.

Facial swelling: Facial swelling can be intense and bothersome to patients but usually does not create a functional problem. The swelling is generally maximal between 24 and 48 hours after surgery and resolves over 1 to 2 weeks.

Blindness: Blindness is extremely rare after periorbital fracture repair, but the vision is always checked immediately after surgery because a retrobulbar hematoma can be evacuated and vision preserved if the condition is diagnosed quickly.

AFTER DISCHARGE

Cosmetic sequelae: Malocclusion, facial scarring, and severe residual disfigurement can occur but are unusual.

BIBLIOGRAPHY

Gwynn PP, Carraway JH, Horton CE, et al. Facial fractures: associated injuries and complications. Plast Reconstr Surg 1971;47:225–230.

Rohrich RJ, Sinn DP. Facial fractures II: lower third. Select Read Plastic Surg 1991;6.

Medical Management of the Surgical Patient, Third Edition,
edited by Michael F. Lubin, H. Kenneth Walker, and Robert B. Smith III.
J.B. Lippincott Company, Philadelphia, PA © 1995.

CHAPTER

FLAP COVERAGE FOR PRESSURE SORES

93

Travis C. Holcombe
M.J. Jurkiewicz

Pressure sores are a common problem in paralyzed or debilitated patients. The surgical indication for treatment of a pressure sore is a wound that is completely through the skin and will not readily close on its own. Reconstruction should be performed only in patients who will be able to avoid placing pressure on these points in the future; otherwise, the problem will quickly recur. Thus, only a few of the many patients with pressure sores are appropriate candidates for reconstruction.

Pressure sores must be completely free of infection and patients must be well nourished before repair. In many instances, patients require hospital admission well in advance of surgery for aggressive wound care and hyperalimentation. Once both the patient and the wound are ready, the operation is performed. General anesthesia is used to prevent a sympathetic response, even in paralyzed patients. In most cases, a nearby flap of soft tissue is turned into the débrided wound. Suction drains usually are placed underneath the flaps to remove excess fluid. Most pressure sore procedures last 1 to 3 hours and blood transfusion usually is not needed.

USUAL POSTOPERATIVE COURSE

Expected postoperative hospital stay: 14 to 28 days

Operative mortality: The operative mortality rate is under 5%. The rare deaths that occur usually are related to the poor general condition of the patients rather than the magnitude of the operation itself.

Special monitoring required: No special monitoring is required.

Patient activity and positioning: Patients are placed in a low-pressure or no-pressure bed for 7 days and are kept on bed rest for a total of 3 weeks without allowing pressure on their flap. They then are permitted to spend brief periods with pressure on the flap (15 minutes every 2 hours) for the next 2 to 3 months.

Alimentation: Fecal soiling of the flap may occur. The problem can be minimized by giving patients enemas 1 or 2 days before surgery and narcotics for 3 or 4 days afterward.

Antibiotic coverage: Only perioperative (24 to 48 hours) antibiotic coverage is provided, using a single broad-spectrum agent.

POSTOPERATIVE COMPLICATIONS

IN THE HOSPITAL

Wound infection: Wound infection occurs in 10% to 20% of patients. Prompt diagnosis depends on the recognition of erythema, persistent spiking fever, or purulent drainage from the wound. Early drainage and broad-spectrum antibiotics minimize systemic effects.

Partial flap loss or dehiscence: Partial flap loss or dehiscence is seen in 10% to 20% of patients. This usually requires early débridement and further flap coverage or, more often, healing by secondary intention.

AFTER DISCHARGE

Recurrence of pressure sores: Recurrence of pressure sores is extremely common (40% to 70%) and can be prevented only by patient compliance or thorough nursing care.

BIBLIOGRAPHY

Colen SR. Pressure sores. In: McCarthy JG, ed. Plastic surgery, vol 6. Philadelphia, WB Saunders, 1990:3834—3835.

Disa JJ, Carlton JM, Goldberg NH. Efficacy of operative cure in pressure sore patients. Plast Reconstr Surg 1992;89:272–278.

Medical Management of the Surgical Patient, Third Edition,
edited by Michael F. Lubin, H. Kenneth Walker, and Robert B. Smith III.
J.B. Lippincott Company, Philadelphia, PA © 1995.

MUSCLE FLAP COVERAGE OF STERNAL WOUND INFECTIONS

Travis C. Holcombe
M.J. Jurkiewicz

Coronary artery bypass grafting is one of the most commonly performed surgical procedures. Wound infections involving the sternum and mediastinum are unusual but do occur and may be life-threatening. One of the most significant contributions that plastic surgery has made to modern medicine has been to greatly reduce the mortality from sternal wound infections by developing the muscle flap closure procedure. Once a sternal wound infection is diagnosed, patients are taken to the operating room, where the infected soft tissues are débrided. A muscle or omental flap is used to cover the sternum and the vital structures of the mediastinum. The chest skin usually can be closed over the flap. These patients can be extremely ill from their sepsis and may require vasopressors and prolonged intubation. Blood transfusion is often required, and the operation is performed under general anesthesia and usually lasts 2 or 3 hours.

USUAL POSTOPERATIVE COURSE

Expected postoperative hospital stay: 1 to 3 weeks

Operative mortality: Operative mortality rate is about 5%. Before the development of muscle flap procedures, mortality from sternal wound infections was 20% to 40%.

Special monitoring required: These patients are usually in an intensive care unit setting and often are intubated with a Swan-Ganz catheter in place.

Patient activity and positioning: Patients are mobilized out of bed as soon as they are hemodynamically stable.

Alimentation: If an abdominal muscle flap or omental flap is used, ileus may delay oral feeding for 2 to 4 days. These patients often are systemically ill to the point that they require hyperalimentation through intravenous or tube feedings.

Antibiotic coverage: Broad-spectrum antibiotic coverage based on Gram stain and culture results usually is continued for 1 to 2 weeks.

POSTOPERATIVE COMPLICATIONS

IN THE HOSPITAL

Respiratory insufficiency: Respiratory insufficiency often is associated with pulmonary sepsis or with the chest wall instability that results from resection of the sternum. Generally, the sternum is not wired back together. Respiratory insufficiency may require prolonged intubation, sometimes necessitating tracheotomy.

Wound problems: Infection and minor dehiscence occur in as many as 10% to 30% of patients but usually can be treated by opening a small part of the wound and providing frequent wet-to-dry dressing changes.

569

AFTER DISCHARGE

Hernias: Hernias can result from the use of abdominal muscle flaps and may be repaired on an elective basis. If a pectoralis muscle flap is used, physical therapy is important to maximize upper extremity function.

Recurrent sternal infection: Recurrence of sternal infection is unusual.

BIBLIOGRAPHY

Nahai F, Rand RP, Hester TR, et al. Primary treatment of the infected sternotomy wound with muscle flaps: a review of 211 consecutive cases. Plast Reconstr Surg 1989;84:434–441.

Stahl RS, Sando WC. Thorax and spine. In: Jurkiewicz MJ, Krizek TJ, Mathes SJ, Ariyan S, eds. Plastic surgery: principles and practice. St Louis, CV Mosby, 1990:1198–1199.

Medical Management of the Surgical Patient, Third Edition,
edited by Michael F. Lubin, H. Kenneth Walker, and Robert B. Smith III.
J.B. Lippincott Company, Philadelphia, PA © 1995.

CHAPTER

SKIN GRAFTING FOR BURNS

95

Travis C. Holcombe
M.J. Jurkiewicz

Skin grafting is a common procedure in the treatment of burn wounds. Wounds that require skin grafting include full-thickness (third-degree) burns, deep partial-thickness (second-degree) burns, and lesser burns that would leave a worse functional or aesthetic result if they were allowed to heal without grafting (eg, hand burns).

The operation usually consists of excising the burn area and covering the excised wound with a skin graft of variable thickness, usually harvested from the thigh. This can be a bloody procedure depending on the size of the burn, and blood transfusions are often needed. The operation generally lasts from 1 to 3 hours and is usually performed under general anesthesia.

USUAL POSTOPERATIVE COURSE

Expected postoperative hospital stay: One day of hospitalization generally can be expected for each percentage point of body area burned. Thus, patients with 25% total body surface area burns can be expected to stay in the hospital about 25 days. This varies greatly, however, according to the presence of coexisting conditions and the location of the burns.

Operative mortality: The operative mortality rate depends on the extent of the burn being treated.

Special monitoring required: For large burns or burns in infants or elderly patients, intensive care unit monitoring is generally advisable.

Patient activity and positioning: Extremities that have undergone skin grafting must be elevated for 5 to 10 days and patients should be kept at strict bed rest. Once the skin graft has become well adherent (usually about a week after the procedure), physical therapy is begun to restore full function. Compression garments reduce swelling and scar formation. Heat lamp therapy is provided to the skin graft donor site to encourage eschar formation, which is painless when dried and heals on its own in 2 to 3 weeks.

Alimentation: Oral alimentation usually is provided immediately after surgery.

Antibiotic coverage: Gram-positive antibiotic coverage generally is adequate unless patients have been hospitalized longer than 2 weeks. In such cases, antibiotics with a broader spectrum of activity are used.

POSTOPERATIVE COMPLICATIONS

IN THE HOSPITAL

Volume depletion: Volume depletion results from fluid losses that occur during the operation and afterward into the widely exposed, inflamed tissues. Close monitoring of the vital signs and hourly urine output is used to guide additional fluid therapy.

Hematoma: Elevation and compressive dressings minimize hematoma development.

Loss of graft: The skin graft can be lost because of motion, hematoma, or infection. If this occurs, the wounds should be treated with local débridement and silver sulfadiazine (Silvadene) wound care. Repeated grafting may be required.

AFTER DISCHARGE

Scarring: Hypertrophic scarring is a common problem. Pressure garments are worn for 6 months to 2 years in an effort to minimize these responses.

BIBLIOGRAPHY

Renz BM, Sherman R. The burn unit experience at Grady Memorial Hospital: 844 cases. J Burn Care Rehabil 1992;13:426–436.

Robson MC, Smith DJ. Thermal injuries. In: Jurkiewicz MJ, Krizek TJ, Mathes SJ, Ariyan S, eds. Plastic surgery: principles and practice. St Louis, CV Mosby, 1990:1383.

SECTION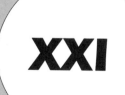

ORTHOPEDIC SURGERY

Medical Management of the Surgical Patient, Third Edition,
edited by Michael F. Lubin, H. Kenneth Walker, and Robert B. Smith III.
J.B. Lippincott Company, Philadelphia, PA © 1995.

CHAPTER

ARTHROSCOPIC SURGERY

96

Jack L. Siegel
Thomas P. Branch

The evolution of arthroscopy, originally called arthroendoscopy, has been dramatic. It is considered to be one of the greatest contributions to orthopedic surgery of the past 100 years. New surgical instrumentation and specialized training have allowed arthroscopic surgery to flourish, and increasing numbers of surgical techniques are being performed under arthroscopic control. Advances in the basic science of joint anatomy and function have led to this rapid evolution. Arthroscopy is both a diagnostic and a therapeutic modality, allowing orthopedic surgeons to document and treat intraarticular pathology using the least invasive treatment method. This approach results in improved patient care. Hospital stays are reduced or eliminated, and rehabilitation times are significantly shorter. Joint stabilization, articular surface procedures, meniscal repair or resection, meniscal transplantation, cruciate ligament reconstruction, joint débridement for infection and degenerative arthritis, and synovectomy can be accomplished using arthroscopic techniques.

All current imaging techniques—magnetic resonance imaging, arthrography, and ultrasound—are measured against joint arthroscopy. Its high accuracy rate affords optimal therapy. According to Dandy and Jackson, the diagnostic accuracy for intraarticular lesions should approach 98% in experienced hands. Clinical findings correlated with a detailed history can and should allow the orthopedic surgeon to proceed directly to arthroscopy for definitive ther-

apy. Some authors believe that magnetic resonance imaging will eliminate the need for diagnostic arthroscopy in acute knee injury. They believe the two procedures to be complementary, each providing definitive information not demonstrated by the other.

It has been clearly shown that degenerative changes in the knee are directly related to the amount of meniscus removed. Thus, the philosophy of meniscal repair has become widely accepted in practice and an overall success rate of over 90% has been documented by some authors. Patients with torn anterior cruciate ligaments and repairable medial menisci should undergo simultaneous ligament reconstruction and meniscal repair. Advances in meniscal transplantation date back to 1971 in association with allografts for tumor reconstruction. In 1981, isolated open meniscal allograft transplantation was carried out; in 1989, the first successful arthroscopic meniscal transplant was performed. Today, meniscal transplantation is continuing to evolve and generally is limited to knees and to grade 1 and 2 articular lesions.

Although the knee has been the joint most amenable to arthroscopic surgery, the use of arthroscopy has also been accepted for the diagnosis and treatment of the small joints (ie, the shoulder, elbow, wrist, and ankle). Shoulder arthroscopy dates back to 1930. Its diagnostic accuracy, as with the knee, is definitive. Several entities (eg, shoulder subluxation or partial rotator cuff tears) can be detected

575

only by arthroscopy even though clinical suspicion may be aroused by the history and physical examination. Surgical treatment using the arthroscope is currently limited to débridement of partial rotator cuff tears and symptomatic flap tears of the glenoid labrum, removal of loose bodies, and stabilization of the shoulder. Shoulder stabilization using arthroscopic techniques is successful only if a specific problem is encountered, such as a Bankart lesion or a bony separation of the anterior ligaments off the anterior glenoid lip.

Although arthroscopic techniques are gaining in popularity, their successful use requires a high level of expertise and surgical skill. There is no one best surgical–arthroscopic approach for a given joint. Strict adherence to principles of visual clarity, minimal trauma, and reliability with reproducibility must prevail. Anesthetic choices include local, regional, or general, each with its specific risks and benefits. Permanent documentation of surgical interaction has become paramount. Photographic techniques, video monitoring, and slide production eliminate doubt about the character of the pathology and surgical treatment, and promote a higher confidence level between surgeons and patients. Surgical drawings and computer data storage provide a scientific foundation for the education of patients and physicians in training. Laser disc imaging will soon replace present methods of documentation.

Obtaining the best possible results from arthroscopic surgery depends closely on patient cooperation with appropriate rehabilitation. Our knowledge of the behavior of grafted and repaired tissues is still incomplete, and many different protocols exist for postoperative rehabilitation designed to optimize cartilage and ligament healing. Biomechanical studies continue to provide information regarding the most reliable and swiftest means of returning patients to their preinjury states. Achieving consistently successful results from arthroscopic surgery depends on appropriate patient selection, sound surgical technique based on known biomechanical and healing principles, and vigilant rehabilitation.

USUAL POSTOPERATIVE COURSE

Expected postoperative hospital stay: Arthroscopic surgery is an outpatient procedure except for patients undergoing complex reconstruction or those with associated medical problems that necessitate admission to the hospital.

Operative mortality: Essentially 0%

Special monitoring required: No special monitoring is required.

Patient activity and positioning: Patients usually require mild narcotic analgesics, and ice wraps are used for 24 to 72 hours after surgery. Rehabilitation protocols are begun and vary according to the surgical procedures performed. Athletic activity is resumed when muscle control and proprioception have returned.

Alimentation: A regular diet is resumed after surgery.

Antibiotic coverage: Antibiotic coverage is provided according to surgeon preference; most administer 1 g of a first-generation cephalosporin before surgery. If hardware is inserted, patients should probably receive intravenous antibiotics for 24 to 48 hours after operation.

POSTOPERATIVE COMPLICATIONS

Joint effusion: a painfully tense effusion frequently develops during the first few postoperative days. It may be relieved by aspiration of the joint.

Thrombophlebitis or pulmonary embolism: Thrombophlebitis and pulmonary embolism are rare complications that are treated with anticoagulant therapy.

Infection: Although it is extremely uncommon, infection should be considered if erythema, excessive pain with motion, and fever are present.

Neurapraxia: Prolonged use of the pneumatic tourniquet may result in neurapraxia. It is managed by observation.

Vascular injury: Vascular injury is rare but may result in compartment syndrome or vascular compromise.

BIBLIOGRAPHY

Dandy DJ, Jackson RW. The impact of arthroscopy and the management of disorders of the knee. J Bone Joint Surg 1975;57B:346–348.

DeHaven KE. Peripheral meniscus repair: an alternative to meniscectomy. (Abstract) J Bone Joint Surg 1981;63B:463.

Delee JC. Complications of arthroscopy and arthroscopic surgery: results of a national survey. Arthroscopy 1985;1:204–220.

Jones RE, Smith EC, Reisch JS. Effects of medial meniscectomy in patients older than forty years. J Bone Joint Surg 1978;60A:783–786.

Noyes FR, Bassett RW, Grood ES, Butler DL. Arthroscopy in acute traumatic hemarthrosis of the knee. J Bone Joint Surg 1980;62A:786–795.

McGinty JB, ed. Operative arthroscopy. New York, Raven Press, 1991.

Medical Management of the Surgical Patient, Third Edition,
edited by Michael F. Lubin, H. Kenneth Walker, and Robert B. Smith III.
J.B. Lippincott Company, Philadelphia, PA © 1995.

CHAPTER

TOTAL KNEE JOINT REPLACEMENT

97

Sam Nasser
J. Robin DeAndrade

Pain from arthritis, either degenerative or inflammatory, is the principal indication for total knee joint replacement. The joint surface is replaced using three components, one for each part of the joint: femur, tibia, and patella. The femoral component is made of metal, is shaped like the distal femur, and fits the bone in much the same manner as a crown fits a tooth. The proximal tibia is replaced with a tray made of either plastic or metal and plastic that is anchored in the bone the way a filling is placed in a tooth. The tray is shaped to accommodate the femoral condyles and may also augment the ligamentous stability of the knee. The patella is replaced with a plastic prosthesis that is convex posteriorly to articulate with the femoral implant. The components are usually affixed with polymethyl methacrylate (acrylic) cement, but biologic fixation is obtained by bony ingrowth in some cases. Although the entire knee is usually replaced, occasionally a "hemiknee" procedure known as a unicondylar knee arthroplasty is performed. In this case, only one femoral condyle and half the tibial plateau are replaced, and the patella is not resurfaced.

The knee is generally approached through an anterior longitudinal incision. A medial flap is raised and the joint capsule is entered through a medial parapatellar incision. The patella is turned "inside out" and displaced laterally, allowing access to the joint. Because the operation is generally done under tourniquet control, blood transfusion is not routinely necessary. The magnitude of surgical stress is moderate. The procedure may be performed using regional (spinal, epidural) or general anesthesia.

USUAL POSTOPERATIVE COURSE

Expected postoperative hospital stay: The postoperative hospital stay ranges from 7 to 10 days, depending on the speed of rehabilitation, the number of other joints affected by arthritis, and the severity of any associated deformity.

Operative mortality: Under 0.1%

Special monitoring required: No special monitoring is required.

Patient activity and positioning: Continuous passive motion is frequently used after this type of procedure. It is carried out by placing patients in motorized splints that gradually flex the knee to a desired angle and then extend it. Pain and morbidity seem to be diminished by this technique. Ambulation is permitted within 1 or 2 days after operation but weight bearing is done with the knee supported in a removable splint or brace for the first 2 to 4 weeks. All immobilization is usually discontinued by 4 weeks after the procedure. The use of crutches or a walker is required for the first 3 to 6 weeks unless patients have other joint problems, in which case additional time may be needed. A cane may be of some use for an additional few weeks or months.

At least 75 degrees of knee flexion usually are obtained within 2 weeks after operation. If this range of motion cannot be regained, manipulation under anesthesia may be required.

Alimentation: No dietary restriction is necessary.

Antibiotic coverage: A prophylactic first-generation cephalosporin is commonly administered intravenously for 48 hours.

Weight bearing: Weight bearing to tolerance, including full weight bearing, is usually allowed after operation as range of motion and comfort permit. The postoperative regimen varies among surgeons, however, and no single best method of management exists.

POSTOPERATIVE COMPLICATIONS

IN THE HOSPITAL

Postoperative bleeding: Because of oozing from the synovium and exposed bone surfaces, postoperative bleeding may reach 200 to 400 mL. Blood transfusion is usually not required.

Wound infection: Infection is a dreaded complication because it can destroy an implanted prosthesis. The use of prophylactic antibiotics has reduced the incidence of infection in the immediate postoperative period to under 0.5%. Wound drainage lasting more than 96 hours requires close examination. If an infection is suspected on other grounds, early exploration is recommended for culture and drainage.

Thrombophlebitis: Swelling of the ipsilateral ankle with pitting edema occurs in about one third of patients. Deep venous thrombosis may be diagnosed clinically in 10% to 25% of patients, whereas diagnostic modalities such as venography, radioiodine-labeled fibrinogen studies, and plethysmography may yield an incidence of 20% to 50%. In untreated patients, the incidence of pulmonary embolus is 10% to 50% and the mortality is 1% to 2%. Accordingly, prophylaxis is essential. Early mobilization and exercises are safe but ineffective measures. Continuous passive motion may decrease the incidence and extent of venous thrombosis. Pharmacologic treatment should be administered, however, especially if there is a history of deep venous thrombosis. A variety of drugs have been used, including heparin, warfarin, and aspirin.

Early postoperative stiffness: With a combination of continuous passive motion and aggressive physical therapy, full extension and 75 to 90 degrees of flexion are generally achieved before patients leave the hospital. This goal is not reached in 10% to 30% of patients, however, and manipulation under anesthesia may be necessary. It is crucial to accomplish at least 75 degrees of flexion by 14 days after the surgical procedure. If this happens, further motion usually is gained over the ensuing weeks and months; if it does not, chronic stiffness is a likely prospect.

AFTER DISCHARGE

Chronic stiffness: If the initial 75 degrees of motion are obtained within 2 weeks, moderate effort will increase movement to 90 or even 110 degrees over the ensuing months. Manipulation under anesthesia after the initial 14 days is less effective because adhesions are difficult to break. With the further passage of time, the chances of success continue to decrease. If stiffness becomes chronic, an open release may be performed after 3 to 6 months, when the acute phase of healing has abated. Final results are inferior, however, compared with those obtained with early mobilization.

Knee instability: Varying degrees of instability may be present. With slight instability, the functional result of the knee replacement is generally acceptable. Stability against varus force is particularly important. Mild anteroposterior and valgus instability are not as likely to compromise function. If significant instability is present, crutches or a walker may be required permanently. Orthoses and braces are awkward and generally do not improve function. Revision surgery is rarely indicated for instability.

Infection: Although the perioperative infection rate is relatively low, the infection rate over the lifetime of the prosthesis remains at least 1%. Spread of sepsis from the gastrointestinal and genitourinary tracts, by either the hematogenous or the lymphatic route, has been demonstrated and appears to be the most common cause of late sepsis. Prophylactic antibiotics should be given if a bacteremia is possible, as with dental manipulation or urethral instrumentation, or if an active bacterial infection is present elsewhere in the body.

Prosthetic loosening: Implant stability, provided by either acrylic cement or biologic fixation, is essential to the success of this procedure. The bone–implant interface is a dynamic one, however, and remodeling eventually occurs. As a result, the relationship between bone and implant obtained at the initial operation may not be maintained over time. The rate of loosening is related to several factors and is difficult to predict accurately. Patients should be informed that loosening eventually occurs and revision may become necessary. Revision surgery is technically more difficult than is initial replacement, often requiring wider exposure, more complex instrumentation such as high-speed drills and specialized chisels, and even custom prostheses. In addition, substantial bone stock may be lost, and banked allograft bone should be available.

BIBLIOGRAPHY

Beckenbaugh RD, Istrup DM. Total hip arthroplasty: a review of 333 cases with long follow-up. J Bone Joint Surg 1978;60A:306–313.

Charnley J. Nine and 10-year results of low friction arthroplasty of the hip. Clin Orthop 1973;95:9–25.

Insall JM, Hood RW, Flawn LB, Sullivan DJ. A five to nine-year follow-up of the first 100 consecutive replacements. J Bone Joint Surg 1983;65A:619–628.

Marshall U. Controversy on total knee arthroplasty. Clin Orthop 1985;192.

CHAPTER

98

SURGERY FOR SCOLIOSIS OR KYPHOSIS IN ADULTS

Medical Management of the Surgical Patient, Third Edition,
edited by Michael F. Lubin, H. Kenneth Walker, and Robert B. Smith III.
J.B. Lippincott Company, Philadelphia, PA © 1995.

Thomas E. Whitesides, Jr.
William C. Horton

The most common indication for surgery in adults with scoliosis or kyphosis is debilitating pain from the deformity or associated spinal stenosis. Other indications include documented progression of the deformity and instability that hinders erect posture or threatens cardiopulmonary function. It is preferable to perform prophylactic surgery during childhood because complications are more frequent, immobilization and rehabilitation are more extensive, and the operative risk is greater in adults. Debility from chronic severe pain may force consideration of surgical intervention in patients with compromised pulmonary function. If cardiac failure is present, however, the prognosis for life is usually not improved by correcting the deformity, and surgery may be ill-advised.

Either a posterior, anterior, or combined operative approach may be used. The principal goals of surgery are decompression of symptomatic neural structures, correction of major imbalance, and fusion. Reconstruction usually includes autologous bone grafting and use of metal internal fixation devices. Regardless of the operative route used, the procedure constitutes a severe surgical stress. Operations last 3 to 10 hours and blood loss may range from 500 to 5000 mL, requiring multiple transfusions.

General endotracheal anesthesia is used, as is somatosensory evoked potential spinal monitoring in most cases.

USUAL POSTOPERATIVE COURSE

Expected postoperative hospital stay: The postoperative hospital stay is about 2 weeks, and patients are fully independent at the time of discharge.

Operative mortality: The operative mortality rate ranges from under 1% in average cases to 10% in compromised patients.

Special monitoring required: Arterial and central venous lines are placed after extensive procedures and blood gases are monitored in the early phase. If pulmonary compromise is significant, the endotracheal tube is retained at the end of the procedure and the volume respirator is used. Patients are rapidly weaned as conditions permit; tracheostomy is rarely required. It is also critical that postoperative monitoring include thorough and well-documented neurologic examinations.

Patient activity and positioning: Patients are usually cared for by "logrolling" on regular hospital beds or, in tenuous situations, on turning frames. Most patients are encouraged to get out of bed and ambulate 3 to 5 days after surgery. Bracing or casts may be necessary, particularly in patients with osteoporosis or major instability.

Alimentation: Paralytic ileus is typical for 1 to 4 days, even in patients undergoing posterior surgical approaches. Oral feedings should be delayed until the ileus is cleared.

Antibiotic coverage: An intravenous cephalosporin is administered for 28 to 48 hours.

Blood loss: Postoperative blood loss is common and results from the raw cancellous bone surface left by the fusion procedure. Such bleeding is monitored by suction drain output and usually decreases rapidly to less than 30 mL per shift by 48 hours after surgery. Postoperative anemia should be anticipated and corrected as medically necessary. Extensive intraoperative and postoperative blood loss is frequently associated with mild to severe coagulopathies. The prothrombin time, partial thromboplastin time, and platelet count are monitored after surgery and any coagulation defects are aggressively reversed while active bleeding is occurring.

Thromboembolism: Some form of prophylaxis for thromboembolism is necessary because bed rest and surgical trauma increase the risk of pulmonary embolism. Early anticoagulation is risky because of associated bleeding from the surgical area. Therefore, elastic stockings, pneumatic compression hose, and early activity in the bed are prescribed. If the risk of venous thrombosis is unusually high in a specific patient, anticoagulants should be administered cautiously until mobilization can be achieved.

Spinal cord and nerve root injury: Spinal cord and nerve root injury is a serious potential problem in all patients undergoing this surgery. Surgeons must make special efforts to prevent such injury and to monitor for its occurrence. Spinal cord monitoring is useful during the operation and may occasionally be necessary in the postoperative phase. Detailed and well-documented serial neurologic examinations (motor, sensory, and rectal) are the keystone of postoperative monitoring. Any complaints of new postoperative numbness, weakness, perianal anesthesia, or incontinence should be rapidly evaluated.

Bladder atony: Postoperative bladder atony is common. A Foley catheter is generally used for 1 or 2 days, followed by intermittent catheterization as needed.

POSTOPERATIVE COMPLICATIONS

IN THE HOSPITAL

Wound infection: Progressive and increasing incisional pain suggests possible infection. Fever, drainage, and an elevated white blood cell count may or may not be present. If infection is suspected, aspiration of the hematoma using meticulous sterile technique is necessary for diagnosis.

Pulmonary insufficiency: The prophylactic use of incentive spirometry and pulmonary physical therapy is important. Poor ventilation and splinting from pain are common after the thoracotomy used in the anterior approach. Appropriate monitoring with physical examinations, serial chest radiographs, and arterial blood gas determinations should be performed.

Pulmonary embolism: If embolism occurs, the standard therapeutic intervention is necessary.

Intestinal or bladder atony: Oral intake is restricted until peristalsis is established. A nasogastric tube may be necessary occasionally for persistent ileus. A urinary catheter may also be required until mobilization has begun.

Anemia secondary to blood loss: Postoperative hematocrit levels are obtained to monitor for anemia related to blood loss, and replacement should be given as necessary. Coagulopathy should also be watched for and corrected.

AFTER DISCHARGE

Bone graft pain: Donor site pain from the harvest of autologous bone is common but gradually dissipates over 1 to 3 months. Increasing pain at the implantation site should raise the suspicion of infection.

Skin ulceration under a brace or cast from pressure and friction: Patients must be closely monitored by personnel with expertise in the care of braces and casts. Cast revision or brace modification may be necessary if skin ulceration occurs.

Implant failure: Internal fixation devices occasionally loosen or break. There frequently is associated new pain and possible deformity, but radiographic examination is necessary for diagnosis. Revision is usually required.

Pseudarthrosis: The bone fusion may fail to heal in any patient. This is most commonly seen after 6 to 8 months in patients who are malnourished, immunocompromised, or noncompliant, or in those who smoke or who have undergone multiple operations.

BIBLIOGRAPHY

Bradford DS. Adult scoliosis: current concepts of treatment. Clin Orthop 1988;229:70–87.

Kostuik JP. Adult scoliosis. In: Rothman RH, Simeone FA, eds. The spine, ed 3, vol 1. Philadelphia, WB Saunders, 1992:897–911.

Moe JH, Winter RB, Bradford DS, Lonstein JE. Scoliosis and other spinal deformities. Philadelphia, WB Saunders, 1978.

Nickel VL, Perry J, Affeldt JE, Dail CW. Elective surgery on patients with respiratory paralysis. J Bone Joint Surg 1957;39A:989–1001.

Medical Management of the Surgical Patient, Third Edition,
edited by Michael F. Lubin, H. Kenneth Walker, and Robert B. Smith III.
J.B. Lippincott Company, Philadelphia, PA © 1995.

CHAPTER

99

TOTAL HIP JOINT REPLACEMENT

James R. Roberson
J. Robin DeAndrade

Pain, stiffness, and limitation of function from arthritis are the primary indications for total replacement of the hip joint. The artificial joint consists of an acetabular component made of high-density polyethylene within a metal shell shaped like a socket and a femoral component made of a high-strength metal alloy fashioned into a spherical head that articulates with the acetabular component. The femoral component is inserted within the intramedullary canal of the femur, and both components are fixed to adjacent bone by either bone cement or tissue ingrowth into a porous coating on the surface of the prosthesis.

Hip joint replacement requires about 2 hours, but the operation can be much longer in complicated cases, such as revision of a failed replacement. The procedure can be done equally well using either general or spinal anesthesia, and epidural anesthesia is used occasionally. The average blood loss is 500 mL, and about half of all patients require transfusions. Preoperative autologous blood donation has become standard, and additional homologous blood transfusion is seldom necessary.

USUAL POSTOPERATIVE COURSE

Expected postoperative hospital stay: 5 to 7 days

Operative mortality rate: Under 1%

Special monitoring required: Neurovascular checking of the extremity should be performed during the early postoperative period and monitoring for clinical signs of deep venous thrombosis conducted during the subsequent hospital stay.

Patient activity and positioning: Mobilization from bed is usually begun on the second postoperative day. Either crutches or a walker is necessary to aid ambulation for about 1 month, and a cane is used for an additional month. Patients are instructed to avoid extremes of hip motion for 3 months to minimize the possibility of dislocation of the artificial joint. The hip should not be hyperextended or flexed more than 90 degrees. Adduction should also be avoided.

Alimentation: Patients are allowed fluids the day of operation, and food intake is advanced as tolerated. Occasionally, the operation results in a temporary ileus, which requires delaying oral intake.

Antibiotic coverage: Prophylactic antibiotics have conclusively been demonstrated to decrease the infection rate after total hip replacement. First-generation cephalosporin is given in the operating room just before the incision is made and then continued for 24 to 48 hours after surgery. Vancomycin is used in patients who are allergic to cephalosporin. Oral penicillin is recommended as prophylaxis before dental work after the hip has been replaced.

POSTOPERATIVE COMPLICATIONS

IN THE HOSPITAL

Elevated temperature: Although fever is a generic complication associated with most surgery, it is ubiquitous after hip replacement. Because of the extensive work done within the marrow of the femur and pelvis, essentially all patients have low-grade fevers as high as 101.5°F for 2 to 4 days. This may be related to marrow fat being filtered in the lungs on a subclinical level without causing changes in the chest radiograph. Embarking on an investigation for infection during this period is expensive and invariably negative if no other clinical findings are apparent.

Deep venous thrombosis: As many as 30% to 50% of patients undergoing hip replacement have been found to have deep venous thrombosis when routine venograms are performed. This incidence can be substantially reduced by prophylactic regimens such as low-dose heparin, warfarin (Coumadin), and sequential compression stockings. Most patients with deep venous thrombosis are asymptomatic, and most clots occur at or below the popliteal vein. Symptomatic pulmonary embolus occurs in about 1% of patients.

Hip dislocation: Hip dislocation occurs in about 3% of primary hip replacements. Closed reduction with or without general anesthesia is usually successful but recurrent dislocations may require reoperation and revision of components.

AFTER DISCHARGE

Dislocation: Dislocation occurs when the joint is placed in the extremes of flexion or extension. The complication becomes much less likely over time, with most cases occurring within the first 6 months after operation.

Infection: Hematogenous seeding of the prosthetic joint is an unlikely, but permanent, possibility. The likelihood of hematogenous seeding is minimal in the absence of immunosuppression or sepsis, but antibiotic prophylaxis is recommended whenever bacteremia is anticipated (ie, dental manipulation or urethral instrumentation).

Loosening of the prosthesis: Firm fixation of the prosthetic components to bone is required for painless function, and loosening can occur over time. Loosening is manifest by limp and pain with weight bearing and by lucent lines around the prosthesis on radiographs.

Polyethylene wear: Repetitive weight-bearing forces on the polyethylene surface result in linear wear of the acetabular component. The microscopic particles produce an inflammatory response that may initiate prosthetic loosening. About 1% of hip replacements each year require revision for various reasons. These revision procedures frequently are technically difficult and are associated with increased operative time, blood loss, and complications.

BIBLIOGRAPHY

Roberson J, Nasser S, eds. Complications of total hip arthroplasty. Orthop Clin North Am 1992;23.

Medical Management of the Surgical Patient, Third Edition,
edited by Michael F. Lubin, H. Kenneth Walker, and Robert B. Smith III.
J.B. Lippincott Company, Philadelphia, PA © 1995.

CHAPTER

100

LUMBAR DISKECTOMY, LAMINECTOMY, AND FUSION

John G. Heller

Posterior lumbar surgery in adults can be divided into three general levels of complexity. Each type of procedure addresses a different consequence of a pathologic spinal motion segment. The simplest and most common disorder is the herniated lumbar disk. If the symptoms produced by a lumbar disk herniation fail to respond to appropriate nonoperative therapy, laminotomy and diskectomy is indicated. Patients are placed either prone or in the knee-chest position on specially designed operating tables. The latter position affords decompression of the abdominal cavity and the epidural veins. The procedure is performed with either loupe magnification or the surgical microscope through a posterior midline incision measuring 3 to 6 cm. The operative level is confirmed radiographically. Blood loss is minimal and the operative time is usually 1 hour or less.

Operative treatment of lumbar stenosis requires a laminectomy. The term refers to the removal of one or more spinous processes and laminae, most commonly for the purpose of decompressing the cauda equina or lumbar nerve roots. Such exposure of the spinal canal allows the removal of facet joint osteophytes and thickened ligamentum flavum, which may contribute to neural compression. Compared with laminotomy and diskectomy, laminectomy takes longer to perform, requires a larger incision, and engenders more blood loss (usually less than 500 mL). Patients with spinal stenosis are older and often have more coexisting medical conditions and operative risk factors.

Under certain circumstances, fusion of a lumbar motion segment may be required. This may be done alone or in combination with either of the decompressive procedures described earlier. If lumbar instability exists before surgery or is created during a laminotomy or laminectomy, a fusion is performed. A posterolateral (intertransverse) fusion requires a far more extensive dissection. Bleeding from the branches of the lumbar segmental vessels can be copious and blood loss increases with each additional level fused. Significant blood loss also occurs from the posterior iliac crest during the harvest of autologous bone graft. Accordingly, intraoperative or perioperative transfusion of blood products should be anticipated. Laminectomy and fusion procedures generally require 3 or 4 hours. If segmental pedicle screw fixation is used as an adjunct to the fusion procedure, operative times increase by 1 or 2 more hours. The use of such instrumentation increases the risk of complications and the volume of blood loss.

USUAL POSTOPERATIVE COURSE

Expected postoperative hospital stay: The expected postoperative hospital stay is 2 to 4 days for laminotomy and diskectomy, 3 to 5 days for laminectomy, and 5 to 7 days for fusion.

Operative mortality: The operative mortality rate generally is under 1% but increases in proportion to the magnitude of the procedure and the preoperative medical status of the patients.

Special monitoring required: Frequent neurologic evaluations should be performed during the first 24 to 48 hours after operation. Any significant change should be reported at once. Bleeding into the paraspinal tissues continues for 2 or 3 days, especially after fusion procedures. The hematocrit decreases after surgery in proportion to the magnitude of the procedure. Platelet counts and coagulation studies should be monitored after large volumes of blood have been lost.

Patient activity and positioning: Ambulation begins on the first postoperative day after laminotomy and laminectomy, and on the second day after fusion procedures. Patients should receive preoperative instruction regarding isometric trunk and lower extremity exercises, body mechanics, and bending and lifting restrictions. A lumbar support may be worn for comfort after laminotomy and laminectomy but is not required. The need for rigid bracing after fusion varies according to the specifics of the procedure and the preference of the surgeon. Unrestricted activity can be expected within 6 to 12 weeks after laminotomy and laminectomy, and within 4 to 6 months after fusion.

Alimentation: Identifiable nutritional deficiencies should be corrected before surgery, especially in patients undergoing fusion. After the operation, food intake is advanced as tolerated. Patients undergoing fusion may have a significant incidence of adynamic ileus. If oral feeding is delayed more than 3 days, parenteral support should be contemplated.

Antibiotic coverage: Prophylaxis with a first-generation cephalosporin is recommended. Additional doses are given during surgery (based on the duration of the procedure and the magnitude of blood loss) and for 24 hours afterward. Antibiotics with a broader spectrum of activity should be used in patients who are compromised hosts, who have colonized urinary tracts, or who require prolonged preoperative hospitalization.

Deep venous thrombosis: Prophylaxis against deep venous thrombosis is recommended. Thigh-high elastic hose should be used in combination with sequential pneumatic compression stockings throughout the operative procedure and for the remainder of the hospitalization.

Blood transfusion: Autologous blood donation is encouraged before fusion procedures and complex or revision laminectomies. Intraoperative red blood cell salvage and reinfusion is practiced during fusion procedures.

Cigarette smoking: Cigarette smoking interferes with bone graft healing. Fusion potential may be maximized by preoperative withdrawal from all tobacco products.

Medications: Medications that impair platelet function should be discontinued 2 to 4 weeks before surgery to minimize intraoperative bleeding, especially when a fusion is planned. Oral narcotics may be appropriate as an alternative analgesic during the preoperative period.

POSTOPERATIVE COMPLICATIONS

IN THE HOSPITAL

Hematoma: Subcutaneous hematomas are most common when the iliac crest is exposed through the same midline incision. Such collections are best prevented through careful wound closure and drainage of dead space; surgical evacuation is seldom necessary. Epidural hematomas usually present within 3 to 5 days as a cause of severe back or leg pain with progressive neurologic deficit. Emergent surgical exploration and decompression is required.

Infection: The incidence of postoperative wound infection varies from 0.5% to 5%, depending on the complexity of the case. The appearance of the wound is often deceptively normal, delaying the diagnosis. Treatment is by immediate surgical débridement, closure over drains, and administration of parenteral antibiotics.

Cerebrospinal fluid leakage: A dural tear should be surgically repaired when it is identified. If primary repair or patching of the dura is not possible, a closed subarachnoid drain should be used to divert the cerebrospinal fluid for 5 days. Strict supine bed rest is maintained for 5 days after a dural repair. The wound dressing should be inspected for cerebrospinal fluid and patients observed for signs of meningitis.

Persistent or recurrent radicular pain or neurologic deficit: Persistent or recurrent radicular pain or neurologic deficit after lumbar decompression may result from operation at the wrong level, incomplete removal of the herniated material or recurrence at the same level, unrecognized or inadequately decompressed foraminal stenosis, or trauma to the neural elements during surgery. Malposition of hooks or pedicle screws may also cause such symptoms after an instrumented fusion. Myelography with computed tomography is recommended to clarify such issues in the immediate postoperative period.

Bowel or bladder dysfunction: Injury to the sacral roots resulting in neurogenic bowel or bladder dysfunction is rare. More often, especially in the elderly, an underlying degree of dysfunction caused by high-grade stenosis and bladder or prostate problems is unmasked under the influence of bed rest and various medications. An intermittent catheterization program should be instituted as soon as possible to minimize the risk of urinary tract infection. Urologic consultation is advisable if the symptoms do not resolve rapidly once patients are ambulatory.

AFTER DISCHARGE

Recurrent radicular pain: If radicular pain recurs after hospital discharge, each of the causes mentioned earlier should be considered again. In addition, postlaminectomy instability or fatigue fractures of the pars interarticularis can cause similar symptoms.

Back pain: The quantity and duration of local wound pain is proportional to the magnitude of the procedure performed. Incisional pain should be managed with analgesics as needed for a reasonable period. Debilitating postdiskectomy back pain may occur in 15% of patients and can be treated by lumbar fusion if warranted. Intervertebral diskitis should also be considered, especially if the pain persists at night. Recurrent or new back pain may also be related to postlaminectomy instability or a failed fusion.

Pseudarthrosis: The incidence of failed fusion varies with the number and location of segments, the use of instrumentation, and the type of bone graft used. The pain is usually related to patients' activity levels. The diagnosis is made with appropriate radiographic studies.

Instrumentation failure: Broken or loose implants are a hallmark of pseudarthroses. Surgical repair of the nonunion is recommended if the symptoms are sufficiently severe.

Wound infection: Wound infection is mentioned again because the diagnosis of a postoperative spinal wound infection is frequently delayed. Increasing back pain in association with malaise, sweats, chills, and an elevated erythrocyte sedimentation rate strongly suggests this diagnosis. Treatment is surgical, followed by the administration of parenteral antibiotics.

Psychosocial dysfunction: For many patients who have undergone back surgery, reentry into the workplace requires a coordinated effort by patients, doctors, therapists, employers, and others. Patients must be strongly motivated to help themselves recover a normal life-style.

BIBLIOGRAPHY

Balderston RA, An HS. Complications in spinal surgery. Philadelphia, WB Saunders, 1991.

Frymoyer JW, ed. The adult spine: principles and practice. New York, Raven Press, 1991.

Garfin SR. Complications of spine surgery. Baltimore, Williams & Wilkins, 1989.

Rothman RH, Simeone FA, eds. The spine, ed 3. Philadelphia, WB Saunders, 1992.

Medical Management of the Surgical Patient, Third Edition,
edited by Michael F. Lubin, H. Kenneth Walker, and Robert B. Smith III.
J.B. Lippincott Company, Philadelphia, PA © 1995.

CHAPTER

SURGERY FOR HIP FRACTURES

101

Mary J. Albert
Thomas E. Whitesides, Jr.

Hip fracture is a general term used in reference to fractures of the femoral neck and peritrochanteric (intertrochanteric or subtrochanteric) regions. These low-energy injuries may result from simple falls in the elderly but are caused by violent trauma in younger persons. Minimally displaced femoral neck fractures in the elderly and all femoral neck fractures in younger patients are treated with percutaneous screw fixation. In patients who are 70 years or older, prosthetic replacement arthroplasty is performed for displaced femoral neck fractures to allow early mobilization and immediate weight bearing. Peritrochanteric fractures are best treated by open reduction with rigid internal fixation. The internal fixation devices used vary widely because of the diverse fracture types that occur in the proximal femur and their individual requirements for establishing stability.

Percutaneous screw fixation requires a small incision, brief anesthesia time, and blood loss of 100 to 300 mL. Prosthetic replacement for displaced femoral neck fractures or internal fixation of peritrochanteric fractures involves a more extensive operative exposure that may require 2 or more hours of operating time, with a blood loss that can exceed 1000 mL.

USUAL POSTOPERATIVE COURSE

Expected postoperative hospital stay: The duration of hospitalization after surgery ranges from 7 to 14 days, depending on the nature and severity of associated medical problems and on premorbid factors such as functional ability, mobility, and social support.

Operative mortality: The anesthetic mortality rate is about 1%, depending on the ASA Classification of Physical Status, but the mortality rates for the first postoperative month and year are as high as 20% and 30%, respectively. Factors related to increased mortality rates include male sex, the presence of dementia, and congestive heart failure.

Special monitoring required: Monitoring requirements are determined by the physical status of the patients. A hematocrit level should be obtained daily for the first 3 days after surgery to assess continuing blood loss from the fracture site and the surgical incision. Mental status should be assessed periodically because acute changes may reflect the onset of infection, overmedication, or hypoxia. Periodic radiographs are used to evaluate fracture healing.

Patient activity and positioning: Most patients are mobilized to chairs within 24 hours of surgery. Physical therapy is then initiated for ambulation with the assistance of a walker or crutches. Wheelchair use should be avoided in patients who can ambulate because it slows rehabilitation and discourages mobility.

Alimentation: After recovery from anesthesia, clear liquids are permitted and food intake is advanced to a regular diet as tolerated. As many as half of elderly patients exhibit findings of malnutrition on hospital admission. Because protein-calorie malnutrition is associated with an increased rate of infection, impaired wound strength, and poor bone

587

healing, postoperative dietary supplements should be provided. Advanced age, diminished physical activity, and narcotic pain medication can result in persistent constipation.

Antibiotic coverage: An intravenous first-generation cephalosporin is administered for 24 to 48 hours or until surgical drains are removed. Supplemental use of an aminoglycoside may be necessary in the face of concomitant infection or a chronic indwelling urinary catheter.

POSTOPERATIVE COMPLICATIONS

IN THE HOSPITAL

Hypotension: Blood loss or dehydration may lead to hypotension. If this occurs, blood and crystalloid replacement is necessary.

Thromboembolism: Deep venous thrombosis occurs in 40% to 50% of patients with hip fractures who do not receive prophylaxis. The incidence of fatal pulmonary embolism in such patients is reported to be 2% to 10%, making it the single most important cause of postoperative death. Measures to decrease the incidence of venous thrombosis include the use of aspirin, pneumatic compression stockings, warfarin, subcutaneous or intravenous heparin, and low-molecular-weight dextran. Even with these therapies, the incidence of venous thrombosis associated with hip surgery is 20%. Low-dose warfarin (Coumadin) therapy should be initiated on the day of operation and the prothrombin time adjusted to 1.5 times control.

Pressure ulcers: As many as 20% to 70% of patients with hip fractures develop pressure sores, most often on the sacrum and heels. Most pressure ulcers appear by the fifth hospital day. Their incidence rises with age, paralysis, sensory impairment, malnutrition, and incontinence. The hospital mortality rate in these patients is reported to be 27%. Preventive measures include the use of egg crate mattresses, heel protectors, frequent turning, and rapid postoperative mobilization.

Urinary retention and urinary tract infection: Urinary tract infections are reported in 10% to 20% of patients and urinary retention occurs in 30% to 50%, possibly related to anesthetic agents and narcotic analgesics. The prophylactic use of an indwelling urinary catheter that is removed within 24 hours of operation decreases the occurrence of retention without increasing the incidence of infection.

Altered mentation: Postoperative confusion has been reported in 30% to 50% of elderly patients. Inciting factors include medications, infection, hypoxemia, electrolyte or glucose abnormalities, and cardiac dysfunction. Such delirium usually abates within 1 week, and prompt return to the prehospital environment may help patients regain their previous mental status.

AFTER DISCHARGE

Recovery time and functional outcome: Mobility before fracture is the strongest predictor of function after fracture; patients who were able to ambulate independently before their fractures have the best outcomes. Poor functional outcome is associated with premorbid dementia and residence in a nursing home. The recovery time is longer for intertrochanteric fractures than for femoral neck fractures.

Prevention of subsequent hip fracture: Because 20% to 25% of patients with hip fractures who survive 5 years sustain fractures in their other hips, preventive measures are recommended, such as using a cane in the opposite hand to assist in proprioception on unfamiliar terrain, and making the home safer by removing obstacles.

Prosthetic dislocation and loosening: Prosthetic dislocation affects 0.3% to 11% of patients and occurs most frequently in the early postoperative period. Loosening is the most common late complication of prosthetic replacement.

Nonunion, malunion, and failure of fixation: Nonunion, malunion, and failure of fixation may occur in as many as 10% of patients who are treated with internal fixation. The need for reoperation depends on the physical status and symptoms of the patients.

BIBLIOGRAPHY

Bray TJ, Smith-Hoefer E, Hooper A, Timmerman L. The displaced femoral neck fracture: internal fixation vs bipolar endoprosthesis: results of a prospective randomized comparison. Clin Orthop 1988;230:127–140.

Ochs M. Surgical management of the hip in the elderly patient. Clin Geriatr Med 1990;6:571–587.

Smith TK. Prevention of complications in orthopedic surgery secondary to nutritional depletion. Clin Orthop 1987;222:91–97.

Versluysen M. Pressure sores in elderly patients. J Bone Joint Surg 1985;67B:10–13.

White BL, Fisher WD, Laurin CA. Rate of mortality for elderly patients after fracture of the hip in the 1980s. J Bone Joint Surg 1987;69A:1335–1340.

Medical Management of the Surgical Patient, Third Edition,
edited by Michael F. Lubin, H. Kenneth Walker, and Robert B. Smith III.
J.B. Lippincott Company, Philadelphia, PA © 1995.

FRACTURES OF THE FEMORAL SHAFT

102

Mary J. Albert

The femur is the longest and structurally strongest bone in the body. Femoral shaft fractures are high-energy injuries resulting from violent trauma. Common causes include motor vehicle accidents, automobile–pedestrian accidents, and gunshot wounds. Isolated femoral shaft fractures can result in significant (2000 to 3000 mL) blood loss into the surrounding tissues. Femur fractures are the most common skeletal injury in patients with multiple trauma and may be associated with life-threatening injuries to the head, chest, and abdomen. Suspected hypovolemic shock necessitates rapid crystalloid and blood replacement, with careful perioperative monitoring of the circulatory status. Open femur fractures demand emergent débridement and stabilization, followed by delayed closure. Because delay of fracture fixation in patients with multiple injuries is associated with an increased incidence of respiratory failure, fat embolism, pneumonia, a longer hospital stay, and more days in the intensive care unit, long-bone fractures should be stabilized within the first 24 hours after injury. Patients are temporarily placed in skeletal traction before operative fixation; extended traction as definitive treatment has no place in the modern care of femoral shaft fractures in adults.

Femoral shaft fractures may be anatomically classified as subtrochanteric, midshaft or diaphyseal, and distal or supracondylar. Fractures at the subtrochanteric level may be treated with intramedullary reconstruction nails or screw-plate devices. The standard of treatment for diaphyseal fractures is closed interlocking intramedullary nailing.

Distal femoral fractures are fixed with blade plates, screw-plate devices, or intramedullary nails. The goals of treatment are rigid fracture fixation, early patient mobilization, and early joint motion. The magnitude of surgical stress, amount of blood loss, and duration of the operative procedure depend on the complexity of the fractures and the overall physical status of the patient. General anesthesia is usually administered. Intraoperative use of autologous blood replacement may be required.

USUAL POSTOPERATIVE COURSE

Expected postoperative hospital stay: The length of hospitalization is highly dependent on the presence of associated injuries, but a 4- to 7-day stay is usual for patients with isolated femoral shaft fractures.

Operative mortality: The operative mortality rate is under 10% for the femoral injury but depends largely on the severity of associated injuries.

Special monitoring required: In the early postoperative period, frequent assessment of the hematocrit, urinary output, level of oxygenation, and systemic neurologic and vascular status is necessary. Periodic radiographs of the fracture are obtained to evaluate stability and healing.

Patient activity and positioning: Rigid fracture fixation permits patients to be mobilized to chairs the day after surgery, with subsequent progression to ambulation using walkers or crutches. Early active range of motion of the hip and knee joints is initiated in physical therapy. The use of a continuous passive motion machine may decrease postoperative pain and speed joint mobilization.

Alimentation: Clear liquids are allowed after operation, and food intake is advanced to a regular diet as tolerated. Patients with multiple injuries have massive metabolic requirements and greatly increased nutritional needs. Central hyperalimentation should be initiated early, with oral supplements provided as the gut becomes functional.

Antibiotic coverage: An intravenous cephalosporin is given for 48 hours after surgery or until surgical drains are removed. Appropriate coverage for open fractures includes first-generation cephalosporin for grade I and II open fractures, with the addition of an aminoglycoside for grade III injuries. For fractures associated with vascular compromise, a massive crush injury, or contamination by grass or soil, intravenous penicillin G, 4 million U every 4 to 6 hours, is added. Adequate tetanus prophylaxis must be provided for all open fractures.

Clinical and radiographic evaluation: Clinical and radiographic examinations are performed monthly to assess fracture healing and progress in rehabilitation.

POSTOPERATIVE COMPLICATIONS

IN THE HOSPITAL

Fat embolism syndrome: The potentially lethal triad of hypoxia, confusion, and petechiae known as fat embolism syndrome typically appears 24 to 72 hours after a fracture. Standard therapy includes pulmonary support, positive-pressure ventilation when necessary, and strict fluid management. Early stabilization of long-bone fractures can reduce the incidence of fat embolism.

Thromboembolism: Deep venous thrombosis is common in patients with lower extremity fractures and may lead to fatal pulmonary emboli. Preventive measures include the use of intermittent compression stockings, aspirin, or anticoagulation with warfarin (Coumadin). Immediate mobilization of patients after surgery, with early ambulation and active joint motion, is important.

Compartment syndrome: Although a compartment syndrome of the thigh is rare, the presence of pain with passive joint extension, pain out of proportion to the injury, pallor, paresthesias, or absence of the pulse must be evaluated with immediate measurement of intracompartmental pressures to determine whether fasciotomy is required.

Nerve paresis: Excessive intraoperative traction may result in a pudendal palsy manifested by decreased or absent sensation on the head of the penis in men or decreased sensation over the labia in women. Peroneal nerve palsy with a footdrop can also occur with excessive intraoperative traction.

AFTER DISCHARGE

Nonunion, delayed union, malunion: The rate of nonunion of femoral shaft fractures treated by closed intramedullary nailing is under 1%. Delayed union is more common and is treated by removal of the locking bolts to allow the fracture to compress or by nail exchange and grafting. Malunion results from any combination of shortening, malrotation, or angular deformity.

Recurrent fracture and hardware failure: Fractures of the fixation device are seen in under 1% of intramedullary nails. The incidence of recurrent fracture at the original fracture site is 5% to 15% when plates are used.

Heterotopic ossification: Small amounts of heterotopic bone may form over the proximal end of the intramedullary nail. This seldom creates a clinical problem. In rare instances, heterotopic bone formation may be so extensive that it interferes with hip motion.

BIBLIOGRAPHY

Bone LB, Johnson KD, Weigelt J, Scheinberg R. Early versus delayed stabilization of femoral fractures. J Bone Joint Surg 1989;71A:336–340.

Gossling HR, Pellegrini V. Fat embolism syndrome: a review of the pathophysiology and physiological basis of treatment. Clin Orthop 1982;165:68–82.

Kuntscher G. Intramedullary surgical technique and its place in orthopaedic surgery. J Bone Joint Surg 1965;47A:809–818.

Seibel R, LaDuca J, Hassett JM, et al. Blunt multiple trauma (ISS 36), femur traction, and the pulmonary failure-septic state. Ann Surg 1985;202:283–295.

Winquist RA, Hansen ST Jr, Clawson DK. Closed intramedullary nailing of femoral fractures: a report of five hundred and twenty cases. J Bone Joint Surg 1984;66A:529–539.

Medical Management of the Surgical Patient, Third Edition,
edited by Michael F. Lubin, H. Kenneth Walker, and Robert B. Smith III.
J.B. Lippincott Company, Philadelphia, PA © 1995.

CHAPTER

103

MAJOR AMPUTATIONS OF THE LOWER EXTREMITY

John D. Henry, Jr.
Lamar L. Fleming

Lower extremity amputations are performed to treat vascular insufficiency, infection, tumors, and severe trauma. The goal of amputation and subsequent rehabilitation is to return patients to an ambulatory, pain-free, independent status. The success of rehabilitation is directly related to the anatomic level of amputation. The more proximal the level of amputation, the higher the energy required for ambulation and the less likely it is that patients will achieve successful independent use of prostheses. Therefore, amputations are generally performed at the most distal site compatible with wound healing to achieve optimum potential for ambulation. Most procedures are performed in elderly patients with vascular insufficiency, and the most common level is below the knee. Several advances, including objective preoperative testing methods to predict healing at proposed levels of amputation, use of the immediate rigid dressing with or without a temporary pylon, and improvements in prosthetic design and materials, have contributed to improved results over the past few years.

Most lower extremity amputations are performed under general anesthesia or regional (spinal or epidural) block. The duration of operation ranges from 45 minutes for a transmetatarsal amputation to 1 hour for a below-knee amputation and as long as 2 hours or more for a hip disarticulation. The magnitude of the surgical stress is directly related to the level of amputation. In procedures in which a tourniquet is used, blood loss is usually minimal. In more proximal amputations, 2 to 4 U of packed red blood cells may be required.

USUAL POSTOPERATIVE COURSE

Expected postoperative hospital stay: Postoperative hospitalization for 5 to 7 days is expected after below-knee amputation if no complications occur.

Operative mortality: The operative mortality depends on the level of amputation and the age and general medical condition of the patient. Mortality rates range from under 0.5% for young patients undergoing amputation for trauma to 20% for elderly patients undergoing above-knee amputation for vascular insufficiency.

Special monitoring required: A well-padded plaster cast or another form of rigid dressing is commonly used after surgery to facilitate wound healing, reduce stump edema, and prevent joint contracture. The cast may be removed for wound inspection if necessary, but should be replaced soon if the wound appears normal to minimize stump swelling. Surgical drains are usually removed 48 hours after operation.

Patient activity and positioning: Patients should be correctly positioned after surgery to prevent joint contractures. In patients with below-knee amputations, the knees are cast in extension to prevent knee flexion contractures. Prolonged hip flexion in bed should be avoided and short periods of lying prone daily are recommended to prevent hip flexion contractures.

Patients are mobilized out of bed on the first postoperative day and physical therapy, including quadriceps, abductor, and hip extension strengthening exercises, is begun on the second day. The cast or rigid dressing is changed 5 to 7 days after surgery both to allow inspection of the wound and to ensure proper cast fitting after the early postoperative edema has subsided. Skin sutures are removed at about 2 weeks. The cast is changed again at 3 to 4 weeks, and a temporary prosthesis is fitted to the limb when the incision has healed. Touch-down weight bearing with the use of crutches or a walker is then increased over the next month to weight bearing as tolerated. To promote stump size stabilization, gentle elastic compression wrapping of the stump is used when the prosthesis is not being worn. When the stump size has not changed in 6 weeks, a permanent prosthesis may be fitted.

Alternatively, younger patients with well-vascularized stumps may be candidates for immediate postoperative prostheses and immediate ambulation as described by Burgess. Immediate weight bearing is not recommended in patients with poor vascularity because of the high risk of wound healing complications.

Alimentation: Because trauma or infection increases energy requirements 30% to 50% above basal values, patients should undergo at least baseline nutritional assessments, including serum albumin and total lymphocyte counts. Nutritional supplementation should be provided as necessary.

Antibiotic coverage: In infected cases, broad-spectrum antibiotics should be used initially until the specific organisms are identified and sensitivities are obtained. Then, antibiotic therapy is tailored to cover the offending organisms. In noninfected cases, prophylactic antibiotics (usually a first-generation cephalosporin) are administered at the time of surgery and continued for 48 hours afterward.

Psychologic effects: The psychologic impact of lower extremity amputation must be addressed. In the postoperative period, grief is the most common emotion expressed. Concerns regarding body image, possible loss of functional independence, and ability to continue with the present job play an important role in adjusting to the loss of a limb. Proper guidance and support by the medical staff are extremely important.

POSTOPERATIVE COMPLICATIONS

IN THE HOSPITAL

Wound necrosis: Insufficient arterial circulation, excessive local pressure, hematoma formation, or skin closure under tension account for most cases of wound necrosis. Small areas of necrosis often heal by secondary intention with local wound care and dressing changes. Flap revision or more proximal amputation may become necessary for the treatment of larger areas of necrosis, especially in patients with poor vascularity.

Joint contracture: Joint contracture is best prevented by early physical therapy and proper positioning. Knee flexion contractures greater than 15 degrees and hip flexion contractures greater than 25 degrees make conventional prosthetic fitting difficult. Severe joint contractures may require serial manipulations and plaster cast applications or surgical releases.

Wound infection: The risk of infection is increased in patients with vascular insufficiency, diabetes, or previous distal infection. Wound débridement, irrigation, and appropriate antibiotic coverage are the usual treatment, although revision of the amputation to a more proximal level is sometimes necessary.

Pulmonary embolism: Deep venous thrombosis and thromboembolism are potential threats to elderly, partially immobilized patients undergoing lower extremity surgery. Prophylaxis with heparin or warfarin (Coumadin) may be appropriate.

AFTER DISCHARGE

Persistent stump edema: Persistent stump edema is one of the most common reasons for delay in permanent prosthetic fitting. The best treatment is prevention through the use of elastic compression dressings or a rigid cast.

Phantom limb sensation: Phantom limb sensation is a nonpainful awareness of the amputated limb. This sensation lasts a variable amount of time and may be permanent in some patients. Patients should be reassured that this is a normal phenomenon and that no specific treatment is necessary.

Phantom pain: Phantom pain occurs in 2% to 10% of adults and is described as burning, cramping, or shooting pain in the amputated limb. The disorder is more common in women and has been reported to occur more frequently in patients who had pain in the limb before surgery. Organic causes such as neuroma, compartment syndrome, and infection should be ruled out. Treatment is individualized, and potentially useful techniques include trigger point injections, paralumbar sympathetic blocks, nerve stimulation, and psychotherapy.

Skin problems: Abrasion of the skin from excessive local pressure or blisters from friction between the skin and the prosthesis may be managed by providing local skin care and temporarily discontinuing use of the prosthesis. Areas of local pressure should be treated by redistributing the pressure over a larger area of the skin through modification of the prosthetic socket liner.

Contralateral limb: Patients with poor vascularity have a 15% to 33% chance of requiring contralateral lower extremity amputation within 5 years. Proper preventive care should be given to their contralateral limbs.

BIBLIOGRAPHY

Bodily KC, Burgess EM. Contralateral limb and patient survival after leg amputation. Am J Surg 1983;146:280–282.

Chapman MW, Madison M. Operative orthopaedics, vol 1. Philadelphia, JB Lippincott, 1988:603–615.

Crenshaw AH. Campbell's operative orthopaedics, ed 8, vol 2. St Louis, CV Mosby, 1992:689–710.

Evarts CM. Surgery of the musculoskeletal system, ed 2, vol 5. New York, Churchill Livingstone, 1990:5121–5161.

Volpicelli LJ, Chambers RB, Wagner FW Jr. Ambulation levels of bilateral lower extremity amputees: analysis of one hundred and three cases. J Bone Joint Surg Am 1983;65:559–605.

Medical Management of the Surgical Patient, Third Edition,
edited by Michael F. Lubin, H. Kenneth Walker, and Robert B. Smith III.
J.B. Lippincott Company, Philadelphia, PA © 1995.

CHAPTER

104

SURGICAL PROCEDURES FOR RHEUMATOID ARTHRITIS

John Gray Seiler III
Sam Nasser

Progressive joint destruction is a characteristic finding in patients with rheumatoid arthritis. The primary indication for surgery in these patients is relief of pain caused by the inflammatory process. Improvement in function also is generally achieved. Operative procedures commonly performed include the following:

- Total joint arthroplasty (joint replacement) of the hip, ankle, shoulder, elbow, wrist, and certain joints of the hand
- Excisional arthroplasty of the metacarpophalangeal, metatarsophalangeal, distal radioulnar, and radiohumeral joints
- Arthrodesis of the spine, ankle, knee, wrist, and hand joints
- Soft tissue procedures to rebalance joints and to débride inflammatory synovium: correction of boutonniére and swan-neck deformities in the fingers and crossed intrinsic transfers in the hand, carpal tunnel release, tendon repairs, and tendon transfers, as well as synovectomy on any joint to débride inflammatory tissue (often resulting in temporary suppression of the disease process)

The surgical stress involved is related to the magnitude of the specific procedure performed. Because multiple surgical procedures are done at the same time in many cases, general anesthesia may be preferred. If a single extremity procedure is planned, however, a regional anesthetic is favored. The length of the procedure also influences the choice of anesthesia. Primary operations usually last no more than 2 to 3 hours, whereas complex revision procedures frequently last 6 hours or more.

Extremity operations performed on joints distal to the shoulder and hip are usually done under tourniquet control, and transfusions are not necessary. Patients undergoing total hip and shoulder replacements may require two or more units of blood or blood products. Donation of autologous blood in anticipation of this need is highly recommended. Typically, two units of autologous blood are stored in coordination with the hospital blood bank or the Red Cross.

Before problems of the appendicular skeleton are addressed, attention should be directed to evaluation of the cervical spine.

A careful general physical examination, including a detailed neurologic examination, should be performed. Preoperative radiographs of the cervical spine, including flexion and extension views, often provide useful information. If significant cervical instability or vertebrobasilar invagination is noted, preoperative consultation with a spine surgeon should be obtained. In addition, multiple levels of spontaneous cervical fusion may occur. In both these situations, the anesthesiologist should be consulted before the operation to prepare for fiberoptic methods of awake intubation.

The staging of operative procedures depends on the specific nature of the joint involvement and pain pattern in affected patients. Generally, operations on the upper extremities are performed after correction of lower extremity problems. The use of canes and crutches during rehabilitation from lower extremity total joint replacement may cause substantial stress on the hands and arms.

In the lower limb, foot and ankle problems should be addressed first to provide a good base of support for the limb during subsequent rehabilitation. This may not require surgical treatment but simply appropriate modification of footwear or bracing. Hip arthroplasty should be performed before knee surgery, not only to facilitate rehabilitation but because knee pain may often be referred from the hip joint. Although bilateral knee arthroplasty during the same period of anesthesia has been shown to be safe and often advantageous, bilateral total hip replacement surgery has an increased complication rate. If severe contracture deformities exist, ipsilateral hip and knee arthroplasty may be indicated.

In the upper limb, patients with significant symptoms in the ipsilateral shoulders and elbows should have the more symptomatic joints addressed at the initial procedure. Either joint may be replaced, with the second procedure done in about 3 months. In general, operations on the wrist should precede operations on the metacarpophalangeal joints. The occasional patients who have primary involvement of the metacarpophalangeal joints should receive initial treatment of those joints. We do not recommend that reconstructive procedures for the metacarpophalangeal joints be performed at one operative procedure.

USUAL POSTOPERATIVE COURSE

Expected postoperative hospital stay: The expected postoperative hospital stay after major joint reconstruction procedures is 7 to 10 days. Compared to patients with other conditions who are undergoing the same procedures, patients with rheumatoid arthritis usually do not require longer hospitalization after upper extremity procedures but may stay longer after lower extremity procedures because of difficulty with physical therapy.

Operative mortality: Under 0.3%

Special monitoring required: Some cases of spinal instrumentation involve the use of intraoperative somatosensory evoked potentials. The general conditions of the patients may necessitate intensive care monitoring during the initial 24 to 48 hours after surgery.

Patient activity and positioning: The postoperative position and level of activity are related to the type of surgical procedure performed. Typically, total shoulder and total elbow arthroplasty require only the use of a sling for a short period. These patients are encouraged to be out of bed the day after surgery. Early and intensive involvement of well-trained occupational and physical therapists is essential to obtaining optimal results.

After hip arthroplasty, an abduction pillow or knee immobilizer is used to help prevent dislocation. Daytime use of these devices generally can be discontinued when patients have regained sufficient muscle control to assist with positioning, but some type of abduction should be maintained at night for about 6 weeks. Total knee replacements should be splinted with a knee immobilizer or other appropriate brace until patients have regained some degree of muscle control of the operated limb, both for comfort and to protect against falls. The use of continuous passive motion after knee arthroplasty has gained considerable popularity, but its timing, duration, and even efficacy are open to debate.

Alimentation: There are no special dietary requirements.

Antibiotic coverage: The administration of first-generation cephalosporin is recommended as prophylaxis for patients with rheumatoid arthritis who are undergoing joint arthroplasty procedures, especially those involving prosthetic replacements. The antibiotic is given just before the procedure is begun and then every 6 hours afterward for 24 to 48 hours or until the drains are removed. For revision procedures, prophylactic antibiotics are not administered until intraoperative cultures have been obtained. During the operation, the wounds are irrigated with an antibiotic solution, typically one containing bacitracin at a concentration of 50,000 U/L.

Corticosteroid therapy: Patients with chronic suppression of the hypothalamic-pituitary-adrenal axis from oral corticosteroid therapy are given intravenous corticosteroids during the perioperative period. One hundred milligrams of intravenous hydrocortisone is given before the procedure, followed by appropriate dosages afterward. Intravenous steroids usually are tapered over a 3-day period until patients are able to resume their usual doses of prednisone

Special care: Procedures involving reconstruction of the hand and wrist often require prolonged periods of splinting and strict compliance with occupational therapy protocols to obtain optimal results.

POSTOPERATIVE COMPLICATIONS

IN THE HOSPITAL

Infection: Wound infection usually presents 5 to 7 days after surgery. Because affected patients are often receiving immunosuppressive agents (antimetabolites, corticosteroids), obvious clinical manifestations of wound infection may be absent and the wound should be observed carefully during the postoperative period. The development of a postoperative infection requires incision and drainage in the operating room. Intraoperative cultures should be obtained and appropriate intravenous antibiotics administered.

Acute adrenal insufficiency: Surgical stress, trauma, or infection may precipitate addisonian crisis in patients with adrenal insufficiency. Because of the potentially severe nature of this condition, initial treatment is begun based on a working diagnosis made from a constellation of signs and symptoms. Patients typically have hypotension, hyperthermia, weakness, nausea, and vomiting. Laboratory testing reveals hyponatremia, hyperkalemia, an elevated blood urea nitrogen level, and a diminished hematocrit. The glucose level is low or normal. The urine sodium concentration is greater than 20 mEq/L, and the plasma cortisol level is low. The treatment of acute adrenal insufficiency requires intravenous glucocorticoid replacement, volume replacement, blood pressure support, and, if infection is suspected, the administration of intravenous antibiotics.

Delayed wound healing: Because of the poor quality of collagen in the skin, periarticular tissues, and bone, postoperative healing may be slowed in patients with rheumatoid arthritis. Therefore, suture removal is delayed longer than customary and the wound is inspected regularly for signs of necrosis or hematoma.

AFTER DISCHARGE

Postoperative fractures: Osteoporosis makes patients with rheumatoid arthritis susceptible to postoperative fractures, especially because the operative procedures may alter mechanical relationships and alignment and may weaken specific areas of bone.

Loosening of the prosthesis: Among patients with total joint replacement, prosthetic loosening is more likely to occur in those with rheumatoid arthritis because of associated osteoporosis. Pain is the usual symptom of loosening.

Disease progression: Both surgeons and patients must bear in mind that operative procedures do not cure the underlying disease process but simply palliate some of its complications. Eventually, progression of the systemic disease may alter the surgical result unfavorably.

BIBLIOGRAPHY

Hollander JL, ed. Arthritis and allied conditions, ed 8. Philadelphia, Lea & Febiger, 1972.

Millender LH, Sledge CB. Symposium on rheumatoid arthritis. (Foreword) Orthop Clin North Am 1975;6:601–602.

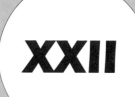

NEUROSURGERY

Medical Management of the Surgical Patient, Third Edition,
edited by Michael F. Lubin, H. Kenneth Walker, and Robert B. Smith III.
J.B. Lippincott Company, Philadelphia, PA © 1995.

CHAPTER

INTRACRANIAL ANEURYSM SURGERY

105

Daniel L. Barrow
Javier Garcia-Bengochea

Intracranial aneurysms are a relatively common disorder found in 2% to 5% of the general population at autopsy. It is estimated that about 20% of these aneurysms become symptomatic, and 25,000 cases of subarachnoid hemorrhage (SAH) resulting from aneurysm rupture occur each year in the United States. Cerebral aneurysms typically are "berry" aneurysms with a well-defined neck and sac distinct from the lumen of the parent vessel, as opposed to the fusiform aneurysms that are encountered in the extracranial peripheral vasculature. Although the etiology of cerebral aneurysms is undetermined, they are thought to arise from defects in the muscularis media, which may be congenital or acquired. Unruptured aneurysms are believed to bleed at a cumulative rate of 3% per year from the time of diagnosis. About 40% to 50% of patients die within the first 2 weeks as a result of the initial hemorrhage, and 35% of those who survive succumb to subsequent hemorrhages in the ensuing 6 months if they do not receive treatment. Thereafter, the risk of rebleeding is once again 3% per year.

The most common presentation of intracranial aneurysms is rupture that results in SAH with or without an intracerebral hematoma or intraventricular blood. Intracranial aneurysms usually come to clinical attention between the fifth and seventh decades of life, and there is a slight female predominance. Less often, aneurysms may exert a mass effect because of their location or size. A common ex-

ample is an aneurysm of the posterior communicating artery that, by virtue of its intimate relationship with the oculomotor nerve, may expand and compress the nerve, resulting in a partial or complete oculomotor nerve deficit. Rarely, a large aneurysm may accumulate thrombus, causing embolization and cerebral infarction. The clinical features of SAH are sudden onset of a severe headache, usually described as the worst headache of the patient's life, often associated with nausea, vomiting, and transient loss of consciousness. In as many as 40% of cases, there may be a history of minor rupture or symptoms referable to the aneurysm.

After the initial history and physical examination have been conducted, a computed tomographic (CT) scan without intravenous contrast is obtained to confirm the diagnosis of SAH or intracerebral hematoma. The results of CT scanning may be negative in 5% to 10% of cases, and these patients require lumbar punctures. Xanthochromia of the cerebrospinal fluid may appear within 6 hours after the hemorrhage and is the hallmark of SAH. Four-vessel cerebral angiography is then performed to identify the aneurysm responsible for the hemorrhage and to search for multiple aneurysms, which occur in about 20% of cases.

Therapeutic intervention is dictated by the clinical conditions of the patients as assessed by the classification of

Hunt and Hess, which grades the severity of meningism and decreasing level of consciousness, both of which may be correlated with surgical outcome. Patients who are not stuporous or who have an intraparenchymal hematoma creating a mass effect are candidates for immediate operation. Otherwise, surgery may be delayed for about 2 weeks until cerebral edema has subsided, patients have stabilized medically, or hydrocephalus, if present, has been treated. The decision regarding timing of surgery is individualized.

The two major potential complications of aneurysmal SAH are rebleeding and cerebral arterial vasospasm. The incidence of rebleeding is estimated to be 4% in the first 24 hours and 1.5% per day over the next 14 days. The risk of rebleeding is decreased by prompt and definitive clip ligation of the aneurysm. Vasospasm usually occurs between 4 and 10 days after SAH and becomes clinically apparent as cerebral ischemia in 30% to 40% of patients during this period, manifested by a decrease in the level of consciousness followed by neurologic deficits that may ultimately result in death. Patients with CT evidence of diffuse SAH in the basal cisterns or major cerebral fissures are at high risk for the development of vasospasm and should be treated accordingly. Antifibrinolytic agents, once used to reduce the risks of rebleeding, accelerate ischemic deficits caused by vasospasm and are no longer used in most patients. Vasospasm is treated by the deliberate inducement of hypertension and by hypervolemic hemodilution in an effort to increase cerebral blood flow. In patients with unclipped aneurysms, this treatment may cause second SAHs. Nimodipine, a selective cerebral calcium channel antagonist that may improve long-term outcomes in patients at risk for vasospasm by reducing the ischemic penumbra through improved collateral circulation, is given intravenously or orally for 3 weeks. Focal vasospasm in the major cerebral arteries may be treated by transluminal cerebral angioplasty in specialized centers, with resultant dramatic clinical improvements in many cases.

During the operative procedure, furosemide, mannitol, and hyperventilation are used to reduce brain size and minimize retraction injury to the brain. Direct surgical obliteration of the aneurysm is accomplished by microsurgical dissection of the aneurysm and its parent vessels. An occlusive clip is then placed across the neck or base of the aneurysm. In the past, hypotensive anesthesia was used to reduce intraluminal pressure during dissection of the aneurysm and thereby decrease the risk of intraoperative rupture. This technique has fallen out of favor, however, and moderate hypertension with temporary clips is more commonly used during critical stages of dissection.

An intraoperative angiogram is performed at many centers to confirm adequate clip placement before closure; otherwise, angiography is performed before patients are discharged from the hospital.

USUAL POSTOPERATIVE COURSE

Expected postoperative hospital stay: 1 to 2 weeks

Operative mortality: The operative mortality rate ranges from 1% to 8%, usually related to patients' preoperative conditions.

Special monitoring required: Intensive care unit observation is necessary, with frequent assessment of vital signs, neurologic status, central venous pressure readings, intake and output, and cardiac monitoring for 48 to 72 hours. If vasospasm is present, 10 to 14 days in the intensive care unit may be required.

Patient activity and positioning: Initially, the head of the bed should be elevated 30 degrees. Patients may get out of bed as soon as possible. If physical therapy is needed, it should be started soon after surgery.

Alimentation: Food intake should be advanced as tolerated. Nasogastric tube feedings may be given if patients are unable to eat or require supplementation.

Antibiotic coverage: No antibiotic coverage is needed.

POSTOPERATIVE COMPLICATIONS

IN THE HOSPITAL

Development of a focal neurologic deficit: The development of a focal neurologic deficit may be related to edema, contusion, or infarction from brain retraction, or to damaged intracranial vessels or nerves. Mannitol or hyperventilation may be required to prevent progressive deterioration or control neurologic deficits. Cerebral vasospasm causing decreased cerebral perfusion can also produce a focal neurologic deficit. If this is suspected, hypervolemic hemodilution treatment should be instituted immediately and a cerebral angiogram obtained to confirm the diagnosis and evaluate for possible transluminal angioplasty.

Subdural or epidural hematoma: Subdural or epidural hematomas can occur after any craniotomy but can be prevented by meticulous intraoperative hemostasis.

Acute hydrocephalus: Intraventricular or subarachnoid blood may prevent either normal circulation or the resorption of cerebrospinal fluid, resulting in acute hydrocephalus. This usually is evident before operation, although only 20% of patients require ventricular cerebrospinal fluid diversionary shunt procedures.

Syndrome of inappropriate secretion of antidiuretic hormone: The syndrome of inappropriate secretion of antidiuretic hormone develops occasionally. The resultant hyponatremia can be associated with an alteration in mentation or with seizures. Fluid restriction usually corrects the problem.

AFTER DISCHARGE

Seizures: Phenytoin is prescribed to prevent seizures for 1 year after operation if the surgeon thinks it advisable.

BIBLIOGRAPHY

Heros RC, Kistler JP. Intracranial arterial aneurysm: an update. Stroke 1983;14:628–631.

Hunt WE, Hess RM. Surgical risk as related to time of intervention in the repair of intracranial aneurysms. J Neurosurg 1968;28:14–20.

Kassell NF, Boarini DJ, Adams HP, et al. Overall management of ruptured aneurysm: comparison of early and late operation. Neurosurgery 1981;9:120–128.

Ojemann RG, Heros RC, Crowell RM, eds. Intracranial aneurysms and subarachnoid hemorrhage: incidence, pathology, clinical features and perioperative management. In: Surgical management of cerebrovascular disease, ed 2. Baltimore, Williams & Wilkins, 1988:147–162.

Winn HR, Richardson AE, Jane JA. The long-term prognosis in untreated cerebral aneurysms. II. Late morbidity and mortality. Ann Neurol 1978;4:418–426.

Medical Management of the Surgical Patient, Third Edition,
edited by Michael F. Lubin, H. Kenneth Walker, and Robert B. Smith III.
J.B. Lippincott Company, Philadelphia, PA © 1995.

CHAPTER

106

SURGERY FOR SPINAL TUMORS

Nelson M. Oyesiku
Roy A.E. Bakay

Spinal tumors may involve the spinal cord, spinal canal, or contiguous structures. These tumors may be classified by their location within the spinal cord as intradural or extradural (Table 106-1). Intradural tumors may be further classified as intramedullary (within the spinal cord) or extramedullary (outside the spinal cord).

INTRADURAL TUMORS

INTRAMEDULLARY

Ependymomas and astrocytomas are the two most common subtypes of intramedullary intradural tumors. Spinal cord ependymomas are twice as common as astrocytomas. Ependymomas usually occur at the cauda equina. Intramedullary tumors are insidious lesions, and their clinical course is variable. Initially, patients may have no symptoms; as the tumors enlarge, segmental dissociated sensory deficits, long tract signs, or weakness may occur. These features make it difficult to distinguish intramedullary tumors from other spinal lesions. Although they are an unusual cause of scoliosis, progressive scoliotic deformity is frequently the first indication of a spinal cord tumor in children.

EXTRAMEDULLARY

Most extramedullary intradural tumors are benign, slow-growing lesions that occur in the fourth to sixth decades of life. Meningiomas and neurilemomas are the most common subtypes. Two thirds of spinal meningiomas are located in the thoracic region, and the lesions occur mostly in women (4:1). They are usually located ventral or lateral to the spinal cord.

Neurilemomas (spinal nerve schwannomas and neurofibromas) usually originate from the dorsal root and may enlarge the foramen and grow into the paraspinal tissues, resulting in a dumbbell-shaped tumor. Unlike meningiomas, they have an equal sex frequency and are uniformly distributed along the spinal canal.

Extramedullary tumors are often in anatomic relation to a nerve root and commonly present with nocturnal radicular pain and dysesthesias. More rostral lesions located near the foramen magnum may present with suboccipital or neck pain and neurologic deficit in the upper extremities. Larger lesions may cause eccentric cord compression and the Brown-Séquard syndrome.

EXTRADURAL TUMORS

Most extradural tumors are malignant and occur in patients with systemic cancer. There is a slight male preponderance, and affected patients generally are in their 60s to 80s. Malignant tumors reach the spine by direct extension or hematogenous spread. The thoracic spine is most commonly involved.

Pain is the initial symptom in 95% of patients; it may be localized or radicular. The pain is relieved by bed rest and aggravated by axial loading or movement. Unfortunately,

TABLE 106–1. Common Spinal Tumors by Location

Location	Common Tumors	Frequent Symptoms
Intradural		
Intramedullary	Ependymomas, astrocytomas	Insidious onset of subtle sensorimotor symptoms and sphincter abnormalities
Extramedullary	Neurilemomas, meningiomas	Nocturnal radicular pain and dysesthesias
Extradural	Metastases, lymphomas	Back pain relieved by lying down

diagnosis is usually delayed until paresis or sphincter dysfunction occurs.

DIAGNOSIS

Magnetic resonance imaging (MRI) with gadolinium enhancement is the study of choice and has supplanted myelography and computed tomographic (CT) scanning. The rostral-caudal extent of the tumor is easily defined by MRI without the need for myelography. MRI also differentiates spinal tumors from nonneoplastic lesions such as syringomyelia and multiple sclerosis. Consequently, the need for diagnostic biopsy has decreased significantly. Furthermore, intramedullary tumors are better visualized with MRI than with other modalities; some tumors, such as lipomas and epidermoids, even have characteristic MRI appearances.

CT is the study of choice for evaluating vertebral bone destruction. CT of the spine combined with contrast enhancement can demarcate the cross-sectional extent of the tumor.

Plain radiographs of the spine may show osteolytic changes in metastatic disease (lung, breast, and kidney) or myeloma, bony erosion with slowly growing tumors, or osteoblastic changes with carcinoma of the prostate and lymphoma. Intraspinal tumors (ependymomas or astrocytomas) may cause interpediculate widening. Enlarged foramina usually indicate a neurofibroma or, less frequently, a meningioma. Rarely, spinal angiography is indicated to exclude a vascular malformation or to plan surgery. Other considerations in the differential diagnosis include spondylosis, herniated disk, hemangioma, syringomyelia, and inflammatory lesions.

TREATMENT

The location of the tumor and the clinical condition of the patient are the two most important factors in determining the goals of surgery and the surgical approach.

Virtually all intradural tumors require surgical treatment. Preoperative treatment with high-dose glucocorticoids is usually required in the form of dexamethasone, 10 mg intravenously or by mouth. Perioperative antistaphylococcic coverage is also given.

Approaches to the spine may be anterior, anterolateral, posterior, or posterolateral, depending on the location of the tumor. In the more common posterior approach, patients are positioned prone on the operating table. A midline skin incision and a regional laminectomy are required to expose the thecal sac. The further course of the operation depends on whether the lesion is intradural or extradural. For intradural lesions, the dura is opened and retracted. Microsurgical dissection, coaxial illumination, ultrasonic guidance probes and aspiration devices, and surgical lasers have enhanced the surgical options for treating tumors within and around the spinal cord. Evoked response monitoring is used to assess long tract function during surgery but its value is controversial.

Intramedullary tumors are usually localized with ultrasound imaging, then a myelotomy is made to expose the lesion. Ependymomas are generally well-defined and more amenable to gross excision than are astrocytomas, which tend to be infiltrating and ill-defined. Adjunctive radiotherapy is usually required for virtually all astrocytomas and for ependymomas with subtotal resections.

To prevent recurrence, meningiomas can be completely removed if the dural attachment is included in the resection. Excision of neurofibromas frequently requires sacrifice of the involved nerve root. A watertight dural closure is important to prevent cerebrospinal fluid leaks.

Indications for surgery in spinal metastases include symptomatic neural compression, instability, progressive deficit despite radiotherapy, neurologic deterioration after maximal radiotherapy, uncertain diagnosis, and recurrent tumor. Current techniques in spinal stabilization provide surgical options for patients with spinal metastases.

Prognostic factors in patients with spinal metastases include tumor histology and pretreatment neurologic status. About 35% of patients with paraparesis and less than 20% of those with paraplegia regain ambulation.

USUAL POSTOPERATIVE COURSE

Expected postoperative hospital stay: Patients usually remain hospitalized for 1 to 2 weeks after surgery. Those who undergo more extensive resections and those who are debilitated can expect more prolonged courses.

Operative mortality: Operative mortality should be minimal except in patients with middle to upper cervical tumors, in whom quadriparesis and respiratory difficulties may arise. Intubation for 24 to 72 hours may be required to ensure an adequate airway.

Special monitoring required: In the early postoperative period, frequent neurologic examinations are necessary to detect deterioration. Patients with severe functional deficits before operation are unlikely to achieve significant improvements.

Patient activity and positioning: A gradual increase in activity and physical therapy are begun as soon as possible to expedite recovery.

Alimentation: No dietary restrictions are required.

Antibiotic coverage: No antibiotic coverage is recommended.

Pain: Acute postoperative pain is treated by a short course of narcotic or nonsteroidal antiinflammatory medication.

Managing prolonged recumbency: Respiratory care is important to prevent atelectasis and pneumonia, especially for patients with prolonged recumbency because of paresis. Pneumatic compression stockings and low-dose heparin are useful in preventing deep venous thrombosis in these patients.

Orthotic devices: Orthotic devices are usually fitted in the hospital, and patients are advised regarding their proper use and care.

Radiotherapy: If radiotherapy is required, it is delayed until the wound is healed.

POSTOPERATIVE COMPLICATIONS

IN THE HOSPITAL

Epidural hematoma: An epidural hematoma may cause spinal cord compression and neurologic deficit in the early postoperative period. Radiologic evaluation by MRI or myelography can identify the lesion. Prompt evacuation is usually required.

Infection: Meningitis is uncommon but superficial or deep wound infections may occur. Reoperation may be required to evacuate a purulent collection. Antibiotics are tailored to the infecting organism.

Cerebrospinal fluid leak: Cerebrospinal fluid leaks are more common in the upper thoracic region. Treatment may involve diversion of cerebrospinal fluid by a lumbar subarachnoid drain or revision of the wound.

Neurologic deterioration: Operative manipulation may cause neural injury or edema resulting in a deficit. The treatment of direct injury depends on the elements involved and the extent of their involvement. Spinal cord edema can be treated with dexamethasone.

AFTER DISCHARGE

Chronic deafferentation pain: The syndrome of chronic deafferentation pain is poorly understood and notoriously difficult to treat.

Spinal instability or deformity: Spinal instability or deformity is a late complication seen after extensive cervical laminectomies and facetectomies, most commonly in children. Operative correction is usually successful.

Cerebrospinal fluid leak: Treatment of cerebrospinal fluid leaks is as outlined earlier.

Neurologic deterioration: Late neurologic deterioration is usually the result of tumor recurrence or complications of radiotherapy.

BIBLIOGRAPHY

Cooper PR. Outcome after operative treatment of intramedullary spinal cord tumors in adults: intermediate and long-term results in 51 patients. Neurosurgery 1989;25:855–859.

Harrington KD. Anterior decompression and stabilization of the spine as a treatment for vertebral collapse and spinal cord compression from metastatic malignancy. Clin Orthop 1988;233:177–197.

Levy WJ, Latchaw J, Hahn JF, et al. Spinal neurofibromas: a report of 66 cases and a comparison with meningiomas. Neurosurgery 1986;18:331–334.

Lunardi P, Missori P, Gagliardi FM, et al. Long-term results of the surgical treatment of spinal dermoid and epidermoid tumors. Neurosurgery 1989;25:860–864.

Siegal T, Siegal T. Current considerations in the management of neoplastic spinal cord compression. Spine 1989;14:223–228.

Sorensen PS, Borgesen SE, Rasmusson B, et al. Metastatic epidural spinal cord compression: results of treatment and survival. Cancer 1990;65:1502–1508.

Sundaresan N, DiGiacinto GV, Hughes JEO, et al. Treatment of neoplastic spinal cord compression: results of a prospective study. Neurosurgery 1991;29:645–650.

Sundaresan N, Schmidek HH, Schiller AL, et al. Tumors of the spine: diagnosis and clinical management. Philadelphia, WB Saunders, 1990.

Medical Management of the Surgical Patient, Third Edition,
edited by Michael F. Lubin, H. Kenneth Walker, and Robert B. Smith III.
J.B. Lippincott Company, Philadelphia, PA © 1995.

CHAPTER

107

CRANIOTOMY FOR BRAIN TUMOR

Jeffrey J. Olson
Andrew Reisner

A myriad of new diagnostic systems and innovative surgical and adjuvant treatments have contributed to the improved morbidity and mortality of patients with brain tumors. Despite these advances, the prime component of almost all therapeutic strategies remains craniotomy with tumor resection. Determination of the need for a craniotomy is based on the suspected tumor pathology; the patient's age, neurologic status, and overall health status; and the relationship of the lesion to eloquent structures of the brain.

The radiographic features of a brain tumor are usually sufficiently specific to proceed with a craniotomy in most cases. It may be impossible to exclude mass lesions that would not ordinarily be treated with a craniotomy, however, such as cerebral infarction, multiple sclerosis, and viral infections. In addition, there are cases of suspected brain tumor in which a craniotomy may not be appropriate treatment. In these cases, stereotactic biopsy is invaluable because it provides a definitive pathologic diagnosis with far less risk to patients than craniotomy. Stereotactic biopsy is purely diagnostic, though, and does not allow tumor resection.

Once the decision is made to perform a craniotomy, the surgeon uses the information obtained from the diagnostic tests to plan the operative approach so as to obtain maximum access to the tumor at minimal risk to the patient. Corticosteroids usually are administered preoperatively to reduce tumor-associated or traumatic brain edema caused by

the surgery. Anticonvulsants are given if patients are at high risk for postoperative seizures. A central venous pressure line, an arterial line, and a Foley catheter are inserted before final operative positioning. Pneumatic stockings are placed to reduce the incidence of venous thrombosis. A spinal drain may be inserted to allow cerebrospinal fluid (CSF) drainage during the operation. Once patients are fully anesthetized, they are carefully positioned on the operating tables with their heads turned and firmly secured in a manner that affords the best exposure of the tumor. Patients who are placed in the sitting position are additionally monitored with a precordial Doppler stethoscope to detect air emboli.

The cranium is entered through bur holes, which are connected with a craniotome. The cranial bone flap is elevated from the field, and epidural hematomas are prevented by securing the exposed dura to the periphery of the skull defect with tack-up sutures. A bulging or tense dura, indicative of raised intracranial pressure, is a common finding in patients with brain tumors. This is treated with elevation of the head to promote venous drainage, hyperventilation to reduce intracranial blood volume, or mannitol infusion to reduce the brain turgor. The dura is then incised and an incision is made in the pia-arachnoid overlying the brain. A path is developed through the brain to the tumor if it is not externally visible. A deep-seated tumor may be localized with intraoperative sonography or stereotaxis. Once the tumor is encountered, tissue samples are submitted for frozen section to provide tumor confirmation and to narrow the differential diagnosis of the type of tumor. This is one of several factors that are important in deciding how extensive the resection should be. Other parameters include the site of the tumor, the age and condition of the patient, and the efficacy of alternate treatment options. The tumor is then partially or completely resected by a variety of sharp and blunt dissection techniques, aided by the surgical laser and ultrasonic aspirator, when appropriate. When the resection is complete, hemostasis of the tumor bed is obtained, the dura is closed, and the bone flap is sutured to the surrounding skull defect. The stress of the procedure is moderate, and blood transfusion may be required.

USUAL POSTOPERATIVE COURSE

Expected postoperative hospital stay: 7 to 10 days

Operative mortality: The operative mortality rate depends on the size and type of the tumor and the condition of the patient but usually is under 5%.

Special monitoring required: The first 2 days after surgery are spent in the intensive care unit. Intracranial pressure monitoring or ventriculostomy may be used during this time.

Patient activity and positioning: Bed rest is necessary until patients are fully conscious. The level of activity is then increased as tolerated. Physiotherapy, speech therapy, and occupational therapy are instituted, if required.

Alimentation: A full, regular diet is provided as soon as possible. Cough and gag reflexes must be present to prevent aspiration.

Antibiotic coverage: Typically, intravenous antibiotics are given immediately postoperatively and then for 24 hours.

Medications: The corticosteroid dosage is tapered on an individual basis, and the administration of anticonvulsants is continued as indicated for tumor type.

POSTOPERATIVE COMPLICATIONS

IN THE HOSPITAL

Hemorrhage: Hemorrhage is a potentially life-threatening complication that usually results from bleeding from the tumor bed and can lead to the formation of an intracerebral hematoma. Because the tumor-associated blood vessels are abnormal, hemostasis is more difficult to achieve than with normal brain tissue. In addition, bleeding may occur into the subdural, epidural, or subgaleal spaces. Systemic hypertension may be a precipitating factor. An intracranial pressure monitor allows early detection of unfavorable changes.

The diagnosis is confirmed by computed tomographic scan, and selected hematomas may require surgical evacuation.

Infection: Infections may be deep or superficial; septic contamination may give rise to cerebritis, intracerebral abscess, meningitis, bone flap infection, or subdural or epidural empyema. All are serious complications. Treatment is enhanced by identification of the offending organism through microbiologic culture and drug sensitivity tests. Appropriate antibiotics always are administered and localized infections are drained surgically.

Cerebral edema: Swelling of the brain may be a function of the brain tumor itself or result from surgical manipulation of the brain tissue. The swollen brain exerts a mass effect that may compromise vital brain stem centers. This is usually well seen on a computed tomographic scan. Treatment includes the use of corticosteroids, hyperventilation, mannitol, and furosemide.

Cerebral infarction: Interruption of the arterial blood supply kills the brain tissue in that particular distribution. The clinical effects are largely dependent on the region that is compromised. It is potentially lethal when the arterial supply to the brain stem is jeopardized. An extensive infarction may occur as a result of venous occlusion, because the venous tributaries typically drain large areas of the brain. Aggravating factors include a low cerebral perfusion pressure, a high hematocrit level, and poor blood oxygenation. Careful control of blood pressure, volume status, and oxygenation are maintained before and after surgery to minimize these factors.

Seizures: Tumors that invade the cerebral cortex and cortical surgical scars are potentially epileptogenic. A seizure that occurs in the immediate postoperative period may raise the intracranial pressure. Therefore, anticonvulsants are routinely administered before surgery as a safeguard. The duration of anticonvulsant therapy is variable and partly dependent on tumor location and pathology. If patients have experienced seizures or are at high risk for them, the medication may be continued indefinitely.

Associated fluid and electrolyte imbalances: Brain tumors adjacent to the hypothalamus and pituitary gland pose special problems, with fluid and electrolyte balances related to the abnormal secretion of antidiuretic hormone. Excessive or insufficient amounts of antidiuretic hormone may result in the syndrome of inappropriate antidiuretic hormone or diabetes insipidus, respectively. These states are managed by a variety of drugs, hormone replacement, or strict fluid control.

Cerebrospinal fluid leaks: The creation of a fistula from the CSF space is of special concern when the paranasal sinuses or ear spaces are breached; this may result in CSF rhinorrhea or otorrhea, respectively. Treatment consists of elevation of the head of the bed, serial spinal taps, continuous

CSF drainage, and, in recalcitrant cases, surgical oblitera-tion of the fistula.

AFTER DISCHARGE

Hydrocephalus: Ventricular enlargement may result from the obstruction of CSF flow along intracerebral pathways (noncommunicating hydrocephalus) or from the obstruc-tion of CSF outflow at the level of the venous sinuses (com-municating hydrocephalus) by tumor, hemorrhage, or sur-gical scars. Placement of a ventriculoperitoneal shunt is the treatment of choice.

Tumor recurrence: Highly malignant tumors inevitably recur despite the use of adjuvant therapies. The most reli-able prognostic indicator of tumor recurrence is the histo-logic type and grade of the tumor at initial presentation. On occasion, a second craniotomy for resection of the tumor re-currence may be considered.

BIBLIOGRAPHY

Cushing H. Intracranial tumors: notes upon a series of two thou-sand verified cases with surgical-mortality percentages pertaining thereto. Springfield, IL, Charles C Thomas, 1932.

Rosenblum ML. The role of surgery in the management of brain tumors. Neurosurg Clin North Am 1990;1.

Russell DS, Rubinstein LJ. Pathology of tumors of the nervous system, ed 5. Baltimore, Williams & Wilkins, 1989.

Salcman M. Neurobiology of brain tumors. In: Wirth FP, Ratche-son RA, eds. Concepts in neurosurgery, vol 4. Baltimore, Williams & Wilkins, 1991.

Schmidek HH, ed. Meningiomas and their surgical manage-ment. Philadelphia, WB Saunders, 1991.

Walters CL, Schmidek HH. Surgical management of intracranial gliomas. In: Schmidek HH, Sweet WH, eds. Operative neurosurgi-cal techniques: indications, methods and results, vol 1. Philadel-phia, WB Saunders, 1988:431–450.

Medical Management of the Surgical Patient, Third Edition,
edited by Michael F. Lubin, H. Kenneth Walker, and Robert B. Smith III.
J.B. Lippincott Company, Philadelphia, PA © 1995.

CHAPTER

108

TRANSSPHENOIDAL SURGERY

George T. Tindall
C. Michael Cawley

Transsphenoidal surgery, originally described by Schloffer in 1907, remains the preferred mode of surgical therapy for most pituitary tumors. Tumors of this region are the most common cause of clinicopathologic syndromes related to the sella, the pituitary gland, and all the surrounding structures, including the optic nerves and chiasm and the cavernous sinus. Tumors of the pituitary generally present with clinical findings related to an endocrinopathy or a mass effect.

Patients with endocrinopathy often have syndromes related to functional secretory pituitary adenomas. The most commonly encountered of these are the Forbes-Albright syndrome (amenorrhea–galactorrhea) from hyperprolactinemia, acromegaly from excessive growth hormone, and Cushing's disease from excessive adrenocorticotropic hormone resulting in hypercortisolism. Patients with symptoms of a mass effect usually are found to have disturbances of visual acuity, visual field defects (bitemporal hemianopsia), cranial nerve palsies, hypopituitarism, headaches, and, rarely, obstructive hydrocephalus or hypothalamic dysfunction. Although any tumor may grow to cause a mass effect, most of those causing mechanical compression are hormonally inactive and, thus, have escaped earlier detection.

Once a diagnosis has been made by clinical examination, various laboratory tests, and modern neuroimaging techniques (most often magnetic resonance imaging), several therapeutic options are available. These include pharmacotherapy, radiotherapy, and surgery. Pharmacotherapy has become an increasingly potent therapeutic option for several of the most common secretory pituitary tumors. Bromocriptine (Parlodel or Pergolide), a dopamine agonist, has been used effectively in the treatment of prolactin-secreting adenomas for more than 10 years. Although the drug has been shown to lower serum prolactin levels and decrease tumor size, it does have certain drawbacks. Bromocriptine shrinks and controls most prolactin-secreting tumors but does not eradicate them. It is tumoristatic, not tumoricidal. If therapy is withdrawn, the tumor returns to its original size. Thus, therapy with bromocriptine has to be continued for life. Another disadvantage of bromocriptine is that it causes fibrosis within the tumor and reduces considerably the cure rate of subsequent surgery (from 80% to 44%) if patients take the drug for more than 1 year.

Bromocriptine has also been used with some success to treat acromegaly caused by growth hormone–secreting adenomas; however, a new somatostatin analogue (octreotide) shows more promise. Octreotide has proved to be effective in lowering growth hormone levels and ameliorating many features of acromegaly. Because significant clinical experience has yet to be accumulated with this therapy, we still recommend surgery in most cases. Major drawbacks to the use of this drug include its expense and dosing schedule (subcutaneously two or three times a day).

Many drugs have been used to treat Cushing's disease, with variable results. In the past, these have included adrenal toxins, serotonin agonists, and dopamine agonists, none of which proved effective. Recently, the antifungal agent ketoconazole has shown some efficacy. Once again, clinical experience with this drug in the treatment of Cushing's disease is limited, and surgery is recommended for proven pituitary-based hypercortisolism.

Radiotherapy has been used widely in the treatment of pituitary tumors for many years. Conventional external-beam therapy found its most useful role as an adjunct to operative or medical therapy. Recent advances in pharmacotherapy and surgical techniques, as well as the recognition of a relatively high incidence of radiation damage to surrounding structures, have led to a decrease in the use of conventional radiation. Generally accepted indications for conventional radiotherapy are now limited to the treatment of recurrent growth hormone or nonsecretory tumors and large tumors invading anatomic structures such as the cavernous sinus. Focused radiation has shown some efficacy in the treatment of pituitary tumors and has proven to be a viable option for pituitary ablation. Good results have been reported in the treatment of acromegaly, Cushing's disease, Nelson's syndrome, and hyperprolactinemia. Drawbacks to radiosurgery include a significant incidence of hypopituitarism and serious damage to surrounding structures such as the optic chiasm, brain stem, and medial temporal lobes because of the high doses of radiation delivered. In addition, this mode of therapy can only be used in tumors that are relatively small and clearly separated in space from delicate surrounding structures. We recommend the use of radiosurgery only as an adjunct to surgical or medical therapy, and even then only in certain circumstances.

Once it has been ascertained that surgery is the most appropriate therapeutic course, a frontotemporal, subfrontal, subtemporal, or transsphenoidal approach to the region of the sella must be selected. Most tumors of the pituitary region can be treated by a transsphenoidal surgical approach. Indications for transsphenoidal surgery include (1) functional intracellular microadenomas for which pharmacotherapy is undesirable or ineffective; (2) infrachiasmatic macroadenomas and other tumors of the pituitary region exhibiting a mass effect that are not amenable to pharmacotherapy; (3) tumors associated with cerebrospinal fluid rhinorrhea; (4) tumors with extension into the sphenoid sinus or bone; (5) cerebrospinal fluid fistulas involving the sphenoid sinus; and (6) biopsy and excision of any lesion in the sphenoid and parasellar areas, including chordoma, nasopharyngeal carcinoma, and sphenoid mucocele or abscess.

The transsphenoidal approach is contraindicated in patients with infectious processes involving the sphenoid sinus, suprasellar masses associated with a normal sella turcica, or "bottleneck" connections between intrasellar tumors and the dumbbell-shaped suprasellar extensions.

Transcranial approaches are usually preferred in patients with significant intracranial extension of pituitary tumors to the subfrontal, retrochiasmatic, or middle fossa regions.

In the past, the transsphenoidal approach was commonly used to perform pituitary ablation, or hypophysectomy. These procedures were carried out in an attempt to relieve pain or to obtain remission from disseminated hormonally active cancers such as those of the breast and prostate. With earlier diagnosis, improved chemotherapeutic agents such as tamoxifen and cisplatin, and improved radiotherapy, the indications for hypophysectomy have almost vanished. The advent of laser photocoagulation in the treatment of diabetic retinopathy has eliminated the role of pituitary ablation in arresting the progression of that condition. The only condition in which hypophysectomy is now indicated is recurrent, refractory Cushing's disease in which a previous transsphenoidal operation revealed a microadenoma.

Transsphenoidal surgery is generally well tolerated in the treatment of pituitary tumors, many of which occur in young patients who are otherwise healthy. General anesthesia is required and the supine position is used. The duration of the procedure ranges from 1 to 3 hours, depending on the size of the tumor and the experience of the surgeon. Previously, a sublabial gingival incision was made to achieve transsphenoidal exposure, but more recently, an endonasal, unilateral transseptal incision has been used to expose the sphenoid sinus and sella. A second incision is usually made in the left lower quadrant of the abdomen for harvesting of fat used to pack the surgical site after the tumor is resected. One unit of blood is ordinarily available for transfusion, but is rarely used.

USUAL POSTOPERATIVE COURSE

Expected postoperative hospital stay: 4 to 6 days

Operative mortality rate: Under 0.5%

Special monitoring required: Intensive care unit observation is required for at least 1 day, with particular attention to fluid balance.

Patient activity and positioning: Coughing, sneezing, and blowing the nose are discouraged. A nasal decongestant is usually prescribed as needed to treat symptoms of congestion.

Alimentation: Clear liquids are permitted the evening of surgery, and food intake is advanced as tolerated.

Antibiotic coverage: Although we do not routinely use prophylactic antibiotics, some neurosurgeons recommend their use.

Corticosteroid therapy: Patients are treated with perioperative corticosteroids (hydrocortisone) to protect against the possibility of adrenal insufficiency as a result of pituitary manipulation. Supplemental steroid therapy is continued until the second postoperative day and then tapered over the next 4 days. Continuation of steroid therapy beyond this point is determined by evidence of residual adrenal axis suppression. This condition should be suspected in patients with persistent headaches and lethargy, and may be confirmed with a morning cortisol measurement taken 24 hours after the last hydrocortisone dose. Corticotropin deficiency should be diagnosed if the serum cortisol level is less than 3 µg/dL and assumed if it is less than 3 to 9 µg/dL. In either case, patients are discharged from the hospital receiving hydrocortisone and return for rapid corticotropin tests 1 month after surgery. If the cortisol level is greater than 9 µg/dL, patients are discharged without further tests or treatment.

POSTOPERATIVE COMPLICATIONS

IN THE HOSPITAL

Persistent diabetes insipidus: Persistent diabetes insipidus must be expected in patients whose urinary outputs exceed 300 mL/h and whose urine specific gravity levels are less than 1.010. The diagnosis is confirmed by measurement of serum sodium (over 146 mEq/L), serum osmolality (over 300 mOsm/L), and urinary osmolality (under 100 mOsm/L). Treatment consists of intramuscular or subcutaneous aqueous vasopressin (Pitressin; 5 U is the usual adult dose), which may be repeated as needed until patients' antidiuretic hormone–secreting mechanisms recover. If this condition persists, intranasal desamino D-arginine vasopressin (DDAVP) may be administered after discharge from the hospital.

Cerebrospinal fluid rhinorrhea: Cerebrospinal fluid rhinorrhea is an uncommon complication seen generally in patients who have undergone hypophysectomy. It can be treated successfully by lumbar punctures or, rarely, reoperation. If the condition is left untreated, meningitis may result.

AFTER DISCHARGE

Delayed cerebrospinal fluid leak: A delayed cerebrospinal fluid leak requires readmission to the hospital for lumbar puncture, lumbar drainage, or reoperation.

Acute or chronic adrenal insufficiency: Failure to take maintenance medications or to increase the dosage during periods of illness or stress may lead to acute or chronic adrenal insufficiency.

BIBLIOGRAPHY

Laws ER, Kern EB. Complications of transsphenoidal surgery. Clin Neurosurg 1976;23:401–416.

Tindall GT, Barrow DL. Disorders of the pituitary. St Louis, CV Mosby, 1986.

Tindall GT, Barrow DL. Tumors of the sellar and parasellar area in adults. In: Youmans JR, ed. Neurological surgery. Philadelphia, WB Saunders, 1990:3447.

Watts NB, Tindall GT. Rapid assessment of corticotropin reserve after pituitary surgery. JAMA 1988;259:708–711.

Medical Management of the Surgical Patient, Third Edition,
edited by Michael F. Lubin, H. Kenneth Walker, and Robert B. Smith III.
J.B. Lippincott Company, Philadelphia, PA © 1995.

CHAPTER

109

VENTRICULAR SHUNT FOR HYDROCEPHALUS IN CHILDREN

Mark S. O'Brien
Andrew Reisner

Hydrocephalus is defined as a condition in which there is a disproportionately large ventricular cerebrospinal fluid (CSF) volume in relation to the total cranial volume. This may or may not be associated with intracranial hypertension, a pathologic state typified by raised intracranial pressure (ICP). Both conditions are manifestations of heterogeneous central nervous system pathologies and, thus, are not in themselves pathognomonic of any specific disease entity. The etiologies of these conditions are multifactorial and encompass congenital, neoplastic, infectious, traumatic, endocrinologic, and iatrogenic causes. Despite the initial insult, the treatment of all children with hydrocephalus or intracranial hypertension is based on similar clinical and surgical tenets.

The natural history of progressive hydrocephalus is well documented. About half of all untreated patients die as a direct result of hydrocephalus. Of the remainder, about 85% have varying cognitive and neurologic abnormalities at follow-up examinations. Therefore, therapeutic intervention is warranted in most cases. There are selected instances when medical treatment of hydrocephalus is appropriate. Numerous drugs have been investigated as treatment agents for hydrocephalus, including those that decrease brain water content or increase CSF absorption, such as carbonic anhydrase inhibitors, mannitol, isosorbide, and urea. These drugs are used in patients who are at high surgical risk and in those who have temporary hydrocephalus. In most cases, however, surgical CSF diversion is the treatment of choice for hydrocephalus.

The chief clinical manifestation of hydrocephalus is macrocephaly. Young children are prone to develop an enlarged head because the cranial vault bony sutures do not fuse until about 10 years of age. In older children and adults, progressive ventricular dilation remains uncompensated by an increase in head size and signs and symptoms of raised ICP ensue more rapidly. Headaches, early morning nausea and vomiting, "sunset" eyes, papilledema, focal neurologic signs, and obtundity are characteristic of intracranial hypertension.

In contemporary neurosurgical practice, ventriculography has been rendered obsolete by neuroimaging technologies such as computed tomography and magnetic resonance imaging, techniques that have become indispensable in the diagnosis and monitoring of patients with hydrocephalus. The surgical indications for hydrocephalus include failed medical treatment, progressive ventricular dilation, and intracranial hypertension. The CSF is usually diverted from the ventricles. There are two types of ventricular shunt procedures: external and internal. External ventricular drainage is used when emergent reduction in ICP is necessary or internal shunt placement is not feasible. External CSF drainage is appropriate in the clinical settings of intracranial hypertension of acute onset, meningitis, or a bleeding diathesis that prohibits more extensive surgery.

External ventricular shunt placement is usually a temporizing procedure and may be performed under local anesthesia. Internal ventricular shunt insertion is performed using general anesthesia and is the definitive surgical treatment of hydrocephalus.

Both external and internal ventricular shunts require the placement of a catheter into the ventricular system of the brain. The ventriculostomy is usually inserted in those areas where the CSF spaces are most capacious, namely the frontal and posterior parietal regions. The right side is preferred because it is usually the nondominant hemisphere and the risk of damage to speech-related areas of the brain is reduced. If the ventricles are asymmetric, the ventriculostomy is inserted into the larger one; in patients in whom the CSF spaces do not communicate, more than one ventriculostomy may be required.

After the skin incision is made, the skull is opened through a bur hole and the underlying dura is incised. A small catheter (about 1.5 mm in diameter) is advanced through the brain substance until a subtle "give" is felt, indicating transition from the brain tissue to the fluid-filled ventricle. Once there is a flow of CSF, the ICP is measured with a manometer and a specimen of CSF is routinely collected for bacteriologic analysis. Correct placement of the ventricular catheter may be confirmed by an intraoperative air ventriculogram. The distal end of the shunt system is then placed in a region to which the CSF is diverted, usually the peritoneal cavity or cardiac atrium. The advantages of peritoneal over atrial placement are as follows: (1) it is technically easier to perform; (2) a longer length of distal catheter may be placed, prolonging the interval for revision; (3) vascular and cardiopulmonary complications may be prevented; and (4) the distal tract is not sacrificed by the child outgrowing the shunt.

Contraindications to a ventriculoperitoneal shunt include peritonitis, peritoneal tumors, a scarred abdomen from previous surgery, and the presence of an enteral stoma. Indirect right atrial placement through the jugular vein, intrapleural placement, and direct atrial placement by thoracotomy are used in that order of preference if intraperitoneal placement cannot be performed. The proximal and distal ends are connected by shunt tubing placed under the skin. A valve is interposed to prevent excessive drainage of CSF with a resultant siphon effect.

In the case of external shunts, the distal end of the tubing is externalized through a separate incision in the scalp and attached to a sterile CSF collection bag. The pressure of CSF outflow may be measured by a simple manometer or electronic pressure transducers. The volume of outflow, and thus the ICP, can be controlled by varying the resistance in the system, which is most easily accomplished by adjusting the relative height of the drainage bag to the patient's head. External ventricular drainage offers the additional advantage of affording easy access to the CSF pathway. This portal may be used to obtain serial fluid samples for diagnostic purposes or to instill drugs directly into the brain. The major encumbrances of external ventricular drainage are restricted patient mobility because of the external shunt components and an infection rate that increases with time. For these reasons, the ventricular drain is either removed or converted to an internal shunt as soon as feasible.

USUAL POSTOPERATIVE COURSE

Expected postoperative hospital stay: Patients are hospitalized overnight if no concomitant problems arise.

Operative mortality: Under 1%

Special monitoring required: The usual pediatric parameters should be monitored, including temperature, intraoperative P_{CO_2} for interpretation of ICP, and intraoperative fluoroscopy for confirmation of catheter placement.

Patient activity and positioning: Patients usually are ambulatory on the first postoperative day. In neonates, pressure on the scalp overlying the shunt system should be avoided by preventing the child from lying on that side of the head and by using a sheepskin pad.

Alimentation: The usual oral feedings are resumed on the day of operation.

Antibiotic coverage: Nafcillin, 25 mg/kg intravenously, is administered at the time of anesthesia induction and every 6 hours for four doses after the operation.

POSTOPERATIVE COMPLICATIONS

IN THE HOSPITAL

Focal neurologic deficits: Ventricular catheters are, by necessity, placed through the brain substance. Usually, this passage is innocuous, with no clinical sequelae. The danger of traumatizing sensitive areas of the brain exists, however. Hemiparesis can be prevented by placing the bur hole either anterior or posterior to the motor region. Similarly, the visual cortex and perisylvian speech areas of the dominant lobe should be avoided.

Seizures: The frequency of seizures in patients with shunted hydrocephalus is higher than in patients with untreated hydrocephalus. This may be the result of cortical injury with ventriculostomy insertion. It is reported to be higher with shunts placed in the frontal regions than with those placed in the parietal areas. Prophylactic anticonvulsant treatment is not indicated, and each case should be assessed and managed individually.

AFTER DISCHARGE

Shunt malfunction: The overall incidence of shunt malfunction is 30%. In the pediatric group, the most frequent cause is proximal catheter obstruction by choroid plexus, ependymal, or glial tissue. Other causes of malfunction are disconnections of the shunt tubing at any point in the system. There is a limit to the amount of catheter that can be inserted into a child's peritoneum, and this length of tubing may be pulled out of the peritoneum with normal growth. The treatment is revision of the malfunctioning components.

Shunt infection: Meticulous aseptic surgical techniques and the use of prophylactic antibiotics have reduced the infection rate to under 5% in major pediatric centers. The most common offending organism is *Staphylococcus epidermidis*. Treatment consists of removal of the entire shunt system; placement of a new, temporary external ventriculostomy; and institution of an appropriate intravenous antibiotic regimen. Once the CSF is sterile, an internal ventricular shunt is reinserted.

Subdural hematoma after shunt placement: The incidence of subdural hematoma after shunt placement is under 3%. This complication is prevented by limiting the amount of CSF that escapes after the proximal catheter is inserted and by using a pressure valve to prevent "overshunting." Small subdural hematomas may reabsorb spontaneously but larger ones require a subdural shunt.

Complications unique to ventriculoperitoneal shunts: Complications unique to ventriculoperitoneal shunts include ascites, pseudocyst formation, viscus perforation, intestinal obstruction, and hernias.

Complications unique to ventriculoatrial shunts: Vascular thrombosis, cardiac arrhythmias, and endocarditis are complications seen only with ventriculoatrial shunts.

BIBLIOGRAPHY

Drake JM, Martin AJ, Henkleman RM. Determination of cerebrospinal fluid shunt obstruction with magnetic resonance phase imaging. J Neurosurg 1991;75:535–540.

Epstein F, Lapras C, Wisoff JH. "Slit-ventricle syndrome": etiology and treatment. Pediatr Neurosci 1988;14:5–10.

Oi S, Matsumoto S, Katayama K, Mochizuki M. Pathophysiology and postnatal outcome of fetal hydrocephalus. Child Nerv Syst 1990;6:338–345.

Scott RM. Hydrocephalus. In: Wirth FP, Ratcheson RA, eds. Concepts in neurosurgery, vol 3. Baltimore, Williams & Wilkins, 1990: 115–121.

Medical Management of the Surgical Patient, Third Edition,
edited by Michael F. Lubin, H. Kenneth Walker, and Robert B. Smith III.
J.B. Lippincott Company, Philadelphia, PA © 1995.

CHAPTER

110

TREATMENT OF HERNIATED DISK

Suzie C. Tindall

CERVICAL LEVEL

The excision of herniated nucleus pulposus in the cervical region is indicated in patients who have neck and radicular arm pain; reflex loss, motor weakness, or sensory changes in a specific nerve root distribution; and radiographic defects on magnetic resonance imaging scans or myelograms or computed tomographic scans consistent with the clinical findings. Patients should have received adequate trials of conservative therapy, including cervical collars, cervical traction, local heat, and muscle relaxants.

Either a posterior or an anterior surgical approach to the lesion may be made. For both, endotracheal anesthesia is used, the operation lasts 1 to 2½ hours, and blood transfusion is rarely required. Results are generally excellent: about 90% of properly selected patients should achieve complete symptomatic improvement.

For the posterior approach, patients are placed prone. Through a midline incision, the paravertebral musculature is dissected away to expose the facet. A foraminotomy is done to expose the nerve root and the soft disk fragment is extracted through an incision in the bulging annulus.

For the anterior approach, patients are placed supine. A small incision is made from the midline to the anterior border of the sternocleidomastoid muscle at the appropriate level and dissection proceeds through the fascial plane, separating the trachea and carotid sheath. The esophagus is retracted and the desired interspace is visualized after separa-

tion of the longus colli muscles. Radiographic confirmation of the correct interspace is obtained and the anterior longitudinal ligament is incised. The disk material is removed using a variety of instruments, including a curette, a Kerrison punch, pituitary forceps, and a high-speed drill. Bony fusion or placement of metallic plates for stabilization may be performed at the surgeon's discretion.

USUAL POSTOPERATIVE COURSE

Expected postoperative hospital stay: 3 to 5 days

Operative mortality: Rare

Special monitoring required: No special postoperative monitoring is required.

Patient activity and positioning: Bed rest is necessary for 12 to 24 hours, followed by progressive ambulation. If a bony fusion has been performed, radiographic confirmation of the bone graft position should be obtained before ambulation is allowed. A cervical collar may be worn.

Alimentation: Food intake is advanced as tolerated.

Antibiotic coverage: Antibiotic coverage is provided at the discretion of the surgeon.

Follow-up: In the case of anterior fusion, follow-up radiographic studies are obtained at 8 weeks. Patients should avoid physical labor, strenuous exercise, or activities predisposing to flexion–extension stresses on the neck for 8 weeks.

POSTOPERATIVE COMPLICATIONS

In the Hospital

Damage to the nerve root or spinal cord from excessive manipulation: When the operation is performed by an experienced surgeon, damage to the nerve root or spinal cord from excessive manipulation is rare.

Inability to obtain good decompression of the nerve root or spinal cord: The surgeon may be unable to obtain good decompression of the nerve root or spinal cord because of the presence of a spondylitic ridge or bar, or pathology that extends too far medially.

Postoperative neck pain from paravertebral muscle spasm: Paravertebral muscle spasm may cause bothersome postoperative neck pain but this generally can be well controlled with analgesics and muscle relaxants.

Intraoperative hemorrhage: Intraoperative hemorrhage usually is caused by dissection that extends too far laterally, resulting in injury to the vertebral artery. A postoperative arteriovenous fistula is possible if the complication is not recognized and properly corrected.

Postoperative wound hematoma: A postoperative wound hematoma should be evacuated immediately because of the possibility of airway obstruction.

Perforation of the pharynx or esophagus: If perforation of the pharynx or esophagus is recognized during the disk procedure, the damaged structure should be repaired and the operation terminated.

Damage to the recurrent laryngeal nerve: Temporary or permanent hoarseness may result from damage to the recurrent laryngeal nerve.

Injuries to the nerve root or cord: Injuries to the nerve root or cord usually are attributable to technical error and are rare with an experienced surgeon.

After Discharge

Disk space or bone graft infection: If disk space or bone graft infections occur, the grafts should be removed and patients treated with traction and appropriate antibiotics.

Extrusion of the bone graft, avascular necrosis, or pseudarthrosis: If bone graft extrusion, avascular necrosis, or pseudarthrosis occurs, treatment includes traction in the supine position and resection and replacement of the graft. Because failure of fusion is much more common in patients

who smoke, many surgeons require that patients quit smoking before they undergo a fusion procedure.

THORACIC LEVEL

Thoracic disk protrusion is unusual. Because of the small diameter of the thoracic spinal canal and the vulnerability of the thoracic cord to traction injury, surgical removal of the disk is usually performed through a costotransversectomy or anterior thoracotomy approach. Conventional laminectomy for a proven, symptomatic thoracic disk herniation is not recommended.

With the advent of magnetic resonance image scanning, thoracic disk herniation is much easier to recognize and the cause of previously unexplained intercostal neuralgias is more easily discerned. Surgical decision making has become more difficult under these circumstances. Because any operation for a thoracic disk herniation is a relatively large undertaking that virtually always leads to significant long-term incisional discomfort, most candidates for surgery should have both pain and neurologic deficits before surgery is considered.

LUMBAR LEVEL

Excision of a herniated nucleus pulposus at the lumbar level is indicated in patients with low back and radicular sciatic leg pain associated with the following:

- Findings on neurologic examination consistent with single nerve root involvement, such as a diminished or absent Achilles or patellar jerk or weakness in the musculature innervated by a specific root
- Positive mechanical signs, including radicular pain with straight-leg raising, pain with opposite-leg raising, and pain on popliteal compression
- Failure to respond to conservative treatment, including bed rest, the use of a lumbosacral corset, and the use of a bed board, heat, analgesics, and muscle relaxants
- Positive results on computed tomographic scanning or myelography showing a defect consistent with the findings on neurologic examination

The procedure is an emergency in patients who have massive midline protrusions with compression of the cauda equina resulting in motor and sensory paresis and loss of sphincter control.

General endotracheal anesthesia is used. Patients are placed prone on supports or in a modified knee–chest position. Through a midline incision over the involved interspace, the paraspinous musculature is retracted to expose the laminal arches laterally to the articular facets. A partial hemilaminectomy is performed, the nerve root is gently retracted medially, the disk fragments are removed, and the disk space is emptied and curetted to loosen and remove degenerated and abnormal disk material. Blood loss should be minimal and transfusion is rarely necessary. The operating microscope may be used at the discretion of the surgeon, thus limiting the size of the incision and the amount of bone removed—a procedure sometimes called a *microdiskectomy*. In experienced hands, the operative results of a standard, conventional lumbar disk operation are as follows: 80% to 85%, good to excellent; 14%, fair; and 5%, no improvement.

USUAL POSTOPERATIVE COURSE

Expected postoperative hospital stay: 2 to 5 days
Operative mortality: Rare
Special monitoring required: No special monitoring is required.
Patient activity and positioning: Bed rest and narcotic analgesic agents are required for 6 to 12 hours after operation, followed by gradual ambulation and reduction in the analgesic dosage. After discharge from the hospital, only bed rest and house activities are permitted for the first 2 weeks, office work is allowed after 2 to 4 weeks, and physical labor can be resumed in 3 months.
Alimentation: Postoperative food intake is permitted as tolerated.
Antibiotic coverage: Antibiotic coverage is provided at the discretion of the surgeon.

POSTOPERATIVE COMPLICATIONS

In the Hospital

Muscle spasms: Muscle spasms are transient and easily controlled with narcotic analgesic agents and muscle relaxants.
Urinary retention in men: Urinary retention may occur in men but usually resolves with ambulation.
Direct surgical injury to neural elements: Surgical trauma may involve nerve root injury or avulsion secondary to improper technique. Cerebrospinal fluid extravasation, fistula, or pseudomeningocele may occur after inadequate repair of a dural tear.

Injury to the great vessels in the pelvis: Piercing the annulus anteriorly with a curette is a technical error that may result in injury to the great vessels in the pelvis. Aortic, iliac, or vena caval injuries usually present with sudden hemodynamic shock at operation, but an iatrogenic arteriovenous fistula may not become apparent until the late postoperative period.

After Discharge

Recurrence of pain leading to reoperation: In 5% of patients, recurrent pain necessitating reoperation may result from inadequate removal of disk fragments, extrusion of more disk material on the same or opposite side, or disk rupture at another level.

Disk space infection: Disk space infection is a rare complication heralded by persistent back, abdominal, and groin pain 5 to 21 days after surgery in association with an elevated sedimentation rate. After 30 days, there is radiographic evidence of destruction of the opposing surfaces of the vertebral bodies, with eventual fusion. Aspiration of the interspace or reoperation with curettage may recover the responsible organism. Treatment involves immobilization and broad-spectrum antibiotic coverage.

Chronic adhesive arachnoiditis: The incidence of chronic adhesive arachnoiditis is not certain because many patients may be asymptomatic. Predisposing factors include not only the surgical procedure but the myelographic contrast agent.

BIBLIOGRAPHY

Gurdjian ES, Ostrowski AZ, Hardy WG, et al. Results of operative treatment of protruded and ruptured lumbar discs based on 1176 operative cases with 82 percent follow-up of 3 to 13 years. J Neurosurg 1961;18:783–791.

Mixter WJ, Barr JS. Rupture of the intervertebral disc with involvement of the spinal canal. N Engl J Med 1934;211:210–215.

Riley LH Fr, Robinson RA, Johnson KA, Walker AE. The results of anterior interbody fusion of the cervical spine: review of ninety-three consecutive cases. J Neurosurg 1969;30:127–133.

Semmes RE. Ruptures of the lumbar intervertebral disc: their mechanism, diagnosis, and treatment. Springfield, IL, Charles C Thomas, 1964.

Wilkins RH, Rengachary SS. Neurosurgery, vol III. New York, McGraw-Hill, 1985:2219–2271.

Medical Management of the Surgical Patient, Third Edition,
edited by Michael F. Lubin, H. Kenneth Walker, and Robert B. Smith III.
J.B. Lippincott Company, Philadelphia, PA © 1995.

CHAPTER

111

EVACUATION OF SUBDURAL HEMATOMAS

Austin R.T. Colohan
Ali F. Krisht

Subdural hematomas can be either acute or chronic. Acute hematomas occur in younger patients and often are related to head trauma. Spontaneous acute subdural hematomas are also common and usually develop in patients with diseases associated with vasculitis or in patients with bleeding disorders. They may also form as extensions of large intracerebral and subarachnoid hemorrhages. Neurosurgical intervention is almost always indicated. Through a craniotomy, the hematoma is evacuated and hemostasis is established.

Chronic subdural hematomas are more common in older patients. They develop gradually after a mild, usually unnoticed, head trauma. They can also occur in children as a complication of shunt surgery. By the time patients are seen, the hematomas are liquefied and can be evacuated readily through a bur hole. After evacuation of a subdural hematoma, the postoperative course can be smooth or extremely complicated.

USUAL POSTOPERATIVE COURSE

Expected postoperative hospital stay: The postoperative hospital stay is usually 3 to 5 days for patients with chronic subdural hematomas and 7 to 10 days for those with acute subdural hematomas, depending on the severity of the injury.

Operative mortality: Patient outcome after the evacuation of acute subdural hematoma has not changed significantly despite recent advances in medical care, largely because of the high incidence of associated severe head injury. The mortality rate varies between 35% and 50%. It may be as high as 65% in older patients and those with a poor level of consciousness, and as low as 9% in young, alert patients. Many survivors are disabled and cannot achieve a full functional state.

The outcome of patients with chronic subdural hematomas is much better. The overall mortality rate is about 10% and drops to 5% in patients who have a mild decrease or no decrease in the level of consciousness at the time of surgery. The functional recovery is good, and 75% of surviving patients resume usual daily activities.

Special monitoring required: Patients are kept in the intensive care unit during the first 24 hours after surgery, where their neurologic status is evaluated hourly and their vital signs (especially blood pressure) are monitored and managed closely. A longer stay may be necessary for patients with poor neurologic status and other associated medical problems. Intracranial pressure (ICP) should be monitored closely in patients with acute subdural hematomas and treated as necessary.

Patient activity and positioning: After the acute period, patients are transferred to regular hospital rooms. Their activity level is determined by their preoperative status but early

617

ambulation is recommended, with the aid of physical therapy if necessary. Comatose patients are usually placed on air mattresses and prescribed aggressive chest physiotherapy to prevent pressure sores and minimize pulmonary complications.

Alimentation: As intravenous fluids are gradually discontinued, an oral diet is resumed. Nasogastric feeding is started on the third postoperative day in comatose patients. Parenteral hyperalimentation may be needed in patients with ileus or associated bowel injuries.

Antibiotic coverage: Antibiotics are not routinely used except in wounds that were contaminated at the time of injury. In such cases, nafcillin, 1 g every 6 hours, is given during the perioperative period (usually for 24 hours).

Other drug therapy: Patients are given anticonvulsant therapy if seizures occur or if there is an associated brain contusion. Corticosteroids are not indicated unless the hematoma resulted from a tumor bleed or from vasculitis related to an autoimmune disease.

POSTOPERATIVE COMPLICATIONS

IN THE HOSPITAL

Immediate Postoperative Complications (0 to 48 Hours)

Increased intracranial pressure: The ICP may increase for several reasons. Removal of the hematoma may lead to swelling of the previously compressed brain. This swelling can be severe and life-threatening, especially when it occurs in a posttraumatically contused and injured brain. The ICP may also increase because of an intracerebral clot that expands after evacuation of the subdural hematoma. In addition, the hematoma itself may recollect. This is more common with hematomas that develop as a result of a bleeding disorder.

Increased ICP should be treated immediately. When a sizable intracranial clot is seen, surgical evacuation should not be delayed. ICP monitors are inserted in injured patients. In addition to monitoring the ICP, the catheters allow cerebrospinal fluid drainage if needed. Patients are intubated and hyperventilated, with the Pco_2 maintained between 26 and 28 mmHg. Mannitol is administered if the ICP remains elevated. It is given initially as a 1-g/kg bolus and then is maintained at a dosage of 0.5 g/kg every 4 to 6 hours, guided by ICP readings. Persistent elevation of the ICP despite these measures usually indicates a poor prognosis. Barbiturate coma has been used in this situation for cerebral protection but the efficacy of this treatment is not well established.

Recurrence of hematoma: Hematomas may recollect after the evacuation of both chronic and acute lesions. This may result from inadequate hemostasis at the initial surgery. It is also common with bleeding disorders. Therefore, all coagulation parameters should be evaluated, including platelet function and coagulation factors.

Late Postoperative Complications (2 to 14 Days)

Neurosurgical complications: Elevated ICP beyond the first 48 hours is most often encountered in hematomas associated with head injury. In these cases, the treatment plan is as outlined earlier. Hydrocephalus may also develop at this stage, especially after an associated subarachnoid hemorrhage. Clinically, the neurologic status worsens and patients become sleepier and less responsive. The computed tomographic scan is usually diagnostic and surgical intervention with a ventriculostomy or a ventriculoperitoneal shunt should not be delayed.

Nonneurosurgical complications: The nonneurosurgical complications that occur at this stage are the same as those seen after any other surgical procedure and include atelectasis, fever, pneumonia, and urinary tract and wound infections. In addition, injured patients are more prone to gastrointestinal bleeding and should be protected with antacids or H_2 blockers.

Electrolyte imbalances become symptomatic during this period. The most common disorder is a dilutional type of hyponatremia caused by the syndrome of inappropriate antidiuretic hormone secretion, which responds to water restriction. Cerebral salt wasting is another electrolyte imbalance that may occur at this stage. It usually responds to replacement of the lost, salt-rich fluid with isotonic or hypertonic infusions.

At this stage, attention should also be paid to the nutritional status. Patients who are unable to swallow or protect the airway should be given enteral nutritional support.

AFTER DISCHARGE

After hospital discharge, possible complications include hydrocephalus and seizure development. Recurrence of the hematoma is unlikely but still possible. If the initial injury involved a contaminated wound, a delayed presentation with headache and low-grade fever should raise the suspicion of a brain abscess, especially if there are associated signs and symptoms of increased ICP. A contrast computed tomographic scan is used to establish the diagnosis and drainage and excision of the abscess should be performed immediately.

BIBLIOGRAPHY

Haselsberger K, Pucher R, Auer LM. Prognosis after acute subdural or epidural haemorrhage. Acta Neurochir (Wien) 1988;90:111–116.

Jamieson KG, Yelland JDN. Surgically treated traumatic subdural hematomas. J Neurosurg 1972;37:137–149.

Mattle H, Kohler S, Huber P, et al. Anticoagulation-related intracranial extracerebral haemorrhage. J Neurol Neurosurg Psychiatry 1989;52:829–837.

Seelig JM, Becker DP, Miller JD, et al. Traumatic acute subdural hematoma: major mortality reduction in comatose patients treated within four hours. N Engl J Med 1981;304:1511–1518.

Tindall GT, Payne NS II, O'Brien MS. Complications of surgery for subdural hematoma. Clin Neurosurg 1976;23:465–482.

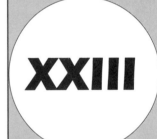
UROLOGIC SURGERY

Medical Management of the Surgical Patient, Third Edition,
edited by Michael F. Lubin, H. Kenneth Walker, and Robert B. Smith III.
J.B. Lippincott Company, Philadelphia, PA © 1995.

CHAPTER

112

MANAGEMENT OF UPPER URINARY TRACT STONES

Harry S. Clarke, Jr.

The last decade has seen the implementation of great technologic advances in both extracorporeal shock wave lithotripsy (ESWL) and endourologic instrumentation. The individual and combined application of these advances has decreased the use of open surgical procedures for the removal of renal calculi to under 1%.

Patients with upper urinary tract stones may have symptoms ranging from asymptomatic microscopic hematuria to severe obstruction requiring hospitalization. Indications for removal of a calculus include unresolving obstruction, decreased renal function, significant bleeding, persistent renal colic, and occupational risk (eg, airline pilot). The size of the stone is important because 80% of all stones measuring 4 mm or less pass spontaneously. Failure of a small stone to progress through the ureter and into the bladder is also an indication for treatment of a renal calculus. Patients with stones larger than 8 mm are candidates for interventional therapy, because only 20% of these calculi pass spontaneously.

The current mainstay in the treatment of both renal and ureteral calculi is ESWL. Numerous clinical series have documented the efficacy of this technique since it was first successfully performed by Chaussy and associates in 1980. The underlying principle of ESWL is that a high-energy amplitude of pressure (shock wave) can be generated in water by the abrupt release of energy in a small space. These sound waves are transmitted through the water and soft tissue with little attenuation because both materials have similar acoustic impedance. When the shock wave comes in contact with a calculus, which has a different density, a compression wave is produced along the anterior surface of the stone, causing it to crumble. As the shock wave traverses the stone to the posterior surface, more energy is reflected, creating stress and fragmentation along this surface. Repeated shock waves focused on the stone eventually reduce it to many small fragments that may be passed spontaneously. All lithotriptors have an energy source, a focusing device, a coupling medium, and a stone-localizing system. Newer devices usually do not require the use of general or regional anesthesia. In many cases, ESWL can be performed as an office procedure, making it both economical and convenient for patients.

The outcome of ESWL is influenced by the size, location, and composition of the calculus. As the volume of the calculus increases, the efficacy of ESWL diminishes significantly. It is for this reason that many clinicians advocate percutaneous nephrolithotripsy as an initial form of therapy for renal calculi exceeding 3 mL in volume. Stone location is also an important consideration. Stone-free success rates are lower after therapy for lower calyceal calculi than for middle or upper calyceal calculi or calculi in the renal pelvis. The success of ESWL monotherapy also decreases as stone hardness increases. More shocks at a higher intensity are required to adequately fragment calcium oxalate monohydrate and cystine stones than calcium oxalate, struvite, or uric acid stones. Pretreatment evaluation of stone composi-

623

tion allows for planned combination therapy with percutaneous nephrolithotripsy, as in the case of a large calcium oxalate monohydrate stone, or with chemolysis, as in the case of a cystine or struvite stone.

The experience with ESWL and its expanding role has redefined the role of percutaneous surgery. Percutaneous procedures are appropriate for many renal and ureteral stones. Patients with large stones or stones associated with obstruction and patients in whom ESWL is contraindicated (eg, because of body size) should be considered for percutaneous lithotripsy. The first use of a percutaneous tract specifically for the removal of a stone was reported in 1977. Since that initial report, the technique has evolved from simple stone extraction through the dilated tract to ureteroscopic fragmentation of stones. There are now three methods of stone fragmentation: ultrasonic, electrohydraulic, and laser lithotripsy. Ultrasonic lithotripsy through a percutaneous tract can be performed with either the 4.5F or 6F hollow probe. These hollow probes have the advantage of removing the stone debris by suction. If all three techniques are available, the ultrasonic probe is used for dense, hard stones, such as calcium oxalate monohydrate, brushite, or cystine calculi, which are more difficult to fracture using the less powerful electrohydraulic or laser lithotripsy.

The pulsed dye laser uses a coumarin green dye to produce laser light of 504 nm for a pulse duration of 1.2 microseconds. The power is adjustable but 60 millijoules per pulse is the recommended and currently allowable limit for lithotripsy. The primary advantage of the laser over the ultrasonic probe is its flexibility. It can be passed through the flexible nephroscope and, thus, reach stones located in posterior calyces other than the one through which the nephrostomy tract has been placed. A second advantage of the laser is that the discharge of energy from the laser directly adjacent to the pelvic and ureteral mucosa causes little or no damage.

Electrohydraulic lithotripsy is performed using flexible probes, which are available in 1.9F and 3F sizes. This technique causes a short-duration electrical discharge within a fluid medium, creating a high-pressure bubble of steam called a cavitation bubble. The expansion and subsequent contraction of this bubble creates a shock wave. Unlike the laser or ultrasound probes, with which the action takes place in contact with the stone, the action of electrohydraulic lithotripsy takes place before the stone with subsequent impaction of the shock wave. The resultant energy is 10 to 100 times that of the laser and injury is much more likely.

The use of percutaneous procedures in combination with ESWL to treat large staghorn calculi has resulted in a much higher stone-free success rate than can be obtained using ESWL alone (66% versus 15%). Studies are being conducted to identify the ideal treatment for all varieties of stones in the genitourinary system.

One other possible therapeutic approach is chemolysis, which involves the establishment of a percutaneous nephrostomy tube as well as a ureteral stent to allow unobstructed flow of an irrigating solution chosen specifically for the composition of the ureteral calculi. Stones composed of struvite, cystine, or uric acid are amenable to dissolution in hemiacidrin, acetylcysteine (Mucomyst), and tromethamine (THAM-E), respectively. The appropriate solution is infused in either an antegrade or a retrograde fashion with a system that is designed to prevent pressure increases greater than 20 cm H_2O. This is necessary to prevent the systemic absorption of the irrigating solution. Chemolysis can be used alone or in conjunction with ESWL. In the latter case, ESWL is performed first to create a greater surface area on which the chemolytic agents may act. Although many clinicians consider chemolysis to be cumbersome and time-consuming, its effectiveness should not be overlooked.

USUAL POSTOPERATIVE COURSE

Expected postoperative hospital stay: ESWL can be performed as an outpatient procedure or with an overnight stay in the hospital. Percutaneous procedures require 3 or 4 days of hospitalization.

Operative mortality: The operative mortality rate of ESWL is 0.01% (sepsis, cardiac arrest) and that of percutaneous procedures ranges from 0.01% to 1%.

Special monitoring required: The blood pressure and electrocardiogram should be monitored during ESWL. To prevent arrhythmias, the electrocardiogram is coupled to the lithotriptor and shock waves are fired during the R wave. For percutaneous procedures, electrolyte and blood urea nitrogen levels should be evaluated to assess the absorption of irrigating fluids and a chest radiograph should be obtained to detect possible pneumothorax from placement of the percutaneous tube.

Patient activity and positioning: The position of patients undergoing ESWL is dictated by the location of their stones. For percutaneous procedures, patients are placed in the supine position and the side undergoing the procedure is elevated as much as 30 degrees. Early ambulation is encouraged after both procedures.

Alimentation: Food intake is promptly advanced to a regular diet in the absence of nausea or ileus.

Antibiotic coverage: For patients without evidence of urinary tract infection, prophylactic oral antibiotics are administered 1 hour before ESWL is performed. Patients with infected urine or a known infected stone should receive intravenous antibiotics at least 24 hours and sometimes 48 hours before the procedure. Antibiotic therapy is continued after ESWL; if fever occurs, intravenous antibiotics are given for at least 24 hours after defervescence takes place and then oral antibiotics are administered. Prophylactic antibiotics are administered 1 hour before percutaneous procedures, which are classified as clean contaminated procedures. Again, if the urine is infected or the stone under treatment is infected, intravenous antibiotics should be administered for 24 to 48 hours before the procedure.

Drains: In patients undergoing ESWL, a ureteral catheter or double-J stent is usually placed for stones larger than 2 cm. Because the newer machines do not require anesthesia, fewer clinicians are placing stents of any kind for smaller stones. For percutaneous procedures, a nephrostomy tube as well as an antegrade ureteral catheter are left in position. If the stones are eliminated and there is no injury to the pelvis or the ureter, the nephrostomy tube is capped on the third or fourth postoperative day and removed the next day. The onset of pain or fever after the tube is capped requires the performance of a nephrostogram to assess for leakage or obstruction. Patients are discharged from the hospital if no pain or untoward symptoms occur after the tube is capped. A ureteral stent is left in place for 1 to 5 days, depending on the site of the stone and the amount of surgical trauma delivered to the ureter. The stent may have a string attached so that patients can remove it at home, or it can be removed in the physician's office.

POSTOPERATIVE COMPLICATIONS

IN THE HOSPITAL

Gross hematuria: Gross hematuria is seen uniformly during and immediately after an ESWL procedure and should clear within 12 to 24 hours. Flank hematoma may also occur and can be painful. All patients undergoing endourologic procedures have some amount of gross hematuria but hemorrhage requiring transfusion occurs in under 5%. Significant hemorrhage can occur from the nephrostomy tube tract. If this persists for more than several minutes, a Foley catheter should be placed through the tract and inflated with 1 to 3 mL of saline solution in the balloon. The outflow tube can subsequently be opened to drainage to assess for cessation of bleeding at hourly intervals. Bleeding from the percutaneous tract is usually self-limiting. Formation of an arteriovenous fistula may result from the placement of a percutaneous nephrostomy tract. This can usually be managed by angiographic embolization.

Fever: Fever is common with infected stones and should be treated with appropriate antibiotics and clinical assessment to ensure adequate drainage.

Stone fragments: ESWL treatment of stones larger than 1.5 to 2 cm usually results in the persistence of several stone fragments, which can cause subsequent obstruction of the ureter by piling up behind the large fragment, creating what is called *steinstrasse*. This can be prevented in most instances by preoperative placement of a ureteral catheter or double-J stent; if it occurs in the presence of a stent, it can be observed and subsequently passes spontaneously. If there is not a patent stent present, drainage must be established with either a percutaneous nephrostomy tube or passage of another stent in exchange for the obstructed stent. Treatment of the steinstrasse is usually achieved by ultrasonic lithotripsy of the lead fragment, allowing passage of the remaining fragments. Residual fragments also may be seen after percutaneous lithotripsy has been performed. Once the nephrostomy tract has been established, it can be reentered subsequently and the fragments removed using flexible ureteroscopy. The combined use of percutaneous procedures followed by ESWL has greatly reduced the number of residual stone fragments.

Pain: Pain is moderate after ESWL and is usually controlled by oral analgesics. Percutaneous procedures are somewhat more painful but also can usually be managed by oral analgesics.

Perforation of the collecting system: The collecting system may become perforated when stents are placed before ESWL in a system with an impacted stone and ureteral mucosa that is highly inflamed. The most vulnerable time for perforation is during placement of the percutaneous tube and subsequent dilation of the tract. Treatment in both instances involves adequate drainage of the collecting system with a percutaneous tube or stent until the urothelium is allowed to heal completely.

AFTER DISCHARGE

Subcapsular hematoma: Subcapsular hematomas can occur after both percutaneous procedures and ESWL but are rare and self-limiting. Computed tomographic scanning after ESWL invariably shows some fluid collection and edema surrounding the treated kidney. This resolves over time without intervention.

Late-onset hypertension: The development of hypertension has been reported after ESWL. This occurs in under 1% to 2% of cases and is being evaluated to determine its true relationship to the procedure.

Urinoma: Urinomas may be seen after percutaneous procedures in which perforation occurs with subsequent obstruction, usually by a retained stone fragment. This results in urinary extravasation into the retroperitoneum, with the formation of a urinoma. Treatment involves draining the collecting system with a percutaneous nephrostomy tube or stent until the urothelium heals and normal drainage is re-established.

Ureteral stricture: Ureteral stricture is rare. When it does occur, it usually appears late after scar formation and can best be delineated by an intravenous pyelogram. Most strictures occurring after percutaneous procedures or stent placement for ESWL can be managed by ureteral dilation.

Recurrent stone formation: Recurrent stone formation should be assessed with a thorough metabolic evaluation. Work-up for an anatomic abnormality should also be performed in an attempt to reduce the recurrence rate.

BIBLIOGRAPHY

Chaussy C, Schmiedt E, Jocham D, et al. First clinical experience with extracorporeally induced destruction of kidney stones by shock waves. J Urol 1982;127:417–420.

Dretler SP. Ureteral stone disease: options for management. Urol Clin North Am 1990;17:217–230.

Motola JA, Smith AD. Therapeutic options for the management of upper tract calculi. Urol Clin North Am 1990;17:191–206.

Segura JW. The role of percutaneous surgery in renal and ureteral stone removal. J Urol 1989;141:780–781.

Segura JW. Current surgical approaches to nephrolithiasis. Endocrinol Metab Clin North Am 1990;19:919–935.

Segura JW. Role of percutaneous procedures in the management of renal calculi. Urol Clin North Am 1990;17:207–216.

Medical Management of the Surgical Patient, Third Edition,
edited by Michael F. Lubin, H. Kenneth Walker, and Robert B. Smith III.
J.B. Lippincott Company, Philadelphia, PA © 1995.

CHAPTER

TRANSURETHRAL RESECTION OF THE PROSTATE

113

Niall T.M. Galloway

Transurethral resection (TUR) of the prostate is indicated for the treatment of bladder outflow obstruction resulting from benign or malignant enlargement of the prostate. Primary symptoms of outflow obstruction include hesitancy and slow flow. Irritative symptoms of frequency, urgency, and nocturia usually reflect bladder problems rather than obstruction but also may be present with obstruction. Chronic retention with overflow incontinence and upper tract damage is a rare, but classic, presentation. Acute retention of urine is common; not all patients need surgery, however, because retention may be transient and caused by factors other than outflow obstruction, such as neurogenic dysfunction. Nonsurgical treatment of such patients with intermittent catheterization is appropriate.

TUR is an endoscopic procedure with direct vision through the instrument or through video endoscopy using a camera and television screen. The resectoscope has an electrically heated wire loop for cutting strips of tissue from the prostate to open the channel for urine flow. The surgical landmarks of the ureteric orifices, bladder neck, and trigone are preserved proximally and the verumontanum (ejaculatory ducts) are preserved distally to prevent injury to the urethral sphincter.

The surgical stress is proportional to the duration of the operation and the size of the prostate resected. Resection usually takes no more than 1 hour, and this corresponds to 45 to 75 g of tissue resected. A spinal anesthetic is preferred to general anesthesia. The irrigating fluid used during transurethral prostatectomy is isosmotic but without elec-

trolyte. Inappropriate absorption of the fluid is possible, particularly if venous channels outside the prostatic capsule are opened during the resection. The resultant fluid shifts provoke minor agitation before other objective signs, and it is helpful to have patients awake. Blood transfusion is rarely required (under 1%); preoperative antibiotic coverage is indicated with agents that have activity against gram-negative organisms. Urine cultures should be done before surgery, particularly in patients who have indwelling catheters, to establish the sensitivity of organisms in the urine.

USUAL POSTOPERATIVE COURSE

Expected postoperative hospital stay: 2 to 4 days

Operative mortality: Operative mortality is under 1%. Risk factors include urinary retention with an indwelling catheter and urinary tract infection; a large prostate with an operation lasting more than 1 hour; and bleeding diathesis or the use of anticoagulants, including aspirin. Renal failure, liver disease, heart disease, and stroke are also associated with higher morbidity and mortality rates.

Special monitoring required: Hemoglobin and hematocrit, creatinine, electrolyte (particularly sodium), and osmolality levels should be monitored.

Patient activity and positioning: The lithotomy position is used for endoscopy. A special drape is available to allow

627

rectal access for manipulation of the prostate during the resection without contamination of the surgical field.

Alimentation: Food intake is permitted as tolerated after the procedure.

Antibiotic coverage: A preoperative antibiotic (a single dose of fluoroquinolone 1 hour before operation) is sufficient for patients who do not have positive urine culture results. If the urine is contaminated or there is an active urinary tract infection, antibiotic treatment should be initiated at least 24 hours before operation and continued for 3 to 5 days.

Instrumentation: A resectoscope of appropriate size for the urethra should be used. If necessary, urethral dilation or a urethrotomy may be performed.

Urodynamic pressure flow studies: Urodynamic pressure flow studies should be done if the clinical features are not typical of outflow obstruction or if endoscopic features are not impressive.

POSTOPERATIVE COMPLICATIONS

IN THE HOSPITAL

Transurethral resection syndrome: Absorption of non-electrolyte fluid (sorbitol or glycine) may provoke the TUR syndrome, which is characterized by restlessness, nausea, vomiting, abdominal pain, pallor, diaphoresis, tachycardia, and dyspnea. There may also be hypotension and alterations on the electrocardiogram. Therapy consists of careful fluid management and the administration of furosemide, 40 to 80 mg. The use of hypertonic saline, 250 to 500 mL of 3% or 5% solution, produces a net loss of water from the intravascular and extravascular spaces. There is some danger in giving hypertonic saline, however, because it temporarily adds more volume to what may be an already compromised circulatory system. Central venous pressure monitoring is indicated when hypertonic saline is administered.

Reactionary hemorrhage: Reactionary hemorrhage may occur after the resection and is usually controlled by gentle traction on the balloon catheter. The balloon should be inflated in the bladder, not in the prostatic fossa, and it should be drawn down to produce tamponade of the vessels at the bladder neck. Three-way irrigation removes blood from the bladder before clotting can occur. If clot retention does develop, it is usually necessary to reinsert the resectoscope and irrigate the bladder free of clots before replacing the catheter. This also provides an opportunity for surgeons to coagulate any persisting arterial bleeders. Venous bleeders are better controlled by conservative measures using balloon traction alone. Continuous bladder irrigation should be done with physiologic saline solution. It is not appropriate to continue using nonelectrolyte solutions after the electrical instruments have been removed.

AFTER DISCHARGE

Secondary hemorrhage: Secondary hemorrhage is seen 10 to 20 days after operation, when the raw surface of the prostate bleeds as the slough is displaced. This often occurs in association with vigorous activity or straining to move the bowels.

Urinary incontinence: The most common form of urinary incontinence is urge incontinence, with difficulty controlling the sudden urinary stream. This usually responds to fluid management and anticholinergic medication, and symptoms often resolve within 3 months. Stress urinary leakage occurs with sphincter weakness, which may be a result of surgery or a manifestation of removal of the passive continence mechanism. Kegel exercises may be helpful.

Urethral stricture: Urethral stricture may be found in 1% to 9% of patients after TUR. The incidence is greater when a larger resectoscope is used. Stricture can occur at the urinary meatus, penoscrotal junction, or bulbar urethra. Bladder neck contraction can also occur. Treatment with dilation or urethrotomy may be required.

Retrograde ejaculation: Retrograde ejaculation is expected after transurethral prostatectomy. Erectile impotence may occur in as many as 30% of patients.

BIBLIOGRAPHY

Holtgrew EWH, Valk WL. Factors influencing the mortality and morbidity of transurethral prostatectomy: a study of 2015 cases. J Urol 1962;87:450–459.

Marshall FF, ed. Urologic complications, ed 2. Complications of transurethral resection of the prostate. Chicago, Mosby–Year Book, 1990:305.

Mebust WK, Holtgrew EWH, Cockett ATK. Transurethral prostatectomy: immediate and postoperative complications. J Urol 1989;141:243–247.

Medical Management of the Surgical Patient, Third Edition,
edited by Michael F. Lubin, H. Kenneth Walker, and Robert B. Smith III.
J.B. Lippincott Company, Philadelphia, PA © 1995.

CHAPTER

RADICAL PROSTATECTOMY

114

Sam D. Graham, Jr.

Radical prostatectomy is the total removal of the prostate and its surrounding tissue, including the seminal vesicles and ampullae of the vas deferens. The operation may be performed using a retropubic, abdominal, or perineal approach. The advantage of the retropubic approach is that it allows simultaneous removal of the pelvic lymph nodes for staging; however, it requires a longer hospitalization and is associated with increased morbidity (blood loss, wound discomfort, prolonged ileus) compared with perineal prostatectomy. The perineal approach allows for an easier anastomosis and reduced perioperative morbidity but requires a separate incision for the pelvic node dissection. With the increased use of laparoscopic lymph node dissection, or the abandonment of nodal dissection in patients with low likelihood of positive nodes, the perineal route is having a resurgence in popularity.

The operative procedure is usually performed after a 36-hour bowel preparation (antibiotic and mechanical) and is done under general anesthesia with endotracheal intubation. Procedure-specific intraoperative risks include hemorrhage (less than 500 mL with perineal prostatectomy and 1100 to 1400 mL with retropubic prostatectomy) and rectal injury (under 1% to 2%). The average operating time is 1½ to 2½ hours for the perineal procedure and 2 to 4 hours for the retropubic approach; laparoscopic node dissection adds 1½ to 2 hours to the procedure.

USUAL POSTOPERATIVE COURSE

Expected postoperative hospital stay: The expected hospital stay is 2 to 4 days after perineal prostatectomy and 4 to 6 days after radical retropubic prostatectomy.

Operative mortality: Under 1%

Special monitoring required: No special monitoring is necessary.

Patient activity and positioning: Patients are ambulatory within 24 to 48 hours of surgery.

Alimentation: Patients undergoing perineal prostatectomy generally are able to eat full diets immediately on recovery from the general anesthetic. Retropubic prostatectomy may result in a short period of ileus, delaying alimentation for several days.

Antibiotic coverage: Because the urinary tract is opened and a catheter is left in place, these patients generally receive antibiotics in addition to those used for the bowel preparation.

Rectal injury: Entry into the rectum is rare but may be closed primarily with no long-term sequelae, providing patients have undergone preoperative bowel preparation. In patients without bowel preparation or patients with extensive lacerations of the rectum (especially those who have undergone radiotherapy), it may be advisable to perform a temporary colostomy.

Drains: Surgical drains are left in place until drainage is minimal (usually 2 to 4 days).

Analgesics: Analgesic requirements are usually minimal in patients undergoing perineal prostatectomy but may be higher in those undergoing radical retropubic prostatectomy.

POSTOPERATIVE COMPLICATIONS

IN THE HOSPITAL

Urocutaneous fistula: Urocutaneous fistula is an uncommon complication because the anastomosis of the bladder to the urethra is generally watertight, but it occurs more frequently when the retropubic approach is used.

Deep venous thrombosis: Clinically evident deep venous thrombosis is uncommon in radical prostatectomy but the true clinical incidence may be much higher, as is probably true in all pelvic surgery.

AFTER DISCHARGE

Incontinence: In most large series, the incidence of urinary incontinence ranges from 2% to 4% in patients without complications. In patients undergoing radical prostatectomy who have had previous surgery or radiation, the incidence increases to 10% to 25%. The incontinence is usually stress type and is generally mild in severity. Patients with neurogenic bladder, morbid obesity, and advanced age have the best chance for definitive correction of their incontinence (including artificial urinary sphincter).

Impotence: The incidence of impotence varies according to the age of the patient and the size of the tumor, as well as the ease with which the neurovascular bundle was dissected off the prostate. The reported incidence of return of potency is 30% to 50% in patients who had at least one neurovascular bundle spared.

BIBLIOGRAPHY

Walsh PC. Radical retropubic prostatectomy. In: Walsh PC, Retik AB, Stamey TA, Vaughan ED, eds. Campbell's urology. Philadelphia, WB Saunders, 1992:2865.

Walsh PC, Lepor H, Egleston JC. Radical retropubic prostatectomy with preservation of sexual function. Prostate 1983;4: 473–485.

Young HH. Cure of cancer of prostate by radical perineal prostatectomy (prostato-seminal vesiculectomy): history, literature and statistics of Young's operation. J Urol 1945;53:188–252.

Medical Management of the Surgical Patient, Third Edition,
edited by Michael F. Lubin, H. Kenneth Walker, and Robert B. Smith III.
J.B. Lippincott Company, Philadelphia, PA © 1995.

CHAPTER

NEPHRECTOMY

115

Sam D. Graham, Jr.

Nephrectomy is indicated in both benign and malignant conditions of the kidney. A simple nephrectomy is the removal of the kidney and a portion of the ureter, usually within Gerota's fascia. Simple nephrectomy is performed for benign diseases such as nonfunctioning kidneys (usually resulting from obstruction or congenital abnormalities); vascular disease (arterial or venous obstruction); infectious processes (pyonephrosis, xanthogranulomatous pyelonephritis, tuberculosis); benign tumors (angiomyolipomas, reninomas); or other miscellaneous indications (nephrocutaneous fistula, trauma). Transplant donor nephrectomy is a variant of simple nephrectomy involving the removal of perinephric tissue and careful dissection of the renal vasculature and ureter for renal transplantation. Transplant nephrectomy is the removal of a renal allograft, usually because of rejection. A radical nephrectomy involves removal of the kidney, adrenal gland, and surrounding perinephric fat within Gerota's fascia. Usually, this operation includes the removal of regional nodes, although some surgeons advocate a wider nodal dissection. If the tumor is locally extensive, radical nephrectomy may be accompanied by splenectomy, partial hepatectomy, partial pancreatectomy, or regional resection of the bowel. Radical nephrectomy is performed in patients with solid renal tumors (usually renal cell carcinoma; occasionally oncocytomas). Nephroureterectomy is the removal of the entire kidney, the ureter (including a cuff of bladder), and surrounding tissues for transitional cell carcinoma of the renal pelvis or upper ureter. Partial nephrectomy is generally performed in patients who are not candidates for total nephrectomy (usually because of poor renal function or a solitary kidney) or in whom total nephrectomy is not indicated because of the presence of an isolated lesion (isolated segmental chronic pyelonephritis).

Surgery of the kidney is almost always performed under general anesthesia. Proper placement of the incision is determined by (1) the planned procedure (malignant lesions require a higher incision than do benign lesions because the dissection is more extensive); (2) extenuating circumstances (removal of a vena caval thrombus with a nephrectomy for renal cell carcinoma may require access to the heart if the thrombus extends into the right atrium and, therefore, may require a midline incision); (3) patient anatomy and body habitus (obese patients are usually better suited to flank incisions because the abdominal wall fat is less extensive in the flank); and (4) surgeon preference. Simple nephrectomy requires 1 to 3 hours of actual surgical time, whereas radical nephrectomy generally takes longer, particularly if the tumor is large or the operation is technically difficult. Simple nephrectomy usually can be performed with a low risk of transfusion, but the likelihood of transfusion increases with more extensive procedures. In patients who require partial nephrectomy or extensive dissection, such as extraction of a tumor thrombus from the vena cava, the probability of transfusion is high because of the potential for sudden and major blood loss. Patients with tumors into the right atrium of the heart may also require cardiopulmonary bypass.

USUAL POSTOPERATIVE COURSE

Expected postoperative hospital stay: For simple or uncomplicated radical nephrectomy, 5 to 7 days of hospitalization is expected. Laparoscopic nephrectomy may result in a shorter hospital stay, although the operative time may be longer. Large or complicated tumors may require 10 days or more of hospitalization, depending on the patient's preoperative physical condition, the extent of the dissection, and possible associated complications.

Operative mortality: For simple nephrectomy, the operative mortality rate is under 1%. Among the older patients who undergo more complex nephrectomies, it increases in proportion to the intricacy of the operation and the presence of metastatic disease or other coexisting conditions and may be as high as 5%.

Special monitoring required: No special monitoring is necessary.

Patient activity and positioning: Patients are usually ambulatory within the first 24 to 48 hours unless the operation was extraordinarily complex.

Alimentation: Food intake is restricted according to the extent of the dissection performed. Retroperitoneal dissection generally results in some degree of ileus and patients must be monitored before their food intake is advanced. The period of ileus may be as short as 24 hours with relatively uncomplicated nephrectomy or as long as 4 days or more if the peritoneum is opened and the bowel is resected.

Antibiotic coverage: Antibiotics usually are not required unless the operation is being performed on an infected or stone-infested kidney, or the surgeon has to open the gastrointestinal tract.

Entry into the chest cavity: Because the pleura is frequently below the 11th rib posteriorly, the possibility of entering the chest cavity in a flank incision is significant and a temporary thoracotomy tube may be required.

Drains: Surgical drains are placed in all patients in whom infection or extravasation is likely. It also may be prudent to place drains in patients who undergo extensive dissection or have the potential for lymphatic or other fluid accumulation. Most drains are removed as soon as it is obvious that the drainage is minimal.

Laboratory values: After a total or partial nephrectomy, patients may experience a brief and usually temporary rise in serum creatinine and blood urea nitrogen levels. Dissection around the pancreas may cause a rise in the serum amylase level, just as liver resection may cause a rise in liver enzyme levels.

Emphysema: Subcutaneous emphysema may be observed after flank cases and should resolve in several days.

Analgesia: Analgesia is required to control incisional pain, which is aggravated when patients become mobile.

POSTOPERATIVE COMPLICATIONS

IN THE HOSPITAL

Wound infection: Wound infection is uncommon in patients undergoing nephrectomy for uninfected kidneys. When infections do occur, they are generally gram-positive unless they are the result of injury to a viscus or an infected kidney, in which case they are more likely to be gram-negative.

Pneumothorax: Pneumothorax usually is recognized in the recovery room and results from operative pleural injury. This complication occasionally may cause significant symptoms but usually is small and detected only by postoperative chest radiography.

Pancreatitis: Dissection around the pancreas in patients with large tumors may result in pancreatitis, which presents as prolonged ileus or unexplained abdominal pain.

Deep venous thrombosis and pulmonary emboli: Deep venous thrombosis and pulmonary emboli are more common in patients who undergo extensive dissection, especially if a vena caval thrombus is removed.

AFTER DISCHARGE

Flank hernia or flank weakness: Hernia or weakness in the flank is more common in obese and elderly patients. Flank hernias are caused by disruption of the fascial closure, whereas flank weakness results from denervation of the flank musculature when the incision divides branches of the intercostal nerves. Hernias frequently require surgical correction but weakness may not be correctable.

Intercostal neuralgia: Entrapment of the sensory branches of the intercostal nerve in the scar may result in intercostal neuralgia. This may be treated with antiinflammatory drugs, nerve blocks, or surgical ablation.

BIBLIOGRAPHY

de Kernion JB, Berry D. The diagnosis and treatment of renal cell carcinoma. Cancer 1980;45:1947–1956.

Schiff M Jr, Glazier WB. Nephrectomy: indications and complications in 347 patients. J Urol 1977;118:930–931.

Medical Management of the Surgical Patient, Third Edition,
edited by Michael F. Lubin, H. Kenneth Walker, and Robert B. Smith III.
J.B. Lippincott Company, Philadelphia, PA © 1995.

CHAPTER

116

CYSTECTOMY AND URINARY DIVERSION

Vahan S. Kassabian

Radical cystectomy is most often performed for muscle-invasive bladder cancer, but additional indications include noncancerous conditions such as radiation cystitis, pyocystis, and other rare entities. In men, the procedure also requires removal of the prostate and is more precisely known as *cystoprostatectomy*. In women, a radical cystectomy is synonymous with anterior pelvic exenteration, which includes removal of the uterus, fallopian tubes, ovaries, bladder, urethra, and anterior vaginal wall. For oncologic indications, a bilateral pelvic lymph node dissection is usually performed before the actual cystectomy is commenced.

Once the bladder has been removed, there are three ways in which a urinary diversion can be performed:

1. An ileal conduit may be formed, which involves isolating a segment of distal ileum and attaching the ureters to form a freely refluxing anastomosis. The ileum is closed on one end and the other end is left open to form a stoma on the anterior abdominal wall, usually on the right side, so that urine may flow continuously from the kidneys into the stoma bag. The stoma location should be chosen carefully before the operation, with the patient standing and sitting, to prevent skin creases or scars. Patients should become familiar with stoma appliances and techniques of care before surgery, and this usually is accomplished by enterostomal therapy practitioners.

2. Continent urinary diversion has the main advantage of not requiring a bag because there is no continuous

exit of urine to the outside. Using small bowel, large bowel, stomach, or any combination of these, a new bladder is surgically created from detubularized bowel and the ureters are anastomosed into this reservoir either in a freely refluxing anastomosis or, usually in the case of large bowel, in an antirefluxing method on the taenia. Fashioning the other end of the neobladder involves the creation of a stomal nipple, usually from intussuscepted bowel, which forms a continent valve mechanism. This requires that patients regularly drain the contents of the reservoir by intermittent catheterization. This procedure is usually reserved for women who do not desire any abdominal wall appliances or for men in whom the urethra has been removed.

3. The technique of orthotopic bladder substitution also involves the use of detubularized bowel to create a new bladder, but in its usual position. No nipple is created; instead, the neobladder is attached to the urethra and the patient's own external sphincter serves as the continent mechanism, allowing voiding through the urethra. This surgical technique most closely resembles a normal bladder both physiologically and aesthetically. It is feasible, however, only in men in whom urethrectomy has not been performed. Candidates must be highly motivated, intelligent, and willing to perform intermittent catheterization if they are unable to empty their neobladders completely.

Many types of continent urinary diversion and orthotopic bladder substitution are possible and each has distinct advantages and disadvantages. The perfect urinary diversion or bladder substitute would be one that has an adequate reservoir, does not reflux, has low voiding pressures, empties adequately, has a low complication rate, and does not promote urinary tract infection, stones, or renal failure. Although none of the available surgical procedures satisfies all these criteria, several have the definite advantage of eliminating external appliances.

All cystectomy procedures are considered to be major surgery. An ileal conduit can be performed in about 4 hours, including the cystectomy and node dissection. A continent urinary diversion or bladder substitute takes an additional 2 hours. All the procedures require mechanical bowel preparation. Blood transfusions may be needed. Parenteral or enteral antibiotics are recommended. Pneumatic compression stockings are recommended to decrease thromboembolic complications.

USUAL POSTOPERATIVE COURSE

Expected postoperative hospital stay: 7 to 14 days

Operative mortality: About 4%

Special monitoring required: Careful monitoring of fluid balance, acid–base balance, and cardiovascular status is essential, especially because many patients are elderly and have associated medical problems.

Patient activity and positioning: Patients should be mobilized to chairs on the first postoperative day because early mobilization is the key to preventing thromboembolic complications.

Alimentation: Nasogastric tube suction or gastric tube placement is continued until there is evidence of good peristalsis and passage of gas, usually after at least 5 days. Abdominal distention must be prevented and the bowel anastomosis protected.

Antibiotic coverage: Perioperative antibiotics are given prophylactically. The first dose is administered before the procedure and treatment is continued for about 48 hours. If the urine is infected before operation, a preoperative course of antibiotics is mandatory.

Fluid requirements: Excessive fluid requirements are usually encountered in the first 3 days because of bowel edema, third spacing, and possible leaks. Enemas, rectal examinations, and suppositories are contraindicated in the early postoperative period because of the danger of perforating the rectal wall. Perforation is rare but may occur if the surgery was difficult or the rectal wall had been thinned.

POSTOPERATIVE COMPLICATIONS

IN THE HOSPITAL

Prolonged ileus: If ileus persists, urinary leakage, enteric leakage, and abscess or infection should be ruled out. Small urinary leaks often heal spontaneously as long as drainage is continued; fecal leakage also usually heals spontaneously with intravenous hyperalimentation and prohibiting oral intake.

Bleeding: Any major bleeding usually occurs within the first 24 hours and may require reoperation if the blood loss does not cease.

Persistent draining: Many surgeons use suction drains in the pelvis; these are removed when drainage is minimal. If leakage persists, the fluid should be analyzed to determine whether it is urine or lymph.

Oliguria or anuria: Insufficient hydration is usually the cause of oliguria or anuria but obstruction caused by edema, blood clot at the ureterointestinal anastomosis, ureteral devascularization, or simple blockage of the drainage catheters should be ruled out.

Ischemia or infarction of the conduit, continent pouch, or neobladder: Ischemia or infarction of the conduit, continent pouch, or neobladder generally is evident during the operation by a change in color of the bowel but can occur after surgery. It is usually related to excessive tension or to hematoma in the mesentery. This complication is rare but requires surgical revision. The stoma normally may appear blue and edematous, especially for the first 24 to 48 hours; nevertheless, it should be observed closely.

Obturator nerve injury: Injury to the obturator nerve should be repaired during the operation because a permanent neurologic deficit can impair adduction of the leg and may disable patients sufficiently to prevent them from driving a car.

Thrombophlebitis and pulmonary embolus: Although subclinical venous thrombosis is common after extensive pelvic surgery, clinical thrombophlebitis and secondary pulmonary embolus are rare. Aggressive therapy is required, with anticoagulation and consideration of a vena caval filter.

Wound infection: Wound infection usually occurs in patients who are debilitated, elderly, and have had previous radiotherapy, bowel injury, or infected urine. Drainage and, possibly, antibiotics are necessary to treat superficial infections; total wound dehiscence usually requires surgery for reclosure.

AFTER DISCHARGE

Acid–base balance: Although the bowel atrophies once it has been isolated from the remaining digestive tract, it still retains a large absorptive capacity. If ileum or colon is used, hyperchloremic metabolic acidosis may occur. If jejunum is used, hyponatremic, hypochloremic, hyperkalemic metabolic acidosis may ensue. If stomach is used, hyponatremic, hypochloremic metabolic alkalosis may result. These abnormalities are related to the degree of preexisting renal insufficiency and usually are not seen with normal renal function.

Mucus production: Small and large bowel initially produce a large amount of mucus, but production decreases over time. This is only a nuisance, causing catheters to plug.

Stomal stenosis: Stenosis is more common in the pediatric population because of disproportionate growth. In adults, stenosis is related to poor skin care. Although proper hygiene may produce some improvement, reconstruction may be necessary.

Peristomal hernia: Peristomal hernias are obvious clinically but often do not cause any obstruction or strangulation. Surgical repair usually is advisable, however.

Hydronephrosis: Persistent reflux of chronically infected urine may be the cause of hydronephrosis but stenosis at the ureteroileal anastomosis must be ruled out. Partial obstruction may result from devascularization or recurrent tumor and usually requires open surgical repair.

Lymphocele: Lymphoceles are common after pelvic lymph node dissection but the lymph is usually well absorbed by the peritoneum. Treatment is only indicated for lymphoceles that cause complications such as infection, obstruction, or edema.

Chronic pyelonephritis: Chronic pyelonephritis is clinically apparent in 10% to 30% of patients who are followed up for 5 years. Among children with ileal conduits, 40% have deterioration of renal function within 10 years. There-fore, in children this may be the chief determinant of life expectancy. Because nonrefluxing conduits theoretically prevent this complication, conversion to a nonrefluxing conduit may be indicated in affected children.

Stones: Urinary stones develop in 10% to 15% of patients within 5 years after the formation of an ileal conduit, usually as a result of chronically infected urine. Hydration is the best prevention. Treatment may include acidification of the urine and control of infection; some stones may require surgical treatment.

Nipple malfunction of continent pouches: Reexploration, catheter drainage, or conversion to a stoma bag may be required for nipple malfunction of continent pouches.

Spontaneous rupture of a continent pouch or bladder substitute: Spontaneous rupture of a continent pouch or bladder substitute is rare and difficult to diagnose but has been reported years after surgery and requires immediate surgical exploration.

Cancer of the continent pouch or bladder substitute: Cancer of the continent pouch or bladder substitute is rare and may occur 15 to 20 years after initial treatment. The finding is usually from ureterosigmoidostomy and, more recently, from bladder augmentation using bowel, because most cancers occur at the anastomotic junction between the bladder and bowel mucosa.

BIBLIOGRAPHY

Benson MC, Olsson CA. Urinary diversion. In: Walsh PC, Retik AB, Stamey TA, Vaughan ED Jr, eds. Campbell's urology, ed 6. Philadelphia, WB Saunders, 1992:2654.

Bricker EM. Symposium on clinical surgery: bladder substitution after pelvic evisceration. Surg Clin North Am 1950;30:1511–1521.

Skinner DG, Crawford ED, Kaufman JJ. Complications of radical cystectomy for carcinoma of the bladder. J Urol 1980;123:690–693.

Medical Management of the Surgical Patient, Third Edition,
edited by Michael F. Lubin, H. Kenneth Walker, and Robert B. Smith III.
J.B. Lippincott Company, Philadelphia, PA © 1995.

CHAPTER

117

RADICAL ORCHIECTOMY AND RETROPERITONEAL LYMPH NODE DISSECTION

Sean P. Heron
Michael A. Witt

Radical inguinal orchiectomy is performed for testicular tumors. An inguinal, rather than a scrotal, approach is used to prevent violation of the superficial inguinal lymphatics.

Ligation of the spermatic cord is undertaken at the internal inguinal ring. High ligation enables resection of the cord structures with the nodal template when retroperitoneal lymph node dissection (RPLND) is performed.

RPLND is an adjuvant operation that is indicated for nonseminomatous germ cell tumors and is required for accurate staging. The traditional RPLND involves the removal of all retroperitoneal lymphatic tissue medial to the ureters, inferior to the renal vessels, and down to the bifurcation of the iliac vessels on the contralateral side and to the internal ring on the ipsilateral side. This surgical approach has been associated with a high incidence of ejaculatory failure. Because the survival of patients with non-seminomatous germ cell tumors has recently increased dramatically as a result of advances in chemotherapy, the rate of ejaculatory failure with traditional RPLND is no longer acceptable. Many centers, therefore, are opting for a more limited dissection to spare at least one sympathetic chain and thereby preserve normal ejaculatory function.

Patients usually have mechanical bowel preparation before RPLND, and perioperative broad-spectrum antibiotic coverage is often used. The operation takes 2 or 3 hours and requires general anesthesia. Blood should be available for transfusion but is generally not needed.

USUAL POSTOPERATIVE COURSE

Expected postoperative hospital stay: Patients are admitted to the hospital on the day of operation and typically remain hospitalized for 5 days afterward.

Operative mortality: Operative mortality is essentially nonexistent.

Special monitoring required: No special monitoring is necessary.

Patient activity and positioning: Ambulation is increased progressively beginning on the day of operation.

Alimentation: Most patients have periods of ileus and require nasogastric tubes, but these may be omitted when a retroperitoneal approach is used and the peritoneal cavities are not violated. When bowel sounds return, the nasogastric tubes are removed and dietary intake is slowly advanced.

Antibiotic coverage: Broad-spectrum antibiotics are continued for 24 hours.

POSTOPERATIVE COMPLICATIONS

IN THE HOSPITAL

Lymphoceles: Lymphoceles occur in less than 5% of cases and may require percutaneous drainage.

Lumbosacral plexus injury: Lumbosacral plexus injury is possible but unusual in patients who undergo a retroperitoneal approach.

Bowel and spinal cord injury: Bowel injury from ligation of the inferior mesenteric artery and spinal cord injury from ligation of lumbar arteries are possible but rarely reported.

AFTER DISCHARGE

Loss of ejaculation: Loss of ejaculation is expected in 40% or more of patients who undergo a complete RPLND. Modified procedures have all but eliminated this complication, with 88% to 100% of patients retaining normal antegrade ejaculation. Imipramine can further reduce ejaculatory disturbances.

Infertility: Infertility is encountered in 25% to 30% of patients with testicular cancer. Sperm banking before testicular or retroperitoneal surgery is advisable for safe preservation of fertility.

BIBLIOGRAPHY

Aass N, Fossa SD, Ous S, et al. Is routine primary retroperitoneal lymph node dissection still justified in patients with low stage nonseminomatous testicular cancer? Br J Urol 1990;65:385–390.

Donohue JP, Foster RS, Rowland RG, et al. Nerve-sparing retroperitoneal lymphadenectomy with preservation of ejaculation. J Urol 1990;144:287–292.

Jewett MA, Torbey C. Nerve-sparing techniques in retroperitoneal lymphadenectomy with low-stage testicular cancer. Semin Urol 1988;613:233–237.

Richie JP. Retroperitoneal lymphadenectomy. In: Glenn JF, ed. Urologic surgery, ed 3. Philadelphia, JB Lippincott, 1983:39.

Richie JP. Clinical stage 1 testicular cancer: the role of modified retroperitoneal lymphadenectomy. J Urol 1990;144:1160–1163.

Sherlag AP, O'Brien DP III, Graham SD Jr. Use of limited retroperitoneal lymphadenectomy in nonseminomatous germ cell tumors. Urology 1989;33:355–357.

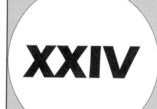

SECTION **XXIV**

OTOLARYNGOLOGIC
SURGERY

Medical Management of the Surgical Patient, Third Edition,
edited by Michael F. Lubin, H. Kenneth Walker, and Robert B. Smith III.
J.B. Lippincott Company, Philadelphia, PA © 1995.

CHAPTER

ENDOSCOPIC SINUS SURGERY

118

Gerald S. Gussack

Surgery of the paranasal sinuses is performed for several specific indications: persistent symptoms after failure of intensive medical therapy, recurrent or chronic infections, and complications of infections, including meningitis, orbital abscess, cellulitis, mucocele, and mucopyocele. In addition, paranasal sinus disease can complicate pulmonary problems such as asthma and cystic fibrosis. These procedures recently have been expanded for use in the treatment of cerebrospinal fluid leak, encephalocele, toxic thyroid exophthalmos, dacryocystorhinostomy, and optic nerve decompression. Since 1985, the techniques of Messerklinger and Wigand using surgical rod lens telescopes have become increasingly popular. These techniques stress the preservation of normal anatomic structures and are aimed at re-creating the normal physiologic pathways of drainage from the paranasal sinuses into the nose. The term *functional endoscopic sinus surgery* has been coined to describe these techniques.

The operations vary in complexity and duration based on the extent of disease. If disease is limited to the anterior ethmoid and maxillary sinuses, the procedure may be performed in as little as 30 to 45 minutes. More extensive sinus disease or nasal polyps may require procedures lasting 2 hours or longer. Blood loss during endoscopic procedures depends on the severity of the disease and is relatively higher for nasal polyps compared with other conditions. Blood loss is usually minimal, however, and cases requiring transfusion are infrequent. The choice of anesthetic techniques for these procedures is evenly divided between general anesthesia and a combination of local anesthesia with intravenous sedation. Patient preference, surgical expertise, and expected duration of the procedure are all considerations in anesthetic decisions.

USUAL POSTOPERATIVE COURSE

Expected postoperative hospital stay: Patients undergo operation on an outpatient basis in about half of uncomplicated sinus procedures. The remaining patients usually can be discharged from the hospital after an overnight admission.

Operative mortality: The operative mortality rate is under 1%. Most of these procedures are performed in an elective setting on patients with few coexisting medical conditions. Sinus procedures are occasionally required in compromised hosts, such as patients with diabetes or patients with leukemia who have fungal infections of the sinuses. These patients can be seriously ill and may have mortality rates exceeding 50%.

Special monitoring required: No special monitoring is necessary.

Patient activity and positioning: Patients are allowed to ambulate on the evening of their procedure. They are advised to avoid straining, bending over, heavy lifting, or vigorous nose blowing. Nasal discharge from sinus drainage

641

and bleeding may persist for several days. Keeping the head elevated at night minimizes bleeding.

Alimentation: A regular diet is permitted as tolerated.

Antibiotic coverage: Perioperative antibiotics are not routinely used. Specimens are usually obtained at the time of the procedure for culture and sensitivity determination, and specific antibiotic therapy can be instituted later based on the results of these studies.

Nasal polyps: Most patients undergoing endoscopic sinus surgery are relatively healthy without significant associated diseases. One subset of patients with the potential for complications are those with nasal polyps. There is a high incidence of patients with nasal polyps, asthma, and aspirin intolerance (French's triad) who must be monitored for pulmonary problems and reactive airway disease. These patients often have taken steroids, such as prednisone, for prolonged periods. Therefore, perioperative "stress dosages" of corticosteroids are required.

POSTOPERATIVE COMPLICATIONS

IN THE HOSPITAL

Bleeding: Bleeding is common after any surgical procedure on the nose. Most bleeding is mucosal in origin and is usually self-limited. Profuse arterial bleeding can arise from the anterior or posterior ethmoid, the sphenopalatine, or, less commonly, the carotid arteries. Bleeding usually responds to nasal packing with expandable Merocel sponges or topical hemostatic agents. Medications with antiplatelet activity, such as salicylates, must not be given.

Nasal drainage: Watery discharge on bending over is a sign of a cerebrospinal fluid fistula. The discharge can be screened for glucose positivity at the bedside but the source is confirmed by testing for the β subunit of transferrin. Small leaks that are intermittent often close spontaneously if patients are kept at bed rest with their heads elevated.

Leaks that fail to close should be investigated for localization with a metrizamide contrast computed tomographic scan. Placement of a lumbar drain, with or without operative exploration, may be required for profuse or persistent leaks. Patients should be carefully monitored for meningitis.

Visual complications: Visual complications result from direct injury to the optic nerve, globe, or extraocular muscles, or from secondary injury related to the formation of an orbital hematoma. Visual acuity and extraocular muscle movements should be checked immediately after surgery and then at frequent intervals to allow prompt recognition of this complication. A lateral canthotomy and orbital exploration may be required to control bleeding. Ophthalmologic consultation is sought in all complications involving the orbit.

AFTER DISCHARGE

Recurrent or persistent sinusitis: Reoperation may be required if symptoms of sinusitis recur or persist despite medical therapy.

BIBLIOGRAPHY

Kennedy DW, Zinreich SS, Rosenbaum NL, Johns ME. Functional endoscopic sinus surgery: theory and diagnostic evaluation. Arch Otolaryngol 1985;111:576–582.

Stammberger H. Endoscopic endonasal surgery: new concepts in treatment of recurring sinusitis. Otolaryngol Head Neck Surg 1986;94:143–147.

Stammberger H. Functional endoscopic sinus surgery. Philadelphia, Decker, 1991:285–320.

Stankiewicz JA. Complications of endoscopic intranasal ethmoidectomy: an update. Laryngoscope 1989;99:686–690.

Wigand ME. Endoscopic surgery of the paranasal sinuses and anterior skull base. New York, Thieme Medical, 1990:78–92.

Medical Management of the Surgical Patient, Third Edition,
edited by Michael F. Lubin, H. Kenneth Walker, and Robert B. Smith III.
J.B. Lippincott Company, Philadelphia, PA © 1995.

TONSILLECTOMY

119

Owen S. Reichman

Until recently, tonsillectomy was the most widely performed surgical procedure in the United States. For many years, it was accepted as a routine part of growing up. Tonsillectomy is now reserved for patients with significant tonsillar pathology. Indications for tonsillectomy are chronic tonsillitis despite medical therapy, hypertrophy causing upper airway obstruction or sleep apnea, and unilateral tonsillar hypertrophy presumed to be neoplastic. The adenoids are often involved with hypertrophy or infection and are usually removed with the tonsils in patients who are younger than 12 years. Adenoidectomy with tympanostomy tube placement is increasingly the treatment of choice for recurrent suppurative or secretory otitis media.

General anesthesia is preferred, but local anesthesia can be used in cooperative patients. The operation usually takes 30 to 60 minutes to perform. Procedures involving general anesthesia are performed with patients supine and their necks extended. Blood loss can be significant, especially in adults, but transfusion is needed in less than 1% of patients. A careful preoperative history should be obtained to rule out hematologic disorders.

Electrocautery or the laser is often used by surgeons to further decrease the amount of blood loss.

USUAL POSTOPERATIVE COURSE

Expected postoperative hospital stay: Most tonsillectomies are performed safely on an outpatient basis, but 1 day of hospitalization may be required.

Operative mortality: The operative mortality rate is under 1%. Deaths are usually attributable to anesthetic problems or severe delayed hemorrhage.

Special monitoring required: No special monitoring is necessary.

Patient activity and positioning: Patients are ambulatory on the day of operation. Activity is slowly increased as tolerated and regular activities are resumed in 2 weeks.

Alimentation: Clear, nonacidic liquids are permitted when nausea has resolved, and a soft diet is provided the next day.

Antibiotic coverage: Antibiotics have been shown to decrease fever, pain, lassitude, foul mouth odor, and poor oral intake. Intravenous ampicillin is usually given at the time of surgery, and then amoxicillin is continued for 1 week. Erythromycin is used in patients who are allergic to penicillin.

Analgesia: Postoperative pain is usually controlled by acetaminophen with codeine.

POSTOPERATIVE COMPLICATIONS

IN THE HOSPITAL

Hemorrhage: The threat of primary (within 24 hours) or delayed (after 24 hours) hemorrhage is present even when the operation is done by the most skilled and experienced surgeons. Postoperative bleeding has been reported to occur in 1% to 14% of patients. It may be manifested by sudden hematemesis of 400 to 500 mL of clot, indicating subclinical constant bleeding. Immediate crossmatching and return to the operating room for ligation of the bleeding vessel are required for any significant bleeding.

Dehydration: Dysphagia caused by pain may prevent adequate oral intake. Intravenous supplementation may be necessary.

Severe pain: Severe pain is especially common in adults. The pain is located in the jaw, throat, and ear. Morphine or meperidine may be required.

Septicemia: Septicemia is most common after an abscess tonsillectomy. Temperature elevations above 38.5°C orally, rapid pulse, somnolence, and anorexia signal the need for blood cultures and intravenous antibiotics.

AFTER DISCHARGE

Hemorrhage: Hemorrhage can occur as late as 19 days after surgery. Patients are instructed to contact their physicians immediately at the onset of any red blood in the saliva, sputum, or secretions.

Prolonged dysphagia: Readmission with intravenous hydration occasionally may be required for prolonged dysphagia.

Voice changes: Scarring of the tonsillar pillars or palate can occur, causing nasopharyngeal stenosis. There can also be some degree of velopharyngeal insufficiency, especially after adenoidectomy. This is usually temporary unless there is an unrecognized submucous cleft palate.

BIBLIOGRAPHY

Chiang TM, Sukis AE, Ross DE. Tonsillectomy performed on an outpatient basis: report of a series of 40,000 cases performed without a death. Arch Otolaryngol 1968;88:307–310.

Gates GA, Avery CA, Prihoda TS, Cooper JC. Effectiveness of adenoidectomy and tympanostomy tubes in the treatment of chronic otitis media with effusion. N Engl J Med 1987;317:1444–1451.

Kornblut A, Kornblut AD. Tonsillectomy and adenoidectomy. In: Paparella MM, Shumrick DA, eds. Otolaryngology, ed 3. Philadelphia, WB Saunders, 1991:2149–2165.

Pratt L. Tonsil and adenoid disorders. In: Gates GW, ed. Current therapy in otolaryngology–head and neck surgery, ed 3. Philadelphia, Decker, 1987:313–315.

Telian SA, Handler SD, Fleisher GR, et al. The effect of antibiotic therapy on recovery after tonsillectomy in children. Arch Otolaryngol Head Neck Surg 1986;112:610–615.

Medical Management of the Surgical Patient, Third Edition,
edited by Michael F. Lubin, H. Kenneth Walker, and Robert B. Smith III.
J.B. Lippincott Company, Philadelphia, PA © 1995.

TRACHEOSTOMY

CHAPTER

120

Owen S. Reichman

Tracheostomy is done to establish an airway in patients with existing or impending upper airway obstruction. Endotracheal intubation has replaced tracheostomy in the initial control of many cases of upper airway obstruction, but emergency tracheostomy is still commonly needed in patients who cannot undergo endotracheal intubation. Tracheostomy is also performed to prevent complications from prolonged endotracheal intubation. Although low-pressure cuffs on endotracheal tubes have decreased such complications, tracheostomy should be considered if airway intubation is still needed after 7 days. Other indications for tracheostomy are inability of patients to manage secretions, severe sleep apnea, and facilitation of ventilation support. Massive facial trauma, direct injuries to the larynx or trachea, and significant pharyngeal trauma are relative contraindications to endotracheal intubation, and tracheostomy should be used.

Direct entrance through the cricothyroid membrane can be used in an emergency, but a procedure below the second tracheal ring should be substituted when proper equipment, lighting, and assistance are available. The use of anesthesia generally depends on the underlying condition. Most procedures are done with standby anesthesia, and they should be performed in the operating room if possible. Patients are placed supine on the operating table with their necks extended. Tracheostomy is more difficult in children and should always be performed in the operating room except in the most dire circumstances. No blood replacement is usually necessary.

USUAL POSTOPERATIVE COURSE

Expected postoperative hospital stay: The duration of hospitalization usually depends on the underlying reason for the tracheostomy. Prolonged or permanent tracheostomy may be needed in cases of laryngeal stenosis, vocal cord lesions, or chronic lung problems. The hospital stay may be shortened by proper patient education and home nursing care.

Operative mortality: The operative mortality rate is 5% for elective procedures and 10% to 50% for emergency procedures.

Special monitoring required: Emergency tracheostomy takes precedence over all monitoring devices. Monitoring for urgent or elective procedures is generally based on the underlying reason for the tracheostomy. Constant pulse oximeter monitoring is required, as well as other usual anesthetic monitoring. A chest radiograph should be done immediately after surgery to evaluate the position of the tube and to assess for subcutaneous emphysema or pneumothorax.

Patient activity and positioning: Patients should have their heads elevated. A high-humidity collar is essential for the first few days. Ambulation is dependent on the underlying condition responsible for the tracheostomy.

Alimentation: Oral intake may be resumed after operation if the oral cavity and gastrointestinal tract are normal. After emergency tracheostomy under adverse conditions, an

645

esophagram or esophagoscopy is advisable to rule out esophageal injury.

Antibiotic coverage: Antibiotics are generally not needed if an elective sterile procedure is carried out in the operating room. Broad-spectrum antibiotic coverage is advisable if sterile technique is not used.

Secretions: Secretions are often copious shortly after the surgery. Constant suction and wound care should be performed diligently. The primary tube is usually changed after 3 days.

Tubes: Synthetic plastic tubes have essentially replaced the classic metal tubes. The new tubes offer advantages in cost, weight, tolerance, maintenance, patient acceptance, and airflow. Retraction sutures are placed in the side of the trachea in infants to permit reinsertion of a displaced tube; in addition, the tube should be sutured to the skin in children until a good tract develops.

POSTOPERATIVE COMPLICATIONS

IN THE HOSPITAL

Displacement of the tube: Coughing is often vigorous during the first few hours; patients should be observed in the intensive care unit or have a constant attendant during the first few hours. A tracheostomy tray should be kept at the bedside for the first 48 hours to facilitate reinsertion.

Bleeding: Venous bleeding from thyroid vessels may occur. This can usually be controlled with surgical gauze packed around the tube.

Local infection: Bacterial tracheitis is common but wound infection seldom becomes a problem.

Crusting: Irrigation with sterile saline solution and use of a high-humidity regimen are helpful. Crusts at the end of the tube may obstruct the airway, necessitating removal of the tube and direct tracheal suctioning.

Pneumothorax: Pneumothorax occurs in 25% of infant tracheostomies because of the high reflection of the pleura into the root of the neck. Chest auscultation and postoperative chest radiographs should identify the condition.

Cervical or mediastinal emphysema: Swelling of the neck structures with crepitus becomes obvious after surgery. Unless it is extensive, no treatment is usually necessary for cervical emphysema. Increased respiratory distress or upper chest pain may signal progressive air accumulation in the mediastinum.

AFTER DISCHARGE

Severe crusting: Home humidifiers and suction should be arranged for all patients before they are discharged from the hospital.

Tube displacement: The family should be taught how to replace the tubes or be instructed to take patients to the nearest emergency department if tubes become displaced.

Erosion of the trachea or major vessels: Erosion of the trachea or major vessels is extremely uncommon but may occur from a long tube or one that presses against an anomalous vessel. Death usually occurs before medical help can be obtained; a few patients are salvaged by emergency operation.

Subglottic stenosis: Subglottic stenosis is generally the result of a tracheostomy that has been performed too high. It may prevent successful decannulation. Tracheal revision is often required.

Maintenance: Prolonged tracheostomy maintenance is difficult for patients and their families. The services of a visiting nurse are usually necessary during the first weeks after discharge from the hospital.

BIBLIOGRAPHY

Seid AB, Gluckman JL. Tracheostomy. In: Paparella MM, Shumrick PA, eds. Otolaryngology, ed 3. Philadelphia, WB Saunders, 1991:2429–2437.

Stock MC, Woodard CG, Shapiro BA, et al. Perioperative complications of elective tracheostomy in critically ill patients. Crit Care Med 1986;14:861–863.

Stowe DG, Kenan PD, Hudson WR. Complications of tracheostomy. Am Surg 1970;36:34–38.

Medical Management of the Surgical Patient, Third Edition,
edited by Michael F. Lubin, H. Kenneth Walker, and Robert B. Smith III.
J.B. Lippincott Company, Philadelphia, PA © 1995.

CHAPTER

121

LARYNGECTOMY AND RADICAL NECK DISSECTION

Owen S. Reichman

Laryngectomy has been the mainstay of surgical therapy for extensive cancer of the larynx. It is an effective procedure for removing the tumor and restoring the ability to swallow. The entire larynx is removed, however, and patients are aphonic and dependent on permanent tracheostomas. If the lesion is not extensive, partial laryngectomy is commonly performed. This is usually referred to as a *supraglottic laryngectomy* for lesions confined to the area above the vocal cords or a *hemilaryngectomy* for lesions confined to one side of the larynx. Partial laryngectomy may permit closure of the tracheostoma some weeks after surgery.

All laryngectomy procedures are performed under general anesthesia with a tracheostomy. The operative time is about 3 hours for laryngectomy, and combined neck dissection takes an additional 1 or 2 hours. Blood transfusion is uncommon with laryngectomy alone but may be required if radical neck dissection also is performed. All laryngeal surgery is semisterile because the pharynx is open to the surgical field.

USUAL POSTOPERATIVE COURSE

Expected postoperative hospital stay: The expected hospital stay is 14 days but depends on the age of the patient, the presence or absence of chronic lung disease, and the availability of home nursing care.

Operative mortality: 1% or less

Special monitoring required: No special monitoring is necessary.

Patient activity and positioning: Patients are usually observed in intensive care units for 24 hours after surgery. Their heads are elevated when they are fully recovered from anesthesia. Closed suction drains are placed at the time of operation and connected to vacuum suction for 24 hours. After that, the drains are placed to bulb suction and removed when the drainage has decreased. Chest radiographs are obtained after operation to rule out pneumothorax.

Alimentation: A feeding tube is inserted at the time of surgery. If bowel function is present, tube feedings are administered in 24 hours and nutritional intake is advanced over the next 1 or 2 days. Clear liquids are usually given by mouth 7 to 10 days after surgery, and food intake is advanced during the next several days to a regular diet. When patients are tolerating a regular diet, tube feedings are stopped. Preoperative radiotherapy or postoperative infections usually prolong this process.

Antibiotic coverage: Because all significant head and neck oncologic surgery is performed through a contaminated field, perioperative broad-spectrum antibiotic coverage is needed. Antibiotics are administered at the time of operation and continued for 2 days. The antibiotic chosen should cover gram-positive aerobic and anaerobic bacteria; some surgeons also choose to add gram-negative coverage.

Humidity: High humidity is necessary throughout the postoperative period. Collar humidification is used in the hospital and a cold mist humidifier is used at home.

Analgesia: Pain is usually controlled with morphine or meperidine for the first 48 to 72 hours. Tylenol with codeine generally is sufficient after that.

POSTOPERATIVE COMPLICATIONS

IN THE HOSPITAL

Pneumonia and bronchitis: Some degree of postoperative bronchitis exists in all patients because of contamination with blood and pharyngeal secretions. About 10% to 15% of patients develop pneumonia. Chest radiographs and careful auscultation are used to monitor for this complication. A ventilator is seldom necessary unless patients had preexisting lung disease. Pulmonary complications are more common in patients who have undergone conservation laryngectomy.

Pharyngeal salivary fistula: The incidence of fistula varies from under 10% in patients undergoing routine laryngectomies to about 40% in those receiving preoperative radiation. Virtually all wound infections are related to salivary leaks through the suture line. If this occurs, the wound is opened and the fistula tract is packed. A large fistula may prolong hospitalization to as much as 6 weeks for packing changes and continued tube feedings.

Major vessel erosion: A fistula in direct contact with a carotid artery or exposure of the vessel by flap necrosis may lead to erosion of the artery wall and rapid hemorrhage. This is much more common in previously irradiated patients. It is treated with ligation of the vessel.

Aspiration: All patients have some degree of aspiration after supraglottic laryngectomy. Most patients overcome this problem within 6 weeks but must learn new swallowing techniques to prevent further aspiration. A percutaneous gastrostomy or feeding tube may be required long-term.

Tracheal stoma dehiscence: Tension on the tracheal stump or local infection may require revision surgery.

Postoperative depression: Patients may experience severe depression on realizing that the voice is gone, that a permanent tracheostoma is necessary, or that prolonged additional treatment and rehabilitation are required. In an effort to avert this, preoperative counseling by speech therapists, vocational rehabilitation counselors, and clinical psychologists is advocated.

AFTER DISCHARGE

Crusting: Severe tracheal crusting with partial obstruction is common unless patients adhere strictly to a high-humidity treatment program.

Pharyngeal stenosis: Pharyngeal stenosis causing dysphagia may develop at any time after surgery. When symptoms occur, it is necessary to rule out tumor recurrence. In the absence of recurrence, periodic dilation with rubber bougies is usually successful in treating stenosis.

Tracheal stenosis: Most patients can discontinue the use of laryngectomy tubes after the stomas have matured. If stenosis occurs, either the use of a silicone stoma stent or surgical revision is required.

Aphonia: Most patients can be rehabilitated. The most common procedure used to restore speech is a tracheoesophageal puncture with a duckbill prosthesis. About 60% to 90% of patients are able to communicate using this method. Others use electronic devices or esophageal speech. Some patients are never able to develop speech, and this can be a great problem, particularly for those who are illiterate.

Hypothyroidism: Mild hypothyroidism is common and seen in 25% to 66% of patients, especially after irradiation.

BIBLIOGRAPHY

Liening DA, Duncan NO, Blakeslee DB, Smith DB. Hypothyroidism following radiotherapy for head and neck cancer. Otolaryngol Head Neck Surg 1990;103:10–13.

Ogura JH, Sessions DG, Specter GS. Conservation surgery for epidermoid carcinoma of the supraglottic larynx. Laryngoscope 1975;85:1808.

Packman RC, Bowen WG, Share BL. Medical management of head and neck surgery patients. In: Thawley SE, Pange WR, eds. Comprehensive management of head and neck tumors. Philadelphia, WB Saunders, 1987:2–13.

Thawley SE. Cysts and tumors of the larynx. In: Paparella MM, Shumick DA, eds. Otolaryngology, ed 3. Philadelphia, Saunders, 1991:2307–2369.

Medical Management of the Surgical Patient, Third Edition,
edited by Michael F. Lubin, H. Kenneth Walker, and Robert B. Smith III.
J.B. Lippincott Company, Philadelphia, PA © 1995.

CHAPTER

COMPOSITE RESECTION OF TONSIL, JAW, AND NECK WITH PEDICLE GRAFTING

122

Owen S. Reichman

In composite resection of the tonsil, jaw, and neck, soft tissue, mandibular bone, and adjacent lymph nodes are resected en bloc for extirpation of tumor. These lesions usually originate in the tonsil or at the base of the tongue and may have invaded the mandible at the time of surgery. If the mandible is not involved with tumor, it may be split for exposure and then plated or wired together at the conclusion of the procedure. The defect that results from a composite resection is usually closed with a myocutaneous or myofascial flap. This may be either a pedicle flap from the shoulder or pectoral region, or a free microvascular graft. Skin grafts are usually taken to close the donor flap site.

The operative time is usually 6 to 8 hours but may be longer if a free microvascular reconstruction is used. Blood loss is generally in the range of 500 to 1500 mL. General anesthesia is always used and a temporary tracheotomy is required. Many patients are malnourished and may need nutritional support before undergoing operation. Most patients who have a tumor requiring this type of surgery need multimodality therapy. Radiation is used either before or after operation. Chemotherapy is not given routinely with this type of cancer, but some regimens show promise and chemotherapy may play an increased role in the future.

USUAL POSTOPERATIVE COURSE

Expected postoperative hospital stay: Patients remain hospitalized after surgery for 10 to 16 days, depending on their age and general condition, the availability of home care, and the rapidity of postoperative healing.

Operative mortality: Usually 1% or less

Special monitoring required: The overall condition of the patient dictates the amount of monitoring required. Rapid hemorrhage may occur, and large intravenous lines should be inserted. A urinary catheter is also necessary. Patients should be observed in the intensive care unit for 24 to 48 hours.

Patient activity and positioning: The head should be elevated and positioned to reduce tension on the reconstructive flap pedicle. Closed suction drains are placed in the wound and kept in place until drainage is decreased. A high-humidity collar and routine tracheotomy maintenance are needed. Care must be taken to avoid tight dressings on the neck to prevent constriction of the flap pedicle. Ambulation is usually possible within 24 hours.

Alimentation: A feeding tube is inserted at the time of operation. Feedings are usually administered when bowel function has returned and are advanced to full strength over 1 or 2 days. When an extensive resection is anticipated and it is likely that dysphagia will be prolonged, a percutaneous endoscopic gastrostomy is often placed before or at the time of surgery. Oral liquids are usually given cautiously about 10 days after operation. If fluids are tolerated, food intake is slowly advanced and the feeding tube is removed. If patients are unable to tolerate tube feedings after operation, intravenous hyperalimentation is required.

Antibiotics: Perioperative antibiotics are administered routinely and continued for 2 days after operation. The agents used must be active against both anaerobes and aerobic

649

gram-positive bacteria. Some surgeons also provide gram-negative coverage.

Analgesia: Meperidine and morphine are used in the immediate postoperative period for pain control. Acetaminophen with codeine is usually sufficient after a few days.

Tracheotomy removal: In most cases, the tracheotomy can be removed 2 to 3 weeks after surgery.

POSTOPERATIVE COMPLICATIONS

IN THE HOSPITAL

Salivary fistula: Salivary fistulas are much more common in patients who have received preoperative radiation. Treatment involves opening the wound and administering local wound care. This complication may prolong the hospitalization and delay alimentation for as long as 6 weeks.

Myocutaneous flap necrosis: When myocutaneous flap necrosis occurs, the flap usually separates from the recipient site and a salivary fistula develops. Drainage, débridement, and secondary repair are required. A new myocutaneous flap may be needed for successful repair.

Major vessel erosion: If the fistula is in direct contact with the vessels in the neck, it may lead to erosion of the arterial wall and rapid hemorrhage. Ligation of the vessel is usually required for treatment.

Dysphagia and impaired deglutition: Depending on the extent of resection, some patients have great difficulty in resuming an oral diet and aspiration is common. It may be necessary to keep the feeding tube in place for several weeks or to insert a percutaneous gastrostomy.

AFTER DISCHARGE

Impaired speech: Tongue immobility and pharyngeal distortion may impair speech. Patients are usually able to compensate for this over several months. Some degree of long-term impairment may persist, but patients' families and close associates are generally able to understand them adequately.

Dysphagia and impaired deglutition: Many patients cannot resume an oral diet for some time. Swallowing therapy with a speech therapist is often of great benefit. Some patients require permanent gastrostomies and are never able to tolerate an oral diet.

Airway obstruction: Airway obstruction is most commonly seen during postoperative radiotherapy. Swelling and irritation from the radiation may impair the already compromised airway and require replacement of the tracheostomy tube.

BIBLIOGRAPHY

Ariyan S. The pectoralis major myocutaneous flap: a versatile flap for reconstruction in the head and neck. Plast Reconstr Surg 1979;63:78–81.

Hidalgo DA. Aesthetic improvements in free-flap mandible reconstruction. Plast Reconstr Surg 1991;88:574–585.

McConnell FMS. Rehabilitation of patients with tumors of the pharynx. In: Thawley SE, Panje WR, eds. Comprehensive management of head and neck tumors. Philadelphia, WB Saunders, 1987:815–857.

Weber RS, Raad I, Frankenthaler R, et al. Ampicillin sulbactan vs clindamycin in head and neck oncologic surgery: the need for gram negative coverage. Arch Otolaryngol Head Neck Surg 1992;118:1159–1163.

Medical Management of the Surgical Patient, Third Edition,
edited by Michael F. Lubin, H. Kenneth Walker, and Robert B. Smith III.
J.B. Lippincott Company, Philadelphia, PA © 1995.

MAXILLECTOMY

CHAPTER

123

Owen S. Reichman

Maxillectomy, in its various forms, is used for the treatment of carcinomas of the maxillary sinus and nasal cavity. Such tumors are often difficult to treat effectively because they may be extensive at the time of diagnosis. The eye, the base of the skull, and other sinuses are frequently involved at the time of initial presentation. Sinus tumors are most common in the sixth and seventh decades, and there is a distinct male predominance.

Multimodality therapy with either preoperative or postoperative radiation is almost always required. The extent of resection depends on the location of the tumor but the basic procedure involves the removal of the entire maxilla, including the hard palate. In more extensive tumors, the orbital floor, orbital contents, and anterior base of the skull may be included in the resected specimen. Because these lesions cause extreme pain and foul necrotic drainage, palliative surgical excision is often desirable even in unresectable tumors.

Maxillectomy generally requires 3 to 6 hours, depending on the extent of disease and the reconstruction techniques used. General anesthesia is always used and blood loss is usually in the range of 800 to 1500 mL. The resulting maxillectomy cavity is generally lined with a split-thickness skin graft, although microvascular free flaps are being used with increasing frequency. A palatal prosthesis is usually created before the operation and inserted into the surgical defect at the time of surgery.

USUAL POSTOPERATIVE COURSE

Expected postoperative hospital stay: The usual postoperative hospital stay is 7 to 14 days.

Operative mortality: The operative mortality rate is 2% or less for a limited maxillectomy but higher for more extensive lesions involving the base of the skull.

Special monitoring required: Vigorous bleeding can occur during the operation as the bone cuts are made and the tumor is removed. Generally, the internal maxillary artery is ligated to control this blood loss. Large intravenous catheters are recommended for volume replacement and central venous pressure monitoring is advised. Oozing from the surgical cavity may continue after the operation, and usual indicators of blood volume status should be observed closely.

Patient activity and positioning: Patients are kept with their heads elevated and are monitored in the intensive care unit overnight. They are usually ambulatory with assistance in 24 hours.

Alimentation: A feeding tube is often placed at the time of surgery and feeding is begun the day after. Skin grafts are held in place with packing, which is usually removed at 5 days. Oral feedings can then be administered and food intake advanced as tolerated, with the feeding tube removed.

Antibiotic coverage: Antibiotics effective against *Staphylo-*

coccus and *Streptococcus* are administered at the time of operation and continued until the packing is removed.

Wound care: The cavity is closely observed each day after the packing is removed, and local cautery and débridement are done as needed. As soon as the packing is removed, irrigation of the cavity is performed to prevent crusting.

Analgesia: Morphine or meperidine is usually needed for pain for at least the first 7 to 10 days.

POSTOPERATIVE COMPLICATIONS

IN THE HOSPITAL

Airway obstruction: Extensive edema of the remaining palate and pharyngeal airway may obstruct the airway. Patients should be completely awake before their endotracheal tubes are removed. If there is any doubt regarding the adequacy of the airway, a tracheotomy should be done at the time of surgery.

Hemorrhage: Sudden soaking of the packing because of nasal hemorrhage may necessitate transfusion and possible reoperation.

Cerebrospinal fluid leak: Cerebrospinal fluid leakage is usually seen after resection of the base of the skull. The head of the bed should be kept elevated and lumbar drains placed. It is occasionally necessary to revise the dural closure.

AFTER DISCHARGE

Diplopia: If the eye is preserved, diplopia can become a problem because of loss of the orbital floor. The orbital floor may be reconstructed at the time of surgery with either a temporalis muscle or a microvascular free flap.

Vocal and deglutition abnormalities: Even with a properly fitted palatal prosthesis, the voice quality is often markedly different and only a soft diet may be manageable.

Cavity crusting, bleeding, and malodorous drainage: Some leakage of food and secretions between the palatal prosthesis and the cavity always occurs. The cavity must be irrigated daily to remove the crust and food particles that accumulate.

Cosmetic disfigurement: The degree of cosmetic disfigurement depends on the extent of resection. The continued care and support of a prosthodontic team are necessary. If the eyelids are not removed, an ocular prosthesis can be used to replace an excised globe.

Pain: Pain is usually a sign of residual tumor and may be difficult to control because of bone and neural invasion.

BIBLIOGRAPHY

Coleman JJ. Microvascular approach to function and appearance of large orbital maxillary defects. Am J Surg 1989;158:337–341.

Krespi YP, Leive TM. Tumors of the nose and paranasal sinuses. In: Paparella MM, Shamrick DA, eds. Otolaryngology, ed 3. Philadelphia, WB Saunders, 1991:1935–1958.

Rice DH, Stanley RB. Surgical therapy of nasal cavity, ethmoid sinus, and maxillary sinus tumors. In: Thawley SE, Pange WR, eds. Comprehensive management of head and neck tumors. Philadelphia, WB Saunders, 1987:368–389.

Terz JJ, Young HF, Lawrence W. Combined craniofacial resection for locally advanced carcinoma of the head and neck. Am J Surg 1980;140:618–624.

Medical Management of the Surgical Patient, Third Edition,
edited by Michael F. Lubin, H. Kenneth Walker, and Robert B. Smith III.
J.B. Lippincott Company, Philadelphia, PA © 1995.

CHAPTER

124

MASTOIDECTOMY OR TYMPANOPLASTY WITH MASTOIDECTOMY

John S. Turner, Jr.

Almost all mastoid procedures are carried out to correct chronic inflammatory diseases such as cholesteatoma. Some attempt virtually always is made to restore hearing (tympanoplasty) at the same time by grafting or inserting prosthetic appliances.

Mastoidectomy alone may take 2 to 4 hours to perform; tympanoplasty adds 30 to 60 minutes of additional operating time. If only tympanoplasty is done, the operation may take 1 to 3 hours. General anesthesia, which permits the use of injectable and topical epinephrine, is required. Blood loss is minimal and transfusion is not needed. Most of the procedure is performed under the operating microscope.

USUAL POSTOPERATIVE COURSE

Expected postoperative hospital stay: The postoperative hospital stay ranges from 1 to 3 days, depending on the presence of nausea, vertigo, pain, and wound drainage.

Operative mortality: Under 1%

Special monitoring required: Cardiac monitoring is necessary during the operation because epinephrine is used.

Patient activity and positioning: Patients get up to go to the bathroom with assistance on the day of operation and usually are ambulatory the next day. They are instructed to keep water out of the operated ear and to avoid blowing the nose to prevent eustachian tube inflation.

Alimentation: Clear liquids are permitted after nausea resolves on the day of operation. Supplementary intravenous fluids may be required for 24 to 36 hours, however, because of labyrinthine stimulation of the emetic center.

Antibiotic coverage: Systemic antibiotics are given because the operation is performed to correct a chronic infection. Intravenous ampicillin is the drug of choice; cephalothin is used in patients with ampicillin allergy. These agents are administered orally after 24 hours. Topical chloramphenicol (Chloromycetin) is usually placed on the mastoid packing.

Skin grafting: Occasionally, a skin graft is used to correct ear canal stenosis.

POSTOPERATIVE COMPLICATIONS

Nausea and vertigo: Excessive nausea, vomiting, and vertigo may be seen, indicating damage to the labyrinth or unusual labyrinthosis. The administration of intravenous fluids may be necessary for several days and antiemetic drugs are usually needed.

Cerebrospinal fluid leak: The dura may be penetrated during the operation, resulting in a cerebrospinal fluid leak that is not detected in the operating room. Head elevation, extended antibiotic therapy with chloromycetin, and lumbar puncture daily to reduce otorrhea may be required.

653

Reoperation for direct closure can be delayed several days to observe the effects of conservative measures.

Facial nerve paralysis from surgical damage: Reoperation for repair should be done immediately if surgical damage causes facial nerve paralysis.

AFTER DISCHARGE

Dizziness: Dizziness may persist for several weeks but this is uncommon. Labyrinthine sedatives such as meclizine, thiethylperazine, or diphenidol may be needed.

Infection: Prolonged infection of the cavity may require frequent cleaning and topical antibiotic treatment.

Stenosis: Revision surgery to correct canal stenosis is infrequently needed.

BIBLIOGRAPHY

Caparosa RJ. An atlas of surgical anatomy and techniques of the temporal bone. Springfield, IL, Charles C Thomas, 1972: 29–78.

Nadol JB, Schuknecht HF. Surgery of the ear and temporal bone. New York, Raven Press, 1992.

Tos M, Thomason J, Peitersen E. Cholesteatoma and mastoidectomy surgery. Berkeley, Kugler & Ghendini, 1989.

Medical Management of the Surgical Patient, Third Edition,
edited by Michael F. Lubin, H. Kenneth Walker, and Robert B. Smith III.
J.B. Lippincott Company, Philadelphia, PA © 1995.

CHAPTER

125

UVULOPALATO-PHARYNGOPLASTY

William G. Grist

Uvulopalatopharyngoplasty (UPPP) is an operation used in the treatment of obstructive sleep apnea (OSA) to enlarge the nasopharyngeal opening into the pharynx by removing redundant or excessive palatal and pharyngeal mucosa and tonsils. In OSA, the airway becomes obstructed partly as a result of passive collapse caused by hypotonicity of the palatal, pharyngeal, and lingual muscles during sleep. In addition, as the airway is narrowed by passive contraction, inspiratory airflow velocity increases and intraluminal pressure decreases in accordance with Bernoulli's principle, further contributing to airway obstruction. If complete obstruction occurs, patients arouse after several seconds to a minute or more. They then take several breaths and drift back to sleep, only to repeat the cycle, frequently as often as 200 to 300 times per night. Patients awaken the next morning feeling unrefreshed and fatigued, and they experience daytime hypersomnolence. The diagnosis of OSA is suggested by these symptoms and by descriptions from the sleeping partner of excessively loud snoring and apnea. Confirmation is obtained by polysomnography, which also quantifies the severity of OSA by measuring the number and duration of apnea events, the degree of hemoglobin-oxygen desaturation, and any associated cardiac events such as bradycardia or arrhythmia. Long-term consequences include a higher incidence of hypertension, stroke, angina, and myocardial infarction in patients with sleep apnea than in control subjects. Loud snoring is usually present in OSA, and UPPP is effective in eliminating or reducing the level of snoring. The procedure may be performed solely for that reason, particularly if the noise is causing marital strife.

Many patients with OSA are excessively overweight, and weight reduction should be encouraged because this will reduce the volume of the tongue, palate, and pharyngeal fat stores and lead to airway enlargement. However, weight reduction in the face of significant sleep apnea is more difficult than normal because of the sedentary behavior of patients with OSA. Thyroid function should also be investigated and treated if hypothyroidism is present.

The treatment of choice for OSA is nasal continuous positive airway pressure (NCPAP). In this method, positive-pressure air is applied to the nose through a tight-fitting mask or nasal appliance. Rather than collapsing with inspiration, the airway is splinted or distended by the positive-pressure inflow. Before NCPAP is used, it is necessary to determine in the sleep laboratory the positive pressure that is required to eliminate the obstruction. The treatment dilemma occurs in patients who fail to respond to NCPAP because of noncompliance, intolerance, nasal obstruction, or mechanical reasons such as poor mask fit. Theoretically, NCPAP should work for most patients, but the failure rate ranges from 20% to 40%.

UPPP serves as an adjunctive treatment of OSA in selected patients. It is not effective in patients who are morbidly obese or in those who have obstruction below the level of the palate (as is the case in patients with macroglossia or mandibular retrognathism). Patients being considered for UPPP must undergo a complete physical examination with emphasis on the nose and the pharynx. Complete or partial nasal obstruction must be corrected before or at the same time as the palatal surgery for UPPP to be successful. Occasionally, nasal airway correction alone is sufficient to produce significant improvement in patients with OSA. The presence and size of tonsils, the length of the soft palate, and the size of the tongue relative to the pharynx are important considerations in the selection of patients for operation.

The goal of UPPP is to enlarge the opening from the nasopharynx to the oropharynx. This is accomplished first by removing the tonsils or, if none are present, by removing the mucosa of the tonsillar fossa. Next, a palatal incision is made connecting the tonsillar wounds along the distal edge of the palatal musculature, and the uvula and palatal mucosa are excised. At this point, the posterior tonsillar pillars, which determine the transverse diameter of the opening from the nasopharynx, are retracted laterally and sutured to the anterior tonsillar pillars. This sets the corners of the opening and increases the transverse diameter about two or three times. The free edge of the palate and tonsillar wounds are then closed.

Ideal candidates for UPPP are patients with large tonsils, a narrow nasopharyngeal outlet, and normal-sized tongue. Patients who have failed to respond to NCPAP and who are not candidates for UPPP should be considered for tracheotomy. In many cases, tracheotomy is excellent treatment because patients can be fitted with self-retaining tracheal buttons that can be occluded during the day and opened at night with little loss of quality of life.

USUAL POSTOPERATIVE COURSE

Expected postoperative hospital stay: The usual postoperative hospital stay is 1 or 2 days. Patients can be discharged when pain control and adequate oral intake are achieved.

Operative mortality: Operative mortality is rare.

Special monitoring required: Pulse oximetry may reveal periods of hemoglobin-oxygen desaturation as a result of persistent OSA caused by swelling at the surgical site and nasal airway obstruction, if nasal surgery was performed at the same setting. A nasopharyngeal airway may be necessary during this period. Intensive care unit observation may be advisable if patients have associated medical conditions that increase their risk during periods of apnea.

Patient activity and positioning: The head should be elevated 30 to 45 degrees. Patients are ambulatory beginning on the day of operation.

Alimentation: Severe pain with swallowing is the most striking feature of the postoperative course. Pain is a function of surgery and not of diet. Patients are usually given

liquids first, and food intake is advanced to solids in the first 24 to 48 hours. Topical anesthetics are not effective in relieving pain, but it is helpful to give systemic analgesics about half an hour before meals.

Antibiotic coverage: Cefazolin is administered intravenously at a dosage of 1 g every 8 hours beginning 30 minutes before surgery and for two doses afterward. In penicillin-allergic patients, clindamycin can be used at a dose of 600 mg every 6 hours.

Palatal incompetence: Patients frequently have mild palatal incompetence immediately after surgery. This improves as postoperative discomfort lessens and palatal edema subsides.

POSTOPERATIVE COMPLICATIONS

IN THE HOSPITAL

Bleeding: Bleeding occasionally occurs in the immediate postoperative period. If it is slight, patients can simply be observed, with their heads elevated. More severe bleeding, in which patients are constantly clearing their throats and coughing, or hematoma formation in the palate may require a return to the operating room because airway obstruction can result.

Associated medical conditions: Many patients with OSA have serious concomitant medical conditions, such as hypertension and cardiac and pulmonary disease. Given the stress of the postoperative course, complications may arise from these associated conditions.

AFTER DISCHARGE

Palatal incompetence: Although palatal incompetence is common in the immediate postoperative period, it rarely persists into the late postoperative period if the surgeon is conservative in the excision of palatal mucosa.

Nasopharyngeal stenosis: Nasopharyngeal stenosis can occur if the posterior pharyngeal wall is denuded at operation. Care should be taken to avoid this error.

BIBLIOGRAPHY

Anad VK, Ferguson P, Schoen L. Obstructive sleep apnea: a comparison of continuous positive airway pressure and surgical treatment. Otolaryngol Head Neck Surg 1991;105:382–390.

Fujita S, Conway W, Zorick F, Roth T. Surgical correction of anatomic abnormalities in obstructive sleep apnea syndrome: uvulopalatopharyngoplasty. Otolaryngol Head Neck Surg 1981;89:923–934.

Hoffstein V, Viner S, Mateika S, Conway J. Treatment of obstructive sleep apnea with nasal continuous positive airway pressure. Am Rev Respir Dis 1992;145:841–845.

Koopmann CF Jr, Moran WB Jr. Surgical management of obstructive sleep apnea. Otolaryngol Clin North Am 1990;23:787–807.

Simons FB, Guilleminault C, Miles LE. The palatopharyngoplasty operation for snoring and sleep apnea: an interim report. Otolaryngol Head Neck Surg 1984;92:375–380.

Westbrook P. Sleep disorders and upper airway obstruction in adults. Otolaryngol Clin North Am 1990;23:727–743.

SECTION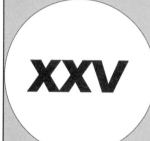

OPHTHALMIC SURGERY

Medical Management of the Surgical Patient, Third Edition,
edited by Michael F. Lubin, H. Kenneth Walker, and Robert B. Smith III.
J.B. Lippincott Company, Philadelphia, PA © 1995.

GENERAL CONSIDERATIONS IN OPHTHALMIC SURGERY

H. Michael Lambert
Pedro F. Lopez
Thomas M. Aaberg

Surgical procedures in ophthalmology are usually minimally invasive, offer a high probability of success, and have a major positive impact on quality of life. Nonetheless, because many patients who need ophthalmic surgery are elderly and have significant systemic diseases, the risks of even low-stress procedures must be balanced against their expected benefits. Optimal preoperative medical management can make surgery safer and more comfortable for patients, as well as improve the final outcome.

ANESTHESIA

Many ophthalmic procedures can be performed under local anesthesia. Exceptions are those cases in which a significant ocular laceration or perforation exists (penetrating trauma, surgical wound dehiscence, perforated corneal ulcer); those that are prolonged (many vitreoretinal and orbital cases); and those that involve adnexal structures that are not easily anesthetized. General anesthesia is indicated for younger patients and those who cannot be relied on to remain motionless and oriented during ophthalmic surgery.

Local anesthesia for intraocular surgery consists of 3 to 5 mL of lidocaine or a longer-acting compound given as a retrobulbar block to immobilize and anesthetize the globe and as a regional seventh nerve block to prevent eyelid closure. The risks of local ophthalmic anesthesia are minimal but include retrobulbar hemorrhage, rupture of the globe, and systemic absorption of the anesthetic agent, the last of which can result in hypertension, apnea, and seizure if the drug is inadvertently injected into a vessel. Appropriate preoperative patient education, mild sedation, and some analgesia allow the local anesthesia to be administered with minimal stress and discomfort.

PATIENT COOPERATION

The patient's internist may have important insight into the level of anxiety and cooperation that can be expected from a particular patient. This information is vital in choosing between local and general anesthesia.

VENTILATION UNDER LOCAL ANESTHESIA

Ophthalmic surgery must be performed on motionless, comfortable patients who are supine. Although oxygen is administered through nasal prongs or a mask, the combination of feeling anxious, lying supine, and being covered with surgical drapes may result in real or perceived dyspnea or disorientation during the operation. Thus, dyspnea and orthopnea are major factors that must be assessed and minimized before ophthalmic surgery is undertaken. Elective operations may need to be postponed until congestive heart failure, severe chronic obstructive lung disease, or other major medical problems are optimally treated. Acute dyspnea and coughing spasms during ophthalmic surgery under local anesthesia can cause hemorrhage and prolapse of intraocular structures, resulting in blindness.

ARTERIAL HYPERTENSION

Acute blood pressure elevation in the operative or early postoperative period can cause intraocular hemorrhage, posing a serious threat to vision. In known hypertensive patients who are undergoing eye surgery under local anesthesia, oral antihypertensive medications should be administered on the morning of surgery. Blood pressure elevation may result from poor preoperative blood pressure control, failure to administer patients' usual medications, excessive anxiety, phenylephrine drops prescribed before operation for pupillary dilation, and epinephrine used as a component of the local anesthetic solution. These factors can be minimized by appropriately evaluating and educating patients before surgery, ensuring continuity of daily medications, using minimal amounts of a low concentration of topical phenylephrine, and substituting newer, longer-acting anesthetic agents to eliminate the need for a vasoconstrictor in the local injection.

COAGULATION

As in any surgical procedure, normal blood coagulation is desirable for ocular surgery. Thus, if medically feasible, patients who undergo therapeutic anticoagulation should be brought back to a normal coagulation level for the ophthalmic procedure. In most cases, anticoagulant therapy can be resumed immediately after the procedure. Aspirin should be withheld for 2 weeks before eye surgery.

For patients in whom normal coagulation cannot be restored even temporarily, some ophthalmic procedures can be modified to minimize the risk of hemorrhage. Cataract procedures and corneal surgery can be performed such that all incisions are placed within the cornea, which is normally an avascular structure. Depending on the severity of the co-agulation defect, however, the risk of retrobulbar hemorrhage associated with the local anesthetic injection may require the use of general anesthesia.

INFECTION

Intraocular infection is both rare and devastating after elective ophthalmic surgery, occurring at a rate of about 1 in 5000 cases. When postoperative infectious endophthalmitis does occur, loss of useful vision is frequent despite aggressive therapy. Thus, it is accepted ophthalmic practice to administer prophylactic topical antibiotics, usually aminoglycoside drops, before and after operation. Dedicating exclusive operating space for ophthalmic procedures may be the best way to prevent eye infections because this precludes contamination from inadequate cleaning after general surgical cases.

Because high antibiotic levels in the anterior segment of the eye are achieved with topical administration, and because subtherapeutic levels in the posterior segment are achieved with systemic administration, topical antibiotics are used more frequently, both for prophylaxis and for therapy, than are systemic antibiotics. Elective intraocular procedures are unlikely to result in significant bacteremia and do not require the use of prophylactic systemic antibiotics to prevent endocarditis.

OPHTHALMIC MEDICATIONS

Dilation of the pupil and cycloplegia are usually necessary before and after surgery, requiring the use of topical phenylephrine (sympathomimetic) and atropine or atropine-like drops (parasympatholytic) such as scopolamine, homatropine, cyclopentolate, and others. Hypertension can be associated with the former, whereas urinary retention and mental disturbances occur with the latter.

Postoperative elevation of intraocular pressure can occur after any intraocular surgery and, if marked and acute, is accompanied by a vagal response that includes nausea, vomiting, and bradycardia. This complication is usually treated with topical β-blocking agents (timolol) and carbonic anhydrase inhibitors (acetazolamide and others), with systemic osmotic agents (mannitol and glycerin) reserved for the most severe cases. Topical β-blockers are absorbed systemically and can result in bronchospasm and heart blockage and can exacerbate congestive heart failure. Acetazolamide (Diamox) is a sulfa derivative that may cause a hypersensitivity reaction in predisposed patients, metabolic abnormalities, gastrointestinal disturbance, paresthesias, lethargy, and, rarely, aplastic suppression of the bone marrow.

Topical corticosteroid preparations are used routinely after many types of eye surgery to minimize inflammation, pain, scarring, and vascularization. Because systemic ab- sorption of such drops and ointments in adults is minimal, adrenal suppression is negligible. When postoperative in- flammation is severe, a short course of high-dose systemic corticosteroids may be used.

Medical Management of the Surgical Patient, Third Edition,
edited by Michael F. Lubin, H. Kenneth Walker, and Robert B. Smith III.
J.B. Lippincott Company, Philadelphia, PA © 1995.

GLAUCOMA SURGERY

H. Michael Lambert
Pedro F. Lopez
Thomas M. Aaberg

The term *glaucoma* refers to a group of disorders in which elevation of the intraocular pressure causes optic nerve damage that is manifested by changes in the optic disc on ophthalmoscopy, loss of visual fields, and ultimate loss of central vision. For primary and secondary open-angle glaucoma, treatment consists of escalating measures, starting with topical medications and carbonic anhydrase inhibitors and progressing to outpatient laser surgery and finally to operative procedures. Outpatient laser iridotomy has replaced operative peripheral iridectomy for uncomplicated angle-closure glaucoma.

Glaucoma surgical procedures performed in the operating room generally include filtering procedures and laser ablation or cryoablation of the ciliary body, the aqueous–producing structure of the eye. Filtration surgery is designed to create a fistula from the anterior chamber to the subconjunctival space, allowing fluid to pass more easily from the eye. Both filtration surgery and cyclocryotherapy can be performed under local anesthesia, but general anesthesia may be preferred.

USUAL POSTOPERATIVE COURSE

Expected postoperative hospital stay: The duration of postoperative hospitalization depends on the severity of the glaucoma and the procedure required.

Operative mortality: Operative mortality is limited to that of the anesthetic used.

Special monitoring required: No special monitoring is required for elective cases. Cardiac monitoring is useful in elderly patients with acute glaucoma because of their increased risk of myocardial ischemia.

Patient activity and positioning: Patients who have undergone filtration surgery wear a protective dressing consisting of eye pads and a shield. Major restrictions on ambulation are unusual. Frequent examinations are necessary after filtration surgery until the anterior chamber begins to reform.

Alimentation: No dietary restrictions are indicated.

Postoperative medications: Frequent applications of topical corticosteroids, topical antibiotics, and atropine-like drops are administered after filtration surgery. After cyclocryotherapy, atropine-like drops and potent oral or intramuscular analgesics are given.

POSTOPERATIVE COMPLICATIONS

Shallow or flat anterior chamber: A shallow or flat anterior chamber frequently results from excessive filtration and flow of aqueous out of the anterior chamber through the surgically created fistula. Corrective measures include special dressings and frequent topical application of cycloplegics and corticosteroid drops. Additional surgery may be required.

Elevated intraocular pressure: Inadequate filtration caused by obstruction of the surgical fistula or scarring of the overlying conjunctiva may lead to elevated intraocular pressure. Rarely, other, more acute types of glaucoma occur during the postoperative course.

Infectious endophthalmitis: Infectious endophthalmitis can occur immediately after operation or may be delayed, especially if the filtering bleb opens.

BIBLIOGRAPHY

Spaeth GL. Glaucoma surgery. In: Tasman W, Jaeger EA, eds. Duane's clinical ophthalmology, vol 5. Philadelphia, JB Lippincott, 1991.

CHAPTER

128

EYE MUSCLE SURGERY

Medical Management of the Surgical Patient, Third Edition,
edited by Michael F. Lubin, H. Kenneth Walker, and Robert B. Smith III.
J.B. Lippincott Company, Philadelphia, PA © 1995.

H. Michael Lambert
Pedro F. Lopez
Thomas M. Aaberg

Eye muscle surgery is performed to straighten horizontally or vertically misaligned eyes, usually in children. Such misalignment may be congenital, acquired, paralytic, or restrictive. Eye muscle surgery may be performed for cosmetic indications or to improve binocular function. In most instances, the muscles are adjusted at surgery; however, a newer technique that is feasible with cooperative patients uses sutures that are adjusted after operation when all anesthetic effect has disappeared.

Eye muscle surgery can be accomplished with general, local, or, in special cases, merely topical anesthesia. Because surgery is extraocular, ocular risk is minimal.

USUAL POSTOPERATIVE COURSE

Expected postoperative hospital stay: Hospitalization is optional, because the procedures can be performed on an ambulatory basis, depending on the constraints of anesthesia.

Operative mortality: Operative mortality is limited to that of the anesthetic used.

Special monitoring required: No special monitoring is necessary.

Patient activity and positioning: If a dressing is used, it consists of eye pads. Generally, there are no restrictions or limitations on activity.

Alimentation: No dietary restrictions are indicated.

Postoperative medications: Topical antibiotics are administered after surgery.

POSTOPERATIVE COMPLICATIONS

Slipped muscle: Slipped muscle is an extraordinarily rare complication resulting when an extraocular muscle detaches from its new site of attachment and retracts posteriorly. It is recognized by a large postoperative misalignment of the eyes and an inability to move the involved eye into the field of action of the detached muscle. Surgical exploration is indicated.

Diplopia: Double vision of varying degrees may occur after surgical alteration of ocular alignment. This is a more prominent postoperative symptom in adults than in young children because the latter demonstrate considerable neurologic plasticity in adapting to altered ocular alignment. The problem is self-limited in most cases.

Failure to achieve desired alignment: Failure to achieve desired alignment is a common complication of eye muscle surgery that takes several weeks to diagnose with certainty and is usually an indication for reoperation.

BIBLIOGRAPHY

Reinecke RD. Muscle surgery. In: Tasman W, Jaeger EA, eds. Duane's clinical ophthalmology, vol 5. Philadelphia, JB Lippincott, 1991.

Medical Management of the Surgical Patient, Third Edition,
edited by Michael F. Lubin, H. Kenneth Walker, and Robert B. Smith III.
J.B. Lippincott Company, Philadelphia, PA © 1995.

CHAPTER

129

ENUCLEATION, EVISCERATION, AND EXENTERATION

H. Michael Lambert
Pedro F. Lopez
Thomas M. Aaberg

Enucleation, or removal, of an eye is indicated and highly therapeutic after severe disease has rendered it blind and painful. A blind eye may be removed within 2 weeks after severe trauma or unsuccessful surgery to prevent sympathetic ophthalmia, an extremely rare condition in which the healthy fellow eye develops granulomatous inflammation from uveal damage and resultant immunologic reaction in the damaged eye. Other processes leading to removal of the eye include large malignant intraocular tumors, advanced and intractable glaucoma, and infectious endophthalmitis.

Three general types of procedures can be performed:

1. In evisceration, the intraocular contents are removed, leaving an intact sclera. Enucleation is the most common eye removal procedure and involves removal of the entire globe, including its scleral coat, leaving the extraocular muscles and a stump of optic nerve.
2. Exenteration, a rarely performed operation in which all orbital contents are removed, is reserved for aggressive ocular and adnexal tumors or infections.
3. A spherical prosthetic implant or dermis fat graft may be used after enucleation or evisceration to replace the volume lost through the removal of ocular contents, thereby giving a better cosmetic appearance and allowing the eventual use of a prosthesis.

The procedures are usually performed under general anesthesia for psychologic as well as physiologic reasons.

USUAL POSTOPERATIVE COURSE

Expected postoperative hospital stay: 1 to 3 days

Operative mortality: Operative mortality is limited to that of the anesthetic used.

Special monitoring required: No special monitoring is necessary.

Patient activity and positioning: The postoperative dressing consists of a plastic conformer to maintain the conjunctival cul-de-sac under a pressure dressing. Minimal restrictions on activity are necessary.

Alimentation: No dietary restricitons are indicated.

Postoperative medications: The use of postoperative medication is typically limited to a topical antibiotic instilled when the dressings are changed.

Psychologic support: Psychologic support is vital because the loss of an eye is a highly emotional event for patients. The treating physician must be fully aware of this need.

POSTOPERATIVE COMPLICATIONS

Swelling of orbital tissue: The use of a pressure dressing minimizes orbital tissue swelling.

Bleeding: Bleeding is usually limited to staining of the pressure dressing.

Extrusion of the implant: In a late complication, the spherical implant may partially or completely extrude through the overlying conjunctiva and connective tissue, usually necessitating additional surgery.

BIBLIOGRAPHY

Ratio GT. Enucleation and evisceration. In: Tasman W, Jaeger EA, eds. Duane's clinical ophthalmology, vol 5. Philadelphia, JB Lippincott, 1991.

CHAPTER

130

Medical Management of the Surgical Patient, Third Edition,
edited by Michael F. Lubin, H. Kenneth Walker, and Robert B. Smith III.
J.B. Lippincott Company, Philadelphia, PA © 1995.

VITREORETINAL SURGERY

H. Michael Lambert
Pedro F. Lopez
Thomas M. Aaberg

The field of vitreoretinal surgery has rapidly expanded in the past two decades. Retinal detachment is caused by a retinal tear or traction from numerous diseases, including diabetes, proliferative vitreoretinopathy, and sickle cell disease. Acute partial retinal detachment, in which the macula remains attached, is a surgical emergency because an excellent visual prognosis is associated with the maintenance of macular attachment. Open eyes resulting from trauma, infectious endophthalmitis, and giant retinal tears are surgical emergencies as well. Other procedures for complete retinal detachment and removal of vitreous (vitrectomy) are usually less urgent.

Repair of retinal detachment caused by a retinal tear (rhegmatogenous retinal detachment) is accomplished by scleral buckling, a procedure in which the sclera is invaginated toward the detached retina by prosthetic elements placed outside the eye. Vitrectomy, a microsurgical technique in which the vitreous gel is slowly removed and replaced by saline, is performed for more complex retinal detachments. Vitrectomy is also the treatment for infectious endophthalmitis and for vitreous hemorrhage and scar tissue formation within the eye. To increase the probability of retinal reattachment in complex cases, sterile room air, other gaseous compounds, or oils may be injected into the eye. Intraoperative laser photocoagulation is often combined with these procedures to provide permanent fixation of the retina.

General anesthesia is used more often for vitreoretinal procedures than for other eye operations. Although local anesthesia can be used for patients with severe medical problems, the prolonged duration of vitreoretinal procedures makes general anesthesia more desirable.

USUAL POSTOPERATIVE COURSE

Expected postoperative hospital stay: The duration of postoperative hospitalization varies according to the severity of the vitreoretinal problem and the response of patients to surgery.

Operative mortality: The only operative mortality is that associated with the anesthetic used.

Special monitoring required: Monitoring requirements are based on the underlying disease.

Patient activity and positioning: Patients must wear eye pads and protective shields to cover the operated eye. Bed rest may be necessary for several days after surgery, especially when inert gaseous compounds are used within the eye, and some patients may have to remain in a particular position for several days to weeks. When gaseous material is left in the eye, air travel is not permitted until the agent has been resorbed to prevent bubble expansion at high altitudes.

Alimentation: No dietary restrictions are indicated.

Postoperative medications: A combination of topical antibiotics, corticosteroids, and atropine-like dilating drops are usually administered after surgery. Systemic corticosteroids may be used to decrease excessive inflammation.

POSTOPERATIVE COMPLICATIONS

Retinal detachment: Reoperation is usually necessary if retinal detachment occurs.

Elevated intraocular pressure: Several mechanisms may result in elevated intraocular pressure. Large increases in intraocular pressure may follow vitreoretinal procedures, commonly accompanied by pain, nausea, and vomiting. Treatment, as discussed in the introductory chapter to this section, may include topical β-blockers, systemic carbonic anhydrase inhibitors, and osmotic agents.

Intraocular infection: Endophthalmitis and infection involving extraocular scleral buckling elements are rare complications of vitreoretinal surgery.

BIBLIOGRAPHY

Benson WE. Vitrectomy. In: Tasman W, Jaeger EA, eds. Duane's clinical ophthalmology, vol 5. Philadelphia, JB Lippincott, 1991.

Curtin VT. Management of retinal detachment. In: Tasman W, Jaeger EA, eds. Duane's clinical ophthalmology, vol 5. Philadelphia, JB Lippincott, 1991.

Medical Management of the Surgical Patient, Third Edition,
edited by Michael F. Lubin, H. Kenneth Walker, and Robert B. Smith III.
J.B. Lippincott Company, Philadelphia, PA © 1995.

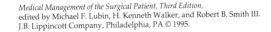

CATARACT SURGERY

H. Michael Lambert
Pedro F. Lopez
Thomas M. Aaberg

Modern cataract surgery is among the most common and successful surgical procedures performed today. Nearly 1 million cataract operations are performed in the United States each year, and well over 90% of patients regain the potential for full visual acuity. Recent technologic advances have improved and accelerated postoperative recovery. Intraocular lenses, replacing cataract spectacles and contact lenses, can be safely implanted in most patients, allowing a rapid return of normal vision. Wound size has been drastically reduced with newer techniques (eg, phacoemulsification) and advances in intraocular lens design. Microsurgical wound closure results in a highly secure incision, allowing immediate ambulation and eliminating the severe limitations formerly placed on patients after cataract surgery.

Refinements in cataract surgery combined with efforts at cost containment are largely responsible for the fact that more of these procedures are being done on an outpatient basis. Because the procedure is brief in duration and most of the patients are elderly and have significant cardiovascular impairment, most cataract extraction is performed under local anesthesia. Patients who can remain comfortable and oriented while they are supine and covered for 30 to 60 minutes are excellent candidates for this approach. The surgical stress is so low and visual rehabilitation so rapid and reliable that severe visual impairment is a reasonable indication for surgery, even in debilitated or terminally ill patients.

USUAL POSTOPERATIVE COURSE

Expected postoperative course: Hospitalization often is not required, although patients must be examined the day after surgery to assess inflammation, intraocular pressure, and wound closure. Several office visits are necessary during the 6 to 8 weeks after operation.

Operative mortality: Operative mortality is limited to that of the anesthetic used.

Special monitoring required: No special monitoring is necessary.

Patient activity and positioning: Restrictions include the use of a rigid eye shield worn at night for several weeks after surgery to prevent direct trauma to the eye. Excessive bending and lifting are discouraged. The hair should not be shampooed for several days, and for several weeks hair washing should be accomplished from behind with assistance so that excess water drips back and away from the operated eye. Dark sunglasses prevent discomfort from the photophobia that is usually present to some degree.

Alimentation: No dietary restrictions are indicated.

Postoperative medications: Postoperative medications are usually limited to topical corticosteroids and antibiotics. Aspirin and other platelet-suppressing agents are cautioned against for the first 3 to 4 weeks after surgery to minimize the risk of expulsive hemorrhage.

POSTOPERATIVE COMPLICATIONS

Wound dehiscence: Wound dehiscence is an increasingly rare complication. A small wound leak without prolapse of intraocular structures generally improves without treatment. More serious degrees of wound disruption, often caused by direct trauma after operation, must be repaired surgically.

Elevation of intraocular pressure: Postoperative glaucoma is common and, if severe, presents with ocular pain, nausea, and vomiting. Treatment includes the administration of topical β-blockers and systemic osmotic agents. Increased intraocular pressure is the most common cause of severe pain in the first 24 hours after surgery.

Postoperative infectious endophthalmitis: Postoperative infectious endophthalmitis is a rare complication that presents with pain and excessive inflammation in the early postoperative course and can result in permanent loss of useful vision despite intensive surgical and antibiotic therapy.

Retinal detachment: Retinal detachment is an unusual and typically late complication of cataract and intraocular surgery. Operative repair is indicated.

BIBLIOGRAPHY

Weinstein GW. Cataract surgery. In: Tasman W, Jaeger EA, eds. Duane's clinical ophthalmology, vol 5. Philadelphia, JB Lippincott, 1991.

Medical Management of the Surgical Patient, Third Edition,
edited by Michael F. Lubin, H. Kenneth Walker, and Robert B. Smith III.
J.B. Lippincott Company, Philadelphia, PA © 1995.

CHAPTER

132

CORNEAL TRANSPLANTATION

H. Michael Lambert
Pedro F. Lopez
Thomas M. Aaberg

Refinements in microsurgical technique and corneal tissue preservation have greatly improved the prognosis for patients undergoing corneal transplantation. Full-thickness corneal transplantation (penetrating keratoplasty) results in a clear graft in over 90% of patients. Decreased visual acuity from corneal opacity, corneal swelling, and abnormalities of corneal shape are the usual indications for surgery. Corneal transplantation can be performed simultaneously with cataract extraction, intraocular lens implantation, and anterior and posterior vitrectomy. Partial-thickness corneal transplantation (lamellar keratoplasty) is sometimes performed for superficial corneal scars or to correct refractive errors.

Although some corneal transplantations are being done in an outpatient setting, many patients are hospitalized for several days. The procedure can be performed with local or general anesthesia and takes about 2 hours. It is vital that patients remain comfortable and motionless throughout the procedure because of the danger of prolapsing intraocular structures through the large, round incision.

USUAL POSTOPERATIVE COURSE

Expected postoperative hospital stay: Hospitalization ranges from 0 to 3 days, depending on the individual patient. Follow-up examinations are frequent during the first few postoperative months.

Operative mortality: Operative mortality is limited to that of the anesthetic used.

Special monitoring required: No special monitoring is necessary.

Patient activity and positioning: Bending and lifting should be minimized for several weeks after surgery. A protective shield must be worn at night to prevent accidental injury and spectacles or sunglasses should be worn during the day to prevent trauma and photophobia. Hair washing precautions should be observed as outlined in Chapter 131. In most cases, ambulation is permitted immediately after surgery.

Alimentation: No dietary restrictions are necessary.

Postoperative medications: Postoperative medications include topical corticosteroids and antibiotics. These are administered more frequently and for a longer period than after cataract surgery. Some patients are maintained on topical corticosteroid therapy indefinitely to prevent rejection. A short course of systemic corticosteroids is occasionally used to treat excessive inflammation.

POSTOPERATIVE COMPLICATIONS

Wound disruption: Wound disruption is an increasingly rare complication with current microsurgical technique. It may be self-limited if it is minor or require surgical correction if aqueous leakage is more profuse.

674

Glaucoma and retinal detachment: Glaucoma and retinal detachment may occur, as discussed in Chapter 131.

Corneal graft rejection: Corneal graft rejection does not occur before the third postoperative week in eyes without previous graft rejection and presents as a painful, photophobic, inflamed eye with loss of visual acuity because of corneal graft edema. Treatment is often successful and consists of frequent applications of topical corticosteroids.

BIBLIOGRAPHY

Stern AL, Taylor DM. Refractive surgery. In: Tasman W, Jaeger EA, eds. Duane's clinical ophthalmology, vol 5. Philadelphia, JB Lippincott, 1991.

Weisenthal RW, Whitson WE, Krachmer JH. Corneal surgery. In: Tasman W, Jaeger EA, eds. Duane's clinical ophthalmology, vol 5. Philadelphia, JB Lippincott, 1991.

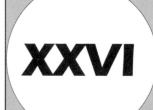

SECTION **XXVI**

GYNECOLOGIC SURGERY

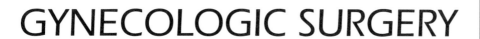

Medical Management of the Surgical Patient, Third Edition,
edited by Michael F. Lubin, H. Kenneth Walker, and Robert B. Smith III.
J.B. Lippincott Company, Philadelphia, PA © 1995.

CHAPTER

UTERINE CURETTAGE

133

Clifford R. Wheeless, Jr.

Uterine curettage is probably the most frequently performed operation in gynecologic surgery. It is used for a variety of indications, including the following:

Polymenorrhea—menstrual cycle interval less than 21 days

Oligomenorrhea—menstrual cycle interval more than 37 days

Metrorrhagia—menstrual bleeding longer than 7 days, or interval bleeding

Menorrhagia—excessive or prolonged menstrual bleeding

Postmenopausal bleeding—uterine bleeding occurring more than 12 months after the last menstrual period in a menopausal woman

Breakthrough bleeding—intermenstrual bleeding in a menstrual cycle that is the result of exogenous hormones

Dysfunctional uterine bleeding—a complex that includes any abnormal uterine bleeding in the absence of pregnancy, neoplasm, infection, or uterine lesion

Abortions—spontaneous abortion, fetal death in utero, septic abortion, legal termination of pregnancy, dilation and evacuation of gestational trophoblastic neoplasias, incomplete abortion, or inevitable abortion

Within this wide range of indications, the most common are incomplete abortion, postmenopausal bleeding, and dysfunctional uterine bleeding. The purpose of curettage of the uterus is to remove endometrial or endocervical tissue for histologic study and to evacuate products of conception.

It is extremely important that dilation and curettage be performed correctly, for proper indications, and with minimal morbidity. If these precautions are disregarded, complications and even death may result. General anesthesia is usually administered because this allows more abdominal relaxation for optimal bimanual examination of the pelvic viscera, but regional and local anesthesia may be used. The operative time for dilation and curettage is less than 15 minutes. Transfusion is rarely indicated unless significant preoperative hemorrhage has occurred, usually associated with pregnancy. It was formerly thought that uterine curettage was contraindicated in the presence of pelvic infection, pyometra, and septic abortion. When indicated, however, and with the use of preoperative antibiotic coverage, dilation and curettage under septic conditions can remove the source of infection (eg, septic abortion, pyometra) and provide valuable histologic information.

During the past 50 years, many instruments have been devised to allow the sampling of endometrial tissue as an outpatient office procedure. These usually are suction devices, such as the Novak curette, which uses a syringe. In patients suspected of having adenocarcinoma, diagnostic confidence in these devices should be maintained only if the biopsy sample shows carcinoma. Otherwise, a classic dilation and curettage should be performed.

USUAL POSTOPERATIVE COURSE

Expected postoperative hospital stay: Most of these procedures are performed on an outpatient basis. Inpatient hospitalization should be reserved for medical or surgical complications.

Operative mortality: The operative mortality rate is under 1% and almost always is associated with an anesthetic complication.

Special monitoring required: No special monitoring is necessary.

Patient activity and positioning: Patients are ambulatory on the day of the procedure.

Alimentation: Food intake is permitted as tolerated on the day of surgery.

Antibiotic coverage: Preoperative antibiotic coverage is indicated for septic abortions and pyometra, and should be directed toward polymicrobial contamination (gram-negative rods, anaerobes, and gram-positive cocci).

Oxytocin: Oxytocin should be administered to patients who have undergone abortion.

POSTOPERATIVE COMPLICATIONS

IN THE HOSPITAL

Perforation of the uterus: Most cases of uterine perforation are associated with the use of sound or cervical dilators and occur in patients with acutely anteflexed or retroflexed uteri. Overnight observation in the hospital is usually required. The two principal dangers of uterine perforation are bleeding and trauma to adjacent abdominal viscera. Lateral perforation through the uterine vessels is especially dangerous. When serious damage from perforation is suspected, a diagnostic laparoscopy should be performed and the damage assessed and repaired.

Hemorrhage: Bleeding may be obvious or concealed within the peritoneal cavity. Hemorrhage generally results from injury to the uterine vein caused by a dilator or curette and requires immediate abdominal exploration, control of bleeding, and, sometimes, hysterectomy.

Intestinal perforation: Intestinal perforation is a rare complication that almost always results from termination of pregnancy and evacuation of products of conception with a suction curette. Lacerated or damaged small intestine can be aspirated through a vacuum curette. Immediate laparotomy is required, with repair or resection of the injured bowel.

AFTER DISCHARGE

Bleeding and fever: If bleeding is copious and sustained, reexploration of the endometrial cavity is indicated. If fever develops, a culture should be obtained from the endometrial cavity and appropriate antibiotics administered.

Asherman's syndrome: Asherman's syndrome predominantly occurs as a consequence of postabortion curettage and should be suspected when there is subsequent amenorrhea. The diagnosis can be confirmed by a hysterosalpingogram and hysteroscopy.

BIBLIOGRAPHY

Thompson JD, Rock JA. Curettage of the uterus. In: Telinde's operative gynecology, ed 7. Philadelphia, JB Lippincott, 1992:307–315.

Ward B. Current concepts of uterine curettage. Postgrad Med J 1960;28:450–456.

Medical Management of the Surgical Patient, Third Edition,
edited by Michael F. Lubin, H. Kenneth Walker, and Robert B. Smith III.
J.B. Lippincott Company, Philadelphia, PA © 1995.

VAGINAL HYSTERECTOMY

Clifford R. Wheeless, Jr.

Some 750,000 hysterectomies were performed in 1979. Assuming constant age-specific hysterectomy rates, the number of such operations will rise over the next 20 years as the population of women aged 30 to 49 years increases. The number of hysterectomies will rise from about 670,000 in 1965 to an estimated 810,000 in 1995 and ultimately to 854,000 by the year 2005.

The most comprehensive recent study on hysterectomy was reported by Wingo and associates from the Centers for Disease Control and Prevention. Among 119,972 women undergoing vaginal hysterectomy, there were 46 deaths. The vaginal approach to hysterectomy was associated with a much lower mortality rate than was the abdominal approach. Excluding pregnancy and cancer-related cases, the mortality rate for abdominal hysterectomy was 8.6 per 10,000 women and that for vaginal hysterectomy was 2.7 per 10,000 women. Hysterectomy should be considered a low-risk operation that can be performed to treat nonpregnant patients and those with benign gynecologic symptoms or disease. Vaginal hysterectomy can be used for many indications, including pelvic relaxation, cervical intraepithelial neoplasia, small leiomyoma, and recurrent dysfunctional uterine bleeding.

The success of a vaginal hysterectomy is directly related to the experience of the surgeon. Surgeons who have any doubt about this procedure should never hesitate to open the abdomen and complete the hysterectomy through the abdominal route or to choose abdominal hysterectomy initially if their operative experience is insufficient to allow proper and safe performance of the vaginal procedure. Vaginal hysterectomy generally takes 1 hour to perform. Transfusion is rarely required. General anesthesia is used most often but spinal or epidural anesthesia also is acceptable.

USUAL POSTOPERATIVE COURSE

Expected postoperative hospital stay: The hospital stay varies from 2 to 4 days, depending on the age and associated medical problems of the patient.

Operative mortality: Under 1%

Special monitoring required: No special monitoring is necessary.

Patient activity and positioning: Patients are ambulatory on the day of operation.

Alimentation: Postoperative food intake is permitted as desired.

Antibiotic coverage: Preoperative antibiotics aimed at polymicrobial contamination, covering gram-negative rods, anaerobes, and gram-positive cocci, should be administered.

Catheterization: Patients who undergo anterior repair of the bladder should have indwelling Foley catheters or suprapubic catheters for several days after surgery. Persistent urinary retention occurs in 10% to 15% of patients but usually responds well to intermittent self-catheterization. Urinary retention should be resolved before the catheter is removed.

Vaginal packing: Vaginal packing with gauze is not required.

POSTOPERATIVE COMPLICATIONS

IN THE HOSPITAL

Excessive vaginal bleeding: Bleeding comes predominantly from two sources. The most serious is a uterine artery pedicle or a uterosacral pedicle that has retracted outside the suture ligature. The next most common site of bleeding is from the posterior vaginal cuff between the uterosacral ligaments. A pelvic examination should be performed in the operating room and the vaginal cuff sutures should be removed. The structures of the broad ligament, the uterine artery pedicle, and the uterosacral pedicle can then be exposed with long Allis clamps applied to the round ligament and to the uterosacral ligament. Bleeding can often be controlled by suture ligature. For surgeons who are less experienced with vaginal surgery, a laparotomy may be required for secure control of bleeding. Cystoscopy should be performed with the intravenous injection of indigo carmine solution to ensure the integrity of the ureters after bleeding from the uterine artery pedicle is controlled. Bleeding from the posterior vaginal cuff is usually controlled with vaginal packing and hemostatic agents.

Intraperitoneal bleeding: When either of the two vascular pedicles described earlier hemorrhages into the peritoneal cavity, tachycardia, low urine output, and low blood pressure are noted. Such bleeding is especially dangerous because the peritoneal cavity can contain several liters of blood before the abdomen appears to be distended. If intraperitoneal bleeding is suspected, patients should be returned to the operating room and exploratory laparotomy should be performed and bleeding controlled. Blood transfusions may be required.

Vaginal cuff abscess: The development of a vaginal cuff abscess is rare if the vaginal cuff has been left open and its margin has been sutured. Most cases are seen in premenopausal women whose vaginal cuffs have been closed. If a vaginal abscess does occur, it should be drained and broad-spectrum antibiotics administered.

Peroneal nerve injury: Peroneal nerve injury is caused by improper positioning of the patient's legs without the usual flexion of the hip and knees. It is manifested by footdrop and a steppage gait. Recovery is slow but almost always complete within 6 to 8 months. Physiotherapy is helpful and a foot brace should be prescribed.

Ureteral injury: Ureteral injury may be asymptomatic but usually causes flank tenderness or spiking fever. It should always be considered when there is persistent ileus or unexplained fever. A ureterovaginal fistula usually presents by the 10th to 14th postoperative day. These patients should undergo immediate intravenous pyelography and cystoscopy to locate the site of the communication. If the fistula is identified in the first 2 or 3 postoperative days and there is no massive tissue necrosis or sepsis in the pelvis, a second exploratory laparotomy and ureteroneocystostomy should be performed. If the fistula is discovered in the second postoperative week, however, when there is a large degree of cellulitis in the pelvis, most patients are better served by having a percutaneous nephrostomy stent inserted by an interventional radiologist. Surgeons should wait 4 to 8 weeks to allow inflammation in the pelvis to subside and then should proceed with exploratory laparotomy and ureteroneocystostomy. Rarely, the percutaneous nephrostomy ureteral stent can be advanced past the ureteral fistula into the bladder. The fistula may then close without stricture, and the problem is solved. Long-term results of ureteral fistula treatment with stents reveal a significant incidence of stenosis with obstruction, however, and most patients require eventual surgical correction.

Vesicovaginal fistula: The principal symptom of vesicovaginal fistula is leakage of urine through the vagina. Methylene blue instilled into the bladder is immediately present in the vagina. Cystoscopy usually confirms the location of the fistula above the ureteric ridge high on the posterior wall of the bladder. If there is no significant cellulitis, edema, or necrosis in the margin of the fistula, immediate repair can be performed and is successful in 80% of cases. With the finding of necrosis or cellulitis in the margin of the fistula, however, it is best to delay treatment until the process has resolved. In most cases, the ideal time is after about 3 months. Foley catheter drainage of the bladder may reduce the distressing flow of urine through the fistula and occasionally allows small fistulas to heal.

AFTER DISCHARGE

Granulation tissue of the vaginal vault: Modern synthetic absorbable suture material has made granulation tissue of the vaginal vault a rare occurrence. It was more common with catgut suture.

Tuboovarian abscess: Tuboovarian abscess is rare but is associated with fever, pain, and a pelvic mass. It usually occurs 10 to 14 days after discharge from the hospital. Although the abscess can sometimes be drained by percutaneous needle and catheter insertion by an interventional radiologist, it often requires surgical incision and drainage.

BIBLIOGRAPHY

Cruikshank SH. Avoiding ureteral injury during total vaginal hysterectomy. South Med J 1985;78:1447–1450.

Dicker RC, Greenspan JR, Strauss LT, et al. Complications of abdominal and vaginal hysterectomy among women of reproductive age in the United States. Am J Obstet Gynecol 1982;144:841–848.

Gray LA. Complications of vaginal surgery. Clin Obstet Gynecol 1982;25:869–881.

Hamod KA, Spence MR, King TR. Prophylactic antibiotics in vaginal hysterectomy: a review. Obstet Gynecol Surv 1982;37:207–216.

Wingo PA, Huezo CM, Rubin GL, et al. The mortality risk associated with hysterectomy. Am J Obstet Gynecol 1985;152:803–808.

Medical Management of the Surgical Patient, Third Edition,
edited by Michael F. Lubin, H. Kenneth Walker, and Robert B. Smith III.
J.B. Lippincott Company, Philadelphia, PA © 1995.

CHAPTER

135

ABDOMINAL HYSTERECTOMY

Clifford R. Wheeless, Jr.

The frequency of abdominal hysterectomy is 1 per 1000 in women younger than 25 years but rises to 16 per 1000 in women older than 35 years. After the age of 35 years, women usually have completed their childbearing and also have a higher incidence of significant gynecologic disease. The mortality risk for hysterectomy in the United States has been studied by the Centers for Disease Control and Prevention. During the years 1979 through 1980, there were 477 deaths among 317,389 women having abdominal hysterectomies. The mortality rate for hysterectomy was higher for procedures associated with pregnancy and cancer than for procedures not associated with these conditions (29.2, 37.8, and 6.0 per 10,000 hysterectomies, respectively). Abdominal hysterectomy had a higher mortality rate than did vaginal hysterectomy. Excluding cases related to pregnancy or cancer, the mortality rate for abdominal hysterectomy was 8.6 per 10,000 women and that for vaginal hysterectomy was 2.7 per 10,000 women.

Simple total abdominal hysterectomy involves the removal of the uterine corpus and cervix through an abdominal incision and is performed for a variety of indications, including uterine leiomyomas, pelvic abscesses, endometriosis, and recurrent dysfunctional uterine bleeding. In addition, simple abdominal hysterectomy is performed for two malignant indications: adenocarcinoma of the endometrium and ovarian cancer. Invasive cancer of the cervix requires a radical abdominal hysterectomy. Transfusion for simple abdominal hysterectomy is rare and the operative time is 1½ to 2 hours. General anesthesia is usually chosen, although spinal anesthesia can be used.

USUAL POSTOPERATIVE COURSE

Expected postoperative hospital stay: 5 to 7 days

Operative mortality: Under 1%

Special monitoring required: No special monitoring is necessary.

Patient activity and positioning: Patients are out of bed on the day of operation and are ambulatory the next day.

Alimentation: Clear liquids are permitted on the first postoperative day, and food intake is progressed to a regular diet by the third day, when bowel function has been demonstrated.

Antibiotic coverage: Preoperative antibiotics aimed at polymicrobial contamination, covering most gram-negative rods, anaerobes, and gram-positive cocci, are administered.

Catheterization: Indwelling Foley catheter drainage is rarely required. Urinary retention is seen in 10% to 15% of patients but can be managed by intermittent self-catheterization.

Vaginal packing: Vaginal packing is not required.

POSTOPERATIVE COMPLICATIONS

IN THE HOSPITAL

Excessive vaginal bleeding: Postoperative vaginal bleeding occurs from predominantly three areas: the infundibulopelvic ligament where an oophorectomy has been performed, the uterine artery pedicle, and the uterosacral ligament pedicle. Vaginal cuff bleeding after abdominal hysterectomy is rare. A pelvic examination should be performed in the operating room and the vaginal cuff sutures removed. The structures of the broad ligament, the uterine artery pedicle, and the uterosacral ligament pedicle can be exposed with long Allis clamps applied to the round ligament and to the uterosacral ligament. Bleeding can often be secured vaginally by reexploration through the vaginal cuff incision but those less experienced with vaginal surgery may need to reopen the abdominal incision. If bleeding occurs from the ovarian artery and vein located in the infundibulopelvic ligament, the vaginal approach is rarely successful and repeated laparotomy is required. The integrity of the ureters is always of concern after bleeding from the pedicles of the uterus is controlled. Indigo carmine dye should be injected intravenously and cystoscopy performed to ensure that the ureters are not obstructed.

Intraperitoneal bleeding: Intraperitoneal bleeding is associated with tachycardia, low urinary output, and low blood pressure. There can be significant loss of blood into the peritoneal cavity before the abdomen becomes significantly distended.

Thromboembolic phenomena: Deep venous thrombosis may be manifested by an unexplained fever and tachycardia. Some patients note swelling and pain in the legs; others do not. Duplex ultrasound evaluation of the legs helps in making the diagnosis but venography may be required if the results are equivocal. The heparin challenge test, which consists of anticoagulation with heparin for 48 hours, produces a significant drop in fever and tachycardia if venous thrombosis is the correct diagnosis.

Dehiscence with or without evisceration: Dehiscence is evidenced by the drainage of serosanguineous fluid through the abdominal incision. These patients should be taken back to surgery and the rectus fascia resutured with a mass closure technique using no. 1 delayed synthetic absorbable suture. A running delayed synthetic absorbable suture has greater strength than does the Smead-Jones suture formerly

advocated for this problem. Dehiscence with evisceration should be managed first by wrapping the intestine in a sterile, moist towel. Patients should then be taken immediately to the operating room, the incision reopened, the intestine replaced in the abdominal cavity, and the wound resutured.

AFTER DISCHARGE

Intestinal obstruction: The location of intestinal obstruction in patients who have undergone gynecologic surgery is almost exclusively in the terminal ileum 24 inches from the ileocecal junction. Obstruction results predominantly from adhesions to a loop of bowel or from the terminal ileum entering an internal hernia and becoming incarcerated. Therapy with long-tube suction decompression can be efficacious. If this method fails, however, patients should be taken to the operating room and reexplored for relief of the intestinal obstruction.

BIBLIOGRAPHY

Dicker RC, Greenspan JR, Strauss LT, et al. Complications of abdominal and vaginal hysterectomy among women of reproductive age in the United States. Am J Obstet Gynecol 1982;144:841–848.

Duff P. Antibiotic prophylaxis for abdominal hysterectomy. Obstet Gynecol 1982;60:25–29.

Jones HW. Evolving aspects of reparative surgery. In: Thompson JD, Rock JA, eds. TeLinde's operative gynecology, ed 7. Philadelphia, JB Lippincott, 1992:739.

Kelly HA. Ligature of the trunks of the uterine and ovarian arteries as a means of checking hemorrhage from the uterus and broad ligaments in abdominal operations. Johns Hopkins Hosp Rep 1890;2:220–223.

Lee RA. Abdominal hysterectomy (simple). In: Breen JL, Osofsky HJ, eds. Current concepts in gynecologic surgery. Baltimore, Williams & Wilkins, 1987:151.

Wingo PA, Huezo CM, Rubin GL, et al. The mortality risk associated with hysterectomy. Am J Obstet Gynecol 1985;152:803–808.

CHAPTER

136

RADICAL ABDOMINAL HYSTERECTOMY

Medical Management of the Surgical Patient, Third Edition,
edited by Michael F. Lubin, H. Kenneth Walker, and Robert B. Smith III.
J.B. Lippincott Company, Philadelphia, PA © 1995.

Clifford R. Wheeless, Jr.

John Clark, working at The Johns Hopkins Hospital, in 1895 published one of the first descriptions of radical hysterectomy for cervical cancer. Wertheim and, later, Meigs published results of their extensive experience with this operation. It is a procedure for stage IB and early stage IIA cancer of the cervix in women who are good operative candidates and wish to avoid the vaginal and ovarian sequelae of pelvic irradiation. Attempts to further delineate radical hysterectomy into classes or types of hysterectomy have not been demonstrated to have significance in prospective trials. Microinvasive carcinoma of the cervix can be treated by simple abdominal hysterectomy with excellent results. Invasive cancers are best treated with the Clark, Meigs, Wertheim radical hysterectomy. Modifications can be made for individual patients requiring special techniques, such as resection of a portion of ureter, bladder, or bowel.

The major focus of the operation is the adequacy of the central dissection. The central cervical tumor must be removed with a sufficient margin of uninvolved normal tissue around it. An adequate central dissection must include the removal of a wide margin of parametrial tissue around the central tumor and total removal of parametria from the bladder, rectum, and lateral pelvic wall; an adequate vaginal cuff must also be removed.

About 16,000 new cases of invasive cervical cancer are reported in the United States each year. About 30% of these are stage IB lesions. If selected cases of early stage IIA cancer are added to the cases of stage IB cancer, potentially 6000 patients per year are candidates for radical hysterec-

tomy. Many of these women, however, are too elderly or ill to undergo an extensive hysterectomy. In addition, the absence of a surgeon properly trained in radical pelvic surgery often means that such patients must be treated with the alternative to radical hysterectomy, namely total pelvic irradiation with brachytherapy.

The 5-year survival of patients with stage IB and early IIA cancers is the same whether they are treated with radical pelvic surgery or with total pelvic irradiation. Treatment complications are also similar. Surgery has three advantages over radiation, however: (1) preservation of the ovary in premenopausal women for ovarian hormone production; (2) preservation of pliable vagina for normal vaginal function; and (3) significantly easier and more successful repair of complications (although the complications of both procedures are minimal).

The operative time for radical hysterectomy ranges from 2½ to 4 hours. General anesthesia is required and blood transfusions should be available and are frequently needed.

USUAL POSTOPERATIVE COURSE

Expected postoperative hospital stay: 8 to 12 days

Operative mortality: Under 1%

Special monitoring required: No special monitoring is usually necessary. Most patients can return to their regular hospital rooms, although a few should be monitored in the intensive care unit for 24 hours.

Patient activity and positioning: Patients are out of bed the day after surgery and completely ambulatory thereafter.

Alimentation: Clear liquids are permitted on the first postoperative day, and food intake is progressed to a regular diet as tolerated, usually by the third day, when bowel function has returned.

Antibiotic coverage: Preoperative antibiotics aimed at polymicrobial contamination, covering gram-negative rods, anaerobes, and gram-positive cocci, are administered. Prolonged antibiotic therapy has not had demonstrable efficacy.

Catheterization: An indwelling Foley catheter is routinely required. It is preferable to leave a suprapubic Foley catheter in place because this allows for a trial of voiding by the sixth postoperative day. A suprapubic catheter is more antiseptic and associated with a lower incidence of urinary tract infection.

Vaginal packing: Vaginal packing is not required.

POSTOPERATIVE COMPLICATIONS

IN THE HOSPITAL

Urinary fistula: The incidence of urinary fistula is the same with both radical surgery and total pelvic radiation and brachytherapy. A ureterovaginal or vesicovaginal fistula should occur in under 3% of cases. Ureterovaginal fistulas are treated by inserting a Silastic stent as a percutaneous nephrostomy that can eventually be internalized, with the proximal portion of the stent in the renal pelvis and the distal portion in the bladder. A cystoscopic approach rarely is successful for retrograde placement of a stent. A stent usually does not result in complete closure of the ureterovaginal fistula without ureteral stricture and upper tract obstruction. Most cases require ureteroneocystostomy 6 to 8 weeks after the original radical hysterectomy, when edema and cellulitis have resolved. In some cases, immediate ureteroneocystostomy can be performed as early as the 10th to 12th postoperative day, but these cases should be selected carefully.

Vesicovaginal fistula is less common than is ureterovaginal fistula. Treatment consists of placing a Foley catheter to decompress the bladder. This occasionally allows for spontaneous closure of a small vesicovaginal fistula, although most such fistulas require surgical repair when the cellulitis and edema surrounding their margins have resolved. This may be as early as 10 days to 2 weeks after surgery but requires 8 to 12 weeks in some cases.

Neurogenic bladder dysfunction: A radical hysterectomy effectively denervates the bladder and upper urethra. The more extensive is the dissection, the greater is the degree of interference with function. All patients have some degree of bladder dysfunction, and the incidence of significant bladder dysfunction may be as high as 50%. In most patients, satisfactory voiding patterns can be established within several months.

Infection: The occurrence of pelvic cellulitis after radical pelvic surgery has been greatly diminished by the use of adequate abdominal drainage of the operative site. The use of prophylactic broad-spectrum antibiotic coverage also has proved effective.

Venous thrombosis and pulmonary embolism: Deep venous thrombosis may lead to pulmonary embolism. In studies using iodine-125–labeled fibrinogen scanning of the lower extremity, as many as 20% of patients undergoing hysterectomies have been found to have venous thrombosis. Good evidence suggests that this complication originates during the surgical procedure in more than half these patients. Prospective, randomized studies by Clarke-Pearson have failed to show that prophylactic anticoagulation with heparin or the use of elastic stockings is helpful in preventing pulmonary embolism from deep venous thrombosis. Therefore, efforts to decrease the frequency of this complication should center around the use of intermittent compression boots on the lower extremities beginning before operation and continuing for at least 5 days afterward.

Intraoperative hemorrhage: Despite the surgeon's technical skills and careful dissection, serious hemorrhage may suddenly appear, especially during retroperitoneal dissections on the lateral pelvic side walls and around the sacrum. The approach to serious hemorrhage in the pelvis should be systematic. First, a finger should be placed on the site of hemorrhage to control the bleeding temporarily. Maximum exposure must then be obtained to allow suture closure of the laceration. Sponge sticks may be used proximal and distal to the laceration to compress the vessels against the vertebra or the pelvic structures and allow proper closure with fine, permanent cardiovascular suture. Vascular clamps may also be placed proximal and distal to the laceration to allow closure of the defect. The application of metal clips to distended major vessels that are actively bleeding is rarely successful and frequently results in further damage to the vessel and greater hemorrhage. Large veins in the pelvis that are extensively damaged should be tied off without attempts at suture repair because the collateral drainage of the pelvis is extensive. If massive hemorrhage is encountered, with the loss of large volumes of blood leading to profound patient deterioration, it is wiser to pack the pelvis with copious bulky packing, close the skin of the abdomen with towel clips, and remove patients to the surgical intensive care unit. After the metabolic, hypothermic, and coagulation defects have been corrected, patients can be returned to the operating room for definitive care.

Postoperative hemorrhage: Postoperative hemorrhage after radical hysterectomy is a rare complication. Because the blood supply in the pelvis during radical hysterectomy is extensively skeletonized as part of the operative procedure, ligatures should be secure. The only exception is when extensive bleeding occurs toward the end of a prolonged radical hysterectomy in which there has been deterioration of the coagulation mechanism associated with metabolic acidosis and hypothermia. If the immediate source of bleeding cannot be recognized and surgically controlled, the pelvis should be packed, the packs brought out through the vagina, and the patients removed to the surgical intensive care unit for stabilization. Patients are returned to the operating room for removal of the packs in 48 hours.

Peripheral nerve injury: Nerve injury with radical hysterectomy is unusual. The most important nerves at risk are the femoral, obturator, perineal, sciatic, genitofemoral, ilioinguinal, iliohypogastric, lateral femoral cutaneous, and pudendal nerves. Most such injuries are not associated with serious or permanent disability, although perineal and sciatic nerve injuries may be persistent.

Dehiscence with or without evisceration: Dehiscence is evidenced by the passage of serosanguineous fluid through the abdominal incision. Patients should be returned to the operating room and the rectus fascia resutured using a mass closure technique. Through-and-through stay sutures involving skin, fat, fascia, muscle, and peritoneum rarely are used any longer.

AFTER DISCHARGE

Intestinal obstruction: Intestinal obstruction rarely occurs after radical hysterectomy. It almost exclusively involves the terminal ileum 24 inches from the ileocecal junction, predominantly from adhesions or an internal hernia. If therapy with long-tube suction decompression fails, patients should be taken to the operating room, where exploration should be performed and the intestinal obstruction relieved.

Leg edema: Leg edema is related to the interruption of regional lymphatics and should be treated with limb elevation and elastic stockings. Late edema may also be a sign of recurrent carcinoma and should be investigated fully to rule out this possibility.

BIBLIOGRAPHY

Clarke-Pearson DL, Jelovsek FR, Creasman WT. Thromboembolism complicating surgery for cervical and uterine malignancy: incidence, risk factors, and prophylaxis. Obstet Gynecol 1983;61:87–94.

Meigs JV. The Wertheim operation for carcinoma of the cervix. Am J Obstet Gynecol 1945;49:542–553.

Morley GW, Seski JC. Radical pelvic surgery vs. radiation therapy for stage I carcinoma of the cervix (exclusive of microcarcinoma). Am J Obstet Gynecol 1976;126:785–798.

National Cancer Institute. Cancer statistics review, 1973–1986. Bethesda, National Institutes of Health, 1989, DHHS Publication No. 2789.

Piver MS, Rutledge F, Smith JP. Five classes of extended hysterectomy for women with cervical cancer. Obstet Gynecol 1974;44:265–272.

Rosenshein NB, Ruth JC, Villar J, et al. A prospective randomized study of doxycycline as a prophylactic antibiotic in patients undergoing radical hysterectomy. Gynecol Oncol 1983;15:201–206.

Symmonds RE. Morbidity and complications of radical hysterectomy with pelvic lymph node dissection. Am J Obstet Gynecol 1966;94:663–678.

Wertheim E. The extended abdominal operation for carcinoma uteri (based on 500 operative cases). Am J Obstet Gynecol 1912;66:169–232.

Wheeless CR. Atlas of pelvic surgery, ed 2. Philadelphia, Lea & Febiger, 1988:421.

Medical Management of the Surgical Patient, Third Edition,
edited by Michael F. Lubin, H. Kenneth Walker, and Robert B. Smith III.
J.B. Lippincott Company, Philadelphia, PA © 1995.

CHAPTER

VULVECTOMY 137

Ira A. Horowitz

Vulvectomy is performed for both preinvasive and malignant conditions of the vulva. This procedure may vary in extent from a skinning procedure performed for multicentric intraepithelial neoplasia to a radical vulvectomy combined with bilateral inguinofemoral lymph node dissections for invasive carcinoma. The radical procedure has changed during the past decade and may range from a hemivulvectomy with unilateral inguinofemoral lymph node dissection to an en bloc resection including bilateral inguinofemoral lymph nodes. Lateralizing stage T1 lesions smaller than 2 cm are treated with a radical hemivulvectomy and ipsilateral lymph node dissection. For larger or midline lesions, attempts are made to perform a radical vulvectomy and bilateral inguinofemoral lymph node dissections through separate incisions. This generally results in fewer postoperative complications (eg, wound infection) and a shorter hospital stay. Depending on the extent of resection, myocutaneous flaps may be needed to fill the operative defect. The time necessary for this operation is 2 to 5 hours and varies according to the extent of resection and reconstruction. General, regional, or combination anesthesia can be equally efficacious. Intraoperative transfusions are not routinely required during radical vulvectomy.

USUAL POSTOPERATIVE COURSE

Expected postoperative hospital stay: The duration of hospitalization ranges from 7 to 21 days, depending on the extent of resection, the required reconstruction, and the rate of wound healing.

Operative mortality: Under 1%

Special monitoring required: Patients undergoing radical vulvectomy do not require specific monitoring. Because most patients are elderly, however, their medical condition, rather than the operative procedure itself, may necessitate intensive care monitoring.

Patient activity and positioning: Bed rest for 48 to 72 hours is recommended to allow the myocutaneous flaps or primary closure to begin healing before increased tension is placed on the suture lines.

Alimentation: Although a regular diet would be tolerated on the first postoperative day, clear liquids or a low-residue diet is recommended to decrease fecal soiling of the wound.

Antibiotic coverage: The perioperative administration of first- or second-generation cephalosporin in the first 24 hours may decrease the risk of wound infection. Some gynecologic oncologists prescribe doxycycline during the immediate postoperative period to reduce the incidence of cellulitis.

Thromboembolism: In the 1986 National Institutes of Health Consensus Report, the use of low-dose heparin and sequential pneumatic compression devices was recommended to decrease thromboembolic phenomena in patients with gynecologic malignancies.

Perineal care: Various philosophies exist regarding perineal care in patients undergoing radical vulvectomy. Most surgeons agree, however, that the wound should be kept dry. This may be accomplished with a heat lamp or hair dryer.

POSTOPERATIVE COMPLICATIONS

IN THE HOSPITAL

Wound separation and necrosis: The most common complication of radical vulvectomy is wound separation and necrosis, which occurs in about 70% to 80% of patients. Although the use of myocutaneous flaps and skin grafts can decrease the incidence of this problem, flaps frequently undergo necrosis at their distal margins. Skin necrosis is treated with aggressive débridement and frequent irrigation. It may take several weeks for complete wound healing to occur. These patients do not require additional skin grafting, and a complete radical vulvectomy can be allowed to granulate in with satisfactory results.

Wound hematoma: In a radical vulvectomy, the saphenous vein is sacrificed. In addition, the various small branching arteries and veins from the femoral vessels may result in a postoperative hematoma. Reexploration may be necessary to evacuate the collection and effect hemostasis.

Cellulitis: Cellulitis is the second most common complication of radical vulvectomy. Patients should be treated with doxycycline or broad-spectrum antibiotics effective against staphylococcal and streptococcal species.

Rupture of femoral vessels: Rupture of femoral vessels is a life-threatening complication that should be treated with local compression to control bleeding until patients can be returned to the operating room for repair of the damaged vessel. Transposition of the sartorius muscle to cover the femoral vessels during the initial operation has almost eliminated this complication.

Femoral neuropathy: The femoral nerve lies lateral to the femoral artery and is only rarely injured during the inguinofemoral dissection.

AFTER DISCHARGE

Edema of the lower extremities: Excision or interruption of the regional lymphatics frequently results in chronic lymphedema. Therapy consists of elastic support stockings and limb elevation. In more severe cases, pneumatic compression devices are used.

Lymphangitis and cellulitis: Lymphangitis and cellulitis require aggressive antibiotic coverage of proper duration.

Vaginal stricture: Cicatricial reaction around the introitus may result in dyspareunia. Vaginal dilators and, occasionally, surgical correction may be required to provide a normal vaginal caliber and restore the ability to have coitus.

Hernia formation: Inguinal and femoral hernias may develop if care is not exercised in closing the respective fascial planes. The incidence of this complication is further decreased by using a sartorius flap at the initial procedure.

Incontinence: Urinary or fecal incontinence may occur after resection of the distal urethra or anal sphincter. Attempts should be made to train patients to achieve increased muscle tone. If efforts prove unsuccessful, or if the resection was extensive, reconstructive surgery is frequently warranted.

BIBLIOGRAPHY

Daly JW, Pomerance AJ. Groin dissection with prevention of tissue loss and postoperative infection. Obstet Gynecol 1979;53:395–399.

DiSaia PJ, Creasman WT, Rich WM. An alternate approach to early cancer of the vulva. Am J Obstet Gynecol 1979;133:825–830.

Hacker NF, Leuchter RS, Berek JS, et al. Radical vulvectomy and bilateral inguinal lymphadenectomy through separate groin incisions. Obstet Gynecol 1981;586:574–579.

Iversen T, Abelet V, Aalders J. Individualised treatment of stage I carcinoma of the vulva. Obstet Gynecol 1981;57:85–89.

Podratz KC, Symmonds RE, Taylor WF. Carcinoma of the vulva: analysis of treatment failures. Am J Obstet Gynecol 1982;143:340–351.

Rutledge FN, Smith JP, Franklin EW. Carcinoma of the vulva. Am J Obstet Gynecol 1970;106:1117–1130.

Way S. Results of a planned attack on carcinoma of the vulva. Br Med J 1954;2:780–782.

Wheeless CR, McGibbon B, Dorsey JH, Maxwell GP. Gracilis myocutaneous flap in the reconstruction of the vulva and female perineum. Obstet Gynecol 1979;54:97–102.

Medical Management of the Surgical Patient, Third Edition
edited by Michael F. Lubin, H. Kenneth Walker, and Robert B. Smith III.
J.B. Lippincott Company, Philadelphia, PA © 1995.

INDEX

Page numbers followed by *f* indicate figures; *t* following a page number indicates a table.